LUMB & JONES'
VETERINARY ANESTHESIA
Third Edition

Edited by

JOHN C. THURMON, D.V.M., M.S., D.A.C.V.A.
WILLIAM J. TRANQUILLI, D.V.M., M.S., D.A.C.V.A.
G. JOHN BENSON, D.V.M., M.S., D.A.C.V.A.

University of Illinois at Urbana–Champaign, College of Veterinary Medicine,
Department of Veterinary Clinical Medicine,
Urbana, Illinois

LUMB & JONES' VETERINARY ANESTHESIA

Third Edition

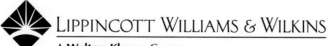

LIPPINCOTT WILLIAMS & WILKINS

A **Wolters Kluwer** Company

Philadelphia • Baltimore • New York • London
Buenos Aires • Hong Kong • Sydney • Tokyo

A Lea & Febiger Book

Executive Editor: Carroll C. Cann
Managing Editor: Tanya Lazar
Production Coordinator: Peter J. Carley
Book Project Editor: Arlene C. Sheir-Allen
Designer: Tom Scheuerman
Typesetter: Graphic World
Printer: Courier
Digitized Illustrations: Graphic World
Binder: Courier

Copyright © 1996 Williams & Wilkins
351 West Camden Street
Baltimore, Maryland 21201-2436 USA

Rose Tree Corporate Center
1400 North Providence Road
Building II, Suite 5025
Media, Pennsylvania 19063-2043 USA

Accurate indications, adverse reactions, and dosage schedules for drugs are provided in this
book, but it is possible that they may change. The reader is urged to review the package
information data of the manufacturers of the medications mentioned.

Printed in the United States of America

Library of Congress Cataloging-in-Publication Data

Lumb and Jones' veterinary anesthesia.—3rd ed. / edited by John C.
 Thurmon, William J. Tranquilli, G. John Benson.
  p. cm.
  Includes bibliographical references and index.
  ISBN 0-683-08238-8
  1. Veterinary anesthesia. I. Thurmon, John C. II. Tranquilli,
 William J. III. Benson, G. John. IV. Lumb, William V. (William
 Valjean). Veterinary anesthesia.
 SF914.L82 1996
 636.089'796—dc20   95-46509
                                            CIP

The Publishers have made every effort to trace the copyright holders for borrowed material.
If they have inadvertently overlooked any, they will be pleased to make the necessary
arrangements at the first opportunity

                                                    99
                              4 5 6 7 8 9 10

Reprints of chapters may be purchased from Williams & Wilkins in quantities of 100 or more.
Call the Special Sales Department, (800)358-3583.

DEDICATION

We dedicate this book to Dr. William V. Lumb and Dr. E. Wynn Jones, pioneers with foresight into the portentous role that anesthesiology would play in the advancement of veterinary surgery and the importance of prevention of pain and suffering of animals, and to all other veterinarians who have dedicated a major portion of their professional careers to establishing and advancing the discipline of veterinary anesthesiology.

John C. Thurmon
William J. Tranquilli
G. John Benson

FOREWORD

Since the initial publication of *Veterinary Anesthesia* in 1973, the science and art of anesthesia have matured immeasurably. Today, a comprehensive book covering the entire field is beyond the capabilities of just two authors such as ourselves. As Founding Diplomates of the American College of Veterinary Anesthesiologists, it is indeed gratifying to us that this new edition has been authored in large part by younger Diplomates of the college.

We are deeply indebted to Drs. Thurmon, Tranquilli, and Benson for assuming editorship of this challenging endeavor. We believe that this new edition will serve as the criterion for education of those who are either learning or practicing animal anesthesia.

William V. Lumb
E. Wynn Jones

PREFACE

The first edition of *Veterinary Anesthesia* by William V. Lumb and E. Wynn Jones was published in 1973. Eleven years later (1984), the second edition was published. The third edition, 12 years later, will mark the text's 23rd anniversary. This edition, as was the second edition, is intended to be a timely revision of this highly respected veterinary anesthesia textbook. The editors have endeavored to conserve as much of the original text as space permits. Some information on the use of older drugs and techniques was purposefully retained for practitioners whose access to newer, more expensive anesthetic drugs and delivery systems/equipment may be limited. Much of this retained information will also provide a historical backdrop to the development of modern anesthetics commonly used by veterinarians in the United States today. Although considerable information, primarily of historic interest, has been deleted, it is still available to the reader in the second edition. A large number of tables have been included to summarize a vast amount of information in a small space. This volume is testimony to the ever-increasing amount of newly published information on veterinary anesthesia.

Although the first and second editions were written by Drs. Lumb and Jones, we have selected a number of experts to assist in this revision. The contributing authors have a wide breadth of clinical experience, national and international reputations, and a willingness to share their knowledge and experience. The authors of individual chapters have been encouraged to pick and choose from basic and clinical material as it impacts on their special area of interest. These authors have also been asked to include personal opinions and experiences. As with the earlier editions, this revision has been prepared for veterinary students, practitioners, and residents. Individuals requiring information on anesthesia for research, zoo, wild, and laboratory animals will also find the text helpful. In addition to chapters on physiologic and pharmacologic principles essential for more than a cursory understanding of animal anesthesia, several new chapters have been added. Among them are specific chapters devoted to: drug interactions, dissociative anesthetics, acid-base balance, fluid and electrolyte therapy, chemical immobilization of terrestrial mammals, perioperative pain and distress, and two multichapter sections on management of anesthesia. Information on the pharmacology of newer anesthetics (eg, propofol and etomidate); anesthetic adjuncts (eg, medetomidine); and anesthetic techniques such as low flow inhalation anesthesia and the use of newly developed injectable anesthetic regimens in a variety of species is presented. Chapters on anesthesia and immobilization of specific species, patients with specific diseases, and the anesthetic management of patients undergoing specific surgical procedures have also been added in this third edition. These chapters are designed to provide practical information for administering anesthesia in domestic, laboratory, wild, and exotic animal species.

In an effort to provide space for new information, we have combined several of the chapters from the second edition. As in earlier editions, we have retained chapter outlines at the beginning of each chapter. The text has further been organized into sections. We believe this arrangement will aid the reader in rapidly locating specific information.

The editors are indebted to the authors for the many hours they have devoted to the preparation of individual chapters. We also extend our thanks to the anesthesia residents and technicians at the University of Illinois for devoting a major amount of time to clinical and instructional duties, which has permitted us to spend more time at author and editorial duties. We acknowledge the assiduous work of the College of Veterinary Medicine Word Processing Center personnel. A special thanks is extended to Joyce Amacher, Elizabeth Erwin, and Shirley Pelmore. The editors are also deeply indebted to Carroll Cann, Susan Hunsberger, Tanya Lazar, Arlene Sheir-Allen, Peter Carley, Susan Rockwell, and Sam Rondinelli of Williams & Wilkins. They have not only been super to work with but have provided sincere encouragement and have played an important inspirational role in completing this task.

John C. Thurmon
William J. Tranquilli
G. John Benson

CONTRIBUTORS

EDWIN J. ANDREWS, V.M.D., Ph.D.
Dean, School of Veterinary Medicine
University of Pennsylvania
Philadelphia, PA

RICHARD M. BEDNARSKI, D.V.M., M.S.*
Associate Professor, Director
The Ohio State University Veterinary Teaching Hospital
Columbus, OH

B. TAYLOR BENNETT, D.V.M.
Laboratory Animal Section
University of Illinois
Chicago, IL

G. JOHN BENSON, D.V.M., M.S.*
University of Illinois at Urbana–Champaign
   College of Veterinary Medicine
Urbana, IL

JOHN R. BOYCE, D.V.M., Ph.D.
Staff Coordinator
American Veterinary Medical Association
Schaumburg, IL

J. DERRELL CLARK, D.V.M., M.S., D.Sc.
Director of Animal Resources
College of Veterinary Medicine
University of Georgia
Athens, GA

LEN K. CULLEN, B.V.Sc., Ph.D.
Murdoch School of Veterinary Studies
College of Veterinary Medicine
Murdoch, Western Australia

H. S. A. DE MORAIS, D.V.M., M.S.
Clinical Instructor
Department of Veterinary Clinical Sciences
The Ohio State University College of Veterinary Medicine
Columbus, OH

A. T. EVANS, D.V.M., M.S.*
Department of Small Animal Medicine and Surgery
Michigan State University College of Veterinary Medicine
East Lansing, MI

STEPHEN A. GREENE, D.V.M., M.S.*
Associate Professor of Anesthesia
Department of Veterinary Clinical Sciences
Washington State University College of
   Veterinary Medicine
Pullman, WA

SANDEE M. HARTSFIELD, D.V.M., M.S.*
Small Animal Medicine and Surgery
Texas A&M University College of Veterinary Medicine
College Station, TX

RALPH C. HARVEY, D.V.M., M.S.*
Department of Urban Practice
University of Tennessee College of Veterinary Medicine
Knoxville, TN

STEVE C. HASKINS, D.V.M., M.S.*
Department of Surgery
University of California, Davis School of Veterinary
   Medicine
Davis, CA

JAMES E. HEAVNER, D.V.M., Ph.D.*
Professor, Anesthesiology and Physiology
Director, Anesthesia Research
Texas Tech University Health Sciences Center
Lubbock, TX

KATHERINE A. HOUPT, V.M.D., Ph.D.
Department of Physiology
College of Veterinary Medicine
Cornell University
Ithaca, NY

JOHN A. E. HUBBELL, D.V.M., M.S.*
Associate Professor of Veterinary Clinical Sciences
Assistant Dean for Academic Affairs
Ohio State University College of Veterinary Medicine
Columbus, OH

HUI CHU LIN, D.V.M., M.S.*
Department of Large Animal Surgery and Medicine
Auburn University College of Veterinary Medicine
Auburn, AL

JOHN W. LUDDERS, D.V.M.*
Associate Professor
Department of Clinical Sciences
Cornell University College of Veterinary Medicine
Ithaca, NY

DAVID D. MARTIN, D.V.M., M.S.
Department of Veterinary Clinical Medicine
University of Illinois College of Veterinary Medicine
Urbana, IL

DIANE MASON, D.V.M., M.S.
Department of Veterinary Clinical Science
Ohio State University College of Veterinary Medicine
Columbus, OH

*Diplomate of the American College
 of Veterinary Anesthesiology.

NORA MATTHEWS, D.V.M.*
Small Animal Medicine and Surgery
Texas A&M University College of Veterinary Medicine
College Station, TX

WAYNE MCDONELL, D.V.M., Ph.D.*
Department of Clinical Sciences
University of Guelph Ontario Veterinary College
Ontario, Canada

W. W. MUIR, D.V.M., Ph.D.*
Department of Veterinary Clinical Science
Ohio State University College of Veterinary Medicine
Columbus, OH

LEON NIELSEN
Wildlife Management Consultant
Safe-Capture International, Inc.
Mount Horeb, WI

KLAUS A. OTTO, D.V.M.*
New York State College of Veterinary Medicine
Cornell University
Ithaca, NY

ROBERT R. PADDLEFORD, D.V.M.*
Department of Small Animal Clinical Sciences
University of Tennessee College of Veterinary Medicine
Knoxville, TN

PETER J. PASCOE, B.V.Sc.*
Department of Surgery
School of Veterinary Medicine
University of California
Davis, CA

THOMAS W. RIEBOLD, D.V.M.*
Oregon State University College of Veterinary Medicine
Corvallis, OR

GORDON W. ROBINSON, V.M.D.
American Society for the Prevention of Cruelty to Animals
New York, NY

*Diplomate of the American College
 of Veterinary Anesthesiology.

JUERGEN SCHUMACHER, D.V.M.
Wildlife and Zoological Medicine Service
Department of Small Animal Clinical Sciences
University of Florida College of Veterinary Medicine
Gainesville, FL

DAVID C. SEELER, D.V.M., M.Sc.*
Associate Professor of Anesthesiology
Atlantic Veterinary College
University of Prince Edward Island
Charlottetown, Price Edward Island, Canada

CHARLES E. SHORT, D.V.M., M.S., Ph.D.*
New York State College of Veterinary Medicine
Cornell University
Ithaca, NY

MICHAEL H. SIMS, D.V.M.
Department of Urban Practice
University of Tennessee College of Veterinary Medicine
Knoxville, TN

ROMAN T. SKARDA, D.M.V., Ph.D.*
Department of Veterinary Clinical Sciences
Ohio State University College of Veterinary Medicine
Columbus, OH

EUGENE P. STEFFEY, V.M.D., Ph.D.*
Department of Surgery
School of Veterinary Medicine
University of California
Davis, CA

JOHN C. THURMON, D.V.M., M.S.*
University of Illinois at Urbana–Champaign
College of Veterinary Medicine
Urbana, IL

WILLIAM J. TRANQUILLI, D.V.M., M.S.*
University of Illinois at Urbana–Champaign
College of Veterinary Medicine
Urbana, IL

CONTENTS

SECTION IX.   EUTHANASIA   861

section I

OVERVIEW OF VETERINARY ANESTHESIA

chapter 1

HISTORY AND OUTLINE OF ANIMAL ANESTHESIA

INTRODUCTION
HISTORY OF ANIMAL ANESTHESIA

DEFINITIONS
   Reasons for Administration of Anesthetics
TYPES OF ANESTHESIA

Introduction

General anesthesia induces immobilization, relaxation, unconsciousness, and freedom from pain. It is indeed one of the miracles of medicine, without which modern surgical techniques could never have developed. The field of anesthesiology has developed into an essential component of veterinary medicine for two major reasons. First is its contribution to the humanitarian care of veterinary surgical patients, and second is its advantage for the veterinarian in protecting personnel while developing modern surgical science.

History of Animal Anesthesia

The earliest recorded attempts to induce anesthesia appear to have been performed in humans. The ancients used opiates, alcohol, asphyxia, and even compression of the carotid arteries to alleviate pain during surgical intervention. In 1540, Paracelsus produced ether and reported it to have a soporific effect on fowl. Despite this, no further progress was made until chemistry was developed and carbon dioxide and several other gases including oxygen were discovered. In 1800, Sir Humphrey Davy suggested that nitrous oxide might have anesthetic properties. Shortly thereafter, H. H. Hickman (1824) demonstrated that pain associated with surgery in dogs could be alleviated by inhalation of a mixture of nitrous oxide and carbon dioxide. He believed that anesthesia was caused by nitrous oxide as a result of carbon dioxide enhancing the rate and depth of breathing. However, recent studies have shown that anesthesia can be induced in

30 to 40 seconds in piglets breathing carbon dioxide (50%) alone in oxygen.(1)

It was not until 1842 that ether was used for human anesthesia. Two years later, a dentist, Dr. Horace Wells (1844), discovered the anesthetic properties of nitrous oxide. Although this finding was neglected for several years, nitrous oxide was reintroduced in man in 1862. Dr. C. P. Jackson, a Boston physician, was the first clinician to employ ether extensively in animals.(2)

Although chloroform was discovered by Liebig in 1831, it was not until 1847 that it was used for general anesthesia in animals by Flourens and in man by Dr. J. Y. Simpson of Edinburgh, Scotland. With the introduction of chloroform, reports began to appear in the veterinary literature of its use in animals. Dadd routinely used general anesthesia in animals and was the first in the United States to advocate humane treatment of animals and the application of scientific principles (i.e., anesthesia) in veterinary practice.(3)

In 1875, Ore published the first monograph on intravenous anesthesia using chloral hydrate; three years later, Humbert described its use in the horse. Pirogoff attempted rectal anesthesia as early as 1847. This route was used later in veterinary patients largely for the administration of chloral hydrate. Intraperitoneal injection was first used in 1892 in France. Thus, the various routes for administration of general anesthetics to animals were established by the end of the nineteenth century.

After the initial isolation of cocaine by Albert Niemann of Germany in 1860, Anrep, in 1878, suggested the possibility of using cocaine for local anesthesia. In 1884, Kohler used cocaine for local anesthesia of the eye, and Halsted described cocaine nerve block anesthesia a year later. Its use was popularized in veterinary surgery by Sir Frederick Hobday, an English veterinarian. G. L. Corning is credited for inducing cocaine spinal anesthesia in a dog in 1885. From his description, however, it would appear that he probably produced epidural anesthesia. In 1898, August Bier of Germany produced true spinal anesthesia in animals and then in himself and an assistant.(4)

While local infiltration was popularized by Reclus in 1890, and Schleich in 1892, conduction anesthesia was introduced by Halsted and Hall in New York in 1884. These techniques became more popular with the discovery of local anesthetics less toxic than cocaine. With these developments, it was possible for Cuille and Sendrail (1901) of France to induce subarachnoid anesthesia in horses, cattle, and dogs. While Cathelin (1901) reported epidural anesthesia in the dog, it remained for Retzgen, Benesch, and Brook to apply the technique of epidural anesthesia in large animal species in the 1920s. Although paralumbar anesthesia was introduced in man by Sellheim in 1909, it was not until the 1940s that Farquharson and Formston applied this technique in cattle. Despite anesthetic developments in the latter half of the nineteenth century, and perhaps owing to unfavorable results, general anesthesia was not readily adopted by the veterinary profession until well into the twentieth century. A heavy hand, without anesthesia, was the stock in trade of the average veterinarian.

In small domestic animals, ether and chloroform were commonly administered in the early part of the twentieth century. However, general anesthesia became more widely accepted after discovery of the barbiturates in the late 1920s and, in particular, with the development of pentobarbital in 1930. Barbiturate anesthesia received an additional boost with introduction of the thiobarbiturates and particularly with thiopental in 1934. Because of rough, prolonged recovery, the acceptance of general anesthesia in large animals was delayed until the introduction of preanesthetics such as the phenothiazine derivatives introduced by Charpentier in France in 1950. General anesthesia of large farm animals was further advanced by the discovery of fluorinated hydrocarbons by Raventos and others and the development of large animal anesthetic equipment for safe administration. Recently, development of new drugs and the safe combinations thereof (e.g., tranquilizers, opioids, alpha$_2$-agonists, dissociatives, muscle relaxants, and inhalant anesthetics) has further advanced our knowledge of veterinary anesthesia in large and small animal species.(5)

In North America, development of veterinary anesthesia as a distinct discipline led to organization of the American Society of Veterinary Anesthesiology in 1970, and in 1975 the American College of Veterinary Anesthesiologists was established. The latter organization establishes criteria for and certifies specialists (diplomates) in veterinary anesthesiology, under the auspices of the American Veterinary Medical Association.

Other groups around the world also promote veterinary anesthesia and include the Association of Veterinary Anaesthetists of Great Britain and Ireland as well as the Anesthesia and Surgery Association in Japan. These associations were instrumental in organizing the International Congress of Veterinary Anaesthesia in order to advance the science of veterinary anesthesiology. The first International Congress was held in Cambridge, England, in 1982, followed by congresses in Sacramento, California, in 1985, in Brisbane, Australia, in 1988, in Utrecht, The Netherlands, in 1991, and in Guelph, Ontario, in 1994.

For further information on the early history of anesthesia, the reader is referred to Clark, Smithcors, and Lee.(6–8) Historical information documenting more recent advances in anesthesiology can be found in Miller.(9)

Definitions

The term *anesthesia,* derived from the Greek *anaisthaesia,* meaning "insensibility," is used to describe the loss of sensation to the entire or any part of the body. Anesthesia is induced by drugs that depress the activity of nervous tissue locally, regionally, or within the central nervous system. From a pharmacologic point of view, there has been a significant redefining of the term *general anesthesia.*(10) Both central nervous stimulants and depressants can be useful general anesthetics.(11) Several terms are used in describing the effects of anesthetic drugs.

1. *Analgesia* refers to freedom from or absence of pain.
2. *Tranquilization* is a state of behavioral change, wherein anxiety is relieved and the patient is relaxed, although aware of its surroundings. In this state, it may appear to be indifferent to minor pain.
3. *Sedation* is a state characterized by central depression accompanied by drowsiness. The patient is unaware of its surroundings.
4. *Narcosis* is a drug-induced state of deep sleep from which the patient cannot be easily aroused. Narcosis may or may not be accompanied by analgesia.
5. *Hypnosis* is a condition of artificially induced sleep, or a trance resembling sleep, resulting from moderate depression of the central nervous system from which the patient is readily aroused. This type of CNS alteration is not commonly attempted by the veterinarian and is rarely achieved in veterinary patients.
6. *Local analgesia* (anesthesia) is a loss of sensation in a circumscribed body area.
7. *Regional analgesia* (anesthesia) is insensibility in a larger, though limited, body area (e.g., paralumbar nerve blockade).

8. *General anesthesia* is drug induced unconsciousness that is characterized by controlled reversible depression of the central nervous system (CNS) and analgesia. In this state the patient is not arousable and sensory, motor, and autonomic reflex functions are attenuated.

9. *Surgical anesthesia* is the stage/plane of general anesthesia that provides unconsciousness, muscular relaxation, and analgesia sufficient for painless surgery.

10. *Balanced anesthesia* is induced by a multiple drug approach. Drugs are targeted to specifically attenuate individual components of the anesthetic state, that is, consciousness, analgesia, muscle relaxation, and autonomic reflexes.

11. *Dissociative anesthesia* is induced by drugs (e.g., ketamine) that dissociate the thalamocortic and limbic systems. This form of anesthesia is characterized by a cataleptoid state in which the eyes remain open and swallowing reflexes remain functional. Skeletal muscle hypertonus persists unless a sedative or muscle relaxant has been given.

REASONS FOR ADMINISTRATION OF ANESTHETICS

First and foremost anesthesia alleviates pain and provides muscle relaxation for surgery. Its use for other purposes is often overlooked. These include restraint, safe transportation of wild and exotic animals, (Chapters 21 and 22), various diagnostic and therapeutic procedures (Chapters 23 and 24), euthanasia, and the humane slaughter of food animals (e.g., carbon dioxide in swine) (Chapter 26).

Types of Anesthesia

The diverse uses for anesthesia; the varying needs for analgesia, immobilization, and muscle relaxation; and the requirements peculiar to species, age, and disease state necessitate the use of a variety of drugs, drug combinations, and methods. Anesthesia is often classified according to type of drug and method or route of drug administration.

1. *Inhalation:* Anesthetic gases or vapors are inhaled in combination with oxygen.

2. *Injectable:* Anesthetic solutions are injected intravenously, intramuscularly, and subcutaneously. Other injectable routes include intrathoracically and intraperitoneally. The latter two routes are not generally recommended.

3. *Oral or rectal:* These routes are occasionally used with liquid anesthetics or suppositories.

4. *Local and conduction:* Anesthetic is applied topically, or injected locally into or around the surgical site (field block), or is injected around a large nerve trunk supplying a specific region (conduction or regional nerve block). In the latter instance, the injection may be perineural (nerve block), or into the epidural or subarachnoid space (true spinal analgesia) (Chapter 16).

5. *Electronarcosis:* An electric current is passed through the cerebrum to induce deep narcosis. This form of anesthesia has never gained popularity in the United States and is rarely used in veterinary practice. Electronarcosis should not be confused with the inhumane practice of electroimmobilization (Chapter 9).

6. *Transcutaneous electric nerve stimulation* (TENS, TNS, TES): Local analgesia is induced by low-intensity, high-frequency electric stimulation of the skin through surface electrodes.

7. *Hypnosis:* A non-drug-induced trancelike state sometimes employed in rabbits and birds.

8. *Acupuncture:* An ancient Chinese system of therapy utilizing long, fine needles to induce analgesia.

9. *Hypothermia:* Body temperature is decreased, either locally or generally, to supplement anesthesia and decrease anesthetic drug requirement. It is primarily used in neonates or in patients undergoing cardiovascular surgery (Chapter 9).

References

1. Thurmon JC, Benson GJ. Anesthesia in ruminants and swine. In: JL Howard, ed. Current veterinary therapy, vol. 3. Food Animal Practice. Philadelphia: WB Saunders, 1993:58–76.
2. Jackson CT. Etherization of animals. Report of the Commissioner of Patents for the Year 1853. Washington, DC: Beverly Tucker, Senate Printer, 1853:59.
3. Dadd GH. The modern horse doctor. Boston: JP Jewett, 1854.
4. Keys TE. The development of anesthesia. Anesthesiology 3:11, 1942.
5. Stevenson DE. The evolution of veterinary anaesthesia. Br Vet J 119:477, 1963.
6. Clark AJ. Aspects of the history of anaesthetics. Br Med J 2:1029, 1938.
7. Smithcors JE. The early use of anaesthesia in veterinary practice. Br Vet J 113:284, 1957.
8. Lee JA. A synopsis of anaesthesia, 4th ed. Baltimore: Williams & Wilkins, 1959.
9. Miller RD. Anesthesia, 2nd ed. New York: Churchill Livingstone, 1986.
10. Heavner JE. Veterinary anesthesia update. J Am Vet Med Assoc 182:30, 1983.
11. Winters WD, Ferrer AT, Guzman-Flores C. The cataleptic state induced by ketamine: A review of the neuropharmacology of anesthesia. Neuropharmacology 11:303, 1972.

chapter 2

CONSIDERATIONS FOR GENERAL ANESTHESIA

Pharmacology

Anesthesia is, of necessity, a reversible process. Knowledge of the factors underlying production of anesthesia, and those that may modify it, is essential to the success of the procedure. The dose of anesthetic and the techniques for its administration are based on the average animal. Because of the many phenomena that modify the effect of an anesthetic, it is unlikely that any given animal will be exactly "average."

Marked variations in response to a standard dose of anesthetic result from the interplay of many factors, especially those related to the metabolic activity of the animal, existing disease or pathology, and the uptake and distribution of the anesthetic.

BIOLOGIC VARIATIONS

Since elimination of anesthetics depends especially on the metabolic processes of the animal, conditions affecting the metabolic rate exert a marked influence on anesthetic effect. Small animals have a higher basal metabolic rate per unit of surface area than large animals; therefore, the smaller the animal, the larger the dose per unit of body weight necessary for anesthesia. Animals with large quantities of fat, which is a relatively inactive nonmetabolizing tissue, have a lower basal metabolic rate per unit of body weight and require less anesthetic than lean muscular animals in good condition. Greyhounds, an example of the latter, are notorious for their tendency toward excitability during induction and for a prolonged period of recovery.(1)

Animals in poor condition also require less anesthetic. Dogs kept on a low food intake resulting in weight losses of 10 to 20% showed a marked increase in duration of anesthesia following a single injection.(2) In the newborn, the basal metabolic rate is low. It gradually increases to its highest point at the time of puberty through early adulthood and then gradually declines. Response to barbiturates varies in dogs of differing ages.(2) Very young animals and older adult animals are most sensitive, whereas dogs in the age range from 3 to 12 months are least sensitive. These age variations are also related to changes in liver enzyme activity.(3) Changes of metabolism with age are not as clear-cut as originally thought. This reflects the fact that gross weight and surface area are not reliable measures of the active tissue mass of the body. In man, at least, data on fat-free body weight indicate little change between the young and aged adult.(4) The basal metabolic rate of males is approximately 7% higher than that of females. In the female, a rise occurs during pregnancy owing to the metabolic activity of the fetuses. Conflicting evidence concerning sex differences in susceptibility to anesthetics has been reported. The anesthetic used may be the determining factor. Sex variance exists in the susceptibility of rats to amobarbital anesthesia.(5) Pregnant females are most susceptible, nonpregnant females less, and male rats least susceptible. In contrast, Kennedy could find no sex variance in the response of mice to hexobarbital anesthesia.(6) Female rats have been shown to be more sensitive to tubocurarine than males of a similar age.(7) Sex hormones may cause differences in response to an anesthetic. Genetic variation in dose response to anesthetics has been reported. A heritable difference in the ability of rabbits to hydrolyze atropine and cocaine (8), genetic variations in response to pentobarbital in mice (7), and strain sensitivity to nitrous oxide (7) and to non-oxygen-dependent reductive biotransformation of halothane in rats have all been reported.(9) In a few people, plasma cholinesterase has been found to be completely absent or replaced by an inactive variant with resultant prolonged action of succinylcholine.(10) Some breeds of swine are susceptible to malignant hyperthermia.(11) Finally, metabolic rate increases with activity; hence, active animals require relatively large doses of anesthetic agents. Mice have been shown to be most sensitive to pentobarbital in the early morning. A seasonal response to morphine has been recorded in the rabbit, and circadian rhythms have been shown to modify minimum alveolar concentrations for halothane and cyclopropane in rats by 5 to 10%.(7)

PHARMACOKINETICS

General anesthesia results from the action of an anesthetic upon the brain and spinal cord. The agent must therefore achieve access to the central nervous tissue.

Although Van Dyke and Chenoweth have demonstrated that significant quantities of some inhalation anesthetics are metabolized within the body (12), for practical purposes they are primarily exhaled. Small amounts are eliminated in feces and urine or diffused through the skin and mucous membranes. Thus, providing respiration and circulation are maintained, inhalants are readily eliminated from the body. In contrast, injectable agents depend upon redistribution within the tissues, detoxification, principally in the liver, and elimination via the kidneys. With injectable anesthetics, anesthetists have less control over the elimination process; for this reason, some consider them to be more dangerous than inhalant anesthetics.

Anesthetics and related drugs are commonly administered by intravenous injection and occasionally by intramuscular, intrathoracic, intraperitoneal, subcutaneous, and even oral or rectal routes. Intravenous administration bypasses the absorption phase of the drug with the consequences that onset and intensity of action are less variable, titration of dose according to response is facilitated, and the risk of toxicity lessens with progressive decline of drug concentration in the plasma.(13)

The body may be considered to have multiple compartments (Table 2–1), which are differentiated by blood supply and tissue-blood partition coefficients.

Table 2–1. Body Compartments Based on Tissue Perfusion

Group	Region	Mass in Kg	% Cardiac Output
Vessel Rich	Brain	1.4	14
	Liver (splanchnic)	2.6	28
	Heart	0.3	5
	Kidney	0.3	23
Intermediate	Muscle	31.0	16
	Skin	3.6	8
Fat	Adipose tissue	12.5	6
Vessel Poor	Residual tissue	11.3	Nil
Total	—	63.0	100

(From Bard, P. Blood suppy of Special Regions. In: Medical Physiology, 11th ed. CV Mosby, St. Louis, 1961. Data on adipose tissue and residual tissue have been added.)

Table 2–2. Factors Influencing Rate of Tissue Equilibration of a Drug Such as Thiopental

Tissue	Blood Flow (l/min)	Tissue Volume (l)	Thiopental Tissue-Blood Partition Coefficient	Capacity*	Time Constant (min)†
Vessel-rich group (VRG)	4.5	6	1.5	9	2
Muscle group (MG)	1.1	33	1.5	50	45
Fat group (FG)	.32	14.5	11.0	160	500
Vessel-poor group (VPG)	.075	12.5	1.5	19	250

*Tissue volume × tissue–blood partition coefficient.
†Capacity/blood flow.
(From Saidman, L.J. Uptake and Distribution of Intravenous Agents: The Thiopental Model. Refresher Courses in Anesthesiology, 3:141, 1975.) (14)

After initial intravenous injection, mixing and dilution rapidly occur, and an initial blood plasma concentration of the drug is established. Blood plasma thus becomes the medium by which the drug is delivered to and removed from its site of action. Factors affecting drug concentration and/or availability in the plasma also affect its concentration and availability at the site of action. Binding of drugs to plasma protein, in which form they cannot readily penetrate cellular membranes, and the removal of drugs by tissues that store, metabolize, and excrete them are all factors that lower the effective concentration of drugs at their site of action.(13, 14) Binding is a reversible fusion of small molecules, such as barbiturates, with protein or other macromolecules, thereby limiting penetration of cellular membranes by molecular size, ionization, and limited lipid solubility. Protein binding varies with the nature of the drug, its concentration, and plasma pH and protein concentration. The fraction of bound ineffective drug increases with decreasing drug concentration and vice versa, and is modified by the presence of other drugs that compete for available binding sites. The rate of clearance of drug from the blood, its distribution to the tissues, and availability to produce its desired effects thus may all be modified by the drug concentration, the plasma pH and protein, the state of body hydration, and the presence of other drugs.(14)

After initial dilution within the vascular system, the drug is distributed to the various tissue compartments according to their perfusion, their capacity for the drug (volume of tissue × tissue-blood partition coefficient), and the partial pressure gradient of drug between blood and tissue. The vessel-rich group of tissues achieves equilibrium with the blood more quickly than do other tissue groups (Table 2–2).(14) Although fat and muscle groups have similar tissue blood flows per unit of tissue, the higher solubility of most anesthetics (e.g., thiobarbiturates) in fat than in muscle accounts for the greater time to achieve equilibrium for fat than for muscle. Changes in tissue blood flow, solubility, and blood-tissue partial pressure gradients thus influence uptake and distribution of intravenous anesthetics. Since the plasma concentration of an intravenous

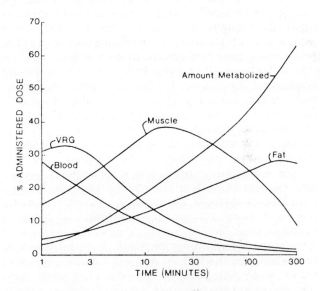

Fig. 2–1. Following an intravenous bolus, the percentage of thiopental remaining in blood rapidly decreases as drug moves from blood to body tissues. Time to attainment of peak tissue levels is a direct function of tissue capacity for barbiturate relative to blood flow. Thus, a larger capacity or smaller blood flow is related to a longer time to reach a peak tissue level. Initially, most thiopental is taken up by the VRG because of its high blood flow. Subsequently, the drug is redistributed to muscle, and to a lesser extent to fat. Throughout this period, small but substantial amounts of thiopental are removed by the liver and metabolized. Unlike removal by the tissues, this removal is cumulative. Note that the rate of metabolism equals the early rate of removal by fat. The sum of this early removal by fat and metabolism is the same as the removal by muscle. (From Eger, E.I., II. Anesthetic Uptake and Action. Williams & Wilkins, Baltimore, 1974.)(15)

anesthetic falls rapidly (Fig. 2–1) (15), and its partial pressure is quickly exceeded by that in the vessel-rich tissues, anesthetic reenters the blood from these tissues to be redistributed to tissues having greater time constants. This redistribution reduces anesthetic concentration in the brain, anesthesia lightens, and anesthetic accumulates in muscle, fat, and vessel-poor tissues.

The ultimate effect of a general anesthetic is contingent upon its ability to cross the blood-brain barrier. This barrier, like the placenta, has permeability characteristics of cellular membranes and therefore limits the penetration of nonlipophilic, ionized, or protein-bound drugs. Penetration of these barriers is, in fact, so slow that little or no drug of the aforementioned types enters the brain or fetus after a single intravenous bolus dose. The barriers are not, however, absolute and slow penetration does occur, becoming significant when the level of drug is maintained over a prolonged period of time.(13) The high lipid-solubility of thiopental relative to pentobarbital accounts for the rapid onset of and recovery from anesthesia induced by the former.(16)

Within moments of tissue uptake and redistribution, elimination of the drug begins. The circulation distributes it to vessel-rich organs able to biotransform and/or excrete it. The liver is the primary site of biotransformation, while the kidney is primarily responsible for excretion. Other organs may occasionally be involved, such as in the elimination of morphine via the gastrointestinal tract.(13) Biotransformation increases the rate of disappearance of the drug from active sites and converts most hypnotics and anesthetics from lipophilic nonpolar compounds to polar water-soluble derivatives capable of excretion by the kidneys. Without such conversion, elimination of lipophilic nonvolatile drugs is markedly prolonged owing to reentry, after glomerular filtration, into the systemic circulation via the tubular epithelium. Although the metabolites resulting from biotransformation are usually less active, more toxic compounds may sometimes result.(17) The rate of biotransformation is determined by the concentration of drug at the site of metabolism (e.g., plasma concentration and hepatic blood flow) and by the intrinsic rate of the process. The latter is determined by such factors as enzymic activity and cofactor availability (e.g., genetics, presence of other drugs, nutrition, hypoxia).(13) Most drug metabolism follows first-order kinetics (a constant fraction is metabolized in a given period). In the event that the concentration exceeds the capacity of the biotransformation process, elimination assumes zero-order kinetics, a constant amount of drug is eliminated (13), and the pharmacologic effect is disproportionately prolonged with increasing or multiple doses.(16) Species variations in biotransformation may also be encountered, for example, lidocaine in man, dog, guinea pig, and rat, and glucuronide conjugation of drugs such as morphine, salicylic acid, and meprobamate in the cat.

Excretion subsequent to or independent of biotransformation is primarily a function of the kidney. Renal excretion is the principal process by which predominantly ionized drugs or those of limited lipid solubility are eliminated (e.g., d-tubocurarine, gallamine triethiodide).(16) The rate of excretion is determined by renal blood flow, glomerular filtration, and tubular secretion and reabsorption. Non-protein-bound drug passes through the glomerulus. Other drugs and metabolites require the active transport processes of tubular secretion, which are sensitive to transport inhibitors and hypoxia. Reabsorption is efficient for those drugs (e.g., nonpolar lipophilics) able to penetrate cellular membranes, and is modified by pH and the rate of tubular urine flow.(13) Intravenous agents used to produce or facilitate anesthesia such as barbiturates, narcotics, tranquilizers, and nondepolarizing relaxants are excreted primarily by the kidneys.(15, 18) Although inhalant anesthetics are primarily eliminated by exhalation, their metabolites are excreted largely by the kidney.

FACTORS MODIFYING PHARMACOKINETICS

It is thus apparent that many factors of common occurrence, such as rate of administration and concentration of anesthetic, physical status, muscular development, adiposity, respiratory and circulatory status, drug permeability coefficients, prior and/or concurrent drug administration, fear, recent feeding, and solubility of inhalant anesthetics in bags and hoses may all modify the uptake, distribution, and elimination of anesthetics.

Concentration and rate of injection of a given dose affect anesthetic action, particularly with short-acting barbiturates. The more dilute the drug or slower the injection, the less effect produced.

Modification of effective ventilation, ventilation-perfusion ratios, and/or alveolar-capillary diffusion from any cause will influence both the uptake and elimination of inhalant drugs, more especially those of greater solubility (Chapter 11). Commonly occurring examples include diaphragmatic hernia, pulmonary edema, pulmonary emphysema or atelectasis, and recumbency in large animals.

Permeation of the blood-brain barrier by narcotics and narcotic antagonists is contingent upon partition coefficients, ionization, and protein binding, and is therefore influenced by hypocarbia and hypercarbia. For example, during hypocarbia higher serum morphine concentrations, higher drug distribution in the lipid phase, and increased ratio of free base:acid salt of morphine facilitates penetration of morphine into the canine brain, in spite of decreased cerebral blood flow.(19)

Variation in distribution of blood to the vessel-rich and vessel-poor tissues, to fat, to muscle, and to the alveoli themselves will modify the pattern of induction and recovery (Chapter 11). In shock, the proportion of the cardiac output flowing to the brain is increased and the potential for redistribution is reduced. Owing to reduced blood volume, dilution of the drug is also diminished, as is hepatic and renal blood flow. The reduction in blood volume diminishes both biotransformation and renal excretion. Induction is thus rapid, the dose required is reduced, and recovery is delayed. Even removal of 2% of the body weight in blood tremendously prolongs the recovery time from thiopental anesthesia in dogs. (2) It may thus be concluded that hemorrhage, such as might accompany a surgical procedure, will significantly increase sleeping time.

When fear, struggling, or fever occur, the decrease in circulation time may delay equilibration of anesthetic concentration between alveoli and pulmonary capillaries, muscle and skin blood flow is increased, induction of anesthesia is delayed, and more anesthetic is required. It is well known that animals showing a period of excitement during induction of anesthesia always require more anesthetic. This causes a tendency toward overdosing with its attendant dangers. For this reason, preanesthetic sedation is often advantageous.

Hounds such as the whippet, greyhound, Afghan, borzoi, wolfhound, and saluki have a low fat-to-body mass ratio, a low muscle-to-body mass ratio, and consequent increased blood levels of unbound drug when anesthetized with barbiturate. Anesthesia is thus characterized by increased sleep times, stormy recoveries, and occasional fatalities. Thin-type muscled or emaciated patients may have similar characteristics.(20)

According to Dukes, a large meal of meat may increase the metabolic rate of dogs as much as 90% above the basal level (specific dynamic effect).(21) Carbohydrate and fat also produce this elevation, though to a lesser extent. It is usually 12 to 18 hours after the last meal before the basal metabolic rate is attained in carnivorous animals. In contrast, the bird is susceptible to starvation. A 6-hour preanesthetic fast may induce hypoglycemia and marked sensitivity to depressant drugs in small birds.(22) Certainly it is important to consider that starvation induces low plasma glucose, mobilized liver glycogen stores, and reduced circulating fatty acids, all of which may alter drug detoxification rates.(7) In addition to altering the metabolic rate, feeding increases chylomicrons in the blood. It has been shown that thiobarbiturates localize in these and the duration of anesthesia is shortened.(23) Feeding also increases blood flow to the abdominal viscera and influences anesthetic distribution.

With the exception of the gastrointestinal tract, nitrogen is the major gas constituent of closed internal body spaces. Owing to the high blood/gas partition coefficient of nitrous oxide relative to nitrogen and the gases of the intestinal tract, administration of nitrous oxide results in transfer of this gas to internal gas spaces of the body. Increased volume or pressure of the gases within these spaces may thus result. Volume increases occur in highly compliant spaces (e.g., intestinal, peritoneal, thoracic) and pressure changes in noncompliant spaces (e.g., sinuses, middle ear).(15) In intestinal loops of dogs anesthetized with halothane-oxygen and 75% nitrous oxide, the intestinal gas volume increased 1.8 times in 2 hours and 2.5 times in 4 hours. In experimental pneumothorax in dogs, the increase was more rapid; a 200 mL pneumothorax was doubled in 10 minutes, tripled in 45 minutes, and quadrupled in 2 hours. In pneumoencephalograms in dogs, the inhalation of 75% nitrous oxide increased cisternal pressure by 60 torr in 10 minutes.(15) Use of nitrous oxide is contraindicated in patients with pneumothorax, in those undergoing pneumoencephalograms, and in intestinal obstructions requiring prolonged anesthesia.

Most noninhaled drugs are weak acids (barbiturates) or weak bases (narcotics, narcotic antagonists, muscle relaxants). Once the drug is injected, equilibrium between ionized and nonionized forms of drug depends on pH of the blood or tissues and the dissociation constant (pKa) of the drug. A difference in pH between tissue and blood may thus result in a drug concentration difference. Plasma acidosis, for instance, increases intracellular barbiturate but decreases intracellular narcotic concentration.(14)

Drug availability at the site of action or of elimination is also modified by the degree of protein binding. Protein binding is diminished by uremia, by hypoproteinemia, and by administration of drugs competing for the binding sites. It may also be impaired by a change in pH or in the nature of the protein secondary to disease, or by dehydration. Decreased binding may make more drug available for specific action, with consequent apparent sensitivity to a normal dose.(14)

Preanesthetic administration of opioid analgesics lower the metabolic rate; atropine causes a slight rise. When they are administered in combination, however, the metabolic rate is decreased. Tranquilizers usually lower the metabolic rate.

It has been demonstrated that administration of various drugs and pesticides stimulates or inhibits hepatic microsomal drug-metabolizing enzymes (enzyme induction, enzyme inhibition). More than 200 drugs are recognized as enzyme inducers (Table 2-3). Maximal enhancement of enzyme levels occurs after approximately 5 days of administration of the inducing agent; levels return to normal 48 to 72 hours after withdrawal of the enzyme inducer.(24) The nature of the induction varies with the type of drug, its dose, and the patient's age, thyroid function, and genetics.(16, 24) Enzyme induction with accelerated biotransformation reduces the pharmacologic activity of drugs normally eliminated by biotransformation, such as certain barbiturates, tranquilizers, hypnotics, and antiinflammatory drugs. Because inhalation anesthetics also undergo biotransformation, their elimination is also influenced by enzyme induction. While this occurrence has little or no effect on the conduct of clinical anesthesia, it is of significance relative to viscerotoxicity. Methoxyflurane biotransformation may be modified quantitatively and qualitatively by enzyme induction to form nephrotoxic metabolites; chloroform hepatotoxicity is similarly induced by biotransformation. The potential for such toxicity in halothane anesthesia is enhanced by hypoxia. Toxicity associated with biotransformation is also enhanced by reduced liver antioxidants, such as glutathione or vitamin E. In all instances, toxicity of the organohalogens depends primarily on formation of reactive intermediates, especially those resulting from non-oxygen-dependent ("reductive") biotransformation (25), and is contingent upon the extent and type of biotransformation, and the metabolic and environmental drug pathways resulting from induction.(24) The extent to which such induced metabolic effects influence clinical animal anesthesia is unknown.

Hepatic microsomal enzymes may also be inhibited, with delay of biotransformation. Inhibitors include organophosphorus insecticides, pesticide synergists of the methylenedioxyphenyl type, guanidine, carbon tetrachloride, chloramphenicol, tetracyclines, and cer-

Table 2–3.   Partial List of Drugs Capable of Producing Microsomal Enzyme Induction

Hypnotics	Antihistaminics
Barbiturates	Diphenhydramine (Benadryl)
Glutethimide (Doriden)	Steroids
Ethanol	Cortisone
Chloral hydrate	Prednisone
Tranquilizers	Norethynodrel (Enovid)
Chlorpromazine (Thorazine)	Methyltestosterone
Promazine (Sparine)	Anesthetics
Meprobamate (Equanil)	Diethyl ether
Chlordiazepoxide (Librium)	Halothane (Fluothane)
Anticonvulsants	Insecticides
Diphenylhydantoin (Dilantin)	DDT
Methylphenylethylhydantoin (Mesantoin)	Chlordane
	o,p'-DDD

(From Brown, B.B. Enzymes of Biotransformation as Related to Anesthesia. ASA Refresher Courses in Anesthesiology, 3:27, 1975.) (17)

tain inhalation anesthetics.(16, 17) Inhibition is illustrated by prolonged plasma half-lives of barbiturates, narcotics, and local anesthetics during halothane anesthesia (17) and prolonged barbiturate anesthesia after a prior or concurrent chloramphenicol medication.(26) Relevant drug interactions may also occur as a result of protein binding and interaction at receptor sites (Table 2–4).

Antibiotics are often administered prior to, during, or immediately after general anesthesia to prevent or treat bacterial infections associated with surgery. In many instances, little consideration is given to adverse responses that may occur from the interaction between antibiotics and drugs commonly used in the operating room.(27) A variety of antibiotics have been shown to cause neuromuscular blockage, the most notable of which are the aminoglycosides (Table 2–4).(27, 28)

The effect of disease on the metabolic rate usually varies with its duration. In the early febrile stage, the rate may be increased; however, as the disease progresses, toxemia may reduce it to low levels. Fever increases the metabolic rate in accordance with van't Hoff's law, which states that for each degree Fahrenheit the temperature rises, the metabolic rate is increased by 7%. When animals suffer from toxemia or liver disease, the functions of this organ are impaired and the ability of the animal to detoxify anesthetics is depressed. Shock lowers the metabolic rate and, because of suppressed cardiovascular function, impairs uptake and distribution of anesthetic agents.

Hepatocellular disease causes reduced protein (primarily albumin) production with consequent limitation of protein binding, increased pharmacologic activity of drugs, and unexpected sensitivity to such drugs as thiopental. Production of specific protein such as pseudocholinesterase may also be impaired, with consequent increased duration of action of succinylcholine. Hepatic disease may delay drug biotransformation because of enzyme inhibition or decreased hepatic blood flow.(29) Some drugs and/or their metabolites (polar, molecular weight > 300) are likely to be excreted in the bile in significant amounts (e.g., morphine, chloramphenicol, digitoxin).(16) The doses of drugs contingent upon hepatic elimination must therefore be modified in the presence of hepatic disease.

Distribution and elimination of anesthetic and related drugs can also be impaired by renal disease with increased potential toxicity. Protein binding of organic acids is reduced in uremic patients, causing increased pharmacologic activity (sensitivity); examples include pentobarbital, phenylbutazone, and cardiac glycosides. The increase of free drug fraction in plasma of patients with renal disease correlates with the degree of hypoalbuminemia.(16) Renal disease may also limit excretion and thereby prolong activity of muscle relaxants such as gallamine and pancuronium.

The degree by which renal disease influences drug protein binding, and therefore its activity and/or excretion, may be modified by fluid therapy (dilution, increased glomerular filtration) and by changes in plasma pH (see protein binding).(15)

Hyperthyroidism is accompanied by an elevated metabolic rate, whereas hypothyroidism is accompanied by lowering of the metabolic rate. Totally thyroidectomized dogs require small doses of anesthetic. Leukemia in some forms increases the metabolic rate, as does severe pain.(30)

Irradiation has been shown to affect (a) potency, onset, duration of action, and brain levels of barbiturate, and (b) activity of the hepatic microsomal enzyme system.(31) Earlier onset of drug action apparently results from radiation-induced modification of the blood-brain barrier. In adult animals, prolongation of drug action occurs, which may be caused by (a) sensitization with a region-specific increase in brain serotonin and (b) partial inhibition of hepatic oxidase. Prenatal irradiation produces impairment of the hepatic microsomal enzyme system in male rats. In young rats postnatally irradiated, a higher radiation dose is necessary to produce the same effect. The anesthetic effect of barbiturates (barbital, hexobarbital, thiopental, pentobarbital) is decreased immediately after irradiation (1 to

Table 2–4.   Interactions at Tissue Receptor Sites

The following agents have neuromuscular blocking properties. They may intensify the effects of nondepolarizing neuromuscular blocking agents (tubocurarine, gallamine, dimethyl tubocurarine), or they may interact with each other.

Antibiotics	*General Anesthetics*
Bacitracin	Ether
Streptomycin, Dihydrostreptomycin	Halothane
Neomycin	Methoxyflurane
Kanamycin	*Other Agents*
Gentamicin	Muscle relaxants
Polymyxin B	Quinine
Oxytetracycline	Promethazine
Lincomycin	Magnesium sulfate
Other tetracyclines	Barbiturates
Colistimethate	Na citrate
Paronomycin	Organophosphorus insecticides
Vancomycin	

The following agents may intensify the neuromuscular blockade produced by succinylcholine.

Anticholinesterase agents
Magnesium sulfate

The following reactions occur at adrenergic receptor sites.

Drug 1	*Drug 2*	*Effect*
Epinephrine	Chloroform	Arrhythmias due to sensitization of the
Levarterenol	Halothane	heart to catecholamines by drug 2
Isoproterenol	Thiamylal	

(From Abbitt, L.E. Drug Interactions. In Drug Interactions, Incompatibilities and Adverse Reactions in Veterinary Practice. Edited by L.E. Abbitt, L.E. Davis, S.D. Farey, and R.D. Scalley. Colorado State University, Fort Collins, Colorado, 1975.)

3 hours). Later, as irradiation sickness develops (tenth to fifteenth day), an increased sensitivity develops.(32)

CELLULAR EFFECTS AND TERATOGENICITY

Interest in mutagenic, carcinogenic, and teratogenic effects of anesthetics increased after an increase in spontaneous abortion of female anesthetists was noted in 1970.(33) It is assumed that this increased rate of abortion was caused by chronic exposure to trace concentrations of anesthetics. Exposure to such anesthetic concentrations in the first trimester of pregnancy should be avoided. Exposure of rats to nitrous oxide on the ninth day of gestation has been shown to cause fetal resorption and skeletal and soft tissue anomalies. Others have also demonstrated that inhalation anesthetics are teratogenic in animals, especially the chick.(33, 34) Corresponding teratogenesis in man has not been conclusively proved.

Epidemiologic studies have suggested an increased incidence of cancer among women, but not men, who work in operating rooms.(34) Commonly used anesthetics, with the exception of fluroxene, have not been shown to be potential carcinogens by in vitro tests. Both general and local anesthetics can inhibit cell division. Anesthetics also affect such immune phenomena as cellular adherence, phagocytosis, lymphocyte transformation, chemotaxis, and the killing of tumor cells.(35)

Assessment of Anesthetic Actions

General anesthesia has simply been defined as complete unconsciousness. When inducing this state, however, the anesthetist requires all the following components: unconsciousness, insensitivity to pain, muscle relaxation, and absence of reflex response. The degree to which these are required for specific procedures varies. The anesthetist must therefore select the most suitable drugs and be able to assess the degree to which the varying effects are induced. Depth of anesthesia is often difficult to assess. Anesthetic drugs that induce adequate anesthesia in one species and operation may not be sufficient at similar doses in another species. Signs characterizing a continuum of progressive increases in CNS depression and analgesia may not occur with some drugs and drug combinations. The dissociatives do not induce ocular signs of increasing CNS depression. Higher doses of propofol do not induce more analgesia commensurate with increased CNS depression. Anesthetists using modern anesthetic drugs must be familiar with their characteristics in order to use them safely.

Historically, the progressive changes resulting from administration of anesthetic drugs have been classified into four stages. Recognizing the signs characteristic of these stages following administration of most anesthetics allows the anesthetist to determine whether the required intensity of CNS depression has been achieved or whether it is insufficient or too much.

STAGES OF GENERAL ANESTHESIA

For descriptive purposes, the levels of CNS depression induced by anesthetics have been divided into four stages depending upon neuromuscular signs exhibited by the patient (Table 2–5). It should be emphasized that no clear division exists between stages, one blending

Table 2–5. Characteristics of the Stages of General Anesthesia

| System Affected | Characteristic Observed | Stage of Anesthesia | | III | | | | |
		I	II	Plane 1 (Light)	2 (Medium)	3 (Medium)	4 (Deep)	IV
Cardiovascular	Pulse*	tachycardia		progressive bradycardia†				weak or imperceptible
	Blood pressure*	hypertension		normal	increasing hypotension			shock level
	Capillary refill		1 sec or less		progressive delay			3 sec or more
	Dysrhythmia probability	+++	+++	++	+	+	++	++++
	Respiratory rate*	irregular or increased		progressive decrease‡			slow irregular	ceased, may gasp terminally
	Respiratory depth*	irregular or increased		progressive decrease			irregular	ceased
	Mucous membrane, skin color			normal			cyanosis§	pale to white
Respiratory	Respiratory action	may be breath holding		thoracoabdominal, abdominal			diaphragmatic	ceased
	Cough reflex	++++	+++	+	lost			
	Laryngeal reflex	+++ may vocalize	+++	lost				
	Intubation possible	no	yes					

Category	Parameter						
Gastrointestinal	Salivation	++++	+++	+	+	diminished, absent, except in ruminants	absent
	Oropharyngeal reflex	++++	+++	+	+	lost	
	Vomition probability	+++	+++	+	very slight		
	Reflux (regurgitation) potential	none		increases with relaxation			++++
	Tympany (rumen, cecum)	none		potential increases with duration of anesthesia			
	Pupils	dilated		normal or constricted, progressive dilation			acutely dilated
Ocular	Corneal reflex	normal	+++		diminishes, lost (horse may persist)		absent
	Lacrimation	normal	+++	+	diminishes, absent		absent
	Photomotor reflex	normal	+++	+	diminishes, absent		absent
	Palpebral reflex	normal	+++	+	diminishes, absent		absent
	Eyeball position	normal	variable		fixed (ventromedial dog and cat)	fixed (central)	
	Nystagmus		++++ especially horse, cow	+		none	
Musculoskeletal	Jaw tone	++++	++++		decreased, minimal		lost
	Limb muscle tone	++++	++++		decreased, minimal		lost
	Abdominal muscle tone	++++	++++	++	decreased, minimal		lost
	Sphincters (anus, bladder)	may void		+	progressive relaxation		control lost
Nervous	Sensorium	+++	+		lost		
	Pedal reflex #	++++	++++	decreased		absent	
	Reaction to surgical manipulation	++++	++++	+		none	

*Surgical stimulation causes increased heart rate, blood pressure, respiratory rate, and depth via autonomic responses that persist in plane 2. Vagal reflexes due to visceral traction persist in plane 3.

†Especially with halothane and methoxyflurane; does not occur with ether.

‡Tachypnea may occur with halothane; rate may be maintained with ether.

#Cyanosis is not apparent until cardiac arrest if O_2 is used.

§Varies with efficiency of analgesia; lost during plane 1 to 2 with methoxyflurane, during plane 3 in barbiturate anesthesia.

+ to ++++ = degree present.

into the next. In addition, variation in response among patients is to be expected. Preanesthetic medication, adequacy of oxygenation, carbon dioxide retention, and physical status of the patient all modify the signs. Patient response is also governed by the anesthetic that is being administered, considerable variation existing between anesthetics.

Stage I. This is termed the *stage of voluntary movement* and is defined as lasting from initial administration to loss of consciousness. Some analgesia may be present in the deeper phases of this stage. In any case, this stage is the most variable. Deviations result from the anesthetic used, from variations in the temperament and condition of the patient, from the manner in which the animal is restrained, and from the rate of induction. A nervous animal is bound to resist restraint. Should the anesthetic necessitate the use of a mask or be irritating to the upper airway, fear with consequent resistance by the patient will be accentuated. Excited, apprehensive animals may struggle violently and voluntarily hold their breath for short periods. Epinephrine release causes a strong rapid heartbeat and pupillary dilation. Salivation is frequent in some species, as are urination and defecation. With the approach of stage II, the animal becomes progressively ataxic, loses its ability to stand, and assumes lateral recumbency. Initially it is able to turn or lift its head without support.

Stage II. This is called the *stage of delirium or involuntary movement*. As the central nervous system (CNS) becomes depressed, the patient loses all voluntary control. This feature marks the change from stage I. By definition, this stage lasts from loss of consciousness to the onset of a regular pattern of breathing. As a result of anesthetic depression of the CNS, reflexes become more primitive and exaggerated. The patient reacts to external stimuli by violent reflex struggling, breath holding, tachypnea, and hyperventilation. Continued catecholamine release causes a fast, strong heartbeat, cardiac arrhythmias may occur, and the pupils may be widely dilated. Eyelash and palpebral reflexes are prominent. Nystagmus commonly occurs in the horse. During this stage, the animal may whine, cry, bellow, or neigh, depending upon the species concerned. In some species, especially ruminants and cats, salivation may be excessive; in the dog, cat, and goat, vomiting may be evoked. The larynx of cats and pigs is very sensitive at this stage, and stimulation may result in laryngeal spasms. Jaw tone is still present, and attempts at endotracheal intubation are met with struggling and may initiate vomition in dogs and cats and active regurgitation in ruminants. In view of the exaggerated reflex responses during this stage, stimulation of any kind should be avoided.

Stage III. This is the stage of *surgical anesthesia* and is characterized by unconsciousness with progressive depression of the reflexes. Muscular relaxation develops, and ventilation becomes slow and regular. Vomiting and swallowing reflexes are lost.

In humans, this stage has been further divided into planes 1 to 4 to give finer differentiation. Others have

suggested the simpler classification of light, medium, and deep. Light anesthesia persists until eyeball movement ceases. Medium anesthesia is characterized by progressive intercostal paralysis, and deep anesthesia by diaphragmatic respiration.(36) A medium depth of unconsciousness or anesthesia has traditionally been considered a light plane of surgical anesthesia (stage III; plane 2) characterized by stable respiration and pulse rate, abolished laryngeal reflexes, a sluggish palpebral reflex, a strong corneal reflex, and adequate muscle relaxation and analgesia for most surgical procedures. Deep surgical anesthesia (stage III; plane 3) is characterized by decreased intercostal muscle function and tidal volume, increased respiration rate, profound muscle relaxation, diaphragmatic breathing, a weak corneal reflex, and a centered and dilated pupil. If CNS depression is allowed to further increase, the patient will progress to stage IV.

Stage IV. In this stage, the CNS is extremely depressed and respirations cease. The heart continues to beat only for a short time. Blood pressure is at the shock level, capillary refill of visible mucous membranes is markedly delayed, and the pupils are widely dilated. The anal and bladder sphincters relax. Death quickly intervenes unless immediate resuscitative steps are taken. If the anesthetic is withdrawn and artificial respiration is initiated before heart action stops, these effects may be overcome and the patient will go through the various stages in reverse.

The stages just described are best seen when inhalant anesthetics are administered, probably because considerable time is required for an anesthetic concentration to accrue in the central nervous system. This allows the various signs to become apparent. With some intravenous anesthetics (e.g., dissociatives) or the concurrent use of preanesthetic sedatives, the assessment of anesthetic-induced depression is difficult and signs of anesthetic depression are not uniformly apparent.

SIGNS OF ANESTHESIA

Respiration. Respiratory minute volume increases during stage I. Breath holding may occur in stage I, especially if preanesthetic sedation is not used. As anesthetic depression increases to stage II, respirations become irregular, and breath holding commonly occurs. With the onset of stage III, breathing once again becomes regular. The depth of respiration at this time depends on the respiratory threshold to stimulation; surgical manipulation, for instance, stimulates, whereas premedication depresses respiration. If barbiturates are used for either preanesthetic sedation or induction, early respiratory depression occurs. During stage III there is progressive weakening of the intercostal muscles and the diaphragm.(37) The depth of respiration declines progressively, thoracic movement decreases, respiration becomes largely or entirely abdominal, and the rate may increase. With an overdose, respiration becomes entirely abdominal and diaphragmatic contraction causes the abdomen to bulge during inspiration and the thorax to collapse. During expiration, the reverse occurs, the anterior excursion of the diaphragm causing the thorax to expand. With progressive overdosage, diaphragmatic movements become smaller, respiratory exchange diminishes further, and respirations are gasping and ultimately cease. In the dog, oral and cervical movements (tracheal tugging) may be observed during this stage.

Circulation. Although blood pressure may be monitored by indirect methods or by direct arterial catheterization, the veterinarian often does not measure pressure but must depend on the pulse rate or bleeding at the surgical site, and on induction of momentary blanching by compressing an exposed mucous membrane (such as the conjunctiva, oral mucosa, or tongue) to give some indication of the circulatory status of the patient. The mucous membranes may show pallor as a result of hemorrhage or shock and cyanosis caused by hypoxia. In rodents, feet, ears, and muzzles are observed for such signs; in poultry, it is necessary to examine the comb and/or wattles; in rats and rabbits, the color of light reflected from the eye is helpful.

During stages I and II, the pulse is strong and accelerated. Arrhythmias sometimes occur during stage II. In stage III, the pulse rate is regular and usually slightly accelerated. During halothane anesthesia, progressive bradycardia occurs. Pain stimulation in light stage III may induce tachycardia or even arrhythmias.

As the depth of anesthesia increases, blood pressure declines, and the pulse weakens.

Ocular signs. These signs include eyeball position and movement, photomotor reflexes and pupillary size, lacrimation, and palpebral, corneal and conjunctival reflexes. Although ocular signs are often helpful, they can be quite variable in most species and should never replace observation of respiratory and circulatory signs. Eyeball movement is especially valuable in horses, in which nystagmus occurs with the onset of stage II and continues through light surgical anesthesia. In cattle, eyeball rotation is very consistent and a reliable indicator of anesthetic depth whether anesthesia is produced by inhalation anesthetics, barbiturates, or combinations of central muscle relaxants, dissociatives, and alpha$_2$-agonists (Fig. 2–2). In light and medium surgical anesthesia in the dog, cat, and pig, the eyeballs are generally turned downward. The eyelids during this time are usually closed, and the third eyelid overlays the medial portion of the cornea. The palpebral reflex becomes sluggish in all species when surgical anesthesia is attained. The pupillary size is modified by the degree of light and by premedication with such drugs as morphine and atropine. The pupils are dilated during stage II, but thereafter constrict. In deep (stage III, plane 4) anesthesia or stage IV, pupillary dilation indicates overdosage. Reflex constriction of the pupil on expo-

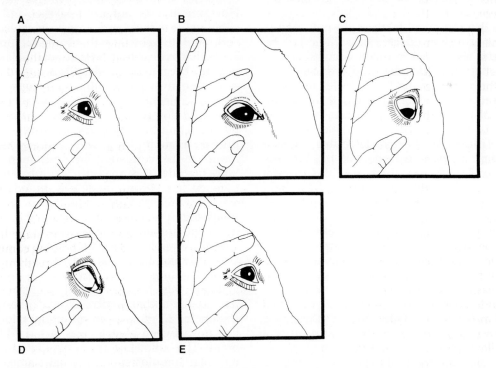

Fig. 2–2. Eyeball position during induction and maintenance of general anesthesia of the cow. A, Position of the cow's eye when unanesthetized and positioned in lateral recumbency. Induction of anesthesia is accompanied by a progressive ventral rotation of the eyeball, becoming partially obscured by the lower eyelid, B and C. As the depth of anesthesia is increased, the cornea becomes completely hidden by the lower eyelid, D. At this time, surgical anesthesia is present. Applying traditional methods of assessing anesthetic depth, the cow would be in stage III, plane 2 to 3. Increasing the depth of anesthesia causes the eye to rotate dorsally, with the cornea becoming centered between the palpebra, E. At this time, deep surgical anesthesia with profound muscle relaxation and CNS depression is present. Eye reflexes have been lost, and the cornea will appear dry and wrinkled. Maintaining this extreme depth of anesthesia can rapidly terminate in death of the patient. Decreasing the depth of anesthesia is accompanied by eyeball rotation occurring in reverse order. (From Thurman JC and Benson EJ. Anesthesia in Ruminants and Swine. Edited by J.L. Howard. In *Current Veterinary Therapy 3, Food Animal Practice.* WB Saunders, Philadelphia, 1993.)

sure to light stimuli (photomotor reflex) is lost on transition from light to medium surgical anesthesia.

Lacrimation is no longer observed in the deeper stages of surgical anesthesia. In the horse, lacrimation is a consistent sign of light surgical anesthesia. Because the eyes may also be open in deep anesthesia, the cornea appears dull and is subject to the adverse effects of drying. To protect against this hazard, ointment should be applied to the eyes or they should be taped closed after anesthesia has been induced. The palpebral reflex, which is a blink induced by touching the eyelids, becomes sluggish or is lost as medium surgical anesthesia develops. Blinking induced by gently touching the cornea (corneal reflex) is variable, but is usually lost shortly after the palpebral reflex. In the horse, the corneal reflex persists into deeper anesthesia.

Pharyngeal and upper airway reflexes. Suppression of these reflexes is of particular importance for endotracheal intubation and for induction of anesthesia in animals with full stomachs, such as ruminants. Coughing and laryngospasm in response to intubation are lost in light surgical anesthesia, but may persist into medium anesthesia in the cat. The intensity of these responses varies with the animal species concerned: especially intense in the cat, and relatively mild in cattle and horses. The swallowing and vomiting reflexes disappear with the onset of stage III; like the laryngeal reflexes, the swallowing reflex persists into medium anesthesia in the cat.

Other signs. After an initial increase during stage II, muscle tone progressively declines, as indicated by relaxation of the abdominal muscles, decreasing efficiency of the intercostal muscles, and reduced resistance to passive flexion of the limbs. In lean animals with shorthaired coats, abdominal muscle relaxation may be such that the profile of viscera is readily apparent. The contour of the rumen may become visible in some ruminants. In cats, detectable extensor tone, in response to passive flexion of the limb by pushing on the digits, persists into medium surgical anesthesia. Generally, limb muscles are relaxed in light anesthesia whereas abdominal muscles are not well relaxed until anesthesia is deep. The tone of the anal sphincter of the horse is a good indicator of relaxation in this species. During stage II the sphincter is tight, but as anesthetic depth increases, the sphincter relaxes so that in deep surgical anesthesia it may gape to such an extent that feces can be observed in the anal canal. Concomitant with progressive dilatation, the anal sphincter gradually loses ability to contract in response to mechanical stimulation in medium to deep surgical anesthesia. Deliberate anal dilation induces an increase in respiratory rate; this respiratory reflex is lost during early stage III.

In dogs, response to opening the jaw is considered to be a useful sign by many veterinarians. During transition from stage II to stage III, passive opening of the mouth may elicit yawning, a response especially likely in barbiturate anesthesia. Resistance to opening the mouth fully is lost in medium anesthesia. The digital (pedal) reflex, in which the limb is flexed in response to painful stimulation of the digits or interdigital region is also a useful guide to the depth of anesthesia in the dog, cat, and rat. This reflex is lost as the transition from light to medium surgical anesthesia occurs. Head shaking in response to ear pinching is a helpful sign in cats, rabbits, and guinea pigs, and is lost with the onset of surgical anesthesia. In cattle and cats, the ear flick reflex in response to tactile stimulation of the hairs within the pinna remains until a medium level of anesthesia is present. Twitching of the whiskers in response to ear pinching is lost as light anesthesia progresses to medium. Response to painful stimulation by pinching the tail of rodents and snakes and the wattles or combs of birds is a useful indicator of the onset of surgical anesthesia. The anal reflex remains until a deeper plane of anesthesia is achieved in birds and is often referred to as the "vent reflex" in this species.

MINIMUM ALVEOLAR CONCENTRATION OF ANESTHETIC (MAC)

In the 1930s, Guedel and several other workers compared anesthetic response and potency. In 1946, Robbins related anesthetic concentration required to induce apnea (LD_{50}) to that which induced loss of righting reflexes.[38] In 1950 Courtin et al. compared anesthetic responses with electroencephalographic changes.[39] However, it was not until Merkel and Eger related stimulus, response, and dose to alveolar partial pressure, and thereby anesthetic partial pressure in the brain, that a consistent indicator of inhalation anesthetic potency became available.[40] As an index of comparison, these investigators utilized the concept of minimal alveolar concentration (MAC) of an anesthetic required to keep a dog from gross movement in response to a painful stimulus.[40] Anesthetic dose was thus expressed as multiples of MAC, an expression that was found to be consistent in both man and animals. Subsequently, this measure of inhalation anesthetic potency has become widely accepted as a means of assessing the effects of increasing anesthetic depths on physiologic processes. For example, the effect of increasing halothane dose as measured in MAC multiples on various physiologic parameters in dogs breathing spontaneously and during controlled ventilation are given in Tables 2–6 and 2–7, respectively.

In animals, MAC is usually determined by maintenance of a consistent end-tidal anesthetic concentration for 15 minutes in an attempt to achieve equilibrium between alveolar gas, arterial blood, and the brain. The animal is then stimulated with a supramaximal stimulus such as a tail clamp, subcutaneous electric current, or surgical incision. If there is no response, the anesthetic concentration is reduced and the procedure repeated. The end-tidal anesthetic concentration midway between that allowing movement and that preventing it is MAC 1.0. In man, the stimulus used is a surgical incision. With this consistent measure

Table 2–6. The Means and Standard Deviations of Various Physiologic Parameters at Different Alveolar Concentrations of Halothane during Spontaneous Respiration in Dogs

	MAC 1.0	MAC 1.5	MAC 2.0	MAC 2.5	MAC 3.0	MAC 3.5	MAC 4.0	R-1.0
Number of dogs represented by data	6	6	6	6	5	4	1	6
Mean arterial pressure (mm Hg)	119 ± 10	96 ± 14	76 ± 10	64 ± 12	67 ± 8	75 ± 16	64	121 ± 3
Mean venous pressure (cm H_2O)	−0.6 ± 2.3	−0.5 ± 2.1	+1.8 ± 3.2	+4.8 ± 4.0	+54 ± 2.5	+11.8 ± 4.5	+9.5	+0.7 + 3.2
Cardiac output (L/min)	1.99 ± 0.52	1.75 ± 0.41	1.66 ± 0.40	1.49 ± 0.48	1.67 ± 0.24	1.06 ± 0.33	1.63	2.20 ± 0.47
Total peripheral resistance (dynes sec/cm^5)	5100 ± 1320	4680 ± 1140	3780 ± 730	3540 ± 1100	3100 ± 520	3750 ± 1000	2800	4580 + 960
Cardiac rate	127 ± 27	124 ± 23	117 ± 22	114 ± 18	124 ± 11	132 ± 20	110	122 ± 13
Respiratory rate	23.3 ± 8.0	22.0 ± 5.7	21.2 ± 4.2	18.7 ± 9.7	19.5 ± 18	3.0 ± 5.2	6.0	32.3 ± 7.5
Tidal volume (mL)	161 ± 39	148 ± 43	120 ± 37	97 ± 50	105 ± 21	15 ± 26	90	143 ± 28
Minute volume (L/min)	3.43 ± 0.66	3.03 ± 0.40	2.86 ± 0.46	2.08 ± 1.02	1.96 ± 1.05	0.18 ± 0.31	0.54	4.50 ± 0.86
Arterial Pco_2 (mm Hg)	41.3 ± 3.2	46.7 ± 2.9	54.5 ± 4.8	69.3 ± 9.5	82.4 ± 12.7	115 ± 31	88	44.5 ± 5.6
Arterial buffer base excess (mEq/L)	−2.25 ± 3.5	−3.1 ± 1.9	−3.7 ± 1.4	−5.5 ± 1.6	−6.0 ± 1.8	−7.4 ± 1.6	−6.0	−4.4 ± 1.7
Arterial pH	7.349 ± 0.103	7.289 ± 0.066	7.228 ± 0.082	7.127 ± 0.071	7.070 ± 0.075	6.950 ± 0.117	7.050	7.281 ± 0.037
Arterial Po_2 (mm Hg)	519 ± 49	503 ± 32	470 ± 41	456 ± 39	460 ± 35	433 ± 45	453	432 ± 63

R-1.0 indicates recovery values at MAC 1.
(From Merkel, G., and Eger, E.I. A Comparative Study of Halothane and Halopropane Anesthesia. Anesthesiology, 24:345, 1963.) (41)

Table 2-7. The Means and Standard Deviations of Various Physiologic Parameters at Different Alveolar Concentrations of Halothane during Controlled Ventilation in Dogs

	MAC 1.0	MAC 1.5	MAC 2.0	MAC 2.5	MAC 3.0	MAC 3.5	MAC 4.0	R-1.0
Number of dogs represented by data	6	6	6	6	5	3	2	6
Mean arterial pressure (mm Hg)	111 ± 22	108 ± 22	91 ± 21	65 ± 26	59 ± 24	65	56	118 ± 10
Mean venous pressure (cm H_2O)	+1.1 ± 0.6	+2.3 ± 2.4	+4.3 ± 1.6	+6.0 ± 0.9	+7.1 ± 0.6	+7.7	+10.5	+3.7 ± 1.1
Cardiac output (L/min)	1.82 ± 0.49	1.45 ± 0.37	1.11 ± 0.32	0.87 ± 0.32	0.75 ± 0.24	0.69	0.53	1.65 ± 0.56
Total peripheral resistance (dynes sec/cm^5)	5490 ± 2440	6230 ± 2100	6870 ± 1600	5800 ± 2210	5050 ± 2300	7070	7330	6003 ± 2000
Cardiac rate	118 ± 27	106 ± 15	109 ± 15	106 ± 9	106 ± 9	120	114	105 ± 14
Respiratory rate	14.2 ± 2.2	13.9 ± 2.8	13.8 ± 2.6	13.4 ± 2.2	12.7 ± 1.7	13.3	12.0	13.3 ± 1.7
Tidal volume (ml)	392 ± 51	372 ± 25	350 ± 28	355 ± 32	361 ± 31	333	345	342 ± 34
Minute volume (L/min)	5.48 ± 0.79	5.12 ± 0.56	4.81 ± 0.57	4.68 ± 0.42	4.54 ± 0.17	4.33	4.14	4.50 ± 0.57
Arterial Pco_2 (mm Hg)	33.2 ± 3.4	32.2 ± 3.6	33.5 ± 4.2	33.4 ± 1.6	33.9 ± 3.3	36.3	32.5	35.8 ± 7.3
Arterial buffer base excess (mEq/L)	-1.4 ± 2.1	-0.25 ± 2.1	+0.7 ± 3.1	+0.3 ± 4.1	-0.3 ± 4.5	+0.3	-2.5	-0.4 ± 2.6
Arterial pH	7.426 ± 0.035	7.451 ± 0.037	7.446 ± 0.070	7.446 ± 0.046	7.430 ± 0.041	7.413	7.413	7.415 ± 0.059
Arterial Po_2 (mm Hg)	434 ± 57	468 ± 31	482 ± 26	469 ± 47	485 ± 22	461	470	482 ± 26

R-1.0 indicates recovery values at MAC 1.0.
(From Merkel, G., and Eger, E.I. A Comparative Study of Halothane and Halopropane Anesthesia. Anesthesiology, 24:346, 1963.) (41)

of potency, it is possible to determine the degree to which various factors affect anesthetic action. For example, the duration of up to 500 minutes of halothane anesthesia in dogs does not affect MAC. However, MAC varies slightly ($\pm 10\%$) during the circadian cycle in rats and mice. Pregnancy reduces inhalant anesthetic requirements as measured by MAC, an effect that is primarily caused by elevated plasma progesterone levels. Levels of $PaCO_2$ of from 15 to 95 torr have no effect on halothane MAC in dogs; higher values are increasingly narcotic. Neither metabolic acidosis nor alkalosis has any marked effect on anesthetic potency as measured by MAC. Halothane MAC significantly increases during ephedrine infusion. This supports the hypothesis that anesthetic requirement is related to the release of CNS catecholamines. Drugs such as alpha-methyldopa and reserpine, which suppress central and peripheral catecholamines, have been shown to produce dose-related reductions in canine halothane MAC values. Conversely, drug-induced increases of CNS catecholamines have been found to increase halothane MAC. Hypothermia ($\leq 28^\circ$ C) in dogs reduces cyclopropane, diethyl ether, fluroxene, halothane, and methoxyflurane MACs rectilinearly. With hyperthermia, halothane MAC increases 8% per degree from 37.3 to 40.7° C; above 42° C MAC decreases. Although potassium levels do not appear to influence halothane MAC in dogs, changes in serum electrolytes or osmolality do appear to alter anesthetic requirements when accompanied by changes in brain sodium (Fig. 2–3).

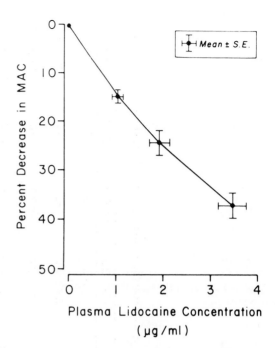

Fig. 2–4. Enflurane MAC in dogs decreases as a function of plasma Lidocaine concentration. (From Himes, R.S., Jr., Munson, E.S., and Embro, J.W. Enflurane Requirement and Ventilatory Response to Carbon Dioxide during Lidocaine Infusion in Dogs. Anesthesiology, 51:131, 1979.)

Nonnarcotic premedicants (amobarbital, barbital, pentobarbital, chlorpromazine, diazepam, hydroxyzine, ketamine) have an inhalation anesthetic sparing effect. Enflurane MAC is decreased by lidocaine (arterial concentrations of 1 to 4 mg/mL in dogs) (Fig. 2–4). Combinations of inhalation anesthetics are generally additive. Further discussion on these and other factors influencing inhalation anesthetic potency (MAC) can be found in Chapter 11.

The curves for anesthetic dose of various inhalant anesthetics versus CNS response are parallel. Thus, the ratios of anesthetic concentrations producing more or less CNS depression than that occurring at MAC 1.0 are relatively constant. In view of the preceding information and the availability of monitors of end-tidal anesthetic concentration, the use of MAC as a guideline for the selection and maintenance of anesthetic concentrations is beneficial. MAC may be used to gauge the margin of safety of an anesthetic relative to the MAC values at which specific effects occur (e.g., the concentration at which the inhalant blocks adrenergic response to surgical stimulation; MAC-BAR). In addition, reductions in the MAC value of specific inhalant anesthetics have been used as a means of quantifying the anesthetic effect of concurrently administered drugs.

SIGNS OF RECOVERY

As anesthetic drugs are eliminated from the brain, the degree of anesthesia lightens and reverse progress through the stages of anesthesia occurs. Induction

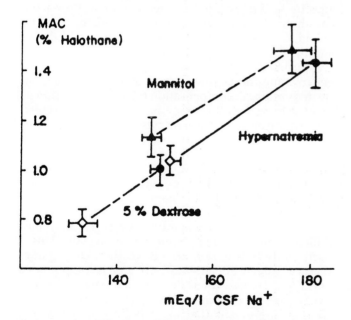

Fig. 2–3. The CSF sodium concentration was altered by intravenous administration of mannitol, hypertonic saline solution, or 5% dextrose. Halothane requirement (MAC) in dogs increased with increasing CSF sodium and decreased with decreasing sodium. (From Tanifuji, Y., and Eger, E.I., II. Brain Sodium, Potassium, and Osmolality: Effects on Anesthetic Requirement. Anesth Analg 57:404, 1978.)

techniques are usually selected and carried out to minimize the duration of stage II, in which excitement and motor activity may occur. During recovery, however, stage II can be prolonged. Every effort should be made to avoid stimulation of the animal at this time. This stage of recovery is of particular concern when large animals are anesthetized. Horses are especially subject to excitement and struggling during this period. The use of short-acting anesthetics and postoperative sedation can do much to minimize this.

During recovery the question arises of how best to judge the recovery from anesthesia, particularly when so many modifying factors must be taken into account. The experienced anesthetist finds himself relying less on classic signs of anesthesia and more on the patient's response to stimuli. Needless to say, effective anesthesia is not only that which just obliterates the patient's response to painful stimuli without depressing vital functions but also that from which recovery is uneventful.

Selection of an Anesthetic

The ideal anesthetic is one that
1. does not depend on metabolism for its termination of action and elimination;
2. permits rapid induction, quick alteration in depth of anesthesia, and rapid recovery;
3. does not depress cardiopulmonary function;
4. is not irritant to any tissue;
5. is inexpensive, stable, noninflammable, and nonexplosive; and
6. requires no special equipment for administration.

No drug available today possesses all of these qualities. Therefore, selection of an anesthetic is a compromise based on appraisal of the situation. Factors to be considered include
1. the patient's species, breed, and age;
2. physical status of the patient;
3. the time required for the surgical (or other) procedure, its type and severity, and the surgeon's skill;
4. familiarity with the proposed anesthetic technique; and
5. equipment and personnel available.

In general veterinarians will have greatest success with drugs they have used most frequently and with which they are most familiar. The art of administration is developed only with experience; therefore, change from a familiar drug to a new one is usually accompanied by a temporary increase in the mortality rate. Clark, speaking of anesthesia in man, stated, "The outstanding fact is that thorough familiarity with a technique is equivalent at least to a 30 percent difference in efficiency. If a person has mastered a technique, it is not worth his while changing to a new and unfamiliar one unless the change promises some big advantage."(41)

Often the length of time required to perform a surgical procedure and the amount of help available during this period dictate the anesthetic that is used. Generally, short procedures are done with short-acting agents, such as thiobarbiturates, propofol, and etomidate, or combinations utilizing dissociative, tranquilizing and/or opioid drugs. Where anesthesia of longer duration is required, inhalation or balanced anesthetic techniques can be safely used.

Species differences may prevent the use of some drugs. For example, procaine is frequently lethal for parakeets, and in high doses morphine can be excitatory in cats. On the other hand, most agents can be used interchangeably among species. Anesthesia in the very young is attended with increased risk owing to size limitations, limited muscular and adipose tissue in which anesthetic may be redistributed, and immature metabolic and excretory mechanisms. For this reason, the use of pentobarbital, and perhaps even thiobarbiturates, in very young patients is contraindicated (Chapter 24).

Aged animals are often poor anesthetic risks because of decreased vitality and the possibility of decreased cardiac, hepatic, and renal function (reserve), which may not be apparent on casual examination (Chapter 24). Drugs should be chosen and administered in doses that result in minimal depression of these systems and that can be easily metabolized and eliminated or reversed with specific antagonists. The same is true of patients in poor physical condition, since the liver and kidneys usually are somewhat affected.

General anesthesia is to be avoided, if at all possible, in animals with renal failure. Local, regional, or epidural anesthesia should be used where possible. If general anesthesia must be used, induction with a short-acting anesthetic such as propofol or etomidate, a potent opioid, or low doses of a thiobarbiturate and inhalant anesthetic are preferred (Chapter 23).

A cardiac murmur per se is not a contraindication for general anesthesia unless it is accompanied by untreated cardiac decompensation (no exercise tolerance). However, such patients may have less cardiac reserve and require more careful supervision during anesthesia. Patients with heartworm infestation and congenital lesions of the heart and great vessels also fall into this category. Balanced techniques utilizing nondepressant drugs such as dissociatives, opioids, etomidate, and isoflurane are preferred (Chapter 23).

Brachycephalic dogs, because of their pendulous soft palate and restricted respiratory passages, may have difficulty in breathing even when awake. This is particularly true in hot, humid weather. During anesthesia, the degree of airway obstruction is compounded, and these animals often die unless a patent airway is maintained via endotracheal intubation. It is wise to use short-lasting agents that are rapidly eliminated (e.g., propofol) so that a prolonged recovery period is avoided and patient control of the airway occurs rapidly (Chapter 23).

In large animals such as horses and cattle, anesthetics should be selected to provide rapid recovery with minimal emergence struggling. Emergence struggling is usually more of a problem in equine anesthesia, while general anesthesia in the ruminant is complicated by the hazards of rumen tympany, regurgitation, and aspiration. These latter complications make the use of regional anesthesia desirable where appropriate. In the event general anesthesia is used, endotracheal intubation is mandatory. In some instances, regional anesthesia in the standing position also presents the advantage that compression of abdominal viscera, as in a recumbent animal, is less likely to impede surgical intervention and respiratory and cardiovascular function (Chapter 20).

The overriding consideration in choosing an anesthetic protocol is one that is safe for the patient. This is based on

1. patient factors likely to influence responses to anesthesia, uptake, distribution and elimination;
2. the physical status of the animal;
3. the specific needs of the species; and
4. the specific needs of the case, including the relative requirements for sedation, immobilization, analgesia, relaxation, and safety.

Secondarily, the anesthetic protocol should be one that provides convenience to the surgeon so that the procedure can be completed efficiently, insures patient comfort, and can be administered with confidence by the veterinarian.

Physical Examination and Patient Preparation

"For every mistake that is made for not knowing, a hundred are made for not looking."

Anonymous

PATIENT EVALUATION

The purpose of the preanesthetic patient evaluation is to determine the patient's physical status. In general, *physical status* refers to the presence or absence of disease and to some extent the reserve of the various systems to withstand the stress of anesthesia and surgery. Specifically, the term refers to the patient's medical condition and the overall efficiency and function of organ systems. The goal is to determine any deviations from the norm that will affect anesthetic uptake, action, elimination and safety. Systems of greatest concern are the nervous, cardiopulmonary, hepatic, and renal. Knowledge of the physical status is an aid to selection of anesthetic drugs and techniques and is an aid in arriving at a preanesthetic prognosis. It is one of the best determinants of the likelihood of cardiopulmonary emergencies occurring during the anesthetic period. As such it is much better than arbitrary predictors such as age. It is axiomatic that the sicker the patient (the poorer the physical status) the greater the likelihood of adverse events or death. Physical status is determined by (a) history; (b) inspection (attitude, condition, conformation, temperament); (c) palpation, percussion, and auscultation; and (d) laboratory determinations and special procedures. Any

abnormalities should be noted. Those that can be corrected should be. If no further improvement can be reasonably corrected by medical treatment, the patient is considered to be medically prepared.

The history and physical exam are the best determinants of the presence of disease. Laboratory tests should be done on the basis of the physical exam and history. The use of extensive laboratory screening of patients has not been found to improve outcome of surgical patients in either human or veterinary medicine. Laboratory screenings frequently fail to uncover pathologic conditions, they detect abnormalities that do not necessarily improve patient care or outcome, and they are inefficient in screening for asymptomatic disease. Moreover, when abnormalities are detected they seldom have any impact on anesthetic protocol or surgical management.(42)

The use of multiple chemical and enzymatic analyses of blood and urine in surgical patients has become common with the advent of automated analyzers and their availability to veterinarians. Their use, as previously noted, has not appreciably improved the outcome of veterinary surgical patients. Frequently, when an abnormal value is reported, surgery is delayed and the test rerun, adding to the total cost of the procedure with little patient benefit. It should be remembered that reference ranges compare the test result with a set of values from a group of similar animals in a defined (determined by physical examination) state of health. The reference range, "normal," is presumed to be within ± 2 standard deviations of the mean. A common error, however, is to assume that the upper and lower limits of this presumed normal range represent a rigid cutoff point between a state of health and disease or normal and abnormal function. Indeed, 5% of normal animals do fall outside this range. Furthermore, a test result in the normal range (within 2 standard deviations of the mean) implies that function is normal, but does not account for the normoglycemic diabetic or the animal with cirrhosis that has normal hepatic enzymes and bilirubin values. Because 5% of nondiseased animals fall outside the normal range as defined, 1 of 20 healthy animals tested will fall outside the range. If multiple tests are performed, the frequency of abnormal tests results in nondiseased animals increases with the number of tests done. As the number of tests increases, the likelihood of an abnormal result in a nondiseased animal increases. In a 10-test profile of independent parameters, there is a 40% chance of at least one test result being outside the reference range. Reference ranges do provide useful standards by which extreme test values can be recognized. However, there is no consistent relationship between the extremes of test results and the presence of a disease. Frequently there is overlap in the distribution of measured test values between healthy and diseased populations. This is caused in part by the statistical nature of the reference ranges, the inherent spectrum of disease (latent to fulminant) and the variable rate of disease progression

Table 2–8. **Classification of Physical Status***

Category	Physical Status	Possible Examples of This Category
I	A normal healthy patient	No discernible disease; animals entered for ovario-hysterectomy, ear trim, caudectomy, castration
II	A patient with mild systemic disease	Skin tumor, fracture without shock, uncomplicated hernia, cryptorchidectomy, localized infection, compensated cardiac disease
III	A patient with severe systemic disease	Fever, dehydration, anemia, cachexia, moderate hypovolemia
IV	A patient with severe systemic disease that is a constant threat to life	Uremia, toxemia, severe dehydration and hypovolemia, anemia, cardiac decompensation, emaciation, high fever
V	A moribund patient not expected to survive 24 hours with or without operation	Extreme shock and dehydration, terminal malignancy or infection, severe trauma

*This classification is the same as that adopted by the American Society of Anesthesiologists.

and host response that the test measures. Thus, test results must be carefully interpreted in light of the physical examination and the history and not rigidly interpreted on a purely empiric basis of being more than 2 standard deviations from the mean of the reference population.(43)

A thorough preanesthetic evaluation of the patient is essential for successful anesthesia and subsequent surgery. Every effort should be made to detect factors that may modify anesthetic action and safety. While such evaluation is important in all patients, it is especially important in the critically ill patient. In addition to body weight and vital signs, the following should be included: The history should include previous and current health; presenting complaint, its severity, and its duration; concurrent symptoms of disease (e.g., diarrhea, vomiting, exercise intolerance, ascites, rales, dyspnea, polyurea-polydipsia, etc.); pregnancy; exposure to drugs; prior anesthetic history; and recent feeding. It is especially important to consider the status of cardiopulmonary function (Chapter 5), the potential of acid-base or electrolyte imbalance (Chapters 18 and 19), the possibility of a full or distended stomach or of hepatic or renal disease, and the prior or concurrent administration of drugs (e.g., organophosphates, diuretics, digitalis preparations, anticonvulsants, corticosteroids, aminoglycoside antibiotics, sulfonamides, and nonsteroidal antiinflammatory drugs).

All body systems should be examined and any abnormalities identified. The physical examination and history will determine the extent to which laboratory tests and special procedures are necessary. In all but extreme emergencies, routine determination of packed cell volume and plasma protein concentration should be performed. Contingent upon the history and physical examination, additional evaluations may include complete blood counts; urinalysis; blood chemistries to identify the status of kidney and liver function, blood gases, and pH; electrocardiography; clotting time and platelet counts; fecal and/or filarial examinations; and blood electrolyte determinations. Tests should not be run unless it is suspected their results could cause a change in anesthetic management. Radiographic and/or fluoroscopic examination may also be indicated, especially in animals susceptible to chronic respiratory infections, such as primates, calves, sheep, and rodents.

Following examination, the physical status of the patient should be classified as to its general state of health according to the American Society of Anesthesiologists (ASA) classification and the information recorded (Table 2–8). This mental exercise forces the anesthetist to evaluate the patient's condition and proves valuable in the proper selection of anesthetic drugs. Classification of overall health is an essential part of any anesthetic record system. The preliminary physical examination should be done in the owner's presence, if possible, so that a prognosis can be given personally. This allows the client to ask questions and enables the veterinarian to communicate the risks of anesthesia and allay any fears concerning management of the patient.

PATIENT PREPARATION

Too often, operations are undertaken with inadequate preparation of the patient. Some foresight here is beneficial. With most types of general anesthesia, it is best to have the patient off feed for 12 hours previously. It should be recalled that some species are adversely affected by fasting. Small mammals and birds and neonates may become hypoglycemic with but a few hours of starvation, and mobilization of glycogen stores may alter rates of drug metabolism and clearance. The latter may be a factor in ruminants. In contrast, feeding in the dog increases the metabolic rate for up to 18 hours. Induction of anesthesia in an animal having a full stomach should be avoided if at all possible, because of the hazards of aspiration. Distension of the rumen in sheep and larger ruminants has been shown to impair ventilation, with consequent hypoxemia and hypercapnia.(44) In the horse, a full stomach may rupture during induction and casting. Although limitation of food does not empty the rumen, the possibility of regurgitation is perhaps reduced if water is withheld for 12 to 24 hours prior to induction.

In most species, especially in the young and aged, water is usually offered up to the time that preanesthetic agents are given. It should be remembered that many old dogs suffer from nephritis. While these animals remain compensated under ideal conditions, the stress of hospitalization, water deprivation, and anesthesia, even without surgery, may cause acute decompensation. To withhold water from these animals, even for short periods, may prove hazardous. Ideally, a mild state of diuresis should be established with intravenous fluids in nephritic patients prior to the administration of anesthetic drugs. In any case, it is good anesthetic practice to administer intravenous fluids during anesthesia to help maintain adequate blood pressure and urine production, and to provide an available route for drug administration.

Systemic administration of antibiotics preoperatively is a helpful prophylactic measure prior to major surgery or if contamination of the operative site is anticipated. Oral antibiotics should be used prior to elective surgery of the gastrointestinal tract. The potential interaction of antibiotics with anesthetic or related drugs should receive careful consideration (Chapter 3). In surgery of the colon, rectum, and anus, preoperative enemas administered a day or two prior to surgery will remove fecal material and facilitate manipulation. On the other hand, an enema just prior to surgery may complicate the situation, since feces will be fluid and the operative site may easily become contaminated.

Dehydrated animals should be treated with fluids and appropriate alimentation prior to operation; fluid therapy should be continued as required. The delay occasioned by administration of fluids is more than compensated by the animal's increased ability to withstand the stress of anesthesia and surgical trespass. An attempt should be made to correlate the patient's electrolyte balance with the type of fluid that is administered (Chapter 19). Anemia and hypovolemia, as determined clinically and by hematologic determinations, should be corrected by administration of whole blood or blood components and balanced electrolyte solutions. Patients in shock without blood loss or in a state of nutritional deficiency will benefit by administration of plasma or plasma expanders. Corticosteroids may be indicated in certain aged or debilitated patients and those undergoing extensive surgery. Preanesthetic administration is more valuable than administration during an operation.

Several conditions may severely restrict effective ventilation. These include upper airway obstruction by masses or abscesses, pneumothorax, hemothorax, pyothorax, chylothorax, diaphragmatic hernia, and gastric or rumen distention. Affected animals are often in a marginal state of oxygenation. Oxygen administration by nasal catheter or mask is indicated if the patient will accept it. Alternatively, a tracheotomy may be performed under local anesthesia prior to induction. Intrapleural air or fluid should be removed by aspiration prior to induction, since the effective lung volume may be greatly reduced and severe respiratory embarrassment may occur on induction. While no attempt should be made to insert an endotracheal catheter in these patients prior to anesthesia, this must be done immediately following induction. Many animals have been lost because the anesthetist was not prepared to carry out all phases of induction—intubation—controlled ventilation in one continuous operation (Chapter 17).

In laboratory animals, especially rats, guinea pigs, mice, and rabbits, chronic respiratory disease may be endemic. In calves, sheep, and swine, lung lesions are common, and in primates tuberculosis may be encountered. Animals having such infections should receive specific therapy prior to anesthesia, and, should resolution not occur, local or regional anesthesia should be strongly considered (Chapter 16).

Decompensated heart disease is a contraindication for general anesthesia. If these animals must be anesthetized, an attempt at compensation through appropriate inotropes, calcium channel blockers, antiarrhythmic drugs, and diuresis should be made prior to anesthesia. If ascites is present, this fluid should be aspirated to reduce excessive pressure on the diaphragm.

In cases of hepatic or renal insufficiency, for instance in many bacterial and viral infections of mice, dogs, or primates, or in parasitism of calves, sheep, and rabbits, the mode of anesthetic elimination should receive strong consideration, with inhalation anesthesia preferred. Under experimental conditions, animals with clinical or subclinical disease of any body system should be identified and rejected from the experiment.

Just prior to induction, it is desirable to encourage defecation and/or urination by giving the animal access to a run or exercise pen. If this attempt is unsuccessful, catheterization or bladder compression may be necessary during surgical preparation.

Once a small animal is anesthetized, the bladder can be emptied by slow steady compression through the abdominal wall or by catheterization. An empty bladder is an advantage in abdominal surgery, particularly in the male, since urination may otherwise contaminate the operative field.

During anesthesia, the patient should, if possible, be restrained in a physiologic position. Compression of the chest, acute angulation of the neck, overextension or compression of limbs, and compression of the posterior vena cava by large viscera can all lead to serious difficulties. Complications include hypoventilation, nerve and/or muscle damage, and impaired venous return. The horse is especially susceptible to myositis and neuritis, resulting from excessive extension, abduction, or compression and ischemia of the muscles. Such complications are more likely to occur when good relaxation is achieved, or blood pressure is depressed and recumbency is prolonged in a lateral position; such a position also adversely affects ventilation-perfusion ratios and thereby the efficiency of gas exchange within the lungs (Chapters 6 and 20). The inefficiency of respiratory exchange is even greater in the supine position.(45) Periodic change of position is therefore recommended.

Tilting the anesthetized patient alters the amount of respiratory gases that can be accommodated in the chest (functional residual capacity; FRC) by as much as 26%.(46) In dogs subjected to hemorrhage, tilting the animal head-up was detrimental, producing lowered blood pressure, hyperpnea, and depression of cardiac contractile force.(47) When the animal was tilted head-down, no circulatory improvement occurred. In pentobarbital-anesthetized dogs lying on a horizontal table, sternal recumbency and left and right lateral recumbency positions consistently produced the least overall change in cardiopulmonary function.(48) The supine position was the least physiologic of the level positions. Prone and supine head-down positions (60°) produced the greatest physiologic derangement.

In all species, the head should be extended to provide a free airway and to prevent kinking of the endotracheal tube. In ruminants, it is desirable to have the head tilted down to permit drainage of saliva. Downward tilting of the hindquarters and abdomen (below the thorax) with minimal compression of the abdomen will limit reflux of rumen contents. On induction, if active regurgitation begins with large volumes of ruminal contents flowing into the pharyngeal cavity, pressure should be applied immediately by externally grasping the esophagus dorsal to the trachea to prevent further flow. Alternatively, an endotracheal tube can be inserted into the esophagus and the cuff rapidly inflated, directing the flow through the tube away from the laryngeal opening while an endotracheal tube is properly placed to protect the airway from contamination. Precautions should also be taken to prevent accumulation of rumen gases during anesthesia. This may be done by passage of a large-bore stomach tube. During emergence from anesthesia, it is desirable to position the ruminant in sternal recumbency. When large species are restrained in recumbency, viscera, restraining ropes, and bands may restrict respiration or compress nerves or muscle groups severely. During restraint in dorsal recumbency, abdominal viscera may compress the large veins and restrict venous return. In all instances, thorough padding beneath the animal is mandatory (Chapter 20).

OPERATIVE RISK

Operative risk refers to uncertainty and potential for misadventure or adverse outcome as a result of anesthesia and surgery. It should be emphasized that physical status, anesthetic risk, and operative risk are entirely different. To determine anesthetic risk, many factors must be considered, including the degree of skill of the anesthetist, the anesthetic to be employed, and the physical status of the patient. To determine operative risk, the foregoing must be appraised and, in addition, the operation to be performed and the skill of the surgeon must also be taken into consideration. Operative risk, then, is determined by factors associated with the patient, anesthesia, and surgery.(49) Patient factors affecting risk include physical status, temperament, age, species and breed, and overall physical fitness. Perioperative morbidity and mortality increase with the severity of preexisting disease. Geriatric and pediatric patients are at increased risk because of limited ability to respond to stress as a result of decreased functional reserves in the former and incomplete development in the latter. Depressed or overly apprehensive or fractious patients are often unstable and difficult to safely induce and maintain. In such patients, careful consideration should be given to preanesthetic management and choice of drugs. Species and breed characteristics can contribute to operative risks. Examples include the increased risk of airway obstruction in brachycephalic dogs, malignant hyperthermia in some strains of swine, increased incidence and severity of myositis in heavy draft horses, and increased incidence of regurgitation and aspiration in ruminants.

Surgical factors that can increase risk include the nature of the procedure itself (i.e., duration, complexity, organ involvement, operating conditions, and emergency). Major surgical procedures and procedures that are complex are associated with increased morbidity and mortality as compared to minor and simple procedures. Involvement of major organs increases risk; central nervous system (CNS), cardiac, and pulmonary procedures have the highest risk, followed by the GI tract, liver, kidney, reproductive organs, muscles, orthopedics, and skin. Procedures done on an emergency basis are more risky because of poorer patient status, that is, unstable or severely compromised patients, decreased ability to prepare or stabilize the patient, and lack of preparation by the surgical and anesthetic team. Operating conditions refer to the physical facilities and equipment and support personnel available. The aggressiveness of the surgical team, experience with the procedure, and frequency of performance are also important. Lastly, the duration of the procedure and fatigue must be considered because patients cannot be operated on indefinitely. The incidence of morbidity and mortality increases with the duration of anesthesia and surgery. Thus, efficiency of the surgical team is important in reducing risk. A related factor is fatigue.(50)

Anesthetic factors that can affect risk include the duration of anesthesia. Many adverse physiologic effects of anesthesia and surgery are time related. The choice of anesthetic can adversely affect the outcome, but more commonly the agents are not so much at fault as the manner in which they are given. Experience of the anesthetist with the protocol is important to its safe administration. Fatigue increases risk because it decreases vigilance. Thus, efficiency of patient monitoring and timely recognition and response to potentially life-threatening events is decreased.(50)

Record Keeping

Death of a patient from any cause is always unpleasant, but a fatality during anesthesia and surgery is even more so because of the obvious practitioner involvement. One will occasionally hear a veterinarian state that he or she has never lost an animal from anesthesia. This is conceivably true, though highly unlikely if a sizable number of animals have been anesthetized. Obviously, the criteria for anesthetic mortality in this instance must be defined. It is human nature to forget the disagreeable and to excuse a fatality by blaming it on something over which the veterinarian has no control. Not all deaths occurring in the perioperative period are anesthetic deaths. Deaths may be caused by (a) anesthesia; (b) surgery; (c) anesthesia primarily, with only a minor surgical contribution; (d) surgery primarily, with only a minor anesthetic contribution; (e) the patient's disease primarily; or (f) indeterminate causes. Deaths related to anesthesia should be recognized and identified. Examples of deaths that are attributable to anesthetic management are (a) death during induction; (b) explosion (rare at this time); (c) pulmonary aspiration; (d) failure to secure the airway; (e) hypoxia; (f) anesthetic overdose; (g) technical mismanagement of the anesthetic system; and (h) maladministration of fluids and air embolism.(50)

As long as anesthetics are administered, the hazard of death can never be eliminated completely; it can, however, be minimized, particularly if one is willing to investigate and to learn from mistakes. Once an anesthetic fatality has occurred, the sequence of the perioperative events preceding the death should be reviewed, their significance should be evaluated, and a necropsy should be performed to piece together its pathogenesis and etiology. Armed with this information, the practitioner can then take steps to prevent a recurrence of this tragedy.

Unfortunately, there is little recorded information concerning mortality in animals anesthetized in clinical practice. This may be because (a) busy practitioners do not have time to collect the necessary data; (b) there is no economic gain to be derived from such collection; and (c) there is lack of interest on the part of individuals best able to obtain these data. To obtain meaningful data concerning anesthesia, certain information must be collected and definite criteria established. A record must be made for each animal anesthetized, with the owner's name and the case number written on it. Among the items that should be recorded are

1. species, breed, age, sex, weight, and physical status of the animal;
2. surgical procedure or other reason for anesthesia;
3. preanesthetic agents given;
4. anesthetic agents used and method of administration;
5. person administering anesthesia (veterinarian, technician, student, lay personnel);
6. duration of anesthesia;
7. supportive measures; and
8. difficulties encountered and methods of correction.

Tabulation of these data will give not only extensive information on anesthesia, but also the incidence of surgical diseases in various species, age groups, and breeds.

Moribund patients are poor anesthetic risks, and if a single agent is used to anesthetize them, the mortality rate for this agent may appear to be disproportionately high. When one is discussing anesthetic mortality, therefore, it is necessary to categorize the physical status of the patient prior to anesthesia to assess risk. The ASA has developed a five-division classification of physical health and therefore anesthetic risk (Table 2–8). A modification of this classification of anesthetic risk can relate severity of patient disease to the occurrence of death. As expected, the mortality rate increases sharply as physical status deteriorates (Table 2–9). There are various reasons for animals undergoing anesthesia with a poor physical status. In some instances, anesthesia and surgery are performed to secure diagnoses on animals that would likely have died within hours. While data is available to define mortality based on patient disease and surgical procedure, percentage figures derived from large patient populations are not necessarily applicable to individual patients or hospitals.

It is necessary that each step of anesthetic administration be recorded in an anesthetic record along with the patient's response (Fig. 2–5). Minimally, the pulse and respiratory rate should be monitored at 5-minute intervals and charted at 10-minute intervals. Trends in these parameters thus become apparent before the patient's condition severely deteriorates, so that remedial steps may be taken.

The diplomates of the American College of Veterinary Anesthesiologists (ACVA) have recently proposed guidelines (1994) for anesthetic monitoring, with the intention of encouraging high-quality care of the anesthetized veterinary patient. The ACVA recognizes that some of the methods may be impractical in certain clinical settings and that it is possible to monitor and manage the anesthetized patient without specialized equipment. The ACVA does not suggest that using any or all of these methods can ensure successful patient outcome, or that failure to use any or all of these methods causes poor outcome. These suggestions are offered only to assist the veterinarian in determining priorities for monitoring and record keeping during anesthesia, surgery, and recovery. These suggestions may be revised as warranted by developing knowledge and technology. The aspects of anesthetic management addressed by the ACVA guidelines that deserve careful attention include patient circulation, oxygenation, and ventilation. Methods of monitoring each of the physi-

Table 2–9. Relationship of Physical Status to Anesthetic Deaths (Colorado State University, 1955–1957)

	Physical Status*	Deaths	Total Anesthetized	Percent Mortality	Ratio
Canine	I	7	1184	0.591	1:169
	II	7	964	0.726	1:138
	III	2	198	1.010	1:99
	IV	11	60	18.333	1:5.4
Feline	I	4	377	1.061	1:94
	II	1	90	1.111	1:90
	III	1	30	3.333	1:30
	IV	3	9	33.333	1:3

*Physical Status		Possible Examples of This Category
I	Healthy No discernible disease	Animals entered for ovariohysterectomy, ear trim, caudectomy
II	Preexisting disease No discernible systemic symptoms	Skin tumor, fracture without shock, uncomplicated hernia, localized infection, compensated cardiac disease
III	Preexisting disease Mild systemic symptoms	Low fever, slight dehydration, slight anemia, slight cachexia
IV	Preexisting disease Severe systemic symptoms	Uremia, toxemia, severe shock, severe dehydration, anemia, cardiac decompensation, emaciation, high fever; includes all moribund animals.

ologic processes are listed here in approximate order of simplest, most economic, and least invasive, to the most complex, expensive, and invasive. Assessment of circulation can be made by palpation of peripheral pulse, palpation of heartbeat by chest wall, auscultation of heartbeat (stethoscope, esophageal stethoscope, or other audible heart monitor), use of an electrocardiogram, use of noninvasive blood flow or blood pressure monitor (e.g., Doppler ultrasonic flow detector, oscillometric flow detector), or the use of an invasive blood pressure monitor (arterial catheter connected to transducer or aneroid manometer). Assessment of oxygenation can be made by observation of mucous membrane color, pulse oximetry (noninvasive estimation of hemoglobin saturation), oxygen analyzer in the inspiratory limb of the breathing circuit, blood gas analysis (PaO_2), or hemoximetry (measurement of hemoglobin saturation in the blood). Assessment of ventilation can be achieved with observation of chest wall movement, observation of breathing bag movement, auscultation of breath sounds, audible respiratory monitor, respirometry (measurement of tidal volume ± minute volume), capnography (measurement of CO_2 in end-expired gas), or blood gas monitoring ($PaCO_2$).

The ACVA further recommends that an anesthetic record should be made on each patient to maintain a legal record of significant events and to enhance recognition of trends in monitored parameters. The record should include all drugs administered, noting the dose, time, and route of administration. Monitored parameters should be recorded on a regular basis (at least every 10 minutes) during anesthesia. Responsible individuals should be aware of the patient status at all times during anesthesia and recovery and be prepared to alert the veterinarian about changes in the patient's condition. If a veterinarian, technician, or other responsible person is unable to remain with the patient

continuously, a responsible person should check the patient's status on a regular basis (at least every 5 minutes) during anesthesia and recovery. The responsible person may be present in the same room although not necessarily solely occupied with the anesthetized patient (for instance, the surgeon may also be responsible for overseeing anesthesia). In either of these situations, audible heart and respiratory monitors are suggested. In the best of situations, a person, solely dedicated to managing and caring for the anesthetized patient, remains with the patient continuously until the end of the anesthetic period.

Insurance Claims Involving Anesthesia. Table 2–10 lists claims presented to the American Veterinary Medical Association Professional Liability Insurance Trust from 1976 through 1982 divided into anesthetic, surgical, and medical claims. For more recent data on anesthetic related claims, the reader is referred to the AVMA Liability Insurance Trust.

Aftercare

Although in most instances recovery from anesthesia is uneventful, the patient should be kept under observation during the recovery period to prevent untoward sequelae. In animal hospitals and laboratory animal facilities, it is wise to have a recovery room for this purpose, since all the necessary equipment, drugs, and materials can be kept in one place, and it is less difficult to observe several animals. In some instances, the "prep" room may also serve as the recovery room; alternatively, recovery and intensive care functions may be combined. Such facilities should be conveniently located for nursing staff.

SMALL ANIMALS

Following removal from the operating room, the animal should be placed in its cage in lateral recumbency.

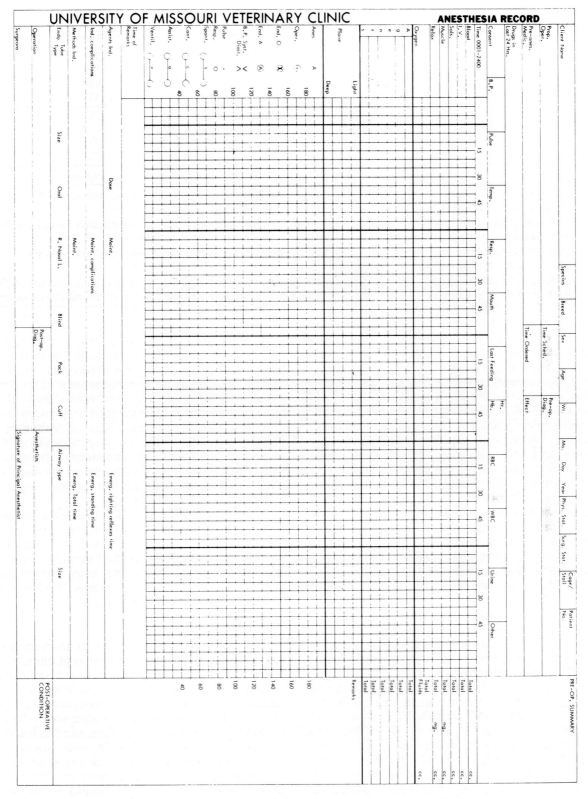

Fig. 2–5. Anesthetic record used at the University of Missouri Veterinary Clinic.

Morph.	Innovar	Barb.	**PRE-MED.**	**PRE-OP. SUMMARY**
Dem.	Atrop.			
I.M.	I.V.			
Rectal	Oral			
Satis.	Inadeq.	Excess	**RELAX**	
d-T-C	Succin.	Over Dose		
Flax.		Antidote		
Epinep.	Nor-ep.	Other	**VASO-CONST.**	
Blood	Plasma	Dextran	**I.V. THERAP.**	
Packed Cells	Albumin			
5 % Gluc. & H₂O	Gluc./Sal.	Saline		
Ringers	Lactate			
1. Good	2. Fair		**PHYSICAL STATUS**	
3. Poor	4. Bad			
5. Emergency (Good)				
6. Emergency (Bad)				
7. Moribund				
Digit.	Antihypert	Endocr.	**PRE-OP. THERAP.**	
Barbit.	Narcot.	Blood		
Fluids	Vasoconst.			
– 1 mo.	– 6 mo.	– 1	**AGE OF PATIENT**	**POST-OP. SUMMARY**
– 2	– 3	– 4		
– 5	– 6	– 7		
– 10	–15	+ 15		
– 5	– 10	– 25	**WEIGHT OF PATIENT**	
– 50	– 100	– 250		
– 500	– 1000	+ 1000		
Nasal	Eye	Dental	**HEAD & NECK**	
Plastic	Ear	Neck		
Superficial	Intracranial			
Cardiac	Great Vessels	Lung	**THORAX**	
Mediast.	Intrapleural	Thor. Cage		
Thor. Superfic.				
Stom. & Duoden.	Colon	Pancreas	**UPPER ABDOMEN**	
Spleen	Rumen	Liver		
Renal	Retro-perit.	Other		
Bowel		U.G. Ops.	**LOWER ABD.**	
Preg. Ops.	Gyn. Ops.	Other		
Inguin.	Lumbar	Abdomen Super.	**ABD. WALL**	
Extra-perit.				
Perin. U.G.	Perin Gyn.	Perin. Obs.	**PERIN.**	
Anorectal	Other			
Column	Cord	Spine	**EXTRE.**	**PREV. ANES. COMPLICATIONS**
Bone	Upper	Joint		
Soft	Lower	Foot		
Supine	Prone	Trendel.	**POSITION**	
L. Lat.	R. Lat.	Flexed		
Head up	Head down			
Heparin	Protomine	Klot		
No bicarbonate	No lactate		**pH**	RESP.　11. Pneu.　12. Hemorrhage　13. Bronch.　14. Trach.　15. Laryng.　16. Empyema
Neo-Syn.	I.V.	Isuprel	**VASO. PRESS**	17. Emphysema　18. Foreign body.
Drip.	Levophed			CARDIO VASC.　19. Cong. H.D.　20. R.H.D.　21. Arterioscle.　22. Hypertens.　23. Hypotens.
Prevent.	Non-prevent	Pt. Disease	**DEATH**	24. Failure　25. Arrhyth.　26. Pulm. Edema　27. Other
Anes.	Surg.	Complic.		NEUROL.　28. Br. Tu.　29. Cd. Tu.　30. Lues　31. Epilep.　32. Paral.
				33. Irrot　34. Other
				G.I.　35. Int. Obst.　36. Perf. Vis.　37. Periton.　38. Ileus　39. Carcinoma
				40. Emesis　41. Other
				G.U.　42. Cystit.　43. Pyel.　44. Nephrit.　45. Anuria　46. Hemat.　47. Album.　48. Glucos.
				49. Acetone　50. Other
				METABOL.　51. Diab.　52. Obese　53. Acid　54. Alkal.　55. Dehydration　56. Other
				HEMATOL.　57. Anemia　58. Hypovol.　59. Polycyth.　60. Leuco.　61. Leucopenia　62. Other
				NO. COMP.　63. No. Pre-op.　64. No. Post-op.　65. Neither　66. Death　67. Autopsy

GENERAL METHODS

Method	Ind.	Main	Emer.	Suppls
O.D.				
NRB				
Mask				
Semi-closed				
Circle				
To & Fro				
Insuff.				
I.V.				
I.M.				
Rectal				
Other				

GENERAL AGENTS

Agent	Ind.	Main	Emer.	Supp.
Ether				
C_HCl_3				
Elect.				
Nitrous Oxide				
Chloral				
Surital				
Pentothal				
Other Barb.				
Metafone				
Fluothane				

ENDO.

L. Nasal	R. Nasal	Oral
Cuff	Pack	↑ Cuff or Pack
Blind	Under Mask	

IND. COMPLIC.

- Excitability
- Cardiac arrest
- Respiratory arrest
- Brady cardia
- Tachy cardia
- Over dosage
- Under dosage

ANES. COMPLIC.

- Cardiac arrest
- Respiratory arrest
- Brady cardia
- Tachy cardia
- Other arrhyth.
- Hypertension
- Hypotension
- Inst. muscle relax.
- Pain
- Alkalosis
- Acidosis
- Hypoxia
- Excitement
- Convulsions
- Paralysis

EMER. COMPLIC.

- Vomiting
- Cyanosis
- Laryngeal spasm
- Laryngeal edema
- Pulmonary edema
- Hemorrhage

STIM.

Mike.	Ritalin	Amph.
Dopram	I.V.	

CARD. CONT.

CaCl₂	Ca Glu	Digit.
Pronestyl	Xylo.	Epinep.
I.V.		

Fig. 2–5 (continued).

Table 2–10. Claims Involving Anesthesia, Surgery, and Medicine Presented to the AVMA Professional Liability Insurance Trust, 1976–1982

Species	Total No. of Claims	Claims Involving:		
		Anesthesia (%)	Surgery (%)	Medicine (%)
Horses	542	13.8	41.7	44.5
Cattle	436	3.9	44.2	51.8
Dogs	1225	13.1	42.5	44.4
Cats	216	6.5	45.8	47.7

(Courtesy of Dinsmore, J.R.: AVMA Professional Liability Insurance Trust, Chicago, Illinois, 1983.)

While the animal remains unconscious or immobile, monitoring deemed necessary in the operating room should be continued. In any case, vital signs should be recorded at 10-minute intervals until the animal regains consciousness. Continued supervision is especially important until extubation and the return of coughing and swallowing reflexes. A blanket, pad, or even newspaper should be placed under and over the patient to conserve body heat. In very small or newborn animals, the ambient temperature should approximate body temperature. Incubators designed for babies are helpful in maintaining body temperature and are used routinely in many laboratories where birds, rodents, and primates are anesthetized. In newborn pigs, an environmental temperature of 90° F has been found desirable.(51) Otherwise, shivering occurs with increased oxygen and energy requirements, and hypoglycemia may result. During recovery, birds should be housed at 100° F; mice, hamsters, and small primates at 95° F; rats, guinea pigs, and rabbits at 90° F; and cats, dogs, and similar carnivores at 77 to 86° F.(7) Depending upon environmental temperatures, heat lamps, heating pads, or warm water blankets may be required. If fluid therapy is used, fluids should be warmed to body temperature.

During recovery, the tongue should be pulled forward to preclude its blocking the pharynx. In brachycephalic breeds or in animals in which respiratory function is compromised, an endotracheal tube should remain in place until upper airway reflexes and jaw movements return. In such animals, sternal recumbency, if practical, is preferred. Care is necessary to assure freedom of the airway from blankets or paper. The water pan should always be removed from the cage to prevent accidental drowning, in the event the semiconscious patient should place its nose and mouth or endotracheal catheter in the container. As soon as the animal regains the righting reflex, the water pan should be returned to the cage and the animal encouraged to drink a small quantity. Food may be offered as soon as the patient can stand.

Predisposition to postoperative respiratory failure may result from continuing drug-induced respiratory depression, postextubation spasm or glottic edema, other respiratory obstructions, diffusion hypoxia, mechanical splinting associated with pain and/or dressings, and persistent hypoventilation and/or atelectasis during anesthesia. Careful evaluation of respiration during the immediate postanesthetic period is therefore essential. If hypoventilation is identified, predisposing causes should be corrected if possible and, if necessary, supportive respiratory therapy should be initiated. Since postoperative hypotension may also occur as a result of a persistent drug effect, hemorrhage, and inadequate volume, adequacy of cardiovascular function should also be carefully and frequently evaluated.

Under no circumstances should an anesthetized animal be placed in the same cage with a conscious one, since the former cannot protect itself. Cannibalism has been known to occur (e.g., in pigs and rats), particularly where the anesthetized patient had an open wound!

When preanesthetic sedation has not been used, animals may thrash and struggle, bruising themselves severely and even breaking teeth during the recovery period. Coursing breeds, such as greyhounds, Russian wolfhounds, and Afghans, are particularly prone to this phenomenon. Judicious use of tranquilizers or opioids in small doses will quiet animals in this condition. Plastic-covered sponge rubber mats or other suitable pads in recovery cages will also afford protection.

Following administration of large doses of barbiturates, some animals will have a prolonged recovery period. Special attention must be given these animals to prevent hypostatic congestion and subsequent pneumonia. They should, of course, be kept warm and turned frequently. In addition, prophylactic antibiotic therapy may be desirable, and a protective ophthalmic ointment placed in the eyes to prevent corneal drying. Intravenous electrolyte solutions in moderate amounts prevent dehydration.

Constrictive bandaging of the head or throat must be avoided because of the danger of asphyxiation. Occasionally cats that have been tightly bandaged around the abdomen show evidence of posterior paralysis on recovery. This condition is apparently caused by decreased circulation to the hindquarters. Removal of the bandage quickly restores them to normal.

It is unwise to send anesthetized animals home, since owners are generally unable to cope with any unusual situation that may arise. In addition, they may become alarmed by the signs of approaching consciousness and may demand service unnecessarily.

LARGE ANIMALS

Like the small animal, the large animal should be removed to a recovery room (stall). The room should be padded to minimize injury during emergence from the anesthetic and recovery of righting reflexes. Availability of oxygen and suction is essential. If a padded floor and pads are not available and it is necessary to use bedding material such as straw, this should be covered with a tarpaulin so that it is kept clear of the external nares or end of the endotracheal tube and the eyes. Using pads beneath the head and limbs is essential. In the horse especially, protection of bony prominences from abrasion is essential. It is an excellent practice to bandage and pad all limbs prior to anesthesia and to keep these in place until recovery is complete. The head of the horse is especially subject to trauma during recovery with resulting abrasions, edema, and even facial paralysis. It should, therefore, be protected with a pad or a padded hood. Halters or headstalls should be used when necessary and should be padded.

Whenever possible, the horse should be allowed to lie quietly in a darkened environment and should be neither restrained nor disturbed. The possibility of emergence struggling and of attempts to stand before coordination is fully recovered is thus less likely. If an endotracheal tube has been used, it should remain in situ until the return of upper airway and swallowing reflexes necessitate its removal. Food and water should be removed from the stall until recovery is complete. If straw or other bedding material is used, the animal should be observed to prevent it from eating. When eye reflexes have fully returned, and nystagmus and pupillary dilatation are absent, the horse is usually able to stand. While the animal is attempting to rise, a steady influence exerted by the handlers in holding up the head and in upward traction on the tail may be helpful.

Some horses, despite preanesthetic sedation, struggle during recovery from anesthesia. Restraint may be required. A "tail rope" or a halter to restrain the head and neck is usually sufficient. Alternatively a sedative (e.g., xylazine) may be administered. Control by medication is preferable, although recovery may be prolonged with large doses. Small amounts of xylazine (100 mg) have proved useful in alleviating pain and calming recovery without unduly lengthening it. Some veterinarians restrain the horse either on the operating table or by ropes and hobbles until they judge the animal is able to stand. Such a practice predisposes to struggling and injuries.

When recovery rooms are not available, it may be necessary to permit recovery in the operating room. Operating rooms having a padded floor, or padded floor with table that lowers to floor level, are suitable. Restraint on the operating table until recovery is complete is undesirable, especially for the horse; struggling is likely and abrasions and nerve injuries are common. Rupture of the colon has been attributed to such restraint in several instances. If a cart is available to transport the animal, a grassy plot is a desirable location for recovery.

Ruminants are handled in a manner similar to that used for horses. Struggling and resulting trauma are usually not problems. Instead, it is necessary to minimize possible regurgitation and aspiration of rumen contents, and ruminal tympany. The endotracheal tube with cuff inflated should therefore remain in position as long as possible. Use of a speculum to prevent damage to or constriction of the tube is helpful. During recovery, the ruminant should be placed in sternal recumbency. If the flexed limbs are abducted slightly, it is usually possible to prop the animal in this position. Padded bolsters, other supports, or even bales of hay can be used to assist in maintaining this position. The head should be down and extended, and the end of the endotracheal tube unobstructed. When anterior epidural anesthesia has been used, the hind legs should be hobbled to a degree sufficient to prevent abduction until muscle control is regained.

The recovering large animal should be protected from temperature extremes. In the absence of heating or air conditioning, blankets, heaters, or fans may be necessary. If an outside recovery area is used, the animal should be shaded from direct sunlight in hot weather and blanketed in cold weather. When recovery is prolonged, the animal should be turned frequently and warmed fluids should be administered intravenously. Vital signs should be continually and routinely monitored until the return of coughing, swallowing, and righting reflexes.

Facilities

All necessary items should be kept in supply and in a state of readiness. When anesthetic emergencies arise, there is no time to hunt for mislaid equipment. The hospital area selected is, in some cases, the operating room itself. It is better, however, to have a separate "prep room" or place for preparing and inducing animals. This contributes to cleanliness in the operating room and leaves the surgeon undistracted. Regardless of the area used, it should be well lighted and equipped to facilitate examination, clipping, washing, and induction of anesthesia. A convenient method for storing clippers is to attach them to the wall or ceiling overhead, using a spring-activated reel. This arrangement will pay for itself over a period of time, since clippers usually break when dropped on the floor. A vacuum cleaner is useful to remove clipped hair from the patient and surroundings. A stainless steel sink with an overlying metal grid is effective for washing the surgical site and for expressing the bladder of small animals. Alternatively, an examination or grooming table with a central trough is also suitable when located adjacent to a sink with both hot and cold water.

The preparation room should also have adequate storage space, a refrigerator, a source of oxygen, nitrous oxide, suction, and a scavenging system for waste gases. The gases and suction should preferably be piped from a central system. If gas cylinders are used, restraint for storage must be provided.

Preparation of large animals for anesthesia and surgery is commonly performed in the operating room itself. This is dictated both by economy of facilities and by the need in many cases for restraint and even anesthesia prior to all but the simplest procedures. Despite this, a preparation room for large animals is essential if thoroughly acceptable aseptic conditions are to be maintained. It can be a stall convenient to the operating room and may also serve as the recovery room, although this is not desirable. In addition to the operating room, the large animal preparation area should be readily accessible to other large animal holding space including a loading and unloading dock. The room or stall should be well lighted and may be equipped with both horse stocks and a cattle chute. The floor should be constructed to minimize slipping and to facilitate drainage and cleaning. As in the small animal preparation room, a sink, hot and cold water, clippers, a vacuum cleaner, oxygen, compressed air, suction, and a scavenging system should be provided. If the preparation room is also to be used as a recovery room, the floor and walls should be padded and the room should be devoid of chute and stocks. An observation window that may be closed and an electric hoist or cart for moving the anesthetized animal should be installed. The room should be arranged to provide a quiet recovery, without light, and with minimal disturbance. Under such conditions, recovery is less likely to be complicated by struggling and excitement.

These facilities may comprise a suite of rooms or may be related functional areas in limited space. In any case, they should provide for an orderly flow of patients and personnel between animal holding space, preparation and induction areas, operating room or radiology, and recovery and/or intensive care. If the animal is induced with an inhalant anesthetic, it is preferable to transport the anesthetic machine with the animal. If this is not done, it will be necessary to equilibrate the gases in the new machine with those in the patient's respiratory tract. Storage space, facilities for washing, cleaning, and, where appropriate, sterilizing anesthetic equipment are essential.

Supplies and Equipment

The following supplies and equipment for anesthesia of animals are useful in the "prep," operating, and recovery rooms:

GENERAL

Anesthetic machine with gas supply
Masks of varying sizes
Endotracheal tubes and connectors of varying sizes
Syringes to inflate endotracheal catheter cuffs
Laryngoscope with assorted blades, spare batteries, and bulbs
Nonrebreathing valves
Carbon dioxide absorbent
Rebreathing bags of assorted sizes
Anesthetics, premedicants, and analeptics
Antiseptics, sterile sponges, "prep" tray
Cotton, gauze, adhesive tape
Anesthetic jelly, topical and local anesthetic solutions
Eye ointment
Sterile syringes; hypodermic and spinal needles of assorted sizes
Clippers with assorted heads
Scissors
Vascular catheters and sterile instruments, suture needles, and suture material for cut-down

Sterile gloves of assorted sizes
Electrolyte solutions, plasma expanders, blood
Fluid-administration sets
Blood-collection and blood-administration sets
Tourniquet
Thermometer (rectal and/or telethermometer)
Stethoscopes (chest and esophageal)
Restraint ropes, straps, or thongs
Heavy gauntleted leather gloves
Small toolkit for minor adjustments (screwdrivers, wrench, Allen wrenches, pliers)
Movable cabinet with lock to store smaller items
Infusion stand
Stool for anesthetist
Suction apparatus with catheters
Kick buckets
Adjustable examination and/or operating lights
Cardiac defibrillator
Cardiac-arrest and emergency kit
Ventilator for assisted or controlled breathing
Monitoring equipment (e.g, electrocardiograph, direct or indirect blood pressure, pulse oximetry, capnography)
Equipment for blood gas and pH determinations
Two- and three-way stopcocks

SMALL ANIMALS

Sandbags for positioning animal
V-shaped trough for table top
Anesthetist's screen
Anesthetic chamber
Small cart or stretcher on wheels and/or transporting cage
Bathroom scale, self-registering
Baby scales and/or balance and weights (metric system) for weighing birds and other small animals
Bath towels and/or blankets
Oxygen therapy cage

LARGE ANIMALS

Restraining ropes
Halters and headstalls
Leg and tail bandages and cotton
Tools for removing shoes and cleaning feet
Pressure sprayer with soap and disinfectant dispenser
Blankets
Oral speculae
Stomach tubes of assorted sizes
Water mattress, padded hood, or rubber pads for head, other body prominences, and limbs
Rubber-covered bolsters or equivalent for positioning animal
Movable cart and/or electric hoist for moving unconscious animal

Ideally, the anesthetized patient is placed in a relaxed, comfortable position. To prevent loss of body heat, an insulation pad beneath the animal is desirable. Alternatively, an absorbent paper cage liner or ordinary bath towels can be put beneath the small animal. The latter items also absorb fluids that drain onto the operating table.

Conventional small animal operating tables suitable for dogs, cats, primates, small ruminants, and swine are poorly designed for optimum positioning of the patient. Tables for humans are more flexible in that they are jointed and can be adjusted to the requirements of the surgeon and comfort of the patient. To overcome the shortcomings of inadequate table design, veterinarians use some additional aids, the least expensive of which is the sandbag. These can be fabricated in several sizes and shapes to fit the needs of various situations.

In many operations, stretching the patient's legs by tying them to the operating table with thongs may complicate the surgical procedure. When a flat-topped operating table is used, it is impossible to tie an anesthetized animal so that it will lie on its back and remain perfectly upright. This is true despite the fact that this is a commonly used position especially in canine and feline operations. This problem may be overcome by the use of adjustable V-top tables or by the use of portable troughs of wood or metal placed on conventional tables. Human operating tables are fitted with body horns that may be used to serve the same purpose.

In larger animals, restraint, induction, and positioning during anesthesia present many physical problems. To overcome these, padded induction and recovery rooms and new types of operating tables have been developed (Fig. 2–6A–D). Large animal operating tables should be padded and should have headrests and movable panels to facilitate access to the animal. Water-filled mattresses, inflated inner tubes, and movable pads are frequently used to protect the body, limbs, and head from undue pressure. The ability to lower the table to floor level or to tilt it to a vertical position facilitates restraint of the animal on the table either prior

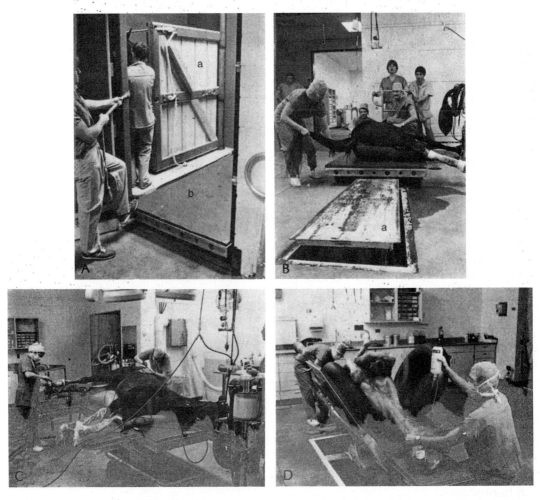

Fig. 2–6. A, Large animal induction stall. Horse is confined behind swinging door (a). Anesthetic is administered in the jugular vein. As animal collapses, it is rolled onto operating table top (b). B, Horse is transported from induction stall to operating room on table top. Top slides onto hydraulic piston in floor (a). C, Table is elevated to proper position and horse is prepared for surgery. Note water-filled mattress under horse for extra padding. Limbs are inserted into plastic sleeves to reduce contamination from feet during surgery. D, Trough-type large animal table. Sides can be raised or lowered with hand cranks. Note inner tubes to protect horse's shoulders.

or subsequent to induction of anesthesia. To assist positioning during anesthesia, tables may be tilted, an overhead hoist may be used, or trough-shaped operating tables may be employed (Fig. 2–6). When permanent facilities are not available, transportable large animal tables can be utilized.

For operations in the standing position, use of a cattle chute or stocks is often indicated. Chutes may be attached to a device that tilts the animal to a laterally recumbent position.

RESTRAINT EQUIPMENT

In addition to the materials previously described, certain equipment is advantageous for handling wild and vicious animals (Chapters 21 and 22). Included among these items are animal control poles, remote injection equipment, and squeeze cages. To handle many species of wild or zoo animals, control poles are very useful. These generally consist of a long wooden or metal pole to which is attached a rope or steel cable, forming a noose that can be controlled by the operator from the opposite end. In use, the animal's head or extremity is caught within the noose, which is then tightened to hold the animal securely. Once the animal is caught, it usually is possible to inject a tranquilizer or anesthetic agent in order to facilitate handling. Caution must be employed in the amount of tension placed on the noose, since it is possible to asphyxiate animals with this device.

An excellent animal control pole is available commercially, either in a standard length or with the ability to be extended to up to 12 feet. An additional advantage of this pole over homemade types is that it has a quick release, allowing an animal to be freed immediately without the operator having to manipulate the noose.

In capture and restraint of wild animals, several devices are used. These include gunpowder and carbon dioxide-powered rifles and pistols, crossbows, blowguns, and pole syringes. With them, it is possible to inject from 1 to 10 mL of any liquid into an animal for varying distances up to approximately 100 yards. The target area is usually the heavy muscles of the hip or neck (Chapter 22).

When zoo and other wild animals are to be anesthetized, the methods used vary with the species, their habitat, the degree of safety required, and the facilities available (Chapters 10, 21, and 22). The animal may be captured, treated, and released in its natural habitat; on the other hand, it may be necessary to premedicate or anesthetize it within its cage or in specially designed devices such as a squeeze cage (Fig. 2–7).

Personnel

Well-trained lay personnel can do much to relieve the veterinarian from some of the more routine aspects of patient preparation and anesthesia. They are also invaluable for restraining and calming nervous animals prior to preanesthetic sedation. The ultimate responsibility for anesthesia rests with the veterinarian, but a lay

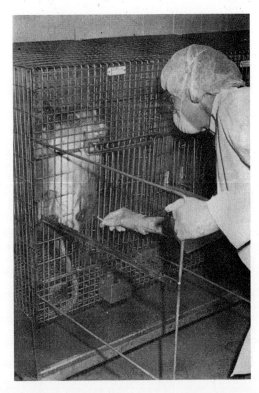

Fig. 2–7. Primate squeeze cage. By pulling on handles, the operator brings a panel at the rear of cage forward, confining the animal against the bars at front. Injection can then be easily performed. Once this is accomplished, the handles are pushed to return the panel to its original position, thus freeing the animal. Note the protective clothing worn by the operator when working with primates. (Courtesy of the Department of Health and Human Services, National Institutes of Health, Bethesda, MD.)

assistant who does not have a working knowledge of these techniques is of little value other than to restrain the animal. For this reason, it is essential that the layperson be taught the signs of anesthesia and of anesthetic emergencies, and be able to initiate steps to cope with the latter. Among the techniques to know are those of subcutaneous, intramuscular, and intravenous injection, endotracheal intubation, oxygen and blood administration, and cardiopulmonary resuscitation.

References

1. Knight GC. Barbiturate anaesthesia in small animals. Proc R Soc Med 42:525, 1949.
2. De Boer B. Factors affecting pentothal anesthesia in dogs. Anesthesiology 8:375, 1947.
3. Kato R, Takanaka A. Metabolism of drugs in old rats. I. Activities of NADPH-linked electron transport and drug metabolizing enzyme systems in liver microsomes of old rats. Jpn J Pharmacol 18:381, 1968.
4. Keys A. Age and the basal metabolism, guidelines to metabolic therapy, vol. 2. Kalamazoo, MI: The Upjohn Company, 1973.
5. Nicholas JS, Barron DH. The use of sodium amytal in the production of anesthesia in the rat. J Pharmacol Exp Ther 46:125, 1932.
6. Kennedy WP. Sodium salt of C-C-cyclohexenylmethyl-N-methyl barbituric acid (Evipan) anaesthesia in laboratory animals. J Pharmacol Exp Ther 50:347, 1934.

7. Green CJ. Animal anaesthesia. London: Laboratory Animals Ltd., 1979.

8. Stormont C, Suzuki Y. Atropinesterase and cocainesterase of rabbit serum: Localization of the enzyme activity in isozymes. Science 167:200, 1970.

9. Gourlay GK, Adams JF, Cousins MJ, Hall P. Genetic differences in reductive metabolism and hepatotoxicity of halothane in three rat strains. Anesthesiology 55:96, 1981.

10. Jenkins J, Balinsky D, and Patient DW. Cholinesterase in plasma: First reported absence in the Bantu: Half-life determination. Science 156:1748, 1967.

11. Jones EW, Nelson TE, Anderson IL, Kerr DD, Burnap TK. Malignant hyperthermia of swine. Anesthesiology 36:42, 1972.

12. Van Dyke RA, Chenoweth MB. Metabolism of volatile anesthetics. Anesthesiology 26:348, 1965.

13. Hug CC. Pharmacokinetics of anesthetics: Intravenous drugs. Annual Refresher Course Lectures, Lecture #225A. Am Soc Anesthesiol, 1978.

14. Saidman LJ. Uptake and distribution of intravenous agents: The thiopental model. Refresher Courses in Anesthesiology 3:141, 1975.

15. Eger EI II. Anesthetic uptake and action. Baltimore: Williams & Wilkins, 1974.

16. Baggot JD. Principles of drug disposition in domestic animals. Philadelphia: WB Saunders, 1977.

17. Brown BR. Enzymes of biotransformation as related to anesthesia. Refresher Courses in Anesthesiology 3:27, 1975.

18. Mazze RI. Renal toxicity of anesthetics. Refresher Courses in Anesthesiology 1:85. 1973.

19. Nishitateno K, Ngai SH, Finek AD, Berkowitz BA. Pharmacokinetics of morphine: Concentrations in the serum and brain of the dog during hyperventilation. Anesthesiology 50:520, 1979.

20. Rouse S. Effects of thiobarbiturate anesthetics on lean dogs. Vet Anesthesiol 5:22, 1978.

21. Dukes HH. The physiology of domestic animals, 6th ed. Ithaca, NY: Comstock, 1947:454.

22. Arnall L. Aspects of anaesthesia in cagebirds. In: O. Graham-Jones, ed. Small animal anaesthesia. Oxford, UK: Pergamon Press, 1974.

23. Anderson EG, Magee DF. A study of the mechanism of the effect of dietary fat in decreasing thiopental sleeping time. J Pharmacol Exp Ther 117:281 1956.

24. Brown BR. Anesthetic hepatic toxicity: A scientific problem? Annual Refresher Course Lectures, Lecture #106B. Am Soc Anesthesiol, 1979.

25. Brown BR. Pharmacogenetics and the halothane hepatitis mystery. Anesthesiology 55:93, 1981.

26. Teske RH, Carter GG. Effect of chloramphenicol on pentobarbital-induced anesthesia in dogs. J Am Vet Med Assoc 159:777, 1971.

27. Adams HR, Teske RH, Mercer HD. Anesthetic-antibiotic interrelationships. J Am Vet Med Assoc 168:409, 1976.

28. Pittinger C, Adamson R. Antibiotic blockade of neuromuscular function. Annu Rev Pharmacol 12:169, 1972.

29. Stoelting RK. Estimation of hepatic function — effects of anesthetic experience. Refresher Courses in Anesthesiology 4:139, 1976.

30. Adriani J. Anesthesia for patients with uncommon and unusual diseases. Anesth Analg 37:1, 1958.

31. Nair V. An ontogenic study of the effects of exposure to x-irradiation on the pharmacology of barbiturates. Chicago Med School Q 28:9, 1969.

32. Saksonov PO, Kozlov VA. Features of the pharmacological action of some anaesthetic drugs in radiation injury. Voen Med Zh 10:40, 1968.

33. Brown BR. Molecular toxicity of inhalation anesthetics. Refresher Courses in Anesthesiology 5:1, 1977.

34. Cullen BF. Cellular effects and toxicity of anesthetics. Refresher Courses in Anesthesiology 6:43, 1978.

35. Duncan PG, Cullen BF. Anesthesiology and immunology. Anesthesiology 45:552, 1976.

36. Lee JA, Atkinson RSA. Synopsis of anaesthesia, 6th ed. Baltimore: Williams & Wilkins, 1968.

37. Gray TC. A Reassessment of the signs and levels of anaesthesia. Irish J Med Sci 419:499, 1960.

38. Robbins BH. Preliminary studies of the anesthetic activity of fluorinated hydrocarbons. J Pharmacol Exp Ther 86:197, 1946.

39. Courtin RF, Bickford RG, Faulconer A Jr. Classification and significance of electroencephalographic patterns produced by nitrous oxide-ether anesthesia during surgical operations. Proc Staff Meetings Mayo Clin 25:197, 1950.

40. Merkel G, Eger EI. A comparative study of halothane and halopropane anesthesia. Anesthesiology 24:346, 1963.

41. Clark AJ. Aspects of the history of anaesthetics. Br Med J 2:1029, 1938.

42. Roizen MF. Routine perioperative evaluation. In: RD Miller, ed. Anesthesia, 2nd ed. New York: Churchill Livingstone, 1986:225–254.

43. MacWilliams PS, Thomas CB. Basic principles of laboratory medicine. In: RJ Murtaugh, ed. Seminars in veterinary medicine and surgery (Small Animal), vol. 7, no. 4 (November), 1992:253–261.

44. Ungerer T, Orr JA, Bisgard GE, Will JA. Cardiopulmonary effects of mechanical distension of the rumen in nonanesthetized sheep. Am J Vet Res 37:807, 1976.

45. De Moor A, Desmet P, Verschooten F. Influence of change of body position on arterial oxygenation and acid-base status in the horse in lateral recumbency. Zentralbl Veterinarmed 21:525, 1974.

46. Kilburn KH, McDonald J, Piccinni FP. Effects of ventilatory pattern and body position on lung volume in dogs. J Appl Physiol 15:801, 1960.

47. Liu CT, Hoff HE, Huggins RA. Circulatory and respiratory responses to postural changes in the hemorrhagic dog. J Appl Physiol 27:460, 1969.

48. DeYoung DW, Lumb WV. Unpublished data, 1971.

49. Collins VJ. Preanesthetic evaluation and preparation. In: Principles of anesthesiology, 2nd ed. Philadelphia: Lea & Febiger, 1976.

50. Collins VJ. Records, mortality and medical legal considerations. In: Principles of anesthesiology, 2nd ed. Philadelphia: Lea & Febiger, 1976.

51. Landy JJ. The use of large germfree animals in medical research. JAMA 178:1084, 1961.

chapter 3

DRUG INTERACTIONS

James E. Heavner

INTRODUCTION
PHARMACOKINETIC INTERACTIONS
PHARMACODYNAMIC INTERACTIONS
NOMENCLATURE

SPECIAL ASPECTS OF DRUG INTERACTION IN
ANESTHESIA
Examples of Drug Interactions Commonly
Encountered in Veterinary Anesthesia

Introduction

It is highly probable that two or more drugs will be used to manage anesthesia in most animals. Medications may be given prior to anesthetic induction to calm the patient, empty the gastrointestinal tract, reduce anesthetic requirements, or counteract side effects of anesthetic drugs or surgery. Then one anesthetic drug or a combination of drugs may be administered to induce anesthesia and another drug used to maintain anesthesia. Neuromuscular blockers may be used, and other drugs may be administered intraoperatively for diagnostic purposes, to provide postoperative analgesia or protection from infection, or to maintain physiologic variables within a target range.

In addition, the patient may be receiving medications for growth promotion or to treat diseases (e.g., bacterial infections, endocrine disturbances, cardiovascular or central nervous system disease, or endo- or ectoparasitism). The person administering the anesthetic may not be the person responsible for the other drug treatments and may not be aware the patient has received other drugs.

In general, estimates of qualitative responses to two or more drugs can be made based on the pharmacologic properties of individual drugs. Predictions of quantitative responses are more difficult. In 1981, Smith stated that research into the quantitation of drug interaction was in a rudimentary state and was rarely useful to the clinician. He further stated that the extent of knowledge of interactions among more than two drugs is discouraging and that even qualitative description of multiple-drug interactions can be overwhelming.[1]

Drug interactions usually result from administration of (a) two drugs in one formulation, as a fixed-dose mixture; (b) two drugs in separate formulations simultaneously; (c) a second drug during prolonged use of the first drug; and (d) two drugs at specific time intervals. Drug interactions are classified as either *pharmacokinetic* or as *pharmacodynamic*. In common parlance, pharmacokinetics refers to what the body does to drugs and pharmacodynamics refers to what drugs do to the body. Pharmacokinetic interactions produce changes in drug concentration at the receptor site by altering absorption, elimination, or distribution.[2] Pharmacodynamic interactions occur when one drug alters the response to another.

Drug interactions may be desirable and used to clinical advantage or may be undesirable and cause therapeutic failure, morbidity or mortality. Orme expressed surprise that adverse drug interactions are not more common given the fact that very many patients receive several drugs concurrently.[3] He cited literature attributing drug interactions to only 6.5 percent of 3600 reported adverse drug reactions.

Pharmacokinetic Interactions

Pharmacokinetic interactions include (a) pharmaceutic incompatibility, (b) alteration of absorption, (c) alteration of drug-biotransformation enzymes, (d) alteration of protein binding, (e) changes in renal or hepatic clearance, (f) changes in excretion through the lungs, and (g) changes in distribution.

Pharmaceutic incompatibility occurs because one drug or drug vehicle reacts chemically or physically with

35

another when two or more drug formulations are mixed. For example, mixing solutions with pH differences can cause the drugs to precipitate from solution or promote drug instability. Barbiturate solutions are quite alkaline (e.g., thiopental Na, pH 10.5), and lowering the pH will cause the barbiturate to precipitate from solution. Epinephrine solution has a very low pH (~1.5), and raising the pH will facilitate oxidation of epinephrine to adrenochrome pigments. Formulations with aqueous vehicle and with organic vehicle usually do not mix well. Diazepam is poorly soluble in water and therefore is formulated in an organic vehicle. It usually forms an emulsion when mixed with aqueous solutions. Single or multiple addition of drugs (e.g., antibiotics) to infusion fluids may result in interaction. Sound practice is to never mix drugs unless one is absolutely certain that no undesirable interaction can occur.

Alteration in absorption as a desirable drug interaction is best demonstrated by the practice of adding epinephrine to local anesthetic solution. Epinephrine prolongs the duration of local anesthetic action by reducing blood flow (secondary to epinephrine-induced vasoconstriction) and thus delaying systemic absorption of the local anesthetic. The second gas effect represents enhanced absorption from the alveoli of volatile anesthetic administered with N_2O. Rapid absorption of N_2O concentrates the other anesthetic in the alveoli, thereby enhancing absorption of the volatile agent.

EMLA cream is an interesting example of a physical change that occurs when two drugs are mixed with a resulting favorable impact on absorption. The cream contains equal parts of the local anesthetics lidocaine and prilocaine that combine to produce a eutectic mixture. Neither local anesthetic is effective when applied to unbroken skin, but the eutectic mixture is effective.

Alterations of drug biotransformation enzymes may either shorten or prolong the duration of action of a drug depending upon (a) the importance of biotransformation in terminating the action of a drug, (b) whether or not an active product is formed, and (c) whether biotransformation is increased or decreased. Many drugs are biotransformed by the mixed-function oxidase systems of the liver, then undergo a conjugation step that enhances excretion in the urine or bile. Plasma esterase also plays an important drug biotransformation role. Biotransformation enzyme changes that may be of clinical importance to anesthesia include enzyme induction produced by chronic drug administration and enzyme inhibition produced by acute or chronic exposure to drugs. Phenobarbital and phenytoin, which may be used to control epilepsy, will induce mixed function oxidases and shorten sleep time (e.g., hexobarbital) or increase the production of toxic products from drugs such as methoxyflurane (organofluorides). Chloramphenicol inhibits hepatic microsomal enzymes of the cytochrome P_{450} complex (4), and thus prolongs the half-life of anesthetic drugs that are metabolized by this system, for example, pentobarbital.(5) Inhibition of

plasma cholinesterase (pseudocholinesterase) by organophosphorus compounds will prolong the duration of action of succinylcholine and reduce the rate of hydrolysis of ester-linked local anesthetics such as procaine and 2-chloroprocaine.

Alteration of protein binding occurs but is rarely of clinical significance.(6) Drugs exist in unbound (free) and bound forms in the blood. The free form is generally immediately available to exert pharmacologic effects but the bound form is not. Many drugs are extensively bound to plasma albumin (acidic drugs) or alpha$_1$-acid glycoprotein (basic drugs). Drug displaced from protein distributes rapidly into tissue and is available for biotransformation and excretion. The net effect of a displacement interaction is usually small, transient, and frequently unrecognized.

Changes in renal or hepatic clearance generally are a consequence of changes in renal or hepatic blood flow, although other actions (e.g., effects on active reuptake by the kidney) can result from one drug influencing the disposition kinetics of another. Blood flow changes are most noted when the liver or kidney extracts a high fraction of drug from the blood presented to it.(7) Lidocaine, meperidine, and morphine are examples of drugs relevant to anesthesia that have high hepatic extractions.(8) Inhalational anesthetics, such as halothane, reduce liver blood flow.

Changes in excretion through the lungs may be important in anesthesia, as pulmonary excretion is a major pathway for elimination of gaseous and volatile inhalation anesthetic agents. Drugs that depress ventilation, such as opioids, may delay pulmonary excretion of inhalation agents.

Changes in distribution can effect the onset and duration of action of many drugs administered intravenously more profoundly than do changes in excretion and metabolism. Intravenous induction agents such as thiopental and thiamylal are typical examples. The concentration of the drug leaving the heart is a function of the rate of injection and the volume into which the drug is injected, that is, the venous return over the period of injection. The rate of delivery to the tissues is determined by the concentration in the arterial blood and the tissue blood flow. Any drug that affects either cardiac output or flow distribution will affect the rate of drug delivery and the total amount delivered, especially to the brain and the myocardium. These two organs are most closely involved with the anesthesia desired and the most serious potential adverse effect, myocardial depression. For a given rate of injection, the concentration of a drug in the arterial blood is a function of cardiac output. Although this is rarely determined before induction, one can make an educated guess as to the cardiovascular status of the patient and the likely changes that may be produced by the drug injected. For example, if thiopental is given to a patient with low cardiac output, a "normal" rate of injection will result in the delivery of a higher-than-normal drug concentration in the brain and myocardium, where most of the output is being distributed. There, the high concentration may further compromise cardiac function, if low output is secondary to reduced cardiac competence.(9)

Pharmacodynamic Interactions

Pharmacodynamic interactions include drug interactions at the same receptor sites or at different sites. In anesthesiology, pharmacodynamic interactions are frequently used clinically, and pharmacokinetic interactions much less often. Pharmacodynamic interactions of marked clinical significance can affect the cardiovascular, respiratory, and central nervous systems as well as the neuromuscular junction and metabolism.

It is common to give a drug (agonist) that binds to a receptor and produces a response and then give another drug (antagonist) that binds to the same receptor and does not produce a response, but terminates the effect of the agonist by displacing it. Examples include the opioids and benzodiazepines and their specific antagonists.

It is also common to give drugs that act at different sites to take advantage of complementary effects, to reduce the side effects of a drug, or to terminate the effect of a drug. Systemic administration of an opioid reduces the concentration of inhalation agent required to prevent the patient from making a directed response to a noxious stimulus. Atropine will reduce or prevent the muscarinic effects (e.g., salivation or bradycardia) of anticholinesterases (e.g., neostigmine) used to counter the action of nondepolarizing neuromuscular blocking agents (e.g., curare or pancuronium). Anticholinesterase compounds antagonize the action of nondepolarizing neuromuscular blocking (ND-NMB) agents by blocking the hydrolysis of endogenous acetylcholine (Ach), allowing Ach to accumulate and compete with ND-MNBs.

Nomenclature

Commonly used terms to describe drug interactions are *addition, antagonism, synergism* and *potentiation*. In purely pharmacologic terms that have underlying theoretical implications, addition refers to simple additivity of fractional doses of two or more drugs, the fraction being expressed relative to the dose of each drug required to produce the same magnitude of response, that is, response to X amount of drug A = response to Y amount of drug B = response to $\frac{1}{2}X_A + \frac{1}{2}Y_B$, $\frac{1}{4}X_A + \frac{3}{4}Y_B$, and so on. Additivity is strong support for the assumption that drug A and drug B act via the same mechanism (e.g., on the same receptors). Confirmatory data is provided by in vitro receptor binding assays. Minimum alveolar concentration (MAC) fractions for inhalational anesthetics are additive.

Synergism refers to the situation where the response to fractional doses as described previously is greater than the response to the sum of the fractional doses (e.g., $\frac{1}{2}X_A + \frac{1}{2}Y_B$ produces more than the response to X_A or Y_B). *Potentiation* refers to the enhancement of action of one drug by a second drug that has no detectable action of its own. *Antagonism* refers to the opposing action of one drug toward another. Antago-

nism may be competitive or noncompetitive. In competitive antagonism the agonist and antagonist compete for the same receptor site. Noncompetitive antagonism occurs when the agonist and antagonist act via different receptors.

Experimental approaches to determine additivity, etc. included dose response analysis (Fig. 3–1) and isobolographic analysis (Fig. 3–2).

Special Aspects of Drug Interaction in Anesthesia

The way anesthetic drugs are usually used raises special considerations with regard to drug interactions.(9) For example, (a) drugs that are rapidly acting are usually used, (b) responses to administered drugs are measured, often very precisely, (c) drug antagonism is often relied upon, and (d) doses or concentrations of drugs are usually titrated to effect. Minor increases or de-

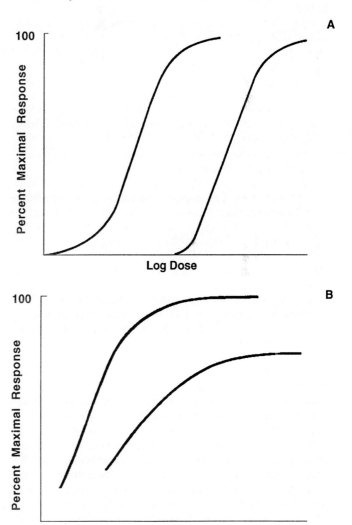

Fig. 3–1. Dose-response curve illustrating competitive antagonism (A) and noncompetitive antagonism (B). In A the dose-response curve is shifted to the right in the presence of an antagonist but the shape of the curve is not changed. In B the dose-response curve is shifted to the right in the presence of an antagonist and the maximal response to the agonist is reduced.

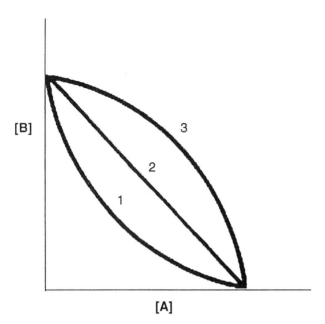

Fig. 3–2. Isobolograms for the response to mixtures of drugs. The sets of concentrations of drugs A and B, which as a mixture produce an effect (e.g., 50% of a maximal response), are plotted. Strict additivity, which means [A] + [B] = a constant results in a curve of slope −1 (2). If the curve is concave (3) some antagonism is present; if the curve is convex (1), synergism is present.

creases in responses are of little consequence and are dealt with routinely.

EXAMPLES OF DRUG INTERACTIONS COMMONLY ENCOUNTERED IN VETERINARY ANESTHESIA

Two or more different kinds of injectable neuroactive agents are frequently used to induce anesthesia with the goal of achieving the highest quality of anesthesia with minimal side effects. The agents frequently have complementary effects on the brain, but one agent may also antagonize an undesirable effect of the other. An example of such a combination is tiletamine and zolazepam (Telazol; an arylcycloalkylamine and a benzodiazepine).

Tiletamine produces sedation, immobility, amnesia, and marked analgesia, but it also may produce muscle rigidity and grand mal seizures. Zolazepam produces sedation, reduction of anxiety, and amnesia, and will prevent muscle rigidity and seizures. Another arylcycloalkylamine-benzodiazepine combination commonly used is ketamine with either midazolam or diazepam. Ketamine is also frequently used in combination with xylazine, a potent hypnotic with central muscle relaxant and analgesic properties.

Acetylpromazine is often used as a preanesthetic agent. In addition to calming the patient, acetylpromazine reduces the dose of anesthetic required to produce anesthesia and reduces the sensitivity of the myocardium to catecholamines, thereby reducing the risk of ventricular arrhythmias. On the other hand, the drug has α-adrenergic blocking activity. This action and the cardiovascular depressant effects of general anesthetics may interact to produce hypotension.

Volatile anesthetics may potentiate cardiovascular depression in patients receiving calcium channel-blocking agents. The gaseous inhalational anesthetic nitrous oxide (N_2O) may be administered along with a potent volatile inhalational anesthetic agent such as halothane or isoflurane. N_2O speeds the induction of anesthesia via the second gas effect, as described earlier. It also reduces the amount of volatile agent required. Because N_2O produces relatively less cardiovascular depression than does an equivalent dose of volatile agent (it may even stimulate), at any given depth of anesthesia, the amount of cardiovascular depression is less with N_2O plus a volatile agent than with the volatile agent alone.

It is becoming increasingly common to combine the use of regionally administered analgesics and light general anesthesia. An example of such an approach is to administer a local anesthetic alone or in combination with an opioid or an alpha$_2$-adrenergic agonist into the epidural or subarachnoid space before or during general anesthesia. Benefits sought with this approach are to reduce the amount of general anesthetic required and to provide preemptive analgesia. Reducing the amount of general anesthetic required reduces the magnitude of systemic side effects of the general anesthetic. Preemptive analgesia (i.e., preventing nociceptive information from going beyond the first synapse in the spinal cord) is thought to reduce postoperative pain and discomfort and thereby improve postoperative comfort (Chapter 4).

Similarly, it is becoming increasingly common to mix local anesthetic and an opioid and/or an alpha$_2$-adrenergic agonist for spinal or epidural anesthesia. The primary goals are (a) to reduce the amount of each drug required and thereby reduce the side effects; and (b) to improve the quality of analgesia. These goals can be achieved because the mechanism of action whereby each component of the mixture produces the desired effect differs and the drugs have different side effects.

The response to neuromuscular blocking agents may be increased or decreased by a number of nonanesthetic drugs that may be administered in the anesthetic or perianesthetic period. For example, anticonvulsants may decrease the response, and an increased response may be present in patients receiving antibiotics or other drugs (e.g., aminoglycosides, polymyxin, or magnesium). Additional information regarding the effects of drug therapy on neuromuscular blocking agents is available elsewhere.(10) For further information, a monograph listing 647 drugs, giving the mechanism of action and potential interaction with anesthetic agents, is available and should be referred to when there is concern about the possibility of specific drug interactions.(11)

References

1. Smith NT. Dangers and opportunities. In: NT Smith, RD Miller, AW Corbasico, eds. Drug interactions in anesthesia. Philadelphia: Lea & Febiger, 1981:1–9.
2. Wood AJJ. Drug interactions and adverse drug reactions. In: M Wood and AJJ Wood, eds. Drugs and anesthesia. Pharmacology for anesthesiologists, 2nd ed. Baltimore: Williams & Wilkins, 1990:73–80.
3. Orme MLE. Drug interactions of clinical importance. In: DM Davis ed. Textbook of adverse drug reactions. Oxford, UK: Oxford University Press, 1991:788–810.
4. Halpert J. Further studies of the suicide inactivation of purified rat liver cytochrome P-450 by chloramphenicol. Mol Pharmacol 21:166–172, 1982.
5. Adams HR, Dixit BN. Prolongation of pentobarbital anesthesia by chloramphenicol in dogs and cats. J Am Vet Med Assoc 156:902–905, 1970.
6. Nies AS. Principles of therapeutics. In: AG Gilman, TW Rail, AS Nies, P Taylor, eds. The pharmacological basics of therapeutics, 8th ed. New York: Pergamon Press, 1990:62–83.
7. Wilkinson GR, Shand DG. A physiological approach to hepatic drug clearance. Clin Pharmacol Therap 18:377–390, 1975.
8. Stanski DG, Watkins WD. Drug disposition in anesthesia. New York: Grune & Stratton, 1982:25.
9. Flacke WF, Flacke JW. Mechanisms: General principles. In: NT Smith, RD Miller and AW Corbasico, eds. Drug interactions in anesthesia. Philadelphia: Lea & Febiger, 1981:11–29.
10. Thornton JA. The effects of drug therapy on the response to anaesthetic agents. In: JA Thornton, ed. Adverse reactions of anaesthetic drugs. New York: Excerpta Medica/Elsevier North-Holland Biomedical Press, 1981:1–27.
11. Mueller RA, Lundberg DBA. Manual of drug interactions for anesthesiology 2nd ed. New York: Churchill Livingstone, 1992.

chapter 4

PERIOPERATIVE PAIN AND DISTRESS

Introduction

The prevention and control of pain is central to the practice of anesthesia. It is essential that the anesthetist have an understanding of the physiologic processes leading to the perception of pain and the responses of the patient to this process. Ultimately, anesthetic patient management is the control of pain and maintenance of homeostasis in the face of pain-inducing insults.

Pain is an unpleasant sensory and emotional experience (perception) associated with actual or potential tissue damage or is described in terms of such damage. Pain arises from the activation of a discrete set of receptors and neural pathways by noxious stimuli that are actually or potentially damaging to tissues. It is an awareness of acute or chronic discomfort occurring in various degrees of severity resulting from injury, disease, or emotional distress as evidenced by biologic or behavioral changes or both. It is a subjective experience accompanied by feelings of fear, anxiety, and panic. Pain elicits protective motor actions, results in learned avoidance, and may modify species-specific traits of behavior including social behavior.(1, 2) *Acute pain* is the result of a traumatic, surgical, or infectious event that is abrupt in onset and relatively short in duration. It is

generally alleviated by analgesic drugs. *Chronic pain* is pain that persists beyond the usual course of an acute disease or beyond a reasonable time for an injury to heal, or that is associated with a chronic pathologic process that persists or recurs for months or years. Chronic pain is seldom permanently alleviated by analgesics, but may frequently respond to tranquilizers or psychotropic drugs combined with environmental manipulation and behavioral conditioning. Acute pain is a symptom of disease, whereas chronic pain itself is a disease. Acute pain has a biologic function in that it serves as a warning that something is wrong and leads to behavioral changes and limits of activity that are protective. Chronic pain does not serve a biologic function and imposes severe detrimental stresses on the patient. Being a perception, pain is always subjective. In people, pain experience has three dimensions — sensory-discriminative, motivational-affective, and cognitive-evaluative — which are subserved by physiologically distinct systems.(3, 4) The sensory-discriminative dimension provides information on the onset, location, intensity, type, and duration of the pain-inducing stimulus. This aspect is subserved primarily by the lateral ascending nociceptive tracts, thalamus, and somatosensory cortex. The motivational-affective dimension disturbs the feeling of well-being of the individual, resulting in the unpleasant effect of pain and suffering, and triggers the organism to action. This dimension is closely linked to the autonomic nervous system, and cardiovascular, respiratory, and gastrointestinal responses are associated with it (although they can occur reflexly as well). This dimension is subserved by the medial ascending nociceptive tracts and their input into the reticular formation and limbic system. The cognitive-evaluative dimension encompasses the effects of prior experience, social and cultural values, anxiety, attention, and conditioning. These activities are largely caused by cortical activity, although cortical activation is dependent on reticular activity. The cognitive-evaluative dimension of the pain experience in lower mammals may be the only one that differs significantly from that in humans. In order to discuss pain physiology and its management, a review of the definitions commonly used to describe this sensation is necessary.

Definitions

Agology is the science and study of pain phenomena.

Allodynia is pain caused by a stimulus that does not normally provoke pain.

Analgesia is the absence of pain in the presence of stimuli that would normally be painful.

Analgesics are drugs that induce analgesia.

Anesthesia is the absence of all sensory modalities.

Anesthetics are drugs that induce regional anesthesia (i.e., in one part of the body) or general anesthesia (i.e., unconsciousness).

Causalgia is a syndrome of prolonged burning pain, allodynia, and hyperpathia after a traumatic nerve lesion, often combined with vasomotor and sudomotor dysfunction and later trophic changes.

Central pain is pain associated with a lesion of the central nervous system.

Deafferentation pain is pain caused by loss of sensory input into the central nervous system, as occurs with avulsion of the brachial plexus or other types of peripheral nerve lesions, or caused by pathology of the central nervous system.

Dermatome is the sensory segmental supply to skin and subcutaneous tissue.

Dysesthesia is an unpleasant abnormal sensation whether spontaneous or evoked.

Hyperesthesia is an increased sensitivity to stimulation, excluding special senses.

Hyperalgesia is an increased response to a stimulation that is normally painful.

Hypoalgesia is a diminished sensitivity to noxious stimulation.

Hypoesthesia is a diminished sensitivity to stimulation, excluding special senses.

Neuralgia is pain in the distribution of a nerve or nerves.

Neuritis is an inflammation of a nerve or nerves.

Neuropathy is a disturbance of function or pathologic change in a nerve.

Nociception is the reception, conduction, and central nervous processing of nerve signals generated by the stimulation of nociceptors. It is the physiologic process that when carried to completion results in the conscious perception of pain.

Nociceptor is a receptor preferentially sensitive to a noxious stimulus or to a stimulus that would become noxious if prolonged.

Nociceptor threshold is the minimum strength of stimulus that will cause a nociceptor to generate a nerve impulse.

Noxious stimulus is one that is actually or potentially damaging to body tissue. It is one of intensity and quality that are adequate to trigger nociceptive reactions in an animal, including pain in people.

Pain (detection) threshold is the least experience of pain that a subject can recognize. The point at which a subject just begins to feel pain when a noxious stimulus is being applied in an ascending trial or at which when pain disappears in a descending trial. The pain detection threshold is relatively constant among individuals and species. In most cases it is higher than the nociceptor threshold.

Pain tolerance is the greatest level of pain that a subject will tolerate. Pain tolerance varies considerably among individuals, both human and animal. It is influenced greatly by the individual's prior experience, environment, stress, and drugs.

Pain tolerance range is the arithmetic difference between the pain detection threshold and the pain tolerance threshold.

Paresthesia is an abnormal sensation, whether spontaneous or evoked. Paresthesias are not painful, as opposed to dysesthesias.

Radiculalgia is pain along the distribution of one or more sensory nerve roots.

Radiculopathy is a disturbance of function or pathologic change in one or more nerve roots.

Radiculitis is an inflammation of one or more nerve roots.

Reflexes are involuntary, purposeful, and orderly responses to a stimulus. The anatomic basis for the reflex arc consists of a receptor, a primary afferent nerve fiber associated with the receptor, a region of integration in the spinal cord or brain stem (synapses), and a lower motor neuron leading to an effector organ such as skeletal muscles (somatic reflexes), smooth muscles, or glands (visceral reflexes).

Reactions are a combination of reflexes designed to produce widespread movement in relation to the application of a stimulus. Reactions are mass reflexes not under voluntary control and therefore do not involve the cerebral cortex.

Responses consist of willful movement of the body or parts of the body. A response cannot occur without involvement of the somatosensory cerebral cortex. A decerebrate animal can give a reaction but not a response. Reflexes and reactions may or may not be perception linked (i.e., the stimulus perceived as painful). Because responses require a functioning somatosensory cortex, the initiating stimulus is perceived.

Somatic is usually used to describe input for body tissues other than viscera.

Suffering is an unpleasant emotional state that is internalized and not expressed outwardly. It is described as an undesirable mental state, an unpleasant emotion that people or animals would normally prefer to avoid. Suffering can refer to a wide range of intense and unpleasant subjective states such as fear and frustration. It can be of either physical or psychologic origin. Suffering can be provoked by pain or by pain-free non-tissue-damaging external stimuli such as denial of the fulfillment of an animal's natural instincts or needs such as maternal deprivation, social contacts, and so on.

Distress is the external expression through emotion or behavior (i.e, fear, anxiety, hyperactivity, aggression or factiousness) of suffering.(5-7)

Nociceptors

Noxious stimuli activate specialized high-threshold receptors, nociceptors, resulting in the generation of impulses in afferent A-delta and C nerve fibers. These nociceptive primary afferent fibers supply skin, subcutaneous tissues, periosteum, joints, muscles, and viscera.(5) Nociceptors located in skin, subcutaneous tissue, and fascia are of three types: mechanical, polymodal, and mechanothermal. In addition, A-delta heat and A-delta and C fiber cold receptors have been described.(8, 9) Mechanical nociceptors are A-delta high-threshold mechanoreceptors or HTMs. HTMs respond only to moderately intense or noxious mechanical stimuli and do not respond to noxious heat or algesic substances, although HTMs can become sensitized to repeatedly applied heat. High-threshold mechanoreceptors have been demonstrated in the skin of the cat, the monkey, and man. The threshold for stimulation is 5 to 1000 times greater than low-threshold mechanoreceptors, which transduce touch via A-beta fibers.(10-12)

C-polymodal receptors (CPM) respond to intense mechanical stimuli (>1 g), thermal stimuli (45–53° C), and often chemical stimuli. Their mechanical threshold is similar to the HTM, but they are also heat sensitive. These receptors respond best to strong, long-lasting stimuli, and have a sustained discharge that slowly adapts. Topical or intradermal acids, histamine, or KCl increases discharge rate for several minutes. C-polymodal receptors are extremely important to nociception, accounting for 50% of sensory C units in the cat, 80 to 90% in the rat and monkey, and 95% in man.(13-15)

Myelinated mechanothermal (MMT; A-delta heat nociceptors) receptors respond to noxious heat as well as strong mechanical stimuli. They are responsible for the first pain of heat and are found in the cat, the monkey, and humans.(10, 11, 13)

Both A-delta and C-fiber nociceptors are essential for perception of acute pain. The rate of discharge of the nociceptor increases with increasing intensity of noxious stimulus. Because of their size and myelinization, A-delta fibers conduct impulses much more rapidly than do the small unmyelinated C fibers. A-delta nociceptors mediate first or fast (pricking) pain, which lasts less than 50 ms following a single stimulus. C polymodal receptors mediate slow (burning) pain, which lasts over a second from a single stimulus.(16) A-delta receptors appear to be specialized for detection of dangerous mechanical and thermal stimuli and for triggering rapid nociceptive responses (first pain). C polymodal receptors respond to strong mechanical, thermal, and chemical stimuli, are sensitized by chemicals released in damaged or inflamed skin, and mediate slow pain.(17) C fibers reinforce the immediate response of A fibers, signal the presence of damaged or inflamed tissue, and promote their protection and rest. All classes of nociceptors become sensitized following mild injury, resulting in hyperalgesia of injured skin.(5)

Nociceptive function in muscle is primarily via C polymodal fibers, which are responsive to bradykinin, histamine, serotonin or KCl, and strong pressure. A-delta mechanoreceptors are also present in muscle, are sensitive to pressure but not stretch, chemical stimulation, and reinforce C polymodal activity.(9)

A-delta and C nociceptors form a plexus in the joint capsule, fat pads, ligaments, and adventitia of blood vessels supplying the joint. They are sensitive to pressure and chemicals including sensitization by prostaglandins.(18) The periosteum and cancellous portion of bone is innervated by both A-delta and C fibers, and appears to have the lowest pain threshold of the deep body tissues. Cortical bone and marrow are not pain sensitive, being supplied primarily by vasomotor fibers. The teeth receive both intradental and periodontal innervation. Pulpal afferents are sensitive to pressure, chemicals, and heat.(5)

Visceral innervation is different from skin in that the ratio of A to C fibers in dorsal roots is 1:2, whereas that in visceral nerves is 1:8 to 1:10. Thus, visceral nociceptive activity is primarily mediated by C polymodal receptors. Visceral afferent nerves have their cell bodies in the dorsal root ganglion, but their axons are primarily associated with sympathetic pathways, are relatively few in number compared to cutaneous afferents, and have large overlapping receptor fields. Mesenteric stretching, inflammation, ischemia, and dilation or spasm of hollow visci result in severe pain, whereas burning, clamping, and cutting do not stimulate visceral pain.(19, 20)

Afferent Nerves

Peripheral nociceptors respond to direct stimulation. Unlike other sensory end organs, nociceptors do not demonstrate fatigue with repeated stimulation, but rather display enhanced sensitivity, lowered threshold of stimulation, and prolonged and enhanced response to stimulation (afterdischarge). Tissue damage caused by injury or disease results in sensitization at the site of injury (i.e., primary hyperalgesia) characterized by lowered pain threshold, increased sensibility to suprathreshold stimuli, and spontaneous pain. Following injury there develops a larger area of hyperalgesia and allodynia around the site of injury called *secondary hyperalgesia.*(5)

Tissue damaged by injury, disease, or inflammation releases endogenous algogenic substances into the extracellular fluid surrounding the nociceptors. These substances include H^+, K^+, serotonin, histamine, prostaglandins, bradykinin, substance P, and many others. In addition to direct excitatory effects on the membranes of nociceptors, they may be indirectly excitatory through their effects on the microcirculation. Serotonin, histamine, H^+, K^+, prostaglandins, and other products of the arachidonic acid cascade are present in tissues, kinins are present in plasma, and substance P in nerve terminals. Histamine is found in mast cells, basophils, and platelets, and serotonin in mast cells and platelets. Substances that directly activate nociceptors include bradykinin, acetylcholine, and K^+; prostaglandins sensitize nociceptors but cannot excite them by themselves. Substance P does not activate or sensitize nociceptors directly but causes extravasation leading to the influx of additional algogenic substances. Although the mechanisms are not well understood, injured primary afferents develop a sensitivity to norepinephrine that can be released from sympathetic postganglionic neurons (sympathetic-dependent hyperalgesia). Norepinephrine may also play a role through stimulation of alpha$_2$ receptors to produce PGE2 and PGI2, which can activate and sensitize nociceptors. Hyperalgesia induced by bradykinin has been shown to be dependent on the sympathetic postganglionic neuron and production of prostaglandins.(17, 21-26)

NOCICEPTIVE AFFERENT NERVES

Nociceptive impulses generated by the nociceptors are carried to the central nervous system by A-delta and C fibers. The afferent nerve, whose cell body is in the dorsal root ganglion, enters the spinal cord via the dorsal nerve root and terminates on cells in the dorsal horn of the gray matter. Alternatively, some nerve fibers may enter the spinal cord via the ventral nerve root or may after entering the ventral root turn back to enter the dorsal root.(9, 27)

The gray matter of the spinal cord can be divided into ten laminae. Laminae I–VI are in the dorsal horn; laminae VII–IX are in the ventral horn, and lamina X is a column of cells immediately surrounding the central canal. Lamina I is called the *marginal layer,* lamina II is called the *substantia gelatinosa* (SG), and laminae III–V make up the *nucleus proprius.* These lamina run throughout the cord and fuse with a similar structure in the medulla, the medullary dorsal horn. On entering the spinal cord, C fibers travel in the most lateral part of the dorsal white matter including Lissauer's tract. A-delta fibers travel in the more medial portion of the dorsal column. The dorsal root afferents give off collateral fibers, most within their segment of entry, but also rostrally and caudally: 3 to 6 segments for A-delta and 2 to 3 for C fibers respectively. A-delta fibers conducting impulses arising from HTM and MMT nociceptors synapse in two areas, laminae I and II, while others synapse in laminae V and X. C-fiber afferents conducting impulses generated by polymodal nociceptors synapse on cells in laminae I, II, and V. A-delta and C fibers mediating visceral nociception synapse predominantly on cells in laminae I and V. Thus, polymodal somatic and visceral nociceptive impulses converge on common cells in laminae I and V.(9, 13, 28-30)

There are many neurotransmitters in the terminals of primary afferent nerves including glutamate, aspartate, sP, somatostatin, vasoactive intestinal peptide, cholecystokinin, gastrin releasing peptide, angiotensin II, calcitonin gene-related peptide (CGRP), enkephalin, dynorphin, and fluoride-resistant acid phosphatate. (9, 31-36)

Dorsal Horn Cells

The primary afferents synapse with cells of three types in the dorsal horn (Fig. 4–1). Nociceptive specific cells (NS) are in high concentration in lamina I but are also found in lamina V. The NS cells receive excitatory input only from nociceptive afferents (HTM, MMT, and CPM), have small receptive fields, and within lamina I are arranged somatotopically. Some NS neurons receive input from all three types of nociceptive afferents; others receive input only from HTMs. Wide dynamic range (WDR) neurons are located in lamina V and receive convergent input from primary afferents innervating skin, subcutaneous tissue, muscle, and viscera. This convergence is the neural basis for referred pain.(37, 38) Wide dynamic range neurons can respond to hair movement and weak mechanical stimuli (touch) but respond maximally to intense potentially or damaging stimuli. Cutaneous nociceptive afferents terminate in laminae I, II, and V. Visceral and muscle nociceptive afferents terminate in laminae I and V but not in lamina II (substantia gelatinosa). Cutaneous and visceral inputs arising from C polymodal nociceptors converge on wide dynamic range neurons in laminae I and V. Likewise, muscle and cutaneous input from A-delta and C fibers converge on neurons in laminae I and V. Cells in the substantia gelatinosa (lamina II) receive input from HTM, MMT, and CPM nociceptors,

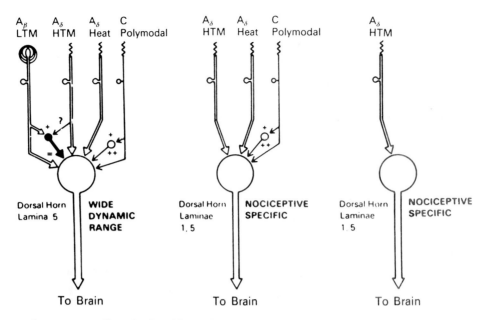

Fig. 4–1. Three types of nociceptive cells in the dorsal horn, their inputs from primary afferents, their location in the spinal cord, and their output to ascending systems. Some wide-dynamic-range (WDR) neurons are also found in lamina I. WDR neurons receive inputs from low-threshold mechanoreceptive primary afferents (LTMs), A-delta thermoreceptive afferents, high-threshold mechanoreceptive afferents (HTMs), and C-polymodal nociceptive afferents. The nociceptive-specific dorsal horn neurons receive input exclusively from nociceptive afferents. (From Price, D.D., and Dubner, R. Invest Dermatol 69:167, 1977.)

and also from low-threshold mechanoreceptors. A variety of responses have been reported from SG cells: excitation by noxious and inhibition by innocuous input; inhibition by both noxious and innocuous input; and excitation by innocuous input and inhibition by noxious input. Thus, cells of the SG function as local interneurons within the dorsal horn to inhibit or facilitate output of NS and WDR neurons as well as influencing neurons in distant parts of the spinal cord and the brain.(13, 39, 40)

Glutamate and aspartate are thought to be the major excitatory neurotransmitters in the CNS. Excitatory amino acids bind to receptors of two types: ionotropic and metabotropic. Ionotropic receptors are (a) N-Methyl-D-Aspartate (NMDA) receptors, (b) a-amino-3-hydroxy-5-methyl-isoxazole-4-propionate/kainate (AMPA/KA) receptors, (c) Kainate (KA) receptors, and (d) 2-amino-4-phosphonobutanoate (L-AP4) receptors. The metabotropic receptors are G-protein or metabotropic glutamate receptors.

N-methyl-D-aspartate receptors appear not to be involved in normal spinal cord function, but only become active after tissue injury. After injury a barrage of C fiber discharges originating from sensitized nociceptors cause release of glutamate, neurokinins, and probably other substances from primary afferent terminals in the spinal cord. These lead to fast synaptic potentials at non-NMDA receptors (i.e., Na-permeable AMPA/KA receptors) and slow synaptic potentials produced by continuous depolarization and the release of peptides (e.g., sP, CGRP). As a consequence, a voltage-dependent magnesium block on NMDA recep-

tors is removed or metabotropic glutamate receptors are activated, resulting in activation of calcium-gated AMPA receptors. These events allow an influx of Ca and activation of early genes, leading to the development and maintenance of hyperalgesia. Only the NMDA receptor subtype is sufficient and needed for development of thermal hypersensitivity; other excitatory amino acid subtypes do not appear to be involved. The NMDA receptor activation has been implicated in the hypersensitivity or "wind-up" associated with repeated C-fiber stimulation and expansion of receptive fields following injury. The NMDA binding sites are found in high concentration in the SG and in low concentration in all other areas of the spinal cord. Aspartate, a proposed NMDA receptor agonist, is released in the dorsal horn by primary afferents. NMDA has been shown to increase the firing rate of nociceptive neurons.

In contrast to thermal hyperalgesia, little is known of mechanical hyperalgesia. Recent studies suggest that coactivation of AMPA and metabotropic receptors, and not NMDA receptors, is both necessary and sufficient to cause mechanical hyperalgesia. As with NMDA and thermal hyperalgesia, the AMPA and metabotropic receptors become active only after tissue injury. Thus, these receptors appear to be responsible for the wind-up associated with peripheral inflammation and mechanical hyperalgesia. AMPA and metabotropic glutamate receptors are found in high concentrations in the SG and in lower concentrations elsewhere in the spinal cord. Cysteine, a possible AMPA and metabotropic glutamate agonist, is released in the dorsal horn by primary afferents.

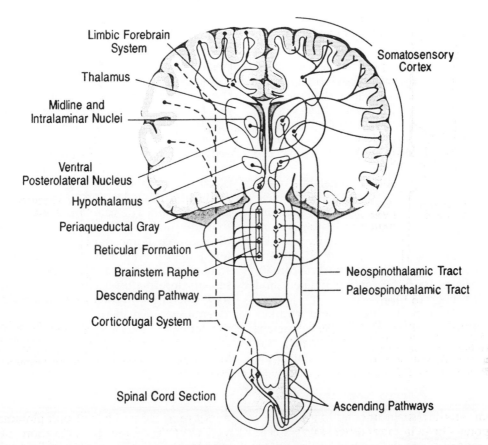

Limbic Forebrain System
Thalamus
Midline and Intralaminar Nuclei
Ventral Posterolateral Nucleus
Hypothalamus
Periaqueductal Gray
Reticular Formation
Brainstem Raphe
Descending Pathway
Corticofugal System
Spinal Cord Section
Somatosensory Cortex
Neospinothalamic Tract
Paleospinothalamic Tract
Ascending Pathways

Fig. 4–2. Ascending pathways in humans. Note that the ascending pathways are contralateral in humans as compared to some ascending ipsilaterally and some contralaterally in the cat. (From Kitchell RL, Guinan MJ. The nature of pain in animals. In: The Experimental Animal in Biomedical Research. vol I. Edited by Rollin BE, Kesel ML. CRC Press, Boca Raton, Fla, 1990.)

While both NMDA and the metabotropic glutamate receptor activation result in activation of second messenger systems, it appears that mechanical and thermal hyperalgesia may be induced by divergent pathways. Activation of NMDA receptors results in an increase in cGMP through the production of nitric oxide (NO) and protein kinase C (PKC). Activation of AMPA and metabotropic glutamate receptors also involve NO, cGMP, and PKC but lead to production of arachidonic acid, which is necessary for the development of mechanical hyperalgesia.(41)

Ascending Pathways

The ascending pathways or tracts are bundles of nerve fibers whose cell bodies are located in the gray matter of the spinal cord or brain stem and terminate by synapsing with cells in the brain, usually in the reticular formation or in the thalamus. The neurons in the dorsal horn whose axons form the fibers of the ascending tracts (NS and WDR neurons) are called *relay or transmitter* (T) *cells* because when excited by afferent nociceptive impulses, they relay or transmit the activity to other parts of the nervous system. Nociceptive information as well as nonnoxious sensory input is conveyed from the spinal cord to the brain by multiple pathways or tracts. These can be divided into lateral and medial groups

(Fig. 4–2). The lateral group includes (a) the neospinothalamic tract, which ascends directly to and terminates in the thalamus; (b) the spinocervical tract, which relays to the thalamus through the lateral cervical nucleus; and (c) the dorsal column-postsynaptic tract, which relays to the thalamus through the dorsal column nuclei. The medial group is comprised of (a) the paleospinothalamic tract, which terminates in the midline intralaminar thalamic regions; (b) the spinoreticular tract, which terminates throughout the reticular formation; (c) the spinomesencephalic tract, which terminates in the mesencephalon; and (d) the propriospinal system, which ascends the spinal cord via a diffuse, polysynaptic network of fibers and synapses to terminate in the reticular system.(42)

There are major differences in these systems among species; however, the similarities outweigh the differences. In humans and subhuman primates the major ascending nociceptive pathway is the neospinothalamic tract. This tract arises in the dorsal horn from NS and WDR cells, crosses the midline, and ascends on the side of the body opposite that from which the impulses arise. The paleospinothalamic tract, arising from WDR neurons, lies just medial (deep) to the neospinothalamic tract. Posterior and deep to the spinothalamic tracts are the spinoreticular tracts, which also arise from WDR neurons. In nonprimates, the nociceptive tracts are more diffuse and often ascend the cord bilaterally. In the cat and pig, unilateral sectioning of the spinal cord does not result in loss of nociception; this may be caused by the relatively large propriospinal system in these animals. Additionally, in the cat the spinothalamic tract arises from cells in the ventral horn (laminae VII and VIII) as opposed to the dorsal horn (laminae I and V) in the rat and monkey. In the rat and monkey most of the fibers cross the midline, while in the cat they project to the ipsilateral thalamus.(7, 43-46)

Subprimates have large spinocervicothalamic tracts, which ascend ipsilaterally and cross the midline near the first cervical segment. This tract primarily contains fibers arising from low-threshold mechanoreceptors, which transmit hair follicle receptor activity but also contains nociceptive fibers. Likewise, in the rat, cat, and monkey, the dorsal column postsynaptic tracts contain a mixture of nociceptive (WDR and NS) fibers and nonnoxious (LTM) fibers.(47-49)

The spinothalamic tracts in the rat and monkey terminate in the ventral posterior lateral (VPL) nucleus of the thalamus, while those of the cat terminate in the shell region of the thalamus dorsal and ventral to the VPL.(50, 51)

Melzack and Casey have postulated that the lateral ascending pathways (i.e., neospinothalamic, dorsal column postsynaptic, and spinocervicothalamic) transmit nociceptive information leading to the sensory-discriminative aspects of pain (Fig. 4–3).(4) In addition, the dorsal column and dorsolateral projection systems are thought to contain large fibers that constitute a "central control trigger" and conduct rapidly to the cortex to activate central control processes prior to the arrival of ascending nociceptive information. The more medial pathways—the paleospinothalamic, spinoreticulothalamic, spinomesencephalic, and propriospinal—convey impulses leading to the motivational-affective aspect of pain. The basis for this concept lies in the fact that the medial pathways are not organized to carry discrete spatial and temporal information; rather, they terminate on brain cells having large receptive fields, sometimes covering half the body. In addition, other sensory information (somatosensory, visual, and auditory) converges on some of these same cells. The medial ascending systems terminate in the reticular formation, the periaqueductal gray matter, and the hypothalamus, and in the midline or intralaminar (nonspecific) thalamic nuclei. People with lesions in these medial ascending tracts state that they can perceive and

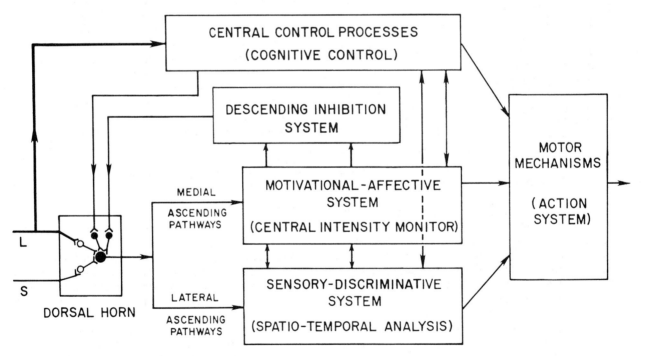

Fig. 4–3. Conceptual model of the sensory, motivational, and central control determinants of pain according to Melzack and Casey. The output of the T-cell in the dorsal horn projects to the sensory-discriminative system via the lateral ascending system and to the motivational-affective system via the medial ascending system. The central control "trigger," composed of the dorsal column and the dorsolateral projection systems, is represented by a heavy line running from the large fiber system to the central control processes, which take place in the brain. These in turn project back to the dorsal horn as well as to the sensory-discriminative and motivational-affective systems. Added to the scheme of Melzack and Casey is the brain stem inhibitory control system activated by impulses in the medial descending system, and which provides descending control on dorsal horn. Moreover, there is much interaction between the motivational-affective and the sensory-discriminative system, as indicated by the arrows. The net effect of all of these interacting systems is activation of the motor (action) system. (Modified from Melzack, R., and Casey, K.L. Sensory, Motivational and Central Control Determinants of Pain. In: The Skin Senses. Edited by D.R. Kenshalo, Jr. Springfield, IL, Charles C Thomas, 1968:423–443.(4)

localize pain, and describe the type of stimulus causing the pain, but that the pain is a stimulus that is not intolerable. In animals, medial tract lesions decrease aversive responses to noxious stimuli from those observed in normal subjects. The lateral pathways terminate in the ventrobasal nucleus of the thalamus, which in turn relays the activity to the somatosensory cortex. Lesions in the lateral ascending pathways interfere with the individual's ability to recognize the type of stimulus and to accurately localize the area being stimulated without affecting the aversive or emotional aspects of the pain experience.(4, 52-54)

The lateral tracts are not as effective as the medial tracts in mediating reflexes or in altering generalized brain function (i.e., general arousal or alertness). The terminations of the medial pathways in the reticular formation and intralaminar thalamic nuclei establish connections with the hypothalamus and other parts of the limbic system. The hypothalamic-limbic system is thought to be responsible for emotional states and reactions.(55) The size of the medial tracts is relatively constant relative to brain size, but the lateral pathways are most highly developed in primates. The lateral ascending nociceptive systems preferentially mediate the onset of sudden changes in noxious stimulation (phasic pain) that relate to the recognition of the life-threatening potential of a noxious stimulus.(56) The lateral system rapidly transmits information regarding the onset and precise location of injury and its intensity and duration, and quickly brings about responses to prevent further injury. The medial system would function to signal persistent or tonic tissue damage. The lateral system would be instrumental in escape responses and eliciting behavioral responses including vocalization to warn other animals of that species to the threat of injury. The medial tracts would appear to be essential for species-specific behavior directed toward minimizing further injury and toward gaining assistance in healing (i.e., being fed, cared for, or groomed).(56)

The differences in numbers of ascending fibers in the lateral tracts of humans compared to that of animals suggest that animals may not be able to receive as much sensory-discriminative information as a person, (i.e., they have a less refined ability to localize and to determine the type of stimulus). In contrast, nonprimates have medial ascending nociceptive tracts that are as large as or larger than those in people, suggesting that they may have greater access to the motivational-affective aspects of the stimulus (i.e., autonomic responses, unpleasant qualities of the stimulus, and life-threatening consequences of the tissue damage). In people whose lateral tracts were sectioned to alleviate intractable pain, the pain often reappeared a year later and was reported as being even more disagreeable than before tractotomy.(57) The return of pain was attributed to propriospinal and dorsal column postsynaptic tracts taking over the functions of the spinothalamic and spinoreticular tracts.(7)

Supraspinal Structures

Nociception involves portions of the medulla oblongata, mesencephalon, diencephalon (thalamus, hypothalamus), and cerebral cortex. The medulla and mesencephalon participate in nociceptive function through their contributions to the reticular system. The thalamus serves as the relay for ascending sensory information entering the cerebral cortex.(58, 59) The thalamus contains a large number of complex nuclei. The thalamic nuclei involved in nociception are divided into several groups. The ventral group consists of the ventral lateral nucleus (VL), ventral posterolateral (VPL) nucleus, and ventral posteromedial (VPM) nucleus; a medial posterior thalamic (POm) complex; an intralaminar group; a midline nuclear group; and a submedius nucleus. The lateral ascending pathways that mediate the sensory-discriminative aspects terminate in the more laterally located nuclei (VPL, VPM, VL, and POm). The medial ascending pathways terminate in the medial nuclei (Fig. 4–2). The VPL and VPM relay sensory information from the body and head respectively to the somatosensory cortex. Lesions in the VPL, the VPM, or the somatosensory cortex result in loss of ability to perceive mechanical stimuli to specific regions of the periphery.(60-62) The cerebral cortex plays a major role in pain perception. The somatosensory cortex functions to provide the sensory-discriminative dimension of pain. The frontal cortex appears to play a significant role in mediating between cognitive activities and the motivational-affective features of pain because it receives input from virtually all sensory and associated cortical areas via intracortical fiber systems and projects to the reticular and limbic systems. The frontal cortex appears to be necessary to the maintenance of the negative affective and aversive motivational aspects of pain. Neocortical processes subserve cognition and psychologic factors, including prior experience, conditioning, anxiety, attention, background, and evaluation of the pain-producing situation.(7)

RETICULAR FORMATION

The reticular formation consists of a core of isodendritic neurons extending through the medulla, pons, and mesencephalon (Fig. 4– 4). The axons of these cells are long, extending along the rostrocaudal axis of the brain stem and brain. The axons send collaterals to the spinal cord, to other reticular neurons, to various sensory and motor nuclei of the brain stem, to the diencephalon, and to the cerebral cortex. It is not a diffuse network of short-axon neurons forming a multisynaptic chain, but rather neurons organized to distribute information rapidly to multiple foci throughout a substantial portion of the neuraxis, extending from the spinal cord to the diencephalon and cerebral cortex. Reticular neurons can mediate motor, autonomic, and sensory function. Within the reticular formation are circumscribed areas of specialized function, but there is substantial interaction providing the basis for unified activity of the reticular core. The reticular formation is essential for

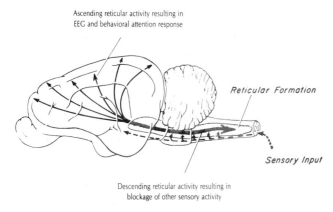

Ascending reticular activity resulting in EEG and behavioral attention response

Reticular Formation

Sensory Input

Descending reticular activity resulting in blockage of other sensory activity

Fig. 4–4. Ascending reticular activity results in an EEG and behavioral attention response. Descending reticular activity results in blockage of other sensory activity. (From Breazile, J.E., and Kitchell, R.L. Pain Perception in Animals. Fed Proc 28:1379, 1969.)

coordination of motor components of behaviors in decerebrate animals. Medullary and pontine reticular neurons regulate various aspects of spinal motor activity and respiratory and other autonomic functions, including those carried out in the spinal cord. The reticular formation has important sensory functions and exerts control over somatic, auditory, and visual sensory systems.(59, 63)

Reticular function appears to be critical to integration of the pain experience and behavior because nociceptive input has such a profound effect on reticular activity. Ascending reticular neurons mediate the affective and motivational aspects of pain via their input into the medial thalamus and hypothalamus, and their projections into the limbic system. Lesions of the limbic system in both humans and animals markedly obtund the aversive quality of noxious stimuli without interfering with the discriminative aspects of somesthesias. The ability of opioids to reduce pain-induced suffering while preserving discriminative function is attributed to their effects on reticular neurons. Among these is the nucleus gigantocellularis, which is most effectively activated by A-delta- and C-fiber activity.(4, 63)

LIMBIC SYSTEM

The limbic system or paleocortex consists of phylogenetically old parts of the telencephalon and subcortical structures derived from them, and parts of the diencephalon and mesencephalon. These structures include the amygdala, hippocampus, septal nuclei, preoptic region, and hypothalamus, and parts of the thalamus and the epithalamus (habenula). The limbic system is concerned with mood and incentives to action (i.e., motivational interactions and emotions). The limbic system endows information derived from internal and external events with its particular significance to the individual and thus determines purposeful behavior.(64) The hypothalamus and limbic structures have an important role in motivated, emotional, and affective

behaviors, which are integral parts of the pain experience.(4) Limbic structures play an important role in the neural basis for aversive drive, and influence the motivational dimension of pain. Electric stimulation of limbic structures (e.g., the hippocampus and amygdala) causes escape behaviors, while ablation results in marked changes in affective behavior and decreased response to noxious stimulation.(65-67)

Descending Control Systems

CORTEX AND DIENCEPHALON

A significant portion of central nervous system activity is concerned with selection, modulation, and control of ascending sensory information by descending fibers from telencephalic structures. These descending supraspinal systems have considerable influence on synaptic transmission in the dorsal horn and all along the ascending somatosensory projection system. Each structure below the brain that projects to the cortex receives descending fibers from the cortex that can influence transmission in the thalamus, reticular formation, trigeminal system, and spinal cord. Similarly, there are descending fibers from these structures that terminate on and influence transmission in lower synapses. These include the rubrospinal, reticulospinal, and raphespinal tracts, which project to several laminae of the spinal cord. Pontine and medullary reticular formation strongly influence synaptic transmission of somatic afferents in the dorsal horn. The descending inhibitory system has been described as being four tiered: (a) cortical and diencephalic systems; (b) mesencephalic periaqueductal gray matter (PAG) and periventricular gray matter (PVG), which are rich in enkephalins and opiate receptors; (c) parts of the rostroventral medulla, especially the nucleus raphe magnus (NRM) and adjacent nuclei, which receive input from the PAG and send serotonergic and noradrenergic fibers in the dorsolateral funiculus to terminate in the spinal and medullary dorsal horn; and (d) the spinal and medullary dorsal horn, which receive axons from the NRM and adjacent nuclei. These mesencephalic axons are serotonergic, terminate on cells in laminae I, II, and V, and selectively inhibit nociceptive neurons and interneurons of the rostrally projecting spinothalamic, spinomesencephalic, and spinoreticular tracts. In addition, noradrenergic neurons arising from the locus ceruleus and other brain-stem nuclei contribute to the endogenous system.(68-71) Axons of corticospinal neurons in the somatosensory cortex follow the major corticospinal tracts passing ipsilaterally in the brain stem, give off fibers to the trigeminal spinal nucleus, cross the midline at the pyramidal decussation, and descend in the dorsolateral funiculus of the cord to terminate in laminae I–VII. Corticospinal fibers in laminae I and II exert postsynaptic control on dorsal horn neurons to inhibit the response of WDR neurons to noxious stimuli.(69) In addition, extrapyramidal somatosensory cortical neurons project to the basal ganglia, thalamus, mesencephalon, and reticular formation to enhance the inhibitory function of the mesencephalic and medullary structures.(68) It is postulated that cortical central control processes activated by large fibers in the dorsal column may initiate descending inhibition of dorsal horn neurons even before nociceptive input reaches the discriminative and motivational systems, and prior to activation of mesencephalic and medullary descending control systems.

MESENCEPHALIC STRUCTURES

The most important anatomic areas contributing to the endogenous analgesia system are concentrated in the PAG and PVG extending from the diencephalon to the medullary raphe nuclei. The nucleus raphe dorsalis (NRD) and the mesencephalic reticular formation are also involved. The PAG receives descending input from the cortex, limbic system, septum, hypothalamus, and amygdala. Ascending input to the PAG is from the nucleus cuneiformis, pontomedullary reticular formation, locus ceruleus, and spinal cord. The PAG has descending connections with the rostral medulla, especially the rostroventral medulla, medullary reticular nuclei, and NRM. Axons of cells in these rostral medullary sites descend in the raphe-spinal and reticulospinal tracts to terminate in laminae I, II, and V of the dorsal horn. In addition, the PAG has direct descending projections to the dorsal horn and ascending projections to the intralaminar nuclei of the thalamus.(68-74)

ROSTROVENTRAL MEDULLA AND PONS

The largest population of brain stem cells that project to the dorsal horn via the dorsal lateral funiculus is in the ventral rostral medulla and caudal pons (RVM). Nuclei included are the NRM, NGC, and nucleus reticularis magnocellularis (NMC). All receive input from the PAG, all send fibers to the spinal cord, and all produce antinociception when stimulated.(30, 60, 75, 76)

Neurochemistry

The PAG contains enkephalin cells and terminals, terminals of beta-endorphin axons, sP, vasoactive intestinal peptide (VIP), and other peptides. Excitation of PAG cells results in descending endogenous analgesia. Because opioids are inhibitory at target neurons, it appears that opioids must be acting at an inhibitory interneuron in the PAG. Substance P induces analgesia when injected into the PAG, presumably by exciting an opioid interneuron, which in turn inhibits an inhibitory interneuron, allowing the PAG output cell to be active.(75)

The RVM nuclei receive convergent input from neurons that contain both enkephalin and 5HT. Neurotensin is a 13-amino-acid peptide that induces analgesia when injected intrathecally. It is derived exclusively from neurons in the CNS. It is released at the RVM nuclei by fibers from the PAG, and by fibers from the dorsolateral pons and ventral lateral medulla. In the RVM are neurons that contain 5HT, enkephalin, sP,

thyrotropin-releasing hormone, and combinations of the four. Furthermore, 5HT, sP, and enkephalin are present in RVM cells that project to the spinal cord. In addition to providing separate pathways to the spinal cord, these parallel systems interact at the brain stem and spinal cord.(30, 75)

Descending systems arising in the raphe nuclei and medulla are primarily monoaminergic, releasing serotonin (5HT) and norepinephrine, and to a lesser degree enkephalins and other peptides. Serotonergic cells are located in the NRM and other medullary and pontine nuclei. NRM-5HT neurons terminate in laminae I, II, IV, and V of the dorsal horn to provide the serotonergic link in descending analgesia from sites in the diencephalon and forebrain. Depletion of 5HT or destruction of 5HT neurons or terminals blocks systemically administered opioid-induced analgesia. Noradrenergic neurons arise from the locus ceruleus and subceruleus and terminate in all laminae of the spinal cord. The descending norepinephrine system mediates analgesia and appears to be critical for opiate-induced analgesia.(30, 34, 39, 69-71, 75, 77-79)

DORSAL HORN

Although some enkephalin axons project to the spinal cord, most of the spinal enkephalin is derived from intrinsic dorsal horn neurons. Most of the enkephalin is found in laminae I, II, and V, and also in VII and X. The predominate opiate binding sites (receptors) are located on the central terminals of small primary afferents and in dorsal horn neurons. The enkephalin terminals synapse with the soma and proximal dendrites of projection neurons (T cells). Incoming nociceptive impulses cause release of enkephalin, which modulates the output of ascending nociceptive neurons. Additionally, there is evidence for a presynaptic enkephalin control of primary afferents through inhibition of release of sP.(9, 28, 32, 77, 80, 81) Dynorphin cells are located in laminae I and V. Dynorphin neurons appear to provide a presynaptic opioid input to primary afferent neurons. Dynorphin synthesis in the cord increases in hyperalgesic states and during peripheral inflammation, and dramatically increases 10 to 20 days following induction of experimental neuropathies. Neurotensin cell bodies are concentrated in laminae II and III, and their processes extend through laminae I, II, and III. Neurotensin terminals form axosomatic and axodendritic synapses with dorsal horn neurons. Neurotensin neurons may activate other intrinsic neurons of the dorsal horn that presynaptically control release of sP from primary afferents. There is a very high concentration of GABA in the dorsal horn, which presynaptically controls primary afferents in laminae I and II.(80) Other peptides that have been identified, primarily in lamina II are sP, somatostatin, cholecystokinin, and avian pancreatic peptide.(32, 73, 77, 80, 82-84)

Serotonin neurons in the dorsal horn originate from descending brain-stem neurons. Serotonergic neurons form axosomatic and axodendritic synapses, and exert postsynaptic control of NS and WDR projection neurons.(9, 34, 75, 79, 80, 82)

Axon terminals of pontine norepinephrine-containing nuclei are localized in laminae I, II, IV–VI, and X. They appear to act on spinothalamic tract neurons via dorsal horn local-circuit neurons.(34)

Because peptides exert action of longer duration than amines or amino acid transmitters, it is thought that their role is one of fine tuning of descending control. It is now apparent that (a) a neuron may receive input from many neurotransmitters; (b) each neurotransmitter may have multiple actions in a given region; and (c) multiple neurotransmitters may exist in a single neuron.(9, 32, 34, 39, 82, 83)

GATE CONTROL THEORY

In 1965, Melzack and Wall proposed a "Gate Theory" to incorporate the concepts of physiologic specialization, spinal and central modulation of nociception, and the psychologic dimensions of the pain experience. This conceptual model has been modified to accommodate newer information, and is still valuable as an aid to understanding nociceptive function and pain. Figure 4–3 represents a modified scheme of the sensory, motivational, and central control determinants of pain.(4) Major points include these:

1. Afferent transmission of nociceptive input to the T cell is modulated in the SG (the gate).
2. Spinal gating is determined by relative activity in large vs small fibers; large fibers inhibit transmission (close the gate), while small fiber activity facilitates transmission (opens the gate).
3. Descending impulses from the brain influence gating.
4. A specialized system of very rapidly conducting large fibers (central control trigger) sets the receptivity of cortical neurons for subsequent afferent volleys and influences the sensory input at the spinal gate and other levels of the neuraxis via descending fibers. This system carries precise information about the location and nature of the stimulus, and allows the brain to identify, localize, evaluate, and selectively modulate sensory input prior to activation of the action system.
5. In the action system, the neural patterns that mediate complex behavior and experience characteristics of pain are activated when output of the T cell exceeds a critical level. Furthermore, the neospinothalamic system functions to process sensory discriminative information about location, intensity, and duration of a stimulus. The paleospinothalamic system and paramedian ascending system activate reticular and limbic structures that subserve the motivational and aversive drive, an unpleasant effect that triggers the individual to action. Higher neocortical processes such as evaluation of the stimulus relative to past experience exert control over both discriminative and motivational systems. The frontal cortex is essential for

maintenance of the negative affective and motivational aspects of pain. Neocortical processes provide cognitive and psychologic factors including prior experience and conditioning, anxiety, attention, suggestion, and evaluation of pain-inducing situations. These processes are undoubtedly responsible for the individual's response to anticipated noxious stimuli—for example, a small dog crying out in anticipation of a painful manipulation prior to any actual physical contact. The complex interaction of sensory, motivational, and cognitive processes determines the behavior characteristic of pain by acting on mechanisms concerned with integrated motor responses. These include the motor cortex, the basal ganglia, and portions of the hypothalamus, brain stem, and ventral horn.

LOCAL AND SYSTEMIC RESPONSES TO NOXIOUS STIMULI

Injury to tissues results in local biochemical changes and autonomic reflex responses intended to be protective. As indicated previously, local biochemical changes are produced by release of intracellular substances from damaged tissue into the extracellular fluid to induce local pain, tenderness, and hyperalgesia. These include hydrogen and potassium ions, serotonin, histamine, prostaglandins, bradykinin, sP, and others. Of these, bradykinin, acetylcholine, and potassium directly activate nociceptors, while the others, especially prostaglandins, sensitize the nociceptors facilitating depolarization. Substance P enhances extravasation and inflammation. Activation of the peripheral nociceptors results in impulses that upon arrival in the dorsal horn undergo peripheral, local, segmental, and suprasegmental descending modification. Transmitted impulses evoke somatomotor and sympathetic segmental autonomic nocifensive reflex responses. The ascending afferent impulses are transmitted to various parts of the brain stem and brain. Impulses reaching the brain stem initiate suprasegmental reflex responses and activate the descending modulating system, while those reaching the cortex stimulate cortical responses.(5, 26, 85)

Segmental reflexes can enhance nociception and produce alterations of ventilation, circulation, gastrointestinal, and urinary function. Stimulation of somatosensory pathways induces increased skeletal muscle tone or spasm, decreasing thoracic and abdominal wall compliance (splinting). In addition, positive feedback loops that initiate nociceptive impulses from the muscles result in reflex spasm, and pain (e.g., pain associated with disc disease).(5, 86)

Stimulation of sympathetic preganglionic neurons causes increased heart rate and stroke volume, and increases myocardial work and oxygen consumption. If pain is severe enough, it can cause severe cardiac dysrhythmias. Sympathetic hyperactivity causes decreased gastrointestinal and urinary function, which can lead to ileus and reduced urinary output.(5)

"WIND-UP"

Injury to peripheral tissues results in both peripheral and central sensitization of nociceptors. Peripheral sensitization is caused by release, and elaboration of algogenic substances from injured and inflamed tissues. Centrally, following a barrage of afferent nociceptive impulses, receptive fields of dorsal horn cells expand and central hypersensitization of dorsal horn cells occurs, resulting in an increased rate of discharge (wind-up). Massive nociceptive input not only sensitizes peripheral nociceptor afferents, it has profound effects on dorsal horn neurons and interneurons, and anterior motor neurons. C fibers from muscles, joints, and periosteum can produce long-latency, long-duration facilitation and very prolonged increased excitability of dorsal horn cells. Receptive fields are expanded, and nociceptive cells become sensitive to nonnoxious stimuli such as light touch. Cells with receptive fields distant from that of the stimulated nerve are also affected. This facilitation, although triggered by peripheral C fibers, is maintained by intrinsic spinal cord processes. This facilitated activity appears to be the basis for widespread prolonged tenderness, hyperalgesia, and bouts of intense skeletal muscle spasm associated with excruciating pain that may persist for days or weeks following injury.(5, 87-89)

Response to Pain and Injury

Nociceptive stimulation of medullary centers of circulation and ventilation, hypothalamic centers of neuroendocrine function (primarily sympathetic), and limbic structures result in suprasegmental reflex responses. These consist of hyperventilation, increased hypothalamic neural sympathetic tone, and increased secretion of catecholamines and other endocrine hormones. Increased neural sympathetic tone and catecholamine secretion add to that induced segmentally to further increase cardiac output, peripheral resistance, blood pressure, cardiac work, and myocardial oxygen consumption. In addition, there is increased secretion of cortisol, ACTH, glucagon, cAMP, ADH, growth hormone, renin, and other catabolically active hormones, and a concomitant decrease in insulin and testosterone. These responses, characteristic of the stress response, cause increased blood glucose, free fatty acids, blood lactate, and ketones, as well as increased rate of metabolism and oxygen consumption. These responses cause substrate mobilization to central organs and injured tissues, and lead to a catabolic state and negative nitrogen balance. The magnitude and duration of these changes parallels that of the degree of tissue damage and may last for days.(5, 82, 90-92)

These nociceptive responses also occur in anesthetized or unconscious patients because the nociceptive neural activity is unobtunded at the spinal and brain stem levels. Nevertheless, the patient is pain-free because the nociceptive activity does not terminate or impinge on a functioning cerebral cortex. These responses can be obtunded or largely prevented by the preoperative administration of analgesic agents (preemptive analgesia).(93) More specifically, when evoked potential responses to somatic stimulation are abolished by epidural or intrathecal local anesthetics, the stress response is inhibited. Peripheral nerve blockade is not as effective at blocking the stress response. Systemic opioids have little effect on the stress response. Epidural or intrathecal opioids when used alone appear to obtund the stress response, but not nearly as effectively as do local anesthetics. In dogs anesthetized with isoflurane for ovariohysterectomy, norepinephrine, epinephrine, ACTH, and cortisol increase intraoperatively corresponding to surgical manipulation and remain increased postoperatively. These endocrine responses were prevented by the preoperative administration of the alpha$_2$-agonist, medetomidine.(94) Administration of analgesics (i.e., morphine or xylazine) has been shown to decrease plasma catecholamine concentrations following onychectomy in cats.(95)

Intense anxiety and fear are an integral part of the pain experience and response. They greatly enhance the hypothalamic responses through cortical stimulation. Pain-free anxiety can cause greater cortisol and catecholamine responses than those resulting directly from nociceptive impulses reaching the hypothalamus.(96, 97) In addition, anxiety causes cortically mediated increases in blood viscosity, clotting time, fibrinolysis, and platelet aggregation.(98-101) Pain-induced responses are summarized in Table 4-1.(102)

These reflex responses induced by tissue damage and pain, while immediately protective for short-term survival of the organism can be deleterious if prolonged. Indeed, in the hospital setting, and specifically in a surgical environment, they may be more deleterious than helpful. More specifically, the stress response results in increased cardiac output, cardiac work, and oxygen consumption at a time when cardiac reserve is diminished. Intense vasoconstriction, especially of the splanchnic beds, leads to ischemia, tissue hypoxia, and release of substances toxic to the myocardium. Renal failure may ensue as a result of intense vasoconstriction and the release of ADH and aldosterone. In many patients with severe posttraumatic or postsurgical pain, these neuroendocrine responses are of sufficient magnitude to initiate and maintain shock.(103)

Attenuation of the stress response through adequate pain relief and supportive therapy should result in improved patient outcome and promote healing. Pain can be controlled initially through systemic administration of analgesics, primarily opioids, and alpha$_2$-adrenergic agonists. Long-term control of pain may include epidural or spinal administration of these agents in combination with local anesthetics. Local and regional nerve blocks (e.g., intercostal, brachial plexus, intraarticular) can play an important role in the perioperative period and as a part of a balanced anesthetic

Table 4–1. Neuroendocrine and Metabolic Responses to Pain

Segmental and suprasegmental reflexes
  Increased sympathetic tone
  Vasconstriction—skin, viscera
  Increased SVR, preload
  Increased SV, HR; CO
  Increased P_a, myocardial work
  Increased metabolic rate, O_2 consumption
  Decreased GI and urinary tone
  Increased skeletal muscle tone
Endocrine responses
  Increased ACTH, cortisol, ADH, GH
    cAMP, catecholamines, renin, angiotensin II
    aldosterone, glucagon, interleukin I
  Decreased insulin, testosterone
Metabolic responses
  Hyperglycemia
    glycogenolysis, gluconeogenesis
  Increased muscle protein metabolism
  Increased lipolysis
Water and electrolytes
  Retention of water and Na^+
  Increased K^+ excretion
  Decreased ECF
Ventilation
  Central hyperventilation
  Segmental hypoventilation
    splinting, bronchospasm
Diencephalic and cortical responses
  Anxiety and fear increase sympathetic responses
  Blood viscosity, clotting time
  Fibrinolysis, platelet aggregation
  Psychologic effects

protocol (Chapter 16).(104) Preemptive analgesia has been shown to be highly effective in preventing wind-up and in reducing the amount of postoperative pain and requirement for analgesics.(93, 105) In addition, the nonsteroidal antiinflammatory drugs (NSAIDs) may be useful in relieving pain resulting from the continued release of algogenic substances from injured and inflamed tissues. Nonpharmacologic treatments such as supportive bandages and splinting should not be overlooked.

Other supportive measures are aimed at countering the segmental, supersegmental, and cortical pain-induced stress responses to ameliorate their effects on major organ function and metabolism such that their impact on homeostasis is minimized. Cardiovascular function can be supported as indicated by crystalloid fluids, blood, and blood products (Chapter 19). Acid-base and electrolyte status must be maintained, and parenteral nutrition may need to be instituted in patients that cannot or will not eat. Cardiac function as determined by arterial pressure, CVP, cardiac output, and EKG should be maintained by inotropes (e.g., dopamine), chronotropes (e.g., isoproterenol), and antiarrhythmics, (e.g., lidocaine) (Chapter 5). Ventilatory function can be supported with supplemental oxygen and control of the airway, and breathing as needed (Chapter 17). Renal function is dependent on adequate fluid administration and cardiac function. In addition, diuretics (i.e., furosemide or mannitol) may be needed to correct oliguria. Corticosteroids, while somewhat controversial, and nonsteroidal antiinflammatories may be helpful in ameliorating the cascade of inflammatory products of tissue breakdown contributing to the shock syndrome. Lastly, the alpha$_2$-adrenergic agonists may be useful for their endocrine effects as well as their potent sedative and analgesic properties. Specifically, these drugs decrease sympathetic tone and inhibit cortisol and ADH while enhancing release of growth hormone.(106) Thus, they may be of value in maintaining renal function, countering the catabolic state, and reducing the stress state detrimental to overall circulatory function.

Concepts in the Management and Control of Pain

Because the anatomic structures and neurophysiologic mechanisms leading to the perception of pain (nociception) are remarkably similar in human beings and animals, it is reasonable to assume that if a stimulus is painful to people, is damaging or potentially damaging to tissues, and induces escape and emotional responses in an animal, it must be considered to be painful to that animal.(107, 108) That animals exhibit signs of distress and learned avoidance behavior, and vocalize in response to noxious (painful) stimuli is further evidence of their capacity to suffer from pain. Pain may not always be overtly expressed and may be evidenced only by subtle changes in behavior or posture. A degree of anthropomorphism is appropriate and desirable, especially in situations that are known to cause pain in people.(109, 110)

Just as antibiotics are administered prophylactically to prevent infection, it is appropriate to administer analgesics to prevent pain where it is likely to occur. The commonly stated reasons for withholding analgesics (e.g., to avoid opioid-induced respiratory depression or because pain relief would result in increased activity leading to self-injury) are seldom valid and should be carefully examined before a decision is made to withhold analgesic drugs. Accurate selection and dosing of analgesic drugs provides relief of pain without severe respiratory depression. Where pulmonary function is compromised, monitoring for signs of respiratory depression will provide all the information that is required to prevent hypoventilation or apnea. Appropriate splinting, bandaging, or confinement will prevent self-injury. Animals should not have to endure pain because of real or imagined sequelae to its relief. Pain-induced alterations in metabolism, endocrine, and cardiopulmonary function are well recognized and of serious consequence to the animal.

Analgesia in the strictest sense is an absence of pain but clinically is the reduction in the intensity of pain perceived. The goal should not be the complete elimination of pain, but to make the pain as tolerable as possible without undue depression of the patient. Analgesia in the clinical setting may be induced by obtunding or interrupting the nociceptive process at one or more points between the peripheral nociceptor and the cerebral cortex. Nociception involves four physiologic processes that are subject to pharmacologic modulation. Transduction is the translation of physical energy (noxious stimuli) into electric activity at the peripheral nociceptor. Transmission is the propagation of nerve impulses through the nervous system. Modulation occurs through the endogenous descending analgesic systems, which modify nociceptive transmission. These endogenous systems (opioid, serotonergic, and noradrenergic) modulate nociception through inhibition of the spinal dorsal horn cells. Perception is the final process resulting from successful transduction, transmission and modulation, and integration of thalamocortical, reticular, and limbic function to produce the final conscious subjective and emotional experience of pain.(111)

Transduction can be largely abolished by use of local anesthetics infiltrated at the site of injury or incision, or by intravenous, postthoracotomy intrapleural or postlaparotomy intraperitoneal injection. Nonsteroidal antiinflammatory drugs will obtund transduction by decreasing production of endogenous algogenic substances such as prostaglandins at the site of injury. Transmission can be abolished by local anesthetic blockade of peripheral nerves or nerve plexuses or by epidural or subarachnoid injection. Modulation can be augmented by subarachnoid or epidural injection of opioids, and/or alpha$_2$-adrenergic agonists. Perception can be obtunded with general anesthetics or by systemic administration of opioids and alpha$_2$-agonists either alone or in combination with tranquilizer-sedatives.(111)

Balanced analgesia results from the administration of analgesic drugs in combination and at multiple sites to induce analgesia by altering more than one portion of the nociceptive process. Thus, transduction could be reduced by nonsteroidal antiinflammatories, transmission decreased by epidural local anesthetics, and modulation increased by epidural or intrathecal opioids and/or alpha$_2$-agonists. Balanced analgesic techniques appear to offer several advantages in the management of postoperative pain. When used preemptively, this approach prevents nociceptive-induced neuroplasmic changes within the spinal cord (windup), prevents development of tachyphylaxis, suppresses the neuroendocrine response to pain and injury more effectively than when single drug regimens are used, and shortens convalescence through improved tissue healing and mobility. Preemptive analgesia refers to the application of balanced analgesic techniques prior to exposing the patient to noxious stimuli (surgical trespass). By so doing, the spinal cord is not exposed to the barrage of afferent nociceptive impulses that induce the neuroplasmic changes leading to hypersensitivity. This concept has

gained acceptance as the most effective means of controlling postoperative pain.(93, 112, 113)

Analgesic Drugs

Analgesics are those drugs whose primary effect is to suppress pain or induce analgesia (Table 4–2). Although actions and effects of most other drugs differ little among mammalian species (114), there are marked differences in response to selected analgesics (e.g., opioids) that are independent of pharmacokinetics among species.(115, 116) The concentration of opioid receptors in the amygdala and frontal cortex of species that are depressed by opioids (e.g., dogs and primates) is nearly twice as great as in those species that become excited in response to opioids (e.g., horses and cats).(117) By decreasing the dose, excitement can be avoided in those species prone to bizarre reactions. Excitement may result indirectly from increased release of norepinephrine and dopamine.(116) This may explain the mechanism whereby dopaminergic and noradrenergic blocking drugs such as phenothiazine and butyrophenone tranquilizers suppress clinical evidence of opioid-induced excitement. Xylazine and detomidine (alpha$_2$-agonists) are effective in preventing opioid-induced excitement in horses, and ruminants. Because analgesia and excitement are mediated by different receptors (i.e., mu-analgesia and phencyclidine-excitement), they can occur concurrently and are not mutually exclusive.

Opioid analgesics induce CNS depression accompanied by miosis, hypothermia, bradycardia, and respiratory depression in primates, dogs, rats, and rabbits. Stimulation occurs in horses, cats, ruminants, and swine characterized by mydriasis, panting, tachycardia, hyperkinesis, and sweating in horses.(115, 116) Systemic effects of opioids include release of ADH, prolactin, and somatotropin; inhibition of the release of luteinizing hormone; increased vagal tone; release of histamine and attendant hypotension; decreased motility and

Table 4–2. Classes of Analgesic Drugs Commonly Used in Animals

Classification	Examples
Opioids	Morphine, meperidine, methadone oxymorphone, pentazocine, butorphanol, nalbuphine, buprenorphine
Salicylates	Aspirin, salicylate
Para-aminophenol derivatives	Acetanilid, acetaminophen, phenacetin
Nonopioid, non-salicylate	Phenylbutazone, dipyrone, meclofenamic acid, flunixin, carprofen, ketoprofen
Local anesthetic agents	Procaine, lidocaine, mepivacaine, tetracaine, bupivacaine
Alpha$_2$-adrenergic agonists	Xylazine, detomidine, medetomidine, romifidine

increased tone of the gastrointestinal tract; spasm of the biliary and pancreatic ducts; spasm of ureteral-smooth muscle and increased bladder tone; and decreased uterine tone.

Opioids raise the pain threshold or decrease the perception of pain by acting at receptors in the dorsal horn of the spinal cord and mesolimbic system (i.e., brain stem-nucleus raphe magnus and locus ceruleus), midbrain periaqueductal gray matter, and several thalamic and hypothalamic nuclei. In the dorsal horn, opioids induce postsynaptic inhibition of nociceptive projection neurons (T cells). In addition, there is some evidence that opioids may act presynaptically to inhibit release of sP from primary afferents. Centrally, at the level of the mesencephalon and medulla, opioids activate the descending endogenous antinociceptive system that modulates nociception in the dorsal horn via release of serotonin and perhaps norepinephrine. Opioids act at the limbic system to alter the emotional component of the pain response, thus making it more bearable. Successful use of opioids requires appropriate selection of the drug and dose for the given species to avoid undesirable side effects. They must be used with caution in animals having impaired pulmonary function because they depress the respiratory and cough centers, decrease secretions, and may induce bronchospasm secondary to histamine release. In species that can freely vomit, nausea and vomiting may occur. Repeated doses can result in constipation and ileus and urinary retention. Mice and rats rapidly develop tolerance and physical dependence to opioid agonists.(118-120) Morphine decreases the number and phagocytic function of macrophages and polymorphonuclear leukocytes in mice and may alter their immune function. Opioids are the analgesic drugs of choice for treatment of severe, acute pain.

While opioids induce analgesia by interfering with nociceptive neural transmission centrally, the nonopioid, nonsteroidal, antiinflammatory analgesics act peripherally to decrease production of algogenic substances, primarily prostanoids, that facilitate generation and conduction of impulses that give rise to pain. When tissues are damaged, mediators are synthesized or released that activate nociceptors and primary afferent neurons, leading to the sensation of pain. When administered prior to tissue damage, the nonopioid analgesics induce analgesia by suppressing inflammation and the production and elaboration of kinins and prostaglandins. These drugs are effective primarily against pain of low to moderate intensity associated with inflammation.(121) They are generally regarded as being useful for treating chronic pain of somatic or integumental origin but of little use for visceral pain. An exception is flunixin, which appears to effectively blunt visceral pain in horses.(122) Recently, the efficacy of NSAIDs has been investigated for acute postoperative pain. In dogs, the preemptive (preoperative) administration of carprofen has been

shown to induce superior postoperative analgesia with less sedation than pethidine (meperidine) following orthopedic surgery.(123) Similarly, carprofen has been shown to induce profound analgesia as effective as that induced by papaveretum with quicker anesthetic recovery and less postrecovery sedation.(124) In horses, administration of carprofen, flunixin, and phenylbutazone at the termination of surgery were equally effective at inducing postoperative analgesia, with flunixin providing the longest duration of action and phenylbutazone the shortest duration.(125) In rats undergoing midline laparotomy, buprenorphine or carprofen administration results in greater food and water consumption and less weight loss than occurs in rats receiving saline.(126)

The pharmacokinetics of these drugs vary widely among species. Following oral administration, wide species variations in plasma concentration result in part from the size of the GI tract and gastric emptying time, which affect the rate of absorption, and also the rate of metabolism and elimination.(127) Toxicity of the nonopioid nonsteroidal antiinflammatory analgesics also varies widely among species and drugs, and deserves some consideration.(122) The most common toxic side effects include gastric and intestinal ulceration, with secondary anemia and hypoproteinemia. Impaired platelet function and delayed parturition have been reported. Nephropathy can occur in patients with hypovolemia, congestive heart failure, or other cardiovascular impairment (anesthesia) caused by inhibition of renal prostaglandin function in the face of increased norepinephrine and angiotensin II. Chronic or repeated use has been associated with chronic interstitial nephritis and renal papillary necrosis. Phenylbutazone and dipyrone have been associated with blood dyscrasias.

Alpha$_2$-adrenergic agonists (e.g., xylazine, detomidine, medetomidine, and romifidine) are generally regarded as sedative-hypnotics and are most commonly administered to induce sedation.(128, 129) They are, however, potent analgesics; xylazine has been shown to be a more potent analgesic agent in the horse for the relief of both visceral and somatic pain than opioids and NSAIDs.(130, 131) These drugs exert their effects through stimulation of alpha$_2$-adrenoceptors in the brain, resulting in decreased norepinephrine release. Sedation results from decreased activity of ascending neural projections to the cerebral cortex and limbic system.(118, 119) Analgesia appears to be the result of both cerebral and spinal effects, possibly in part mediated by serotonin and the descending endogenous analgesia system.(120) Alpha$_2$-adrenergic and opioid receptors appear to interact in ways that are not fully understood.(120, 128, 132) Administration of alpha$_2$-agonists (i.e., clonidine) has been shown to relieve symptoms of withdrawal in opioid-dependent humans.(133, 134) They have also been used to "rescue" opioid-induced analgesia that has waned following chronic administration. The combination of an opioid and an alpha$_2$-agonist enhances and prolongs analgesia in dogs and cats.(136-138) They have been used in combination for some years in horses.(139, 140)

Although xylazine is the most commonly used sedative-analgesic in veterinary medicine, its comparative pharmacokinetics have not been studied extensively.(129) When administered intravenously, xylazine has a rapid onset of action and short duration. There is a wide variation in species sensitivity and response to xylazine. Detomidine is more potent and longer acting than xylazine. Medetomidine and romifidine are currently under investigation. Medetomidine is the most potent and selective alpha$_2$-agonist to date, being capable of reducing the minimal alveolar concentration of halothane in dogs by more than 85%. In addition to having profound sedative and analgesic activity, alpha$_2$-agonists induce cardiovascular and metabolic responses also related to their peripheral adrenergic effects. Following their administration, arterial blood pressure increases then decreases; cardiac output is decreased.(141) Insulin release is inhibited, resulting in hyperglycemia.(142-144) Urinary output is increased as a result of decreased ADH and vasopressin release and decreased water reabsorption by nephrons.(142, 145-147)

True analgesia can be induced by neural blockade of the nociceptive nerves or tracts by local infiltration, by regional nerve blocks, or by epidural or intrathecal injection of local anesthetic agents. Analgesia so induced is complete in the area blocked. Intercostal nerve blockade and intrapleural local anesthetic administration have been advocated to relieve pain following thoracotomy and presumably result in better alveolar ventilation postoperatively than when opioid-induced analgesia is present.(148, 149) Lastly, nonpharmacologic methods of pain relief can be utilized to good effect. These include immobilization and support with casts, splints, or bandages; appropriate use of hot or cold packs; and physical therapy such as massage and stretching.(150)

When pain is severe and acute, opioids are some of the most effective analgesics under most circumstances. These drugs do, however, have relatively short half-lives and so require supplemental dosing. Most will provide analgesia within 30 minutes of administration. Duration of action varies but is usually on the order of 2 to 4 hours. The agonist-antagonists butorphanol and buprenorphine appear to induce longer periods of analgesia (i.e., 4 to 5 hours for butorphanol and up to 8 to 12 hours for buprenorphine).(151) In order to provide long-term analgesia, transdermal formulations of fentanyl have been developed and utilized by veterinarians to control chronic pain in dogs and cats. Transdermal patch (Duragesic, 25 µg) application should be performed at least 12 hours prior to surgical stimulus to ensure adequate blood concentration of fentanyl. Surgically induced pain may require the use of opioids for 24 to 48 hours postoperatively. Recently, morphine intraarticular admin-

istration following joint surgery has been shown to effectively relieve pain for many hours postoperatively.(152) The nonsteroidal antiinflammatory drugs generally are not sufficient by themselves to relieve severe postoperative pain. Studies in our laboratory have shown that morphine 0.1 mg/kg intravenously effectively reduces catecholamines in cats following declawing, while 40 mg/kg salicylate had no effect. Nevertheless, NSAIDs can be used in combination with opioids postoperatively to good effect because they have differing mechanisms and sites of action. Further, they can be continued when opioids are no longer necessary. NSAIDs provide good analgesia where pain is induced by inflammation or is chronic and of integumentary or musculoskeletal origin. These drugs may be selected for a given species such that they may be administered at 12- to 24-hour intervals.

While the foregoing discussion has focused on the use of analgesics to control pain in conscious patients, one must not ignore their use in patients that are chemically restrained. Animals are frequently anesthetized for diagnostic and manipulative procedures that are otherwise difficult or not possible in the awake patient. Where pain is not present or caused by the procedure (e.g., radiology), only muscle relaxation and hypnosis or sedation are required for patient management. However, when the procedure is painful or invasive, the protocol should be chosen to ensure that analgesia is sufficient to prevent the patient from perceiving pain. In the unconscious patient, pain cannot be perceived because the cerebral cortex and thalamus are not functioning. Therefore, inhalation agents and barbiturates are adequate analgesics when appropriately dosed because they induce dose-dependent levels of unconsciousness and muscle relaxation. Where anesthesia is maintained with these drugs, intraoperative analgesia is assured so long as the patient is relaxed and not responsive (i.e., in surgical anesthesia). However, analgesia is lost upon recovery. Postoperative pain will need to be controlled with analgesics. The situation is more complex when muscle relaxants are included in the protocol. Because these drugs paralyze the patient, they prevent movement even though pain may be experienced. It is inhumane to perform invasive procedures in immobilized animals without analgesia or unconsciousness. Likewise, the use of muscle relaxants in conjunction with subanesthetic doses of anesthetics must be avoided when painful procedures are to be performed. When muscle relaxants are used, analgesia must be assured through adequate depth of general anesthesia and/or the administration of analgesic drugs, such as morphine or oxymorphone. Signs of inadequate analgesia/anesthesia in paralyzed patients include sudden alterations in arterial blood pressure and heart rate, usually hypertension and tachycardia, cardiac dysrhythmias, dilated pupils, and sweating in horses.

The phencyclidine derivatives, ketamine and tiletamine, induce a dissociative cataleptoid state, somatic analgesia, and altered consciousness. The patient is immobilized but not relaxed or fully unconscious, and analgesia is incomplete. The dissociative state is poorly understood, but it is believed that somatic analgesia results from the interruption or dissociation of ascending nociceptive input as it traverses the thalamoneocortical system. The dissociatives are excellent for chemical restraint and immobilization but must be supplemented with an analgesic for invasive procedures and particularly those involving visceral manipulation. Several recent studies have also assessed and documented the analgesic efficacy of epidurally administered ketamine.(153, 154)

Recommended doses and dose intervals (where available) for selected analgesics used to treat acute and chronic pain of some common domestic species are given in Tables 4-3, 4-4, and 4-5. As with any therapeutic regimen, the response should be moni-

Table 4–3. Doses (mg/kg) of Analgesics That Have Been Used to Ameliorate Pain in Common Domestic Species*

	Swine	Sheep/Goat	Cattle	Dog	Cat	Horse
Acetaminophen	NA	NA	NA	10–15 PO q 8 hr	NR	NA
Aspirin	10 PO q 4 hr	100 PO q 12 hr	100 PO q 12 hr	10 PO q 8–12 hr	10 PO q 48–72 hr	25 PO q 12 hr then 10 PO q 24 hr
Buprenorphine	0.005–0.01 IM q 12 hr	0.005 IM q 12 hr	NA	0.01–0.2 SQ/IM q 8–12 hr	0.005–0.01 IM q 12 hr	0.004–0.006 IV
Butorphanol	NA	NA	NA	0.05–0.2 IV 0.2–0.5 SQ q 3–4 hr	0.1–0.4 IM q 6 hr	0.022 IM q 2–4 hr
Fentanyl	NR		NR	0.04–0.08 IM/IV q 1–2 hr	NR	0.002 IM
Meperidine	2 IM q 4 hr	Do not exceed 200 mg total dose.	2 IM	2–6 IM q 1 hr 10 IM 10 SQ/IM q 2 hr	5 IM 10 SQ/IM q 2 hr	2–4 IM/IV
Morphine	0.2 IM	Do not exceed 10 mg total dose IM.	NR	0.05–1 IM/SQ q 4 hr 0.25 IM q 6 hr 0.5–5 SQ/IM q 2–4 hr	0.05–0.1 IM/SQ q 4 hr 0.1 SQ q 4 hr	0.22 IM
Oxymorphone□	0.02 IM	NR	NR	0.04 IM 0.2 IV/IM/SQ q 4–6 hr	0.2 IV/IM/SQ q 4–6 hr	0.022 IM
Pentazocine	2 IM q 4 hr	NA	NR	2 IM 1.5–3 IM q 4 hr	2–3 IM/IV q 4 hr	0.33 IV
Phenylbutazone	NA	10 PO	NA	22 PO 9 PO q 8 hr	NR	5 PO q 24 hr 3–6 IV q 12 hr
Xylazine	1.0 IM	0.05–0.1 IM	0.1 IM	1.1 IM	1.1 IM	2.2 IM q 30–60 min
Innovar-Vet (mL/kg)	0.07 IM	NA	NA	0.05 IM	NA	NA

NR = Not recommended.
NA = Not available.
□Calculated as 0.1 dose of morphine.
*These doses have been compiled from many sources. (10, 11, 12, 34–37, 56–58) The wide variability of recommended doses appears related to the variety and severity of stimuli used to establish the individual drug's analgesic activity in a given species. Doses are intended as guidelines only. Clinical judgment must be exercised to provide effective analgesia in a given situation.

Table 4–4. Nonsteroidal Antiinflammatory Analgesics Used to Manage Mild Pain in Dogs and Cats

Drug	Dose (mg/kg)	Animal	Route	Dose Interval
Aspirin	10–20	Dog	PO	8–12 hours
	10–20	Cat	PO	48 hours
Phenylbutazone	10–20	Dog	PO	8–12 hours
Meclofenamic Acid*	1.0–2.5	Dog	PO	24 hours
Piroxicam*	0.2–0.44	Dog	PO	48 hours
Naproxen*	1.5–3.0	Dog	PO	24 hours

*The probability of gastrointestinal irritation cautions that these drugs not be used for extended periods of time.

Table 4–5. Opioids Used to Control Chronic Pain in Dogs and Cats

Drug	Dose (mg/kg)	Animal	Route	Dose Interval
Aspirin plus Codeine	8–10	Dog	PO	8–10 hours
	1.5–3.0			
Codeine	2–3	Dog	PO	4–8 hours
Morphine*	0.5–4.0	Dog	PO	4–5 hours
Morphine SR†	0.5–4.0	Dog	PO	12 hours
Fentanyl Transdermal Patch Formulation	(Duragesic; 25μg)●	Dog and cat	Skin	several days
Butorphanol	0.2–1.0	Cat	PO	4–5 hours

*Morphine may be given to cats at one tenth the dog dose.
†Sustained release morphine tablets.
●Small dogs and cats require ⅓ to ½ patch; large dogs can be given whole patch.

tored, and where an adequate response showing relief of pain has not occurred, additional drug or drugs should be given. Extrapolation of data from one species to another should be avoided where specific information is available.

References

1. Wright EM Jr, Marcella KL, Woodson JF. Animal pain: Evaluation and control. Lab Anim (May/June):20–36, 1985.
2. Zimmerman M. Behavioural investigations of pain in animals. In: Duncan IJH and Molony V, eds. Agriculture: Assessing pain in farm animals, 1986:16.
3. Melzack R. Neurophysiological foundations of pain. In: RA Sternbach, ed. The psychology of pain. New York: Raven Press, 1986:1.
4. Melzack R, Casey KL. Sensory, motivational and central control determinants of pain. In: D. Kenshalo, ed. The skin senses. Springfield, IL: Charles C Thomas, 1968:423.
5. Bonica JJ. General considerations of acute pain. In: JJ Bonica, JD Loeser, CR Chapman, and WE Fordyce, eds. The management of pain, 2nd ed. Philadelphia: Lea & Febiger, 1990:159–179.
6. International Association for the Study of Pain. Pain terms: A list with definitions and notes on usage. Pain 6:249, 1979; 14:205, 1982
7. Kitchell RL, Guinan MJ. The nature of pain in animals. In: BE Rollan and ML Kesel, eds. The experimental animal in biomedical research. Boston: CRC Press, 1990:85.
8. Basbaum AI. Anatomical substrates of pain and pain modulation and their relation to analgesic drug action. In: M Kuhar and G Pasternak, eds. Analgesics: Neurochemical, behavioral, and clinical perspectives. New York: Raven Press, 1984:97–123.
9. Willis WD. The pain system: The neural basis of nociceptive transmission in the mammalian nervous system. Basel: S Karger, 1985.
10. Burgess PR, Perl ER. Cutaneous mechanoreceptors and nociceptors. In: A Iggo, ed. Handbook of sensory physiology, vol. 2. New York: Springer-Verlag, 1973:29–78.
11. Adriaensen H, Gybels J, Handwerker HO, Van Hees J. Response properties of thin myelinated (A-delta) fibers in human skin nerves. Pain 1(suppl):S89, 1981.
12. Lynn B. The detection of injury and tissue damage. In: PD Wall and R Melzack, eds. Textbook of pain. New York: Churchill Livingstone, 1984:19–31.
13. Dubner R, Bennett GJ. Spinal and trigeminal mechanisms of nociception. Annu Rev Neurosci 6:381, 1983.
14. Hallim RG, Torebjork HE, Wiesenfeld Z. Nociceptors and warm receptors innervated by C fibers in human skin. J Neurol Neurosurg Psychiatry 44:313, 1981.
15. Van Hees J, Gybels JM. Pain related to single afferent C fibers from human skin. Brain Res 48:397, 1972.
16. LaMotte RH, Campbell JN. Comparison of responses of warm and nociceptive C-fiber afferents in monkey with human judgements of thermal pain. J Neurophysiol 41:509, 1978.
17. Perl ER. Sensitization of nociceptors and its relation to sensation. In: JJ Bonica and D Albe-Fessard, eds. Advances in pain research and therapy, vol. 1. New York: Raven Press, 1976:17–28.
18. Coggeshall RE, et al. Discharge characteristics of fine medial articular afferents at rest and during passive movements of inflamed knee joints. Brain Res 272:185, 1983.
19. Cervero F. Mechanisms of visceral pain. In: Persistant pain, vol. 4. New York: Grune & Stratton, 1983:1–19.
20. Janig W, Morrison JFB. Functional properties of spinal visceral afferents supplying abdominal and pelvic organs with special emphasis on visceral nociception. In: F Cervero and JF Morrison, eds. Visceral sensation. Amsterdam: Elsevier, 1986:87–114.
21. Brodal A. Neurological anatomy in relation to clinical medicine, 3rd ed. New York: Oxford University Press, 1981.
22. Langford LA, Coggeshal RE. Branching of sensory axons in the peripheral nerve of the rat. J Comp Neurol 203:745, 1981.

23. Gasser HS. Pain-producing impulses in peripheral nerves. Proc Annu Res Nerv Ment Dis 23:44, 1943.
24. Hokfelt T et al. Neuropeptides and pain pathways. In: JJ Bonica, U Lindblom, and A Iggo, eds. Advances in pain research and therapy, vol. 5. New York: Raven Press, 1983:227–246.
25. Keele CA, Armstrong D. Substances producing pain and itch. In: H Barcroft, H Davson, and WDM Paton, eds. Monographs of the physiological society, vol. 12. London: Edward Arnold, 1964:1–374.
26. Morrison DC, Henson PM. Release of mediators from mast cells and basophils induced by different stimuli. In: MK Bach, ed. Immediate hypersensitivity: Modern concepts and developments. New York: Marcel Dekker, 1978:431–511.
27. Coggeshall RE et al. Unmyelinated axons in human ventral roots. A possible explanation for the failure of dorsal rhizotomy to relieve pain. Brain 98:157, 1975.
28. Rexed B. The cytoarchitectonic organization of the spinal cord in the cat. J Comp Neurol 96:415, 1952.
29. Light RA, Perl ER. Spinal termination of functionally identified primary afferent neurons with slowly conducting myelinated fibers. J Comp Neurol 186:133, 1979.
30. Coggeshall RE, Chung K, Chung JM, Langford LA. Primary afferent axons in the tract of lissauer in the monkey. J Comp Neurol 196:431, 1981.
31. Melzack R, Wall PD, Ty TC. Acute pain in an emergency clinic: Latency of onset and descriptor patterns related to different injuries. Pain 14:33, 1982.
32. Willis WD, Coggeshall RE. Sensory mechanisms of the spinal cord. New York: Plenum Press, 1978.
33. Bessou P, Perl ER. Response of cutaneous sensory units with unmyelinated fibers to noxious stimuli. J Neurophysiol 32:1025, 1969.
34. Nieuwenhuys R, Voogd J, van Huijzen C. The human central nervous system, 2nd ed. New York: Springer-Verlag, 1981.
35. Ruda MA, Bennett GJ, Dubner R. Neurochemistry and neurocircuitry in the dorsal horn. Prog Brain Res 66:219, 1986.
36. Yaksh TL. The central pharmacology of primary afferents with emphasis on the disposition and role of primary afferent substance P. In: TL Yaksh, ed. Spinal afferent processing. New York: Plenum Press, 1986:165–195.
37. Pomeranz B, Wall PD, Weber WV. Cord cells responding to fine myelinated afferents from viscera, muscle and skin. J Physiol 199:511, 1968.
38. Price DD, Dubner R. Neurons that subserve the sensory-discriminative aspects of pain. Pain 3:307, 1977
39. Dubner R et al. Neural circuitry mediating nociception in the medullary and spinal dorsal horn. In: L Kruger and JC Liebeskind, eds. Advances in pain research and therapy, vol. 6. New York: Raven Press, 1984:151–166.
40. Cervero F, Iggo A, Molovny V. An electrophysiological study of neurones in the substantia gelatinosa of rolandi of the cat's spinal cord. Q J Exp Physiol 64:297, 1979.
41. Meller ST: Mechanism of hyperalgesia. In: DI Bryden, ed. Animal pain and its control. Post Graduate Committee in Veterinary Science, University of Sydney, Sydney, Australia, 1994:205–209.
42. Dennis SG, Melzack R. Pain signalling systems in the dorsal and ventral spinal cord. Pain 4:97, 1977.
43. Kennard MA. The course of ascending fibers in the spinal cord of the cat essential to the recognition of painful stimuli. J Comp Neurol 199:511, 1954.
44. Breazile JA, Kitchell RL. Ventrolateral spinal cord afferents to the brain stem in the domestic pig. J Comp Neurol 133:363, 1968.
45. Trevino DL, Coulter JD, Willis WD Jr. Location of cells of origin of the spinothalamic tract in lumbosacral enlargement of the monkey. J Neurophysiol 36:750, 1973.
46. Carstens E, Trevino DL. Laminar origins of spinothalamic projections in the cat as determined by the retrograde transport of horseradish peroxidase. J Comp Neurol 182:151, 1978.
47. Trevino DL, Carstens E. Confirmation of the location of spinothalamic neurons in the cat and the monkey by retrograde transport of horseradish peroxidase. Brain Res 98:177, 1975.
48. Brown AG, Franz DN. Responses of spinocervical tract neurons to natural stimulation of identified cutaneous receptors. Exp Brain Res 7:231, 1969.
49. Cervero F, Iggo A, Molony V. Responses of spinocervical tract neurones to noxious stimulation of the skin. J Physiol 267:537, 1977.
50. Boivie J. An anatomical reinvestigation of the termination of the spinothalamic tract in the monkey. J Comp Neurol 186:343, 1979.
51. Berkley KJ. Spatial relationships between the terminations of somatic sensory and motor pathways in the rostral brainstem of cats and monkeys. J Comp Neurol 193:283, 1980.
52. Mitchell CL, Kaebler WW. Effect of medial thalamic lesions on responses elicited by tooth pulp stimulation. Am J Physiol 210:263, 1966.
53. Mitchell CL, Kaebler WW. Unilateral vs bilateral lesions and reactivity to noxious stimuli. Arch Neurol 17:653, 1967.
54. Kaebler WW, Mitchell CL, Yarmat AJ, Affifi AK, Lorens SA. Centrum medianum-parafasciculus lesions and reactivity to noxious and non-noxious stimuli. Exp Neurol 46:282, 1975.
55. Cassem NH. Current topics in medicine. II. Pain. In: E Rubenstein and DD Federman, eds. Scientific American Medicine, November 1983. New York: Scientific American, 1987:1.
56. Dennis SG, Melzack R. Perspectives on phylogenetic evolution of pain expression. In: RL Kitchell, HH Erickson, E Carstens, and LE Davis, eds. Animal pain: Perception and alleviation. Bethesda, MD: American Physiological Society, 1983, 151.
57. White JC, Sweet WH. Pain and the neurosurgeon: A forty year experience. Springfield, IL: Charles C Thomas, 1969:850.
58. Bowser D. Role of the reticular formation in responses to noxious stimuli. Pain 2:361, 1976.
59. Casey KL. The reticular formation and pain: Towards a unifying concept. In: JJ Bonica, ed. Pain Research Publications: Association for reseach in nervous and mental disease. New York: Raven Press, 1980:63.
60. Willis WD. Thalamocortical mechanisms of pain. Adv Pain Res 9:245, 1985.
61. Willis WD Jr. The origin and destination of pathways involved in pain transmission. In: PD Wall and R Melzack, eds. Textbook of pain. New York: Churchill Livingstone, 1984:88.
62. Willis WD Jr. Nociceptive transmission to the thalamus and cerebral cortex. In: The pain system. The neural basis of nociceptive transmission in the mammalian nervous system. Basel: S Karger, 1985.
63. Casey KL. Supraspinal mechanisms and pain. The reticular formation. In: HW Kosterlitz and LY Terenius, eds. Pain and society. Verlag Weinheim, Chemie, 1980:183–200.
64. Janig W. The autonomic nervous system. In: RF Schmidt and G Thews, eds. Human physiology. New York: Springer-Verlag, 1983:111–144.
65. Price DD, Hayes RL, Ruda MA, Dubner R. Spinal and temporal transformations of input to spinothalamic neurons and their relation to somatic sensation. J Neurophysiol 41:933, 1978.
66. Schreiner L, Kling A. Behavioral changes following rhinencephalic injury in the cat. J Neurophysiol 15:643, 1953.
67. Folz EL, White LE. Pain "relief" by frontal cingulumotomy. J Neurosurg 19:89, 1962.
68. Kerr FWL. Neuroanatomical substrates of nociception in the spinal cord. Pain 1:325, 1975.
69. Gebhart GF. Modulatory effects of descending systems on spinal dorsal horn neurons. In: TL Yaksh, ed. Spinal afferent processing. New York: Plenum Press, 1986:391–416.
70. Hammond DL. Control systems of nociceptive afferent processing: The descending inhibitory pathways. In: TL Yaksh, ed. Spinal afferent processing. New York: Plenum Press, 1986:363–390.
71. Westlund KN, Coulter JD. Descending projections of the locus coeruleus and subcoeruleus/medial parabrachial nuclei in monkey: Axonal transport studies and dopamine-beta-hydroxylase immunocytochemistry. Brain Res Rev 2:235, 1980.
72. Snyder RL. The organization of the dorsal root entry zone in cats and monkeys. J Comp Neurol 174:47, 1977.

73. Sindou M, Quoex C, Baleydier C. Fiber organization at the posterior spinal cord-rootlet junction in man. J Comp Neurol 153:15, 1974.

74. Frykholm R, Hyde J, Norlen G, Skogland CR. On pain sensations produced by stimulation of ventral roots in man. Acta Physiol Scand 29(suppl 106):455, 1953.

75. Yaksh TL, Hammond DL. Peripheral and central substrates in the rostral transmission of nociceptive information. Pain 13:1, 1982.

76. Mantyh PW. Connections of midbrain periaqueductal grey in monkey. II. Descending efferent projections. J Neurophysiol 49:528, 1983.

77. Basbaum AI, Fields HL. Endogenous pain control systems: Brainstem spinal pathways and endorphin circuitry. Ann Rev Neurosci 7:309, 1984.

78. LaMotte C. Distribution of the tract of lissauer and the dorsal root fibers in the primate spinal cord. J Comp Neurol 172:529, 1977.

79. Hammond DL. Pharmacology of central pain-modulating networks (biogenic amines and nonopioid analgesics). In: HL Fields, R Dubner, and F Cervero, eds. Advances in pain research and therapy, vol. 9. New York: Raven Press, 1985:499–511.

80. Basbaum AI. Functional analysis of the cytochemistry of the spinal dorsal horn. In: HL Fields, R Dubner, and F Gervero, eds. Advances in pain research and therapy, vol. 9. New York: Raven Press, 1985:149–175.

81. LaMotte C, Pert CB, Snyder SH. Opiate receptor binding in primate spinal cord: Distribution and changes after dorsal horn section. Brain Res 112:407, 1976.

82. Melzack R, Wall PD. The challenge of pain. New York: Basic Books, 1982.

83. Dubner R. Specialization in nociceptive pathways: Sensory discrimination, sensory modulation, and neural conectivity. In: HL Fields, R Dubner, and F Cervero, eds. Advances in pain research and therapy, vol. 9. New York, Raven Press, 1985: 111–137.

84. Iadorola MJ et al. Enhancement of dynorphin gene expression in spinal cord following experimental inflammation: Stimulus specificity, behavioral parameters, and opioid receptor binding. Pain 35:315, 1988.

85. Kitchell RL, Johnson RD: Assessment of pain in animals, in animal stress, Bethesda, MD: American Physiologic Association, 1985:113.

86. Zimmerman M. Peripheral and central mechanisms of nociception, pain and pain therapy; Facts and hypotheses. In: JJ Bonica, JC Liebeskind, and DC Albe-Fessard, eds. Advances in pain research and therapy, vol. 3. New York: Raven Press, 1979:3–32.

87. Thompson SWN, King AE, Woolf CJ. Activity-dependent changes in rat ventral horn neurons in vitto; Summation of prolonged afferent evoked postsynaptic depolarizations produce a D-2-amino-5-phosphonovaleric acid sensitive windup. Eur J Neurosci 2:638, 1990.

88. Cook AJ et al. Dynamic receptive field plasticity in rat spinal cord dorsal horn following C-primary afferent input. Nature 325:151, 1987.

89. Woolf CJ, Wall PD. The relative effectiveness of C-primary afferents of different origins in evoking a prolonged facilitation on the flexor reflex in the rat. J Neurosci 6:1433, 1986.

90. Kehlet H. Pain relief and modification of the stress response. In: MJ Cousins and GD Philips, eds. Acute pain management. New York: Churchill Livingstone, 1986:49–65.

91. Wilmore DW, Long JM, Mason AD, Pruitt BA. Stress in surgical patients as a neurophysiologic reflex response. Surg Gynecol Obstot 142:257, 1976.

92. Bessman FP, Renner VJ. The biphasic hormonal nature of stress. In: RA Crowley and BF Trump, eds. Pathophysiology of shock, anoxia and ischemia. Baltimore: Williams & Wilkins, 1982: 60–65.

93. Woolf CJ, Chong MS. Preemptive analgesia—treating postoperative pain by preventing the establishment of central sensitization. Anesth Analg 77:362, 1993.

94. Benson GJ (manuscript in preparation), 1995.

95. Benson GJ, Wheaton LG, Thurmon JC, Tranquilli WJ, Olson WA, Davis CA. Postoperative catecholamine response to onychec-

tomy in isoflurane-anesthetized cats: Effect of analgesics. Vet Surg 20:222, 1991.

96. Hume DM, Egdahl RH. The importance of the brain in the endocrine response to injury. Ann Surg 150:697, 1959.

97. Hume DM. The endocrine and metabolic response to injury. In: SE Schwartz, ed. Principles of surgery. New York: McGraw-Hill, 1969.

98. Schneider RA. The relation of stress to clotting time, relative viscosity, and certain biophysical alterations of the blood in normotensive and hypertensive subjects. In: HG Wolff, SG Wolff, and CC Hare, eds. Life stresses and bodily disease. Baltimore: Williams & Wilkins, 1950:818–831.

99. Dreyfuss F. Coagulation time of the blood, level of blood eosinophiles and thrombocytes under emotional stress. J Psychosom Res 1:252, 1956.

100. Ogston D, McDonald GA, Fullerton HW. The influence of anxiety in tests of blood coagulability and fibrinolytic activity. Lancet 2:521, 1962.

101. Zahavi J, Dreyfuss F. Adenosine diphosphate-induced platelet aggregation in myocardial infarction and ischemic heart disease. Presented at Second Congress of Thrombosis and Hemostasis, Oslo, July 13, 1971.

102. Wright EM Jr, Woodson JF. Clinical assessment of pain in laboratory animals. In: BE Rollin and ML Kesel, eds. The experimental animal in biomedical research, Boca Raton: CRC Press, 1990, 205.

103. Roizen MF. Should we all have a sympathectomy at birth? Or at least postoperatively? [Editorial] Anesthesiology 68:482, 1988.

104. Kehlet H. Influence of epidural analgesia on the endocrine-metabolic response to surgery. Acta Anesthesiol Scand 70:39, 1978.

105. Woolf CJ. Recent advances in the pathophysiology of acute pain. Br J Anaesth 63:139, 1989.

106. Maze M, Tranquilli WJ. Alpha-2-adrenoceptor agonists: Defining the role in clinical anaesthesia. Anesthesiology 74:581–605, 1991.

107. Rowan A, Tannenbaum J. Animal rights. In National Forum 66, 30, 1986.

108. Kitchell RL. Problems in defining pain and peripheral mechanisms of pain. J Am Vet Med Assoc 191:1195, 1987.

109. Soma LR. Behavioral changes and the assessment of pain in animals. In: J Grady, S Hildebrand, and W McDonnell, eds. Proc Second International Congress of Veterinary Anesthesia, Chap. 34. Sacramento, California, 1985.

110. Breazile JE, Kitchell RL, Naitok Y. Neural basis of pain in animals. In: Proc Fifteenth Research Conference of the American Meat Institute Foundation, Chap. 53. Chicago, 1963.

111. Katz N, Ferrante FM. Nociception. In: FM Ferrante and TR VadeBoncouer, eds. Postoperative pain management. New York: Churchill Livingstone, 1992.

112. Woolf CJ. Recent advances in the pathophysiology of acute pain. Br J Anaesth. 63, 1989, 139–146.

113. Woolf CJ, Thompson SWN. The induction and maintenance of central sensitization is dependent on N-methyl-D-aspartic acid receptor activation: Implications for the treatment of post-injury pain hypersensitivity states. Pain 44:293–299, 1991.

114. Davis LE, Neff-Davis CA, Wilke JR. Monitoring drug concentrations in animal patients. J Am Vet Med Assoc 176:1156, 1980.

115. Jaffe JH, Martin WR. Opioid analgesics and antagonists. In: AG Gilman, LS Goodman, and TW Rall, eds. The pharmacologic basis of therapeutics, 7th ed. New York: Macmillan, 1985:491.

116. Booth NH. Neuroleptanalgesics, narcotic analgesics, and analgesic antagonists. In: NH Booth and LE McDonald, eds. Veterinary Pharmacology and Therapeutics, 5th ed. Ames, IA: Iowa State University Press, 1982:267.

117. Simon EJ. The opiate receptors. In: JR Smythes and RJ Bradley, eds. Receptors in pharmacology, Chap. 257. New York: Marcel Dekker, 1977.

118. Martin PR, Ebert MH, Gordon EK, et al. Effects of clonidine on central and peripheral catecholamine metabolism. Clin Pharmacol Ther 35:322, 1984.

119. Stenberg D. The role of alpha-adrenoceptors in the regulation of vigilance and pain. Acta Vet Scand 82:29. 1986.

120. Lewis JW, Liebeskind JC. Pain suppressive systems of the brain. Trends Pharmacol Sci 73, 1983.
121. Benson GJ, Thurmon JC. Species differences as a consideration in alleviation of animal pain and distress. J Am Vet Med Assoc 191:1227, 1987.
122. Jenkins WL. Pharmacologic aspects of analgesic drugs in animals: An overview. J Am Vet Med Assoc 191:1231, 1987.
123. Lascelles BD, Butterworth SJ, and Waterman AE. Postoperative analgesic and sedative effects of carprofen and pethedine in dogs. Vet Rec 134(8):189–191, 1994.
124. Nolan A, Reid J. Comparison of the postoperative analgesic and sedative effects of carprofen and papaveretum in the dog. Vet Rec 133(10):240–242, 1993.
125. Johnson CB, Tailor PM, Young SS, Brearley JC. Postoperative analgesia using phenylbutazone, flunixin or carprofen in horses, Vet Rec 133(14):136–138, 1993.
126. Lyles JH, Flecknell PA. The comparison of the effects of buprenorphine, carprofen and flunixin following laparotomy in rats, J Vet Pharmacol Ther 17(4) 284–290, 1994.
127. Davis LE. Species differences in drug distribution vs. factors in alleviation of animal pain. In: RL Kitchell and HH Erickson, eds. Animal pain—perception and alleviation. Bethesda, MD: American Physiological Society, 1983:161.
128. Short CE. Neuroleptanalgesia and alpha-adrenergic receptor analgesia. In: CE Short, ed. Principles and Practice of Veterinary Anesthesia. Baltimore: Williams & Wilkins, 1987:47.
129. Garcia-Villar R, Toutain PL, Alvineric M et al. The pharmacokinetics of xylazine hydrochloride: An interspecific study. J Vet Pharmacol Ther 4:87, 1981.
130. Pippi NL, Lumb WV. Objective tests of analgesic drugs in ponies. Am J Vet Res 40:1082, 1979.
131. Muir WW, Robertson JT. Visceral analgesia: Effects of xylazine, butorphanol, meperidine and pentazocine in horses. Am J Vet Res 46:2081, 1985.
132. Browning S, Lawrence D, Livingston A et al. Interactions of drugs active at opiate receptors and drugs active at alpha-2 receptors on various test systems. Br J Pharmacol 11:487, 1982.
133. Bakris GL, Cross PD, Hammarstem JE. The use of clonidine for management of opiate abstinence in a chronic pain patient. Mayo Clin Proc 57:657, 1982.
134. Lal H, Fielding S. Clonidine in the treatment of narcotic addiction. Trends Pharmacol Sci 70, 1983.
135. Tranquilli WJ, Maze M. Clinical pharmacology and use of alpha 2 agonists in veterinary anesthesia. Anaesth Pharmacol Rev 3:297–309, 1993.
136. Benson GJ, Thurmon JC, Tranquilli WJ. Intravenous sedation-analgesia (neuroleptanalgesia?) induced by morphine or butorphanol and xylazine in pointer dogs. In: Proc American College of Veterinary Anesthesiologists. Las Vegas, Nevada, 1986.
137. Duke T, Komulainen A, Remedios A et al. The analgesic effects of administering fentanyl or medetomidine in the lumbosacral epidural space of cats. J Vet Surg 23:143, 1994.
138. Branson K, Ko JCH, Tranquilli WJ et al. Duration of analgesia induced by epidurally administered morphine and medetomidine in the dog. J Vet Pharm Therap 16:369, 1993.
139. Klein LV, Baetjer C. Preliminary report: Xylazine and morphine sedation in horses. Vet Anesthesiol 1:2, 1974.
140. Tranquilli WJ, Thurmon JC, Turner TA et al. A preliminary report: Butorphanol tartrate as an adjunct to xylazine-ketamine in the horse. Equine Pract 5:26, 1983.
141. Klide AM, Calderwood HW, Soma LR. Cardiopulmonary effects of xylazine in dogs. Am J Vet Res 36:931, 1975.
142. Thurmon JC, Steffey EP, Zinkl JG, et al. Xylazine causes transient dose-related hyperglycemia and increased urine volumes in mares. Am J Vet Res 45:224, 1984.
143. Thurmon JC, Neff-Davis CA, Davis LE et al. Xylazine hydrochloride-induced hyperglycemia and hypoinsulinemia in thoroughbred horses. J Vet Pharmacol Ther 5:241, 1982.
144. Benson GJ, Thurmon JC, Neff-Davis CA et al. Effect of xylazine hydrochloride upon plasma glucose and serum insulin concentrations in adult pointer dogs. J Am Anim Hosp Assoc 20:791, 1984.
145. Thurmon JC, Nelson DR, Hartsfield SM et al. Effects of xylazine hydrochloride on urine in cattle. Aust Vet J 54:178, 1978.
146. Greene SA, Thurmon JC, Tranquilli WJ et al. Effect of yohimbine on xylazine-induced hypoinsulinemia and hyperglycemia in mares. Am J Vet Res 48:676, 1987.
147. Greene SA, Thurmon JC, Benson GJ et al. ADH prevents xylazine-induced diuresis in mares [abstract]. Veterinary Midwest Anesthesia Conference (VMAC). Urbana, Illinois, May 31, 1986.
148. Haskins SC. Use of analgesics postoperatively and in a small animal intensive care unit. J Am Vet Med Assoc 191:1266, 1987.
149. Berg RJ, Orton EC. Pulmonary function in dogs after intercostal thoracotomy: Comparison of morphine, oxymorphone, and selective intercostal nerve block. Am J Vet Res 47:471, 1986.
150. Crane SW. Perioperative analgesia: A surgeon's perspective. J Am Vet Med Assoc 191:1254, 1987.
151. Flecknell PA. The relief of pain in laboratory animals. Laboratory Animals 18:147, 1984.
152. Day TK, Pepper WT, Tobias TA, et al. Comparison of intra-articular and epidural morphine administration for analgesia following stifle arthrotomy in dogs [abstract]. Veterinary Midwest Conference (VMAC). Columbus, OH, June 17, 1995.
153. Klimscha W, Brinkmann H, Plattner O, et al. Epidural ketamine and clonidine for postoperative analgesia after lower limb surgery. Anesthesiology 79:A805, 1993.
154. Martin D, Tranquilli WJ, Thurmon JC et al. Hemodynamic effect of the epidural injection of ketamine in isoflurane anesthetized dogs [abstract]. Veterinary Midwest Anesthesia Conference (VMAC). Columbus, Ohio. June 17, 1995.

section II

PHYSIOLOGY

chapter 5

CARDIOVASCULAR SYSTEM

W. W. Muir and Diane Mason

Introduction

A fundamental understanding and appreciation of the role of the cardiovascular system and circulatory dynamics is paramount for safe anesthetic practice. The uptake, delivery, distribution, redistribution, metabolism, and clearance of anesthetic drugs is dependent upon blood flow. The importance of the cardiovascular system to patient well-being and the diverse effects of drugs used in the practice of anesthesia on hemodynamics emphasize the need to have a working knowledge of hemodynamics in order to adequately assess patient status using monitoring devices that focus on the cardiovascular system. The cardiovascular system is composed of the heart, blood vessels, and blood volume, and is designed to supply a continuous flow of oxygen and nutrients to all tissues of the body. Oxygen and nutrient supply and waste removal are facilitated by major exchange organs, including the lungs, where blood becomes oxygenated and carbon dioxide is removed; the gastrointestinal system, where foodstuffs are absorbed and solid and liquid wastes are eliminated; and the kidneys, where additional byproducts of ingestion and cellular metabolism are excreted. More specifically, the principal function of the heart is to pump blood, of the vasculature to carry blood to and from the heart and facilitate exchange processes in the peripheral tissues, and of the blood to function as the transport medium, or solvent, for all the body homeostatic and exchange processes. Oxygenated blood returning from the lung enters the left atrium and subsequently the left ventricle, and is ejected into the aorta, which, through an elaborate array of major arteries, distributes blood to all the tissues of the body. The end branches of these major arteries, the arterioles, give rise to a vascular bed of exchange vessels, the capillaries, where oxygen and nutrients are exchanged for the byproducts of cellular metabolism. The capillaries, in turn, reunite to form venules and veins that return blood to the right atrium, right ventricle, and lungs (Fig. 5–1). The continuous circulation of blood is dependent upon a functional heart, normal blood vessels, and adequate blood volume, and serves to maintain a constant internal environment for all living cells.

The purpose of this chapter is to discuss the pertinent aspects of the physiology of the cardiovascular system that are of particular relevance or importance to the veterinary anesthetist. A stepwise approach is taken that describes the structure and function of the heart, blood vessels, lymphatic system, and blood. This is followed by a discussion of the neural, humoral, and local control of mechanisms that regulate cardiovascular function. Methods for assessing cardiovascular function and a general discussion of diseases of the cardiovascular system are briefly reviewed.

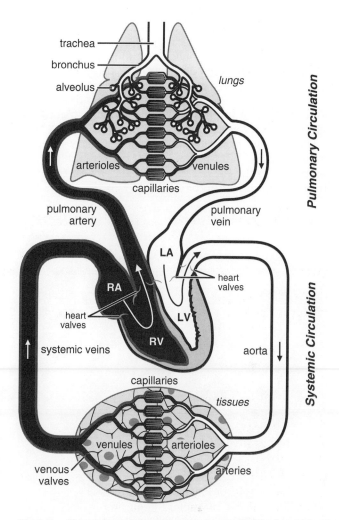

Fig. 5–1. The cardiovascular system is comprised of the heart, blood, and two parallel circulations (pulmonary, systemic). *Pulmonary Circulation:* The pulmonary artery carries blood from the right ventricle (RV) to the lungs where carbon dioxide is eliminated and oxygen is taken up. Oxygenated blood returns to the left atrium (LA) via pulmonary veins. *Systemic Circulation:* Blood is pumped by the left ventricle (LV) into the aorta which distributes blood to the peripheral tissues. Oxygen and nutrients are exchanged for carbon dioxide and other byproducts of tissue metabolism in capillary beds, after which the blood is returned to the right atrium (RA) through venules and large systemic veins. (Modified from Shepherd, J.T., and Vanhoutte, P.M. The Human Cardiovascular System: Facts and Concepts, 1st ed. Raven Press, New York, 1979:3.)

Functional Anatomy of the Heart and Circulation

HEART

The structure of the cardiovascular system is well suited for its function: the delivery of oxygen and nutrients to peripheral tissues and removal of the byproducts of cellular metabolism. The heart, as one key component of the cardiovascular system, functions to pump blood throughout the body. The heart is composed of four chambers: two thin-walled atria separated by an interatrial septum and two thick-walled ventricles separated by an interventricular septum. The boundaries of the various chambers are easily defined by the great veins (cranial and caudal vena cava), which return blood to the right atrium; the smaller pulmonary veins, which return oxygenated blood from the lung to the left atrium; the coronary sulcus, which separates the atria from the ventricles; and the anterior and posterior interventricular (longitudinal) sulci, which separate the right and left ventricles (Fig. 5–2A).

The left anterior interventricular coronary artery, a branch of the left main coronary artery, frequently referred to as the *left anterior descending coronary artery* in humans, provides the blood supply to the ventricular septum and left ventricular free wall. The left posterior interventricular coronary artery, most frequently an extension of the left circumflex coronary artery (the other major branch of the left main coronary artery), occasionally arises from the right coronary artery and provides the blood supply to the posterior left ventricle. The right coronary artery provides the blood supply to the right ventricular free wall and infrequently the posterior wall of the left ventricle (Fig. 5–2B). The atria receive blood returning from the systemic (right atrium) and pulmonary (left atrium) circulations, and to a limited degree act as storage chambers. The ventricles, the major pumping chambers of the heart, are separated from the atria by the tricuspid valve on the right side and the mitral valve on the left side. The ventricles receive blood from their respective atria and eject it across semilunar valves—the pulmonic valve between the right ventricle and pulmonary artery and the aortic valve between the left ventricle and aorta—into the pulmonary (right ventricle) and systemic (left ventricle) circulations. Once the process of cardiac contraction is initiated, almost simultaneous contraction of the atria is followed by nearly synchronous contraction of the ventricles, which results in pressure differences between the atria, ventricles, pulmonary and systemic circulations. Cardiac contraction produces pressure differences, which are responsible for atrioventricular and semilunar valve opening and closing and the production of heart sounds. When the heart relaxes, for example, pressure changes within the heart, pulmonary artery, and aorta cause the semilunar valves to close (producing the second heart sound; S_2) and the atrioventricular valves to open prior to the cycle repeating itself. Chordae tendineae originating from papillary muscles located on the inner wall of the ventricular chambers are attached to the free edges of the atrioventricular valve leaflets and help to maintain valve competence and prevent regurgitation of blood into the atrium during ventricular contraction. Alteration in heart chamber volume (stretch) produced by changes in blood volume, deformation (pericardial tamponade), or disease can have profound effects upon myocardial function, as do the effects produced by neurohumoral, metabolic, and pharmacologic perturbations.

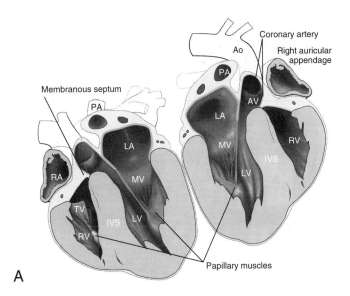

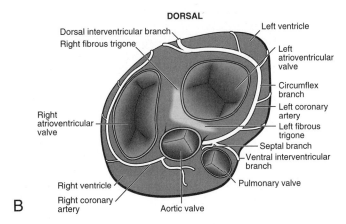

Fig. 5–2. The heart is a pump comprised of two thin-walled and two thick-walled chambers and a highly reactive and diffuse vascular network (coronary circulation). The thin-walled right (RA) and left (LA) atrium are separated from each other and the two thick-walled right (RV) and left (LV) ventricles by a membranous septum (between the right and left atrium) and the tricuspid (TV) and mitral (MV) valves. The interventricular septum (IVS) lies between the right and left ventricles. The pulmonary and aortic (AV) valves separate the RV and LV from the pulmonary artery (PA) and aorta (AO) respectively (A, above). The right and left coronary arteries emerge from the base of the aorta to supply blood to all the chambers of the heart including the heart valves (B, below).

BLOOD VESSELS

The principal role of blood vessels and the vascular network is to carry blood to and from oxygen and nutrient exchange sites: the capillaries.(1) The large and small vessels of the pulmonary and systemic circulations are excellently designed to facilitate the delivery of blood to the exchange sites in the pulmonary and systemic capillary beds and to return blood to the heart. The aorta and other large arteries compose the high-pressure portion of the systemic circulation and are relatively stiff compared to veins, possessing a high proportion of elastic tissue in comparison to smooth muscle and fibrous tissues. This histologic difference causes the aorta to stretch following ventricular contraction and the ejection of blood. The potential (stored) energy that is produced in the stretched aorta following cardiac contraction is returned as kinetic (motion) energy and blood flow during cardiac relaxation. The highly elastic vessel architecture of the aorta facilitates the continuous, albeit nonuniform, flow of blood to peripheral tissues throughout the cardiac cycle (contraction-relaxation-rest) and has been termed the *Windkessel effect*. The Windkessel effect is believed to be responsible for as much as 50% of peripheral blood flow in most species during normal heart rates. Tachyarrhythmias and vascular diseases (stiff nonelastic vessels) hamper the Windkessel effect and produce distinctive changes in the arterial pressure waveform. More distal larger arteries contain greater percentages of smooth muscle compared to elastic tissue and act as conduits for the transfer of blood under high pressure to peripheral tissues. The most distal small arteries, terminal arterioles and arteriovenous anastomoses, contain a predominance of smooth muscle, are highly innervated, and function as sphincters that regulate the distribution of blood flow, aid in the regulation of systemic blood pressure, and modulate tissue perfusion pressure. The capillaries are the functional exchange sites for oxygen, nutrients, electrolytes, cellular waste products, and other substances. These vessels are generally no more than one or two cell layers thick and comprise that portion of the vasculature with by far the largest surface area. Capillaries are of three different types: continuous (lung, muscle), fenestrated (kidney, intestine), and discontinuous (liver, spleen, bone marrow). All capillaries are highly porous and are found in varying numbers in different tissue beds depending on tissue metabolism and the importance of fluid exchange. Postcapillary venules are composed of an endothelial lining and fibrous tissue and function to collect blood from capillaries. Some venules act as postcapillary sphincters, and all venules merge into small veins. Small and larger veins contain increasing amounts of fibrous tissue in addition to smooth muscle and elastic tissue, although their walls are much thinner than comparably sized arteries. Many veins contain "valves" that act in conjunction with external compression (contracting muscles and pressure differences in the abdominal and thoracic cavities) to facilitate the flow of blood toward the heart. Collectively, the venules and small and large veins function to return blood to the right atrium; more important, they act as a major blood reservoir. Indeed, 60 to 70% of the blood volume may be stored in the venous vasculature during resting conditions (Fig. 5–3).

Two additional structural components that are important during normal circulatory function are arteriovenous anastomoses and the lymphatic system. Arteriovenous anastomoses, as the name implies, bypass capillary beds. They possess smooth muscle cells throughout their entire length and are located in most if not all tissue beds. Most arteriovenous anastomoses

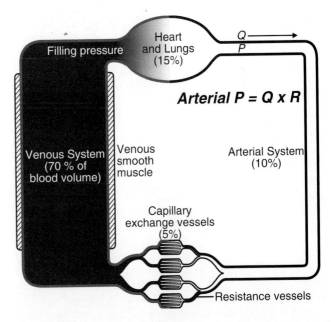

Fig. 5–3. Blood is unevenly distributed throughout the circulatory system. The largest portion of the blood volume is contained within the systemic veins. Relatively small changes in venous capacity can alter the heart's filling pressure dramatically, resulting in predictable changes in cardiac output (Q), peripheral vascular resistance (R) and arterial blood pressure (P). Decreases in filling pressure, for example, decrease Q and P and increase R. (Modified from Shepherd, J.T., and Vanhoutte, P.M. The Human Cardiovascular System: Facts and Concepts, 1st ed. Raven Press, New York, 1979:11.)

are believed to be extremely important in regulating blood flow to highly vascular tissue beds (skin, feet). Their role in maintaining normal homeostasis, however, is speculative other than for thermoregulation.

The peripheral lymphatic system is not anatomically connected to the circulatory system but nevertheless is integrally involved in maintaining normal circulatory dynamics, especially interstitial fluid volume (approximately 10% of the capillary filtrate). Lymphatic capillaries collect interstitial fluid, lymph, which is eventually returned to the cranial vena cava and right atrium after passing through a series of lymph vessels, lymph nodes, and the thoracic duct. Lymph vessels have smooth muscle within their walls and contain valves similar to those in veins. Contraction of skeletal muscle (lymphatic pump) and lymph vessel smooth muscle, in conjunction with lymphatic "valves," are responsible for lymph flow.

BLOOD

Blood is the fluid (approximately 60% plasma and 40% cells) responsible for carrying oxygen, nutrients, and other blood-borne substances to all the tissues of the body and for delivering carbon dioxide, the byproducts of cellular metabolism, and foreign substances (e.g., anesthetic drugs) to the appropriate organs of elimination. This suspension of red and white blood cells and platelets in plasma is also responsible for maintaining a normal cellular environment (homeostasis), prevention of hemorrhage (clotting), and defense against foreign substances (immunity).(2) Red blood cells contain hemoglobin, which binds and carries oxygen to peripheral tissue sites.(3) The amount of oxygen carried by blood is called the arterial oxygen content (CaO_2). The CaO_2 can be calculated by knowing the hemoglobin concentration (Hb; g/dL) of red blood cells, the binding of oxygen to hemoglobin (normally 1.34 ml/g/dL), the percentage saturation of hemoglobin (SaO_2), which is a function of the PO_2, and the oxygen dissolved in plasma (PaO_2 mm Hg × 0.003 mL/mm Hg) such that CaO_2 = Hb × 1.34 × SaO_2 + (PaO_2 × 0.003). The rate of oxygen transport or delivery (DO_2) to tissues is the product of blood flow (Q) and CaO_2:

$$DO_2 = Q \times CaO_2$$

Binding of oxygen to hemoglobin depends upon the partial pressure of oxygen (PO_2) and the shape of the oxyhemoglobin dissociation curve (Chapter 6). The oxyhemoglobin dissociation curve is generally sigmoid and is influenced by pH, PCO_2, temperature, and 2,3-diphosphoglycerate (DPG) concentration. Increases in pH and decreases in PCO_2, temperature, and 2,3-DPG in the lung all shift the oxyhemoglobin curve to the left, thereby increasing oxygen binding to hemoglobin and decreasing oxygen availability. The opposite changes occur in peripheral tissues, where hemoglobin divests itself of oxygen in proportion to the decrease in PO_2. Once the amount of deoxygenated hemoglobin (unsaturated hemoglobin) exceeds 5 g/100 mL, the blood changes from a red to a blue color (cyanosis). Carbon dioxide produced by metabolizing tissues binds to deoxygenated hemoglobin and is eliminated by the lung during the oxygenation process prior to the blood returning to the systemic circulation and the cycle repeating itself.

The plasma is composed of about 90% water by weight, plasma proteins (7%), and other organic (carbohydrates, fats) and inorganic (Na, K^+, Cl^-, etc.) substances. Although there are molecules including electrolytes in the plasma that contribute to the total osmotic pressure, their importance in the exchange of water between the circulation and the tissues is minimized by their small size and their relatively free permeability across capillaries. The relevant osmotic pressure influencing water exchange between capillaries and tissues is the colloidal osmotic pressure (COP), which is primarily caused by the relatively large molecular weight of plasma proteins. The COP is approximately 25 mm Hg, and it and the capillary fluid pressure (hydrostatic pressure) are the two key forces (see Starling's law of the capillary) that govern water exchange in the capillaries and the acute maintenance of the plasma volume and therefore blood volume. The day-to-day regulation of blood volume is also dependent upon the balance of fluid intake by the gastrointestinal system and fluid losses by the kidneys, lungs, and skin. Neural and hormonal factors, including osmore-

ceptors in the hypothalamus, antidiuretic hormone released by neurons in the supraoptic and paraventricular nuclei, aldosterone and renin produced by the kidney, and the release of atrial natriuretic peptide by atrial receptors sensitive to stretch, are all integrally involved in maintaining plasma and therefore blood volume. The one mechanism above all others, however, that dominates the control of plasma and blood volume is the effect of blood volume on arterial blood pressure and the consequences of arterial blood pressure upon the urinary excretion of sodium and water (Fig. 5–4A).(4) Alterations in arterial blood pressure, therefore, can have profound effects upon fluid exchange and blood volume (natriuresis, pressure diuresis). The interplay of these mechanisms ultimately controls

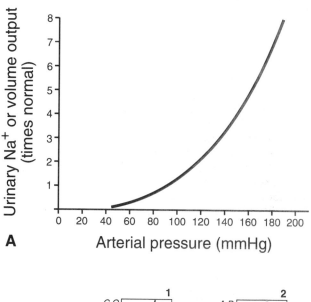

A

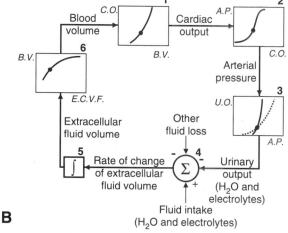

B

Fig. 5–4. The effect of arterial blood pressure on the urinary excretion of Na^+ and urine volume (A, top), and a scheme for a basic feedback mechanism which controls blood volume and extracellular fluid volume (B, bottom). Cardiac output (C.O.); arterial blood pressure (A.P.); urine output (U.O.); extracellular fluid volume (E.C.F.V.); blood volume (B.V.). (Modified from Guyton, A.C. Textbook of Medical Physiology, 8th ed. WB Saunders, Philadelphia, 1991:321.)

arterial blood pressure, blood volume, extracellular fluid volume, and renal excretion of salt and water (Fig. 5–4B).

Hemorrheology

PRESSURE, RESISTANCE, FLOW

In an electric system, the current flow (I) or charge ($+$) is determined by the electromotive force or voltage (E) and the resistance to current flow (R) according to Ohm's law:

$$I = \frac{E}{R} \qquad 5-1$$

The flow of fluids (Q) through nondistensible tubes depends upon pressure (P) and the resistance to flow (R). Therefore, and in the most general terms,

$$Q = \frac{P}{R} \qquad 5-2$$

Hemorrheology is the study of blood flow in the vascular system.(5, 6) The resistance to blood flow is determined by blood viscosity (η) and the geometric factors of blood vessels (radius, length). The steady, nonpulsatile, laminar flow of Newtonian fluids (homogenous fluids in which viscosity does not change with flow velocity or vascular geometry), like water, saline, and, under physiologic conditions, plasma, can be described by the popular and frequently quoted Poiseuille-Hagen law, which states:

$$Q = \frac{(P_1 - P_2)\, r^4 \pi}{8L\eta} \quad R = \frac{8L\eta}{r^4 \pi} \qquad 5-3$$

where $P_1 - p_2$ is the pressure difference, r^4 is the radius to the fourth power, L is the length of the tube, η is the viscosity of the fluid, and $\pi/8$ is a constant of proportionality.(7) The maintenance of laminar flow is a fundamental assumption of the resistance offered to steady-state fluid flow in the Poiseuille-Hagen equation. This law, although frequently used for assessing blood flow in the vascular system, is descriptive only, and must be kept in perspective when considering the real-life situation, since blood is not a homogenous fluid and blood flow is not steady but pulsatile and is not always laminar. These differences from the idealized steady laminar flow of Newtonian fluids through nondistensible tubes of constant radius have important consequences on the quantity of blood flow to peripheral tissue beds, oxygen delivery, and the distribution of blood flow between tissue beds.

The relationship between vessel (or chamber when describing the heart) distending pressure, vessel diameter, vessel wall thickness, and vessel wall tension is described by Laplace's law:

$$P = \frac{2Th}{r} \quad \text{or} \quad T = \frac{Pr}{2h} \qquad 5-4$$

where T is wall tension, P is developed pressure, r is the internal radius, and h is the wall thickness. This relationship is extremely important because it relates pressure and vessel dimension to changes in developed tension, which is known to be an important determinant of ventricular-vascular coupling (afterload), myocardial work, and myocardial oxygen consumption.(8)

VISCOSITY

Since blood is a non-Newtonian fluid that is delivered through progressively narrowing blood vessels in a pulsatile nonlaminar or even turbulent manner, how can blood flow be accurately characterized? More specifically, how can the resistance (R) to blood flow be thought of in functional terms? First, the major factors influencing blood flow resistance (R_p) are blood viscosity (η) and vascular hindrance or impedance (Z): (9, 10)

$$R_p = \eta \times Z$$

It should be noted that the term R_p is not the same as R in Ohm's law or the equivalent thereof in the Poiseuille-Hagen equation ($8L\eta/r^4\pi$) but represents the resistance to blood flow in a pulsatile (R_p; p = pulsatile) or oscillatory non-steady-state or, simply stated, more physiologic system. The resistance (R) term in the two previous examples is more correctly thought of in terms of a nonpulsatile, nonoscillatory, and nonphysiologic system.

The viscosity term (η), although of lesser importance than Z in determining R_p, is dependent upon red blood cell concentration or hematocrit, red blood cell aggregability and deformability, plasma viscosity, temperature, and blood flow conditions.(6) The rheologic term that characterizes blood flow conditions is shear rate, which is a function of blood flow velocity, and vascular geometry. The viscosity of blood is shear rate dependent. Viscosity decreases as shear rate increases according to the equation

$$\eta = \frac{\text{shear stress (dynes/cm}^2)}{\text{shear rate(sec}^{-1})} \qquad 5-5$$

where shear stress is the force applied during pulsatile blood flow between theoretic layers of blood in the blood vessel. It is interesting that shear rate gradually increases and η decreases as large arteries become smaller, is greatest in the capillaries regardless of low flow rates, and then decreases in venules and large veins. This phenomenon, known as the *Fahraeus-Lindquist effect*, is attributed to "plasma skimming" and red blood cell deformability; that is, viscosity in capillaries is low because red blood cells may only be able to pass through capillaries single file, permitting the development of a cell-free layer of plasma next to the capillary wall that, in conjunction with red blood cell folding, increases the cell-free component of blood compared to the situation in

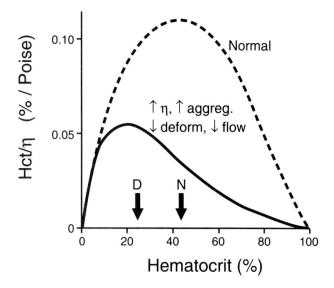

Fig. 5–5. The effects of changes in hematocrit (Hct; %) on an index of oxygen transport (Hct/η). The arrow marked N represents a relatively normal Hct. The arrow marked D represents a patient with anemia or hemodilution. The dashed line represents the normal situation when Hct is the only variable. The solid line represents the response to changes in Hct when plasma viscosity (η) is increased, red cell aggregation is increased, red cell deformability is decreased, or blood flow rate is decreased. (Modified from Lasala, P.A., Chien, S., and Michelson, C.B. Hemorheology: What Is the Ideal Hematocrit? In: Askanasi, J., Starker, R.M., and Weissman, C., eds. Fluid and Electrolyte Management in Critical Care, 1st ed. Butterworth, Boston, 1986:210.)

larger blood vessels.(9) The smaller the vessel, the greater the effect. Under normal circumstances, the most important variable in determining η is the hematocrit.

The optimum hematocrit for transporting the most oxygen per unit time to tissues varies between species (e.g., man 47%, dog 46%, cow 32%, horse 42%, camel 27%) because of differences in anatomy and circulatory dynamics. High hematocrits (polycythemia), low blood flow conditions (shock), increased red blood cell aggregability and rouleaux formation (sepsis), and hyperproteinemia (dehydration) can all cause η to increase, resulting in a decrease in oxygen delivery to tissues (Fig. 5–5). Hematocrits greater than 65% lead to sludging of blood in capillaries and venules and dramatically increase the work of pumping blood. Hemodilution (fluid administration) is often beneficial in treating these previous conditions and has been used during anesthesia to reduce red blood cell loss and improve oxygen delivery during low blood flow states.(11, 12) Indeed, the optimum hematocrit for dogs subjected to hemorrhagic shock and an arterial blood pressure of 50 mm Hg is 20 to 25%.(9)

IMPEDANCE

The impedance (Z) term, the second key factor in determining blood flow in pulsatile systems, is a measure of the opposition to flow presented by pulsatile

blood flow in an elastic vascular system.(10) Quantitatively, impedance is the relationship between pulsatile pressure and pulsatile flow in arteries:

$$Z_L = \frac{P_1 - P_2}{Q} \; (Z_L = R_P + R) \qquad 5\text{–}6$$

where Z_L represents longitudinal impedance, which is the sum of the pulsatile (R_p) and steady nonpulsatile resistive (R) components of longitudinal arterial resistance. Under normal (nonstressed) conditions the steady nonpulsatile resistive component represents 90% of the total impedance to blood flow while the pulsatile component comprises 10%. This fact (R = 90% of Z_L) is the principal reason so many investigators and clinicians calculate vascular resistance from Ohm's law. The components of Z_L may change considerably, however, in diseased animals or during pharmacologic manipulation, with R_p becoming much more important.

Impedance is determined by the various frequency components that comprise the arterial pressure and flow waveforms, is measured by applying a Fourier or harmonic analysis to these waveforms, and is expressed as a ratio or modulus and phase (Fig. 5–6). A positive phase value indicates that flow harmonics lag behind pressure harmonics, and vice versa, the

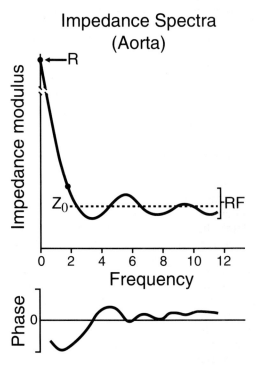

Fig. 5–6. The impedance modulus and phase of a hypothetic aortic impedance spectra. The impedance modulus decreases from 0 Hz (R; peripheral vascular resistance) to a low value that oscillates around a characteristic value (Z_0) because of pulse wave reflections (RF). Negative phase values indicate that flow harmonics lead pressure harmonics and vice versa.

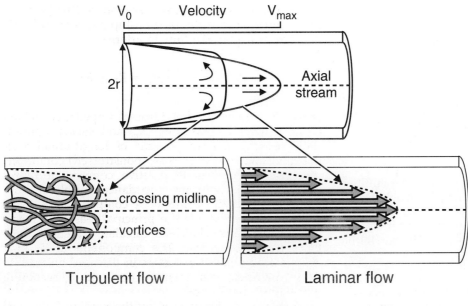

$$RN = \frac{pD_v}{\eta}$$

Fig. 5–7. Velocity profiles for laminar and turbulent blood flow. Note that during turbulent blood flow vortices develop and that both axial and mean velocity are lower than during laminar flow. Maximal velocity (V_{max}); Reynolds number (RN); blood density (p); vessel diameter (D_v); viscosity (η).

key point being that impedance is a frequency-dependent, not time-dependent, index. Input impedance (Z_i), the ratio of pressure and flow at an arterial site that is considered to be the input to the vascular tree (e.g., the aortic root), is dependent upon local arterial properties (elastance, compliance), the properties of all the vessels beyond the point of measurement down to the points where pulsations and pulse wave reflections from narrowing arteries (particularly arterioles) and vessel bifurcations disappear. Impedance to blood flow, therefore, is viewed as having a resistive (steady-state) component due primarily to the arterioles and a reactive (pulsatile) component due to vessel wall properties (compliance, elastance, and pulse wave reflection). Low systolic arterial pressure permits more complete ventricular ejection, maintains low myocardial oxygen demands and provides little stimulus for hypertrophy. High diastolic pressure ensures adequate coronary blood flow and myocardial perfusion because the majority of myocardial blood flow occurs during ventricular relaxation. Increases in arterial stiffness increase pulse pressure amplitude and systolic pressure, and decrease diastolic pressure. Poorly timed wave reflections generally decrease diastolic pressure. The totality of these effects increases myocardial work, oxygen consumption, and energy requirements, and decreases myocardial perfusion. Ideally, the best match between the heart's pumping activity and the vascular response to the ejection of blood (ventricular-vascular coupling) is obtained when myocardial work is kept as low as possible (low systolic pressure) while maintaining adequate perfusion of the heart and peripheral tissues (high diastolic pressure).(13-15) Within perfusing limits, a reduction in mean arterial pressure (a characteristic of most anesthetic drugs) improves arterial distensibility, delays pressure wave reflections, and causes a smaller reduction in diastolic pressure than hypovolemia. Anesthesia and anesthetic drugs also produce variable effects upon hematocrit, red blood cell deformability, and plasma protein concentrations, leading to alterations in η, which, when combined with changes in Z, may favorably affect ventricular-vascular coupling, providing hypotension (50–60 mm Hg) does not occur.(9, 16, 17)

TURBULENCE

Pulsatile blood flow may be laminar with a longitudinal velocity that takes the form of a parabola or may be irregular or turbulent (Fig. 5–7). More pressure or myocardial energy (work) is required to pump blood when the flow is turbulent. The potential for turbulence to develop in blood vessels can be predicted by a dimensionless number called the Reynolds number (RN): (18)

$$RN = \frac{pDv}{\eta} \qquad 5\text{–}7$$

where p is fluid density, D is vessel diameter, and v is the mean blood flow velocity. The blood viscosity (η) is inversely proportional to the Reynolds number, and is an important determinant of turbulent blood flow. Turbulence usually produces vibrations of the surrounding tissue structures, leading to murmurs and, with time, vascular dilation caused by weakening of the supporting elements of the vessel wall. Chronic or acute hemodilution (fluid therapy) reduces hematocrit and therefore η, leading to an increase in RN and the production of "functional" cardiac murmurs. Cardiac (pulmonic and aortic stenosis) and vascular (coarctation of the aorta) diseases that narrow valve openings or blood vessels increase v and are important causes of murmurs.

The Heart

The purpose of the heart is to pump blood in quantities sufficient to meet the body's metabolic demands. To achieve this function requires a highly integrated series of electric, mechanical, and metabolic events that culminate in repetitive contraction and relaxation of the myocardium.

ELECTROPHYSIOLOGY OF THE HEART

Normal cardiac electric activity is essential for normal cardiac contractile function (excitation-contraction coupling). Indeed, myocardial contraction is preceded by and will not occur without electric activation, although normal or near-normal electric activity is possible without myocardial contraction (electric-mechanical uncoupling; electric-mechanical dissociation). The cardiac cell membrane (sarcolemma) is a highly specialized lipid bilayer that contains protein-associated channels, pumps, enzymes, and exchangers in an architecturally sophisticated yet fluid (reorganizable, movable) medium. Most drugs and many anesthetic drugs produce important direct and indirect effects on the cell membrane and intracellular organelles, ultimately altering cardiac excitation-contraction coupling.

The molecular composition and fluidity of cardiac membranes determine their ion transport and membrane-associated electric properties. The unequal distribution of different ions, especially sodium, potassium, and chloride, is responsible for the development of the resting membrane potential of cardiac cells as predicted by the Nernst equation or, more accurately, the Goldman-Hodgkin-Katz constant-field equation.(19-21)

Nernst equation:

$$E = \frac{-61 \text{ mV}}{Z \log (C_i/C_o)} \qquad 5\text{-}8$$

$$-61 = 2.303 \frac{RT}{F}$$

where

E = electromotive force
C_i, C_o = ion concentration inside (i) and outside (o) the cell membrane
Z = valence
R = gas constant

T = absolute temperature
F = Faraday constant
2.303 = conversion of ln to log 10
Goldman-Hodgkin-Katz equation:

$$E_m = -61 \text{ mV} \log \frac{[\text{K}]_i + (P_{\text{Na}}/P_\text{K}) [\text{Na}]_i}{[\text{K}]_o + (P_{\text{Na}}/P_\text{K}) [\text{Na}]_o} \qquad 5\text{-}9$$

where

E_m = resting membrane potential
P_{Na}/P_K ratio = relative permeability of membrane Na to K, normally 0.04 in myocardial cells

The transmembrane electric potential generated by cardiac cells is the result of transmembrane ion fluxes (active properties) through "gated" membrane pores or "channels" (Table 5–1).(21) Ion channels are characterized by their ionic selectivity, conductance, gating characteristics, and density. The channel-gating mechanisms control ion passage and are composed of both activation and inactivation gates, which are voltage and frequently time dependent. The functional configuration of the gates determines channel state: activated or open, inactivated or closed, and resting (capable of being activated). The directional movement (inward, outward) of the various ions is ultimately dependent upon channel state and the electromechanical driving force (equilibrium potential minus membrane potential) for each ion. The electromechanical driving force, as illustrated by the Nernst equation, is composed of an electric force and a concentration gradient. It should be noted that in the presence of many anesthetic drugs, particularly local anesthetics (lidocaine, mepivacaine), and inhalation anesthetics (halothane, isoflurane), these same channels may demonstrate use-dependent block.(22, 23) Use-dependent block is the phenomenon exhibited by cardiac cells wherein, in the presence of a drug, increases in stimulation rate (e.g., heart rate) produces a more pronounced drug effect upon the electric properties of the heart than during slower stimulation.

Excitability or the ability of the cardiac cell membrane to generate an electric potential (action potential) is a fundamental intrinsic property of cardiac cells.(19) The action potential of cardiac muscle varies considerably from that of nerves and skeletal muscle. The cardiac action potential arises from a more negative membrane potential (90 vs. 65 mV), is greater in magnitude (130 vs. 80 mV), and is much longer in duration (150–300 vs 1 ms). Five characteristic phases of the cardiac action potential are discernable in most cardiac cells; phase 0, or the phase of rapid depolarization, is due to the rapid flux of sodium ions (fast inward current) into the cell; phase 1, the early phase of repolarization, is caused by the transient outward movement of potassium ions; phase 2, the plateau phase, is attributed to the continued but decreased entry of sodium ions and a large but slow influx of calcium ions (slow inward current) into

Table 5–1. Currents Associated with the Cardiac Action Potential

Current	Abbreviation	Qualities
Fast inward sodium current	I_{Na}	Responsible for upstroke of action potential; abolished by tetrodotoxin; inhibited by class I antiarrhythmic agents
Slow inward calcium current	I_{Ca}, I_{si}	Important for plateau phase of cardiac action potential; involved in excitation-contraction coupling; increased by β-stimulation; inhibited by calcium antagonist
Subtype T	$I_{Ca(t)}$	Transient calcium current, opening at low voltages (-60 to -50 mV); may be important in sinus node depolarization
Subtype L	$I_{Ca(l)}$	Long-duration calcium current, inhibited by calcium antagonists
Other currents		
Diastolic pacemaker current in Purkinje fibers	I_f or I_h	Inward funny sodium (and potassium) current responsible for initial phase of spontaneous depolarization in Purkinje tissue; increased by β-stimulation; may contribute to SA node automaticity
Sodium/calcium exchange	I_{Na-Ca}	May contribute to late phase of cardiac action potential plateau (controversial)
Voltage-operated K currents		
Background potassium current with inward reactification	I_{K1} or I_{Krec}	Generates resting membrane potential; depolarization shuts the channel off, hence voltage-gated; current flows again during repolarization to help end the action potential, therefore rectifies; absent in pacemaker cells
Delayed reactifier potassium current	I_K	Time-dependent outward potassium current; activated by depolarization (fully active at $+10$ mV) and deactivated by repolarization; voltage-gated; responsible for repolarization in nodal cells and contributes to spontaneous depolarization; divided into I_{Kr} (r = rapid) and I_{Ks} (s = slow)
Early transient outward potassium current	I_{to}	Transient outward early potassium current, previously called *chloride current*; prominent in epicardial ventricular cells, Purkinje fibers and atrial cells, causes phase 1; may also shorten action potential duration
Ligand-operated G-dependent K currents Acetylcholine-sensitive	I_{KACh}	Activated by acetylcholine muscarinic receptors in nodal, Purkinje, and atrial cells; not in ventricles; time independent; when current switched on in nodal cells, spontaneous depolarization is delayed
Adenosine-sensitive	I_{KADO}	Probably same as I_{KACh}; adenosine stimulates time-independent background potassium current
Ligand-gated Non-G-dependent K current ATP-regulated	I_{KATP}	Lack of ATP activates (e.g., ischemia); inhibited by sulfonylureas, activated by K-channel activators (pinacidil)

(Modified from Opie, L.H. The Heart: Physiology and Metabolism, 2nd ed. Raven Press, New York, 1991:88–89.)

cells; phase 3 is the phase of repolarization during which the membrane potential returns to its resting value due to potassium efflux (outward current) from the cell; and phase 4 is a resting phase in atrial and ventricular muscle cells prior to the initiation of the next action potential (Fig. 5–8; Table 5–2). The magnitude and rate of sodium influx into cardiac cells determines the magnitude and rate of change in membrane potential (dV/dt) during phase 0 of the cardiac action potential. The greater the dV/dt, the more rapid the transmission and conduction of the cardiac impulse through cardiac tissue.[20] Cardiac cells that normally possess a more negative membrane potential (atrial and ventricular muscle cells, Purkinje cells) demonstrate greater excitability and a more rapid conduction velocity than those with less negative membrane potentials (sinoatrial and atrioventricular nodes; diseased myocardium).(23) Calcium entry into cardiac cells during phase 2 triggers intracellular calcium release, which is important for normal cellular contraction and, with potassium, determines action potential duration in atrial and ventricular myocytes. Since calcium enters the cell slowly and at a less negative membrane potential, cardiac cells with a reduced resting membrane potential (sinoatrial and atrioventricular nodes) demonstrate a considerably decreased dV/dt and slow conduction velocity compared to atrial and ventricular muscle and Purkinje cells.(20) Potassium efflux from cardiac cells is controlled by a variety of mechanisms, including concentration differences across the membrane and the changing permeability (diffusional) characteristics of the cell membrane to potassium (Table 5–1). Collectively, the channels responsible for phase 3 repolarization are also the major determinants of cardiac action potential duration, cardiac cell refractoriness, and the duration of the supernormal period (Fig. 5–8). The duration of the cardiac action potential has important clinical implications relative to the amount of calcium entry and the potential for arrhythmia development.(22) Longer cardiac action potentials permit more

calcium entry into the cell and prolong cellular refractoriness. Arrhythmias develop if there are large disparities or inhomogeneities in the action potential duration and refractoriness of adjacent cardiac cells due to reentry of electric impulses and reexcitation of the heart (see "Cardiac Arrhythmias").(24) Reentry is one mechanism whereby the ultra-short-acting barbiturates and inhalation anesthetics are known to produce cardiac arrhythmias.

Phase 4 diastolic depolarization (pacemaker potential) occurs in the sinoatrial and atrioventricular nodes and atrial and ventricular (Purkinje network) specialized tissues.(20, 21) Diastolic depolarization imparts the unique property of automaticity to the heart. The resting membrane potential depolarizes toward a threshold potential in tissues with this property, which when reached triggers the development of an action potential. The ionic processes responsible for phase 4 or diastolic depolarization vary between the various specialized tissues of the heart primarily because of differences in their resting or maximum diastolic potential and cell type (e.g., sinoatrial vs atrioventricular node vs Purkinje cell). Cells in the sinoatrial and atrial ventricular nodes have comparatively less negative

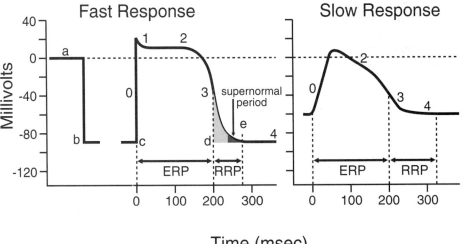

Fig. 5–8. Cardiac transmembrane potential changes associated with fast and slow response action potentials. Note that slow response action potentials originate from a less negative resting membrane potential and have a much slower rate of rise (phase 0). During the supernormal period a subthreshold stimulus can elicit a normal action potential. See text for an explanation of the action potential phases 1 through 4. Effective refractory period (ERP); relative refractory period (RRP).

Table 5–2. Major Ion Fluxes During the Cardiac Action Potential

Name	Ion	Movement	Current	Phase of Action Potential
I_{Na}	Na^+	In	Inward	0 (depolarization)
I_{Cl}	Cl^-	In	Outward	1 (early repolarization)
I^{to}	K^+	Out	Outward	1 (early repolarization)
I_{Ca}	Ca^{2+}	In	Inward	2 (plateau)
I_{K1}^a	K^+	Out	Outward	2 (plateau)
I_k	K^+	Out	Outward	3 (repolarization)
I_f	Na^+	In	Inward	4 (depolarization in automatic cells)

Open I_{K1} channels in resting cells are the major contributor to the equilibrium responsible for the Nernst potential during phase 4 (resting potential).

(Modified from Katz, A.M. Physiology of the Heart, 1st ed. Raven Press, New York, 1977:246.)

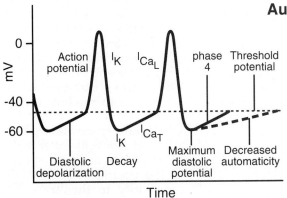

Automaticity Increased by:

↑ Heart rate

↑ Temp

Mild O$_2$ deficiency

↓ K$_0$

↑ Ca^{2+}

Catecholamines

Thyroxine

Fig. 5–9. The transmembrane potential of cardiac tissue within the sinoatrial node (pacemaker tissue) is characterized by a less negative maximum diastolic potential, which depolarizes toward threshold (phase 4 diastolic depolarization), a slow phase 0 caused primarily by activation of I_{CaL}, and a relatively rapid repolarization due to I$_K$. The rate of phase 4 diastolic depolarization (automaticity) can be increased by increases in heart rate, temperature, calcium, catecholamines and thyroxine and decreases in oxygen tension and extracellular potassium concentration.

maximum diastolic potentials (-65 mV) than Purkinje cells and are dependent upon the entry of calcium ion (slow inward current) and a progressive decrease in membrane permeability to potassium efflux for their automaticity (Fig. 5–9). Automatic cells in atrial specialized pathways and the ventricular Purkinje network have a more negative maximum diastolic potential (-90 mV) and are dependent upon a hyperpolarizing-induced "funny" inward current, termed I_f, carried mainly by sodium ions and a decrease in potassium efflux for their automaticity (Table 5–1). Because potassium ions normally leave cardiac cells in order to restore or maintain the resting membrane potential, any decrease in potassium efflux facilitates the depolarization process. The principal mechanisms responsible for altering automaticity are changes in the threshold potential, the rate of phase 4 depolarization, and the maximum diastolic potential following repolarization. The cardiac tissue with the most rapid rate of phase 4 depolarization (normally the sinoatrial node) is termed the *pacemaker* and determines the heart rate. The cardiac pacemaker normally depresses the automaticity of slower or subsidiary pacemakers (overdrive suppression), preventing more than one pacemaker from controlling heart rate. In mechanical terms, overdrive suppression in subsidiary pacemakers is due to activation of the Na$^+$-K$^+$ pump, leading to membrane hyperpolarization and a longer time to reach threshold.(20, 22) Subsidiary pacemakers are most suppressed at fast heart rates because the Na$^+$-K$^+$ pump is more active at faster rates, resulting in a more negative maximum diastolic potential. Automaticity is also influenced by local factors, including temperature, pH, and blood gases (PO$_2$, PCO$_2$), extracellular potassium concentration, catecholamines, and various hormones (Fig. 5–9).

The algebraic sum of all the action potentials produced by each cardiac cell following activation by the sinoatrial node is responsible for the body surface electrocardiogram (ECG; Fig. 5–10). Initiation of an electric impulse in the sinoatrial node is followed by rapid electric transmission of the impulse through the atria, giving rise to the P wave. Repolarization of the atria gives rise to the TA wave, which is most obvious in large animals (horses, cattle), where the total atrial tissue

mass is substantial enough to generate enough electromotive force to be electrocardiographically recognizable. Repolarization of the atria in smaller species (dogs, cats) and depolarization of the sinoatrial and atrioventricular nodes does not generate a large enough electric potential to be recorded at the body surface. Once the wave of depolarization reaches the atrioventricular node, conduction is slowed because of the atrioventricular node's low resting membrane potential (approximately -60 mV) and the relatively depressed rate of phase 0 (decremental conduction). Increased parasympathetic tone can produce marked slowing of atrioventricular nodal conduction leading to first-, second-, and third-degree heart block. Many drugs used in anesthesia, including opioids, alpha$_2$-agonists and occasionally acepromazine, increase parasympathetic tone, causing heart block and bradyarrhythmias (see "Cardiac Arrhythmias"). The anticholinergic drugs atropine and glycopyrrolate are generally effective therapy in these situations.

Under normal conditions conduction of the electric impulse through the atrioventricular node produces the PR or PQ interval of the electrocardiogram and provides time for the atria to contract prior to activation and contraction of the ventricles. This delay is functionally important, particularly at faster heart rates, because it permits atrial contraction to contribute to ventricular filling. It is worth remembering that cells of the atrioventricular node are extremely dependent upon calcium ion for the generation of an action potential and conduction of the electric impulse. Cells of the atrioventricular node are extremely sensitive to drugs that block transsarcolemmal calcium flux (large doses of anesthetics, of barbiturates, inhalants, etc.; the so-called calcium antagonists verapamil and diltiazem). These and other drugs and cardiac disease can produce atrioventricular block and postrepolarization refractoriness that are not responsive to anticholinergic drugs. Postrepolarization refractoriness is the phenomenon wherein cardiac cells remain refractory to electric activation after complete repolarization.(22, 24) This phenomenon is most likely to produce atrioventricular block as the rate of atrial depolarization is increased. Increases in parasympathetic tone, therefore, particularly in the presence of drugs or disease (ischemia) that interfere with conduction of the electric impulse through the atrioventricular node, can lead to electrocardiographic evidence of first- (prolonged PR interval), second- (blocked P wave), or third-degree (dissociation of P and QRS complex) atrioventricular block.

Once the electric impulse has traversed the atrioventricular node, it is rapidly transmitted to the ventricular muscle by specialized muscle cells commonly referred to as *Purkinje fibers*. Purkinje fibers conduct the electric impulse at relatively rapid speeds (3–5 m/s) based upon their size and electric properties (Fig. 5–10). Purkinje fibers have a much longer action potential duration and refractory period than ventricular muscle cells, which normally prevents reentry of the electric impulse and reactivation of the ventricles (see "Cardiac Arrhythmias"). Anatomically, Purkinje fibers originate from the bundle of His and divide into the left and right bundle branches. The left bundle branch divides further into the left anterior and left posterior divisions of the conduction system. These fibers serve as electric conduits for the transmission of the electric impulse, first to the ventricular papillary muscles, which are activated and contract just prior to electric activation of the remaining ventricular myocardium. The activation and contraction of the ventricular papillary muscles cause their attached chordae tendineae to tense, helping to prevent prolapse of the atrioventricular valves into their respective atria during ventricular contraction. Ventricular depolarization (activation) produces the QRS complex of the ECG and is immediately followed by ventricular

repolarization, giving rise to the T wave. It is important to remember that, although the transmission of the electric impulse has, by analogy, been compared to dropping a pebble in water leading to a concentric wave front, or, in the case of the heart, a concentric wave of depolarization—the conduction of the electric impulse in the heart is ultimately dependent upon uniform ("isotropic") cell-to-cell resistive and capacitive (passive) membrane properties that are largely determined by low-resistance gap or nexus junctions between cells and the spatial variation in myocardial cell refractoriness.(25–27) The configuration and magnitude of the T wave vary considerably between species and are influenced by changes in heart rate, blood temperature, and the extracellular potassium concentration. Hyperkalemia, for example, produces T waves that are of large magnitude, generally spiked or pointed, and of short duration (short QT interval).

The interval beginning immediately following the S wave of the QRS complex (J point) and preceding the T wave is referred to as the *ST* or *STT segment* and is important clinically. Elevation or depression of the STT segment (±0.2 mV or greater) from the isoelectric line is usually an indication of myocardial hypoxia or ischemia, low cardiac output, anemia, or cardiac contusion, and suggests the potential for arrhythmia development. Rarely, "U waves" can be distinguished immediately following the completion of the T wave, and are believed to represent repolarization of Purkinje cells. Like TA waves, U waves are more frequently observed in larger species (horses, cattle) during electrolyte (hypokalemia, hypocalcemia) imbalances or drug (quinidine, digitalis) therapy (Fig. 5–10).

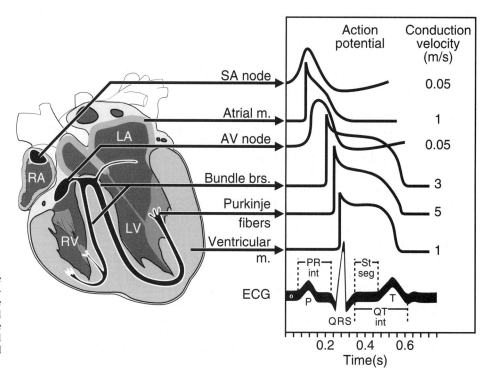

Fig. 5–10. The transmembrane potential (action potential) recorded from all the tissues of the heart (specialized tissue and muscle) summate to produce the P-QRS-T complex (ECG) recorded at the body surface. Sinoatrial (SA); atrioventricular (AV).

In summary, the cardiac cell membrane possesses both active (ion movement) and passive (resistive, capacitive) properties that determine the heart's excitability, automaticity, rhythmicity, refractoriness, and ability to conduct an electric impulse. Anesthetic drugs, via their effects on both the active (e.g., lidocaine, a sodium channel blocker; barbiturates, and inhalants suppress calcium currents) and passive (e.g., halothane and isoflurane change membrane fluidity and depress gap junctions) properties of the heart, can produce significant alterations in cardiac excitability and conduction of the electric impulse, ultimately predisposing to cardiac arrhythmias and mechanical contraction abnormalities.(28-33)

EXCITATION-CONTRACTION COUPLING

Excitation-contraction coupling refers to the process wherein electric activation of the heart is transformed to muscle contraction. The process begins with the cardiac action potential and the depolarization process, and ends with the interaction of the contractile proteins in the individual sarcomeres. The normal extracellular calcium ion concentration is 10^{-3} M compared to an intracellular calcium ion concentration of 10^{-7} M. The electric activation of the sarcolemma and transverse tubule (T-tubule) membranes by the cardiac action potential causes an influx of a small quantity of calcium ions during phase 2 of the cardiac action potential, triggering the release of a much greater quantity of calcium (calcium-induced calcium release) from calsequestrin-bound calcium sources in the sarcoplasmic reticulum. Calcium-induced calcium release raises the intracellular calcium concentration from 10^{-7} M to 10^{-5} M and results in cellular contraction (Fig. 5–11). The importance of calcium influx during phase 2 of the action potential in the contractile process of cardiac muscle compared to other muscles (skeletal, smooth) cannot be overemphasized, because cardiac contraction is more dependent upon and responds instantaneously to changes in the extracellular calcium concentration. Most calcium ions entering the cardiac cell do so through voltage-dependent calcium channels, although some calcium ions enter via the calcium-sodium exchange reaction.(34) Calcium channels are located throughout the T-tubule system, which penetrates deep into the cell interior. The T-tubules abut large terminal cisternae, which are the terminal portion of a diffuse intracellular longitudinal tubular system, the sarcoplasmic reticulum. Voltage-dependent calcium channels are of two types (Table 5–1): a slow, long-lasting (L-type) channel that is opened by complete cellular depolarization, and a fast but transient (T-type) channel that is activated earlier than L-type channels and at more negative potentials (Fig. 5–9). The exact mechanism whereby the calcium channels (both L- and T-type) of the T-tubules communicate with the calcium release channels of the sarcoplasmic reticulum remains unresolved. It is generally accepted that the majority of calcium entering the cardiac cell during each action potential does so through the L-type channel, also termed the *dihydropyridine* (DHP) *receptor* due to its sensitivity to specific types of calcium antagonists (verapamil, diltiazem, nifedipinelike compounds).(35) Whether or not the amount of calcium passing through the DHP receptor (L-type channel) is essential for initiating the series of events leading to cellular contraction, however, remains controversial, since it is known that the rate of change of intracellular calcium concentration is the most effective activator of intracellular calcium release from the sarcoplasmic reticulum. This latter observation suggests that the rapid T-type channels may be important in the excitation-contraction process. It is interesting that T-type channels activate at more negative potentials than L-type channels and are insensitive to sodium channel blockers (lidocaine, tetrodotoxin) and calcium antagonist drugs.(34) Taken together, these observations suggest that T-type channels account for the early phase of calcium channel opening and may be important in initiating intracellular calcium release and electrical depolarization of less polarized tissues such as the sinoatrial and atrioventricular nodes.(21, 22) The L-type (DHP receptor) channels are more prevalent in atrial and ventricular muscle cells than T-type channels, open at less negative potentials, and may account for the latter phases of calcium channel opening.(34) Both channels, however, are physiologically linked via specialized proteins termed *feet*, which are bridging or spanning proteins connecting them to the calcium release mechanism in the sarcoplasmic reticulum. The "foot" proteins are a part of a large molecular weight protein complex in the sarcoplasmic reticulum, termed the *ryanodine receptor* because of its affinity for ryanodine.(35) The ryanodine receptor functions as a type of sarcoplasmic reticulum calcium releasing channel; low concentrations of ryanodine enhance calcium release, whereas large concentrations inhibit calcium release from the sarcoplasmic reticulum.

To summarize, the large extracellular (10^{-3} M) intracellular (10^{-7} M) calcium ion gradient facilitates the transarcolemmal flux of calcium ions through calcium channels (T- and primarily L-type) during the depolarization process. The L-type channel can be blocked by dihydropyridine (DHP) drugs and is therefore called a *DHP receptor*. The increase in intracellular calcium triggers the release of calcium (calcium-induced calcium release) from specialized calcium channels (ryanodine receptors in the sarcoplasmic reticulum), resulting in an increase in intracellular calcium ion concentration (10^{-5} M), which causes myocardial cellular contraction.

CARDIAC CONTRACTION AND RELAXATION

Contraction. Heart muscle cells are composed of contractile units termed *sarcomeres,* which contain thick (myosin) and thin (actin) contractile proteins, regulatory proteins (troponin and tropomyosin), and various structural proteins. The thick myosin filaments are composed of approximately 300 molecules, each ending in a bilobed head. Half (150) of the myosin bilobed

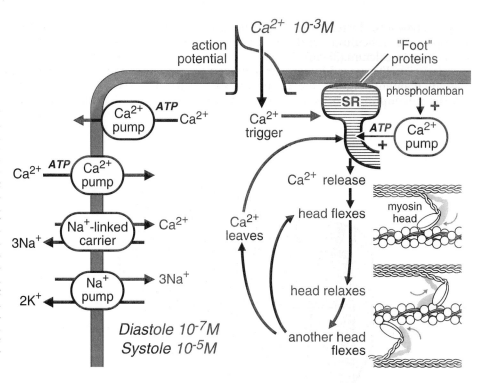

Fig. 5–11. Calcium can enter the cardiac cell during the cardiac action potential (slow response), via an energy-dependent calcium pump or in exchange for intracellular sodium. Increases in intracellular calcium trigger the release of calcium from the sarcoplasmic reticulum (SR) by a process termed *calcium-induced* calcium release. Increases in intracellular calcium (10^{-7} to 10^{-5} M) in the vicinity of the contractile apparatus causes the myosin heads to flex, resulting in sarcomere shortening. The utilization of ATP and formation of ADP and inorganic phosphate, in combination with reuptake of calcium by the SR, causes the myosin head to relax. Phospholamban modulates the pump responsible for the reuptake of calcium into the SR.

heads are located at each end of the sarcomere and project from the thick filament toward the thin filaments (serve as crossbridges). The thin filaments are attached at one end to structural proteins (Z-line) that separate each sarcomere. Each thin filament contains two helical strands of actin intertwined with tropomyosin, which has periodic troponin complexes (Fig. 5–12). Increases in intracellular calcium initiated during phase 2 of the cardiac action potential and amplified by subsequent calcium-induced calcium release serve as the catalyst for actin-myosin interaction and sarcomere shortening. More specifically, calcium ions bind to the regulatory protein Troponin-C (C for calcium), which removes the inhibitory function of Troponin-I (I for inhibitor) on the chemical interaction between actin and myosin. Transformation of chemical energy into sarcomere shortening and mechanical work centers around ATP hydrolysis by myosin ATPase. Hydrolysis of ATP to ADP with the release of inorganic phosphate (Pi) results in a strong attachment between actin and myosin and a conformational change in the bilobed myosin head that causes the head to flex and the actin filaments to move centrally, resulting in sarcomere shortening (Fig. 5–12). Increases in intracellular calcium facilitate this chemical process by increasing myosin ATPase activity. Therefore, by combining with Troponin-C and increasing intracellular myosin ATPase activity, calcium serves as the principal factor in determining the rate at which crossbridges attach and detach. The rate of crossbridge interaction is the basis for the force-velocity relationship in isolated tissue experiments studying cardiac muscle contractile activity (Fig 5–13). The rate of crossbridge attachment deter-

mines the velocity of sarcomere shortening and has been termed *cardiac contractility*. Furthermore, by increasing the number of interacting crossbridges, intracellular calcium increases the maximum force attainable. Clinically, the rate of pressure change (*dP/dt*) and the rate of force development (*dF/dt*) in intact animals have been used as indirect, albeit crude, measures of cardiac contractility.(36, 37)

Optimal sarcomere length for actin myosin interaction is approximately 2.2 microns. Lengths shorter or greater than this were once thought to decrease the force of cardiac contraction by theoretically decreasing the number of available myosin heads for interaction with actin.(36) The concept of optimal sarcomere length relative to the velocity of sarcomere shortening serves as the explanation for the Frank-Starling law of the heart, which predicts an increase in contractile force when sarcomeres are stretched (increased ventricular volume) to their optimal length (Fig. 5–13). It is unlikely, however, that this explanation is totally correct, since sarcomeres rarely change in length (or only minimally so) when loaded, even during dilated forms of heart failure.(35) The more accepted and probable explanation for Starling's law of the heart (length-dependent changes in force development) is that sarcomere loading (increased tension) increases troponin-C affinity for calcium, leading to increased activation of the myofilament and sarcomere shortening without increases in sarcomere length or additional increases in intracellular calcium.(37) Many intravenous anesthetic drugs (barbiturates, ketamine, propofol) and in particular the inhalation anesthetics are known to decrease cardiac contractility by decreasing calcium influx through

L-type channels, decreasing calcium release from the sarcoplasmic reticulum, and decreasing troponin-C sensitivity to calcium.(38-46)

Relaxation. Decreased interaction between actin and myosin filaments signals the beginning of the actin-myosin uncoupling process and myocardial relaxation, and is directly related to a decrease in intracellular calcium ion concentration. Three principal mechanisms are important in reducing intracellular calcium ion concentration and the subsequent decrease in cardiac contractile force. The depolarization-triggered increases in intracellular calcium increase the activity of the

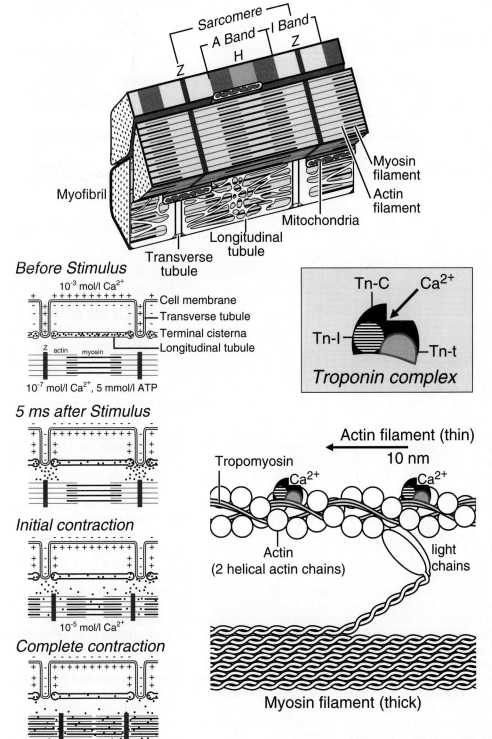

Fig. 5–12. A cardiac muscle fiber contains an overlapping array of thin (actin) and thick (myosin) contractile proteins that produces various bands (Z, A, H, I) within each sarcomere when viewed microscopically. Note that both the transverse (T tubule) and longitudinal tubule system facilitate the presence of relatively large amounts of extracellular calcium (10^{-3} M) in the vicinity of the contractile proteins (top). Membrane depolarization initiates calcium entry into the cardiac cell, contractile protein interaction, and sarcomere shortening (left). More specifically, the binding of calcium with troponin-C (Tn-C) removes the inhibitory function of troponin-I (Tn-I) on actin-myosin interaction. Troponin-t (Tn-t) links the tropinin complex to tropomyosin (right).

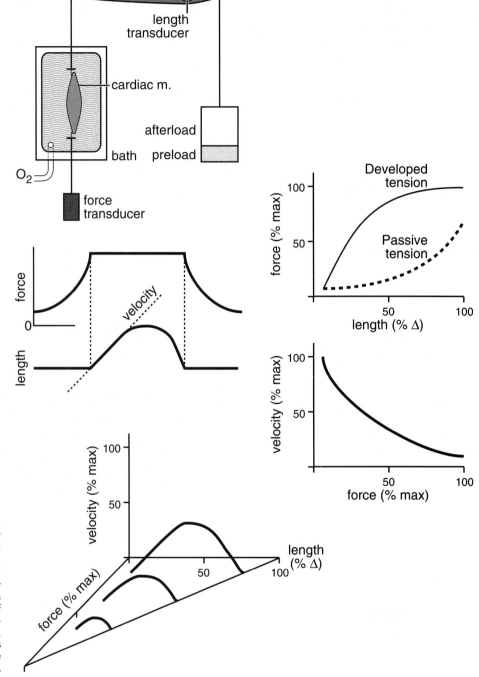

Fig. 5–13. The relationship between force development, velocity of muscle fiber shortening and muscle length in an isolated cardiac muscle experiment. Within physiologic limits, force and velocity increase as muscle length increases (Frank-Starling effect) and velocity decreases as developed force increases. Isolated muscle experiments are used to determine the direct effects of drugs upon cardiac mechanics without neurohumoral influences. Although preload is frequently equated to ventricular filling pressure and afterload is clinically thought of in terms of arterial blood pressure, the transfer of experimental data obtained from isolated muscle experiments to intact animals must be done knowledgeably and cautiously.

calcium regulatory protein calmodulin. Calmodulin serves as an intracellular calcium sensor and, when activated (calmodulin-calcium complex), stimulates the active extrusion of calcium by pumps in the sarcolemma, increases the activity of a phospholamban-modulated calcium pump (increasing calcium uptake by the sarcoplasmic reticulum), and enhances the activity of the sodium-calcium exchanger.(37) Notably

halothane (and other inhalants) interferes with the reuptake of calcium by the sarcoplasmic reticulum, thereby interfering with the relaxation process and ultimately leading to intracellular calcium depletion.(43, 44) The calmodulin-calcium complex also inhibits the release of calcium from the sarcoplasmic reticulum. Mitochondrial uptake of calcium ion only minimally buffers increases in intracellular calcium concentration (Fig. 5–11). From this series of events it is clear that increases in intracellular calcium first enhance (through the calcium-induced calcium release mechanism) then decrease (through the formation of the calmodulin-calcium complex and related mechanisms) the concentration of intracellular calcium, leading to cyclic sarcomere shortening and lengthening and ultimately myocardial contraction (systole), relaxation, and rest (diastole) before the next electric event triggers the mechanical process to repeat itself (Fig. 5–11).

THE CARDIAC CYCLE AND PRESSURE-VOLUME LOOP

Historically, the cardiac cycle has been used as a diagrammatic attempt to describe the electric (ECG), mechanical (pressure, volume, flow) and acoustic (heart-sound) events associated with cardiac contraction and relaxation as a function of time (Fig. 5–14A). Just as important (but not as descriptive) as the time-varying cardiac cycle is the time-independent representation of the cardiac cycle, the ventricular pressure-volume loop (Fig. 5–14B). The advantage of the pressure-volume

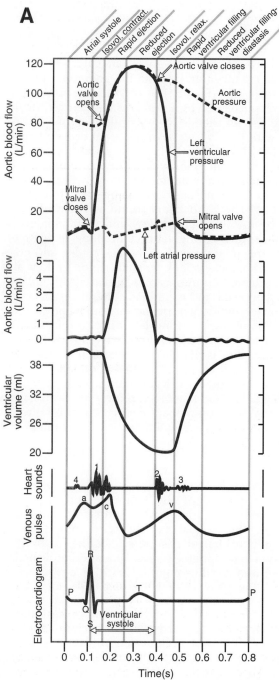

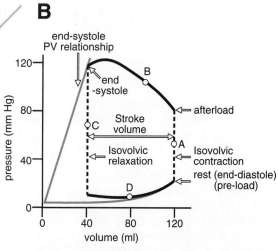

Fig. 5–14. The cardiac cycle (A) diagrammatically illustrates the relationship between mechanical, acoustical and electrical events as a function of time. The pressure-volume loop (B) is a time-independent illustration of the cardiac cycle that can be used to derive load-independent indices of cardiac function. (Modified from Berne, R.M., and Levy, M.N. Principles of Physiology, 1st ed. CV Mosby, St. Louis, 1990:222, 224.)

loop compared to the cardiac cycle is its ability to be used to assess load-independent indices of ventricular systolic and diastolic performance, ventricular vascular interaction (coupling), and myocardial energetics. Changes in the pressure-volume loop can also be used to illustrate and quantitate the determinants of changes in cardiac function: preload, afterload, and cardiac contractility.(5, 7, 15, 36) The various qualitative components of the cardiac cycle and pressure-volume loop are essentially identical for both the right and left ventricles, although the sequence of electric activation and the pressure changes are different.

Because electric activity precedes mechanical activity, the P wave of the surface ECG is a reasonable starting point to begin a description of the cardiac cycle (Fig. 5–14A). Electric activation of the atria produces the P wave of the ECG and results in almost simultaneous contraction of the atria. Atrial contraction increases intraatrial pressure, producing the "a" wave of the atrial pressure curve. The atria (both right and left) normally function as blood reservoirs and conduits for blood transfer, and upon contraction prime the ventricles by contributing approximately 10 to 30% (more at faster heart rates) of the blood volume that fills the ventricles. The atrial contribution to ventricular filling is frequently referred to as the atrial "kick." The atrial kick brings the atrioventricular (mitral, tricuspid) valves into relatively close apposition prior to ventricular contraction and is responsible for the fourth heart sound (S_4). Ventricular contraction is signaled by the R wave of the ECG and begins after a variable delay (PR interval) during which the electric impulse traverses the atrioventricular node and Purkinje network. Once the ventricular pressure increases to a value greater than that in the atrium, the atrioventricular valves close, actually bulging into their respective atria and giving rise to the "C" wave of the atrial pressure curve. The atrioventricular valves are prevented from completely prolapsing into the atrial chambers by chordae tendineae. The sudden development of tension in the contracting myocardium and tensing of the chordae tendineae coincident with atrioventricular valve closure are responsible for the first heart sound (S_1). The rapid increase in ventricular pressure while both the atrioventricular (mitral, tricuspid) and semilunar (aortic, pulmonic) valves are closed is termed *isovolumic contraction* because the volume of the ventricle remains constant (Figs. 5–14A and B). Once ventricular pressure exceeds that in the aorta or pulmonary artery, the semilunar valves open and ejection begins (Fig. 5–14A). The ejection phase of the cardiac cycle is characterized by a rapid increase in ventricular pressure, aortic and pulmonic pressures, and an abrupt decrease in ventricular volume. These changes coincide with a large increase in aortic flow and a decrease in the venous pressure curve as the atrioventricular valves are drawn towards the apex of the heart. Ventricular pressure exceeds aortic pressure during the first third of ventricular ejection (rapid ejection period), reaches equilibrium with aortic pres-

sure, and thereafter, because of the onset of ventricular relaxation, declines more rapidly than aortic pressure (decreased ejection period). Blood continues to be ejected from the ventricle until the semilunar valves close because of the momentum of blood flow. Closure of the semilunar valves marks the end of ventricular systole (by most definitions) and is associated with the development of the second heart sound (S_2). The second heart sound is composed of both aortic (A_2) and pulmonic (P_2) components and is frequently split (10–15 ms) during slow heart rates and in larger species (horses, cattle).(47) Rarely is the volume of blood ejected (stroke volume; SV) by the normal ventricle greater than 50% (ejection fraction; EF) of its total volume.

The period between closure of the semilunar valves and opening of the atrioventricular valves is termed *isovolumic relaxation* and marks the beginning of ventricular relaxation (Figs. 5–14A and B). Isovolumic relaxation is characterized by a rapid decrease in ventricular pressure and no change in ventricular volume, and coincides with the "V" wave of the atrial pressure curve (Fig. 5–14A). Once ventricular pressure falls below atrial pressure, the semilunar valves open, initiating the phase of rapid ventricular filling (possibly facilitated by ventricular suction) and producing the third heart sound (S_3). The third heart sound is believed to be caused by turbulent blood flow and vibrations in the ventricular walls during ventricular filling, is relatively easily heard in larger species (horses, cattle), and gives rise to the characteristic ventricular gallop in dogs and cats with dilated forms of cardiac disease.(48) Ventricular filling proceeds more gradually after the initial rapid filling phase, while ventricular pressure and volume increase nonlinearly during late diastole (Fig. 5–14B). The slope of the pressure-volume curve (dP/dV) during ventricular filling is an index of ventricular stiffness, and its inverse (dV/dP) is used to assess ventricular compliance.(49) The slow ventricular-filling phase is termed *diastasis* and continues as blood returns to the atria from the systemic and pulmonary circulations until the cardiac cycle is reinitiated by the next electric impulse.(50)

DETERMINANTS OF CARDIAC PERFORMANCE AND CARDIAC OUTPUT

The cardiac cycle and pressure volume loop provide a descriptive picture of the temporal and sequential events that occur during cardiac contraction and relaxation. The ultimate goal of the heart's pumping activity, however, is to deliver adequate quantities of oxygenated blood to peripheral tissues. This is accomplished by the continuous adjustment of cardiac output (CO), which is the product of heart rate (HR) and stroke volume (SV):

$$CO = HR \times SV$$

Decreases in ventricular filling time and vascular autoregulatory effects limit cardiac output at faster heart rates.(7) Stroke volume is the amount of blood

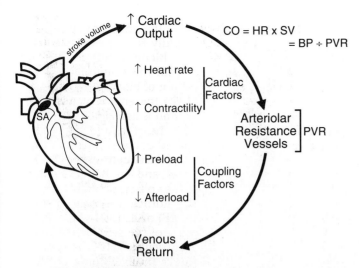

$$CO = HR \times SV$$
$$= BP \div PVR$$

Fig. 5–15. Cardiac output is equal to heart rate (HR) times stroke volume (SV), or arterial blood pressure (BP) divided by peripheral vascular resistance (PVR). Increases in heart rate, cardiac contractility, and preload, and decreases in afterload increase cardiac output. Preload and afterload are considered to be coupling factors because they are dependent upon vascular resistance, capacitance, and compliance.

ejected from the ventricle during contraction and therefore represents the difference between the end-diastolic and end-systolic ventricular volumes (SV = EDV – ESV, Fig. 5–14B). Traditionally, stroke volume has been considered to be primarily determined by one intrinsic property, cardiac contractility, and two vascular coupling factors, preload and afterload.(15) The refinement and development of more descriptive methods for the assessment of cardiac function, however, have led to the consideration of relaxation (lusitropic) effects upon stroke volume.(50, 51) Lusitropic properties are those that are responsible for ventricular chamber stiffness (*dP/dV*) or its inverse, compliance (*dV/dP*). Finally, ventricular wall motion abnormalities caused by ischemia, cardiac arrhythmias, myocardial inflammation, and space-occupying lesions (tumors; pericardial effusion) may influence stroke volume. It should be remembered that changes in preload, afterload, or myocardial contractile (inotropic) and relaxant (lusitropic) properties can influence each other and therefore influence stroke volume. These factors in turn are all influenced by heart rate, leading to a complex interplay of variables that collectively determine cardiac output (Fig. 5–15).(5, 7, 8)

The terms *preload* and *afterload,* described earlier in this section as two determinants of cardiac output, originated from isolated muscle experiments in which preload represented the original load, length, or stretch placed upon the muscle prior to its stimulation and contraction, and afterload represented the force or tension developed before the muscle contracts (Fig. 5–13). Isolated cardiac muscle studies continue to be essential for understanding and describing cardiac muscle physiology, metabolism, and muscle re-

sponses to various perturbations (hypoxia, ischemia, drugs), and are usually presented as three-dimensional plots of force, velocity, and length (Fig. 5–13). Cardiac function in intact animals is unlike isolated cardiac muscle, however, because ventricular performance is determined by intrinsic and vascular coupling factors and modulated by neurohumoral influences, the autonomic nervous system, pericardial and intrathoracic constraints, ventricular-vascular interaction, and atrial contraction.(13, 52, 53) Regardless, the terms *preload* and *afterload* remain popular jargon when describing ventricular performance in the intact animal.

Preload. Preload in the intact animal is usually explained in terms of the Frank-Starling relationship or as heterometric autoregulation; increases in myocardial fiber length (ventricular volume) (Figs. 5–15 and 5–16) increase the force of cardiac contraction and cardiac output.(8, 15) Whether or not individual sarcomeres actually increase in length (stretch) with increases in ventricular volume is controversial (see "Cardiac Contraction"); more likely, the myofilaments develop an increased sensitivity to calcium, resulting in an increase in contractile force.(35) Regardless of individual sarcomere length changes, the Frank-Starling relationship serves as an important compensatory mechanism for maintaining stroke volume when ventricular contractility and afterload are acutely changed. Because of the difficulty in accurately determining ventricular volume in the clinical setting, ventricular diameter (echocardiography) ventricular end-diastolic pressure, pulmonary capillary wedge pressure, and occasionally mean atrial pressure are used as measures of preload.(50) The substitution of pressure for volume, although common, must be done with the understanding that there are many instances (stiff or noncompliant hearts) when pressure does not accurately represent changes in

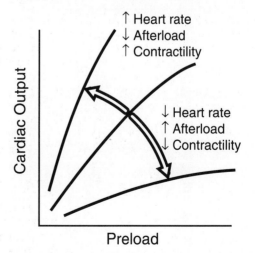

Fig. 5–16. Cardiac output increases as preload increases (Frank-Starling effect). The steepness of the Frank-Starling curve is also affected by changes in heart rate, cardiac contractility, and afterload.

ventricular volume and therefore is not an accurate index of preload.

Afterload. The term *afterload* is used throughout the basic and clinical cardiology literature to describe the force opposing ventricular ejection.(7, 15) One major reason for the great interest in this physiologic determinant of cardiac function is its inverse relationship with cardiac output and its direct correlation with myocardial oxygen consumption (Fig. 5–15).(15, 54) Although conceptually straightforward, clinical descriptions and use of the term *afterload* have suffered from an incomplete understanding of what the term actually represents. Afterload in isolated tissues is the force generated "after" the preload in order for the muscle to shorten. The total load in isolated muscle experiments is therefore represented by the preload plus the afterload. In contrast to isolated muscle, afterload in intact animals changes continuously throughout ventricular ejection and is more accurately described by the tension (stress) developed in the left ventricular wall during ejection or as the arterial input impedance (Z_i).(55) Ventricular wall stress or tension has traditionally been estimated from the Laplace relationship:

$$\text{Tension } (T) = \frac{Pr}{2h} \qquad 5\text{--}10$$

It is noteworthy that using this assessment of ventricular afterload assumes a spherical ventricular geometry. A much more accurate yet technically more difficult method for assessing afterload in the intact animal is to measure arterial input impedance.(55) Arterial input impedance is an expression of the arterial system's response to pulsatile blood flow and is a function of arterial pressure, arterial wall elasticity, vessel dimensions down to the point where pulsations are attenuated, and blood viscosity (see "Hemorrheology: Impedance"). As such, arterial input impedance incorporates time-varying resistance (pressure, flow) and reactance (intrinsic vessel wall characteristics) components. The measurement of arterial input impedance requires the simultaneous and instantaneous measurement of aortic root pressure and flow.(10, 55) Both waveforms are subjected to a Fourier transformation from which a series of sine waves and frequencies are derived. The amplitude ratios of the pressure-flow components at each frequency are calculated and plotted versus frequency as impedance moduli. Any phase shift between pressure and flow (pressure leading flow or vice versa) occurring during the ejection phase is also plotted at each frequency (Fig. 5–6). From this relationship the characteristic impedance (Z_o) can be determined by averaging the impedance moduli at high frequencies. The characteristic impedance is the pressure-flow relationship when pressure and flow waves are not influenced by wave reflection (it approximates input impedance during maximal vasodilation). Characteristic impedance is approximately 5% of the

total arterial resistance and is generally an exquisitely sensitive indicator of vessel wall elasticity or compliance. The impedance modulus at zero frequency (nonpulsatile flow) is equivalent to vascular resistance (R) and is usually described as total peripheral resistance (TPR) or systemic vascular resistance (SVR). The SVR can be calculated (with appropriate values) by a rearrangement of the mechanical equivalent of Ohm's law:

$$\text{SVR} = 80 \times \frac{(\text{MAP} - \text{VP})}{\text{CO}} \qquad 5\text{--}11$$

where MAP is mean arterial pressure, VP is venous pressure, CO is cardiac output, and 80 is a conversion factor used to change measurements in L/min and mm Hg to dynes $\cdot$ s $\cdot$ cm^{-5}. Although much less accurate than the determination of impedance moduli, particularly when assessing the effects of progressive cardiac disease or drugs that change both cardiac and vascular properties simultaneously, the measurement of SVR is used clinically as a measure of afterload because it is technically simple to obtain and intuitively easier to understand.

Inotropy. Cardiac contractility (inotropy) is the intrinsic ability of the heart to generate force, and as such relates directly to physicochemical processes and the availability of intracellular calcium (see "Excitation-Contraction Coupling").(35, 36) The term *homeometric autoregulation* is frequently applied to those factors other than muscle fiber length that influence the force of cardiac contraction.(7) Contractility is generally described in isolated muscle preparations by shifts of the force, velocity—length relationship (Fig. 5–13), or in intact animals by shifts in the ventricular function curve (e.g., shifts in the Frank-Starling relationship; Fig. 5–16). It is generally believed that a decrease in cardiac contractility is the key cause of heart failure in patients with cardiac disease or following the administration of potent negative inotropic drugs (e.g., anesthetics).(43, 44, 56-59)

Ideal indices of cardiac contractility should be independent of changes in heart rate, preload, afterload, and cardiac size—in other words, be load independent. Many indices of contractility have evolved in an attempt to develop a truly load-independent measure of cardiac contractile activity. These indices vary considerably in their load dependency, sensitivity, and specificity as measures of cardiac contractility, and generally fall into one of four broad categories: (1) isovolumic contraction phase indices; (2) ejection phase indices; (3) pressure-volume relationship indices; and (4) stress-strain relationship indices (Table 5–3).(49, 59, 60) Although many approaches for assessing cardiac contractility are useful experimentally and clinically, only the isovolumic phase indices (because of their ease of measurement), the pressure-volume relationship indices (because of their load independence), and the ejection phase index, preload recruitable stroke work,

Table 5–3. Hemodynamic Indices of Systolic and Diastolic Function

Systolic Function
1. Isovolumic indices
   a. dP/dt_{max}; dP/dt_{40}; $dP/dt/V_{ed}$
   b. V_{max}
   c. Power; rate of charge of power
2. Ejection phase indices
   a. Cardiac output
   b. Ejection fraction, (EDV − ESV)/EDV
   c. Stroke work
   d. Maximum velocity of circumferential shortening
   e. LV ejection time
   f. Preejection period
3. Pressure volume indices
   a. E_{es} and E_{max}
   b. End-systolic pressure-volume ratios
   c. T_{max} (time to E_{max})
4. Stress-strain indices
   a. Elastic stiffness (stress/strain)
   b. End-systolic stress-volume ratio

Diastolic Function
1. Isovolumic relaxation indices (pressure derived)
   a. dP/dt_{min}
   b. Time constant of LV pressure fall (T)
   c. Relaxation time
   d. $-dT/dt$ (tension fall)
2. Diastolic filling indices
   a. dP/dV
   b. Peak filling rate (dV/dt_{max})
   c. Chamber stiffness (dP/dV v P)
3. End-diastolic indices
   a. End-diastolic pressure
   b. End-diastolic P/V ratio
4. Interval-derived indices
   a. Time to $-dP/dt_{min}$; time to 50% $-dP/dt_{min}$
   b. Diastolic filling time
   c. Isovolumic relaxation period
   d. Time from minimal left ventricular dimension to mitral valve opening

diastole states that relaxation begins with the closure of the aortic valve, which is heralded by the second heart sound (S_2; Fig. 5–14A).(50, 51) Diastole is thereafter divided into four phases: isovolumic relaxation, early rapid ventricular filling, slow ventricular filling (diastasis), and atrial systole (during sinus rhythm). Mechanical factors, loading factors, inotropic activity, heart rate, and asynchronicity (patterns of relaxation) are the major determinants of diastole. Factors and interventions that specifically alter the ventricular end diastolic volume versus pressure relationship, called lusitropic factors, are of special interest because of their importance in determining ventricular compliance or stiffness. A partial list of methods used to quantitatively describe relaxation includes pressure, volume-derived, and interval indices (Table 5–3). All of these indices provide useful information but must be carefully applied in order to properly analyze the appropriate phase of relaxation. Indices of isovolumetric relaxation (rate of ventricular pressure decline, $-dP/dt$, and the time constant for relaxation) are useful for measuring the active phase of relaxation and reflect the dissociation of actin-myosin linkages because of reuptake of cytoplasmic calcium by the sarcoplasmic reticulum (Fig. 5–11). These indices are particularly influenced by myocardial systolic function, ventricular loading conditions (preload, afterload), and heart rate. Indices of diastasis or slow ventricular filling (chamber stiffness, dP/dV, and myocardial stiffness) are used to determine the passive properties of diastolic function and are principally influenced by viscoelastic properties, ventricular interaction, coronary blood flow, and pericardial restraint.

have gained acceptance.(59) Additionally, the measurement of the pressure-volume relationship can be used to assess myocardial energetics.(15, 49) This is because the amount of oxygen consumed by the heart for mechanical work is proportional to the area within the pressure-volume loop, while the oxygen consumed for basal metabolism is proportional to the area enclosed by the end-systolic pressure-volume relationship, the diastolic pressure-volume curve, and the isovolumic relaxation phase of the pressure-volume loop (Fig. 5–17).

Lusitropy. A description of the relaxation phases following cardiac contraction are often omitted from textbooks of cardiovascular physiology but are fundamentally important to an understanding of cardiac performance.(50) Two reasons for the lack of attention are the inability to agree upon a definition of when diastole begins and disagreement over acceptable indices for the assessment of the various phases of diastole. The most popular and clinically relevant definition of

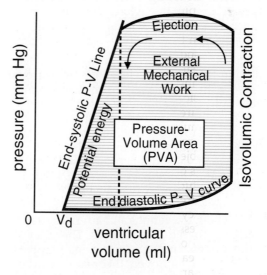

Fig. 5–17. The ventricular pressure-volume loop and the end-systolic P-V line can be used to determine the pressure volume area (PVA). The area within the pressure-volume loop (within the dotted lines) represents the external work done by the heart and is proportional to myocardial oxygen consumption. The triangular area between the end-systolic P-V line and isovolumic relaxation represents the end-systolic potential energy and is proportional to the oxygen consumed for basal metabolism.

Table 5–4.   Common Hemodynamic Effects of Anesthetic Drugs in Intact Animals

Drug	Heart Rate	Cardiac Output	Contractility	Blood Pressure	Right Atrial Pressure	Myocardial Oxygen Consumption
Anticholinergics	↑	↑	↑	NC- ↑	↓	↑
Phenothiazines	↑	↑	↓	↓	↓	NC- ↑
Butyrophenones	↑	NC- ↑	↓	Slight ↓	↓	NC- ↑
Benzodiazepines	NC	NC	NC	NC	NC	↓
Alpha$_2$- agonists	↓	↓	NC- ↓	Initial ↑, then ↓	↑	↑
Opioids	↓	↓	NC- ↓	NC- ↓	NC	NC
Barbiturates	↑	↓	↓	↓	↓	NC- ↑
Propofol	NC- ↑	↓	↓	↓	↓	NC- ↑
Etomidate	NC- ↑	NC- ↓	NC- ↓	NC- ↓	NC- ↓	NC- ↑
Dissociative drugs	↑	↑	↑	↑	↓	↑
Inhalation anesthetics	↓	↓	↓	↓	↓	↓
Skeletal muscle relaxants						
1. Pancuronium	↑	↑	NC	↑	NC	↑
2. Atracurium	NC- ↑	NC	NC	May ↓ (histamine)	NC	NC
3. Vecuronium	NC	NC	NC	NC	NC	NC

↑, increase; ↓, decrease; NC, no change.

Regardless of the care in picking an index to evaluate cardiac systolic or diastolic performance, it is clear that even greater thought must be given to the factors (determinants of performance) that influence the index. Drugs used as preanesthetic medication or for intravenous or inhalation anesthesia can produce profound effects upon indices of cardiac performance and are often much more complex in their actions than originally surmised (Table 5–4).(50, 56, 61-63)

Ventricular-Vascular Coupling

The concept of ventricular-vascular coupling is not new but is rarely discussed or adequately described by most textbooks.(14) The principal reason for inadequate treatment is the historical focus on pressure-derived measurements and the cardiac cycle, which stems from the relative ease with which pressure measurements can be made. Sphygmomanometry-based measurements and their derivations are undoubtedly important, but by themselves lead to an overly simplistic and often erroneous understanding of cardiovascular function. New technology (M-mode and 2-D color flow Doppler echocardiography) and theory have made it possible to expand our understanding of cardiac mechanical activity and begin to appreciate the relevance, dependence, and importance of both the venous and arterial systems and their coupling to the heart.(5, 52) The clinical relevance of this understanding is increasingly apparent from the new and improved theories of cardiovascular disease (congenital or acquired), myocardial metabolic disturbances (ischemia, hypoxia), and the mechanisms of drug effects (anesthetics, etc.) on the cardiovascular system. Indeed, the clinical application of the principles of ventricular-vascular coupling has resulted in new and improved therapies for cardiovascular disease.(13, 16)

Ventricular-vascular coupling, as the name implies, concerns the interrelationship or coupling of the heart to the venous and arterial systems. Thus, loading conditions (preload, afterload) and vascular dynamics (resistive, reactance, and viscoelastic properties) ultimately influence ventricular performance and blood flow.(14, 49) Coronary blood flow and myocardial perfusion are also important components of ventricular-vascular coupling because normal function and the viability of the heart are dependent upon adequate myocardial perfusion, which occurs almost exclusively during diastole.

VASCULAR FUNCTION CURVE

The modern concept of ventricular-vascular coupling has been popularized by Guyton, who used the "vascular function curve," and more precisely the venous return curve and cardiac (ventricular) function curve, to predict changes in cardiac output (Fig. 5–18A).(5) Guyton's ventricular-vascular coupling diagrams emphasize that the important independent variables in the determination of cardiac output are the sums of vascular resistances and capacitances and cardiac contractility. The venous return curve describes an inverse relationship between venous return and cardiac output. The horizontal (abscissa) intercept of the venous return curve or the venous pressure at zero cardiac output is the mean circulatory filling pressure, which is a function of venous capacitance and the total blood volume and has been directly correlated to survival from hemorrhagic and septic shock. Variations in the venous return curve can be produced by altering venous resistance, capacitance, or blood volume (Fig. 5–18B). Equilibrium of the venous return—ventricular function curve is reached when venous return at a given pressure is matched by the ability of the ventricle, when distended to the same pressure, to pump the venous return. Thus, an increase in venous pressure

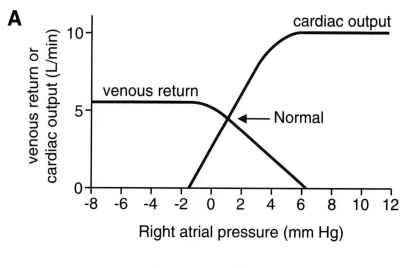

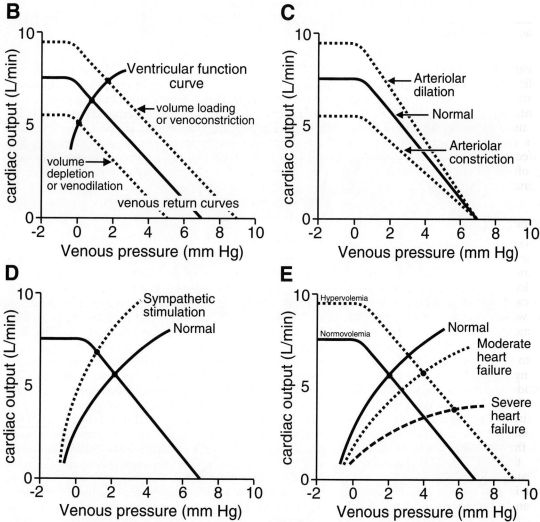

Fig. 5–18. Ventricular-vascular coupling curves. Venous return and cardiac output are determined by the opposing effects of right atrial pressure (A). For example, increases in right atrial pressure increase cardiac output but decrease venous return. Alterations in blood volume (B), sympathetic tone (C), vascular tone (D), and cardiac function (E) produce predictable effects upon the coupling of venous return to cardiac output at a given venous pressure. Note that during heart failure (E) cardiac output is preserved at the expense of increases in venous pressure. (Modified from Berne, R.M., and Levy, M.N. Principles of Physiology, 1st ed. CV Mosby, St. Louis, 1990.)

increases cardiac output during the next cardiac cycle, as defined by the ventricular function curve. Increases in cardiac output in turn transfer blood from the venous to the arterial circulation, thus decreasing venous pressure. This process continues in progressively decreasing steps until a new equilibrium for cardiac output and venous return is reached, realizing that only one equilibrium point for cardiac output and venous return exists. Similar rationalizations can be used for other perturbations: changes in blood volume, arterial resistance, and cardiac contractility.(8, 52) It can be argued that this type of presentation of hemodynamics and cardiovascular function results in circular reasoning, since a change in cardiac output can be used to explain the change in venous return and vice versa. Indeed, since both venous return and cardiac output are equal to the flow around the circuit, the point that a given cardiac output is obtained is determined by a myriad of venous return and ventricular function

curves and their determinants (venous and arterial capacitance and resistance, blood volume, cardiac contractility).(5, 7, 8)

VENTRICULAR-ARTERIAL COUPLING

More recent evaluations of ventricular-vascular coupling have focused upon the left ventricular pressure-volume relationship and the ejection of blood into the ascending aorta (ventricular-arterial coupling) (Fig. 5–19A).(13) This approach, first popularized and validated by Suga and Sunagawa in isolated and intact dog hearts, has been applied clinically using noninvasive (echocardiographic) techniques.(15, 49, 53, 64) The power of this approach stems from its clinical applicability and the ability to derive a multitude of important indices for assessing cardiovascular function in intact animals.(49)

The inscription of the instantaneous pressure-volume loop permits the calculation of load-dependent and

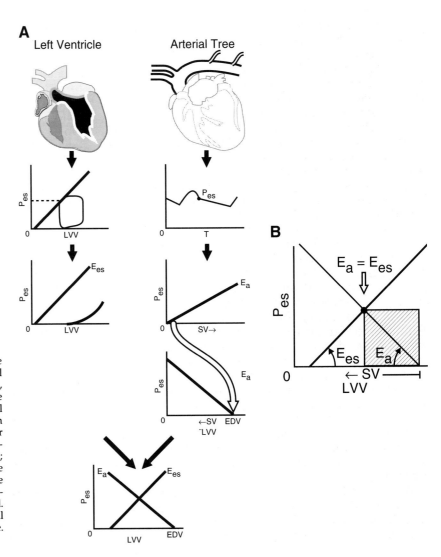

Fig. 5–19. Ventricular-arterial coupling. The coupling of the ventricle with the arterial system (A) produces an equilibrium point (A, bottom) at which the ventricle functions. The shaded area in B represents the maximal stroke work during optimal coupling when the slopes of the arterial and ventricular relationships are the same. End-systolic pressure (P_{es}); left ventricular volume (LVV); stroke volume (SV); end diastolic volume (EDV); end-systolic elastance (E_{es}); effective arterial elastance (E_a). (Modified from Sunagawa, K., Maughan, W.L., Burkhoff, D., et al. Left Ventricular Interaction with Arterial Load Studied in Isolated Canine Ventricle. Am J Physiol 245:H733, 1983.)

independent indices of cardiac contractility, myocardial oxygen requirements, and myocardial efficiency.(15) For example, the ratio of ventricular pressure to ventricular volume (dP/dV) varies throughout the cardiac cycle (time-varying elastance) and inscription of the pressure-volume loop. Acute reductions in preload are used to produce progressively smaller pressure-volume loops and construct a straight line by connecting all the end-systolic points. This line is known as the *end-systolic pressure-volume relationship*, the slope of which is the end-systolic ventricular elastance (E_{es}), a load-independent index directly proportional to ventricular contractility (Figs. 5–17 and 5–19A). The mechanical work (stroke work; SW) performed by the heart is proportional to the pressure-volume area (PVA; work = pressure-volume), which is linearly related to myocardial oxygen consumption (MVO_2), and which, when plotted against the end-diastolic volume, derives another sensitive and load-independent index of cardiac contractility termed *preload recruitable stroke work* (PRSW). Mechanical efficiency (ME) of the heart, which is the ratio of SW to MVO_2, is therefore derived by dividing SW by PVA (ME = SW/PVA).

The ejection of blood into the ascending aorta is governed by the same resistive and reactive (viscoelastic) properties that govern venous return. These arterial loading properties (afterload) influence stroke volume.(55) The difference between the end-diastolic and end-systolic volumes of the pressure-volume relationship is stroke volume, which, when plotted versus end-systolic pressure (P_{es}) during decreases in stroke volume, renders a line, the slope of which is the effective arterial elastance (E_a). In practice, E_a is generally approximated by the ratio of P_{es} to SV (P_{es}/SV = E_a). This parameter is particularly powerful because it incorporates the principal elements of vascular load (afterload), including peripheral resistance, total vascular compliance, characteristic impedance (see "Determinants of Cardiac Performance and Cardiac Output"), and alterations induced by heart rate changes. It is noteworthy that the purely resistive components of vascular load are adequately accounted for by determining the steady-state or nonpulsatile parameter total peripheral resistance, which accounts for approximately 90% of vascular load under normal conditions. The pulsatile or dynamic component of vascular load generally accounts for approximately 10% of vascular load under normal conditions, adds to the resistive component, and becomes increasingly important during cardiovascular disease, changes in blood volume, or following the administration of drugs that affect the cardiovascular system.(49, 57, 58, 60) Other methods for accurately analyzing arterial afterload have been described (see "Determinants of Cardiac Performance and Cardiac Output").

Because both E_{es} and E_a have the measurement of P_{es} and ventricular volume in common, they can be plotted on a single graph to yield the "ideal" ventricular-arterial coupling point for any set of cardiovascular circumstances (Fig. 5–19B). Stated another way, if end-diastolic volume (preload), E_a, and E_{es} are known, stroke volume and therefore cardiac output (CO = SV – HR) can be predicted. Furthermore, this analysis predicts that SW should be maximized when this relationship is equal to 1 ($E_{es} = E_a$) and that maximal mechanical efficiency (ME) is attained when $E_a = E_{es}/2$, since ME = SW/PVA = $1/(1 + E_a/E_{es}/2)$.

The ideal ventricular-arterial coupling point in intact animals occurs when mean arterial pressure is adequate for organ flow (approximately 60–70 mm Hg) and systolic pressure is low while diastolic pressure is high (small pressure pulse). Low systolic pressure facilitates maximal ventricular ejection and low oxygen demands by the myocardium, whereas high diastolic pressure ensures adequate coronary perfusion. Ideal ventricular arterial interaction is impaired by anything that decreases cardiac contractility (decreased E_{es}) or increases arterial stiffness (increased E_a). Increases in arterial stiffness increase pulse amplitude, increasing systolic pressure and thereby decreasing SV for a given cardiac contractility and increasing MVO_2. Diastolic pressure usually falls, thereby reducing coronary blood flow and myocardial perfusion. Furthermore, alterations in the timing of pulse wave reflection, principally initiated by increases in arteriolar tone, could augment systolic pressure and reduce diastolic pressure, exacerbating the situation.(10, 55, 65)

Cardiac Metabolism

The maintenance of normal cardiac activity is dependent upon the metabolic pathways by which ATP is generated. Even a superficial description of these pathways is far beyond the scope and purpose of this chapter and is more appropriately described in texts specifically designed to discuss this subject.(54) Suffice it to say that the heart generates ATP by two primary methods: glycolysis and oxidative phosphorylation. These processes are continually modified by the energy requirements of the cell and by neural and hormonal inputs. The ATP produced supplies energy for cardiac contraction, relaxation, and related activities (Fig. 5–20).

The Vascular System

The purpose of the vascular system (arteries, capillaries, veins) is to transport and facilitate the exchange of a wide range of nutrients and waste products. Originating from the heart, the circulatory system consists of two separate circulations connected in series (Fig. 5–1). The pulmonary circulation receives its blood supply from the right ventricle, perfuses the lung, and empties into the left atrium. The systemic circulation receives its blood supply from the left ventricle, perfuses most of the body's organs and tissues, and empties into the right atrium. More specifically, the systemic circulation (and the pulmonary) undergoes repeated division into smaller and smaller parallel vascular beds that terminate in the arterioles (the smallest arteries), which further subdivide to form the capillary bed.(7) During

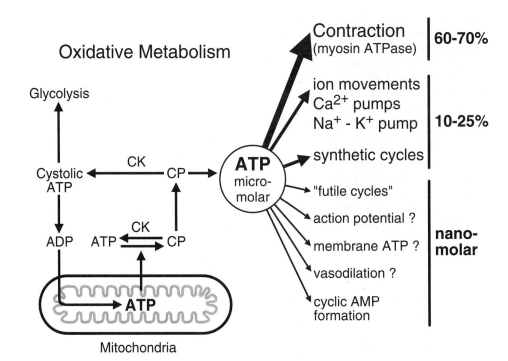

Fig. 5–20. Oxidative metabolism produces ATP, which supplies energy for cardiac contraction and other cellular activities. Note that over 60% of the ATP generated by oxidative metabolism is used for contraction. Creatine kinase (CK); creatine phosphokinase (CP).

this process of repeated division, the overall cross-sectional area of the circulation increases dramatically, reaching a maximum in the capillaries (Fig. 5–21).(1, 66)

Structurally, all blood vessels contain an endothelial layer (tunica intima) on their inner surface that provides a smooth surface and prevents clotting. All but capillaries also contain varying proportions of elastic fibers, smooth muscle, and collagen (Fig. 5–22). These three tissue types comprise the tunica media, which is composed mostly of smooth muscle and elastic connective tissue, and the tunica externa (adventitia), which contains fibrous collagen fibers. The proportion of elastic connective tissue to smooth muscle determines the vessel's principal function (i.e., conduit, resistive, or capacitive). The amount of smooth muscle also determines the vessel's resting tone, myogenic basal tone (spontaneous contractions), and the amount of "stress relaxation" (delayed capacitance), and "reverse stress relaxation" exhibited by the vessel. Stress relaxation is characterized as a rapid initial increase in resting tone caused by an increase in vascular volume that declines gradually during the next several minutes. Pressure decreases because of smooth muscle myofilament rearrangement. Reverse stress-relaxation is the reverse of this process.

VASCULAR SMOOTH MUSCLE CONTRACTION

Vascular smooth muscle is considerably different from cardiac muscle, both structurally and functionally.(37) Vascular smooth muscle cells are small, 5 to 10 μm in diameter, and spindle-shaped. They do not contain regular sarcomeric units or Z-bands, or possess the same key regulatory proteins (absence of troponin C and troponin N) as cardiac cells. Functionally, depolarization is not essential for initiation of muscle contraction

in vascular smooth muscle. The contraction process is slow and tonic, is prolonged, and intracellular increases in cAMP cause vascular smooth muscle cells and vessels to dilate, not contract. One thing that is similar between cardiac and vascular smooth muscle cells is that they are both dependent upon increases in intracellular calcium for contraction.

A multitude of pathways are available by which vascular smooth muscle cells can increase intracellular calcium ion concentration and contract, including calcium influx through voltage (slow calcium channels) and receptor-operated ion channels, calcium release from the sarcoplasmic reticulum by calcium (calcium-induced calcium release) or some other activator (inositol triphosphate; IP$_3$), and by reversal of the sodium-calcium exchange mechanism. Regardless of the mechanism responsible, increases in intracellular calcium serve as the second messenger for smooth muscle actin-myosin interaction. Once intracellular calcium concentration increases beyond a critical threshold, calcium ions combine with the ubiquitous calcium-binding protein calmodulin, forming a calcium-calmodulin complex, which in turn binds to myosin light-chain kinase and activates ATP-dependent phosphorylation of myosin, resulting in actin-myosin interaction (Fig. 5–23). The formation of the actin-myosin crossbridge in vascular smooth muscle (in contrast to cardiac muscle) produces a sustained tonic type of contraction. The slow cycling or noncycling cross-bridges formed in vascular smooth muscle are called *latchbridges*. Relaxation occurs when myosin light chain kinase is dephosphorylated by the enzyme myosin light chain phosphatase. The regulation of myosin light chain phosphatase is poorly understood but is probably affected by many drugs used to produce chemical restraint and anesthesia.(37, 67) Other mechanisms that facilitate relaxation of vascular smooth muscle center around decreases in intracellular calcium concentration due to reuptake of calcium ion by the sarcoplasmic reticulum, exchange of intracellular calcium for extracellular sodium, stimulation of the calcium-ATPase calcium pump, and termination of calcium influx into the cell (Fig. 5–23). It is interesting that increases in intracellular cyclic AMP and GMP produce vasodilatory, not contractile, effects in vascular smooth muscle. Cyclic AMP inhibits myosin light chain phosphorylation. The effects of cyclic GMP are incompletely understood, but it may produce an effect similar to cyclic AMP or accelerate the ejection of calcium ions from vascular

smooth muscle cells. Finally, vascular smooth muscle contraction can occur without an initial influx of extracellular calcium or the release of intracellular calcium.(37) Alpha-adrenoceptor stimulation, for example, can act through a G-protein to form diacylglycerol (DAG) and IP_3. IP_3 causes the release of calcium from the sarcoplasmic reticulum, initiating the contraction process. Diacylglycerol can also activate a protein kinase, which may phosphorylate myosin light chain kinase to initiate tonic contractions.

VESSEL TYPES

From a purely functional standpoint, vessels can be categorized as primarily elastic Windkessel types or conduits (large arteries), resistance vessels (small arter-

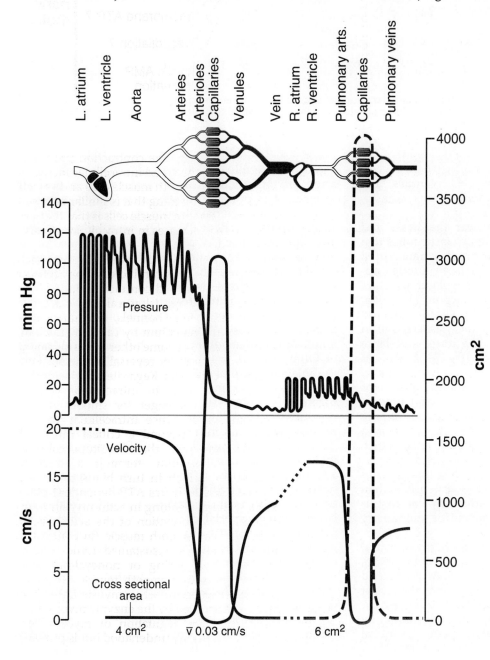

Fig. 5–21. The relationship between blood pressure, blood flow velocity, and cross-sectional area of the cardiovascular system. Note that as blood approaches the capillaries, blood pressure and blood flow velocity decrease and cross-sectional area increases. (Modified from Witzleb E. Functions of the Vascular System. In: Schmidt, R.F., and Thews, G., eds. Human Physiology, 1st ed. Springer-Verlag, New York, 1983:408.)

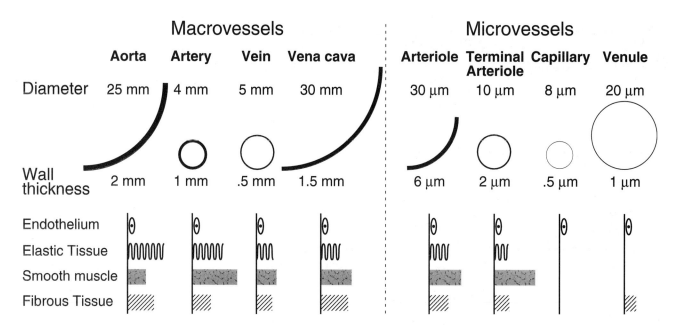

Fig. 5–22. The relative amounts of the various components (elastic, smooth muscle, fibrous tissue) of macro- and microvessels are illustrated. Note the differences with changes in vessel diameter and between arteries and veins. (Modified from Berne, R.M., and Levy, M.N. Principles of Physiology, 1st ed. CV Mosby, St. Louis, 1990:195.)

ies), sphincter vessels (arterioles), exchange vessels (capillaries), capacitance vessels (venules and veins), and shunt vessels (arteriovenous anastomoses).(1, 68)

Large arteries. Large arteries near the heart and throughout the extremities are highly elastic tubes that serve as conduits through which blood is transported to the periphery. The elasticity of large arteries opposes the stretching effect that the blood pressure produces following ventricular contraction. The initial stretching of the aorta produced by ventricular ejection, for example, is opposed by the elastic tissue in the vessel walls, which returns the aorta and large arteries to their original dimension (Fig. 5–22). As was previously mentioned, this squeezing phenomena of large arteries is termed the *Windkessel effect* and helps to convert the discontinuous (cyclic, phasic) flow of arterial blood associated with ventricular pumping into a continuous although somewhat nonuniform flow to the peripheral arteries. The degree to which the larger arteries can be stretched is dependent upon the ratio of elastic to collagen fibers. Systemic arteries are in general six to ten times less distensible than systemic veins. The pulmonary artery, by contrast, is about half as distensible as systemic or pulmonary veins (Fig. 5–24).(69)

Blood pressure in arteries (arterial pulse pressure and blood pressure), whether obtained directly or indirectly, is frequently assessed during anesthesia. Arterial blood pressure measurement in particular is one of the fastest and most informative means of assessing cardiovascular function, and when done correctly and frequently provides an accurate indication of drug effects, surgical events, and hemodynamic trends. The most important

vascular determinant of arterial blood pressure is arteriolar tone, which can be modified by almost all drugs used to produce anesthesia.(5, 7, 68) The factors that determine arterial blood pressure are heart rate, stroke volume (HR × SV = Q), vascular resistance, arterial compliance ($\Delta V/\Delta P$), and blood volume. Blood volume is one of the major variables affecting the mean circulatory pressure, which is defined as the equilibrium pressure of the circulation when blood flow is zero. The mean circulatory filling pressure is approximately 7 mm Hg when blood volume is normal (90 mL/kg). Increases in mean circulatory filling pressure augment ventricular filling and cardiac output. From the mechanical analog of Ohm's law ($E = IR$) we know that $P = QR$. This formula predicts that if either cardiac output or peripheral vascular resistance increase either individually or together, so will arterial blood pressure. Arterial blood pressure is a key component in determining perfusion pressure (upstream minus downstream pressure) and the adequacy of tissue blood flow. Perfusion pressures greater than 60 mm Hg are generally thought to be adequate for perfusion of tissues. Structures like the heart (coronary circulation), lung (pulmonary circulation), kidneys (renal circulation), and fetus (fetal circulation) contain special circulations where changes in perfusion pressure can have immediate effects on organ function. In the coronary circulation, for example, if perfusion pressure (determined by the difference between arterial diastolic and ventricular end diastolic pressures) decreases, subendocardial ischemia develops.(7)

Clinically, arterial blood pressure is generally measured as mean arterial pressure. When mean arterial blood pressure cannot be directly assessed, it is esti-

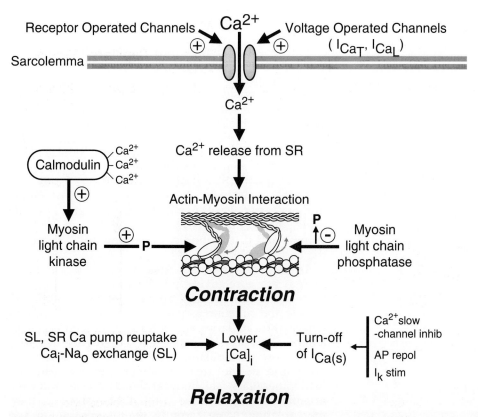

Fig. 5–23. The excitation-contraction coupling process in vascular smooth muscle. Calcium enters cardiac cells through two types of voltage-dependent calcium channels (L, T) and several types of receptor-operated channels, which triggers the release of intracellular calcium (calcium-induced calcium release) from the sarcoplasmic reticulum (SR). Not shown is that some agonists act on smooth muscle membrane receptors to stimulate phosphatidylinositol turnover and the production of inositol triphosphate (IP_3) and diacylglycerol (DAG). IP_3 releases calcium from the SR and DAG activates protein kinase C, which stimulates the activity of the voltage-dependent slow calcium channels. Increases in intracellular calcium also interacts with calmodulin to form a calcium-calmodulin complex stimulating myosin light chain kinase, which together with intracellular calcium facilitates actin-myosin interaction. Contraction terminates when myosin light chain phosphatase dephosphorylates the myosin light chain and intracellular calcium is reduced by sarcolemmal (SL) and SR reuptake, intracellular calcium-extracellular sodium exchange, and the turning off of the slow calcium channels.

mated by the formula $P_m = P_d + \frac{1}{3}(P_s - P_d)$ where P_m, P_s, and P_d are mean (m), systolic (s), and diastolic (d) blood pressures, respectively (Fig. 5–25).(4, 5) Both P_s and P_d can be measured indirectly using either Doppler or oscillometric techniques (Chapter 15). Most drugs used to produce anesthesia decrease cardiac output and peripheral vascular resistance. It should be remembered that if peripheral vascular resistance is elevated, the arterial blood pressure may be within normal limits, regardless of low blood flow to peripheral tissues. Several anesthetic drugs (ketamine, low doses of thiobarbiturates) can increase peripheral vascular resistance (producing no change or increases in arterial blood pressure) while decreasing cardiac output (Table 5–4).

The arterial pulse pressure $(P_s - P_d)$ and pulse pressure waveform can provide valuable information regarding changes in vascular compliance and vessel tone. Generally, drugs (phenothiazines) or diseases (endotoxic shock) that produce marked arterial dilating effects increase vascular compliance, causing a rapid rise, short duration, and rapid fall in the arterial waveform while increasing the arterial pulse pressure.

Situations that produce vasoconstriction decrease vascular compliance, resulting in a longer duration pulse waveform and a slower fall in the systolic blood pressure to diastolic values.(68) The pulse pressure may contain secondary and sometimes tertiary pressure waveforms, particularly if the measuring site is in a peripheral artery some distance from the heart.(65) Secondary and tertiary pulse waves are an indication of normal or elevated vascular tone in response to sympathetic nervous system stimulation or the vascular effects of drugs (ketamine, catecholamines).

Resistance vessels. Resistance vessels include the terminal (small) arteries, arterioles, and metarterioles, and to a much lesser extent the capillaries and venules. Under normal conditions, the arterioles provide over 50% of the total systemic vascular resistance whereas large and small arteries account for 20%, capillaries 25%, and veins 5%. As indicated earlier, the Hagen-Poiseuille equation describes resistance as:

$$R = \frac{8 \cdot 1 \cdot \eta}{\pi r^4} \qquad 5\text{--}12$$

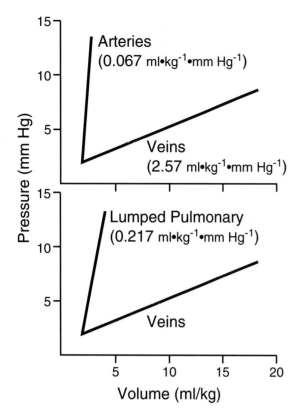

Fig. 5–24. Compliance (volume-pressure) curves for systemic arteries and veins and the lumped pulmonary vascular beds. Note that a small increase in volume causes a much larger increase in arterial pressure than venous pressure, suggesting a much lower compliance. (Modified from Green, J.F. Fundamental Cardiovascular and Pulmonary Physiology, 2nd ed. Lea & Febiger, Philadelphia, 1987:66–67.)

where l is length, η is blood viscosity, π is the constant 2.13, and r is the vessel radius. From this relationship, it should be clear that as vessel radius decreases and vessel length and blood viscosity increase, vascular resistance increases.

Sphincter vessels. Sphincter vessels represent a specific type of resistance vessel that is anatomically the absolute terminal portion of the precapillary arteriole. Functionally, sphincter vessels help to regulate the number of open capillaries and therefore the size of the capillary bed that is available for exchange processes. The relatively thick-walled muscular arterioles and sphincter vessels are influenced by a variety of neural, humoral, and local metabolic factors, and are the principal determinants for the regulation of both the volume and distribution of blood flow to all tissues of the body (Table 5–5).

Arteriovenous shunts. Arteriovenous anastomoses (AVAs) are a relatively poorly understood group of vessels that contain large amounts of vascular smooth muscle and function as pathways by which blood can bypass the capillaries and return to the venous circulation. These vessels can reduce or totally interrupt blood flow to capillaries. Arteriovenous anastomoses are found in the greatest numbers in the skin and extremities (ears, feet, hooves) of most species and were originally thought to be primarily involved in thermoregulation. More recently, their identification and verification in the intestinal wall, kidney, liver, and skeletal muscles have increased interest in their role as a separate blood flow regulatory mechanism for controlling nutrient blood flow to these tissues. The

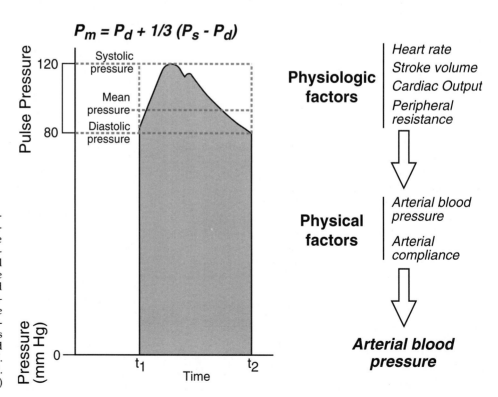

Fig. 5–25. Arterial blood pressure is determined by both physiologic and physical factors. The mean arterial pressure (P_m) represents the area under the arterial pressure curve divided by the duration of the cardiac cycle and can be estimated by adding one-third the difference between the systolic (P_s) and diastolic (P_d) arterial pressure to P_d. P_s minus P_d is the pulse pressure. (Modified from Berne, R.M., and Levy, M.N. Principles of Physiology, 1st ed. CV Mosby, St. Louis, 1990:259.)

Table 5–5. Distribution of Cardiac Output to
Peripheral Tissues

Organ	% of Total
1. Heart	4
2. Brain	14
3. Kidneys	20
4. Gastrointestinal tract	22
5. Skeletal muscle	20
6. Skin	8
7. Other organs	12

influence of anesthetic drugs on AVAs is poorly understood and largely unknown.(68, 70)

Capillaries. The capillaries are functionally the most important portion of the circulatory system, since they are the exchange units for elements between the blood and interstitial fluid. They penetrate nearly every tissue of the body, their numbers per gram of tissue and ultrastructure being dependent upon tissue metabolic rate and tissue function. Structurally, capillaries are one layer of endothelial cells surrounded by reticular fibers. There are three types of capillaries. Capillaries located in striated and smooth muscle, connective tissue, and the pulmonary circulation are uninterrupted or continuous, although they contain a large number of pores. Capillaries in the glomeruli of the kidney and in the intestine are fenestrated because of the high levels of metabolism and importance of active exchange of fluids. Capillaries in the liver, spleen, and bone marrow are discontinuous, containing intercellular gaps through which fluid and blood cells can easily pass.(68) Regardless of the type of capillary examined, the exchange of fluid, nutrients, and cellular waste products between blood and interstitial fluid is their primary function. Capillary exchange is governed by two primary processes, *diffusion* and *filtration*. Fick's law of *diffusion* describes solute exchange (J_s) as

$$J_s = \frac{DA}{M_T}\Delta C \qquad 5\text{–}13$$

where D is the diffusion coefficient, A is the capillary surface area, M_T is the membrane thickness, and ΔC is the concentration gradient or difference. The diffusion coefficient is determined by the diffusion medium and qualities characteristic to the diffusion particle such as molecular weight, ionic charge, and lipid solubility. Exchange by *filtration* is determined by four primary factors (P_c, P_i, π_c, π_i) according to a dynamic equilibrium equation, first proposed by Starling and Landis and modified by Pappenheimer and Soto-Rivera, wherein

$$Q_c = K\,[(P_c - P_i)] + \sigma(\pi_c - \pi_i)$$

where Q_c is fluid flow across the capillary (positive for filtration, negative for reabsorption), P_c and P_i are capillary and interstitial hydrostatic pressures, π_p and π_i are the plasma and interstitial colloid osmotic pressures of proteins, K is the capillary filtration coefficient, and σ

is the osmotic reflection coefficient for all plasma proteins.(71, 72) The filtration coefficient (K) indicates the resistance of the capillary wall to fluid flow and is determined by the exchange surface area, the number and radius of capillary pores, the capillary wall thickness, and the viscosity of the filtering fluid. The osmotic reflection coefficient (σ) is an indicator of transvascular protein transport and is usually assumed to be 1 or close to 1 in normal animals, since most capillary beds are impermeable to colloids. Providing all factors can be measured, calculated, or estimated in Starling's equation, net fluid flux across the capillary wall can be accurately quantitated.(71) Under normal conditions these factors are responsible for fluid filtration at the arterial end of the capillary and fluid reabsorption at the venous end of the capillary (Fig. 5-26). Any excess fluid that is filtered during the exchange process is carried away by lymph vessels. Increases in P_c (volume overload, venous obstruction, heart failure) and K (histamine, cytokines, kinins) or decreases in π_p (hypoproteinemia) cause excess fluid to accumulate in the interstitial space, resulting in edema. Excessive fluid accumulation in the lung, intestine, and liver (so-called "overflow organs") can result in fluid collection in the alveoli, intestinal lumen, and peritoneal cavity.(72) Decreases in P_c (hypotension, hypovolemia) and increases in π_p (hyperproteinemia, dehydration) result in net reabsorption of fluid from the interstitial space and an increase in plasma volume. Anesthesia, anesthetic drugs, quantity and type of fluid administered, and the type of anesthetic techniques used can have important effects upon the Starling forces.(72) For example, most anesthetic drugs and anesthetic techniques decrease P_c, resulting in net fluid reabsorption from the interstitial space and hemodilution. If the anesthetic drug or technique produces significant cardiac depression, P_c may increase, resulting in edema (e.g., pulmonary edema). Finally, several drugs, including the opioids (morphine, meperidine) and steroidal anesthetics (alphaxolone-alphadolone) can cause histamine release, thereby increasing K, resulting in interstitial fluid accumulation (Table 5–6).(68)

Veins and Venules. The veins and venules comprise the final component of the vascular system and, although structurally similar to arteries, are relatively devoid of elastic tissue and possess comparatively less smooth muscle (Fig. 5–22). Veins in general have a greater radius and thinner walls than arteries and functionally serve to return blood to the heart and as capacitance (volume storage) vessels (Fig. 5–3). The relationship between vascular volume (V) and vascular transmural pressure (P) is termed *vascular compliance* ($C = \Delta V/\Delta P$), which is the inverse of elasticity and for the low-pressure veins is several orders of magnitude greater than most arteries (Fig. 5–24A).(69) It is interesting that the lumped compliance of the pulmonary vascular bed is less than that of the systemic circulation, implying that the blood storage capability of the lungs compared to the systemic circulation, particularly the systemic small veins and venules, is small (Fig. 5–24B).

Venous return is facilitated by venous one-way valves, contraction of skeletal muscle (muscle pump), the negative intrathoracic pressure during breathing (respiratory pump), increases in intraabdominal pressure (abdominal pump), and the suction effect of the heart during rapid ventricular filling.(68) Hydrostatic pressure ·(gravity), increased intrathoracic pressure (IPPV, PEEP), and venous occlusion or obstruction initially impair or inhibit venous return. The capacious venous vessels of the liver, splanchnic viscera, and skin (in many species), together with the sinusoids of the spleen, can be considered blood reservoirs, as are the pulmonary vessels, although to a much lesser extent.

Table 5–6.   Causes of Increased Interstitial Fluid Volume and Edema

Increased Filtration Pressure
  Arteriolar dilation
  Venular constriction
  Increased venous pressure (heart failure, incompetent valves, venous obstruction, increased total ECF volume, effect of gravity, etc.)
Decreased Osmotic Pressure Gradient Across Capillary
  Decreased plasma protein level
  Accumulation of osmotically active substances in interstitial space
Increased Capillary Permeability
  Substance P
  Histamine and related substances
  Kinins, etc.
Inadequate Lymph Flow

Lymphatics. The lymphatic system constitutes a closed-ended, separate, yet parallel drainage system through which interstitial fluid (normally <10% of filtered fluid) is returned to the blood vascular system (Fig. 5–26).(72) Lymphatic channels are thin-walled (generally one cell layer thick) vessels that contain one-way valves that facilitate the transfer of lymph (interstitial fluid) via lymph vessels of increasing size first to lymph nodes, and eventually to the lymphatic duct and heart. Skeletal muscle contraction facilitates lymph flow (lymphatic pump) to the heart similar to its effect upon venous blood flow.(68)

Nervous, Humoral, and Local Control of the Cardiovascular System

The regulatory control of the cardiovascular system is integrated through the combined effects of the central and peripheral nervous systems, the influence of circulating (humoral) vasoactive substances, and local tissue mediators that modulate vascular tone.(73–77) These regulatory processes maintain blood flow at an appropriate level while distributing blood flow to meet the needs of tissue beds that have the greatest demand.

The autonomic nervous system exerts a major influence upon the regulation of cardiovascular function.(76) Peripheral receptors—including baroreceptors, mechanoreceptors, and chemoreceptors—respond to changes in blood pressure, volume, or gas tensions, respectively, and send information to the central nervous system through afferent nerves. These sensory signals are integrated in "control centers" located in the

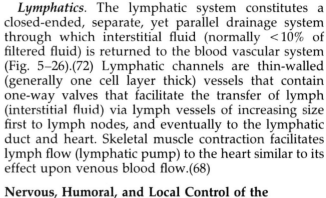

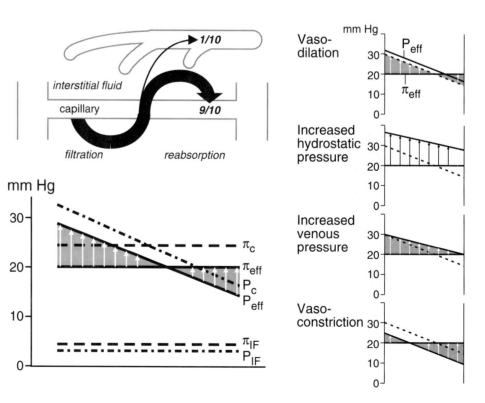

Fig. 5–26. Starling's law of the capillary suggests that fluid movement between the capillary and the interstitial space can be predicted by changes in capillary (P_c) and interstitial (P_i) hydrostatic pressure and capillary (π_c) and interstitial (π_c) colloid osmotic pressure. The algebraic sum of these pressures produces an effective transmural filtration pressure (P_{eff}) and effective colloid osmotic pressure (π_{eff}), which determine capillary filtration and reabsorption. Only about 10% of the plasma filtrate enters the lymphatic system during health. Filtration-reabsorption is shifted toward increased filtration during vasodilation, increased hydrostatic and venous pressure, and toward increased reabsorption during vasoconstriction. These diagrams assume the filtration coefficient and the osmotic reflection coefficient (see text) are minimally affected. (Modified from Witzleb, E. Functions of the Vascular System. In: Schmidt, R.F., and Thews, G., eds. Human Physiology, 1st ed. Springer-Verlag, New York, 1983:419–420.)

hypothalamus, pons, and medulla into responses carried by efferent sympathetic or parasympathetic nerves to the periphery. The autonomic nervous system also modulates the release of various peptides providing a generalized humoral influence on cardiac contractile performance and vascular tone.(66) Minute-to-minute changes in blood flow are regulated by local control mechanisms, which are somewhat independent from nervous system input. Vasodilator substances, primarily the byproducts of tissue metabolism, act on small vessels, producing vasodilation proportional to the amount of metabolite produced. In addition, the vascular endothelium is known to modulate both local and neural control mechanisms through the release of prostaglandins and endothelial-derived factors, such as nitric oxide (NO). Anesthetic drugs can and do interfere with the sensory (input), neural integration (processing) and effector (output) mechanisms that control cardiovascular function.(78-82)

NEURAL CONTROL OF CARDIOVASCULAR FUNCTION

Nervous system regulation of the cardiovascular system depends upon three components within the nervous system: afferent input, central integration and processing, and efferent output.(76, 83)

Afferent Input. Afferent input to the central nervous system is received from peripheral sensors that respond to acute changes in blood pressure, blood volume, and tissue metabolism. These peripheral sensors are the first step in a reflex arc in which the effector organs are the heart and vasculature. The reflex arc generally operates as a negative feedback system, designed to maintain a variable blood pressure at a fixed value, or "set point."(83)

Arterial baroreceptors are stretch receptors (mechanoreceptors) located in the carotid sinus and aortic arch that respond to increases in arterial blood pressure by incremental increases in the firing rate of sensory fibers, which are carried by the glossopharyngeal and vagus nerves.(76) These impulses travel to the nucleus tractus solitarius within the central nervous system, are processed, and initiate an effector response that returns blood pressure to its normal range (Fig. 5–27). This response is accomplished by parasympathetic activation, which decreases heart rate and inhibition of sympathetic vasoconstrictor output to arterioles and veins. Baroreceptors become inoperative at an arterial blood pressure below 60 mm Hg, but the frequency of nerve impulses increases progressively as pressure rises above 60 mm Hg, reaching a maximum at approximately 180 mm Hg.(4, 83) Most baroreceptors have a set point of approximately 100 mm Hg. However, if arterial blood pressure changes to a new value and remains static, the baroreceptors "reset" to this new set point

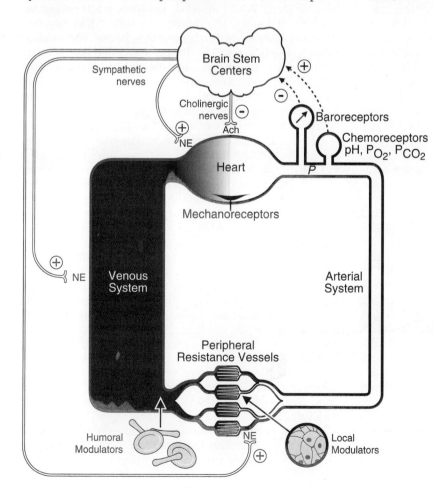

Fig. 5–27. Nervous, humoral and local (tissue) regulatory factors insure that blood flow and pressure are maintained within physiologic limits. Mechanoreceptors and chemoreceptors sense changes in wall tension (stretch) and pH and blood gases (PaO$_2$, PaCO$_2$) respectively. Substances produced in peripheral tissues and released into the circulation by endocrine glands also modulate blood vessels and the distribution of blood flow. Nervous impulses generated by the heart, vasculature, and peripheral sensors are transmitted to and integrated in the brain stem, which alters sympathetic and parasympathetic tone in order to make appropriate adjustments. The release of norepinephrine (NE) by sympathetic nerves stimulates the heart and constricts blood vessels. The release of acetylcholine (Ach) by parasympathetic nerves depresses the heart. Stimulatory (+); inhibitory (−). (Modified from Shepherd, J.T., and Vanhoutte, P.M. The Human Cardiovascular System: Facts and Concepts, 1st ed. Raven Press, New York, 1979:12.)

within 24 to 48 hours. This is why baroreceptors are only effective for short-term control of blood pressure. Most, if not all, anesthetic drugs interfere with baroreceptor responsiveness. Inhalation anesthetics in particular depress normal baroreflex responsiveness and diminish sympathetic output from the central nervous system. The degree of baroreceptor depression is dependent on both the depth of anesthesia and the patient's physical status.(84, 85)

Cardiac mechanoreceptors are located in the right and left atria and ventricles and help to minimize changes in systemic blood pressure in response to changes in blood volume. These cardiac stretch receptors differ from the baroreceptors in that they respond to comparatively small changes in stretch or pressure as do pressure receptors within the pulmonary circulation. The atria contain two types of receptors located at the venoatrial junctions.(83) Atrial A receptors react primarily to changes in heart rate, whereas B receptors respond to short-term changes in atrial volume. An increase in atrial volume activates both the A and B atrial mechanoreceptors, sending impulses to the medulla via vagal afferents. Depending upon the prevailing heart rate and arterial blood pressure, heart rate may increase (Bainbridge reflex) or decrease (baroreflex, activation of atrial depressor [C] fibers). Atrial distension also decreases sympathetic output to renal afferent arterioles, resulting in vasodilation, while the hypothalamus receives neural input, which decreases the release of vasopressin (antidiuretic hormone) both of which act to increase urine flow.(76) A rapid loss of free water into the urine helps return circulating blood volume to normal values. In addition to these neural responses, atrial natriuretic peptide (ANP) is released into the bloodstream by atrial cardiocytes in response to atrial distension. Atrial natriuretic peptide increases sodium excretion by the kidney with an accompanying increase in water loss.(74)

Ventricular mechanoreceptors located in the ventricular endocardium discharge in parallel with changes in ventricular pressure and produce effects that help to regulate systemic blood pressure and myocardial work. Ventricular distension, however, also stimulates powerful depressor reflexes that decrease heart rate and peripheral vascular resistance, resulting in bradycardia and hypotension (Bezold-Jarisch reflex).(83) The activation of ventricular nonmyelinated C fibers serves as the basis for this reflex response. It is interesting that impulses initiated by either ventricular distention or the injection of certain chemicals (capsaicin, serotonin) into the coronary arteries can produce the Bezold-Jarisch reflex, which is also called the *coronary chemoreflex.*

The carotid artery and aortic arch contain specialized sensory chemoreceptors termed the *carotid and aortic bodies* (Fig. 5–27).(76) The carotid and aortic bodies receive the highest blood flow per gram of tissue weight of any organ within the body. These chemoreceptors are sensitive to changes in arterial oxygen and carbon dioxide tension, hydrogen ion concentration (pH), and temperature. The chemoreceptors of the carotid and aortic bodies help to regulate respiratory function in response to decreases in pH and the arterial partial pressure of O_2 and increases in the arterial partial pressure of CO_2. Afferent activity from the carotid body is carried by the glossopharyngeal nerve and from the aortic body by the vagus. These sensors are most sensitive to changes in hydrogen ion concentration and respond proportionally to the magnitude of the change from their set point. The set point for activation is a pH below 7.40. The approximate set point for CO_2 is 40 mm Hg and for O_2 80 mm Hg. Increases in afferent activity from the chemoreceptors increase minute ventilation restoring arterial blood pH, CO_2, and/or O_2 to normal. Hypoxia, hypercarbia, and nonrespiratory acidosis may cause bradycardia, coronary vasodilation, and an increase in systemic arteriolar resistance. This effect is most pronounced if the normal increase in ventilation is prevented, for example, during anesthesia. Chemoreceptors located within the ventricular epicardium respond to hypoxia or ischemia by initiating the coronary chemoreflex (Bezold-Jarisch reflex), producing bradycardia and hypotension.

Central nervous system integration. No single brain nucleus or center controls cardiovascular function; rather, multiple regions modulate the autonomic nervous system. When afferent impulses from peripheral sensors arrive in the brain, they are integrated to produce a neural and/or humoral response. The nucleus tractus solitarius (NTS) in the medulla is the relay station for afferent impulses from peripheral sensors (Fig. 5–28). Neurons originating in the NTS send information to the vagal nucleus and to various regions collectively referred to as the *vasomotor center.* Vagal nuclei send nerve fibers directly to the heart. Nerve cell bodies for the sympathetic nervous system are located in the thoracolumbar spinal cord and are linked to the NTS through axons traveling in the bulbospinal tract (Fig. 5–29). The bulbospinal tract contains both excitatory and inhibitory axons that cause either increases or decreases in sympathetic output. Centers in the hypothalamus link the somatic and autonomic responses necessary for the animal to adapt to its environment. They initiate adrenergic constriction of resistance and capacitance vessels and cholinergic dilation of vessels supplying skeletal and cardiac muscle during the fight-flight response. Hypothalamic centers modulate the cardiovascular response (cutaneous vasoactivity) to body temperature changes during shivering, sweating or panting. The hypothalamus also modulates the cardiovascular response to exercise and may be involved in blood pressure regulation.(76) Finally, the cerebral cortex influences cardiovascular function by modulating the cardiovascular response to exercise, emotion, ischemia and hypoxia.(83)

Efferent output. The autonomic nervous system is the efferent link between the central nervous system and the cardiovascular system, providing rapid control of

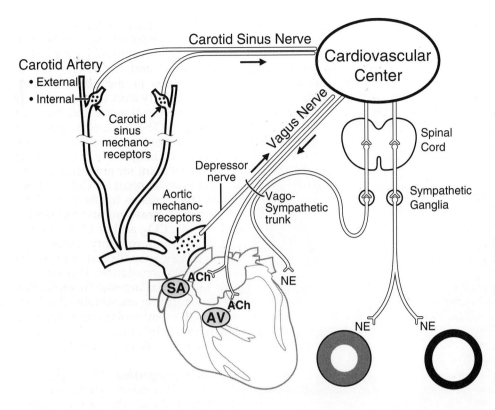

Fig. 5–28. Mechanoreceptors in the carotid sinus and aortic arch send impulses via the carotid sinus nerve, a branch of the glossopharyngeal nerve, and the vagosympathetic trunk, respectively, to the solitary tract nucleus in the brain stem (cardiovascular centers). Changes in the activity of these mechanoreceptors caused by changes in arterial blood pressure result in adjustments in sympathetic and parasympathetic outflow to the heart and resistance (arterial) and capacitance (veins) vessels. Sinoatrial (SA) and atrioventricular (AV) nodes; norepinephrine (NE); acetylcholine (Ach). (Modified from Shepherd, J.T., and Vanhoutte, P.M. The Human Cardiovascular System: Facts and Concepts, 1st ed. Raven Press, New York, 1979:132.)

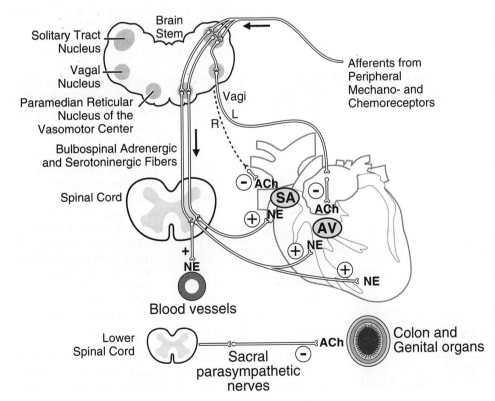

Fig. 5–29. Distribution of sympathetic and parasympathetic nerves to the cardiovascular system. The solitary tract nucleus is the main receiving point in the brain stem for afferent input arriving from peripheral sensors and higher centers in the brain. Interneurons connect the solitary tract nucleus to the vasomotor center, from which bulbospinal tract fibers descend to the spinal cord and synapse with preganglionic sympathetic nerves to the heart and blood vessels. Interneurons also connect the solitary tract nucleus to the vagal nucleus in the brain stem, where they synapse with preganglionic parasympathetic nerve fibers, which are carried by the vagus nerve to the heart. Parasympathetic nerve fibers to the blood vessels of the colon and genital organs arise from centers in the sacral portion of the spinal cord. (Modified from Shepherd, J.T., and Vanhoutte, P.M. The Human Cardiovascular System: Facts and Concepts, 1st ed. Raven Press, New York, 1979: 124.)

Table 5–7. Mechanism of Action of Selected Neurotransmitters

Transmitter	Receptor	Second Messenger	Net Channel Effects
Acetylcholine	N_G and N_s	—	↑Na^+, other small ions
	m_1	↑IP_3, DAG	↑CA^{2+}
	m_2 (cardiac)	↓Cyclic AMP	↓Ca^{2+}
	m_3	↑IP_3, DAG	
	m_4 (glandular)	↓Cyclic AMP	
	m_5	↑IP_3, DAG	
Dopamine	D_1	↑Cyclic AMP	
	D_2	↓Cyclic AMP	↑K^+, ↓Ca^{2+}
Norepinephrine*	α_1	↑IP_3, DAG	↓K^+
	α_2	↓Cyclic AMP	↑K^+, ↓Ca^{2+}
	β_1	↑Cyclic AMP	
	β_2	↑Cyclic AMP	
	β_3	↑Cyclic AMP	
5HT	$5HT_{1A}$	↓Cyclic AMP	↑K^+
	$5HT_{1B}$	↓Cyclic AMP	
	$5HT_{1C}$	↑IP_3, DAG	
	$5HT_{1D}$	↓Cyclic AMP	↓K^+
	$5HT_2$	↑IP_3, DAG	↓K^+
	$5HT_3$	—	↑Na^+
	$5HT_4$	↑Cyclic AMP	
Adenosine	A_1	↓Cyclic AMP	
	A_2	↑Cyclic AMP	
Glutamate, aspartate	NMDA	—	↑Na^+, Ca^{2+}
	AMPA	—	↑Na^+
	Quisqualate	↑IP_3, DAG	—
	Kainate	—	↑Na^+
GABA	$GABA_A$	—	↑Cl^-
	$GABA_B$	↑IP_3, DAG	↑K^+, ↓Ca^{2+}

*Three subtypes of α_1 and 3 subtypes of α_2 receptors have been identified.
(Modified from Ganong, W.F. Review of Medical Physiology, 16th ed. Appleton-Lange, East Norwalk, CT, 1993:86.)

both blood pressure and blood flow.(76) Efferent impulses are carried by sympathetic and parasympathetic nerves. Adrenergic and cholinergic receptors in target organs initiate the intracellular changes that result in a cellular response to the signals arriving from the CNS (Table 5–7).

SYMPATHETIC NERVOUS SYSTEM

Sympathetic pathways originate in the intermediolateral columns of the thoracolumbar segments of the spinal cord.(74, 76) Both inhibitory and excitatory input arrives at preganglionic sympathetic nerve cell bodies via axons traveling in the bulbospinal tract (Fig. 5–29). Descending inhibitory pathways are serotoninergic; descending excitatory pathways are adrenergic. The balance between these two types of input determines the prevailing level of sympathetic tone to the periphery.

Preganglionic sympathetic nerves send axons via the ventral roots of the spinal cord to paravertebral ganglia located just outside of the vertebral column. Many of the preganglionic fibers ascend the paravertebral chains and synapse with postganglionic neurons in the cranial, middle, and caudal (stellate) cervical ganglia (Fig. 5–30). Here they synapse with postganglionic sympathetic neurons, which send their fibers to the heart, blood vessels, and viscera. Postganglionic cardiac sympathetic nerve fibers innervate the sinoatrial node, the atrioventricular node, and the atrial and ventricular myocardium (Fig. 5–29). Postganglionic sympathetic fibers release the neurotransmitter norepinephrine, which binds to adrenoceptors on cardiac cell membranes (Table 5–7).

Postganglionic sympathetic nerve fibers also leave the paravertebral ganglia via spinal nerves to innervate vessels throughout the body. Normally, sympathetic tone maintains a partial state of contraction in vascular smooth muscle, providing the resistance necessary to maintain adequate systemic blood pressure and aid in the control of the fractional distribution of cardiac output to body tissues.(73, 76) The extent of innervation to the resistance vessels (arterioles) varies with tissue type. The kidney, spleen, gastrointestinal tract, and skin are extensively innervated by the sympathetic nervous system. Redistribution of blood flow away from these tissues during times of crisis preserves blood flow to the brain, heart, and skeletal muscle.

Sympathetic neurotransmission. The vast majority of sympathetic postganglionic fibers are adrenergic, releasing norepinephrine at their neuroeffector junctions. The amino acid tyrosine is the substrate used by these nerves to produce norepinephrine. Tyrosine is actively transported across the nerve cell membrane into the neural axoplasm, where it is converted by tyrosine hydroxylase and decarboxylation to dopamine, which is stored in vesicles within the nerve. Inside the storage vesicles a final hydroxylation step takes place to produce the neurotransmitter norepinephrine. Nerve action potentials increase intracellular calcium, causing the vesicles to fuse with the nerve cell membrane and release norepinephrine into the synaptic cleft, where it binds to a variety of adrenoceptors (Table 5–7). There are presynaptic receptors on the nerve cell membrane and postsynaptic receptors located on the effector organ. Postsynaptic receptor binding of nor-

epinephrine triggers a cascade of intracellular events that ultimately produce a cellular action. The effective half-life of norepinephrine after release into the synaptic cleft is very short. Norepinephrine is degraded locally at the neuroeffector junction by the enzymes, monamine oxidase (MAO) and catechol-O-methyltransferase (COMT). Most of the norepinephrine released into the synaptic cleft undergoes reuptake into adrenergic nerve terminals where it reenters storage vesicles. This neuronal amine-uptake system is designated *uptake-1* and has a high affinity for norepinephrine, a lower affinity for epinephrine and little affinity for the synthetic beta-agonist, isoproterenol. Norepinephrine may rapidly diffuse out of the synaptic cleft,

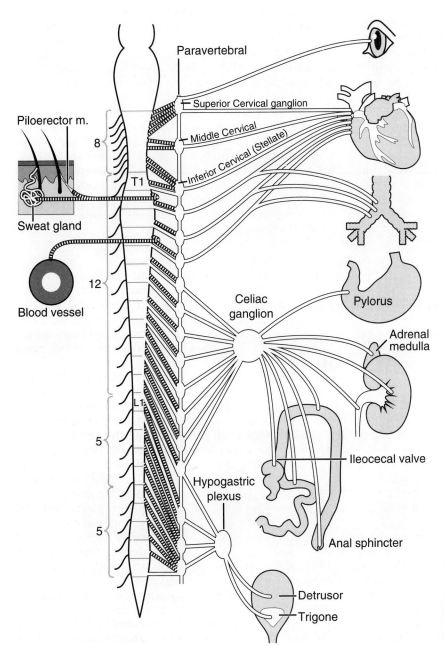

Fig. 5–30. The sympathetic nervous system. Note the location of the stellate and hypogastric ganglia. (Modified from Guyton, A.C. Textbook of Medical Physiology, 8th ed. WB Saunders, Philadelphia, 1991:668.)

where it undergoes reuptake at extraneuronal sites or is carried into the venous blood and metabolized in the lung. The extraneuronal reuptake pathway has been designated *uptake*-2 and has a low affinity for norepinephrine, a higher affinity for epinephrine, and a very high affinity for isoproterenol. Uptake-2 is of the greatest physiologic significance in the elimination of circulating catecholamines, primarily epinephrine, released by the adrenal gland, and has little physiologic significance for norepinephrine released at postganglionic sympathetic nerve terminals.

Adrenoceptors. The sequence of intracellular events initiated by receptor binding of norepinephrine is determined by the type of adrenoceptor stimulated. The classification of adrenoceptors continues to evolve based upon both pharmacologic and molecular criteria.(83-85) All adrenoceptors have a similar homology of structure and produce intracellular events by binding to membrane guanine nucleotide-regulatory proteins (G proteins).(88) The structure of the G protein–coupled receptor consists of a single subunit protein with seven hydrophobic transmembrane segments, three hydrophilic extracellular sequences, and three hydrophilic intracytoplasmic loops. These membrane-associated regulatory proteins serve to convert the signal arriving at the cell membrane into a specific enzyme system response or ion channel activity that produces a cellular response. Autonomic transmission in the cardiovascular system is initiated by stimulation of three different G proteins. G_s stimulates adenylate cyclase, causing a rise in intracellular cAMP. G_i inhibits

adenylate cyclase, decreasing the concentration of intracellular cAMP (Fig. 5–31). G_p activates phospholipase C, which hydrolyzes phosphoinositol to inositol triphosphate (IP_3) and diacylglycerol (DAG). Inositol triphosphate causes the release of Ca^{2+} from the sarcoplasmic reticulum. DAG activates protein kinase C, which phosphorylates contractile proteins in the myocardium and vascular smooth muscle.

Beta adrenoceptors are classified pharmacologically into three types: beta$_1$, beta$_2$, and beta$_3$, based upon their relative affinities for various agonists.(87) The physiologic significance of the beta$_3$ receptor is unclear. Beta$_1$ and beta$_2$ receptor subtypes, when activated by norepinephrine, epinephrine or other beta-agonists, stimulate the formation of the enzyme adenylate cyclase through the G protein, G_s, causing an increase in intracellular cAMP. Beta receptors also activate L-type Ca^{2+} channels in myocardial and vascular tissue, thereby increasing intracellular calcium concentration (Table 5–7). Both beta$_1$ and beta$_2$ adrenoceptors are found in the heart and are responsible for increases in heart rate and contractility during sympathetic stimulation (Table 5–8). Beta adrenoceptor stimulation increases the slope of phase-4 diastolic depolarization in pacemaker tissues and subsidiary automatic cells. Increases in intracellular cAMP and Ca^{2+} increase cardiac contractility and facilitates cardiac relaxation. Although both beta$_1$ and beta$_2$ adrenoceptors are present in the heart, beta$_1$ adrenoceptors predominate during health, especially in the ventricular myocardium.

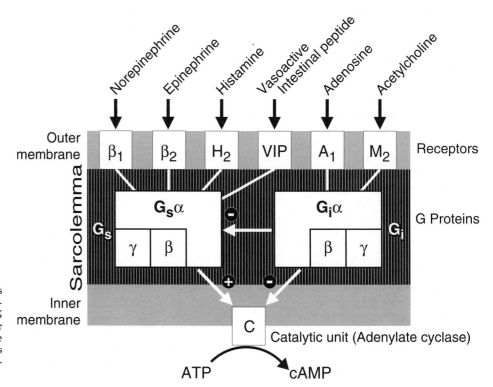

Fig. 5–31. Stimulation of various types of receptors in the myocardial cell membrane activates the G proteins G_s or G_i, which either promote (G_s) or inhibit (G_i) the catalytic subunit that causes cAMP synthesis. See text for discussion.

Table 5–8.   G Protein–Coupled Receptor Superfamily of Genes and Gene Products in Cardiac Tissue*

Receptor Type and Subtype	Location	G Protein	Biologic Response
Adrenergic			
β_1	Myocardium	G_s	AC stimulation, positive inotropic and chronotropic responses
	Coronary vascular	G_2	AC stimulation, vasodilation(?)
β_2	Myocardium	G_s	AC stimulation, positive inotropic and chronotropic responses
	Coronary vasculature(?)	G_s	AC stimulation, vasodilation(?)
α_1	Myocardium	G_P	PI hydrolysis stimulation, positive inotropic response(?)
	Coronary vasculature	G_P	PI stimulation, vasoconstriction
Muscarinic			
m_2	Myocardium	G_i	AC inhibition, negative inotropic and chronotropic responses
m_2'	Myocardium	G_P	PI stimulation, positive inotropic response
m_3(?)	Coronary vasculature	G_P(?)	PI stimulation, vasoconstriction(?)
m_3(?)	Coronary endothelium	G_P(?)	EDRF production, GC stimulation, vasodilation

*AC, Adenylate cyclase; PI, phosphatidylinositol; EDRF, endothelium-derived relaxing factor or NO; GC, guanylate cyclase (Modified from Opie, L.H. The Heart: Physiology and Metabolism, 2nd ed. Raven Press, New York, 1991:164.)

Beta$_2$ adrenoreceptors relax smooth muscle in vascular, bronchial, gastrointestinal, and genitourinary tissues. Beta$_2$ adrenoceptors in the vasculature are not innervated and therefore produce vasodilation in response to circulating catecholamines. Their location in specific vascular beds suggests a role in the distribution of blood flow, especially during exercise.

Three alpha$_1$ receptor subtypes have been classified according to their affinity to adrenergic agonists.(86, 87) The receptor subtypes are designated alpha$_{1A}$, alpha$_{1B}$, and alpha$_{1C}$, but their distribution is not universal across species or within specific tissue beds. All alpha$_1$ receptor subtypes currently identified produce their intracellular effect by activation of the enzyme phospholipase C via the G protein G$_p$. Phospholipase C hydrolyzes phosphoinositol and releases Ca^{2+} from intracytoplasmic stores, causing the contractile response seen in myocardial or vascular smooth muscle cells (Tables 5–7 and 5–8).

Three subtypes of alpha$_2$ receptors, alpha$_{2A}$, alpha$_{2B}$, and alpha$_{2C}$, have been identified by pharmacologic studies, although the tissue distribution of these subtypes is unclear.(89) Alpha$_2$ receptors inhibit adenylate cyclase through the G protein G$_i$. Inhibition of adenylate cyclase attenuates cAMP production in target cells. This mechanism is important in platelets and renal tubules; however, in vascular smooth muscle an alternative signal transduction mechanism is responsible for the vasoconstrictor response. Alpha$_2$ receptors are located presynaptically and extrasynaptically in vascular smooth muscle. Stimulation of extrasynaptic alpha$_2$ adrenoceptors by alpha-adrenergic agonists activates a receptor-operated calcium channel that increases the concentration of calcium intracellu-

larly, producing vascular smooth muscle contraction, complementing the contractile effect of alpha$_1$ receptors activated by stimulation of sympathetic nerves. Because of their extrasynaptic location, alpha$_2$ receptors respond to circulating catecholamines, such as epinephrine and norepinephrine, and aid in maintaining generalized sympathetic vasoconstriction in response to catecholamine output from the adrenal gland. This later response is important in the fight-flight response that occurs in crisis situations such as trauma or hemorrhage.

Alpha$_1$ and alpha$_2$ receptors coexist in the vasculature as described earlier.(87) There is a greater response to alpha$_2$ stimulation on the venous side of the circulation compared to the arterial side. Therefore, alpha$_2$-mediated vasoconstriction may be most important in mobilizing blood volume from veins, leading to an increase in cardiac filling, an important first step in increasing cardiac output during stress situations such as exercise or hemorrhage. Receptor-operated calcium channels in vascular smooth muscle can be blocked by calcium antagonists (verapamil, diltiazem, nifedipine).(89)

Alpha$_1$ and alpha$_2$ adrenoceptors can cause complimentary or antagonistic responses depending on their location. For example, norepinephrine stimulates alpha$_1$ adrenoceptors located on the postsynaptic cell membrane, causing contraction of vascular smooth muscle and vasoconstriction. Norepinephrine also binds to presynaptic alpha$_2$ receptors, producing a negative feedback effect that decreases the release of norepinephrine from the nerve terminal. Thus, alpha$_2$ receptors help to modulate the vasoconstrictor response initiated by alpha$_1$ postsynaptic receptor stimulation. Alpha$_2$ adrenoceptors help to ensure that only a short-term vasoconstrictor response occurs after sympathetic nerve stimulation.

Dopamine is the immediate metabolic precursor of norepinephrine in adrenergic nerves and functions as a neurotransmitter in the central nervous system (Table 5–7).(90) Disorders of dopamine transmission in the CNS are recognized clinically as Parkinson's disease. Peripheral dopamine receptors (DA_1 and DA_2) are particularly important in regulating blood flow to the mesenteric and renal vascular beds. Postsynaptic DA_1 receptors in the renal and mesenteric vascular beds cause vasodilation, increasing perfusion to renal and splanchnic tissues. DA_2 receptors, located presynaptically on postganglionic sympathetic nerves, inhibit the release of norepinephrine, much like the presynaptic $alpha_2$ receptors.

Stimulation of postganglionic sympathetic fibers supplying vascular smooth muscle not only causes the release of the neurotransmitter norepinephrine but in addition the release of the cotransmitter neuropeptide Y.(90, 91) Neuropeptide Y is present in vesicles contained in postganglionic sympathetic nerve terminals, is synergistic with the effects of norepinephrine on the peripheral vasculature, and produces vasoconstriction. Neuropeptide Y is also found in the adrenal medulla. Circulating levels of neuropeptide Y inhibit renin release and stimulate the release of atrial natriuretic peptide. The role of neuropeptide Y in cardiovascular regulation has not been fully characterized; however, it may be an important mediator in the central control of blood pressure.

Sympathetic cholinergic nerve fibers originate in the cerebral cortex and send descending fibers to the spinal cord. These nerve fibers synapse in the sympathetic ganglia and send postganglionic fibers to precapillary vessels in skeletal muscle.(83) Postganglionic cholinergic sympathetic nerve fibers are activated only during times of high sympathetic tone (fear, pain, or exercise) and release acetylcholine, which produces vasodilation in skeletal muscle.

PARASYMPATHETIC NERVOUS SYSTEM

The parasympathetic nervous system (PNS) originates from two sites (cervical, sacral) within the central nervous system (Fig. 5–32). Long preganglionic parasympathetic nerve fibers located in the central nervous system synapse with relatively short postganglionic parasympathetic neurons in ganglia located in the target organ. The cranial portion of the parasympathetic nervous system originates in the medulla oblongata. Axions travel via the vagus nerve to synapse with postganglionic parasympathetic nerves that terminate in the heart and blood vessels.(76, 83)

Parasympathetic neurotransmission. Acetylcholine is the neurotransmitter released at autonomic ganglia and from postganglionic parasympathetic nerves. Cholinergic nerves actively transport choline from the extracellular fluid into the neural axoplasm, where it is acted upon by the enzyme choline acetyltransferase, combined with acetyl coenzyme A, and converted to acetylcholine, which like norepinephrine is stored in vesicles within the nerve. Cholinergic nerve action potentials increase intracellular calcium, resulting in vesicular and nerve cell membrane fusion and the release of acetylcholine into the synaptic cleft. Acetylcholine binds to specific receptors, mediating a cellular response that varies with the tissue innervated and the type of cholinergic receptor involved. The actions of acetylcholine are rapidly terminated by hydrolysis into choline and acetic acid by the enzyme acetylcholinesterase. The acetylcholine that diffuses out of the synaptic cleft and into the extracellular fluid or plasma is hydrolysed by plasma butyrylcholinesterase (pseudocholinesterase). The choline produced from this metabolism is rapidly taken up by the nerve cell and used in the resynthesis of acetylcholine.

Cholinoceptors. Cholinergic receptors are either nicotinic or muscarinic and are totally unrelated in location, structure, and function (Tables 5–7 and 5–8). Nicotinic receptors are located in autonomic ganglia, in the adrenal medulla, and at the neuromuscular junction of skeletal muscle. Muscarinic receptors are located at postganglionic parasympathetic nerve terminals.(92)

Nicotinic receptors are pentameric membrane proteins that form a nonselective ion channel in the cell membrane. Postsynaptic nicotinic receptors, located in the autonomic ganglia or the neuromuscular junction, when stimulated by acetylcholine, open their ion channel, allowing the flow of cations into the nerve or muscle cell resulting in depolarization and ultimately nerve cell transmission of an electric impulse or muscular contraction. Nicotinic receptors are subclassified into N_G receptors, located at autonomic ganglia, and N_S receptors located in the neuromuscular junction and within the CNS.

Muscarinic receptors are located in the autonomic effector organs of the parasympathetic nervous system, for example, the heart, smooth muscle, and the exocrine glands.(92) They are G protein—coupled and show more homology to adrenergic and dopaminergic receptors than to the nicotinic cholinergic receptors. Five different cholinergic receptors have been distinguished through molecular binding techniques. Muscarinic receptors m_1, m_3, and m_5 are functionally similar and when bound to their respective G proteins stimulate phosphoinositol hydrolysis through activation of phospholipase C (Table 5–8). Muscarinic receptors m_2 and m_4 show similarity in that they both attenuate the actions of adenylate cyclase intracellularly.

The vagus nerve innervates the sinoatrial node, the atrial myocardium, the atrioventricular node, and to a much lesser extent the ventricular myocardium. Stimulation of m_2 receptors by acetylcholine activates several different membrane G proteins, resulting in

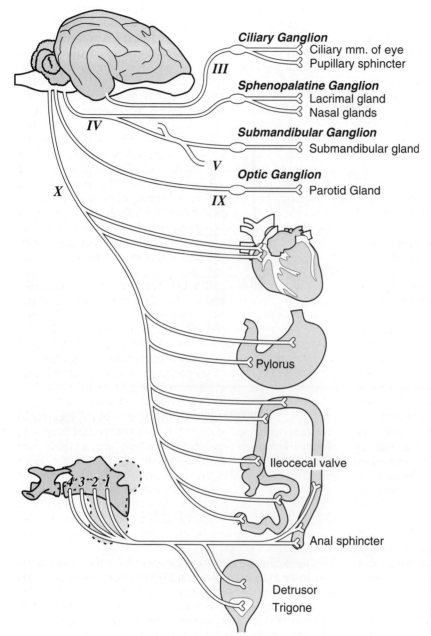

Ciliary Ganglion
Ciliary mm. of eye
Pupillary sphincter

III

Sphenopalatine Ganglion
Lacrimal gland
Nasal glands

IV

Submandibular Ganglion
Submandibular gland

V

Optic Ganglion
Parotid Gland

X

IX

Pylorus

Ileocecal valve

4 3 2 1

Anal sphincter

Detrusor

Trigone

Fig. 5–32. The parasympathetic system. Note the distribution of cranial nerves III, IV, V, IX and X. (Modified from Guyton, A.C. Textbook of Medical Physiology, 8th ed. WB Saunders, Philadelphia, 1991:669.)

inhibition of adenylate cyclase, activation of potassium channels, and activation of phospholipase C, which hydrolyzes phosphoinositol. These effects result in a decrease in the slope of phase 4 diastolic depolarization in pacemaker and subsidiary automatic tissues, and hyperpolarization of cardiac cell membranes through activation of membrane potassium channels. Heart rate is decreased, as are the rate of conduction of impulses through the AV node and cardiac contractility. High levels of parasympathetic tone can result in atrioventricular dissociation (first-, second-, and third-degree heart block) and temporary cardiac asystole. Stimulation of the parasympathetic nervous

system produces minimal effects on peripheral blood vessels. Acetylcholine binds to m_2 receptors in vessels, which mediates an endothelial-dependent vasorelaxation (Fig. 5–33).

The sacral division of the parasympathetic nervous system has preganglionic nerve cell bodies located in the intermediolateral column of the spinal cord.(76, 83) Parasympathetic nerves in this region congregate to form the nervi erigentes or pelvic nerves that innervate the intestines, colon, rectum, bladder, and genitalia (Fig. 5–32). Stimulation of the parasympathetic nerves also causes increased blood flow to salivary glands and genital erectile tissue.

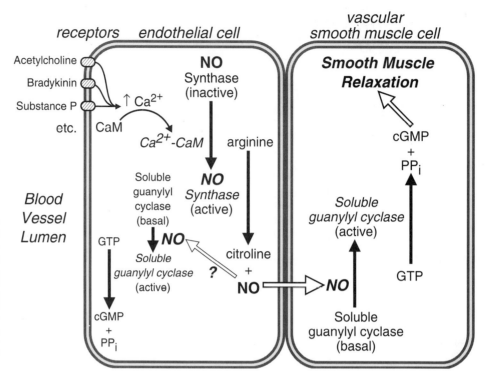

Fig. 5–33. Various agonists (acetylcholine, bradykinin, substance P) stimulate receptors on the vascular endothelium leading to the formation of nitric oxide (NO), which modulates the formation of soluble guanylyl cyclase which in turn facilitates the formation of cGMP and smooth muscle relaxation. (Modified from Guyton, A.C. Textbook of Medical Physiology, 8th ed. WB Saunders, Philadelphia, 1991.)

Humoral Mechanisms of Cardiovascular Control

The autonomic nervous system functions to produce acute changes in cardiovascular function that can be large in magnitude but are generally short in duration. Sustained changes in cardiopulmonary function are produced by humoral mechanisms.(75-77) The adrenal medulla is a modified sympathetic ganglion innervated by preganglionic sympathetic fibers, and is part of the sympathetic nervous system. The "neuronal" cells of the adrenal medulla, rather than sending axons to target organs, release the "neurotransmitters," epinephrine and norepinephrine, into the circulation. Precipitating factors for the release of catecholamines from the adrenal medulla include pain, trauma, hypovolemia, hypotension, hypoxia, hypothermia, hypoglycemia, exercise stress and fear (fight-flight). Circulating catecholamines produce a variety of effects, including increases in metabolic rate, glycogenolysis in the liver and skeletal muscle, gluconeogenesis in the liver, and an increase in the availability of free fatty acids, an important nutrient source for the myocardium. Circulating catecholamines increase heart rate and cardiac contractility, dilate vascular beds in skeletal and cardiac muscle, and constrict splanchnic and cutaneous arterioles, diminishing blood supply to organs that are less essential.(66) The actions of the adrenal medulla are complementary to the effects of sympathetic nerve stimulation. Together the autonomic nervous system and humoral mechanisms provide both rapid (nervous system) and sustained (humoral) responses to stressful situations.(75, 76, 83)

Table 5–9.   Stimuli that Increase Renin Secretion

Sodium depletion
Diuretics
Hypotension
Hemorrhage
Upright posture
Dehydration
Constriction of renal artery or aorta
Cardiac failure

The kidney is the major site for activation of the renin-angiotensin system.(75) Renin is produced in the kidney during sodium depletion, decreases in the extracellular fluid volume, or increases in sympathetic output (Table 5–9). Secretion of renin into the systemic circulation converts circulating angiotensinogen, produced by the liver, to angiotensin I. Angiotensin I is converted to angiotensin II by an angiotensin converting enzyme that is present in pulmonary vascular endothelium. Angiotensin II produces arteriolar constriction, resulting in increases in blood pressure, and stimulates the adrenal cortex to release aldosterone, a hormone that causes renal reabsorption of Na^+ and water, effectively increasing the extracellular fluid volume (Fig. 5–34).

The hypothalamus is directly involved in the central neural control of cardiovascular responses, but it also plays an important role in the humoral regulation of cardiovascular function. Arginine vasopressin (antidiuretic hormone, ADH) is produced in the hypothalamus and is transported through nerve cell axons to the

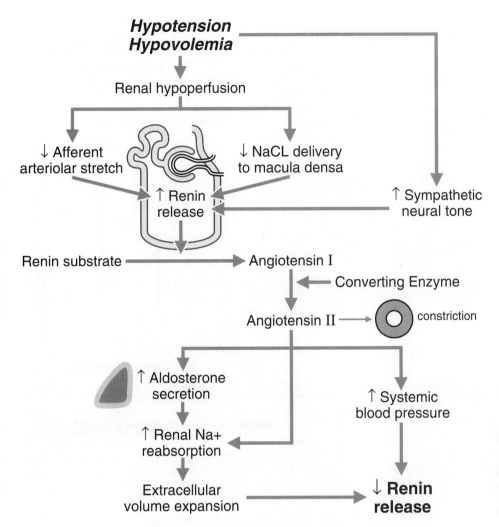

Hypotension Hypovolemia

Renal hypoperfusion

↓ Afferent arteriolar stretch

↓ NaCL delivery to macula densa

↑ Renin release

↑ Sympathetic neural tone

Renin substrate ⟶ Angiotensin I

⟵ Converting Enzyme

Angiotensin II ⟶ ⟶ constriction

↑ Aldosterone secretion

↑ Systemic blood pressure

↑ Renal Na+ reabsorption

Extracellular volume expansion ⟶ **↓ Renin release**

Fig. 5–34. The renin-angiotensin system. Note that either hypotension or hypovolemia can result in renal hypoperfusion and activation of the sympathetic nervous system, which increase renal renin release.

posterior pituitary.(75) Under normal circumstances the pituitary releases vasopressin in response to increases in plasma solute, resulting in an increase in circulating vasopressin. Vasopressin acts on the collecting ducts of the kidney, where it stimulates water conservation, thereby returning plasma osmolality (and volume) to normal. Vasopressin is a vasoconstrictor, especially in mesenteric vessels; therefore, the presence of circulating vasopressin is influential in the redistribution of systemic blood flow. Vasopressin release by the pituitary can also occur in the absence of changes in plasma osmolality. Examples of nonosmotic stimuli that cause the release of vasopressin are pain, stress, hypoxia, heart failure, and volume depletion. A number of anesthetic drugs are associated with increased circulating levels of arginine vasopressin, including opioids (morphine, Demerol) and barbiturates.(75)

Local Control Systems in the Vasculature

Autoregulation is the ability of blood vessels to adjust blood flow in accordance with metabolic need and to maintain blood flow despite extreme changes in tissue perfusion pressure (Fig. 5–35).(66) Most tissues are capable of regulating their own bloodflow during physiologic changes in perfusion pressure.(68)

Neurogenic basal tone exists in many vessels. Non-neurogenic (intrinsic) basal tone is additive to neurogenic basal tone and is present in vessels of the skin and skeletal muscle. A reduction in vasomotor tone in these vessels usually represents a reduction in the neurogenic component. *Active dilation* is a term applied when vascular tone decreases below the nonneurogenic basal level and is the result of two components, a pressure-sensitive mechanism termed the *myogenic component* and a metabolic mechanism, influenced by local oxygen tension.(66, 68) Both mechanisms are linked to the release of local vasodilatory mediators. This phenomenon, also termed *reactive hyperemia*, occurs in arterioles less than 25 μm in diameter. The myogenic mechanism is responsible for reactive hyperemia after short occlusion periods (30 seconds). As flow returns to the previously occluded arteriole, blood flow velocity increases, which increases wall shear stress, causing the release of nitric oxide (NO) from the vascular endothelium. The metabolic component of reactive hyperemia occurs after longer periods of occlusion (>30 seconds).

Decreases in oxygen tension release a vasodilatory prostaglandin that maintains blood flow until normal oxygen tension is reestablished. Endothelial damage in small arterioles eliminates the reactive hyperemic response altogether, since both NO and prostaglandins are products of vascular endothelial cells.(66, 79, 82) Hyperbaric oxygen conditions also eliminate the metabolic component of reactive hyperemia, by maintaining elevated oxygen tensions in tissues despite vascular occlusion. Stretch of vascular smooth muscle opposes the myogenic vasodilator response seen in larger vessels (Bayliss effect).(66) The proposed mechanism for the Bayliss effect is a pressure-induced depolarization of the endothelial cell mediated through an inwardly rectifying potassium channel. The effects of anesthetic drugs on reactive hyperemia and the Bayliss effect are incompletely understood and highly variable.

Capillary blood flow is linked to the rate of tissue metabolism and oxygen tension. The exact mechanism involved in this linkage is not completely understood, although a number of mechanisms may be responsible for regulating capillary blood flow.(68) The number of open precapillary sphincters is approximately proportional to the level of metabolic activity in the tissue supplied. As metabolic activity increases, the local oxygen tension decreases until a critical level of tissue hypoxia occurs, resulting in vasodilation. Precapillary sphincters are also responsive to mediators that are released as byproducts of tissue metabolism, such as lactic acid, carbon dioxide, and potassium.

Peptides and other substances are important in regulating tissue blood flow (Table 5–10). The actions of local enzymes produce kinins such as bradykinin from the substrate kallikrein. Kinins produce vasodilatory effects that are short lived because of rapid inactivation by peptidases in the plasma. Arachidonic acid metabolism produces a variety of prostaglandins that tend to be compartmentalized and produce very specific local effects. Stimulation of arachidonic acid metabolism in the pulmonary vasculature results in the production of the vasodilatory prostaglandin prostacyclin (PGI_2). Renal hypoperfusion results in the production of PGI_2, which acts to restore renal blood flow, urine volume and sodium excretion. There are specific receptor sites on vascular endothelium for a variety of agonists (including acetylcholine, bradykinin, and histamine) that when bound by the appropriate agonist induce the formation and release of NO. Nitric oxide is rapidly deactivated by hemoglobin and therefore is only important as a local mediator. Nitric oxide relaxes vascular smooth muscle through stimulation of guanylate cyclase, increasing intracellular cGMP (Fig. 5–33). Vascular endothelial cells also produce a potent vasoconstrictor substance

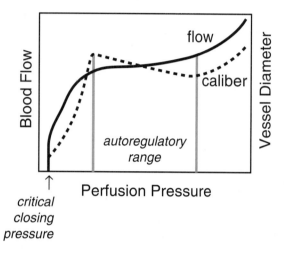

Fig. 5–35. The relationship between blood flow and perfusion pressure in peripheral vascular beds is characterized by an autoregulatory range over which blood flow changes very little regardless of increases or decreases in perfusion pressure. The normal autoregulatory range for most vascular beds is between 60 and 180 mm Hg. Some vascular beds (brain, gut, skeletal muscle) acutely collapse when the perfusion pressure approximates 15 to 30 mm Hg (critical closing pressure). (Modified from Shepherd, J.T., and Vanhoutte, P.M. The Human Cardiovascular System: Facts and Concepts, 1st ed. Raven Press, New York, 1979:95.)

Table 5–10.　Summary of Factors Affecting the Caliber of the Arterioles

Constriction	Dilation
Increased noradrenergic discharge	Decreased noradrenergic discharge
Circulating catecholamines (except epinephrine in skeletal muscle and liver)	Circulating epinephrine in skeletal muscle and liver
	Circulating ANP
Circulating angiotensin II	Activation of cholinergic dilators in skeletal muscle
Circulating AVP	Histamine
Locally released serotonin	Kinins
Decreased local temperature	Substance P (axon reflex)
Endothelin-I	$CGRP_\alpha$
Neuropeptide Y	VIP
Circulating Na^+-K^+ ATPase inhibitor	EDRF or NO
	Decreased O_2 tension
	Increased CO_2 tension
	Decreased pH
	Lactate, K^+, adenosine, etc.
	Increased local temperature

known as *endothelin* that acts upon endothelin receptors on vascular smooth muscle cells.(66, 83) Endothelin is released by the endothelium in response to increased intraluminal pressure, contributing to the Bayliss effect, and is selective for certain vascular beds including coronary vessels, renal afferent arteries, and venous capacitance vessels. It is both a positive inotrope and a chronotrope. Endothelin increases plasma levels of other humoral mediators, such as atrial natriuretic factor, renin, aldosterone, and circulating catecholamines. Endothelin receptors have been located in several areas of the brain involved in modulation of autonomic nervous system efferent activity (Table 5–10).

Diseases of the Cardiovascular System

HEART DISEASE

Historically, heart disease has been categorized based upon duration of disease, cause, structural defect, and functional changes. One clinically useful method for categorizing heart disease is based upon clinical signs (exercise intolerance, ascites, edema, cough, etc.). *Acute* and *chronic heart disease* are differentiated on the basis of the rapidity of development of clinical signs. Chronic heart failure usually takes many months to years to develop and is associated with a variety of compensatory neuroendocrine, physiologic, and pathophysiologic adjustments. *Congenital* or *acquired heart disease* identifies the condition as being present since birth or developing in association with a specific developing cardiac lesion. Congenital or acquired heart disease can be acute or chronic. *Right-* or *left-sided heart failure* identifies the right or left ventricle as the primary cause of heart failure. *Systolic* and *diastolic dysfunction* refer to the phase of the cardiac cycle that is most severely compromised. *Forward heart failure* refers to cardiac diseases that result in a low cardiac output secondary to an impediment to ventricular ejection (increased afterload), decreased inotropy, or both. *Backward failure* refers to situations that result in pulmonary and systemic venous congestion (congestive heart failure). *Low output failure* occurs when cardiac output is below normal and *high output failure* when (and regardless of cardiac contractile function) cardiac output is above normal (e.g., septic shock). It should be clear that the terms that have evolved to categorize heart failure (*congenital, acquired; acute, chronic; right-sided, left-sided; systolic, diastolic; forward, backward; low output, high output*) are for the most part descriptive and that an appreciation of their meaning must be considered in association with the pathophysiologic compensatory changes that occur.

Heart disease from any cause usually progresses through three phases: overload (excessive work), compensatory, and pathologic.(93) Whatever the inciting cause, ventricular overload brought about by excessive work leads to increases in both the oxygen and nutrient requirements of the heart. Initial compensatory changes include increases in sympathetic tone and a variety of neurohumoral responses that act to sustain or increase cardiac inotropy and promote the retention of salt and water (Fig. 5–36). These responses are usually followed by compensatory ventricular hypertrophy associated with decreases in both the rate of ventricular pressure development and rate of relaxation. The pathologic phase of heart failure exists when an abnormality in cardiac function is responsible for a decrease in cardiac output to a degree that is insufficient to meet the oxygen and nutrient requirements of metabolizing tissues. It is important to realize that this definition incorporates situations in which the heart may be contracting normally or be hypercontractile. For example, cardiac output may be decreased during sinus tachycardia or bradycardia, cardiac arrhythmias, and the initial stages of valvular insufficiency (mitral insufficiency). Decrease in cardiac contractile performance is only one potential cause for a decrease in cardiac output and should be differentiated from other potential causes of heart failure in order to provide appropriate therapy and prevent drug-induced complications.

Ultimately, failure of the ventricular myocardium is caused by pressure overload, volume overload, or primary myocardial disease (cardiomyopathy). The cardiomyopathies have been further categorized as hypertrophic, dilated, restrictive (infiltrative myocardial disease), or constrictive (pericardial disease).(93) The cause for many forms of hypertrophic and dilated cardiomyopathy remains unknown. The signal for ventricular hypertrophy, although uncertain, is probably multifactorial, involving stretch-activated ion channels, increased ventricular tension, adrenergic factors, increased oxygen consumption (oxygen supply/demand imbalance) and ATP utilization or increases in the quantity of metabolic breakdown products. Regardless of stimulus, increased work initiates the production of growth factors that, through various proto-oncogenes (c-fos, m-myc), and in conjunction with the production of heat shock proteins (HSP-70), stimulate transcription, change myofibrillar isoform ratios from fast to slow (V_1 to V_3), and increase cell growth.(93, 94) Clinically and experimentally, diseases that produce sustained pressure overload (aortic and pulmonic stenosis, hypertension) result in concentric ventricular hypertrophy. Concentric ventricular hypertrophy is characterized by marked increases in ventricular wall thickness without increases in ventricular volume. Heart disease that is caused by volume overload is generally the result of valvular regurgitation (aortic or mitral incompetence) or congenital defects (atrial or ventricular septal defect, patent ductus arteriosus) and results in longitudinal or so-called eccentric hypertrophy. Longitudinal hypertrophy is characterized by increases in chamber volume without an increase in wall thickness. The type of ventricular hypertrophy that develops is governed by processes that minimize myocardial oxygen consumption and work and maintain or maximize ventricular efficiency. Regardless, myocardial hypertrophy results in cellular changes that interfere with normal cellular metabolism and predisposes to systolic and diastolic dysfunction (Table 5–11). These intracellular changes and resultant abnormalities in ventricular function are further exacerbated by a decrease in capillary surface area to cell volume (capillary inadequacy), thereby limiting oxygen delivery, which increases myocardial fibrosis. Decreases in oxygen delivery, whether brought about by capillary

inadequacy, low cardiac output, or anemia, can result in myocardial ischemia. Subendocardial ischemia is particularly common in patients with heart failure because subendocardial perfusion is influenced by the difference between aortic diastolic pressure and ventricular end-diastolic pressure and the ventricular wall tension. Myocardial ischemia in turn results in abnormal cellular

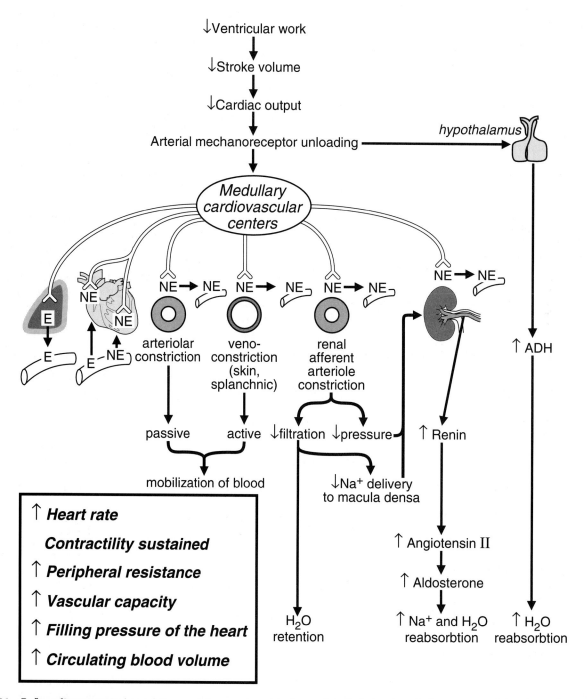

Fig. 5–36. Reflex adjustments to heart failure and decreased ventricular work include increases in heart rate, peripheral vascular resistance, vascular capacity, filling pressure of the heart and circulating blood volume. Cardiac contractility is sustained by increases in sympathetic tone. These changes help to maintain cardiac output. (Modified from Shepherd, J.T., Vanhoutte, P.M. The Human Cardiovascular System: Facts and Concepts, 1st ed. Raven Press, New York, 1979:259.)

Table 5–11. Receptors and Signaling Systems in Heart Failure

1. Receptors
   β_1-adrenergic receptors downgraded, i.e., density decreased
   β_2-adrenergic receptor density unchanged, function uncoupling
   α_1-adrenergic receptors relatively increased in density
   VIP receptors decreased in density, but affinity considerably increased
2. G-proteins
   G_i increased with inhibition of adenylate cyclase
   G_s normal or decreased
3. Adenylate cyclase
   Decreased cyclase activity with less production of cAMP, related to G_i increase; still responds directly to forskolin
4. cAMP
   Production impaired, presumably due to adenylate cyclase inhibition
5. Calcium transients
   Transients with low peak and delayed fall in diastole
   Calcium uptake by sarcoplasmic reticulum unchanged or decreased in situ
   Calcium release by sarcoplasmic reticulum increased
   Decreased myofibrilae
   Sensitivity to calcium ion
   Single calcium channels activity normal
   Amount of calcium entry via calcium channel may be abnormal

(Modified from Opie, L.H. The Heart: Physiology and Metabolism, 2nd ed. Raven Press, New York, 1991:409.)

calcium cycling, intracellular calcium overload, oxygen wastage, cardiac arrhythmias, sarcomere contracture, and eventually cell death. Familiarity with the pathophysiologic mechanisms of heart failure and cellular metabolism during heart failure and ischemia aids in the selection of appropriate preanesthetic and anesthetic drugs and suggests potential approaches for therapy.(44)

Cardiac arrhythmias. Cardiac arrhythmias include abnormalities in cardiac rate, rhythm, site of origin of the cardiac impulse, or pattern of atrial or ventricular depolarization. The cause for cardiac arrhythmias in intact hearts is attributed to abnormalities in automaticity, conduction, or both (Table 5–12). Ultimately, all changes in cardiac electric activity can be thought of in terms of alterations in one or more of the active or passive electrophysiologic properties of the cell membrane.(24) Increases or decreases in normal automaticity in spontaneously beating hearts, for example, result from changes in phase 4 depolarization, which is electrically initiated by calcium (I_{Ca}) and sodium (I_f) currents in sinoatrial and atrioventricular node or sodium (I_f) and potassium (I_{K1}) currents in Purkinje tissue. The electrocardiographic appearance of abnormal impulses due to abnormal automaticity, however, are most likely caused by changes in I_K or I_{Ca}. Abnormal electric impulses that occur as a direct result of prior electric activity are referred to as "triggered" and are in most instances caused by defects in I_{Ca}, leading to the development of both early (prior to repolarization) or

Table 5–12. Classification of Arrhythmogenic Mechanisms at the Cellular Level in Terms of Vulnerable Parameters

Mechanisms of Arrhythmia	Vulnerable Parameter (Antiarrhythmic Effect)	Ionic Currents Most Likely to Modulate Vulnerable Parameter
Automaticity:		
A. Enhanced normal automaticity	Phase 4 depolarization (decrease)	I_f, I_{Ca-T} (block)
B. Abnormal automaticity	Maximum diastolic potential (hyperpolarize) or	I_{KACh} (activate) I_X; I_{KACh} (activate)
	Phase 4 depolarization (decrease)	I_{Ca-L}; I_{Na} (block)
Triggered activity based on		
A. Early afterdepolarizations (EAD)	Action potential duration (shorten) or EAD (suppress)	I_X; (activate)
B. Delayed afterdepolarizations (DAD)	Calcium overload (unload) or DAD (suppress)	I_{Ca-L}; I_{Na} (block) I_{Ca-L} (block) I_{Ca-L}; I_{Na} (block)
Conduction:		
Reentry dependent on Na channels		
A. Primary impaired conduction (long excitable gap)	Excitability and conduction (decrease)	I_{Na} (block)
B. Conduction encroaching on refractoriness (short excitable gap)	Effective refractory period (prolong)	I_K (block)
Other:		
Reentry dependent on Ca channels	Excitability and conduction (decrease)	I_{Ca-L} (block)
Other mechanisms		
Reflection	Excitability (decrease)	I_{Na}; I_{Ca-L} (block)
Parasystole	Phase 4 depolarization (decrease)	I_f (block) (If MDP high)

(Modified from The Task Force of the Working Group on Arrhythmias of the European Society of Cardiology. The "Sicilian gambit": A new approach to the classification of antiarrhythmic drugs based on their actions on arrhythmogenic mechanisms. Eur Heart J 12:1112–1131, 1991.)

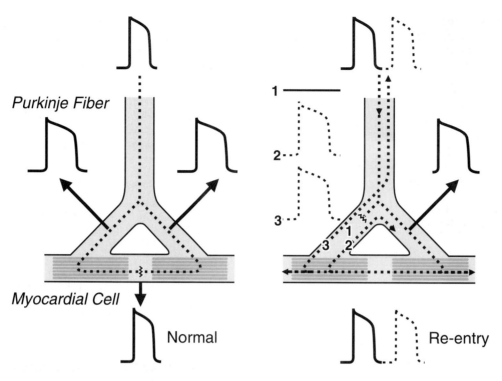

Fig. 5–37. Reentry. During normal conditions the cardiac action potential is transmitted through modified muscle fibers (specialized fibers) to the atrial and ventricular muscle cells, resulting in depolarization followed by repolarization. The action potential is not perpetuated because the surrounding tissues at the end point of activation remain refractory to reactivation (normal). During various disease processes (ischemia, hypoxia, inflammation, fibrosis) and in the presence of some drugs (intravenous and inhalation anesthetics) the action potential may be blocked (unidirectional block) as it travels in an antegrade direction through cardiac tissue, 1. If the electrical impulse is delayed (conduction delay) as it travels through adjacent tissue, it may reenter and be conducted in a retrograde direction (retrograde conduction), thereby reactivating the same tissue segment, 2, or more peripheral tissue segments, 3 (left). The longer the conduction delay the more likely the electric impulse will find the tissue to be reentered excitable (not refractory) and the greater the likelihood for reentry (dotted lines). Continuous reentry of cardiac tissue is called *circus movement* and can lead to sustained cardiac rhythm disturbances including ventricular fibrillation. Reentry involving a small amount (several square millimeters) of cardiac tissue is called *microreentry*, whereas reentry that incorporates the specialized conducting system of the heart is called *macroreentry*.

delayed (after repolarization) afterpotentials arising from the cell membrane.(22) Abnormal heart rhythm resulting from abnormal conduction and random or ordered reentry can be caused by spatial differences in membrane refractory periods or discontinuous anisotropic (dissimilar in all directions) propagation (Fig. 5–37). The latter electrophysiologic abnormality can occur as a result of cellular "uncoupling" owing to a decreased number of effective cellular connections (gap junctions) caused by fibrosis, ischemia, or drug therapy.(24, 26, 27) Regardless of cause, changes in either the active (ion current movements) or passive (membrane characteristics) properties of the cardiac cell membrane can result in a wide array of cardiac rate or rhythm disturbances that are recordable at the body surface. Anesthetic drugs and various anesthetic techniques produce marked changes in cardiac cellular active and passive electrophysiologic properties, resulting in the development of cardiac arrhythmias (Table 5–13). The inhalation anesthetics in particular are known to shorten action potential duration and decrease refractoriness, thereby predisposing to conduction abnormalities and reentry. Halothane and, to a

lesser extent, methoxyflurane, enflurane, and isoflurane "sensitize" the myocardium to catecholamines. Both alpha$_1$ and beta$_1$ adrenoceptors are involved in the cardiac sensitization phenomena. Finally, most anesthetic drugs can produce pronounced effects upon cardiac rate and rhythm because of the general membrane depressant effects.

VASCULAR DISEASE

Primary diseases of the vascular system are not well recognized in veterinary medicine.(95) Arterial hypertension occurs in dogs and cats secondary to renal disease or endocrine disorders. Systemic hypertension is defined as a systolic blood pressure above 160 mm Hg and a diastolic blood pressure above 95 mm Hg. Chronic renal disease, especially glomerular disease, can be associated with systemic hypertension secondary to a decrease in renal blood flow and activation of the renin-angiotensin system, release of aldosterone, and an increase in sympathetic tone.(75) Systemic vasoconstriction and renal retention of sodium water contribute to the elevation of arterial blood pressure. Hyperadrenocorticism may cause systemic hypertension because mineralocorticoids cause retention of sodium and water, expanding the circulating blood volume. Pheochromocytomas secrete an excess of circulating catecholamines and perhaps neuropeptide Y, which induces systemic vasoconstriction, elevating blood pressure. No matter what the cause of systemic hypertension, myocardial work increases and can induce left ventricular hypertrophy and a decrease in cardiovascular reserve.

Canine heartworm disease is a disease affecting dogs and rarely cats.(95) Myointimal proliferation occurs in the pulmonary arteries, narrowing their lumen. Cellular

Table 5–13. Cardiac Arrhythmias Produced by Preanesthetic and Anesthetic Drugs

Drugs	Arrhythmia
Anticholinergics	
Atropine	Sinus tachycardia
Glycopyrrolate	Sinus tachycardia
Phenothiazine	
Acepromazine	Sinus tachycardia
	Sinus bradycardia (rarely)
Alpha₂- Agonists	
Xylazine	Sinus bradycardia; first-, second-degree atrioventricular block; third-degree atrioventricular block (rarely); sinus arrest (rarely)
Detomidine	
Medetomidine	
Opioids	
Morphine	Sinus bradycardia
Oxymorphone	First-, second-degree atrioventricular block
Fentanyl	
Butorphanol	
Benzodiazepines	
Diazepam	Arrhythmias rarely observed; sinus bradycardia, temporary cardiac arrest
Midazolam	
Intravenous Anesthetics	
Thiobarbiturates (Thiamylal, Thiopental)	Bradyarrhythmias; Premature ventricular depolarizations; Ventricular tachycardia; Sinus tachycardia; ventricular arrhythmias; Sinus tachycardia, bradyarrhythmias (rarely); Sinus tachycardia, bradyarrhythmias (rarely)
Inhalation Anesthetics	
Methoxyflurane	Sinus bradycardia
Halothane	Bradyarrhythmias
Isoflurane	Premature ventricular depolarizations; Ventricular tachycardia; Ventricular fibrillation or cardiac arrest (Note: Halothane and methoxyflurane sensitize the myocardium to catecholamines.)

debris from dying worms form thromboemboli that obstruct pulmonary arteries. Pulmonary vascular endothelial damage results in pulmonary vasoconstriction secondary to the loss of endothelial-derived relaxant factors. Right-sided congestive heart failure often develops secondary to the elevated pulmonary vascular resistance. Oxygen therapy (preoxygenation) and cardiovascular support may be required for heartworm patients prior to anesthesia.

Arteriovenous (AV) malformations result in an elevation in venous pressure that ultimately contributes to dilation and tortuosity of the vein. The arterial pressure downstream from the fistula may be decreased, impairing tissue perfusion. Arteriovenous malformations increase myocardial work by producing volume overload, similar to a ventricular septal defect or mitral insufficiency. The surgical correction of an AV fistula can result in reflex bradycardia (Branham's sign) at the time of shunt ligation. The same phenomenon is seen at the time of ligation of a patent ductus arteriosus due to the sudden increase in arterial pressure and the response of arterial baroreceptors. The administration of anticholinergics can minimize or prevent bradycardia.

BLOOD COMPONENTS AND BLOOD VOLUME

Preservation of the integrity of the circulation is a responsibility that many humoral factors share. The effects of drugs used for chemical restraint and anesthesia (phenothiazines, butyrophenones, barbiturates, inhalation anesthetics) upon clotting time and bleeding time are incompletely understood but generally considered to be of importance in most animals. Exaggeration of bleeding disorders most frequently occurs in animals with thrombocytopenia or hereditary coagulation factor deficiencies (von Willebrand's disease). Many drugs inhibit platelet aggregation, which normally contributes significantly to hemostasis.(96) Phenothiazines, barbiturates, and halothane decrease platelet numbers and inhibit platelet aggregation, although little change in gross hemostasis is observed. Decreases in platelet and other circulating cell (red and white cells) numbers has been attributed to hemodilution secondary to hypotension, margination of white blood cells along vessel walls, and sequestration of red blood cells in the spleen. Finally, it should be recognized that most intravenous and inhalation anesthetics are known to suppress the immune system, an effect that is generally short lived but may become clinically relevant in immunosuppressed animals.(97)

The most important function of the cardiovascular system is to deliver oxygen and nutrients to metabolizing tissues.(3) The blood volume and hematocrit are of primary concern in maintaining adequate oxygen delivery, providing cardiac output and the distribution of blood flow are maintained within normal limits. The importance of adequate oxygen delivery (DO_2) cannot be overemphasized, because reduced oxygen consumption (VO_2) is known to be the common denominator in all forms of shock, including hemorrhagic and anemic shock (Chapter 24C, "Trauma Patients"). There are multiple reasons for this: First, oxygen transport is the major function of the cardiovascular system; second, oxygen is the most flow-dependent blood constituent because it has the highest extraction ratio of any substance carried in the blood; third, oxygen cannot be stored; and finally, oxygen transport and consumption are related to survival. Indeed, mortality is virtually 100% assured when the cumulative VO_2 deficit following hypoxemia, hemorrhage, or anemia exceeds 140 mL/kg.

Experimentally, hemorrhagic and anemic shock models are used to mimic clinical conditions where DO_2 and VO_2 are decreased. Popular models include a 50 to 75% decrease in blood volume (40–60 mL/kg; fixed volume model), withdrawal of blood to a predetermined blood pressure (e.g., 40 mm Hg) and maintenance of this pressure for 2 hours (fixed pressure or Wigger's model) and a decrease of the hematocrit to 8 to 12% by acute exchange transfusion with crystalloid (lactated Ringer's) or colloidal (6% Dextran 70) solutions (normoxic isovolemic hemodilution). These models produce acute reductions in DO_2 and a marked reduction in VO_2, which, if not treated, result in death (irreversible shock). Reductions in VO_2 therefore can be viewed as the ultimate regulatory factor responsible for cardiovascular compensatory responses, including increases in heart rate, cardiac contractility, cardiac output, and vascular tone. Other changes in cardiovascular function are determined by the primary precipitating event. Hemodilution, for example, produces increases in stroke volume, a redistribution of blood flow to the coronary and cerebral blood vessels, and a marked decrease in blood viscosity.(17) The last effect, decrease in blood viscosity, facilitates capillary blood flow and can increase cardiac output by decreasing afterload. These hemodynamic changes have resulted in the clinical use of mild to moderate normovolemic hemodilution prior to anesthesia and surgery (Hb = 6–10 g/dL) in order to improve cardiac output, peripheral perfusion, and DO_2. The effects of anesthetic drugs on VO_2, DO_2, cardiac output, and the distribution of blood flow must be considered prior to their use in any hypovolemic, anemic, or normovolemic anemic patients.(98)

References

1. Mulvany MJ, Aalkjaer C. Structure and function of small arteries. Physiol Rev 70:921–961, 1990.
2. Burton AC. Composition of blood. In: Burton AC, ed. Physiology and biophysics of the circulation, 2nd ed. Chicago: Year Book, 1972:15–21.
3. Snyder JV. Oxygen transport: the model and reality. In: Snyder JV, Pinsky MR, eds. Oxygen transport in the critically ill. Chicago: Year Book, 1987:3–15.
4. Guyton AC. Dominant role of the kidneys in long-term regulation of arterial pressure and in hypertension: the integrated system for pressure control. In: Textbook of medical physiology, 8th ed. Philadelphia: WB Saunders, 205–220, 1991.
5. Guyton AC. Overview of the circulation, and medical physics of pressure, flow, and resistance. In: Textbook of medical physiology, 8th ed. Philadelphia: WB Saunders, 1991:150–158.
6. Lasala PA, Chien S, Michelsen CB. Hemorrheology: what is the ideal hematocrit? In: Askanasi J, Starker RM, Weissman C, eds. Fluid and electrolyte management in critical care. Boston: Butterworth, 1986:203–213.
7. Berne RM, Levy MN. Hemodynamics. In: Principles of physiology. St. Louis: CV Mosby, 1990:245–254.
8. Berne RM, Levy MN. Control of cardiac output: coupling of the heart and blood vessels. In: Principles of physiology. St. Louis: CV Mosby, 1990:287–299.
9. Burton AC. Viscosity and the manner in which blood flows. In: Physiology and biophysics of the circulation, 2nd ed. Chicago: Year Book, 1972:39–48.
10. Nichols WW, O'Rourke MF. Vascular impedance. In: Nichols WW, O'Rourke MF, eds. McDonald's blood flow in arteries: theoretical, experimental and clinical principles, 3rd ed. Philadelphia: Lea & Febiger, 1990:283–329.
11. Chapler CK, Cain SM. The physiologic reserve in oxygen carrying capacity: studies in experimental hemodilution. Can J Physiol Pharmacol 64:7–12, 1986.
12. Leone BJ Spahn DR. Anemia, hemodilution, and oxygen delivery. Anesth Analg 75:651–653, 1992.
13. Little WC, Cheng C. Left ventricular-arterial coupling in conscious dogs. Am J Physiol 261 (Heart Circ Physiol 30):H70–H76, 1991.
14. Shroff SG, Weber KT, Janicki JS. Coupling of the left ventricle with the systemic arterial circulation. In: Nichols WW, O'Rourke MF, eds. McDonald's blood flow in arteries: theoretical, experimental and clinical principles, 3rd ed. Philadelphia: Lea & Febiger, 1990:343–359.
15. Suga H, Igarashi Y, Yamada O, Goto Y. Mechanical efficiency of the left ventricle as a function of preload, afterload, and contractility. Heart Vessels 1985:1:3–8.
16. Nichols WW, O'Rourke MF, Avolio AP, Yaginuma T, Murgo JP, Pepine CJ, Conti CR. Age-related changes in left ventricular/arterial coupling. In: Yin FCP, ed. Ventricular/Vascular coupling: clinical, physiological, and engineering aspects. New York: Springer-Verlag 1987:79–114.
17. Bowens C, Spahn DR, Frasco PE, Smith R, McRae, RL, Leone BJ. Hemodilution induces stable changes in global cardiovascular and regional myocardial function. Anesth Analg 76:1027–1032, 1998.
18. Burton AC. Kinetic energy in the circulation; streamline flow and turbulence; measurement of arterial pressure. In: Burton AC, ed. Physiology and biophysics of the circulation, 2nd ed. Chicago: Year Book, 1972:104–114.
19. Berne RM, Levy MN. Electrical activity of the heart. In: Principles of physiology. St. Louis: CV Mosby, 1990:197–213.
20. Kutchai HC. Generation and conduction of action potentials. In: Berne RM, Levy MN, eds. Principles of physiology. St. Louis: CV Mosby, 1990:27–39.
21. Opie LH. Channels, pumps, and exchangers. In: Opie LH, ed. The heart: physiology and metabolism, 2nd ed. New York: Raven Press 1991:67–101.
22. Boyden PA. Cellular electrophysiologic basis of cardiac arrhythmias. In: Tilley LP, ed. Essentials of canine and feline electrocardiography: interpretation and treatment, 3rd ed. Philadelphia: Lea & Febiger, 1992: 274–286.
23. Turner LA, Polic S, Hoffmann RG, Kampine JP, Bosnjak ZJ. Actions of volatile anesthetics on ischemic and nonischemic Purkinje fibers in the infarcted canine heart: regional action potential characteristics. Anesth Analg 76:726–733, 1993.
24. The Task Force of the Working Group on Arrhythmias of the European Society of Cardiology. The "Sicilian gambit": a new approach to the classification of antiarrhythmic drugs based on their actions on arrhythmogenic mechanisms. Eur Heart J 12:1112–1131, 1991.
25. Burt JM, Spray DC. Volatile anesthetics block intercellular communication between neonatal rat myocardial cells. Circ Res 65:829–837, 1989.
26. Spach MS, Dolber PC. Discontinuous anisotropic propagation. In: Rosen MR, Janse MJ, Wit AL, eds. Cardiac electrophysiology: a textbook. Mount Kisco, NY: Futura Publishing, 1990:517–534.
27. Spach MS, Dolber PC, Heidlage JF. Influence of the passive anisotropic properties on directional differences in propagation following modification of the sodium conductance in human

atrial muscle. A model of re-entry based on anistropic discontinuous propagation. Circ Res 62:811–832, 1988.

28. Baum VC. Distinctive effects of three intravenous anesthetics on the inward rectifier (I_{K1}) and the delayed rectifier (I_K) potassium currents in myocardium: implications for the mechanism of action. Anesth Analg 76:18–23, 1993.

29. Boban M, Atlee JL, Vicenzi M, Kampine JP, Bosnjak ZJ. Anesthetics and automaticity in latent pacemaker fibers: IV. Effects of isoflurane and epinephrine or norepinephrine on automaticity of dominant and subsidiary atrial pacemakers in the canine heart. Anesthesiology 79(3):555–562, 1993

30. Eskinder H, Supan FD, Turner LA, Kampine JP, Bosnjak Z. The effects of halothane and isoflurane on slowly inactivating sodium current in canine cardiac Purkinje cells. Anesth Anal 77:32–37, 1993.

31. Hatakeyama N, Ito Y, Momose Y. Effects of sevoflurane, isoflurane, and halothane on mechanical and electrophysiologic properties of canine myocardium. Anesth Analg 76:1327–1332, 1993.

32. Polic S, Bosnjak ZJ, Marijic J, Hoffmann RG, Kampine JP, Turner LA. Actions of halothane, isoflurane, and enflurane on the regional action potential characteristics of canine Purkinje fibers. Anesth Analg 73:603–611, 1991.

33. Turner LA, Polic S, Hoffmann RG, Kampine JP, Busnjak ZJ. Actions of halothane and isoflurane on Purkinje fibers in the infarcted canine heart: conduction, regional refractoriness, and reentry. Anesth Analg 76:718–725, 1993.

34. Balke CW, Gold MR. Calcium channels in the heart: an overview. Heart Dis Stroke 1:398–403, 1992.

35. Opie LH. Intracellular calcium fluxes and sarcoplasmic reticulum. In: Opie LH, ed. The heart: physiology and metabolism, 2nd ed. New York: Raven Press. 1991:127–146.

36. Katz AM. Contractile proteins: mechanisms and control of the cardiac contractile process, series elasticity, "active state", length-tension relationship and cardiac mechanics. In: Katz AM, ed. Physiology of the heart. Raven Press. 1977:119–136.

37. Paul RJ, Ferguson DG, Heiny JA. Muscle physiology: molecular mechanisms. In: Spearlakis N, Banks RO, eds. Physiology. Little, Brown & Co. 189–208, 1993.

38. Blanck TJJ, Chiancone E, Salviati G, Heitmiller ES, Verzili D, Luciani G, Colotti G. Halothane does not alter Ca^{2+} affinity of tropinin C. Anesthesiology 76:100–105, 1992.

39. Bosnjak ZJ, Supan FD, Rusch NJ. The effects of halothane, enflurane, and isoflurane on calcium current in isolated canine ventricular cells. Anesthesiology 74:340–345, 1991.

40. Bosnjak ZJ, Aggarwal A, Turner LA, Kampine JM, Kampine JP. Differential effects of halothane, enflurane, and isoflurane on Ca^{2+} transients and papillary muscle tension in guinea pigs. Anesthesiology 76:123–131, 1992.

41. Frazer MJ, Lynch C. Halothane and isoflurane effects on Ca^{2+} fluxes of isolated myocardial sarcoplasmic reticulum. Anesthesiology 77:316–323, 1992.

42. Kongsayreepong S, Cook DJ, Housmans PR. Mechanism of the direct, negative inotropic effect of ketamine in isolated ferret and frog ventricular myocardium. Anesthesiology 79:313–322, 1993.

43. Pagel PS, Kampine JP, Schmeling WT, Warltier DC. Reversal of volatile anesthetic-induced depression of myocardial contractility by extracellular calcium also enhances left ventricular diastolic function. Anesthesiology 8:141–154, 1993.

44. Rusy BF, Komai H. Anesthetic depression of myocardial contractility: a review of possible mechanisms. Anesthesiology 67:745–766, 1987.

45. Schmidt U, Schwinger RHG, Uberfuhr P, Kreuzer E, Reichart B, Meyer LV, Erdmann E, Böhm M. Evidence for an interaction of halothane with the L-type Ca^{2+} channel in human myocardium. Anesthesiology 79:332–339, 1993.

46. Wilde DW, Davidson BA, Smith MD, Knight PR. Effects of isoflurane and enflurane on intracellular Ca^{2+} mobilization in isolated cardiac myocytes. Anesthesiology 79:73–82, 1993.

47. Welker FH, Muir WW. An investigation of the second heart sound in the normal horse. Eq Vet J 22:403–407, 1990.

48. Ettinger SJ, Suter PF. Heart sounds and phonocardiography. In: Canine cardiology. WB Saunders. 1970:12–39.

49. Sagawa K. The end-systolic pressure-volume relation of the ventricle: definition, modifications and clinical use . Circulation 63:1223–1227, 1981.

50. Brutsaert DL, Rademakers FE, Sys SU, Gillebert TC, Housmans PR. Analysis of relaxation in the evaluation of ventricular function of the heart. Prog Cardiovasc Dis 28:143–163, 1985.

51. Little WC, Downes TR. Clinical evaluation of left ventricular diastolic performance. Prog Cardiovasc Dis 32:273–290, 1990.

52. Freeman GL, Colston JT. Role of ventriculovascular coupling in cardiac response to increased contractility in closed-chest dogs. J Clin Invest 86:1278–1284, 1990.

53. Hayashida K, Sunagawa K, Noma M, Sugimachi M, Ando H, Nakamura M. Mechanical matching of the left ventricle with the arterial system in exercising dogs. Circ Res 71:481–489, 1992.

54. Opie LH. Ventricular function. In: The heart: physiology and metabolism, 2nd ed. New York: Raven Press. 1991:301–338.

55. Nichols WW, O'Rourke FO, Auolio AP, Yaginuma T, Murgo JP, Pepine CJ, Conti CR. Age-related changes in left ventricular arterial coupling. In: Yin CP, ed. Ventricular/Vascular coupling: clinical, physiological, and engineering aspects. New York: Springer-Verlag. 1987:79–714.

56. Bonow RO, Udelson JE. Left ventricular diastolic dysfunction as a cause of congestive heart failure: mechanisms and management. Ann Intern Med 117:502–510, 1992.

57. Pagel PS, Kampine JP, Schmeling WT, Warltier DC. Comparison of end-systolic pressure-length relations and preload recruitable stroke work as indices of myocardial contractility in the conscious and anesthetized, chronically instrumented dog. Anesthesiology 73:278–290, 1990.

58. Pagel PS, Kampine JP, Schmeling WT, Warltier DC. Ketamine depresses myocardial contractility as evaluated by the preload recruitable stroke work relationship in chronically instrumented dogs with autonomic nervous system blockade. Anesthesiology 76:564–572, 1992.

59. Swanson CR, Muir WW. Simultaneous evaluation of left ventricular end-systolic pressure-volume ratio and time constant of isovolumic pressure decline in dogs exposed to equivalent MAC halothane and isoflurane. Anesthesiology 68:764–770, 1988.

60. Pagel PS, Kampine JP, Schmeling WT, Warltier DC. Comparison of the systemic and coronary hemodynamic actions of desflurane, isoflurane, halothane, and enflurane in the chronically instrumented dog. Anesthesiology 74:539–551, 1991.

61. Moffitt EA, Sethna DH. The coronary circulation and myocardial oxygenation in coronary artery disease: effects of anesthesia. Anesth Analg 65:395–410, 1986.

62. Pagel PS, Kampine JP, Schmeling WT, Warltier DC. Alteration of left ventricular diastolic function by desflurane, isoflurane, and halothane in the chronically instrumented dog with autonomic nervous system blockade. Anesthesiology 74:1103–1114, 1991.

63. Pagel PS, Schmeling WT, Kampine JP, Warltier DC. Alteration of canine left ventricular diastolic function by intravenous anesthetics in vivo: ketamine and propofol. Anesthesiology 76:419–425, 1992.

64. Asanoi H, Sasayama S, Kameyama T. Ventriculoarterial coupling in normal and failing heart in humans. Circ Res 65:483–493, 1989.

65. Milnor WR. The normal hemodynamic state: vascular impedance and wave reflection. In: Hemodynamics, 2nd ed. Baltimore: Williams & Wilkins. 1989:142–224.

66. Bevan JA, Bevan RD. Changes in arteries as they get smaller. In: Vanhoutte P, ed. Vasodilatation: vascular smooth muscle, peptides, autonomic nerves and endothelium. New York: Raven Press. 1988:55–60.

67. Tsuchida H, Namba H, Yamakage M, Fujita S, Notsuki E, Namiki A. Effects of halothane and isoflurane on cytosolic calcium ion concentration and contraction in the vascular smooth muscle of the rat aorta. Anesthesiology 78:531–540, 1993.

68. Witzleb Z. Functions of the vascular system. In: Schmidt RF, Thews G, eds. Human physiology. New York: Springer-Verlag. 1983:397–455.

69. Green JR. Circulatory mechanics. In: Fundamental cardiovascular and pulmonary physiology, 2nd ed. Philadelphia: Lea & Febiger. 1987:59–80.

70. Yano H, Takaori M. Effect of hemodilution on capillary and arteriolovenous shunt flow in organs after cardiac arrest in dogs. Crit Care Med 18:1146–1151, 1990.

71. Pappenheimer JR, Soto-Rivera A. Effective osmotic pressure of the plasma proteins and other quantities associated with the capillary circulation in the hindlimbs of cats and dogs. Am J Physiol 152:471–491, 1948.

72. Taylor AE. Capillary fluid filtration: starling forces and lymph flow. Circ Res 49:557–575, 1981.

73. Guyton AC. Local control of blood flow by the tissues and humoral regulation. In: Textbook of medical physiology, 8th ed. Philadelphia: WB Saunders, 1991:185–193.

74. Levy MN. Neural and reflex control of the circulation. In: Garfein O, ed. Current concepts in cardiovascular physiology. San Diego: Academic Press, 1990:133–207.

75. Mirenda JV, Grissom TE. Anesthetic implications of the renin-angiotensin system and angiotensin-converting enzyme inhibitors. Anesth Analg 72:667–683, 1991.

76. Shepherd JT, Vanhoutte PM. Neurohumoral regulation. In: The human cardiovascular system: facts and concepts. New York: Raven Press, 1979:107–155.

77. Oparil S, Katholi R. Humoral control of the circulation. In: Garfein O, ed. Current concepts in cardiovascular physiology. San Diego: Academic Press, 1990:210–287.

78. Arimura H, Bosnjak ZJ, Hoka S, Kampine JP. Modifications by halothane of responses to acute hypoxia in systemic vascular capacitance, resistance, and sympathetic nerve activity in dogs. Anesth Analg 73:319–326, 1991.

79. Hart JL, Jing M, Bina S, Freas W, Van Dyke RA, Muldoon SM. Effects of halothane on EDRF/cGMP-mediated vascular smooth muscle relaxations. Anesthesiology 79–323–331, 1993.

80. McCallum JB, Stekiel TA, Bosnjak ZJ Kampine JP. Does isoflurane alter mesenteric venous capacitance in the intact rabbit? Anesth Analg 76:1095–1105, 1993.

81. Toda H, Nakamura K, Hatano Y, Nishiwada M, Kakuyama M, Mori K. Halothane and isoflurane inhibit endothelium-dependent relaxation elicited by acetylcholine. Anesth Analg 75:198–203, 1992.

82. Uggeri MJ, Proctor GJ, Johns RA. Halothane, enflurane, and isoflurane attenuate both receptor- and non-receptor-mediated EFRF production in rat thoracic aorta. Anesthesiology 76:1012–1017, 1992.

83. Blaustein AS, Walsh RA. Regulation of the cardiovascular system. In: Spearlakis N, Banks RO, eds. Physiology. Little, Brown & Co. 1993:351–372.

84. Greisheimer FM. The circulatory effects of anesthetics. In: Hamilton WF, ed. Handbook of physiology circulation, sec. 2, vol. 3. Am Physiol Society. 1965:2477–2510.

85. Hellyer PW, Bednarski RM, Hubbell JAE, Muir WW. Effects of halothane and isoflurane on baroreflex sensitivity in horses. Am J Vet Res 50:2127–2134, 1989.

86. Harrison JK, Pearson WR, Lynch KR. Molecular characterization of alpha-1 and alpha-2 adrenoceptors. Trends Pharm Sci 12:62–67, 1991.

87. Van Zwieten PA. Adrenergic and muscarinic receptors: classification, pathophysiological relevance and drug target. J Hypertens 9(suppl 6):S18–S27, 1991.

88. Schulz S, Yuen PST, Garbers DL. The expanding family of guanylyl cyclases. Trends Pharm Sci 12:116–120, 1991.

89. Maze M, Tranquilli W. Alpha-2 adrenoceptor agonists: defining the role in clinical anesthesia. Anesthesiol 74:581–605, 1991.

90. Lokhandwala MF, Hegde SS. Cardiovascular pharmacology of adrenergic and dopaminergic receptors: significance in congestive heart failure. Am J Med 90(suppl 5B):2S–9S, 1991.

91. Walker P, Grouzmann E, Burnier M, Waeber B. The role of neuropeptide Y in cardiovascular regulation. Trends Pharm Sci 12:111–115, 1991.

92. Hosey MM. Diversity of structure, signaling and regulation within the family of muscarinic cholinergic receptors. FASEB J 6:845–852, 1992.

93. Drexler H. Reduced exercise tolerance in chronic heart failure and its relationship to neurohumoral factors. Eur Heart J 12:21–28, 1991.

94. Opie LH. Ventricular overload and heart failure. In: The heart: physiology and metabolism, 2nd ed. New York: Raven Press. 1991:396–424.

95. Bonagura J, Stepien R. Vascular diseases. In: Birchard SJ, Sherding RG, eds. Saunders manual of small animal practice. Philadelphia: WB Saunders. 1993:494–499.

96. Barr SC, Ludders JW, Looney AL, Gleed RD, Erb HN. Platelet aggregation in dogs after sedation with acepromazine and atropine and during subsequent general anesthesia and surgery. Am J Vet Res. 1992:53:2067–2070.

97. Lewis RE, Cruse JM, Hazelwood J. Halothane induced suppression of cell-mediated immunity in normal and tumor-bearing C3H$_f$/He mice. Anesth Analg 59:666–671, 1988.

98. Van der Linden P, Gilbart E, Engelman E, Schmartz D, Vincent JL. Effects of anesthetic agents on systemic critical O_2 delivery. J Appl Physiol 1994:71:83–93.

chapter 6

RESPIRATORY SYSTEM

Wayne McDonell

Introduction

Maintenance of adequate respiratory function is a prime requirement for safe anesthesia. Inadequate tissue oxygenation may lead to an acute cessation of vital organ function, especially of the brain or myocardium, and an anesthetic fatality. Excessive elevations in arterial carbon dioxide tensions ($PaCO_2$) or sustained moderate hypoxemia may produce lesser degrees of organ dysfunction, which contribute to a less than optimum postanesthetic recovery. Delayed recovery of consciousness, postanesthetic myopathy in large animals, and postanesthetic renal, hepatic, or cardiac insufficiency can all originate from inadequate respiratory function during anesthesia.

During general anesthesia there is always a tendency for arterial oxygen tensions (PaO_2) to be less than observed with the same species while conscious and breathing the same inspired oxygen concentration (F_IO_2).(1–3) There is also a tendency for $PaCO_2$ to be elevated above the conscious resting values if the anesthetized animal is breathing spontaneously, and for increases in airway resistance to occur unless an endotracheal tube is utilized. Some differences are seen depending on the actual anesthetic regime used, but the

115

depth of anesthesia is often more of a factor. Species and breed differences exist, and some of these are illustrated in this chapter. Positioning during anesthesia, concurrent drug utilization, and the magnitude of preanesthetic cardiorespiratory dysfunction all affect respiratory function.

Respiratory dysfunction during general anesthesia and the postoperative period is caused by the disruption of many physiologic mechanisms and, in the larger species especially, an exaggeration of anatomic and mechanical factors.(1, 4) An understanding of respiratory function as it relates to anesthesia requires consideration of (a) the neural control of respiration and its effect on alveolar ventilation ($\dot{V}_A$); (b) the influence of anesthesia on the airway, chest wall, and lung volumes; and (c) the alterations in ventilation/perfusion (V/Q) relationships during anesthesia.(1, 3)

It is assumed that the reader is already reasonably knowledgeable regarding basic pulmonary physiology, which is considered in detail elsewhere.(5–7) Much of the information that is available about the effects of anesthesia on respiration comes from studies in humans. However, there are important differences in how veterinarians generally administer anesthetics to animals when compared to anesthesia of humans. In veterinary practice intravenous anesthetics are often used without oxygen supplementation, at least under field conditions. There is much less use of peripheral-acting muscle relaxants in veterinary anesthesia, and generally intermittent positive pressure ventilation (IPPV) is utilized on a "need to" rather than routine basis. During general anesthesia with inhalants, 100% oxygen is usually used as the carrier gas, whereas a 2:1 mixture of nitrous oxide and oxygen is commonly used as the carrier gas in human anesthesia. Dogs and cats have frequently been utilized for investigations of neural control and mechanical alterations associated with anesthesia, but often under experimental situations that differ quite markedly from how anesthetics are administered to veterinary patients.

Definitions

Respiration is the total process whereby oxygen is supplied to and utilized by body cells and carbon dioxide is eliminated by means of gradients. *Ventilation* is the movement of gas in and out of alveoli. The ventilatory requirement for homeostasis varies with the metabolic requirement of the animal, and it thus varies with body size, the level of activity, body temperature, and the depth of anesthesia. Pulmonary ventilation is accomplished by expansion and contraction of the lungs. Several terms are used to describe the various types of breathing that may be observed.

1. *Eupnea* is ordinary quiet breathing.
2. *Dyspnea* is labored breathing.
3. *Tachypnea* is increased respiratory rate.
4. *Hyperpnea* is fast and/or deep respiration, indicating "overrespiration."

5. *Polypnea* is a rapid, shallow, panting type of respiration.
6. *Bradypnea* is slow regular respiration.
7. *Hypopnea* is slow and/or shallow breathing indicating "underrespiration."
8. *Apnea* is transient (or longer) cessation of breathing.
9. *Cheyne-Stokes respirations* increase in rate and depth, and then become slower, followed by a brief period of apnea.
10. *Biot's respirations* are sequences of gasps, apnea, and several deep gasps.
11. *Kussmaul's respirations* are regular deep respirations without pause.
12. *Apneustic respiration* is long gasping inspirations with several subsequent ineffective exhalations.

To describe the events of pulmonary ventilation, air in the lung has been subdivided into four different volumes and four different capacities (Fig. 6–1). Only tidal volume and functional residual capacity can be measured in conscious noncooperative animals.

1. *Tidal volume* (V_T) is the volume of air inspired or expired in one breath.
2. *Inspiratory reserve volume* (IRV) is the volume of air that can be inspired over and above the normal tidal volume.
3. *Expiratory reserve volume* (ERV) is the amount of air that can be expired by forceful expiration after a normal expiration.
4. *Residual volume* (RV) is the air remaining in the lungs after the most forceful expiration.

Another term frequently used is the minute respiratory volume or *minute ventilation* ($\dot{V}_E$). This is equal to V_T times the *respiratory frequency* (f). Occasionally, it is desirable to consider two or more of the aforementioned volumes together. Such combinations are termed *pulmonary capacities*.

1. *Inspiratory capacity* (IC) is the tidal volume plus the inspiratory reserve volume. This is the amount of air that can be inhaled starting after a normal

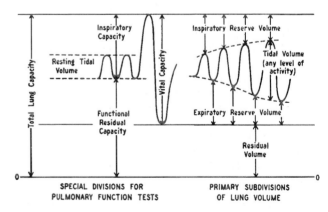

Fig. 6–1. Lung volumes and capacities. (From Standardization of Definitions and Symbols in Respiratory Physiology. Fed Proc 9:602, 1950.)

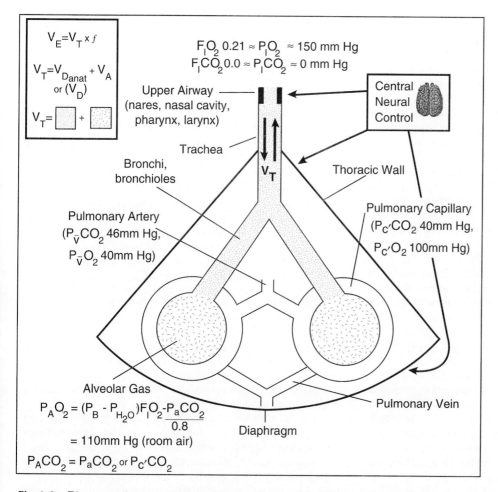

$$V_E = V_T \times f$$

$$V_T = V_{D_{anat}} + V_A$$
or (V_D)

$$V_T = \boxed{} + \boxed{}$$

$F_IO_2 \; 0.21 \approx P_IO_2 \approx 150 \text{ mm Hg}$
$F_ICO_2 \; 0.0 \approx P_ICO_2 \approx 0 \text{ mm Hg}$

Upper Airway (nares, nasal cavity, pharynx, larynx)

Central Neural Control

Trachea

Bronchi, bronchioles

V_T

Thoracic Wall

Pulmonary Artery
$(P_{\bar{v}}CO_2 \; 46\text{mm Hg},$
$P_{\bar{v}}O_2 \; 40\text{mm Hg})$

Pulmonary Capillary
$(P_{c'}CO_2 \; 40\text{mm Hg},$
$P_{c'}O_2 \; 100\text{mm Hg})$

Alveolar Gas
$$P_AO_2 = (P_B - P_{H_2O})F_IO_2 - \frac{P_aCO_2}{0.8}$$
$$= 110\text{mm Hg (room air)}$$
$$P_ACO_2 = P_aCO_2 \text{ or } P_{c'}CO_2$$

Pulmonary Vein

Diaphragm

Fig. 6–2. Diagrammatic representation of the neural control, bellows mechanism (diaphragm and thoracic wall) and matching of pulmonary artery blood and alveolar gas in the lung. F_I refers to fraction of inspired gases and f is respiratory frequency. Tidal volume (V_T), anatomic dead space ($V_{D \, anat}$), alveolar volume (V_A), and representative inspired (P_I), alveolar (P_A), pulmonary arterial ($P_{\bar{v}}$), and end-capillary ($P_{c'}$) partial pressures of oxygen and carbon dioxide are also illustrated. See the text for detailed explanation.

expiration and distending the lungs to the maximum amount.

2. *Functional residual capacity* (FRC) is the expiratory reserve volume plus the residual volume. This is the amount of air remaining in the lungs after a normal expiration.

3. *Vital capacity* (VC) is the inspiratory reserve volume plus the tidal volume plus the expiratory reserve volume. This is the maximum amount of air that can be expelled from the lungs after first filling them to their maximum capacity.

4. *Total lung capacity* (TLC) is the inspiratory reserve volume plus the tidal volume plus the expiratory reserve volume plus the residual volume, or the maximum volume to which the lungs can be expanded with the greatest possible inspiratory effort.

Ventilation and Gas Exchange in Conscious Animals

From the anesthetist's viewpoint, it is useful to consider the ventilatory system in terms of its major components:

neural control, the bellows mechanism (chest wall and diaphragm), upper airway, and lung parenchyma (Fig. 6–2). Alterations of (a) the neural control of ventilation by sedative, opioid, or anesthetic depression; (b) upper or lower airway patency by muscle relaxation or spasm; or (c) the bellows mechanism of the thorax through neuromuscular paralysis, space-occupying lesions of the thorax, or a change in the diaphragm shape, location, or function may all appreciably affect ventilatory adequacy and the efficiency of gas exchange. Within the parenchyma less than optimum matching of fresh alveolar gas with pulmonary capillary blood will produce blood gas alterations, particularly in regard to PaO_2.

CONTROL OF RESPIRATION

With the aid of the circulation (Chapter 5), respiration regulates the oxygen, carbon dioxide, and hydrogen ion environment of the cell. Respiratory function is controlled by central respiratory centers, central and peripheral chemoreceptors, pulmonary reflexes, and nonrespiratory neural input. Control of respiration has been described as an integrated feedback control system.(6, 7) The central neural "controller" includes specialized groups of neurons located in the cerebrum, brain stem, and spinal cord that govern both voluntary and automatic ventilation through regulation of the activity of the respiratory muscles. The respiratory muscles by contracting give rise to alveolar ventilation, and changes in alveolar ventilation affect blood gas tensions and hydrogen ion concentration. Blood gas tensions and hydrogen ion concentrations are monitored by peripheral and central chemoreceptors that return signals to the central controller to provide necessary adjustments in ventilation. Mechanoreceptors in the lungs and stretch receptors in the respiratory muscles monitor, respectively, the degree of expansion or stretch of the lungs and the "effort" of breathing, feeding back information to the central controller to alter the pattern of breathing. Adjustments also occur to accommodated nonrespiratory activities such as thermoregulation and vocalization.

Overall, this complex control system produces a combination of respiratory frequency and depth that is best suited for optimum ventilation with minimal effort for the particular species, and that adjusts oxygen supply and carbon dioxide elimination so as to maintain homeostasis (reflected by stable arterial blood gas levels) over a wide range of environmental and metabolic situations. Sedatives, analgesics, anesthetics, and the equipment used for inhalational anesthesia may profoundly alter respiration and the ability of the animal to maintain cellular homeostasis.

MECHANICAL FACTORS

Transfer of gases to and from the lungs is dependent upon developing a pressure gradient between the atmosphere and the alveoli, and is modified by the resistance to flow between these two regions and the elasticity of the lungs and chest wall. With spontaneous respiration, during inspiration active muscular effort serves to enlarge the pleural cavity through expansion of the thoracic wall and contraction of the diaphragm (Fig. 6–2). Intrapleural pressure is thereby reduced to a more subatmospheric pressure, and a mouth/nostril to alveolar pressure gradient is established. In contrast to inspiration, expiration is normally passive and depends upon the return of the chest wall and lungs to a resting position, that is to FRC. The horse is a notable exception in that abdominal muscle contraction plays a part in normal expiratory activity, producing a biphasic mode of exhalation.(5) As the size of the pleural space decreases, intrapleural and consequently alveolar pressures are elevated, and the pressure gradient is reversed so that air flows from the alveoli to the atmosphere. Thus, fluctuating pressure gradients between the atmosphere and the alveoli cause air to flow in and out of the lungs. The factors that contribute to these pressure gradients and the measurement of their magnitude are referred to as *pulmonary mechanics.*

During assisted or controlled artificial or mechanical ventilation, atmospheric to alveolar pressure gradients also occur, but mouth pressure is more positive than alveolar pressure on inspiration, hence the term *positive pressure ventilation.* This has important circulatory consequences (Chapter 17). Both the lungs and chest wall provide an elastic resistance to expansion on inspiration. The relationship between the pressure gradient (P) and the resultant volume increase (V) in liters (L) of the lungs and thorax is known as *total compliance* (C_T).(3)

$$C_T \text{ (L/cm } H_2O) = \Delta V \text{ (L)}/\Delta P \text{ (cm } H_2O)$$

The relationship of C_T to the individual compliances of the lungs (C_L) and chest wall (C_{CW}) is additive, as the lungs and chest wall are arranged concentrically and can be expressed as

$$1/C_T = 1/C_L + 1/C_{CW}$$

To measure C_T, V and the transthoracic pressure (that is the pressure at the alveolus minus ambient pressure) must be known. In anesthetized animals, this is often done by measuring the inspiratory volume delivered from a ventilator bellows or rebreathing bag while recording the change in airway (taken to be alveolar) pressure between end-exhalation and end-inspiration. If the lungs and/or chest wall are less compliant (i.e., stiffer), then higher transthoracic pressures are required to deliver a given tidal volume. The experienced anesthetist can often sense this change as an increased force required to mechanically squeeze a set volume from a rebreathing bag by hand. This may provide the first clue that an animal is developing a space-occupying problem in the thorax or abdomen (e.g., accumulation of air or blood), or that the end of the endotracheal tube has become repositioned in one main bronchus and is only inflating one lung.

Dynamic C_T is the volume change divided by the transthoracic pressure change at the point of zero airflow (end-inspiration) when the previous inflow of air has been sufficiently rapid for dynamic factors to influence the distribution of air throughout the lung. For practical purposes dynamic C_T is equal to the tidal volume divided by the peak airway pressure. *Static* C_T is determined when the preceding inflow of air has been sufficiently slow for distribution throughout the lung to be solely in accord with regional elasticity. Under these conditions gas distribution to alveoli with faster and slower filling rates is equivalent, and as a result the static C_T (or C_L) value is usually greater than dynamic C_T (or C_L).

To determine the elasticity of the lung per se (C_L), V and the transpulmonary pressure gradient (that is, pressure at the alveolus minus pressure at the pleural space) must be known. This measurement is harder to determine accurately. In practice the transpulmonary pressure gradient is generally determined using a differential pressure transducer to simultaneously determine mouth (considered equal to alveolar) and pleural pressure changes. Pleural pressure changes are estimated from intrathoracic esophageal pressure swings recorded with a balloon-tipped catheter. Lungs develop a low compliance (become stiffer) with a reduction in lung volume or regional atelectasis; as a result of pulmonary edema or fibrosis; and, in the case of dynamic C_L, with regional differences in airway resistance.

For air to flow into the lungs, a pressure gradient must also be developed to overcome the nonelastic (airway) resistance to airflow. The relationship between the pressure gradient across the pulmonary system (P_L) and the rate of airflow ($\dot{V}$) is known as *airway resistance* (R_L):(3)

$$R_L \text{ (cm H}_2\text{O/L/s)} = \Delta P_L \text{ (cm H}_2\text{O)} /\dot{V} \text{ (L/s)}$$

The caliber of the airway and rate and pattern of airflow all contribute to the pressure gradient along the airway. According to the Hagen-Poiseuille law, laminar gas flow through a tube is proportional to the pressure gradient across the tube, the fourth power of the diameter of the tube, and inversely to the viscosity:

pressure loss = constant × viscosity × length of tube × flow rate/diameter^4 × flow rate

The significance of this equation relative to anesthesia is to realize that changes in airway (or apparatus) diameter may markedly affect the resistance to airflow. If the diameter of the airway is reduced by 50%, for instance by using too small an endotracheal tube, the resistance goes up 16-fold.

At higher flow rates that exceed the critical velocity of the system, or in the face of sudden changes in airway diameter, airflow will no longer be laminar and becomes turbulent in nature. The significance of a transition from laminar to turbulent flow is illustrated by the fact that, at rates approximating critical flow, the resistance to flow increases by about 50% if the flow becomes turbulent. Measurements of airway resistance are carried out by a variety of methods, most of which involve the simultaneous determination of instantaneous airflow with a pneumotachograph and of transpulmonary pressure (P_L) as described earlier.

Airway resistance increases with the rate of respiration and with narrowing of the airway by reflex contraction of the bronchiolar muscles, with small airway disease where there is edema of the airway wall and mucous accumulation, with a reduction in lung volume, or through aspiration of foreign material. Airway resistance during anesthesia can be minimized by using an airway that is as wide as possible and in which sudden alterations in direction or diameter are minimized.

PULMONARY VENTILATION

The important factor in pulmonary ventilation is the rate at which *alveolar air* is exchanged with atmospheric air. This is not equal to the minute ventilation volume because a large portion of inspired air is used to fill the respiratory passages, rather than alveoli, and no signif-

icant gaseous exchange occurs in this air (Fig. 6–2). The *respiratory frequency* (f) and volume of each breath, *tidal volume* (V_T), determine the *minute ventilation* ($\dot{V}_E$). The portion of each V_T that only reaches the upper airway and tracheobronchial tree fills the *anatomic dead space* and is referred to as *dead space volume* ($V_{D\,anat}$). The $V_{D\,anat}$ is fairly constant; therefore slow, deep breathing is more effective than rapid, shallow breathing. This is especially so during general anesthesia and with IPPV. The "effective" volume, or portion of V_T that contributes to gas exchange, is the *alveolar volume* (V_A), usually referred to as *minute alveolar ventilation* ($\dot{V}_A$). Nonperfused alveoli do not contribute to gas exchange and constitute *alveolar dead space* (V_{DA}). In conscious, unsedated healthy animals V_{DA} is minimal, whereas during general anesthesia it may increase owing to a fall in cardiac output ($\dot{Q}$) and/or pulmonary artery blood pressure. *Physiologic dead space* (V_D) includes $V_{D\,anat}$ and V_{DA} (Fig. 6–2), and is usually expressed as a minute value ($\dot{V}_D$) along with $\dot{V}_A$, or as a ratio of V_D/V_T. In unsedated tracheostomized dogs breathing quietly through a standard endotracheal tube, V_D was 5.9 mL/kg and the ratio of V_D/V_T was 35%.(8) This ratio of V_D/V_T is similar to that found in humans, but the V_D figure is larger, reflecting the increased $V_{D\,anat}$ in dogs on a body weight basis. During methoxyflurane anesthesia with spontaneous respiration, V_D increased very little (about 0.5 mL/kg) but V_D/V_T increased to over 50% because V_T decreased. Others have shown similar results with other anesthetics. In larger species such as the horse and cow, the ratio V_D/V_T in conscious animals is about 50%.(9) Higher proportions of dead space have been reported, but such values probably reflect a tachypneic state or failure to subtract the added dead space associated with the use of the mask in gas collection. In unsedated cows V_D is about 3.7 mL/kg and in horses about 5.2 mL/kg.(9) Representative normal ventilation, blood gas, and acid-base values for a range of species are shown in Tables 6–1 and 6–2.

LUNG VOLUMES

The subdivisions of lung volume are shown in Figure 6–1. Most of these volumes cannot be measured in conscious animals, as they require cooperation of the test subject. Measurements of V_T and FRC can be obtained in conscious animals, while estimates of total lung capacity (TLC) are generally made by inflation of the lung to above 30 cm H$_2$O inflation pressure in anesthetized animals. Values for TLC are reasonably similar between the domestic species when compared on a body weight basis, but the total volume varies from less than 2.0 mL in a mouse to over 45 L in horses and cows (Table 6–3). This factor and the variation in V_T observed across species (Table 6-1) have quite significant implications relative to the design of suitable inhalant anesthetic apparatus and the relative importance of added mechanical dead space. A liter of apparatus dead space in a healthy conscious horse or cow constitutes only a small portion of the V_T and has little effect on $\dot{V}_A$ or blood gases (38), whereas a dead space of even 15 mL in a cat amounts

Table 6–1. Breathing Frequency (f), Tidal Volume (V_T), and Minute Ventilation (V̇_E) of Various Species

Species	Mean Body wt (kg)	n	Conditions[b]	f (breaths/min)	V_T (ml)	V_T (ml/kg)	V̇_E (ml/min)	V̇_E (ml/kg/min)	References
Mice	0.02	NS[a]	Awake, prone	163.4	0.15	7.78	24.5	1239	10
	0.032	NS	Anesthetized	109	0.18	5.63	21.0	720	10
Rats	0.113	NS	Awake, prone	85.5	0.87	7.67	72.9	646	10
	0.305	NS	Awake, pleth	103	2.08	6.83	213	701	10
Cats	3.8	4	Unanesthetized, pleth	22	30	7.9	664	174	11
	3.7	NS	Anesthetized	30	34	9.2	960	310	10
Dogs	18.6	6	Awake, prone, chronic trach, intubated	13	309	16.6	3818	205	12
	18.8	8	Awake, standing, chronic trach, intubated	16.5	314	16.9	4963	264	8
Sheep	32–37	4	Awake, standing mask	38	289	8.3	10,400	297	13
Goats	36.3	3	Awake, standing mask	13.6	470	12.9	6313	174	14
	46.4	6	Awake, standing mask	26	483	10.4	11,900	256	15
	47.6	6	Awake, standing mask	17.6	602	12.6	10,540	221	16
Pigs	12.9	4	Awake, standing	13.1	209	15.9	2731	208	17
Cows	517 Holstein	7	Awake, standing mask	23.7	3676	7.1	85,977	166	9
	405 Jersey	11	Awake, standing mask	28.6	3360	8.3	94,870	234	18
Calves	43–73 Hereford	8	4–6 wk old, standing sling	26.7	403	15.1	10,290	385	19
Horses	402	6	Awake, standing mask	11.8	4253	10.6	49,466	123	9
	483	6	Awake, standing mask	15.5	4860	10.1	74,600	154	20
	486	15	Awake, standing mask (some sedated) (mask V_D not removed)	10	7300	15.0	79,000	163	21
Ponies	147	19	Awake, standing mask	19.0	1370	9.3	26,380	180	22

[a]Not specified
[b]pleth = whole body plethysmograph = trach, tracheostomy

Table 6–2. Arterial Blood Gas and Acid-Base Values for Various Species

Species	Body wt (kg)	n	Conditions	pHa	Pa_{CO_2}	Pa_{O_2}	HCO_3^-	References
Rats	0.207	10	Awake, chronic catheter	7.44	32.7		21.5	23
	0.305	8	Awake, prone, chronic catheter	7.467	39.8		28.7	24
Rabbits	3.1	NS[a]	Awake, catheter	7.388	32.8	86	21	25
	3.5	20	Awake, catheter	7.47	28.5	89.2	20.2	26
Cats	2.5–5.1	8	Unsedated, chronic catheter, prone	7.41	28.0	108	18	27
	3–8	10	Unsedated, not restrained, chronic catheter	7.426	32.5	108	22.1	28
Dogs	18.8	8	Chronic tracheostomy, catheter, unsedated, standing	7.383	39.0	103.8	22.1	8
	12.2	22	Chronic catheters lateral recumbency	7.40	35	102	21	29
Sheep	33	NS	Awake, catheter	7.44	40.9	96	27.6	25
	24.5	11	Unsedated, prone, carotid loop	7.48	33	92		30
Goats	18	6	Unsedated, standing	7.46	36.5	101		14
	47.6	6	Unsedated, standing catheter	7.45	35.3	94.5	24.1	16
Calves	46.6	6	Unsedated, standing	7.45	41.1	87.1	27.6	15
	31–57	4	Standing, unsedated, aortic catheter	7.39	40	81	24	31
	48–66	20	Unanesthetized, catheter	7.37	42.8	93.6	23.6	32
Cows	517	7	Awake, unsedated, standing	7.40	39.6	83.1	24.4	9
	641	7	Awake, unsedated, standing	7.435	38.7	95.1	25.5	b
Horses	402	6	Awake, unsedated, standing	7.39	41.1	80.7	24.5	9
Ponies	147	19	Standing, aortic catheter	7.40	40	88.7	24.4	22

[a]Not specified
[b]Warren, R., and McDonell, W.N. (unpublished observations)

Table 6–3. Lung Volumes of Various Mammalian Species; Total Lung Capacity (TLC), Functional Residual Capacity (FRC), and Residual Volume (RV)

Species	Body wt (kg)	n	Conditions	TLC		FRC (mL/kg)	RV (mL/kg)	References
				mL	mL/kg			
Mice	0.020	NSᵃ	Anesthetized	1.57	78.5	25.0	19.5	10
Rats	0.31	NS	Anesthetized, prone	12.2	39.4	6.8	4.2	10
Rabbits	3.14	NS	Anesthetized, supine	111	35.4	11.6	6.4	10
Cats	3.7	4	Anesthetized			17.8		33
Dogs	18.6	6	Awake, prone	2090	112.4	53.6	16.7	12
	9.2	140	Unsedated, 1 year old			44.8		34
Sheep	24.5	4	Unsedated, prone, nasal endotracheal tube			45.3		30
Goats	46.4	6	Unsedated, standing, facemask			49.6		15
Cows	517	7	Awake, standing			39.4		35
	537	5	Anesthetized, prone	45,377	84.5	31.9	16.1	35
Horses	485		Anesthetized, prone	44,800	92.4	36.3	19.0	36
	402	6	Awake, standing			51.3		35
	394	4	Anesthetized, prone, lung inflated to 35–40 cm H₂O, starved 18 h	45,468	115.4	37.9		35
Ponies	(450–822)	6	Conscious, standing			35.6		37
	(164–288)	8	Conscious standing			39.9		37

ᵃNot specified

to 50% of V_T and will quite likely alter alveolar ventilation and $PaCO_2$ levels. In the smallest mammals virtually all mask systems will lead to some rebreathing of carbon dioxide during anesthesia, unless a loose fitting mask is used with a flow through system.

The volume of gas remaining in the lungs at the end of a normal expiration, that is, the FRC, varies considerably as the position of the diaphragm, in particular, changes. Abdominal tympany from any source (e.g., near-term gravid uterus, bowel distension, obesity, tumor etc.) will tend to move the diaphragm forward and lessen the FRC. Few actual measurements have been made of this phenomenon in relation to animals, but the consequences on ventilation and respiratory function during anesthesia are consistent with a decrease in FRC.

INTRAPULMONARY MATCHING OF BLOOD AND GAS

Matching of alveolar gas and pulmonary capillary blood flow is influenced by gravitational factors and the fact that the pulmonary artery circulation is a low-pressure system. Intrapleural pressure is more subatmospheric in the uppermost part of the thorax than in the lowermost portion (39), partly due to the "weight" of the lung in the thorax. Alveolar size is largest in the uppermost areas of the lung and smallest in the ventral regions. Since the larger alveoli have a lower compliance (they are less distensible), they expand less on inspiration and air preferentially enters the more compliant lower alveoli, producing a vertical gradient of ventilation in the standing animal breathing quietly.(40, 41) The tendency for preferential ventral ventilation in the lung may also be associated with regional chest wall and diaphragmatic movement. During anesthesia, the distribution of ventilation becomes more uneven and may even reverse so that the uppermost lung of the laterally recumbent horse is receiving most of the ventilation.

The major effect of gravity on the lung is to produce a vertical perfusion gradient in the pulmonary circulation, with the lower region being perfused more. The distribution of these gravitational effects on lung perfusion is commonly divided and functionally described as a three- or four-"zone" system.(41, 42) At rest the uppermost alveoli may be minimally perfused (Fig. 6–3, zone I) with alveolar pressure (P_A) greater than pulmonary artery (P_{pa}) and vein (P_{pv}) pressures. In zone II, P_{pa} is greater than P_A, and the difference between the two is the driving pressure for blood flow at the front end of the capillaries. The relationship between P_A and P_{pv} governs flow through the terminal aspect of the capillaries. In zone III, P_{pa} and P_{pv} both exceed P_A and the vessels are fully distended, with the perfusion being determined by the pressure difference between P_{pa} and P_{pv}. In zone IV, the weight of the lung increases the interstitial pressure to a point that blood flow is reduced toward that of zone II, or less. These factors are important during anesthesia in that cardiac output is often reduced and P_{pa} may fall. Moreover, when the body position is altered and an animal becomes recum-

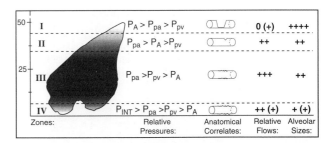

Fig. 6–3. Diagrammatic illustration of pulmonary artery (P_{pa}), pulmonary vein (P_{pv}), pulmonary interstitial (P_{INT}) and alveolar (P_A) pressure-flow relationships in the lung. (Modified with permission from Porcelli, R.J. Pulmonary Hemodynamics. In: Treatise on Pulmonary Toxicology. Edited by R.A. Parent. CRC Press, Boca Raton, FL, 1992:243.) See text for detailed explanation.

bent, there is thought to be a realignment of the pulmonary blood flow along gravitational lines consistent with the new body position.(3) However, these relationships are not necessarily straightforward, especially in the larger species, perhaps because of the large decrease in FRC that accompanies recumbency and the generation of a larger zone IV area in the thorax.

A simplified diagrammatic representation of altered V/Q is shown in Figure 6–4.(43) One extreme is to have a perfused alveolus or area of the lung with no ventilation so that the blood is not oxygenated while passing the region. Other extremes are for the alveolus to be ventilated but not perfused, or alternately for an alveolus or region to be neither ventilated nor perfused. Often the alteration of V/Q within the lung is somewhere in between these extremes and is characterized by alveoli throughout the lung that are only relatively underventilated or underperfused, producing an increase in the alveolar-to-arterial oxygen gradient. Since carbon dioxide is more diffusible across the alveolar capillary membrane, diffusion and V/Q problems commonly lead to decreased PaO_2 levels before there is a $PaCO_2$ change. It is possible to compensate for nonventilation of portions of the lung through increased ventilation of the rest of the lung in terms of carbon dioxide clearance, as occurs with the tachypneic pneumonic animal. The same increase in ventilation of "good" lung areas will never compensate completely for areas where there is inadequate oxygen uptake. The hemoglobin oxygen saturation curve is sigmoid shaped (Fig. 6–5), and hemoglobin is nearly fully saturated with oxygen at a PaO_2 of 90 to 100 mm Hg. Consequently, an increase in ventilation to the "good" areas of the lung cannot increase the oxygen content of blood very much, even though the alveolar partial pressure of oxygen (P_AO_2) increases. The clinical significance of this is that many pulmonary problems present as hypoxemia rather than hypercapnia.

EFFECT OF ALTERED ALVEOLAR VENTILATION

For any given metabolic output $PaCO_2$ and $\dot{V}_A$ are directly and inversely related: if $\dot{V}_A$ falls by 50%, $PaCO_2$

doubles, while if $\dot{V}_A$ is increased by 100% (say by IPPV) $PaCO_2$ levels will fall by 50% once equilibrium is established (Fig. 6–6). This is an important concept to grasp in that it explains how an experienced anesthetist is able to make fairly good approximations about the

resultant $PaCO_2$ level he or she will produce when an animal is put on a volume-limited ventilator at a particular f and V_T setting. For instance, in most anesthetized dogs with a body weight that is average for the breed, $PaCO_2$ will be near eucapnic levels when f is set at 8 to 10 per minute and V_T at 20 mL/kg. In anesthetized adult horses and cows a comparative eucapnic setting would be f at 5 per minute and V_T at 15 mL/kg.

Hyperventilation occurs when $\dot{V}_A$ is excessive relative to metabolic rate; as a result, $PaCO_2$ is reduced. Hyperventilation may or may not be accompanied by an increased respiratory rate, referred to as *tachypnea*. *Hypoventilation* is present when $\dot{V}_A$ is small relative to metabolic rate and $PaCO_2$ rises: hypoventilation may be accompanied by a slow (bradypnea), normal, or rapid f. A lowered $PaCO_2$ level is referred to as *hypocapnia* and an elevated level as *hypercapnia*, while normal $PaCO_2$ is termed *eucapnia*. Most, but not all, of the common species have a normal resting $PaCO_2$ level close to 40 mm Hg (Table 6–2). Hypercapnia and hypocapnia produce *respiratory acidosis* and *alkalosis*, respectively, since carbon dioxide in the body is in dynamic equilibrium with carbonic acid, and ultimately hydrogen ion concentration $[H^+]$:

$$CO_2 + H_2O \rightleftarrows H_2CO_3 \rightleftarrows H^+ + HCO_3^-$$

Acidemia and alkalemia are respectively defined as a plasma pH significantly below or above the normal arterial or venous value for the species in question (Chapter 18). Concurrent metabolic acid-base disturbances and the presence or absence of compensation through renal excretion will determine the actual degree of pH change accompanying hypocapnia or

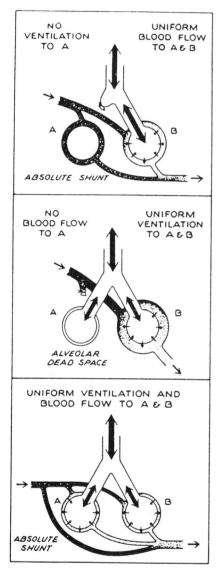

Fig. 6–4. Uneven ventilation and pulmonary blood flow. The alveoli, where rapid gas exchange occurs, are represented by rounded areas. Leading into these are tubes depicting the conducting airways of anatomic dead space in which no effective gas exchange occurs. Arrows entering the alveoli show distribution of total inspired gas (large arrow) to various alveoli. Small arrows crossing alveolar walls show the process of diffusion of O_2 out of the alveoli into the blood and of CO_2 from the blood into the alveoli. The shaded channel surrounding the alveoli represents pulmonary blood flow. It enters the capillary bed as mixed venous blood (dark) and emerges as arterialized blood (light). Top, lung A has no ventilation but normal blood flow, while lung B has normal ventilation and blood flow. Center, lung A has normal ventilation but no blood flow, while lung B has normal ventilation and increased blood flow. Bottom, a shunt of venous to arterial blood completely bypasses the lung. (Reproduced with permission from Comroe, J.H. Physiology of Respiration, 2nd ed. Year Book, Chicago, 1974.)

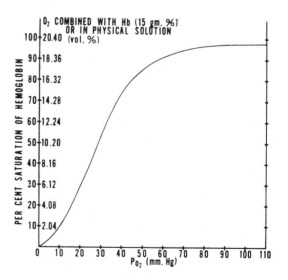

Fig. 6–5. Oxygen-hemoglobin dissociation curve of dog blood at pH 7.40. The percentage HbO_2 and O_2 content changes little when the PO2 changes from 100 mm Hg (normal) to 60 mm Hg, as may occur during cardiopulmonary dysfunction or disease. (With permission from Gillespie, J.R., and Martin, D.B. Long-term oxygen cage therapy for hypoxemic dogs. J Am Vet Med Assoc 156:717, 1970.)

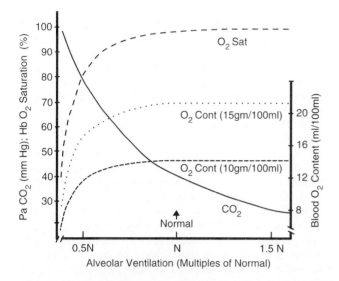

Fig. 6–6. Effect of altered alveolar ventilation on hemoglobin saturation, blood oxygen content, and $PaCO_2$ levels. As alveolar ventilation is halved, the $PaCO_2$ level doubles, illustrating the inverse and direct relationship between alveolar ventilation and carbon dioxide clearance. Note the difference in oxygen content with anemia (hemoglobin 10 g/100 mL instead of 15 g/100 mL), and the eventual sharp drop in hemoglobin oxygen saturation and oxygen content as alveolar ventilation decreases to less than 50% of the normal value. (See text for further explanation.)

hypercapnia. During general anesthesia hypoventilation and hypercapnia are far more likely to occur in spontaneously breathing animals, while hyperventilation and hypocapnia most often occur when tidal volumes are too large in smaller animals during IPPV.

The relationship between $\dot{V}_A$ and oxygen saturation (and in turn the oxygen content of arterial blood) is not linear because of the sigmoid shape of the hemoglobin saturation curve (Fig. 6–5). This factor has important clinical applications for the anesthetist. With a 50% decrease in $\dot{V}_A$, hemoglobin is still 80% saturated and the actual oxygen content of blood (if hemoglobin concentration is 15 g/dL) will have only fallen from 21.2 to 16.8 mL/dL. Such an animal would not likely demonstrate cyanotic mucous membranes, or even cardiovascular signs (tachycardia/bradycardia, increased/decreased blood pressure) associated with respiratory insufficiency. However, as the level of $\dot{V}_A$ decreases further, there is a sharp and potentially catastrophic decrease in the oxygen content of arterial blood so that at a $\dot{V}_A$ that is 40% of normal, hemoglobin saturation is 50% and the oxygen content has fallen to 7.04 mL/dL. This degree of hypoxemia may well lead to cardiorespiratory collapse quite suddenly. An understanding of this nonlinear effect of $\dot{V}_A$ deficiency on oxygen content helps to explain why an apparently "okay" animal on an intravenous general anesthetic breathing room air can suddenly stop breathing or go into cardiovascular collapse without any apparent change in the depth of anesthesia.

Figure 6–6 illustrates the important interrelationship between a lower hemoglobin level (e.g., 10 g/dL) and

blood oxygen content with altered ventilatory homeostasis. The blood oxygen content is reduced by nearly 7 mL/dL with a decrease in hemoglobin from 15 to 10 g/dL even when hemoglobin saturation is 100%, and dangerously low blood oxygen contents occur with further ventilatory depression.

Hypoxia refers to any state in which the oxygen in the lung, blood, and/or tissues is abnormally low, resulting in abnormal organ function and/or cellular damage. *Hypoxemia* refers to insufficient oxygenation of blood to meet metabolic requirement. In spontaneously breathing animals hypoxemia is characterized by PaO_2 levels lower than the normal level for the species. Resting PaO_2 levels in domestic species generally range from 80 to 100 mm Hg in healthy, unsedated animals (Table 6–2). Some clinicians consider a PaO_2 below 70 mm Hg($\sim$ 94% hemoglobin saturation) as hypoxemia in an animal at or near sea level, although the clinical significance of this degree of blood oxygen tension would vary depending upon factors such as the health and age of the animal, hemoglobin concentration, and the duration of low oxygen tension in relation to the rate of tissue metabolism (e.g., hypothermic patients). The causes of hypoxia and hypercapnia during anesthesia are given in Chapter 15.

Oxygen Transport in the Blood

Under normal conditions, oxygen is taken into the pulmonary alveoli and carbon dioxide is removed from them at a rate that is sufficient to maintain the composition of alveolar air at a relatively constant concentration. The composition of respiratory gases in man is shown in Table 6–4. At body temperature, alveolar air is saturated with water vapor, which has a pressure at 37° C of 48 mm Hg. If the pressure in the alveolus is 760 mm Hg, then the pressure due to dry air is 760 - 48 = 712 mm Hg. Knowing the composition of alveolar air, one can calculate the pressure of each gas in the alveolus.

Pressure of respiratory gases in the alveolus:

$$O_2 = (760 - 48) \times 0.14 = 100 \text{ mm Hg}$$
$$CO_2 = (760 - 48) \times 0.056 = 40 \text{ mm Hg}$$
$$N_2 = (760 - 48) \times 0.80 = 570 \text{ mm Hg}$$

Oxygen pressure in the lungs at sea level is approximately 100 mm Hg at 38° C. Under these conditions, 100 mL of plasma will hold 0.3 mL of oxygen in physical

Table 6–4. Composition of Respiratory Gases in Humans

Gas	Inspired Air (%)	Expired Air (%)	Alveolar Air (%)
O_2	20.95	16.1	14.0
CO_2	0.04	4.1	5.6
N_2*	79.0	79.2	80.0

*There is no change in the absolute concentration of N_2. The change in percent occurs because more oxygen is used than carbon dioxide produced.

solution. Whole blood, under the same conditions, will hold 20 mL of oxygen, or about 60 times as much as plasma. Carbon dioxide is similarly held by blood. Thus, it is apparent that oxygen and carbon dioxide in blood are transported largely in chemical combination, since both are carried by blood in much greater quantities than would occur if simple absorption took place.

In the lung, gas exchange occurs across both the alveolar and capillary membranes. The total distance across which exchange takes place is less than 1 micron; therefore, it occurs rapidly. Equilibrium almost develops between blood in the lungs and air in the alveolus, and the PO_2 in the blood almost equals the PO_2 in the alveolus. At complete saturation, each gram of hemoglobin combines with 1.36 mL of oxygen. This is the total carrying capacity of hemoglobin, or four oxygen molecules combined with each hemoglobin molecule. The ability of hemoglobin to combine with oxygen depends on the partial pressure of oxygen in the surrounding environment. The degree to which it will become saturated at various oxygen partial pressures varies considerably (Fig. 6–5). It is adjusted so that, even when ventilation is inefficient or the supply of oxygen is sparse as at higher altitudes, the degree of saturation still approaches 100%. For instance, although it is probably not fully saturated until it is exposed to a PO_2 of 250 mm Hg, hemoglobin is $\sim 94\%$ saturated when the oxygen partial pressure is only 70 mm Hg.

Although there is relatively little change in saturation between 70 and 250 mm Hg partial pressure of oxygen, a marked change occurs between 10 and 40 mm Hg, a partial pressure characteristic of actively metabolizing tissues. Thus, as hemoglobin is exposed to tissues having partial pressures of oxygen within this range, it must yield its oxygen to the tissues. The lower the PO_2 of these tissues, the greater the amount of oxygen that hemoglobin must give up. The degree to which hemoglobin gives up its oxygen is influenced by environmental pH, PCO_2, and temperature—all mechanisms that protect the metabolizing cell. As the pH decreases and the PCO_2 and local temperature increase, at any given PO_2 value, especially in the range of 10 to 40 mm Hg, hemoglobin releases oxygen to the surrounding environment more readily. It is also interesting to note that nature has adapted for the relatively lower oxygen environment of the fetus, since fetal hemoglobin carries a greater percentage of oxygen at a lower partial pressure.

Certain enzyme systems aid dissociation of oxygen from hemoglobin, the most completely studied being the enzyme system producing 2,3-diphosphoglycerate (2,3-DPG). This system enhances dissociation of oxygen from hemoglobin by competing with oxygen for the binding site. Lowered levels of enzyme increase the affinity of hemoglobin for oxygen and thus act as if the curve is shifted to the left. The oxygen tension at which 50% saturation of hemoglobin is achieved (P_{50}) is used to measure affinity of hemoglobin for oxygen. Reduced P_{50} occurs in septic patients and in carbon monoxide poisoning. The reverse has been encountered in chronic anemia. Since tissues require a given volume of oxygen

per unit of time, the hemoglobin concentration of blood has a significant influence upon oxygen content and delivery to the tissues.

Although an increase in the partial pressure of alveolar oxygen above normal results in only a small increase in oxygen carried by hemoglobin, plasma carries oxygen in an amount directly proportional to the partial pressure of oxygen in the alveoli. At normal atmospheric pressure, when the animal is breathing air at 38° C, 0.3 mL of oxygen is carried in solution in 100 mL of blood. If pure oxygen is administered, the partial pressure of oxygen in the alveoli is raised from 100 to almost 650 mm Hg. Plasma oxygen is thus elevated almost seven times, that is, from 0.3 to 1.8 mL per 100 mL of blood. The result is an increase of about 10% in oxygen content of the blood. This is of some importance, since oxygen transfers from blood to tissues by diffusion, and the process occurs at a rate proportional to the difference in oxygen tension between plasma and body tissues.

A common misconception is that oxygenation of a patient can be improved by increasing the *pressure* at which oxygen is administered. Except in hyperbaric chambers, improved oxygenation of the patient is obtained not by increasing the pressure of the gas mixture, but by increasing the *proportion* of oxygen in the mixture. At a positive pressure exceeding 40 mm Hg, the capillary circulation in the lungs is inhibited; therefore, it is not practical to administer oxygen at a pressure exceeding this pressure.

The partial pressures of oxygen in various portions of the cardiopulmonary system are as follows: Nasal air = 160 mm Hg; alveolar air = 100 mm Hg; arterial blood = 90–95 mm Hg; interstitial fluid = 30 mm Hg; intracellular fluid = 10 mm Hg; venous blood = 40 mm Hg. Little oxygen is lost in large blood vessels. A continuous pressure gradient is present from the alveolus to the tissue cell.

Oxygen has a weak covalent link with hemoglobin. Four factors influence oxygen uptake: (a) change in pH due to carbon dioxide, (b) the specific effect of carbon dioxide, (c) temperature, and (d) the effect of salts and enzymes. Decreasing the carbon dioxide tension in blood raises the pH and causes hemoglobin to bind more oxygen; when the carbon dioxide tension increases, the oxygen dissociation curve shifts to the right. Carbon dioxide reacts with hemoglobin to form carbaminohemoglobin, which has much less affinity for oxygen than does hemoglobin. Thus, it also exerts a specific effect. Increased temperature also favors dissociation of oxyhemoglobin. As metabolic rates increase, there is increased heat in the tissue, which, in turn, enhances dissociation of oxygen from hemoglobin. The salt and electrolyte concentrations of blood have also been shown to affect oxygenation, although the mechanism of action is obscure. Ordinarily, variations in electrolyte concentration of blood have little effect on oxygen transport.

Several factors increase the availability of oxygen to tissues:

1. *Increased circulation.* Up to five times as much blood may flow through the tissues.
2. *Increased respiratory rate.* The carbon dioxide tension of the blood regulates the respiratory center.
3. *Increased deoxygenation of a given volume of blood.* This may be caused by (a) lowered oxygen tension in the cells, (b) increased temperature with increased dissociation, and (c) increased amounts of metabolic byproducts, such as carbon dioxide and lactic acid, which are acidic. These factors favor local vasodilation with the consequent benefit of increased oxygen supply in instances of increased tissue metabolism.

When combined, these factors can increase oxygen availability to tissues over the resting state by a factor of 10. The rate of muscular activity is not limited by oxygen supply, since muscle can incur an oxygen deficit.

Carbon Dioxide Transport

Carbon dioxide is an end product of glucose oxidation. During severe exercise, the production of carbon dioxide is increased enormously, whereas during anesthesia production likely decreases. In the tissues, carbon dioxide in the presence of carbonic anhydrase reacts with water to form carbonic acid. Because of the blood buffer systems, transport of carbon dioxide to the lungs for excretion is effected with little change in blood pH. The importance of the lungs in excreting this volatile acid is illustrated by the fact that, in man, the kidneys eliminate 40 to 80 mEq per day, while the lungs eliminate 13,000 mEq per day.(43)

$$CO_2 + H_2O \rightleftarrows H_2CO_3 \rightleftarrows H^+ + HCO_3$$
$$\text{Carbonic Anhydrase}$$

Under ordinary circumstances, the pH of venous blood is only 0.01 to 0.03 pH units lower than that of arterial blood. The carbon dioxide pressure gradient, opposite to that of oxygen, exists from the tissues to the atmospheric air: Tissues = 50 mm Hg (during exercise may be higher); venous blood = 46 mm Hg; alveolar air = 40 mm Hg; expired air = 32 mm Hg; atmospheric air = 0.3 mm Hg; and arterial blood = 40 mm Hg (equilibrium with alveolar air). Some carbon dioxide is carried dissolved in the plasma. This is divided into (a) H_2CO_3, and (b) carbon dioxide in simple solution. These are referred to as *carbonic acid.* The amount of carbon dioxide transported as carbonic acid is about 10% of the total and is found in the plasma. The greater portion of carbon dioxide transport is achieved in the form of *bicarbonate.* This may occur (a) in plasma through buffering action with plasma protein (this accounts for 5% of carbon dioxide transport), or (b) by formation of bicarbonate in the red blood cell accompanied by the chloride shift (this accounts for approximately 70%) (Fig. 6–7). The excellent buffering capacity of hemoglobin allows changes in hydrogen ion content to occur during this process with minimal change in pH.

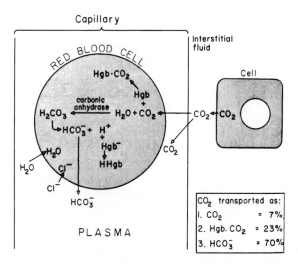

Fig. 6–7. Transport of carbon dioxide in the blood. (With permission from Guyton, A.C. Textbook of Medical Physiology, 6th ed. WB Saunders, Philadelphia, 1981.)

As blood passes to the venous side of the vascular system, carbon dioxide is absorbed and diffuses into the red blood cell (Fig. 6–7). Here it is converted to carbonic acid. Reduced hemoglobin, a weaker acid, gives up its alkali, chiefly potassium, to carbonic acid. As bicarbonate is thus formed and accumulates in the erythrocyte, the ionic equilibrium between cell and plasma is upset. The corpuscular membrane is impermeable to potassium, but bicarbonate diffuses through into the plasma. Chloride ions, in turn, shift into the cell to restore ionic equilibrium and balance the potassium. The chloride shift enables carbon dioxide to be carried without any change in blood pH and is the main method of transport.

A third method by which carbon dioxide is carried is in the form of carbamino compounds. Amino acids and aliphatic amines combine with carbon dioxide to form unstable carbamino compounds. Hemoglobin is the main protein acting in this manner, though many can do so. The efficiency of this reaction is greater with Hb than with HbO_2. Thus, as HbO_2 dissociates, its capacity to carry CO_2 increases.(2, 43) The mechanisms of carbon dioxide and oxygen transport are integrated in the blood in at least three ways.

1. The acidity of carbonic acid produced in the tissues favors release of oxygen without a change in oxygen tension. The release of carbon dioxide in the lungs favors oxygen uptake (Bohr effect).
2. Release of oxygen favors carbon dioxide uptake and vice versa in the carbamino mechanism. Upon the release of oxygen, hemoglobin becomes a weaker acid and is more capable of accepting hydrogen ions, thereby facilitating its buffering effect (Haldane effect).
3. The two acid forms of the hemoglobin molecule favor dissociation by shifting from one form to the other. Oxygen uptake favors carbon dioxide loss and vice versa.

Just as the amount of oxygen transported by the blood depends on the partial pressure of oxygen to which the blood is exposed, so is carbon dioxide transport likewise affected; however, the carbon dioxide dissociation curve is more or less linear. Thus, in contrast to the minimal effects on oxygen content (Fig. 6–6), hyper- and hypoventilation may have marked effects on carbon dioxide content of blood and tissues.

Upper Airway Obstruction

With the onset of general anesthesia there is a relaxation of the nasal alar and pharyngeal musculature and, in deeper planes, abolishment of the cough reflex. The net effect is to predispose toward upper airway obstruction. This is particularly evident in brachycephalic dogs suffering from stenotic nares, an elongated soft palate, everted lateral laryngeal ventricles, and/or a hypoplastic trachea. In these animals the onset of general anesthesia may produce serious and potentially fatal upper airway obstruction unless the trachea is intubated. Experience has shown that it is preferable to perform endotracheal intubation in all anesthetized dogs, partly to protect against upper airway obstruction, but also to protect against possible aspiration of secretions or refluxed gastric contents from the stomach. It is important, however, that the endotracheal intubation be done atraumatically. Routine use of a laryngoscope reduces trauma during intubation. In many domestic and laboratory species the decision as to whether to utilize an endotracheal tube or not is a risk/benefit decision that must be determined by the species involved, the anesthetic regimen employed and the experience of the anesthetist, the intended operation, the health of the animal, and the duration of anesthesia (Chapter 20).

In ruminants endotracheal intubation is required for all but the shortest anesthetics, such as diazepam premedication with low-dose ketamine in sheep, calves, and goats, which only lasts about 5 minutes. The prime reason for endotracheal intubation is to protect against aspiration of rumen contents after active or passive regurgitation. In swine endotracheal intubation is comparatively difficult and requires considerable experience if trauma is to be avoided. Swine have inherently small airways, and they are more likely to develop apnea than other domestic species. Nevertheless, for most relatively short-duration surgeries (e.g., hernia repair, cryptorchidectomy) the risk/benefit balance is better served by not intubating swine, but instead by paying careful attention to the depth of anesthesia and to the character of respiration and head position so as to minimize the chance of serious upper airway obstruction. In most species the best airway is provided when the head is kept in a somewhat extended position: The pig is unusual in that the best airway is provided with the head at a normal angle to the neck (Chapter 20).

If significant upper airway obstruction occurs in any species, and the depth of anesthesia is not excessive, the animal usually develops an exaggerated respiratory effort that is primarily abdominal in character. The chest wall may even move inward on inspiration (paradoxical respiration) if the degree of upper airway obstruction is moderate or severe. The only other clinical situation that produces this subtle but distinctive change in the character of respiration is extremely deep anesthesia. This usually occurs at an anesthetic plane just before complete cessation of respiratory drive, that is apnea, ensues (Chapter 2).

In rodents–such as mice, gerbils, hamsters, and guinea pigs–and in rabbits, endotracheal intubation may be difficult unless the anesthetist is experienced with the technique and has special equipment. In these species, longer, well-controlled periods of anesthesia for experimental purposes may well require endotracheal intubation. Shorter procedures carried out in a veterinary practice may often be done without using an endotracheal tube. A suitable face mask and nonrebreathing administration system may be used for oxygen administration (in the case of injectable anesthesia) or for administration of an oxygen/inhalant regimen using a precision vaporizer. When the anesthetist is capable of doing atraumatic endotracheal intubation and has suitably small tubes (3 to 4 mm), it is preferable to intubate ferrets and rabbits, since surgical anesthetic planes produce considerable respiratory depression in both species, and it is much easier to deal with apnea if an endotracheal tube is already in place (Chapter 21).

There is some controversy as to whether or not an endotracheal tube should always be placed in cats for short-duration procedures (e.g., neutering). Cats tend to maintain a patent airway somewhat more effectively than do other species, unless drugs are used (e.g., ether) that increase the incidence of secretions and/or laryngospasm. Laryngospasm is comparatively rare when halothane or isoflurane are administered by mask, or when ketamine is used along with diazepam, acepromazine, or low-dose xylazine for injectable anesthesia. Moreover, endotracheal intubation requires a deeper level of anesthesia than is needed for some minor surgery/diagnostic procedures. Laryngospasm is more likely to occur postanesthesia when the larynx has been traumatized during intubation or when the endotracheal tubes have been cleared with some sort of detergent or disinfectant between animals without adequate rinsing. In a large morbidity/mortality study carried out in the United Kingdom, postanesthetic airway obstruction was one of the more frequently encountered problems in cats (45), and the suspicion is that this might well be associated with trauma during insertion of an endotracheal tube into the airway. On the other hand, there can be no denying the many advantages associated with endotracheal intubation in the cat, as with other species. A patent airway is immediately available if the animal needs IPPV because of apnea or respiratory insufficiency, the risk of aspiration of gastric contents is markedly reduced, and it is easier to scavenge anesthetic waste gases if an inhalant anesthetic is being used. In cats, laryngeal desensitization with lidocaine will help to reduce spasm and

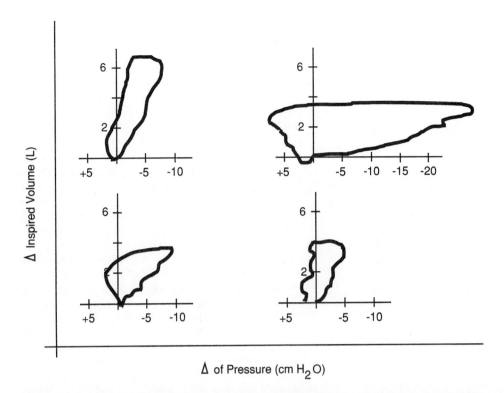

Δ Inspired Volume (L)

Δ of Pressure (cm H₂O)

Fig. 6–8. Changes in nonelastic work of breathing with the onset of general anesthesia (thiobarbiturate) in a spontaneously breathing horse. The change in transpulmonary pressure (airway opening to esophageal balloon) is shown as the abscissa, and the change in volume (tidal volume) is shown on the ordinate scale. The area within the loops is a measure of the nonelastic work of breathing and is a reflection of the airway resistance as well as a small component of tissue resistance. The upper left loop was obtained from the conscious horse breathing quietly; the upper right loop was obtained after 15 minutes of anesthesia with the horse in lateral recumbency and breathing without an endotracheal tube in place; the lower left loop is after the horse was intubated with a 25-mm tube; and the lower right loop was obtained once the horse stood in recovery with the tube removed. Note the large increase in nonelastic work of breathing during anesthesia until an endotracheal tube is inserted, and that fairly large negative pressures (10 to 15 cm H₂O) must be generated before there is an appreciable volume of inspired gas. This is indicative of upper airway obstruction. (W. McDonell, unpublished observations.)

trauma associated with the placement of a tube. Endotracheal tube placement for shorter procedures is not mandatory, providing that emergency airway and oxygen are readily available and the patency of the airway is being continuously monitored.

Veterinary anesthesia textbooks have hitherto placed little emphasis on the need to provide for a secure airway in horses, primarily because regurgitation is very rare. While it is true that short-duration, injectable field anesthetic techniques have been carried out for many years without the use of an endotracheal tube, a considerable degree of upper airway obstruction does occur in the horse (Fig. 6–8), primarily because the nostrils no longer flare during inspiration. As such, placement of an endotracheal tube may be considered desirable.(46)

This tendency toward upper airway obstruction increases when a horse has been anesthetized for longer than 1 or 2 hours, especially when in dorsal recumbency. It is thought that passive congestion and tissue swelling occur because the nasopharynx structures are lower than the heart in the anesthetized animal, and that this predisposes the animal to airway obstruction in the recovery period when the endotracheal tube is removed. As a result, many equine anesthetists now secure an orotracheal, nasotracheal or nasopharyngeal airway during the recovery process whenever horses have been anesthetized for any extended length of time (i.e., over 30–45 minutes).(47, 48) Clinically, it appears that the insurance of an adequate diameter patent airway while the horse is trying to get up (and is breathing vigorously) prevents the "panic" associated with partial or complete airway obstruction and leads to more controlled recoveries. There is a need for large-scale morbidity/mortality studies that address the issue of when and where endotracheal tubes should be used during routine veterinary anesthesia, especially in a practice setting.

Anesthetic Alteration of the Control of Respiration

Respiratory drive and the adjustment of f, V_T, and $\dot{V}_A$ are achieved in the conscious animal through a complex neural regulatory mechanism. Respiratory rhythm originates in the medulla and is modified by inputs from higher brain centers and the activity of chemoreceptor, pulmonary, and airway receptors. The central neural control mechanisms regulate the activity of the primary and accessory respiratory muscles, producing gas movement into and out of the lung and tracheobron-

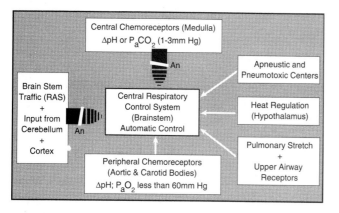

Fig. 6–9. Schematic diagram of the control of ventilation in conscious and anesthetized animals. In the conscious animal the level of alveolar ventilation is primarily determined by the P_aCO_2 level (as sensed by the central chemoreceptors) and the level of brain-stem traffic, with the apneustic and pneumotoxic centers and the stretch receptors governing the relationship between tidal volume and frequency to achieve the required alveolar ventilation. General anesthesia (An) reduces brain-stem traffic and the chemoreceptor response to carbon dioxide, leading to an increase in P_aCO_2. In most species the peripheral chemoreceptors begin to influence the level of alveolar ventilation if P_aO_2 falls below 60 mm Hg.

chial tree. These control mechanisms are described in detail elsewhere.(5, 6, 49) Although there is certainly a similarity in the respiratory control mechanism between species, it is important to realize that various components may assume greater importance in different species.(1, 50)

NORMAL CONTROL MECHANISMS

As important as the detailed information referred to earlier is in helping us understand the respiratory adaptations to high altitude, disease, and exercise, for the successful management of clinical anesthesia a much simplified understanding of the control of respiration will suffice (Fig. 6–9). In conscious animals $\dot{V}_E$ and $\dot{V}_A$ are primarily determined by central chemoreceptor responsiveness to $PaCO_2$ levels. The *central chemoreceptors*, located on the ventral surface of the medulla and bathed by cerebrospinal fluid, are exquisitely sensitive to changes in $PaCO_2$ levels because CO_2 is readily diffusible into cerebrospinal fluid and the central chemoreceptor cell. The changes in $PaCO_2$ are probably ultimately detected as a change in the pH within the chemoreceptor cell. This ventilatory response to CO_2 is often presented as a response curve wherein $\dot{V}_A$ or $\dot{V}_E$ are plotted against $PaCO_2$, P_ACO_2, the end-tidal carbon dioxide partial pressure ($P_{ET}CO_2$), or the inspired carbon dioxide level (Fig. 6–10A). An increase in $PaCO_2$ of 3 to 5 mm Hg will produce a rapid doubling or tripling of $\dot{V}_A$ in an effort to return $PaCO_2$ to eucapnic levels. This response is a little less sensitive in horses(51, 52), and a lot less sensitive in burrowing and diving mammals.(53) In ruminants, the gas produced in the rumen may consist of more than 60% carbon dioxide, and when it is eructated a significant proportion of this gas is inhaled, contributing to a cyclic breathing pat-

tern.(49) A fall in arterial pH will also stimulate respiration through the central and peripheral chemoreceptors, as seen with metabolic acidosis: this response is slower. The central chemoreceptors are not responsive to alterations in PaO_2 levels.

Peripheral chemoreceptors are located in the carotid and aortic bodies, and these receptors generally only play a significant part in respiratory drive when PaO_2 levels fall below 60 mm Hg.(6, 52) This is illustrated in Figure 6–10B, drawn from a study on conscious horses.(54) As the F_IO_2 was decreased from 1.0 (100% inspired oxygen) down to 0.16, there was no change in $\dot{V}_E$. At an F_IO_2 of 0.16 the alveolar oxygen tension (P_AO_2) would be 60 to 65 mm Hg at sea level. In sheep, goats, calves, and ponies, however, carotid body denervation results in some hypoventilation, hypoxemia, and hypercapnia, and it is estimated that carotid body receptor activity is responsible for up to 30% of the resting $\dot{V}_A$ drive in calves at sea level (55), and up to 40% in miniature pigs.(17)

The activity of the central neural systems and the level of ventilatory drive are also influenced by the general level of central nervous system activity, especially by traffic through the reticular activating system (RAS). This is evidenced by the decrease in $\dot{V}_A$ and small increase in $PaCO_2$ that accompany sleep, and by the fact that exercising animals commonly become hypocapnic even if tissue oxygen delivery is adequate. Anesthetists make good use of this link between RAS activity and respiratory drive by using an increase in sensory stimulation (limb flexion, twisting a horse's ear, rolling a dog or cat over, or vigorously rubbing the body surface) to increase ventilatory drive during emergence from inhalation anesthesia, thereby speeding inhalant drug elimination and recovery.

The apneustic and pneumotaxic centers, and pulmonary and airway receptors, are primarily responsible for adjusting the balance between f and V_T to achieve a given level of $\dot{V}_A$, usually in a way that minimizes the energy cost of breathing. Although the function of these receptors is generally not considered to be greatly influenced by the action of anesthetic and perianesthetic agents, they may play a part in some of the species differences we see in response to a particular drug or group of drugs. In smaller species as the dose of an inhalant agent increases, f often remains constant or increases (56, 57), while in the horse f remains more or less constant as the depth of halothane or isoflurane anesthesia increases.(58) Respiratory rate is usually less with isoflurane than with halothane at an equipotent dose, while V_T is larger.(58) The barbiturates usually decrease f and V_T as the dose is increased, while the primary response to increasing inhalant doses is to reduce V_T (ether is an exception). In ruminants general anesthesia is often associated with tachypnea and very shallow breathing.(59, 60) All of these differences might well originate from species and/or drug differences in the central inspiratory/expiratory switching mechanisms or lung receptor activity (stretch receptors, irritant receptors, C-fibers), but so far the evidence is primarily speculative. Irritant airway receptor activity, especially in the larynx and tracheal regions, appears to differ quite markedly between species. The horse, for instance, has a weak laryngeal reflex and it is rather easy to insert a nasoendotracheal tube in the conscious animal, even without the aid of local anesthesia (Chapter 20). In contrast, swine and cats have a strong laryngeal reflex, and fairly deep anesthesia is required for easy endotracheal intubation unless local desensitization is produced using a topical anesthetic. Dogs are intermediate in their response (Chapter 17).

Apneic Threshold. The *apneic threshold* is the $PaCO_2$ level at which ventilation becomes zero, that is, where spontaneous ventilatory effort ceases (Fig. 6–10A). If the $PaCO_2$ is reduced by 5 to 9 mm Hg from normal values through voluntary hyperventilation (conscious human), or by artificial ventilation of sedated or anesthetized animals, apnea is produced. The distance between the resting $PaCO_2$ level and the apnea threshold is relatively constant (i.e., 5–9 mm Hg) irrespective of the anesthetic depth.(58) The veterinary anesthetist makes use of the apneic threshold to "gain control" of respiration (i.e. abolish spontaneous efforts) when putting an animal on a ventilator, or to temporarily provide for a quiet surgical field without having to resort to the use of muscle relaxant drugs.

DRUG EFFECT ON CONTROL OF VENTILATION

Anesthetics and some perianesthetic drugs alter the central and peripheral chemoreceptor response to carbon dioxide and oxygen in a dose-dependent manner.(61-63) This has important clinical implications in terms of maintaining homeostasis during the peri-operative period. There will also be a diminution in external signs in an hypoxemic or hypercarbic anesthetized animal. Whereas unsedated animals usually demonstrate obvious tachypnea and an increase in V_T or respiratory effort in response to serious hypoxemia or hypercapnia, these external "signs" of an impending crisis may well be absent or greatly diminished in the anesthetized animal.

General anesthesia. All of the general anesthetic agents in current use produce a dose-dependent decrease in the response to carbon dioxide.(24, 62) With the commonly used inhalant agents (enflurane, halothane, isoflurane) the carbon dioxide response is almost flat at 2.0 MAC (Fig. 6–11).(64) The reduced sensory input and central sensitivity to carbon dioxide produces a marked fall in $\dot{V}_A$, usually through a dose-related fall in V_T with f being reasonably well maintained. A proportional increase in V_D/V_T occurs, since V_{Danat} is more or less constant. As a result of these changes, $PaCO_2$ levels increase as the anesthetic dose is increased when animals breathe spontaneously (Fig. 6–12A). In light anesthetic planes (e.g., 1.2 MAC) $PaCO_2$ will generally remain moderately elevated, but stable, over many hours of anesthesia, whereas at higher concentrations or in ruminants there is a progressive increase in $PaCO_2$ over time. The degree of hypercarbia at equipotent doses of inhalant (and intravenous) anesthetic agents varies with the species and the degree of surgical stimulation (Figure 6–12B).

In ruminants the degree of hypercarbia is greater with equipotent inhalant anesthetic doses than for horses and dogs (Fig. 6–12B). Clinically swine and rabbits also seem to be more prone to hypercarbia, while

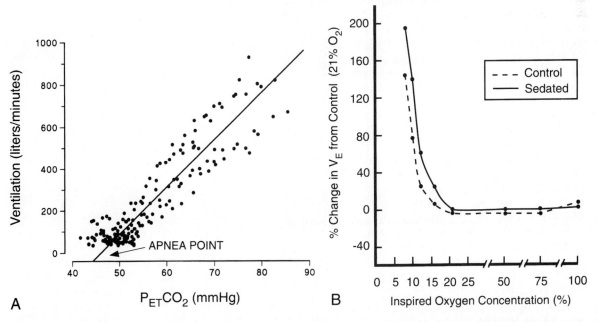

Fig. 6–10. A, A carbon dioxide response curve for six horses showing individual data points, the regression line and the theoretical apnea point. Minute ventilation is plotted against end-tidal CO_2. The horses were permitted to rebreathe carbon dioxide from a large spirometer filled with 30% oxygen. (Data modified from Gauvreau et al.[51]) B, An oxygen response curve for unsedated horses and horses sedated with acepromazine. The percentage change in ventilation is plotted against the inspired oxygen concentration. (Data modified from Muir and Hamlin.[54])

deep-diving seals may become totally apneic during light levels of anesthesia, or even just opioid sedation.(70) When surgery is being carried out, the level of respiratory depression is usually less and the differences between drugs may disappear. In dorsally recumbent, spontaneously breathing pregnant mares induced with xylazine and thiamylal sodium and maintained on halothane or isoflurane for laparotomy surgery, $PaCO_2$ levels increased from 53.8 to 58.3 mm Hg during halothane, and were 60.7 to 60.5 mm Hg during isoflurane anesthesia. There was no significant difference in $PaCO_2$ (or PaO_2) levels with the two agents from 30 to 90 minutes, although f was lower (4 to 5/min) with isoflurane than with halothane (8 to 10/min).(71)

Barbiturates, propofol, and the cyclohexamines (ketamine, phencyclidine, tiletamine) also produce a similar dose-related alteration of the carbon dioxide response, which may, in the case of barbiturates, outlast the period of actual anesthesia by some time.(72) Although it is generally considered that ketamine is not as much of a respiratory depressant as the barbiturates (63), clinical experience and survey studies have shown that safe, clinically effective doses of ketamine may induce apnea in some susceptible individuals.(45) The typical response to increasing doses of barbiturates is for both V_T and f to decrease. When injectable anesthetics are used before inhalation agents, as is commonly done in clinical veterinary anesthesia, the respiratory depressant effects of both drugs are at least additive.(72)

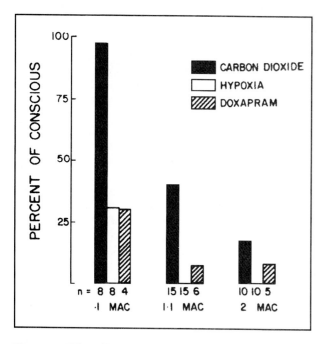

Fig. 6–11. Effect of halothane sedation (0.1 MAC) and anesthesia (1.1 and 2.0 MAC) on depression of the ventilatory response to hypoxia, hypercapnia, and doxapram expressed as a percentage of the awake control response. (Reproduced with permission from Knill, R.L., and Gelb, A.W. Ventilatory response to hypoxia and hypercapnia during halothane sedation and anesthesia in man. Anesthesiology 49:244-251, 1978.

Although the control of ventilation during anesthesia is primarily determined by central carbon dioxide responsiveness (albeit reduced), during very deep barbiturate anesthesia CO_2 ventilatory drive may disappear and the drive becomes hypoxic. Hypoxic drive sensitivity is also lessened appreciably by general anesthetics (at least inhalants) in a dose-related manner (Fig. 6–11).(64) It is interesting to note that, although the peripheral chemoreceptor response to PaO_2 at physiologic levels (80–110 mm Hg) is virtually nonexistent in conscious animals, in anesthetized horses, dogs, and ducks it has been shown that $PaCO_2$ levels are greater at F_IO_2 1.0 than F_IO_2 0.3.(50, 73, 74) It is therefore possible that the high oxygen levels used in most inhalant regimens contribute somewhat to depression of ventilation while helping to ensure that the level of oxygenation is adequate.

Opioids. When given alone, opioids shift the carbon dioxide response curve to the right with little change in slope, except at very high doses. This means that the resting $PaCO_2$ level might be a little higher in an animal receiving a therapeutic dose of an opioid for premedication or postoperative recovery, but that the response to further carbon dioxide challenge (from metabolism, airway obstruction, etc.) will not be abolished. Clinically, when opioids are used at high doses as part of a balanced anesthetic regimen there is an additive effect of the opioid depression of the respiratory center and the general anesthetic, and apnea may be produced.(75) In addition, the mu opioids in particular tend to produce rapid shallow breathing in dogs (76), which may interfere with the subsequent uptake of an inhalant anesthetic.

At the doses commonly employed for routine opioid premedication or postoperative analgesia in veterinary practice, significant respiratory depression is very rarely seen, at least in terms of producing hypercapnia.(76-78) Frequency of ventilation may decrease owing to a decrease in apprehension. In fact, effective alveolar ventilation may well improve when opioid analgesics are employed for postoperative pain relief.(79) The postoperative use of opioids has been implicated in the development of an increased incidence of postoperative atelectasis and hypoxemia in humans, especially during sleep.(80) Clinical evidence would suggest that the incidence of similar problems in veterinary patients is rare, but it is an area that warrants further study.

The historical tendency to minimize the use of opioids for postoperative analgesia because of the fear of serious respiratory problems is simply not based on facts, as is now well recognized.(81) There is a ceiling effect and less respiratory depression associated with opioid agonists/antagonists (e.g., pentazocine, butorphanol, nalbuphine, buprenorphine) when used at high doses than with the pure mu-agonists (meperidine, morphine, oxymorphone).(82) Using the epidural route of administration helps to ensure that there is minimal postoperative respiratory depression with high-risk cases.(83, 84)

Tranquilizers. The phenothiazine and benzodiazepine sedatives often reduce the respiratory rate,

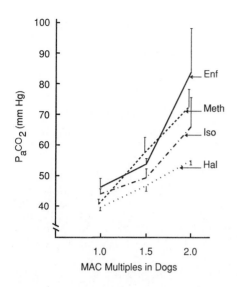

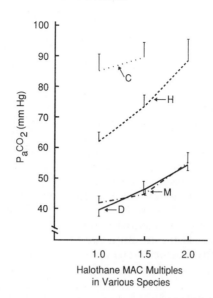

Fig. 6-12. A, Influence of increasing anesthetic dose (multiples of MAC) on $PaCO_2$ in spontaneously breathing dogs anesthetized with enflurane (Enf), methoxyflurane (Meth), isoflurane (Iso) or halothane (Hal). (Data compiled from a series of studies done by Steffey and co-workers.)

B, Differences in the $PaCO_2$ with spontaneous breathing and increasing halothane levels (multiples of MAC) in calves (C), horses (H), monkeys (M), and dogs (D). (Data compiled from a series of studies done by Steffey and co-workers.)

especially if the animal is somewhat excited prior to administration, but they do not appreciably alter arterial blood gas tensions.(77, 85, 86) There are few studies of the effect of these drugs on carbon dioxide responsiveness, especially in animals. Horses sedated with acepromazine (0.65 mg/kg IV) responded similarly, in terms of $\dot{V}_E$ change, to unsedated horses until the level of hypoxia or hypercapnia was quite severe (F_IO_2 0.1 or F_ICO_2 0.06), at which time the response was lessened.(54) When used alone diazepam (0.05 to 0.4 mg/kg IV) does not produce significant changes in PaO_2 or $PaCO_2$ in horses.(87) The respiratory protective nature of these drugs is such that when they are combined with a general anesthetic, and the required dose of the general anesthetic is thereby lessened, ventilation is better than when an equipotent dose of the general anesthetic (barbiturate, inhalant) is used alone. This may be one of the reasons why phenothiazine and benzodiazepine tranquilizers are widely employed as preanesthetic drugs in clinical practice.

Sedatives/hypnotics. The alpha$_2$-adrenoceptor agonists produce a more complicated effect on respiration. The usual clinical doses of xylazine and detomidine produce laryngeal relaxation in the horse and an alteration in pulmonary mechanics (dynamic compliance and pulmonary resistance).(88, 89) Some, but not all, of this effect is produced by the change in position of the head with sedation.(90) Certainly, the degree of laryngeal dysfunction produced by alpha$_2$-agonist sedation in the horse precludes using this type of sedation when carrying out diagnostic examination of the larynx. Although most studies have failed to demonstrate a significant increase in $PaCO_2$ levels after sedation of the horse with xylazine, detomidine, or romifidine (91, 92), a fall in PaO_2 of 10 to 20 mm Hg is often (88, 90, 91), but not always seen.(88)

In sheep it is apparent that clinically useful sedative doses of xylazine (93) and other alpha$_2$-agonists (94) produce significant hypoxemia without producing hypoventilation. Sheep remain eucapnic or even become hypocapnic from the hypoxic stimulus. This response is associated with an increased "stiffness" (decrease in compliance) of the respiratory system (chest wall and lung together), even when an endotracheal tube is in place (95), and with an increase in the maximum change in transpulmonary pressure during tidal breathing.(94) It appears that there is an increase in lower airway resistance in sheep after alpha$_2$-agonist sedation for yet unexplained reasons. It is not clear if this response also occurs in other ruminants, partly because the effect of a change in body position was not taken into consideration in many studies. When healthy adult Holstein cows ($n = 7$) positioned in left lateral recumbency (on a tilt table) were given 0.2 mg/kg xylazine IV, mean PaO_2 levels decreased from 79.0 ± 4.5 (SEM) to 54.5 ± 2.7 mm Hg at 5 minutes and to 58.4 ± 2.6 at 15 minutes postxylazine. There was also a significant increase in $PaCO_2$ levels from 34.9 ± 2.0 mm Hg to more normal levels of 45.0 ± 2.1 and 45.6 ± 1.4 mm Hg at 5 and 15 min (Warren and McDonell, unpublished data). In another study carried out on dorsally recumbent adult cows, PaO_2 levels were significantly lower in xylazine-sedated cows (0.05 mg/kg IV) when compared to unsedated cows, but the reduction in arterial oxygen tension was no different from that seen with acepromazine or chloral hydrate sedation.(96)

In cats, xylazine sedation does not apparently produce hypercapnia or hypoxemia (97), whereas in dogs the respiratory effects of xylazine have not been definitively documented. Some investigators have demonstrated fairly large reductions in arterial oxygen tension without hypercapnia in dogs (98), while others have not observed this response using a similar dose of xylazine.(99, 100) Decreases in PaO_2 occur when ketamine (10 mg/kg) and xylazine are given to dogs breathing room air.(100) It is fair to say that further investigations in dogs are needed to assess the respiratory depressant effects of alpha$_2$-agonists when used in various drug combinations and dosages before any definitive recommendations on their use in this species can be made.

Changes in Ventilation/Perfusion Relationships During Anesthesia

The onset of general anesthesia (3, 4), or in the case of larger animals even a change in body position (101-104), often produces lower PaO_2 levels than expected for the delivered concentration of inspired oxygen. This change can occur even without hypoventilation and during both spontaneous and controlled breathing. Lower PaO_2 is produced by altered ventilation/perfusion ratios within the lung. Much of what we know about this phenomenon of altered gas exchange is derived from studies of the human response to anesthesia, some experiments in dogs, and many studies on anesthetized horses. It is obvious when one looks at the collective results that there are important species differences, although the reason(s) for these differences are not always obvious.

VENTILATION/PERFUSION SCATTER UNDER NORMAL CONDITIONS

To understand how anesthesia alters ventilation/perfusion (or V/Q) relationships, it is first necessary to appreciate the scatter of V/Q ratios in the normal lung of unanesthetized animals, and to appreciate the

mechanisms by which regional matching of pulmonary blood flow and alveolar ventilation are optimized.(3, 41) A schematic representation of V/Q relationships in the conscious and anesthetized animal is shown in Fig. 6–13.

Intrapleural pressure is more subatmospheric over the uppermost areas of the lung than adjacent to dependent regions because of the "weight" of the lung within the thoracic cavity.(39, 105) Partly because of differences in lung density between species and partly because of differences in chest wall configuration, the total vertical gradient of intrapleural pressure over the whole lung apparently does not differ much between species, despite large differences in lung size and height. This is fortuitous, because otherwise there would be a tendency for too great a discrepancy between the size of the uppermost and lowermost alveoli. The gradient of intrapleural pressure means that in the unanesthetized animal the uppermost alveoli (A in Fig. 6–13) are larger than alveoli in the middle and lower regions of the lung (C and D). Since the pressure-volume curve of the lung is sigmoid, the larger alveoli tend to be on the flat part of the curve and thus distend less for any given change of intrapleural pressure during inspiration.(3, 106) Thus, the more dependent alveoli (D) receive proportionally

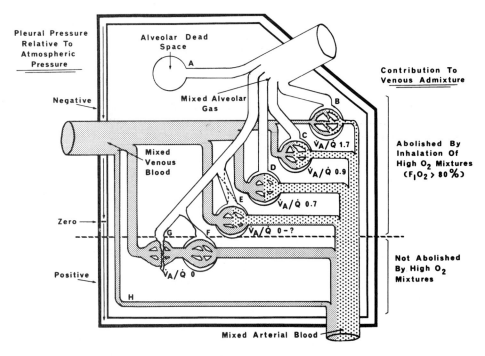

Fig. 6–13. Schematic diagram of ventilation/perfusion relationships in the lung and the primary mechanisms whereby venous admixture and the $P_{(A-a)}O_2$ gradient increases during anesthesia. The gradient of pleural pressure is shown with the uppermost aspect of the pleural space more subatmospheric than the dependent region, which may even become positive relative to atmosphere if lung volume decreases enough. The inflow of gas is represented by the unshaded area in the tracheobronchial tree. This inspired gas may reach alveoli that are not perfused (A), may reach alveoli that are variably perfused (B, C, D), or may intermittently reach alveoli (E) through airways that only open later during the inspiration. Nonventilated alveoli (F) will usually become atelectatic (G), especially when high inspired oxygen levels are used. The fine shaded area represents the flow of mixed venous blood from the pulmonary artery, and the coarse shaded area represents postcapillary oxygenated blood. Blood flow from alveoli with low V/Q ratios (E), from nonventilated alveoli, or from anatomic shunt areas (H) will all contribute to the venous admixture effect and increase the $P_{(A-a)}O_2$ gradient. The venous admixture effect of low V/Q areas is abolished when high-oxygen mixtures are inhaled, as even poorly ventilated alveoli will have sufficient oxygen to oxygenate the blood going past.

more of an inspired tidal volume, unless there is a disease process (e.g., chronic airway obstruction, pneumonia) or decrease in lung volume that leads to intermittent or complete airway closure (E and F), or actual atelectasis (G).

At the same time there is a vertical gradient of pulmonary blood flow, since the pulmonary artery is a low-pressure system affected by hydrostatic pressure.(42, 107) Some alveoli may receive no perfusion (A) and constitute an alveolar dead space, while in Fig. 6–13 alveolus D receives more perfusion than B. In most species the increased ventilation of alveolus D is not sufficient to match the higher perfusion, and the V/Q ratio of alveolus D is 0.7, versus the V/Q ratio of 1.7 for alveolus B. Overall, the collective scatter of V/Q ratios for the normal lung in the resting individual is 0.8 to 0.9.

Based on radioisotope distribution evidence, the vertical gradient of perfusion and ventilation is minimal in the standing dog with a horizontal lung (108), and matching of vertical perfusion and ventilation gradients in the conscious horse is such that there is little difference in V/Q in different lung regions.(109) More recent studies in horses using a multiple inert gas washout method suggest the scatter of V/Q ratios in the conscious horse is very similar to that seen in humans.(110) No regions of low V/Q were identified, but a minor shunt component (< 3% of cardiac output) was observed. A high V/Q area was observed (constituting 3 to 17% of the total), and the extent of this area was correlated with lower pulmonary artery pressures.(110)

When pulmonary artery blood flows through vascular channels not adjacent to alveoli (Fig. 6–13H) or passes nonventilated alveoli (G and F), unoxygenated blood will pass from the right side of the circulation into the left side, leading to a lower PaO_2.

In the conscious, unsedated animal, if regional ventilation is decreased there is a local vasoconstriction (hypoxic pulmonary vasoconstriction, or HPV) that tends to divert blood flow away from underventilated areas of the lung.(107) There is an apparent difference in the strength of the HPV response to whole lung hypoxia in various species (111), based on high-altitude and excised lung studies.(112, 113) Cattle and swine have a strong reflex, while ponies, cats, and rabbits have an intermediate response. Sheep, cats, and dogs show less response. It appears, however, that under normal conditions even species with a weak hypoxic pulmonary reflex are capable of considerable blood flow diversion in response to regional areas of low alveolar O_2 content.(111, 114)

MEASUREMENT OF V/Q MISMATCH

When the barometric pressure, inspired oxygen concentration, $PaCO_2$, and respiratory quotient are known, it is possible to calculate the partial pressure of oxygen in the alveolus (P_AO_2) using one form of the alveolar air equation (Fig. 6–2). The difference between this value and the PaO_2, that is, the alveolar-to-arterial gradient or the $P_{(A-a)}O_2$, provides a convenient and practical mea-

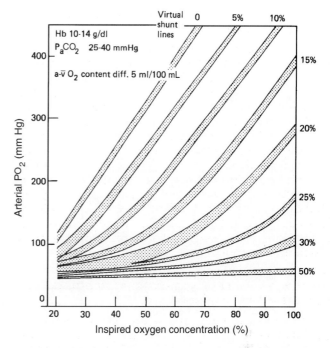

Fig. 6–14. An isoshunt diagram depicting the relationship between inspired oxygen concentration, arterial PO_2 and various degrees of venous admixture or pulmonary shunt. Shunt flow is expressed as a percentage of cardiac output. The arteriovenous oxygen content difference is assumed to be 5.0 mL per 100 mL blood, reflecting a normal cardiac output. The shunt bands have been drawn to include the range of hemoglobin and $PaCO_2$ levels shown. (Redrawn from Benetar, S.R., Hewlett, A.M., and Nunn, J.F. The use of iso-shunt lines for control of oxygen therapy. Br J Anaesth 45:713, 1973 with permission.)

sure of the relative efficiency of gas exchange. This measurement is commonly utilized in anesthetic studies. The measured $P_{(A-a)}O_2$ value increases as F_IO_2 goes up for any given V/Q situation, and it is imperative that the F_IO_2 level be taken into account when comparisons are made. In practice most $P_{(A-a)}O_2$ determinations are made at oxygen concentrations of 21% or near 100%.

Determinations of the amount of venous admixture or pulmonary shunt flow can be made if mixed venous (pulmonary artery) and arterial blood oxygen contents are obtained along with a measurement of cardiac output and calculated P_AO_2. The terms *venous admixture* and *shunt flow* do not mean exactly the same thing, although they are often used interchangeably in the literature causing some confusion. *Venous admixture* refers to the degree of admixture of mixed venous blood with pulmonary end-capillary blood that would be required to produce the observed difference between the arterial and the end-capillary PO_2.(2) The end-capillary PO_2 is assumed to equal the "ideal" alveolar PO_2. Venous admixture (QS) is a calculated amount, that is a proportion of cardiac output, and it includes the PaO_2 lowering effect of low V/Q areas, blood flow past nonventilated areas, and true *anatomic shunt flow* (bronchial and thebesian venous blood flow). When the inspired oxygen level is high, blood passing low-V/Q

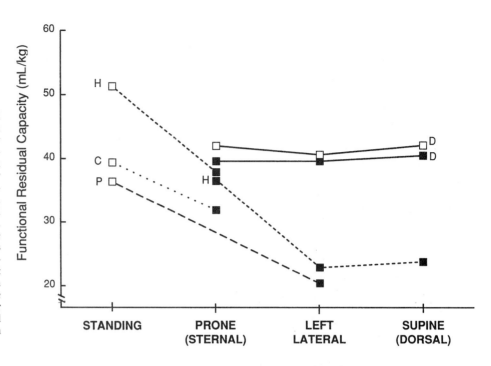

Fig. 6–15. Effect of positional changes and general anesthesia on functional residual capacity (FRC) in dogs (D), cattle (C), ponies (P), and horses (H). FRC in the conscious state is shown by the open symbol and in the anesthetized state by a closed symbol. All measurements were obtained during barbiturate anesthesia. Note that FRC does not change appreciably in anesthetized dogs with positional changes and decreases markedly with the onset of anesthesia and recumbency in the larger species. In the horse FRC is markedly less in dorsal or lateral recumbency, versus sternal recumbency. Data taken from various studies.(35–37, 117)

areas will be oxygenated (Fig. 6–13), and the $P_{(A-a)}O_2$ gradient and determination of venous admixture is a measure of all the total blood flow not contributing to gas exchange, hence the term *pulmonary shunt flow*. Note that this flow includes both anatomic shunt flow and flow past nonventilated or collapsed alveoli.

If one knows the inspired oxygen concentration and the PaO_2, and makes an assumption that the arterial-venous oxygen extraction is normal, it is possible to use an isoshunt diagram to provide a convenient and reasonably accurate estimate of the magnitude of pulmonary shunt flow (Fig. 6–14).(115) This diagram also illustrates the poor response, in terms of improving PaO_2, that will occur with increased inspired oxygen concentrations when shunt flows are over 30%.

EFFECT OF POSITIONAL CHANGES

Very few thorough studies of the respiratory consequences of positional changes have been carried out in conscious domestic animals because of the technical difficulties in doing such studies in an uncooperative animal. In conscious humans positioned in lateral recumbency there is proportionately more ventilation to the lowermost lung.(116) There is a slight fall in FRC, but in individuals with normal lungs and body confirmation there is little change in PaO_2. Conscious dogs positioned in sternal (prone), lateral, and dorsal (supine) recumbency showed no positional change in FRC (Fig. 6–15).(117) Unsedated sheep (101), cattle (104), and ponies (102) develop some degree of hypoxia when put into lateral recumbency, although this finding was not present in another group of ponies.(118) Mean PaO_2 levels in unsedated adult cattle positioned in dorsal recumbency are in the range of 60 to 70 mm Hg, with some animals experiencing marked hypoxemia. (103, 104)

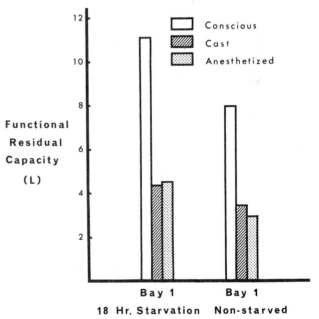

Fig. 6–16. Functional residual capacity (FRC) in a xylazine-sedated pony (273 kg) while standing (conscious), after positioning in left lateral recumbency with hobbles (cast), and following induction of anesthesia with thiopental (anesthetized). The study was done twice, once after an 18-hour period of starvation and once without starvation. FRC was measured by helium dilution.(139)

Although the evidence in conscious animals is mainly circumstantial and meager, it does appear that the main determinant of FRC is a decrease in lung volume in the recumbent animal (Fig. 6–16), as has been reported in anesthetized animals.(36, 37) It is interesting that when conscious, sedated 1400- to 4000-kg elephants voluntarily moved from a standing position to left lateral recumbency, PaO_2 levels only decreased from 96.2 to 83.8 mm Hg (at 10 minutes).(119) This relative protection against positional hypoxemia may be related to anatomic differences in the lung parenchyma, chest wall, and lung adhesion to the chest wall.(120)

In standing cows and sheep, rumen distension and the associated increase in abdominal pressure produce a decrease in PaO_2, and at very high rumenal pressures a reduction in $\dot{V}_E$ and cardiac output.(121, 122) In four standing ponies (two starved for 18 hours and two nonstarved) FRC as measured by helium dilution decreased by 13.4% (range 11.6–14.7%) after sedation with 0.04 mg/kg acepromazine given intramuscularly. In another study, overnight starvation increased the FRC of standing, unsedated ponies ($n = 5$) by about 16%.(37)

EFFECT OF ANESTHESIA AND SPECIES DIFFERENCES

As mentioned earlier, deep sedation and general anesthesia commonly produce a fall in PaO_2 levels even in healthy animals. Some of this decrease can be associated with hypoventilation (Fig. 6–6), but even when $PaCO_2$ levels are eucapnic, PaO_2 is generally decreased. The anesthetic-induced change in PaO_2 is associated with increases in the scatter of V/Q ratios, the $P_{(A-a)}O_2$ gradient, and the level of venous admixture.(2, 3) In the case of larger mammals there may even be gross V/Q mismatch.(1, 123) It is generally appreciated that increased $P_{(A-a)}O_2$ gradients are always increased during general anesthesia in the horse.(1, 4, 124, 125) Healthy horses may have low PaO_2 levels when anesthetized with injectable drugs.(126) In horses with diseased lungs or depressed cardiopulmonary function (e.g., anesthesia) it may be impossible to maintain PaO_2 levels above 70 mm Hg even with 100% inspired oxygen.(127) The same response to 100% oxygen administration may be observed in adult cattle.(60)

Recumbency per se does not produce significant hypoxemia in healthy dogs, cats, or people, and in the case of larger mammals produces less of an increase in the $P_{(A-a)}O_2$ gradient than is seen after the onset of anesthesia. What are the factors that produce hypoxemic changes in anesthetized animals? Research on the respiratory effects of anesthetics has focused on their influence on HPV; on lung volume, chest wall, and pulmonary mechanical factors; and on the resultant distribution of regional pulmonary blood and gas flow.

Hypoxic Pulmonary Vasoconstriction. It appears that this important protective mechanism to optimize V/Q in the lung is obtunded by many anesthetics. Investigations in intact animals and with excised lungs have established that all inhalational agents reduce HPV, and that none of the examined injectable agents (narcotics, barbiturates, or benzodiazepines) have any detectable effect.(107) The onset of the interference with HPV is rapid with inhaled anesthetics and persists throughout the duration of the anesthetic. The end result of this interference with HPV is that, for any given level of altered intrapulmonary gas distribution caused by reduced lung volume, intermittent airway closure, or

regional atelectasis, a greater degree of hypoxemia exists. With an animal breathing 100% oxygen and HPV abolished, it has been estimated that PaO_2 would be only 100 mm Hg with 30% of the lung atelectatic, versus a PaO_2 level of over 400 mm Hg with the same degree of atelectasis and an intact HPV response.(107) There have been no clinically relevant, controlled comparisons of $P_{(A-a)}O_2$ gradients using intravenous anesthesia versus inhalational anesthesia in veterinary patients. There is some evidence that PaO_2 is better maintained in horses when a xylazine/ketamine/guaifenesin infusion is used to maintain anesthesia instead of halothane.(128)

In the anesthetized horse there is evidence that pulmonary perfusion does not linearly increase from the uppermost lung areas to the lowermost areas solely on a gravitational basis, even when HPV is abolished.(129, 130) It has been demonstrated that the gravity-dependent pulmonary blood flow of conscious horses is altered when positioned in sternal, lateral, or dorsal recumbency during halothane anesthesia.(131) There was a reduction of blood flow to the cranioventral areas of the lung and a proportional increase in flow to dorsocaudal regions, irrespective of body position. Recently a nongravitational pulmonary blood flow pattern in pentobarbital-anesthetized ponies has been demonstrated.(132) It is possible that at least some of this diversion of pulmonary blood flow from the most dependent areas of the horse lung is related to creation of a zone IV area of blood flow from reduced lung volume and an increase in interstitial fluid pressure (Fig. 6–3). This sort of diversion has been observed in persons at low lung volumes (133), and in dogs when interstitial fluid pressures were elevated.(134) Whatever the cause, in the laterally recumbent horse, the redistribution of pulmonary blood flow away from relatively nonventilated lower lung to better ventilated upper lung has a beneficial effect in reducing the degree of venous admixture.(130) It is important to appreciate that redistribution is far from complete, and venous admixture or shunt flows in horses are often in excess of 20%.

Functional Residual Volume. In recumbent humans FRC is reduced by about 0.5 L with the induction of general anesthesia (106), which is 15 to 20% of the normal FRC. The mechanisms underlying this reduction in FRC remain unclear. Atelectasis, increased thoracic or abdominal blood volume, and loss of some inherent tone in the diaphragm at end-exhalation all seem to be involved.(80, 106, 116) Irrespective of the cause, there is evidence of a correlation between changes in FRC and the $P_{(A-a)}O_2$ gradient after induction of anesthesia.(135) There is little information regarding FRC changes in dogs and cats, but in one well-controlled study, the onset of general anesthesia did not alter FRC significantly in sternal, lateral, or dorsally recumbent dogs (Fig. 6–15).(117) These were medium-sized mongrel dogs (13–28 kg), and it is possible that larger dogs might show a different response. Differences in V/Q ratios during anesthesia have been noted between beagles and greyhound-type dogs.(136)

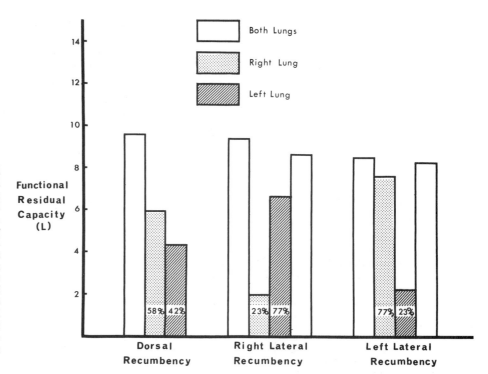

Fig. 6–17. Functional residual capacity (FRC) of the left and right lungs, and both lungs, in a horse positioned in dorsal and right and left lateral recumbency. The horse was maintained under stable intravenous anesthesia and FRC was determined by helium dilution using a double-lumen endotracheal tube to separate the two lungs.(139) Note that the FRC of the dependent lung decreases from the proportion measured during dorsal recumbency and becomes a small percentage of the total FRC, irrespective of which lung is dependent.

In the horse and cow, the decrease in FRC with the onset of recumbency and general anesthesia may be quite marked, as much as 50 to 70% (Fig. 6–15). This has been radiographically demonstrated (137, 138) and directly measured by helium dilution (37, 140) or nitrogen washout.(35) This change in FRC seems to be primarily related to the positional change from an upright posture to recumbency (Fig. 6–16) and, in horses at least, is greater in lateral or dorsal recumbency than in the prone position (Fig. 6–15).(36) In the laterally recumbent animal the dependent lung is poorly aerated radiographically (137, 138) and has a smaller FRC (as measured by helium dilution) (Fig. 6–17). Recent studies using nuclear scintigraphy (123) and computed tomography (141) have clearly demonstrated that there is markedly less ventilation of the dependent lung of the horse in lateral recumbency during anesthesia. This reduction in lower lung volume is accompanied by actual atelectasis (Fig. 6–18).

It is possible to increase the FRC of anesthetized horses through the use of high (20 to 30 cm H_2O) positive end-expiratory pressures (PEEP), and in so doing to reduce the $P_{(A-a)}O_2$ gradient.(127, 142) If PEEP of this magnitude is introduced there is a marked decrease in venous return to the heart and in cardiac output. The mechanism whereby PEEP reduces the $P_{(A-a)}O_2$ gradient and venous admixture is probably by increasing total and/or regional FRC, with subsequent prevention of the intermittent airway closure and reversal of the atelectasis that is represented diagrammatically by al-

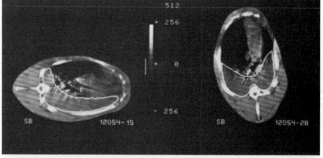
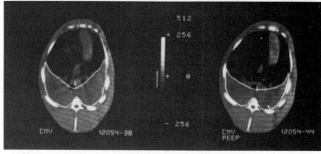

Fig. 6–18. Transverse computed tomography scans of the thorax of a pony during anesthesia with thiopental/halothane in left lateral recumbency (left upper panel) and in dorsal recumbency during spontaneous respiration (right upper panel), mechanical ventilation (left lower panel), and mechanical ventilation with PEEP of 10 cm H_2O (right lower panel). Note the appearance of large dense areas encircled by a white line in dependent lung regions. The heart is visible as a white area in the middle of the thorax. (Reproduced with permission from Nyman, G. et al. Atelectasis causes gas exchange impairment in the anaesthetized horse. Equine Vet J 22:317–324, 1990.)

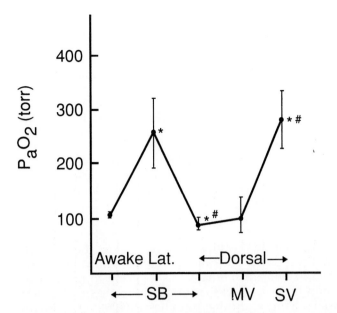

Fig. 6–19. Arterial oxygen tension (mean ± SEM) in the awake standing horse (F_IO_2 = 0.21), and during anesthesia in the lateral (Lat.) and dorsal recumbent positions (F_IO_2 > 0.92). SB, spontaneous breathing; MV, general mechanical ventilation; SV, selective mechanical ventilation of dependent lung regions with PEEP 20 cm H_2O; *, significantly different from awake value; #, significantly different from the previous value. (Reproduced with permission from Nyman G., et al. Selective mechanical ventilation of dependent lung regions in the anesthetized horse in dorsal recumbency. Br J Anaesth 59:1027–1034, 1987.)

veolus F and G in Fig. 6–13. Recently, Moens and colleagues utilized a double-lumened endotracheal tube and differential IPPV (higher V_T and PEEP of 10 to 20 cm H_2O) to the lowermost lung of quite large laterally recumbent horses (420–660 kg).(143) This technique increased PaO_2 levels by over 100% and decreased pulmonary shunt perfusion by 33%. Similar beneficial effects have been reported using PEEP and selective mechanical ventilation of dependent areas of the lungs in dorsally recumbent ponies (Fig. 6–19).(144) With the onset of general anesthesia and positioning in lateral recumbency PaO_2 levels were only elevated to about 250 mm Hg, rather than the expected above 500 mm Hg that should occur if there was no problem with gas exchange. When the horses were moved into dorsal recumbency their mean PaO_2 level fell to below 100 mm Hg. Conventional IPPV of the whole lung did little to improve PaO_2, whereas selective mechanical ventilation of the dependent areas of the lung with 20 cm H_2O restored PaO_2 to the level measured in lateral recumbency.

Chest Wall and Pulmonary Mechanics Changes. The evidence implicating alteration of chest wall (including diaphragm) and lung mechanical factors as causative agents in the increase in $P_{(A-a)}O_2$ during anesthesia is often conflicting. Certainly there is a difference in the chest wall mechanics between humans and dogs during general anesthesia.(106) It appears that most dog breeds (and probably cats) have a more compliant lateral chest wall that tends to contribute relatively little to the inspiratory effort compared to the diaphragm with clinical doses of most anesthetics. In all species dangerously deep planes of anesthesia are commonly associated with flaccidity of the thoracic wall and paradoxical inward movement during inspiration ("paradoxical" inspiration). If one watches closely, this same type of respiration may be seen in cats, ferrets, and other small mammals even with light levels of anesthesia (Chapter 2).

In the horse and cow, with the onset of anesthesia and movement into lateral recumbency, there is radiographic evidence of a marked change in the two-dimensional lung silhouette and the position of the diaphragm.(137, 138) In ponies anesthetized with halothane the diaphragmatic outline moved forward rather uniformly in sternal (prone) or lateral recumbency, but the forward shift was considerably greater in lateral recumbency.(137) When the ponies were positioned in dorsal (supine) recumbency, the diaphragmatic outline "sagged" toward the now-dependent spine region. With minor variations, Watney's observations in 315- to 400-kg cattle were very similar.(138) The positional alteration of the diaphragmatic silhouette agrees nicely with the reduction in FRC noted by Sorenson and Robinson when ponies were moved from sternal to lateral or dorsal recumbency.(36) In lateral recumbency the dorsal areas of the diaphragm moved more during inspiration than the more ventral sternal area, while the uppermost crural movement exceeded that of the lowermost crural segment.(145) This is in contrast to awake and anesthetized recumbent persons, where it is the most dependent portions of the diaphragm that are most active.(146) The tonic activity of the lateral chest wall, especially that provided by the serratus ventralis muscle, is greatly decreased in anesthetized horses, and it is postulated that this reduces the stabilization of the lateral chest wall.(147)

While it is generally accepted that halothane and isoflurane produce bronchodilation in man (148, 149), general anesthesia produces an apparent increase in the elastic recoil of the lung.(106) In anesthetized ponies, halothane, isoflurane, and enflurane had a mild bronchodilating effect (150), while in cows (151) and in standing horses at subanesthetic concentrations (152) halothane did not produce bronchodilation.(151) Interpretation of measurements of pulmonary resistance and compliance during anesthesia are made difficult because changes in lung volume per se will alter these values (3, 151), as was demonstrated when nonstarved cows were studied over a 3-hour anesthetic.(153) It would appear, however, that the chest wall and lung volume changes play a much larger part in the generation of increased $P_{(A-a)}O_2$ gradients during anesthesia than any true alteration of lung mechanics.

Clinical Implications of Altered Respiration During Anesthesia

The complexity of the respiratory response to anesthesia in veterinary patients may seem more than a little daunting to the novice anesthetist, and to the veterinary practitioner of necessity functioning without the benefit of appreciable advanced training in the discipline. This is made so, in part, because of the variety of species that we attend to, as well as the wide range of drugs and environments in which veterinarians find that they must sedate, chemically restrain, or anesthetize animals. In this section an attempt will be made to summarize the most important clinical considerations relative to respiratory management on a species basis for the typical patient. This overview is based to a large extent on personal experience from anesthetizing such cases and from discussions over the years with academic colleagues and practicing veterinarians. Unfortunately, there are exceedingly few morbidity/mortality surveys of relevant case material upon which one might base more objective conclusions. It is important to appreciate that there may be exceptions to these generalizations, based on the inherent health of the animal being treated, and due to the fact that the anesthetic response in an individual animal is not always "typical." There is simply no safe alternative other than ongoing careful monitoring of the respiratory system during anesthesia (Chapter 15).

HUMANS

Since so much of our knowledge of the altered physiology of anesthesia is derived from the human literature, it helps to understand how human anesthesia differs from veterinary anesthesia. In anesthetized humans there is an increase in alveolar dead space of about 70 mL and venous admixture constitutes approximately 10% of the cardiac output, versus 2 to 3% in unanesthetized individuals.(154) With this degree of venous admixture, an inspired oxygen concentration of about 35% will usually restore a normal PaO_2 (Fig. 6–14). Thus, the upper limit for nitrous oxide in an oxygen/nitrous oxide mixture is commonly 66%, that is, a 1:2 ratio of $O_2:N_2O$. Muscle relaxants and comparatively high doses of opioids (on an "effect," not mg/kg basis) are commonly incorporated into the anesthetic regimen, so IPPV is very commonly employed.(2, 3) The target when ventilating anesthetized subjects is usually to produce eucapnia or slight hypocapnia. This was originally done because of an apparent potentiation effect of the anesthetic dose, but now is done primarily to prevent sympathetic stimulation with resultant tachycardia and hypertension, both of which are dangerous in a patient population prone to atherosclerotic disease. Eucapnia also minimizes the risk of increased intracranial or intraocular pressure, which is especially important in trauma patients, the elderly, or those with ocular and/or central nervous system disease.

Some form of airway protection (oropharyngeal or endotracheal tube) is almost always utilized, and continuous airway pressure monitoring is employed to ensure that there is no inadvertent disconnection from the anesthetic circuit of a paralyzed patient that cannot breathe spontaneously. Continuous end-tidal CO_2 and hemoglobin saturation monitoring is now widely employed, using capnography and noninvasive pulse oximetry, respectively.(155) The reasons for the increased use of these monitoring devices are that the equipment is now cost-effective and user friendly, provides medicolegal protection, and provides an early warning system of cardiorespiratory failure that decreases the mortality rate associated with general anesthesia.(156, 157)

DOGS AND CATS

In reasonably healthy dogs and cats the $P_{(A-a)}O_2$ gradient and the degree of venous admixture is less than in humans. Perhaps this is owing to the smaller lungs in these species or to the difference in the chest wall changes during anesthesia (106), or perhaps because there is excellent collateral pulmonary ventilation in these species.(111) A high degree of collateral ventilation means that if an alveolus is not ventilated via the airway, it may well receive gas exchange through passages (pores of Kohn) leading to other alveoli that are ventilated.

Despite the relatively favorable situation in regard to V/Q mismatch in these species, a minimum inspired oxygen level of 30 to 35% is still recommended. For the first few minutes after a barbiturate induction PaO_2 may be as low as 50 mm Hg in nonventilated healthy dogs (158), with less change in cats.(158) The degree of hypoxemia is somewhat less after a ketamine induction, but venous admixture still may be 20 to 25% for a few minutes after induction.(85, 86) Obese, deeply anesthetized animals, animals with a distended abdomen (e.g., pregnancy, bowel obstruction), or those with pulmonary disease or space-occupying lesions of the thorax (tumor, pneumothorax, hemothorax, or diaphragmatic hernia) are particularly at risk. Oxygen supplementation is needed nearly as much in deeply sedated animals as in those receiving a general anesthetic (intravenous or inhalant). As can be seen in Figure 6–20, increasing the inspired oxygen level also provides protection against hypoxemia caused by hypoventilation, and again adequate protection is generally achieved with 30 to 35%. This is why simple maneuvers such as placing a face mask with oxygen on a high-risk patient before and during induction or use of a nasal oxygen catheter in the postoperative period are beneficial.

When 100% oxygen mixtures are utilized with the common inhalant anesthetics, in dogs and cats free of serious cardiopulmonary disease, the arterial PaO_2 level is generally 450 to 525 mm Hg whether the animal is breathing spontaneously or being ventilated (56, 65, 160, 161), and irrespective of body position. With such high inspired oxygen levels, hypoxemia usually only occurs through disconnection of the animal from the

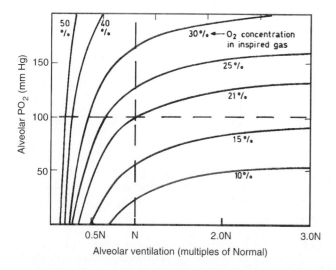

Fig. 6–20. Protective effect of increased inspired oxygen concentrations with various degrees of alveolar hypoventilation and hyperventilation. With 30% inspired oxygen alveolar PO_2 levels are above 100 mm Hg even when alveolar ventilation is half normal. (Modified with permission from Nunn, J.F. Applied Respiratory Physiology, 3rd ed. Butterworth, London, 1987:111.)

anesthetic machine, or with faulty placement of the endotracheal tube, cardiac arrest, or total apnea for over 5 minutes. Nevertheless, even with such high PaO_2 levels, tissue hypoxia can occur if hemoglobin levels are low or there is inadequate circulation (low cardiac output).

The decision to institute assisted or controlled IPPV is generally made to prevent or treat hypercapnia, rather than to achieve oxygenation. Nearly all spontaneously breathing dogs and cats show some degree of hypoventilation and hypercapnia ($PaCO_2$ of 45–55 mm Hg). The clinical importance of this in the nonneurologic case is open to debate. Dogs and cats do not have atherosclerosis, and over the years hundreds of thousands of dogs and cats have been successfully anesthetized in practice while breathing spontaneously. From a practical viewpoint, with short-duration anesthetics (less than 1 hour) in relatively healthy animals, the important aspects are to ensure that the airway is patent, that the animal is oxygenated, and that the animal does not become apneic; the development of moderate levels of hypercapnia is likely to be well tolerated. The need for IPPV increases as the depth of anesthesia has to be increased for certain types of surgery (e.g., hip replacement) unless local supplementation is used (e.g., epidural opioid or local anesthetic). It also increases when opioids are used as a major component of the anesthetic regimen; for the obese, neonate, geriatric, or neurologic patient; with certain body positions (e.g., perineal hernia repair, dorsal laminectomy); with prolonged operations; or when dealing with a poor-risk patient (Chapters 23 and 24).

A few guidelines relative to the respiratory component of anesthesia for dogs and cats are given here.

1. Nearly all canine anesthetics are better done with an endotracheal tube in place, and in many situations cats should be intubated (Chapter 17).
2. Use at least 30 to 35% inspired oxygen in all anesthetized dogs and cats, even those on an injectable anesthetic mixture, or when deeply sedated.
3. Hypoxemia is rare in spontaneously breathing dogs and cats if breathing an oxygen mixture approaching 100%.
4. After a prolonged period of anesthesia in cats and smaller dogs, and with shorter anesthetics in larger dogs with deep chests, it is advisable to inflate the lungs to 30 cm H_2O airway pressure (that is to "sigh" the lungs) periodically and at the end of anesthesia.
5. Prolonged immobility and excessive fluid administration can lead to increased venous admixture and a fall in PaO_2 in addition to that produced by anesthesia per se.(162)

SMALL RUMINANTS AND SWINE

Ruminants are especially prone to the development of regurgitation and aspiration, along with tachypnea and hypoventilation, during general anesthesia.(60) For shorter procedures (45 to 60 minutes) hypoventilation and hypercapnia often may be safely ignored if an adequate oxygen supply is maintained. Often sedation and local analgesia are utilized to maintain a secure airway and adequate respiration.(163) During clinical anesthesia in pigs, especially if a barbiturate is used in a field situation, particular care must be taken to ensure that the airway is patent and that apnea does not occur.

The degree of ventilation/perfusion mismatch and venous admixture is intermediate in these animals, and of such a magnitude that virtually all anesthetized animals breathing room air will have PaO_2 levels somewhat below normal. In dorsally recumbent, ventilated sheep anesthetized with pentobarbital-halothane, atelectasis of the dependent lung regions developed quite quickly.(164) The magnitude of this atelectasis was much less than the same group of researchers observed in ponies.(141) Pulmonary disease is not uncommon in small ruminants and swine, and will lead to V/Q mismatch in addition to that induced by anesthesia, lowering PaO_2 levels further. Abdominal distension caused by the development of rumenal tympany, or in the case of swine a full stomach, will add to the degree of pulmonary dysfunction (Chapter 20).

During inhalation anesthesia with 100% oxygen, PaO_2 is usually in the range of 200 to 350 mm Hg–well within safe limits.(67, 165) In spontaneously breathing sheep changes in body position (dorsal, left and right lateral) do not seem to alter the PaO_2 appreciably, and the $P_{(A-a)}O_2$ gradient is rather constant when the sheep are sighed every 3 to 5 minutes.(165) Clinical experience would suggest the situation is similar in goats and pigs. The following are guidelines for respiratory management during anesthesia.

1. General anesthesia in sheep, goats, and calves with a developed rumen (i.e., by 2–4 weeks) requires placement of an endotracheal tube if protection against regurgitation and aspiration is to be ensured. This is best done for all but the shortest and lightest anesthetics.

2. Endotracheal intubation is not advised for swine unless the operation is complex or prolonged, or the operator is skilled with the technique.

3. During intravenous anesthesia of more compromised animals, application of a face mask or insertion of a nasal or tracheal oxygen catheter and insufflation of 2 to 5 L/min oxygen will help to ensure that hypoxemia does not occur.

4. Ketamine-based anesthesia is less likely to lead to apnea or severe respiratory depression than barbiturate anesthesia.

5. Prolonged inhalation anesthesia (longer than 45 to 60 minutes) may require IPPV to prevent hypercapnia and may be required to maintain a stable plane of anesthesia due to the tachypneic breathing pattern.

6. Mild to moderate hypercapnia is well tolerated, and serious hypoxemia is rare if inhalation anesthesia with 100% oxygen is used.

7. The combination of progressive abdominal tympany (even in animals starved for up to 24 hours) and the rapid, shallow respiration tend to produce a progressive increase in $P_{(A-a)}O_2$ gradients. Periodic "sighing" of the lungs (every 10 to 15 minutes) by inflating them to 30 cm H_2O seems to minimize the progressive increase in venous admixture, and is particularly advisable at the end of an operation before extubation and return to a room air environment. Placement in sternal recumbency during recovery benefits pulmonary function, and in the case of ruminants, helps to protect against regurgitation and aspiration.

ADULT CATTLE AND HORSES

Adult cattle (153, 166) and horses (1, 4, 125, 167) develop very significant increases in $P_{(A-a)}O_2$ gradients and venous admixture when they are anesthetized and become recumbent. On the basis of inspired oxygen concentration and PaO_2 levels, it can be calculated that spontaneously breathing halothane-anesthetized horses have pulmonary shunt flows of 20 to 25%, with a reduction to about 15% in the ventilated horse.(168) These were healthy horses, positioned in lateral recumbency and subjected to no surgery. Over the intervening 25 years others have reported PaO_2 levels and $P_{(A-a)}O_2$ gradients from many studies in other healthy horses that are reflective of pulmonary shunt flows of at least the same magnitude.(144, 170-172) The degree of V/Q mismatch is greater in dorsal than in lateral recumbency (169, 172-175), in larger horses, and perhaps in older horses.(169) Researchers have consistently noted that the actual variability between PaO2 levels in similar horses receiving similar anesthetics is quite large (Fig. 6–21).(170) The reasons for this variability are not clear,

but probably relate to body confirmation and perhaps the level of abdominal distension due to obesity, gas distension or ingesta in the large bowel. The $P_{(A-a)}O_2$ gradient does not generally increase over time in healthy starved animals (170, 174), but there will be a progressive fall in PaO_2 if the degree of abdominal distension increases. This was clearly illustrated in an interesting study carried out on fed and nonfed cows, where the failure to starve the cows before the general anesthetic lead to a progressive increase in $P_{(A-a)}O_2$ and pulmonary resistance, and a fall in PaO_2 and dynamic compliance (Figs. 6–22A and B).(153)

When an anesthetized horse (usually a colic surgery or cesarian section) inhales 100% oxygen and has a resultant PaO_2 value of less than 70 mm Hg, it is clear from Figure 6–14 that over 50% of the cardiac output is being shunted through the lungs without contributing to gas exchange. While adult cattle also demonstrate fairly large $P_{(A-a)}O_2$ gradients during inhalational anesthesia, serious hypoxemia seems to be confined to very large animals, especially if they must be positioned in dorsal recumbency. Chronic pulmonary disease and lung consolidation is relatively common in cattle as an aftermath of juvenile respiratory disease. It is surprising that such animals do not demonstrate large increases in $P_{(A-a)}O_2$ levels during inhalant anesthesia, perhaps because pulmonary blood flow is also decreased in the nonventilated lung areas.

When adult cattle are positioned in dorsal recumbency using rope restraint, with or without sedation, some of them become quite hypoxemic.(103, 104) The same is true of horses anesthetized with the common injectable mixtures for short-duration field anesthesia. Admittedly, the vast majority of animals so anesthetized

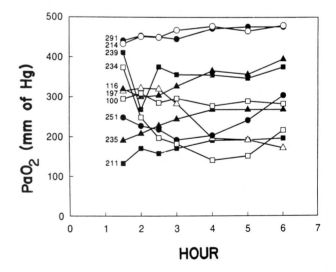

Fig. 6–21. Arterial PO_2 values in ten spontaneously breathing, normal horses anesthetized with halothane over 5.0 hours in lateral recumbency. Note the wide variability in the PaO_2 levels between horses and the relative stability of the value for an individual horse over time. The horses were starved overnight before the onset of anesthesia. (Reproduced from Steffey, E.P. et al. Time-related responses of spontaneously breathing, laterally recumbent horses to prolonged anesthesia with halothane. Am J Vet Res 48:952–957, 1987.)

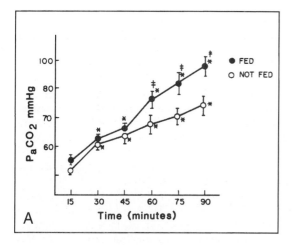

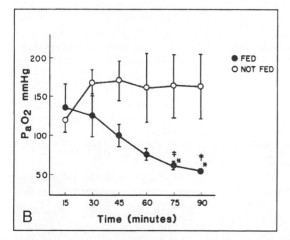

Fig. 6–22. Change in P_aCO_2 (A) and P_aO_2 (B) levels in spontaneously breathing cows with and without prior starvation. Note the greater degree of hypercapnia in the fed animals and the progressively lower P_aO_2. This change was accompanied by an increase in the $P_{(A-a)}O_2$, an increase in airway resistance, and a fall in compliance. These changes were probably associated with a decrease in lung volume from the development of abdominal tympany. (Reproduced from Blaze, C.A. et al. Effect of withholding feed on ventilation and the incidence of regurgitation during halothane anesthesia of adult cattle. Am J Vet Res 49:2126–2129, 1988.)

survive with no obvious adverse after effects. This is more a credit to the inherent safety reserve the animal has relative to oxygen supply and to the underlying good health status of most patients than to the anesthetic regimes per se. Nasal or nasotracheal oxygen insufflation (15 L/min) markedly improves the safety factor in restraining and anesthetizing such animals, and is always desirable if circumstances permit such treatment. Some guidelines relative to respiratory support of anesthetized adult cattle and horses include the following:

1. General anesthesia requires endotracheal intubation in adult cattle as the risk of regurgitation and aspiration is high, even with prior starvation (Chapter 20). There is some risk of regurgitation and aspiration when cattle are restrained in a recumbent position with sedatives, including xy-

lazine. The incidence of regurgitation, however, is fairly low, and routine intubation of nonanesthetized cattle is not practical.

2. Longer-duration anesthetics in horses are better carried out with an endotracheal tube in place, and this also facilitates oxygen insufflation (Chapter 20).

3. Oxygen insufflation with 15 L/min, especially if the tip of the oxygen catheter tube is placed in the trachea, will usually prevent any serious hypoxia in relatively healthy horses and cattle during general anesthesia or recovery. This flow rate down the trachea will even maintain sufficient oxygenation to keep apneic animals alive for at least 10 minutes.(167)

4. If oxygen supplementation is not possible, adult cattle and horses are better positioned in lateral than in dorsal recumbency (if the surgery permits the choice).

5. When preoperative starvation can be utilized, it is desirable, as it improves ventilation and oxygenation after the induction of anesthesia.

6. Nitrous oxide use is generally not advisable for cattle or in dorsally recumbent horses, and if used to supplement analgesia for orthopedic surgery in laterally recumbent horses should not exceed an inspired concentration of 50% (4 L O_2:4 L N_2O minimum).(176)

7. Inhalant general anesthetics lasting longer than 45 minutes in cattle almost always require IPPV to prevent excessive $PaCO_2$ elevations. In horses, operations over 1 or 2 hours will generally need IPPV if the need has not developed earlier. It should be appreciated that in dorsally recumbent horses breathing spontaneously, arterial hypoxemia is not always improved with initiation of IPPV, which may actually decrease PaO_2 and seriously decrease oxygen delivery to tissues.(177) Moderate increases in $PaCO_2$ levels actually produce useful hemodynamic stimulation without apparent adverse effects (178) and seem to be well tolerated.

8. Treatment of low PaO_2 levels with high levels of PEEP (20 to 30 cm H_2O) is feasible if the blood volume is adequate and inotropic support is utilized.(127, 142) While differential lung ventilation with PEEP reduces hypoxemia experimentally (143, 144), it is hard to see how this can be utilized clinically on those animals that actually need treating.

9. Periodic "sighing" of the lungs in adult cattle and horses probably does no harm, nor does it probably do much good. Full inflation of the lungs after the abdomen has been decompressed surgically, or when the animal is positioned in sternal recumbency in recovery can be quite useful in restoring adequate PaO_2 levels.

EXOTIC SPECIES

It is very difficult to generalize how to best optimize respiratory function during anesthesia for the diverse range of exotic animals. Even if not used routinely, supplemental oxygenation and the means to establish an airway should be available if at all possible. Chemical stimulation of respiration (e.g., doxapram) or the availability of receptor-specific antagonist drugs can be lifesaving in the case of an inadvertent anesthetic overdose. Respiration is generally better supported with dissociatives than with barbiturate anesthetics (Chapters 10, 21, and 22). The larger the species, the more likely recumbency and positional changes may seriously interfere with cardiopulmonary homeostasis, although exceptions may exist (e.g., the elephant). In general, it is desirable to keep larger terrestrial mammals in sternal rather than lateral or dorsal recumbency during restraint and/or anesthesia, unless such positioning is going to lead to excessive pressure on the limbs for a prolonged period.

References

1. Soma LR. Equine anesthesia: Causes of reduced oxygen and increased carbon dioxide tensions. Comp Cont Ed 11:S57–63, 1980.
2. Nunn JF. Applied Physiology, 3rd ed. London: Butterworths, 1987.
3. Benumof JL. Respiratory physiology and respiratory function during anesthesia. In: Anesthesia, 3rd ed. Vol 1. Edited by R.D. Robinson. New York: Churchill Livingstone, 1990:505–550.
4. Hall LW. General anesthesia: Fundamental considerations. Vet Clin North Am Large Anim Pract 3:3–15, 1981.
5. Robinson NE. The respiratory system. In: Equine Anesthesia: Monitoring and Emergency Therapy. Edited by W.W. Muir and J.E. Hubbell. St. Louis: Mosby Year Book, 1991:7–38.
6. Ruckebusch Y, Phaneuf Y-P, Dunlop R. Physiology of Small and Large Animals. Philadelphia: BC Decker, 1991:53–91.
7. Leff AR, Schumacker PT. Respiratory Physiology: Basics and Applications. Philadelphia: WB Saunders, 1993.
8. McDonell WN. Ventilation and Acid-Base Equilibrium with Methoxyflurane Anesthesia in Dogs [MSc. Thesis]. University of Guelph, Guelph, Ontario, 1969.
9. Gallivan GJ, McDonell WN, Forrest JB. Comparative ventilation and gas exchange in the horse and cow. Res Vet Sci 46:331–336, 1989.
10. Lai Y-L. Comparative ventilation of the normal lung. In: Treatise of Pulmonary Toxicology. Vol. 1. Comparative Biology of the Normal Lung. Edited by R.A. Parent. Boca Raton, FL: CRC Press 1992:219–224.
11. Fordyce WE, Tenney SM. Role of carotid bodies in ventilatory acclimation to chronic hypoxia by the awake cat. Respir Physiol 58:207–221, 1984.
12. Gillespie DJ, Hyatt RE. Respiratory mechanics in the unanesthetized dog. J Appl Physiol 35:98–102, 1974.
13. Hales JRS, Webster MED. Respiratory function during thermal tachypnea in sheep. J Physiol (Lond) 190:241–260, 1967.
14. Bakima M, Gustin P, Lekeux P, Lomba F. Mechanics of breathing in goats. Res Vet Sci 45:332–336, 1988.
15. Mesina JE, Bisgard GE, Robinson GM. Pulmonary function changes in goats given 3-methylindole orally. Am J Vet Res 45:1526–1531, 1984.
16. Forster HV, Bisgard GE, Klein JP. Effect of peripheral chemoreceptor denervation on acclimatization of goats during hypoxia. J Appl Physiol 50:392–398, 1981.
17. Verbrugghe C, Laurent P, Bouvert P. Chemoreflex drive of ventilation in the awake miniature pig. Respir Physiol 47:379–391, 1982.
18. Keith IM, Bisgard GE, Manohar M, Klein J, Bullard YA. Respiratory effects of pregnancy and progesterone in Jersey cows. Respir Physiol 50:351–358, 1982.
19. Bisgard GE, Ruis AV, Grover RF, Will JA. Ventilatory control in the Hereford calf. J Appl Physiol 35:220–226, 1973.
20. Willoughby RA, McDonell WN. Pulmonary function testing in horses. Vet Clin North Am Large Anim Pract 1:171–196, 1979.
21. Gillespie JR, Tyler WS, Eberly VE. Pulmonary ventilation and resistance in emphysematous and control horses. J Appl Physiol 21:416–422, 1966.
22. Orr JA, Bisgard GE, Forster HV, Rowlings CA, Buss DD, Will JA. Cardiopulmonary measurements in nonanesthetized, resting normal ponies. Am J Vet Res 36:1667–1670, 1975.
23. Libermann IM, Capano A, Gonzalez F, Bruzzana H. Blood acid-base status in normal albino rats. Lab Anim Sci 23:862–865, 1973.
24. Lai Y-L, Tsuya Y, Hildebrandt J. Ventilatory response to acute CO_2 exposure in the rat. J Appl Physiol 45:611–618, 1978.
25. Lahiri S. Blood oxygen affinity and alveolar ventilation in relation to body weight in mammals. Am J Physiol 229:529–536, 1975.
26. Neutze JM, Wyler F, Rudolph AM. Use of radioactive microspheres to assess cardiac output in rabbits. Am J Physiol 215:486–495, 1968.
27. Dyson DH, Allen DG, Ingwersen W, Pascoe PJ, O'Grady M. Effects of Saffan on cardiopulmonary function in healthy cats. Can J Vet Res 51:236–239, 1987.
28. Herbert DA, Mitchell RA. Blood gas tensions and acid-base balance in awake cats. J Appl Physiol 30:434–436, 1971.
29. Horwitz LD, Bishop VS, Stone HL, Stegall HF. Cardiovascular effects of low-oxygen atmospheres in conscious and anesthetized dogs. J Appl Physiol 27:370–373, 1969.
30. Wanner A, Reinhart ME. Respiratory mechanics on conscious sheep: Response to methacholine. J Appl Physiol Respir Environ Exercise Physiol 44:479–482, 1978.
31. Bisgard GE, Vogel JHK. Hypoventilation and pulmonary hypertension in calves after carotid body excision. J Appl Physiol 31:431–437, 1971.
32. Donawick WJ, Baue AE. Blood gases, acid-base balance, and alveolar-arterial oxygen gradient in calves. Am J Vet Res 29:561–567, 1968.
33. Crosfill ML, Widdicombe JG. Physical characteristics of the chest and lungs and the work of breathing in different mammalian species. J Physiol (Lond) 158:1–14, 1961.
34. Mauderly JL. Effect of age on pulmonary structure and function of immature and adult animals and man. Fed Proc 38:173–177, 1979.
35. Gallivan GJ, McDonell WN, Forrest JB. Comparative pulmonary mechanics in the horse and the cow. Res Vet Sci 46:330, 1989.
36. Sorenson PR, Robinson NE. Postural effects on lung volumes and asynchronous ventilation in anesthetized horses. J Appl Physiol Respir Environ Exercise Physiol 48:97–103, 1980.
37. McDonell WN, Hall LW. Functional residual capacity in conscious and anaesthetized horses. Br J Anaesth 46:802–803, 1974.
38. Gallivan GJ, Bignell W, McDonell WN, Whiting TL. Simple nonrebreathing valves for use with large mammals. Can J Vet Res 53:143–146, 1989.
39. Derksen FJ, Robinson NE. Esophageal and intrapleural pressures in the healthy conscious pony. Am J Vet Res 41:1756–1761, 1980.
40. Amis TC, Pascoe JR, Hornof W. Topographic distribution of pulmonary ventilation and perfusion in the horse. Am J Vet Res 45:1597–1601, 1984.
41. West JB. Ventilation-perfusion relationships. Am Rev Respir Dis 116:919–943, 1977.
42. Porcelli RJ. Pulmonary Hemodynamics. In: Treatise on Pulmonary Toxicology. Vol 1. Comparative Biology of the Normal Lung. Edited by R.A. Parent. Boca Raton, FL: CRC Press, 1992:241–270.
43. Comroe JH. Physiology of Respiration, 2nd ed. Chicago, Year Book, 1974.
44. Gillespie JR, Martin DB. Long-term oxygen cage therapy for hypoxemic dogs. J Am Vet Med Assoc 156:717, 1970.
45. Clarke KW, Hall LW. A survey of anesthesia in small animal practice: AVA/BSAVA report. J Assoc Vet Anaesth 17:4–10, 1990.
46. Daunt DA. Supportive therapy in the anesthetized horse. Vet Clin North Am Equine Pract 6:557–573, 1990.

47. Kelly AB, Steffey EP. Inhalation anesthesia: Drugs and techniques. Vet Clin North Am Equine Pract 3:59–71, 1981.
48. McDonell WN, Dyson DH. Management of anesthetic emergencies. In: Current Practice of Equine Surgery. Edited by N.A. White and J.N. Moore. Philadelphia: JB Lippincott, 1990: 103–114.
49. Lekeux P, Rollin F, Art T. Control of breathing in resting and exercising animals. In: Pulmonary Function in Healthy, Exercising and Diseased Animals. Edited by P. Lekeux. Gent, Belgium, Vlaams Diergeneeskundig Tijdschrift (Special Issue), 1993:123–145.
50. Gaudy JH, Sicard JF, Boitier JF. Ventilatory effects of oxygen in the dog under thiopentone anesthesia. Br J Anesth 60:456–460, 1988.
51. Gauvreau GM, Wilson BA, Schnurr DL, Young SS, McDonell WN. Oxygen cost of ventilation in the horse. Res Vet Sci 1993: 59; 171.
52. Muir WW, Moore CA, Hamlin RL. Ventilatory alterations in normal horses in response to changes in inspired oxygen and carbon dioxide. Am J Vet Res 36:155–159, 1975.
53. Boggs DF. Comparative control of respiration. In: Treatise on Pulmonary Toxicology. Vol 1. Comparative Biology of the Normal Lung. Edited by R.A. Parent. Boca Raton, FL: CRC Press, 1992:314–315.
54. Muir WW, Hamlin RL. Effects of acetylpromazine on ventilatory variables in the horse. Am J Vet Res 36:1439–1442, 1975.
55. Bisgard GE, Vagel JH. Hypoventilation and pulmonary hypertension in calves after carotid body excision. J Appl Physiol 31:431–437, 1971.
56. Steffey EP, Farver TB, Woliner MJ. Circulatory and respiratory effects of methoxyflurane on dogs: Comparison of halothane. Am J Vet Res 45:2574–2579, 1984.
57. Gautier H, Bonora M, Zaoui D. Influence of halothane on control of breathing in intact and decerebrated cats. J Appl Physiol 63:546–553, 1987.
58. Steffey EP, Howland D. Comparison of circulatory and respiratory effects of isoflurane and halothane anesthesia in horses. Am J Vet Res 41:821–825, 1980.
59. Trim CM. Sedation and general anesthesia in ruminants. Calif Vet 35:29–36, 1981.
60. Steffey EP. Some characteristics of ruminants and swine that complicate management of general anesthesia. Vet Clin North Am Food Anim Pract 2:507–516, 1986.
61. Hornbein TF. Anesthetics and ventilatory control. In: Effects of Anesthesia. Edited by B.G. Covino, H.A. Fozzard, K. Rehder, and G. Strichartz. Bethesda, MA: American Physiological Society, 1985:75–90.
62. Pavlin EG, Hornbein TF. Anesthesia and the control of ventilation. In: Handbook of Physiology, sec. 3: The Respiratory System. Vol 11, Control of Breathing, part 2. Edited by A.P. Fishman, Bethesda, MA: American Physiological Society. 1986:793–813.
63. Hirshman CA, McCullough RE, Cohen PJ, Weil JV. Hypoxic ventilatory drive in dogs during thiopental, ketamine, or pentobarbital anesthesia. Anesthesiology 43:628–634, 1975.
64. Knill RL, Gelb AW. Ventilatory response to hypoxia and hypercapnia during halothane sedation and anesthesia in man. Anesthesiology 49:244–251, 1978.
65. Steffey EP, Howland D. Isoflurane potency in the dog and cat. Am J Vet Res 38:1833–1836, 1977.
66. Steffey EP, Howland D. Potency of enflurane in dogs: Comparison with halothane and isoflurane. Am J Vet Res 39:573–577, 1978.
67. Steffey EP, Howland D. Halothane anesthesia in calves. Am J Vet Res 40:372–376, 1979.
68. Steffey EP, Gillespie JR, Berry JD, Eger EI, Rhode EA. Cardiovascular effects of halothane in the stump-tailed Macque during spontaneous and controlled ventilation. Am J Vet Res 35:1315–1319, 1974.
69. Steffey EP, Howland D, Giri S, Eger EI. Enflurane, halothane, and isoflurane potency in horses. Am J Vet Res 38:1037–1039, 1977.
70. McDonell W. Anesthesia of the harp seal. J Wildl Dis 8:287–295, 1972.
71. Daunt DA, Steffey EP, Pascoe JR, Willits N, Daels PF. Actions of isoflurane and halothane in pregnant mares. J Am Vet Med Assoc 201:1367–1374, 1992.
72. Brandstater B, Eger EI, Edelist G. Constant depth halothane anesthesia in respiratory studies. J Appl Physiol 20:171–174, 1965.
73. Cuvelliéz SG, Eicker SW, McLauchlin C, Brunson DB. Cardiovascular and respiratory effects of inspired oxygen fraction in halothane-anesthetized horses. Am J Vet Res 51:1226–1231, 1990.
74. Seaman GC, Ludders JW, Erb HN, Gleed RD. Effects of low and high fractions of inspired oxygen on ventilation in ducks anesthetized with isoflurane. Am J Vet Res 55:395–398, 1994.
75. Nolan AM, Reid J. The use of intraoperative fentanyl in spontaneously breathing dogs undergoing orthopaedic surgery. J Vet Anaesth 18:30–39, 1991.
76. Copeland VS, Haskins SC, Patz DJ. Oxymorphone: Cardiovascular, pulmonary, and behavioral effects in the dog. Am J Vet Res 48:1626–1630, 1987.
77. Turner DM, Ilkiw JE, Rose RJ, Warren JM. Respiratory and cardiovascular effects of five drugs used as sedatives in the dog. Aust Vet J 50:260–265, 1974.
78. Berg RJ, Orton EC. Pulmonary function in dogs after intercostal thoracotomy: Comparison of morphine, oxymorphone and selective intercostal nerve block. Am J Vet Res 47:471–474, 1986.
79. Katz J, Kavanagh BP, Sandler AN. Preemptive analgesia: Clinical evidence of neuroplasty contributing to post-operative pain. Anesthesiology 77:439–446, 1992.
80. Jones JG, Sapsford DJ, Wheatley RG. Post-operative hypoxaemia: Mechanisms and time course. Anaesthesia 45:566–573, 1990.
81. Taylor PM, Houlton JEF. Post-operative analgesia in the dog: A comparison of morphine, buprenorphine, and pentazocine. J Small Anim Pract 25:437–451, 1984.
82. Jacobson JD, McGrath CJ, Smith EP. Cardiorespiratory effects of induction and maintenance of anesthesia with ketamine-midazolam combination, with and without prior administration of butorphanol or oxymorphone. Am J Vet Res 55:543–550, 1994.
83. Popilskis S, Kohn D, Sanchez JA, Gorman P. Epidural versus intramuscular oxymorphone analgesia after thoracotomy in dogs. Vet Surg 20:462–467, 1991.
84. Pascoe PJ, Dyson DH. Analgesia after lateral thoracotomy in dogs. Epidural morphine versus intercostal bupivacaine. Vet Surg 22:141–147, 1993.
85. Haskins SC, Farver TB, Patz JD. Cardiovascular changes in dogs given diazepam and diazepam-ketamine. Am J Vet Res 17:795–798, 1986.
86. Farver TB, Haskins SC, Patz JD. Cardiopulmonary effects of aceepromazine and of the subsequent administration of ketamine in the dog. Am J Vet Res 47:631–635, 1986.
87. Muir WW, Sams RA, Huffman RH, Noonan JA. Pharmacodynamic and pharmacokinetic properties of diazepam in horses. Am J Vet Res 43:1756–1762, 1982.
88. Reitemeyer H, Klein HJ, Deegen E. The effect of sedatives on lung function in horses. Acta Vet Scand 82:111–120, 1986.
89. Lavoie JP, Pascoe JR, Kurpershoek CJ. Effects of xylazine on ventilation in horses. Am J Vet Res 53:916–920, 1992.
90. Lavoie JP, Pascoe JR, Kurpershoek CJ. Effect of head and neck position on respiratory mechanics in horses sedated with xylazine. Am J Vet Res 53:1653–1657, 1992.
91. Wagner AE, Muir WW, Hinchcliff KW. Cardiovascular effects of xylazine and detomidine in horses. Am J Vet Res 52:651–657, 1991.
92. Clarke KW, England GCW, Goossens L. Sedative and cardiovascular effects of romifidine, alone and in combination with butorphanol, in the horse. J Vet Anaesth 18:25–29, 1991.
93. Doherty TJ, Pascoe PJ, McDonell WN, Monteith G. Cardiopulmonary effects of xylazine and yohimbine in laterally recumbent sheep. Can J Vet Res 50:517–521, 1986.
94. Celly C, McDonell W, Black W, Young S. Cardiopulmonary effects of alpha-2 adrenoceptor agonists in sheep. Proc 5th Int Cong Vet Anesth [Abstract]. Guelph, Ontario, 1994:117.
95. Nolan A, Livingston A, Waterman A. The effects of alpha$_2$ adrenoreceptor agonists on airway pressure in anaesthetized sheep. J Vet Pharmacol Ther 9:157–163, 1986.

96. Adetunji A, McDonell WN, Pascoe PJ. Cardiopulmonary effects of xylazine, acetylpromazine and chloral hydrate in supine cows. Proc 2nd Int Cong Vet Anesth [Abstract]. Sacramento, Calif., 110, 1985.
97. Allen DG, Dyson DH, Pascoe PJ, O'Grady MR. Evaluation of a xylazine-ketamine hydrochloride combination in the cat. Can Vet Res 50:23–26, 1986.
98. McDonell WN, Van Gorder J. Cardiopulmonary effects of xylazine/ketamine in dogs. Proc Annu Sci Mtg Am Coll Vet Anesth [Abstract]. 1982.
99. Klide AM, Calderwood HW, Soma LR. Cardiopulmonary effects of xylazine in dogs. Am J Vet Res 36:931–935, 1975.
100. Haskins SC, Patz JD, Farver TB. Xylazine and xylazine-ketamine in dogs. Am J Vet Res 47:636–641, 1986.
101. Mitchell B, Williams JT. Respiratory function changes in sheep associated with lying in lateral recumbency and with sedation by xylazine. Proc Assoc Vet Anaesth Great Br Ir 6:32–36, 1977.
102. Hall LW. Cardiovascular and pulmonary effects of recumbency in two conscious ponies. Equine Vet J 16:89–92, 1984.
103. Klein L, Fisher H. Cardiopulmonary effects of restraint in dorsal recumbency on awake cattle. Am J Vet Res 49:1605–1608, 1988.
104. Wagner AE, Muir WW, Grospitch BJ. Cardiopulmonary effects of position in conscious cattle. Am J Vet Res 51:7–10, 1990.
105. Agostoni E. Mechanics of the pleural space. Physiol Rev 52:57–128, 1972.
106. Rehder K. Anesthesia and the mechanics of respiration. In: Effects of Anesthesia, Edited by B.G. Covino, H.A. Fozzard, K. Rehder, and G. Strichartz. Bethesda, MA: American Physiological Society, 1985:91–106.
107. Marshall BE, Marshall C. Anesthesia and pulmonary circulation. In: Effects of Anesthesia, Edited by B.G. Covino, H.A. Fozzard, K. Rehder, and G. Strichartz. Bethesda, MA: American Physiological Society, 1985:121–136.
108. Amis TC, Jones HA, Hughes JMB. A conscious dog model for study of regional lung function. J Appl Physiol Respir Environ Exercise Physiol 53:1050–1054, 1982.
109. Amis TC, Pascoe JR, Hornof W. Topographic distribution of pulmonary ventilation and perfusion in the horse. Am J Vet Res 45:1597–1601, 1984.
110. Hedenstierna G, Nyman G, Kvart C, Funkquist B. Ventilation-perfusion relationships in the standing horse: An inert gas elimination study. Equine Vet J 19:514–519, 1987.
111. Robinson NE. Some functional consequences of species differences in lung anatomy. Adv Vet Sci Comp Med 26:1–33, 1982.
112. Tucker A, McMurtry IF, Reeves JT, Alexander AF, Will DH, Grover RF. Lung vascular smooth muscle as a determinant of pulmonary hypertension at high altitude. Am J Physiol 228:762–767, 1975.
113. Elliott AR, Steffey EP, Jarvis KA, Marshall BE. Unilateral hypoxic pulmonary vasoconstriction in the dog, pony and miniature swine. Respir Physiol 85:355–369, 1991.
114. Marshall BE, Marshall C, Benumof J, Saidman LJ. Hypoxic pulmonary vasoconstriction in dogs: Effects of lung segment size and oxygen tension. J Appl Physiol Respir Environ Exercise Physiol 51:1543–1551, 1981.
115. Benetar SR, Hewlett AM, Nunn JF. The use of iso-shunt lines for control of oxygen therapy. Br J Anaesth 45:711–718, 1973.
116. Froese AB. Effects of anesthesia and paralysis on the chest wall. In: Effects of Anaesthesia, Edited by B.G. Covino, H.A. Fozzard, K. Rehder, and G. Strichartz. Bethesda, MA: American Physiological Society, 1985:107–120.
117. Lai YL, Rodarte JR, Hyatt RE. Respiratory mechanics in recumbent dogs anesthetized with thiopental sodium. J Appl Physiol Environ Exercise Physiol 46:716–720, 1979.
118. Rugh KS, Garner HE, Hatfield DG, Herrold D. Arterial oxygen and carbon dioxide tensions in conscious laterally recumbent ponies. Equine Vet J 16:185–188, 1984.
119. Honeyman VL, Pettifer GR, Dyson DH. Arterial blood pressure and blood gas valves in normal standing and laterally recumbent African (Loxodonta Africana) and Asian (Elephas maximus) elephants. J Zoo Wild Med 23:205–210, 1992.
120. Engel S. The respiratory tissue of the elephant (Elephas indicus). Acta Anat (Basel) 5:105–111, 1963.
121. Ungerer T, Orr JA, Bisgard GE, Will JA. Cardiopulmonary effects of mechanical distension of the rumen in nonanesthetized sheep. Am J Vet Res 37:807–810, 1976.
122. Musewe VO, Gillespie JR, Berry JD. Influence of ruminal insufflation on pulmonary function and diaphragmatic electromyography in cattle. Am J Vet Res 40:26–31, 1979.
123. Hornof WJ, Dunlop CI, Prestage R, Amis TC. Effects of lateral recumbency on regional lung function in anesthetized horses. Am J Vet Res 47:277–282, 1986.
124. Thurmon JC. General clinical considerations for anesthesia in the horse. Vet Clin North Am Equine Pract 6:485–494, 1990.
125. Stegman GF. Pulmonary function in the horse during anesthesia. A review. J S Afr Vet Assoc 57:49–53, 1986.
126. Wan P, Trim CM, Mueller PO. Xylazine-ketamine and detomidine-tiletamine-zolazepam anesthesia in horses. Vet Surg 21:312–318, 1992.
127. Wilson DV, McFeely AM. Positive end-expiratory pressure during colic surgery in horses: 74 cases (1986–1988). J Am Vet Med Assoc 199:917–921, 1991.
128. Young LE, Bartram DH, Diamond MJ, Gregg AS, Jones RS. Clinical evaluation of an infusion of xylazine, guaifenesin and ketamine for maintenance of anaesthesia in horses. Equine Vet J 25:115–119, 1993.
129. Staddon GE, Weaver BMQ. Regional pulmonary perfusion in horses: A comparison between anesthetized and conscious standing animals. Res Vet Sci 30:44–48, 1981.
130. Stolk PWT. The effect of anesthesia on pulmonary blood flow in the horse. Proc Assoc Vet Anaesth Great Br Ir 10:119–129, 1982.
131. Dobson A, Gleed RD, Meyer RE, Stewart BJ. Changes in blood flow distribution in equine lungs induced by anesthesia. Q J Exp Physiol 70:283–297, 1985.
132. Jarvis KA, Steffey EP, Tyler WS, Willits N, Woliner M. Pulmonary blood flow distribution in anesthetized ponies. J Appl Physiol 72:1173–1178, 1992.
133. Hughes JMB, Glazier JB, Maloney JE, West JB. Effect of lung volume on the distribution of pulmonary blood flow in man. Respir Physiol 4:58–72, 1968.
134. Hughes JMB, Glazier JB, Maloney JE, West JB. Effect of extra-alveolar vessels on distribution of blood flow in the dog lung. J Appl Physiol 25:701–712, 1968.
135. Hewlett AM, Hulands GH, Nunn JF, Milledge JS. Functional residual capacity during anesthesia. III. Artificial ventilation. Br J Anaesth 46:495–503, 1974.
136. Clerex C, VandenBrom WE, deVries HW. Comparison of inhalation-to-perfusion ratio in anesthetized dogs with barrel-shaped thorax vs dogs with deep thorax. Am J Vet Res 52:1097–1103, 1991.
137. McDonell WN, Hall LW, Jeffcott LB. Radiographic evidence of impaired pulmonary function in laterally recumbent anaesthetized horses. Equine Vet J 11:24–32, 1979.
138. Watney GCG. Radiographic evidence of pulmonary dysfunction in anesthetized cattle. Res Vet Sci 41:162–171, 1986.
139. McDonell WN. The effect of anesthesia on pulmonary gas exchange and arterial oxygenation in the horse (Dissertation). University of Cambridge, 1974.
140. Watney GCG. Effects of xylazine/halothane anaesthesia on the pulmonary mechanics of adult cattle. J Assoc Vet Anaesth 14:16–28, 1986/87.
141. Nyman G, Funkquist B, Kvart C, Frostell C, et al. Atelectasis causes gas exchange impairment in the anaesthetized horse. Equine Vet J 22:317–324, 1990.
142. Wilson DV, Soma LR. Cardiopulmonary effects of positive end-expiratory pressure in anesthetized, mechanically ventilated ponies. Am J Vet Res 51:734–739, 1990.
143. Moens Y, Largerweij E, Gootjes P, Poortman J. Differential artificial ventilation in anesthetized horses positioned in lateral recumbency. Am J Vet Res 55:1319–1326, 1994.
144. Nyman G, Frostell C, Hedenstierna G, Funkquist B, Kvart G, Blomqvist H. Selective mechanical ventilation of dependent lung regions in the anesthetized horse in dorsal recumbency. Br J Anaesth 59:1027–1034, 1987.

145. Benson J, Manohar M, Kneller SK, Thurmon JC, Steffey EP. Radiographic characterization of diaphragmatic excursion in halothane anesthetized ponies: Spontaneous and controlled ventilation systems. Am J Vet Res 43:617–621, 1982.

146. Froese AB, Bryan AC. Effects of anesthesia and paralysis on diaphragmatic mechanics in man. Anesthesiology 41:242–255, 1974.

147. Hall LW, Aziz HA, Groenendyk J, Keates H, Rex MAE. Electromyography of some respiratory muscles in the horse. Res Vet Sci 50:328–333, 1991.

148. Aviado DM. Regulation of bronchomotor tone during anesthesia. Anesthesiology 42:68–80 1975.

149. Heneghan CPH, Bergman NA, Jordan C, Lehane JR, Catley DM. Effect of isoflurane on bronchomotor in man. Br J Anaesth 58:24–28, 1986.

150. Watney GCG, Jordan C, Hall LW. Effect of halothane, enflurane and isoflurane on bronchomotor tone in anaesthetized ponies. Br J Anaesth 59:1022–1026, 1987.

151. Watney GCG. Effect of halothane on bronchial calibre of anaesthetized cattle. Vet Rec 20:9–12, 1987.

152. Hall LW, Young SS. Effect of inhalation anesthetics on total respiratory resistance in conscious ponies. J Vet Pharmacol Ther 15:174–179, 1992.

153. Blaze CA, LeBlanc PH, Robinson NE. Effect of withholding feed on ventilation and the incidence of regurgitation during halothane anesthesia of adult cattle. Am J Vet Res 49:2126–2129, 1988.

154. Nunn JF. Anesthesia and pulmonary gas exchange. In Effects of Anesthesia. Edited by B.G. Covino, H.A. Fozzard, K. Rehder, and G. Strichartz. Bethesda, MA: American Physiological Society, 1985:137–147.

155. Barker SJ, Tremper KK. Respiratory monitoring, blood-gas measurement, oximetry, and pulse oximetry. Curr Opin Anaesth 5:816–825, 1992.

156. Cullen DJ, Nemeskal AR, Cooper JB, Zaslavsky A, Dwyer MJ. Effect of oximetry, age, and ASA physical status on the frequency of patients admitted unexpectedly to a postoperative intensive care unit and severity of their anesthetic-related complications. Anesth Analg 74:181–188, 1992.

157. Cote CJ, Rolf N, Lui LM, Goudsouzian HG, Ryan JF, et al. A single blind study of combined pulse oximetry and capnography in children. Anesthesiology 74:980–987, 1991.

158. Turner DM, Ilkiw JE. Cardiovascular and respiratory effects of three rapidly acting barbiturates in dogs. Am J Vet Res 51:598–604, 1990.

159. Dyson DH, Allen DG, Ingwersen W, Pascoe PJ. Evaluation of acepromazine/meperidine/atropine premedication followed by thiopental anesthesia in the cat. Can J Vet Res 52:419–422, 1988.

160. Steffey EP, Farver TB, Woliner MJ. Cardiopulmonary function during 7 h of constant-dose halothane and methoxyflurane. J Appl Physiol 63:1351–1359, 1987.

161. Ingwersen W, Allen DG, Dyson DH, Pascoe PJ, O'Grady, M.R. Cardiopulmonary effects of a halothane/oxygen combination in healthy cats. Can J Vet Res 52:386–391, 1988.

162. Ray JF, Yost L, Moallem S, Sonoudos GM, et al. Immobility, hypoxemia, and pulmonary arteriovenous shunting. Arch Surg 109:537–541, 1974.

163. Ewing KK. Anesthesia techniques in sheep and goats. Vet Clin North Am Food Anim Pract 6:759–778, 1990.

164. Hedenstierna G, Lundquist H, Lundh B, Tokies L, et al. Pulmonary densities during anaesthesia. An experimental study on lung morphology and gas exchange. Eur Respir J 2:528–535, 1989.

165. Fujimoto JL, Lenchan TM. The influence of body position on the blood gas and acid-base status of halothane anesthetized sheep. Vet Surg 14:169–172, 1985.

166. Semrad SD, Trim CM, Hardee GE. Hypertension in bulls and steers anesthetized with guaifenesin-thiobarbiturate-halothane combination. Am J Vet Res 47:1577–1582, 1986.

167. Blaze CA, Robinson NE. Apneic oxygenation in anesthetized ponies and horses. Vet Res Comm 11:281–291, 1987.

168. Hall LW, Gillespie JR, Tyler WS. Alveolar-arterial oxygen tension differences in anaesthetized horses. Br J Anaesth 40:560–568, 1968.

169. de Moor A, van den Hende C. Inspiratory concentrations of O_2, N_2, and N_2O, arterial oxygenation and acid-base status during closed system halothane anaesthesia in the horse. Zentralbl Veterinarmed 19:1–7, 1972.

170. Steffey EP, Kelly AB, Woliner MJ. Time-related responses of spontaneously breathing, laterally recumbent horses to prolonged anesthesia with halothane. Am J Vet Res 48:952–957, 1987.

171. Nyman G, Hedenstierna G. Comparison of conventional and selective mechanical ventilation in the anaesthetized horse. J Vet Med 35:299–315, 1988.

172. Gleed RD. Improvement in arterial oxygen tension with change in posture in anaesthetized horses. Res Vet Sci 44:255–259, 1988.

173. Nyman G, Funkquist B, Kvart C. Postural effects on blood gas tension, blood pressure, heart rate, ECG and respiratory rate during prolonged anaesthesia in the horse. J Vet Med , 35:54–62, 1988.

174. Steffey EP, Kelly AB, Hodgson DS, Grandy JL, Woliner MJ, Willits N. Effect of body posture on cardiopulmonary function in horses during five hours of constant-dose halothane anesthesia. Am J Vet Res 51:11–16, 1990.

175. Stegmann GF, Littlejohn A. The effect of lateral and dorsal recumbency on cardiopulmonary function in the anaesthetized horse. J S Afr Vet Assoc 58:21–27, 1987.

176. Young LE, Richards DLS, Brearly JC, Bartram DH, Jones RS. The effect of a 50% inspired mixture of nitrous oxide on arterial oxygen tension in spontaneously breathing horses anaesthetized with halothane. J Vet Anaesth 19:37–40, 1992.

177. Day TK, Gaynor JS, Muir WW, Bednarski RM, Mason DE. Blood gas values during intermittent positive pressure ventilation and spontaneous ventilation in 160 anesthetized horses positioned in lateral and dorsal recumbancy. Vet Surg 24:266–276, 1995.

178. Wagner AE, Bednarski RM, Muir WW. Hemodynamic effects of carbon dioxide during intermittent positive-pressure ventilation in horses. Am J Vet Res 51:1922–1928, 1990.

chapter **7** *A*

NERVOUS SYSTEM: THE CENTRAL NERVOUS SYSTEM

CENTRAL NERVOUS SYSTEM
  Brain
  Cranial Nerves
  Spinal Cord
  Cerebrospinal Fluid
PERIPHERAL NERVOUS SYSTEM
  Spinal Nerves
AUTONOMIC NERVOUS SYSTEM
  Parasympathetic System
  Sympathetic System
FUNCTION OF NEURONS

Axonal Conduction
Neuroregulators
Transmission at the Myoneural Junction
Cholinergic Transmission
Adrenergic Transmission
RECEPTORS
  Cholinergic
  Adrenergic
THEORIES OF ANESTHESIA
  Sites of Action of General Anesthetics

Central Nervous System

Because anesthetics preferentially affect the nervous system, a general knowledge of its parts and functions is essential. Anatomically, the nervous system can be divided into central and peripheral divisions. The central division, composed of the brain and spinal cord, contains all of the important nerve centers or nuclei. The peripheral division is composed of nerves and ganglia that supply the different organs and tissues.

Functionally, the nervous system can be divided into somatic and visceral (autonomic) divisions, each with efferent and afferent tracts. The somatic efferent fibers terminate in the motor end plates of skeletal muscle. The afferent somatic fibers convey three sensory modalities from the periphery: pain, temperature (both warm and cold), and light and deep touch (pressure). In addition, somatic afferents conduct impulses arising in the eye and ear to provide sight and hearing.

Autonomic efferents innervate smooth muscle, cardiac muscle, and glands and the muscles of mastication, the pharynx, and the larynx. Autonomic afferents carry impulses from receptors in mucous membranes or in the walls of organs stimulated by distension or by the chemical composition of the substances contained in the

organ. In addition, autonomic afferent fibers mediate the sensations of smell and taste. The somatic division is primarily concerned with peripheral sensations and voluntary movement, and the autonomic system is concerned with maintenance of visceral function and homeostasis, including regulation of heart rate and blood pressure, temperature, glandular secretion, peristalsis, sphincter tension, and pupil size. Anesthesia is concerned with both physiologic divisions, since analgesia, relaxation of skeletal muscle, and maintenance of cardiopulmonary function are essential (Chapters 4 through 6).

BRAIN

The brain can be divided into the cerebrum and the brain stem. The cerebrum consists of telencephalic and diencephalic portions. The telencephalic portion is comprised of the cerebral hemispheres, which consist of an outer cortical layer of gray matter containing nerve cell bodies or neurons and an inner medullary core of white matter consisting mainly of myelinated nerve fibers. The basal ganglia (corpus striatum, amygdaloid, and claustrum) are large masses of gray matter at the base of each cerebral hemisphere. The corpus striatum

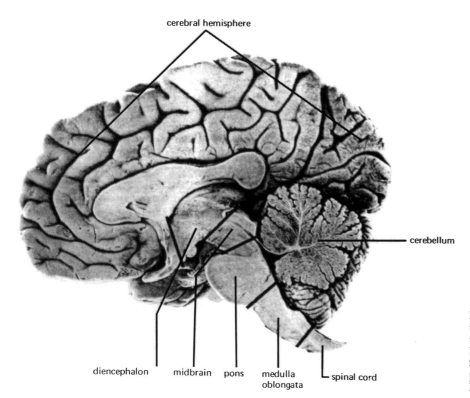

cerebral hemisphere

cerebellum

diencephalon   midbrain   pons   medulla   spinal cord
                                      oblongata

Fig. 7A–1. Regions of the mature human central nervous system in sagittal section. From Barr M.L. The Human Nervous System: An Anatomic Viewpoint. Harper & Row Publishers, Hagerstown, Md, 1979.

and claustrum are poorly understood but appear to contribute to the extrapyramidal motor system. Their primary function appears to be inhibition of motor function and maintenance of balance between opposing muscles at both the cortical and brain-stem levels. Dopamine and GABA are the primary inhibitory neurotransmitters released. The amygdaloid nucleus is a component of the olfactory and limbic systems. The cerebral cortex is where sensory, motor, and associational activity occur. The white matter of the cerebrum consists of corticocortical fibers and projection fibers. The corticocortical fibers connect different areas in the same hemisphere (association fibers) and in the opposite hemisphere (commissural fibers). Fibers connecting the cortical areas of the two hemispheres cross the midline in a large commissure, the corpus callosum. Projection fibers originate or terminate in the cortex and connect it with the basal ganglia, brain stem, or spinal cord. The fibers passing between the cortex and subcortical centers converge to form a compact internal capsule (Fig. 7A–1).

The diencephalic portion of the cerebrum forms the central core of the cerebrum and is surrounded by the hemispheres. It consists of the thalamus, subthalamus, epithalamus, and hypothalamus, and is positioned between the cerebrum and the brain stem. The thalamus receives fibers from all sensory systems except the olfactory and projects to sensory areas of the cerebral cortex. The cerebral cortex is an outgrowth of the lower centers, especially the thalamus. As a result, for each area of the cortex, there is a smaller corresponding area within the thalamus. Portions of the thalamus are involved in reverberating circuits with nonspecific

cortical areas concerned with complex mental processes. Thalamic nuclei participate in neural circuits related to emotional aspects of brain function (limbic system), are part of the ascending reticular activating system, and are incorporated into motor pathways from the cerebellum and corpus striatum to the motor cortex.

The subthalamus is comprised of a motor nucleus, sensory tracts that terminate in the thalamus, and tracts from the cerebellum and corpus striatum to the thalamus. The epithalamus is composed of the pineal gland and tracts concerned with autonomic responses to olfactory and emotional changes. The hypothalamus is the primary center for integrative control of the autonomic nervous system. Parasympathetic responses, including slowing of the heart rate, vasodilation, decreased blood pressure, salivation, increased gastrointestinal peristalsis, contraction of the urinary bladder, and sweating, are elicited by stimulation of the anterior hypothalamus. Stimulation of the posterior and lateral hypothalamus elicits sympathetic responses, including increased heart rate and blood pressure, cessation of gastrointestinal peristalsis, dilation of the pupils, and hyperglycemia. The hypothalamus plays a major role in maintaining homeostasis through control of temperature, thirst, and appetite. Nervous control of the endocrine system is via the hypothalamic neurohypophyseal hormones. Only the adrenal medulla is regulated by direct nervous connections (i.e., the preganglionic sympathetic fibers). The hypothalamus plays a major role in producing responses to emotional changes, to needs signaled by hunger and thirst, and to maintenance of homeostasis.

The brain stem consists of the midbrain, pons, and medulla oblongata (Fig. 7A–2). The midbrain contains sensory and motor pathways, the nuclei of the third and fourth cranial nerves (oculomotor and trochlear), and two major motor nuclei, the red nucleus and the substantia nigra. The dorsal part of the midbrain is primarily involved with auditory function and visual reflex movements of the eyes and head. The cerebellum is connected to the midbrain by the superior cerebellar peduncles.

The pons consists of two distinct parts. The dorsal portion, like the rest of the brain stem, has both sensory and motor tracts. In addition, the dorsal pons contains the nuclei of the fifth, sixth, seventh, and eighth cranial nerves (trigeminal, abducens, facial, and acoustic). The ventral pons functions as a large synaptic region, providing a connection between the cerebral motor cortex and the contralateral cerebellar hemisphere via the middle cerebellar peduncles.

Caudal to the pons is the medulla oblongata, and posterior to it is the spinal cord. In addition to nerve tracts, the medulla contains vital nerve centers that regulate respiration and circulation. Four pairs of cranial nerves connect to it: the glossopharyngeal (ninth), vagus (tenth), spinal accessory (eleventh), and hypoglossal (twelfth). The cerebellum is connected to the medulla by the inferior cerebellar peduncles.

The cerebellum lies dorsal to the brain stem and is formed by two hemispheres separated by a central portion, the vermis. The cerebellum receives input from the sensory systems and the cerebral cortex. The cerebellum integrates muscle tone in relation to equilibrium, locomotion, posture and nonstereotyped movements based on experience. It is chiefly concerned with muscular coordination (Fig. 7A–2).

CRANIAL NERVES

Cranial nerves consist of (a) a peripheral portion, (b) a nuclear center in the brain stem (except olfactory and optic nerves), and (c) central connections with other parts of the brain (Fig. 7A–3). All twelve cranial nerves are paired.

Functionally, cranial nerves can be divided into those carrying impulses away from the brain (efferent), those carrying impulses toward the brain (afferent), and those performing both functions (mixed):

Afferent Nerves	*Efferent Nerves*	*Mixed Nerves*
1. Olfactory	3. Oculomotor	5. Trigeminal
2. Optic	4. Trochlear	7. Facial
8. Acoustic	6. Abducens	9. Glossopha-
	11. Spinal	ryngeal
	Accessory	10. Vagus
	12. Hypoglossal	

The *olfactory, optic,* and *acoustic* nerves are afferent and therefore sensory, providing the senses of smell, sight, and hearing, and balance respectively.

The efferent cranial nerves include the *oculomotor nerve,* which innervates muscles of the eye: dorsal, medial, and ventral rectus muscles; ventral oblique; levator palpebrae superioris; ciliary muscle; and the sphincter pupillae. The *trochlear nerve* innervates the dorsal oblique muscle of the eye, and the *abducens nerve* supplies the lateral rectus and retractor oculi muscles. The *spinal accessory nerve* arises from the medulla and also has fibers from all seven cervical nerves that run cranially to combine with the medullary roots. The spinal accessory nerve contributes some fibers to the vagus nerve, then runs caudally to innervate the muscles of the neck and shoulder. The *hypoglossal*

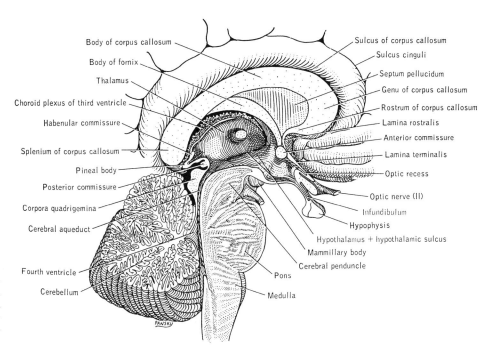

Fig. 7A–2. Median sagittal section through the brain stem. From House E.L. and Pansky B. A Functional Approach to Neuroanatomy. 2nd Ed. McGraw-Hill, Blacklick, OH.

Body of corpus callosum
Body of fornix
Thalamus
Choroid plexus of third ventricle
Habenular commissure
Splenium of corpus callosum
Pineal body
Posterior commissure
Corpora quadrigemina
Cerebral aqueduct
Fourth ventricle
Cerebellum

Sulcus of corpus callosum
Sulcus cinguli
Septum pellucidum
Genu of corpus callosum
Rostrum of corpus callosum
Lamina rostralis
Anterior commissure
Lamina terminalis
Optic recess
Optic nerve (II)
Infundibulum
Hypophysis
Hypothalamus + hypothalamic sulcus
Mammillary body
Cerebral penduncle
Pons
Medulla

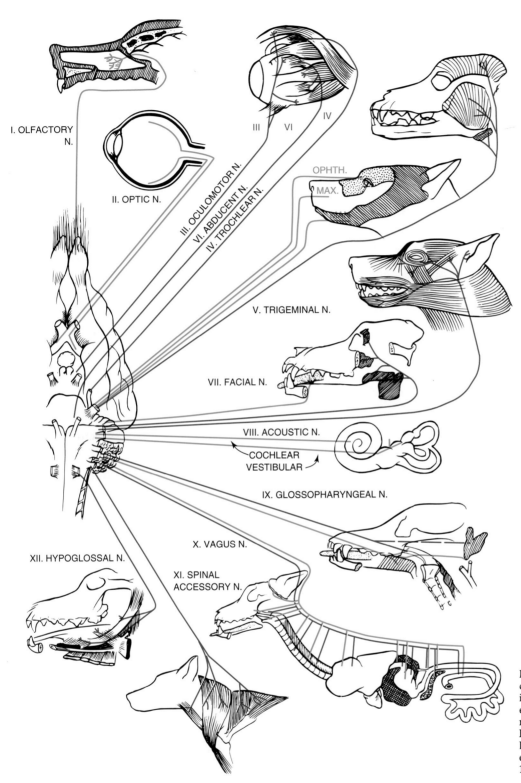

I. OLFACTORY N.

II. OPTIC N.

III. OCULOMOTOR N.
VI. ABDUCENT N.
IV. TROCHLEAR N.

V. TRIGEMINAL N.

VII. FACIAL N.

VIII. ACOUSTIC N.

COCHLEAR
VESTIBULAR

IX. GLOSSOPHARYNGEAL N.

X. VAGUS N.

XI. SPINAL ACCESSORY N.

XII. HYPOGLOSSAL N.

OPHTH.
MAX.

III VI IV

Fig. 7A–3. The origin and major distribution of the cranial nerves in the dog. Red lines represent efferent fibers, and green lines represent afferent fibers. From Hoerlein B.F. Canine Neurology, Diagnosis and Treatment. 3rd ed. W.B. Saunders, Philadelphia, 1978.

nerve innervates the muscles of the pharynx and the larynx, and the intrinsic muscles of the tongue.

The *trigeminal nerve* is sensory to the skin of the muzzle and head and motor to the muscles of mastication. It has three main branches, the ophthalmic, maxillary, and mandibular. The ophthalmic is sensory to skin of the forehead, the eyeball (corneal and palpebral reflexes), and the skin of the lower eyelid; the maxillary is sensory to the skin of the muzzle, nose, and upper lip; the mucous membrane of the nose and nasopharynx, the hard and soft palate, and the teeth of the upper jaw. The mandibular branch supplies sensation to the lower part of the face, side of the head, lower lip and teeth, ear, and tongue, and is motor to the muscles of mastication.

The *facial nerve* is motor to all the cutaneous muscles of the face, lips, nose, cheeks, ears, and ventral neck, and to the submandibular and sublingual salivary glands and the lacrimal gland. It is sensory to the taste buds and to the skin of the external ear.

The *glossopharyngeal nerve* is motor to the stylopharyngeus muscle and to the parotid and zygomatic salivary glands. It is sensory to the pharynx, tonsil, tongue (touch, temperature, pain and taste) and carotid body and sinus (chemoreceptors and baroreceptors).

The *vagus nerve* supplies organs and muscles of the neck, thorax, and abdomen. Preganglionic parasympathetic fibers are supplied to the heart, smooth muscle, and glands of the thorax and abdominal viscera. Motor innervation is supplied to the pharynx, cricothyroideus muscle of the larynx, intrinsic muscles of the larynx, and striated muscle of the esophagus. The sensory component of the vagus nerve supplies the base of the tongue (touch, temperature, pain, and taste), pharynx, esophagus, stomach, intestines, larynx, trachea, bronchi, lungs, heart, aortic baroreceptors, and other viscera.

SPINAL CORD

From the medulla, the spinal cord runs posteriorly in the vertebral canal. In the dog and cat the spinal cord terminates at the level of the last lumbar vertebra; in the horse, ruminants, and swine the cord terminates in the midsacrum. The caudal portion of the vertebral canal contains the cauda equina, which is composed of descending spinal nerves. The cord is surrounded by the meninges, which support and protect it. From without inward, they are the dura mater, arachnoid,

and pia mater. The spinal fluid is found in the subarachnoid space (Fig. 7A–4).

The spinal cord is the least differentiated portion of the central nervous system. It is segmental in nature, having paired spinal nerves at each vertebral segment that attach to the cord by a dorsal sensory root and a ventral motor root (Bell-Magendie Law) and exit the canal via the intervertebral foramen. In the fetus, all spinal nerves exit at right angles to the spinal cord. In the adult, however, owing to differential growth rates between the spinal cord and the bony vertebral canal, the nerves must run posteriorly to reach their respective intervertebral foramina. This fact is significant and affects the level of analgesia induced by the deposition of analgesic drug within the spinal canal.

The cord has an H-shaped central core of gray matter containing nerve cell bodies. The gray matter functions as the initial site for processing of incoming sensory information and as a relay station for transmission of these signals to the brain. It also serves as the final site for processing descending motor impulses from the brain to the skeletal muscles. The gray matter can be divided into dorsal, ventral, and lateral horns. The dorsal horn is the gate through which impulses in sensory nerve fibers are processed, initiating impulses in ascending tracts. Afferent tactile, temperature, and pain impulses are processed and transmitted in the substantia gelatinosa of the dorsal horn (Chapter 4). The lateral horns of the thoracolumbar segments contain the cell bodies of the preganglionic sympathetic nerves. The ventral horn of the gray matter contains the alpha and gamma motor neurons, which leave the cord via

Fig. 7A–4 A cross section of the spine in the dog. (1) spinous process, (2) cranial articular process, (3) caudal articular process, (4) accessory process, (5) transverse process, (6) nucleus pulposus, (6') fibrous ring or annulus fibrosus, (6") dorsal longitudinal ligament, (7) epidural space, (8) subarachnoid space, (9) dura mater, (10) arachnoid, (11) longitudinal venous sinus, (12) ventral nerve root, (13) dorsal root ganglion, (14) spinal nerve, (15) dorsal branch of spinal nerve, (16) ventral branch of spinal nerve, (17) ramus communicans, (18) sympathetic trunk ganglion. (From Worthman, R. The Nerve of That Dog. Washington State University, 1960.)

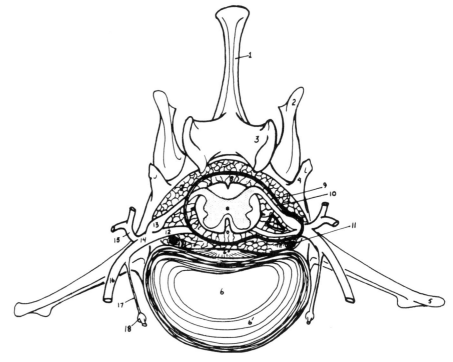

the ventral nerve roots to innervate the skeletal muscles. Cells of Renshaw in the ventral gray matter are intermediary neurons that synapse in the ventral horn with ventral motor neurons to inhibit their activity and prevent excessive activity. There are three types of cells in the gray matter. Internuncial cells are the smallest and are most prevalent in the dorsal and intermediate zones. Internuncial cells receive afferents from dorsal root fibers and fibers in descending tracts of the white matter. Axons of internuncial cells terminate on motor and tract cell bodies and modulate their activity by releasing inhibitory or excitatory neurotransmitters. Motor cells are found in the ventral horn and consist of alpha and gamma motor neurons. Axons of tract cells constitute the ascending fasciculi of the lateral and ventral white columns. Tract cells (transmitter cells) are located primarily in the dorsal and intermediate zones of the gray matter. Cells of the lateral horn and the sacral autonomic nucleus are preganglionic neurons of the sympathetic and parasympathetic systems respectively.

The gray matter is surrounded by the white matter, the myelinated axons of intermediate longitudinally running nerve fibers. This outer white matter is divided into three major columns: dorsal, lateral, and ventral. Within these columns are ascending and descending tracts. The nerve fibers of the white matter are organized into ascending afferent tracts that convey sensory information to the brain and descending efferent motor tracts that convey impulses to peripheral effector organs. The spinal cord contains nerve circuits that subserve important spinal reflexes. Afferent fibers arriving at the cord through the dorsal nerve roots carry sensory impulses, which can initiate spinal reflexes and are also transmitted to the brain stem and cerebellum, where they enter various circuits including those that influence movement. Sensory information is also transmitted through the brain stem to the thalamus and cerebral cortex, where it becomes part of the conscious experience (perception) colored with emotional overtones and where immediate or delayed behavioral responses are initiated. Some descending tracts arising from the cortex and brain stem carry efferent motor impulses; others excite or inhibit spinal circuits. Thus, the spinal cord is much more complex than a mere cable or conduit and plays a much larger role in regulatory CNS function than was previously thought.

Efferent fibers, passing from the cord in the ventral nerve roots, transmit motor impulses from higher centers or from reflex centers within the cord to muscles and glands. Ascending and descending tracts within the cord connect the higher centers and the various cord segments with each other. For a more complete description of the spinal tracts in the dog, the reader is referred to Hoerlein.(1)

The meninges (dura mater, arachnoidea, and pia mater) surround the spinal cord (Fig. 7A–4). Various spaces are associated with the meninges and are important in understanding spinal anesthetics and nomenclature. The dura mater has two layers within the cranial vault, an inner or visceral layer and an outer layer adherent to the cranial periosteum. The inner or visceral layer invests the spinal cord and ventral and dorsal nerve root; the outer layer is absent in the vertebral canal of some species. The epidural space is that space within the spinal canal outside the visceral layer of the dura mater. It has also been referred to as the *extradural space* and, in those species having both layers of dura, the *intradural space.* The dura adheres to the periosteum of the foramen magnum, thereby preventing communication between the cranial and vertebral epidural spaces. The epidural space contains blood vessels, lymphatics, and fat, and communicates with the paravertebral tissues via the intervertebral foramina. This communication may be interrupted in older animals by fibrous connective tissue and bony malformations associated with spinal arthritis, and in obese patients by fat.

The subarachnoid space is located between the arachnoidea and pia mater. The subarachnoid space contains cerebrospinal fluid and is continuous between the cranial and vertebral segments. There is no direct communication between the epidural and subarachnoid spaces. The pia mater is one cell layer thick and lies directly on the brain and spinal cord.

At each segment, dorsal and ventral nerve roots emerge from the cord to form the bilateral spinal nerves. The thoracolumbar nerves contain sympathetic fibers. As the nerve roots leave the spinal cord, they pierce the meninges and carry a layer of each with them. These nerve roots with their meningeal covers unite to form the spinal nerves. The meningeal covers fuse at the junction of the roots and extend no farther peripherally.

CEREBROSPINAL FLUID

The cerebrospinal fluid (CSF) is found in both an internal (ventricular) system and an external (subarachnoid) system. The internal system consists of the paired lateral ventricles within the cerebral hemispheres, the third ventricle medially between the thalamus and hypothalamus and the fourth ventricle, lying beneath the cerebellum and within the medulla. Cerebrospinal fluid is produced by the choroid plexus, a fringelike fold of pia mater found on the floor of both lateral ventricles and in the fourth ventricle, and also by the ependymal epithelium lining the ventricles.(2) Fluid in the lateral ventricles empties into the third ventricle through the paired foramina of Monro. The third ventricle, in turn, empties into the fourth through the aqueduct of Sylvius. The central canal of the spinal cord is continuous with the fourth ventricle. The external or subarachnoid system overlies the brain and spinal cord. The bilateral foramina of Luschka allow fluid to pass between the ventricular and subarachnoid systems. In animals phylogenetically below the ape, the foramen of Magendie is not found. Absorption of CSF occurs at the arachnoid villi or granulations located primarily in the subdural venous sinuses. The arachnoid villi are fingerlike projections of the arachnoidal membrane that penetrate the venous sinuses. Their endothelium is porous and highly permeable, allowing free passage of

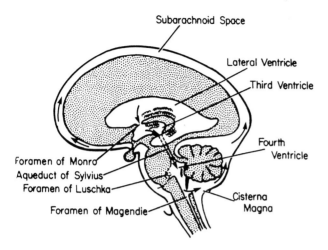

Suborachnoid Space
Lateral Ventricle
Third Ventricle
Fourth Ventricle
Foramen of Monro
Aqueduct of Sylvius
Foramen of Luschka
Cisterna Magna
Foramen of Magendie

Fig. 7A–5. Circulation of cerebrospinal fluid. From Stoelting, R.K. The Pharmacology and Physiology in Anesthetic Practice, 2nd. ed., J.B. Lippincott, Philadelphia, 1991.

water, electrolytes, proteins, and even red blood cells (Fig. 7A–5).

Cerebrospinal fluid functions to cushion the brain within the cranial vault. It is formed from the blood by secretory and filtration processes. Normal pressure of the CSF is 10 mm Hg. The concentration of sodium is equal to that of plasma, the concentration of chloride in the CSF is 15% greater, and the concentration of potassium and glucose is 40% and 30% less than in plasma respectively. The specific gravity of CSF is 1.002 to 1.009. The pH of CSF is closely maintained at 7.32. Carbon dioxide but not hydrogen ion readily crosses the blood-brain barrier. Bicarbonate ion is actively transported. As a result, the pH of CSF is rapidly altered by changes in $PaCO_2$ but not by changes in arterial pH. In general, the choroid plexus and the capillary membranes are highly permeable to water, oxygen, carbon dioxide, and most lipid-soluble substances such as anesthetics and alcohol; slightly permeable to electrolytes such as sodium, potassium, and chloride; and nearly impermeable to plasma proteins and large organic molecules. Glucose is actively transported across the capillary endothelium (blood-brain barrier). Conversely, the pia mater, which covers the brain and spinal cord, and the ependyma, which lines the ventricles, are freely permeable to many substances. Thus, drugs that cannot gain access to tissues of the CNS when administered systemically may penetrate nervous tissues when administered into the subarachnoid space.

The brain–blood–cerebrospinal fluid volume is constant because the skull forms an inelastic box. A volume increase in any one component occurs at the expense of one or both of the other two (Monro-Kellie hypothesis). Normal intracranial pressure is less than 15 mm Hg. As the pressure of cerebrospinal fluid increases, it may reach a point at which it inhibits blood flow to the brain. Increased cerebral or spinal fluid pressure produces a reflex increase in heart rate and blood pressure.(3) It has been hypothesized that the increase in cerebrospinal fluid pressure creates ischemia of neurons, and that this

is the stimulus for increased sympathetic activity. Hypotensive drugs, osmotic diuretics, hypothermia, and hyperventilation may all be used to decrease intracranial pressure. Effects of various anesthetics and anesthetic adjuncts on overall CNS function are discussed in Section 3, "Pharmacology" (see the specific anesthetics) and Chapter 23.

Peripheral Nervous System

SPINAL NERVES

Spinal nerves supply motor and sensory innervation to most of the body (somatic nervous system), with the exception of the head and viscera. They also form part of the autonomic nervous system, which controls visceral functions. Spinal nerves vary in number depending on species. Anatomically, the spinal nerves are formed by a combination of dorsal and ventral spinal roots arising from the spinal cord. These join and leave the spinal canal through the intervertebral foramina. The dorsal root carries afferent fibers whose nuclei are in the dorsal root ganglion. The ventral roots contain efferent fibers. The efferent motor fibers travel in the ventral nerve roots that originate from axons of the ventral and lateral horns of the gray matter.

Nerves can be classified by their size and degree of myelination, which determines speed of impulse transmission. Large, heavily myelinated fibers have the highest conduction velocities, while small nonmyelinated fibers have lower conduction rates (Table 7A–1). The largest Type A fibers are subclassified as A-alpha, A-beta, A-gamma, and A-delta fibers. A-alpha fibers innervate skeletal muscles and also subserve proprioception. A-beta fibers subserve touch and pressure. A-gamma fibers innervate the skeletal muscle spindles to maintain muscle tone. A-delta fibers subserve temperature, fast pain, and touch. Type B fibers are preganglionic autonomic fibers. Type C fibers are smallest and are postganglionic sympathetic fibers or transmit slow pain, touch, and temperature sensations.

The spinal cord is divided into segments for descriptive purposes, there being in the dog 8 cervical, 13 thoracic, 7 lumbar, 3 sacral, and 4 or 5 coccygeal segments. The segmental distribution of the motor roots in the dog is set forth in Table 7A–2.

After leaving the intervertebral foramen, each spinal nerve divides into dorsal and ventral branches. The dorsal branches generally supply the muscles and skin of the back, while the ventral branches supply the muscles and skin of the thorax, abdomen, and extremities. Branches from several spinal nerves may combine to form plexuses such as the brachial plexus or major nerves such as the sciatic nerve (Figs. 7A–6 and 7A–7).

A myotome is the mass of musculature innervated from one ventral spinal nerve root (motor). It is derived from the somite of an embryonic segment and forms the skeletal musculature originating from that segment. The area supplied by a single dorsal nerve root (sensory) is called a *dermatome*. There is considerable overlap of areas supplied by adjacent roots. Knowledge

Table 7A–1. Classification of Nerve Fibers

		Terminology	Fiber Diameter	Conduction Speed (meters/second)
Myelinated somatic fibers	A	Alpha Beta Gamma Delta Epsilon	20 μ ↓ (3–4μ) 2 μ	120 ↓ (6–30)→pain fibers 5
Myelinated visceral fibers (preganglionic autonomic)	B		<3 μ	3–15
Nonmyelinated somatic fibers	C		<2 μ	0.5–2→pain fibers

(From Wylie, W.D., and Churchill-Davidson, H.C.: A Practice of Anaesthesia. Lloyd-Luke, Ltd., London, 1966, and Gasser, H.S.: Pain Producing Impulses in Peripheral Nerves. Assoc Res Nerv Dis Proc, 23:44, 1943.)

Table 7A–2. Segmental Distribution of Motor Roots in the Dog

C3-4-5	Distributed in segmental manner to most of the neck musculature.
C5	May send a branch to the phrenic nerve.
C6 (usually 7)	Phrenic nerves to the diaphragm.
C6-7-8, T1 (occasionally 2)	Brachial plexus to the forelimb.
T2-8	Intercostal nerves to the thorax.
T9-13	Nerves to the muscles of the ventral and lower lateral parts of the abdominal wall.
L1-2 (occasionally 3)	Nerves to the muscles of the caudolateral abdominal wall and the thigh in the region of the stifle.
L4-5-6-7, S1-2-3	Lumbosacral plexus to the hindlimb.
L4-5-6 (occasionally 3)	Femoral nerve to extensors of the stifle.
L5-6 (occasionally 4)	Obturator nerve, the abductor of the hip.
L6-7, S1	Sciatic nerve supplying all other muscles of the hindlimb.

(From McGrath, J.T.: Neurologic Examination of the Dog, 2nd ed. Lea & Febiger, Philadelphia, 1960.)

of myotomes and dermatomes is essential for regional anesthesia of the thorax, abdomen, and limbs.

Branching off the spinal nerves in the thoracic and lumbar areas are rami communicantes, which connect the spinal nerves with a chain of ganglia lying lateral to the vertebral bodies, termed the *vertebral sympathetic ganglia* (Fig. 7A–8).

Automatic Nervous System

The autonomic nervous system is often called the *vegetative, visceral,* or *involuntary nervous system* because its action requires no conscious control. In this respect, it contrasts with the somatic nervous system supplying the striated muscles. The autonomic nervous system is comprised of the efferent and afferent nerves inner-

vating the viscera. Thus, its primary efferent role is in maintenance of homeostasis through control of circulation, breathing, excretion, and maintenance of body temperature. These regulatory functions are subject to modification by input from higher brain centers, especially as a result of reactions to the environment. Visceral efferents consist of two neurons rather than a single motor neuron as occurs in the somatic system. The cell body of the first neuron is in the brain stem or spinal cord. Its axon terminates on the cell body of the second, located in an autonomic ganglion. The axon of the ganglion cell terminates in the effector cell.

Autonomic visceral afferents are primarily sensory neurons similar to those in somatic tissues. They elicit reflex responses in viscera and a feeling of fullness of hollow organs such as the stomach, large intestine, and bladder. Afferent impulses contribute to feelings of well-being or malaise and conduct impulses for pain. Special visceral afferents mediate the special senses of taste and olfactory function. The general visceral afferents have their cell bodies in the sensory ganglia of the cranial and spinal nerves that include the autonomic outflow. These neurons are of two types: physiologic afferents and pain afferents. Physiologic afferents are present in both sympathetic and parasympathetic divisions, while pain afferents are almost exclusively sympathetic. The most important visceral physiologic afferents are associated with the parasympathetic division and mediate cardiovascular, respiratory, and gastrointestinal reflexes (e.g., baroreceptor, chemoreceptor, Hering-Breuer, emptying of the rectum and bladder subject to conscious control, and feelings of fullness or hunger).

Visceral pain afferents are associated with the sympathetic division. Cell bodies are located in the thoracolumbar dorsal root ganglia. Their peripheral processes reach the sympathetic trunk via the white rami communicantes (Fig. 7A–8), run in the sympathetic trunk, and reach the viscera through the cardiac, pulmonary, or splanchnic nerves. Central terminations are on transmitter cells in the substantia gelatinosa. The ascending pathway for visceral pain coincides at least in part with that for somatic pain (Chapter 4).

both pre- and postganglionic neurons. Each preganglionic fiber synapses with 1 to 3 postganglionic neurons, which terminate on a limited number of effector cells. Acetylcholine is rapidly inactivated by acetylcholinesterase at the synapse resulting in a short duration of discharge. Thus, parasympathetic activity is highly localized. Preganglionic fibers of the parasympathetic system arise in three areas: the midbrain (tectal outflow), the medulla (medullary outflow), and the sacral spinal cord (sacral outflow) (Fig. 7A–9). These efferent fibers generally are long and synapse with one or two postganglionic fibers in a ganglion on or within the organ supplied. The tectal outflow originates in the Edinger–Westphal nucleus of the third (oculomotor) cranial nerve and synapses at the ciliary ganglion in the orbit to innervate the pupillary

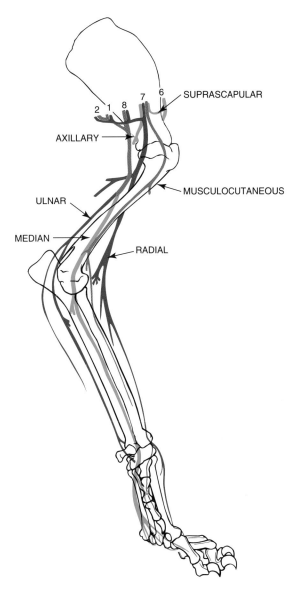

Fig. 7A–6. A medial view of the front limb of the dog illustrating the relative course and distribution of the major nerves to the leg. Note the spinal nerves making up the brachial plexus, C6-7-8 and T1-2. (From Hoerlein, B.F. Canine Neurology, Diagnosis, and Treatment, 3rd ed. WB Saunders, Philadelphia, 1978.)

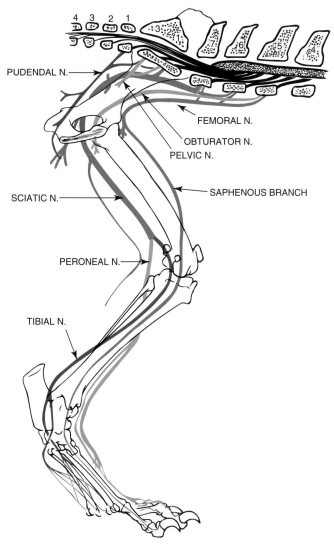

Fig. 7A–7. A medial view of the canine hind limb illustrating the relative course and distribution of the major nerves. Note the spinal nerves making up the sciatic nerve. (From Hoerlein, B.F. Canine Neurology, Diagnosis, and Treatment, 3rd ed., WB Saunders, Philadelphia, 1978.)

The hypothalamus is the primary area of the brain that controls the autonomic nervous system. The autonomic system can be further subdivided into the craniosacral or parasympathetic division and the thoracolumbar or sympathetic division (Fig. 7A–9). A characteristic of the autonomic nervous system is that both divisions are constantly active, resulting in a basal level of sympathetic and parasympathetic tone. Thus, each division can increase or decrease its effect at a given organ to more closely regulate function.

PARASYMPATHETIC SYSTEM

The parasympathetic system functions to conserve and restore energy. Acetylcholine is the neurotransmitter at

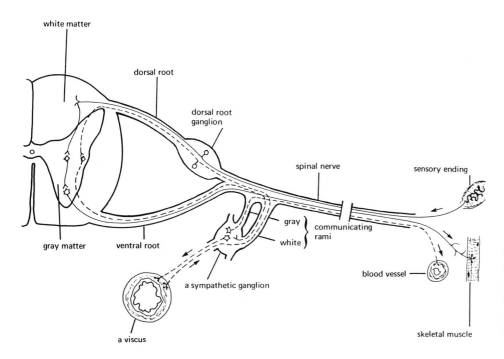

Fig. 7A–8. Components of a spinal nerve between the first thoracic and second or third lumbar segments. From Barr M.L. The Human Nervous System: An Anatomic Viewpoint. Harper & Row Publishers, Hagerstown, Md, 1979.

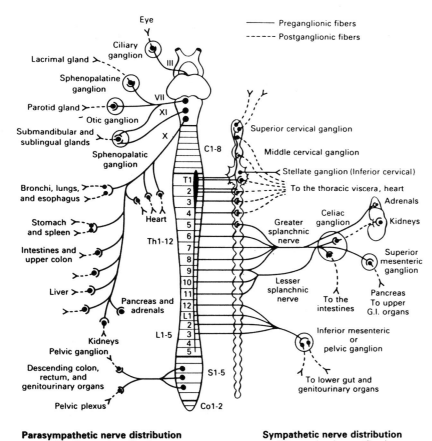

Parasympathetic nerve distribution
(Craniosacral outflow)

Sympathetic nerve distribution
(Thoracolumbar outflow)

Fig. 7A–9. Schematic distribution of the craniosacral (parasympathetic) and thoracolumbar (sympathetic) nervous system. Parasympathetic preganglionic fibers pass directly to the organ that is innervated. Their postganglionic cell bodies are situated near or within the innervated viscera. This limited distribution of parasympathetic postganglionic fibers is consistent with the discrete and limited effect of parasympathetic function. The postganglionic sympathetic neurons originate in either the paired sympathetic ganglia or one of the unpaired collateral plexi. One preganglionic fiber influences many postganglionic neurons. Activation of the sympathetic nervous system produces a more diffuse physiologic response rather than discrete effects. (From Barash, P.G., Cullen, B.F., and Stoelting, R.K. Clinical Anesthesia. JB Lippincott, Philadelphia, 1989.)

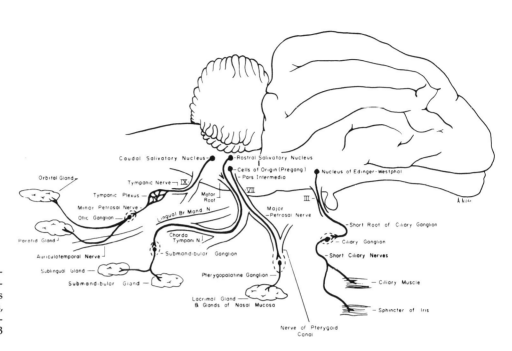

Fig. 7A–10. Routes of distribution of preganglionic and postganglionic parasympathetic fibers in the head region. (From Evans, H.E., and Christensen, G.C. Miller's Anatomy of the Dog. WB Saunders, Philadelphia, 1979.)

sphincter and ciliary muscles (Fig. 7A–10). The medullary outflow is comprised of the parasympathetic components of the seventh (facial), ninth (glossopharyngeal), and tenth (vagus) cranial nerves. The facial nerve synapses at the submandibular ganglion to supply the submaxillary and sublingual glands, and at the pterygopalatine ganglion to innervate the lacrimal and nasal glands. The autonomic fibers of the glossopharyngeal nerve travel to the otic ganglion, where they synapse to innervate the parotid and orbital salivary glands.

The vagus nerves contain approximately 80% of the parasympathetic nerve fibers in the body. The preganglionic fibers are long and synapse in small ganglia that lie directly on or in the viscera of the thorax and abdomen. Fibers are supplied to the heart, lungs, esophagus, stomach, small intestine, proximal colon, liver, gallbladder, pancreas, kidneys, and upper ureters. In the heart, they are distributed to the SA and AV nodes, and to a lesser extent to the atria. There are few or no vagal parasympathetic fibers in the ventricles. In the intestinal wall, they form the plexuses of Meissner and Auerbach. The vagus also carries afferent fibers, arising from the nodose ganglion, that produce visceral reflexes but apparently not pain.

The sacral outflow originates in the second, third, and fourth sacral segments of the spinal cord. Preganglionic fibers form the pelvic nerves (nervi erigentes), which synapse in ganglia near the bladder, distal colon, rectum, and sexual organs. The vagus and pelvic nerves thus provide secretory, vasodilator, and motor fibers for the thoracic, abdominal, and pelvic organs.

Autonomic nerve endings in the effector organ may terminate within cells or on the cell membrane. Smooth muscle cells may have protoplasmic bridges so that neural stimulus of one causes many to react. No distinctive nerve ending exists comparable to somatic nerve endings within the myoneural junction.

SYMPATHETIC SYSTEM

The sympathetic nervous system mediates activities that accompany expenditures of energy. Thus, sympathetic activity is greatest during stress or times of emergency. Sympathetic activity is necessary for normal responses to stimuli in the external environment (stressors). As in the parasympathetic system, acetylcholine is the neurotransmitter between pre- and postganglionic neurons. The neurotransmitter between postganglionic neurons and effector cells is norepinephrine. An exception is the sweat gland, whose sympathetic terminals are cholinergic. In contrast to the parasympathetic division, strong sympathetic stimulation produces generalized effects. This occurs because each preganglionic neuron synapses with 20 to 30 postganglionic neurons, each of which terminates on many effector cells. This results in a divergence of stimuli. In addition, norepinephrine at postganglionic synapses and norepinephrine and epinephrine secreted by the adrenal medulla in response to sympathetic stimulation are deactivated rather slowly.

The sympathetic nervous system arises from cells in the intermediolateral columns of the first thoracic to the fourth or fifth lumbar cord segments (canine) (Fig. 7A–9). Their axons pass through the ventral spinal roots and synapse in sympathetic ganglia with postganglionic nerve cells (Fig. 7A–8).

There are three types of sympathetic ganglia: vertebral, prevertebral, and terminal. *Vertebral ganglia* are paired and lie in the lateral sympathetic chains paralleling the vertebral column (Fig. 7A–9). They are connected to each other by nerve trunks and to the spinal cord and spinal nerves by rami communicantes. White rami carry the preganglionic outflow from the spinal cord in myelinated fibers. These synapse with nonmyelinated fibers in the vertebral ganglia. The nonmyelinated fibers exit via the gray rami to join the spinal nerves supplying the blood vessels of skeletal muscle and the sweat glands, pilomotor muscles, and blood vessels of the skin (Fig. 7A–8).

Prevertebral ganglia are located in the abdomen and pelvis and consist mainly of the celiac, aorticorenal, and anterior and posterior mesenteric ganglia. The bladder and rectum are supplied by *terminal ganglia* located in close proximity to these organs.

Preganglionic fibers from the upper thorax form the cervical sympathetic chain and synapse with postganglionic fibers to form the sympathetic supply to the head and neck (sudomotor, pilomotor, vasomotor, secretory, and pupillodilator innervation). The upper thoracic chain supplies postganglionic fibers that form the cardiac, esophageal, and pulmonary plexuses. The splanchnic nerves are formed from preganglionic fibers, which do not synapse until they reach the celiac ganglion. Postganglionic fibers from this and other prevertebral ganglia ramify widely to supply the abdominal viscera.

The adrenal medulla is unique in that it is embryologically, anatomically, and functionally homologous to the sympathetic ganglia. Chromaffin cells within the medulla originate from the neural crest and are innervated by preganglionic fibers. Activation of the sympathetic nervous system results in release of epinephrine and norepinephrine (80% and 20% respectively), which act as systemic hormones, from the adrenal medulla. The response is similar to but of longer duration (10–30 seconds) than occurs with release from nerve terminals. Circulating norepinephrine causes vasoconstriction, gastrointestinal inhibition, increased cardiac activity, and pupillary dilation. Circulating epinephrine has greater cardiac and metabolic effects than norepinephrine, and because of beta$_2$ receptor activity induces vasodilation in skeletal muscle. In addition, circulating norepinephrine and epinephrine have generalized metabolic effects in tissues that do not receive sympathetic innervation. Basal sympathetic tone is caused in part by adrenal medullary activity.

In contrast to the parasympathetic system, preganglionic sympathetic fibers may synapse with many postganglionic nerve cells, and are thus capable of producing massive sympathetic discharge. The sympathetic and parasympathetic systems continually modulate each other's effects on organ function. Homeostasis is achieved through a balance of vital organ activity regulated by the stimulatory and inhibitory activities of these two nervous systems.

Function of Neurons

AXONAL CONDUCTION

Nerve impulses are electric currents. They pass along the axon to the presynaptic membrane. From a pharmacologic standpoint, there is an important distinction between electric conduction of a nerve impulse along an axon and chemical transmission of this signal across the synapse. Local anesthetic agents block conduction, whereas a much larger group of drugs, including local anesthetics, alter transmission.

Using electrodes, it can be shown that the internal resting potential of an axon is approximately 70 millivolts (mV) negative to the exterior of the axon. This is termed the *internal resting potential* (RP) and is caused by (a) a higher internal concentration of potassium and (b) selective permeability of the resting axonal membrane to potassium.

When a resting axon is stimulated electrically, a nerve action potential (NAP) is produced that will travel the full length of the neuron in either direction (Fig. 7A–11). Most general anesthetics (isoflurane, halothane, and nitrous oxide) have little effect on nerve conduction velocity.(4, 5)

NEUROREGULATORS

Neuroregulators play a key role in communication among nerve cells (Table 7A–3). They may be subdivided into two groups. Small molecule neurotransmitters are synthesized in the cytosol of the presynaptic terminal, absorbed into the transmitter vesicles, and released into the synaptic cleft in response to the arrival of an action potential at the nerve ending. Release of neurotransmitters is voltage dependent and requires calcium influx into the presynaptic terminal (Fig. 7A–12). Following its release, the transmitter binds with the postsynaptic receptor. Excitation of the postjunctional membrane results from increased sodium conductance; inhibition occurs when potassium or chloride conductance is enhanced. Some transmitters bind to receptors that activate enzymes, thus altering cellular function.

Neuropeptide modulators are synthesized in the neuronal cell body and are transported to the nerve terminal by axonal streaming. They are released in response to an action potential, but in much smaller quantities than are the small molecule transmitters. The neuropeptides induce prolonged effects to amplify or dampen neuronal activity. They exert their effects through a variety of mechanisms, including prolonged closure of calcium channels, alteration of cellular metabolism, activation or inactivation of specific genes, and prolonged alteration in the numbers of excitatory or inhibitory receptors. Although only a single small molecule neurotransmitter is released by each type of neuron, the same neuron may release one or more neuropeptide modulators at the same time. The latter

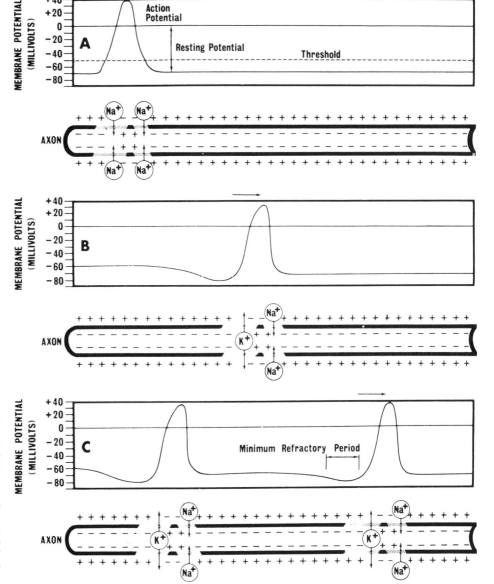

Fig. 7A–11. Schematic representation of nerve impulse. A, Depolarizing electrotonic effects result in sodium ions entering the axon. The resting potential is gradually altered until threshold is reached. At this time sodium ions enter the axon in great numbers, resulting in an action potential. B and C, Propagation of the nerve impulse is illustrated. Sodium ions enter the axon in advance of the nerve impulse, and potassium ions flow out after the impulse has passed. The outflow of potassium ions results in a brief refractory period. (Modified from Katz, 1961. From Miller, M.E., Christensen, G.C., and Evans, H.E. Anatomy of the Dog. WB Saunders, Philadelphia, 1964.)

can be released from within the brain or from other parts of the body to act on neurons distant from the release site.(6) In terms of anesthesia, many neuroregulators are known to be of great importance, whereas the significance of others may not be appreciated at this time.

When an impulse reaches a peripheral nerve ending, one of two chemical substances is released. Acetylcholine (ACH) is the chemical effector at (a) all preganglionic autonomic endings, (b) all postganglionic parasympathetic endings, (c) all motor nerve endings to skeletal muscle (somatic), (d) some central nervous system neurons, and (e) some postganglionic sympathetic fibers (sweat glands). Norepinephrine (noradrenalin) is the effector at most postganglionic sympathetic endings. Small amounts of epinephrine may also be released here. Many neurohumoral transmitters are

active in the central nervous system. These include acetylcholine, norepinephrine, 5–hydroxytryptamine (5–HT or serotonin), gamma-aminobutyric acid (GABA), and others (Table 7A–3).

Acetylcholine is secreted in many areas of the brain but is primarily found in the motor cortex, basal ganglia, and motor nerves of the skeletal muscles, and at autonomic ganglia, postganglionic parasympathetic, and some postganglionic sympathetic endings. Acetylcholine is an excitatory neurotransmitter except at certain peripheral parasympathetic endings such as the vagal cardiac fibers.

Norepinephrine is secreted by neurons having their cell bodies in the brain stem and hypothalamus. In particular, neurons in the locus ceruleus of the pons send nerve fibers to widespread areas of the brain to control overall activity and mood. In most areas these fibers are excitatory, but in some are inhibitory. Norepinephrine is secreted by most postganglionic sympathetic fibers and may be excitatory or inhibitory.

Dopamine is secreted primarily by neurons in the substantia nigra and basal ganglia and is inhibitory. Glycine is an inhibitory neurotransmitter in the spinal cord and in the retina. Gamma-aminobutyric acid (GABA) is an inhibitory neurotransmitter that is secreted in the spinal cord, cerebellum, basal ganglia, and many areas of the cerebral cortex. As much as one third of all synapses in the brain may be GABAergic. The alpha and beta subunits of the GABA receptor constitute the chloride channel. When two molecules of GABA bind to these receptor sites, the chloride channel opens,

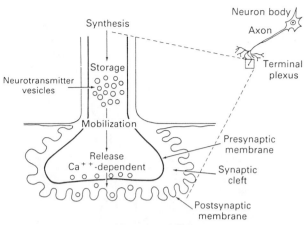

EFFECTOR CELL

Fig. 7A–12. Anatomy and physiology of the terminal postganglionic fibers of sympathetic and parasympathetic fibers are similar. (From Barash, P.G., Cullen, B.F., and Stoelting, R.K. Clinical Anesthesia. JB Lippincott, Philadelphia, 1989.)

allowing chloride to enter the cell, resulting in hyperpolarization and decreased neuronal activity. Glutamate is an excitatory neurotransmitter secreted by presynaptic terminals in sensory pathways. Serotonin is secreted by neurons originating in the brain stem and projecting to many areas, especially the hypothalamus and the dorsal horn. Serotonin inhibits pain pathways at the spinal level and is believed to alter mood and cause sleep through its inhibitory activity in the brain. Substance P is an excitatory neurotransmitter released by pain fibers in the substantia gelatinosa. Endorphins are neurotransmitters released in the spinal cord, brain stem, thalamus, and hypothalamus. Endorphins activate descending tracts that inhibit transmission of pain impulses in the spinal cord. Histamine is present in high concentrations in the hypothalamus and reticular activating system, where it is thought to be inhibitory via a cyclic AMP second messenger.

TRANSMISSION AT THE MYONEURAL JUNCTION

The terminal axon connects with the sarcoplasm of the muscle fiber by the presynaptic terminal membrane. Facing it is a second membrane, the postjunctional membrane. The two are separated by a space, the subneural space. The area where the nerve meets the muscle is termed the *motor end plate* (Fig. 7A–13).

The postjunctional membrane is preferentially permeable to sodium and potassium ions. The interior, facing the muscle, is negatively charged; the exterior, facing the nerve, is positively charged. This polarity is caused by an excess of sodium ions outside and potassium ions inside. The electrostatic difference in potential between sides is approximately 90 mV.

When a nerve impulse reaches the end of the axon, it releases acetylcholine from its bound form in the synaptic vesicles. It is immediately absorbed on the cholinergic receptors of the postjunctional membrane.

Table 7A–3. Neuroregulators and Modulators

Small-Molecule, Rapidly Acting Neurotransmitters
Class I
 Acetylcholine
Class II: Amines
 Norepinephrine
 Epinephrine
 Dopamine
 Serotonin
 Histamine
Class III: Amino Acids
 Gamma-aminobutyric acid (GABA)
 Glycine
 Glutamate
 Aspartate

Neuropeptide, Slow Acting Transmitters
 Hypothalamic-releasing hormone
 Thyrotropin-releasing hormone
 Luteinizing-releasing hormone
 Somatostatin

Pituitary Peptides
 ACTH
 Beta-Endorphin
 Alpha-Melanocyte stimulating hormone
 Prolactin
 Luteinizing hormone
 Thyrotropin
 Growth hormone
 Vasopressin
 Oxytocin

Peptides That Act on Gut and Brain
 Leucine enkephalin
 Methionine enkephalin
 Substance P
 Gastrin
 Cholecystokinin
 Vasoactive intestinal polypeptide
 Neurotensin
 Insulin
 Glucagon

Peptides That Act on Other Tissues
 Angiotensin II
 Bradykinin
 Carnosine
 Sleep peptides
 Calcitonin

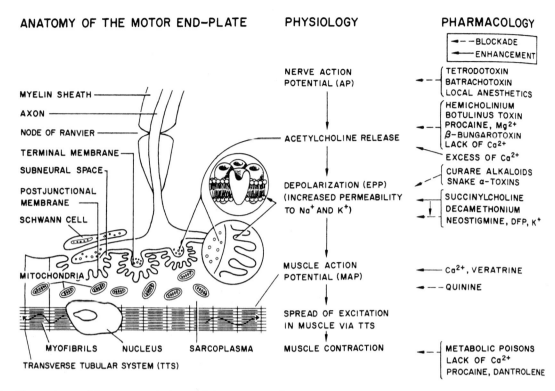

Fig. 7A–13.   The anatomy of the motor end plate and the sequence of events from the nerve action potential to the contraction of a muscle fiber. (From Gilman, A.G., Goodman, L.S., and Gilman, A., eds. The Pharmacological Basis of Therapeutics, 6th ed. Macmillan, New York, 1980.)

This changes the configuration of proteins in the membrane and its permeability. Sodium migrates inward and potassium outward, with a decrease in negativity within the postjunctional membrane termed *depolarization.* From -90 to -45 mV nothing occurs. This range (-90 to -45) is termed the *end plate potential* (EPP) (Fig. 7A–14). Below -45 mV, electric activity spreads to the muscle around the end plate and is termed the action potential (AP). This reaches a positive value of up to +30 mV.

Depolarization requires 0.2 to 0.4 ms. During this time, acetylcholine is hydrolyzed to acetic acid and choline by acetylcholine esterase present in the postjunctional membrane. As acetylcholine is hydrolyzed, the membrane permeability is restored to its normal state and the ions return to their respective sides (repolarization). Muscle contraction is delayed 2 to 3 ms; hence, repolarization is already complete when contraction occurs. Through action of cholineacetylase, acetic acid and choline recombine to form acetylcholine. Acetylcholine is then absorbed as a protein of one of the end plate membranes.

CHOLINERGIC TRANSMISSION

When a nerve impulse reaches the synapse, acetylcholine is released. It almost instantly crosses the synaptic cleft and unites with receptors on the postjunctional membrane causing a local increase in ionic permeability of the membrane (Fig. 7A–15). Two types of permeability change may occur: (a) a generalized increase in

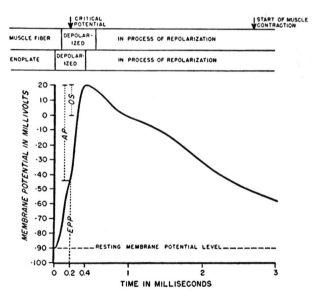

Fig. 7A–14.   EPP, end plate potential; AP, action potential; OS, overshoot. Owing to the release of acetylcholine by the nerve impulse at the end plate at zero time, the end plate potential is generated, and in about 0.2 ms the resting membrane potential of the end plate (-90 mV) decreases to -45 mV). When this critical level is reached, the potential change, from here on termed *action potential,* becomes propagated, and within another 0.2 ms, overshoots and becomes electropositive (+15–20 millivolts). Within the next 2 to 3 ms, the end plate becomes repolarized, and when the polarization process is almost complete, the contraction of the muscle fiber starts. (From Adriani, J. The Chemistry and Physics of Anesthesia, 2nd ed. Charles C Thomas, Springfield, IL, 1962.)

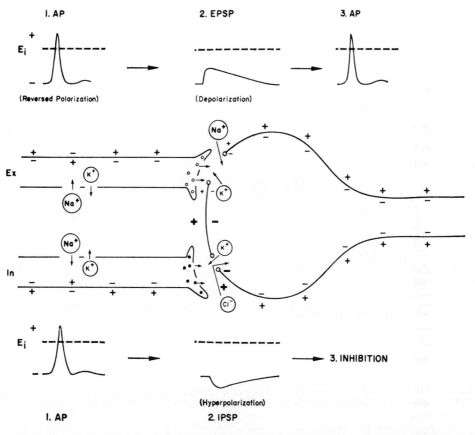

Fig. 7A–15. Steps involved in excitatory (Ex) and inhibitory (In) neurohumoral transmission. 1, The nerve action potential (NAP), consisting in a self–propagated reversal of negativity (the internal potential, E_i, goes from a negative value, through 0 potential, indicated by the broken line, to a positive value) of the axonal membrane, arrives at the presynaptic terminal and causes release of the excitatory (o) or inhibitory (•) transmitter. 2, Combination of the excitatory transmitter with postsynaptic receptors produces a localized depolarization, the excitatory postsynaptic potential (EPSP), through an increase in permeability to all ions (Na^+ and K^+ being chiefly involved). The inhibitory transmitter causes a selective increase in permeability to the smaller ions (K^+ and Cl^- being chiefly involved), resulting in a localized hyperpolarization, the inhibitory postsynaptic potential (IPSP). 3, The EPSP initiates a conducted NAP in the postsynaptic neuron; this can, however, be prevented by the hyperpolarization induced by a concurrent IPSP. The transmitter is dissipated by enzymatic destruction or by diffusion. (From Gilman, A.G., Goodman, L.S., and Gilman, A., eds. The Pharmacological Basis of Therapeutics, 6th ed. Macmillan, New York, 1980.)

permeability to all ions producing a depolarized membrane and an excitatory postsynaptic potential (EPSP), and (b) a selective increase in permeability only to small ions (K^+, Cl^-), resulting in stabilization of the membrane and an inhibitory postsynaptic potential (IPSP).

If an EPSP exceeds the threshold level, it initiates a nerve action potential (NAP) in a postsynaptic neuron or a muscle action potential (MAP) in skeletal or cardiac muscle. In smooth muscle, propagated impulses do not occur and a local contractile response is initiated; in glands, secretion results. An IPSP tends to oppose an EPSP, and the ultimate result is the algebraic sum of the reactions. Impulses can be transmitted across junctions at frequencies up to several hundred per second.

Nicoll and Iwamoto (7) demonstrated that ganglionic transmission was approximately twenty times more sensitive to pentobarbital than was axonal conduction. The fast excitatory postsynaptic potential (EPSP) was approximately ten times more sensitive to pentobarbital than were the slow potentials (slow EPSP and slow

IPSP). Halothane, ether, chloral hydrate, chloralose, and phenobarbital also exert some degree of selectivity toward the fast EPSP. Ethanol and urethan reduced all potentials indiscriminately.

Two cholinesterases are present in the body and are capable of hydrolyzing acetylcholine. Acetylcholine esterase (AChE), true, specific, "e"–type ChE, is found principally in neurons and at neuromuscular junctions, but also in erythrocytes, thrombocytes, and the placenta. It is responsible for terminating the action of acetylcholine by hydrolysis to acetic acid and choline. Practically all pharmacologic actions of anti–ChE agents are due to inhibition of AChE.

Butyrocholinesterase (BuChE, nonspecific, pseudo, plasma, or "s"–type ChE) occurs in glial cells of nervous tissue, in liver, plasma, and other organs. Its specific physiologic function is unknown; it can hydrolyze ACh but so slowly as to be unimportant physiologically. Inhibition by drugs of pseudocholinesterase produces no functional derangement.

ADRENERGIC TRANSMISSION

The catecholamines (dopamine, norepinephrine, and epinephrine) all function as neurotransmitters. They are synthesized by a series of enzymes (Fig. 7A–16). The first step in the pathway is conversion of the amino acid tyrosine to L-dopa. This reaction is followed by conversion of L-dopa to dopamine, which is subsequently converted to norepinephrine (noradrenalin). In specific nuclei of the central nervous system and in the adrenal medulla, norepinephrine is further converted to form epinephrine (adrenalin). The catecholamines are taken up and stored within vesicles in sympathetic nerves and in the adrenal medulla (Fig. 7A–17). They are released in response to nerve stimulation by a process of exocytosis, during which the vesicle opens to the exterior of the cell and discharges its contents into the synaptic cleft. They cross the cleft and unite with adrenoreceptors on the effector cell to produce the appropriate response. The neurotransmitter actions of catecholamines are terminated principally by a process termed *uptake-1* (Fig. 7A–17). A second uptake into nonneural cells has been designated *uptake-2*. Neither of these processes is the same as the vesicular amine uptake that occurs within the neuron.

Generally, enzymatic degradation of catecholamines is not as important as neural membrane uptake in termination of neurotransmitter activity, although in some tissues metabolism of amines does play an important role. The two most important metabolic enzymes are catechol–O–methyltransferase (COMT)

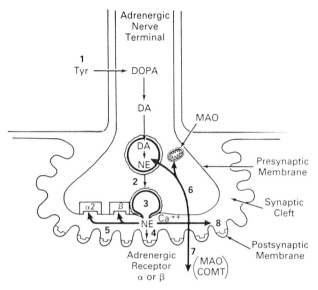

EFFECTOR CELL

Fig. 7A–17. Schematic of the synthesis and disposition of NE in adrenergic transmission: 1, synthesis and storage in neuronal vesicles; 2, action potential permits Ca entry; 3, exocytosis of NE into synaptic gap; 4, NE reacts with receptor on effector cell; 5, NE may react with presynaptic alpha$_2$ receptor to inhibit further release or, 6, with presynaptic beta receptor to enhance reuptake of NE (uptake-1). 7, Extraneuronal uptake (uptake-2) absorbs NE into the effector cell with overflow occurring systemically, 8. MAO, monoamine oxidase; COMT, catechol-O-methyltransferase; Tyr, tyrosine; DOPA, dihydroxyphenylalanine; NE = norepinephrine. (From Barash, P.G., Cullen, B.F., and Stoelting, R.K. Clinical Anesthesia. JB Lippincott, Philadelphia, 1989.)

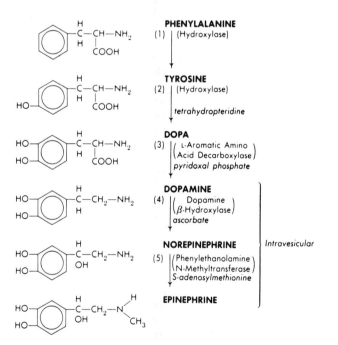

Fig. 7A–16. Steps in enzymatic synthesis of norepinephrine and epinephrine. (After Holtz et al., 1938; Blaschko, 1939; Gurin and Delluva, 1947; Levin et al., 1960.) (From Goodman, L.S. and Gilman, A. The Pharmacological Basis of Therapeutics, 4th ed, Macmillan, New York, 1970.)

and monoamine oxidase (MAO). MAO is associated with mitochondria, whereas COMT is primarily a cytoplasmic enzyme.

Receptors

CHOLINERGIC

Receptors are the target site on the cell membrane to which agonists bind and activate to induce a response in the effector cell. Receptors appear to be macromolecular proteins in the plasma membrane. Acetylcholine is the neurotransmitter at three distinct classes of receptors, which can be differentiated by anatomic location and affinity for various agonists and antagonists. Anatomically, cholinergic receptors are found (a) in the parasympathetic system, (b) in the brain and the ganglia of the sympathetic system, and (c) at the myoneural junction of voluntary striated skeletal muscle. Pharmacologically, the acetylcholine receptors are classified as muscarinic or nicotinic based on their selectivity for muscarine or nicotine, and further subtyped based on affinity for selected antagonist drugs. Each type has at least two subtypes. Thus, nicotinic receptors are classed as N_1 and N_2, N_1 being located at both sympathetic and parasympathetic ganglia and N_2 at the myoneural junction. Muscarinic receptors are designated M_1, M_2, and M_3. The M_1 receptor is located

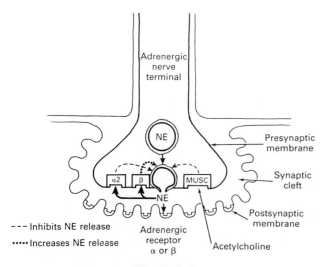

Effector Cell

--- Inhibits NE release

····· Increases NE release

Fig. 7A–18. Schematic of some of the presynaptic adrenergic receptors thought to exist. Agonist and antagonist drugs are clinically available for these receptors. The alpha$_2$ receptors serve as a negative feedback mechanism whereby NE stimulation inhibits its own release. Presynaptic beta stimulation increases NE uptake, augmenting its availability. Presynaptic muscarinic receptors (Musc) respond to ACh diffusing from nearby cholinergic terminals, inhibit NE release, and can be blocked by atropine. (From Barash, P.G., Cullen, B.F., and Stoelting, R.K. Clinical Anesthesia. JB Lippincott, Philadelphia, 1989.)

at cholinergic synapses within the CNS, primarily in the hippocampus (M_{1a}) and at sympathetic ganglia and nerve endings (M_{1b}). M_2 receptors are located at the postganglionic parasympathetic terminals in heart and smooth muscle throughout the body. Activation of M_2 receptors results in bradycardia, decreased strength of contraction, and smooth muscle contraction. M_3 receptors are primarily located at exocrine glands and smooth muscle, where they induce contraction. M_2 and M_3 muscarinic receptors are also found on the presynaptic membrane of sympathetic nerve terminals in the myocardium, coronary vessels, and peripheral vasculature. These adrenergic muscarinic receptors are stimulated by acetylcholine and inhibit release of norepinephrine in a manner similar to that of the alpha$_2$ receptor stimulation (Fig. 7A–18) They also occur prejunctionally on cholinergic neurons and inhibit release of acetylcholine. Prejunctional M_1 receptors have been demonstrated in some tissues of selected species (guinea pig ileum) and found to facilitate rather than inhibit subsequent release of neurotransmitter.(8)

ADRENERGIC

Ahlquist (9) first proposed that catecholamines produced their effects by interaction with cell surface receptors, which he termed *alpha* or *beta adrenoceptors*. He classified receptors on the basis of their ability to combine with the chemical structure of a series of adrenergic agonists. He further pointed out that neither the tissue site of the receptors nor the physiologic

response (excitation or inhibition) was related to this recognition function. Thus, a drug may have entirely different actions from tissue to tissue, depending upon the type of receptor and the biochemical change that occurs on binding of the receptor.

Ahlquist's original classification was expanded by Lands et al. (10), who proposed that beta receptors could be subdivided into and beta$_1$ and beta$_2$. Beta$_1$ receptors are found in the heart and control contractility and rate; in adipose tissue they control lipolysis. Beta$_2$ receptors mediate relaxation in smooth muscle, control lipolysis in skeletal muscle, and control glycolysis in the liver. Catecholamines acting on cardiac beta$_1$ adrenoceptors produce a positive inotropic and chronotropic effect. Vascular smooth muscle in some blood vessels and bronchial smooth muscle have beta$_2$ receptors that mediate vasodilation or bronchodilation (Table 7A–4).

Berthelsen and Pittinger (11) demonstrated alpha$_1$ and alpha$_2$ receptors. Stimulation of alpha receptors located on the nerve terminal itself (presynaptic receptors) results in decreased exocytotic release of norepinephrine by the nerve (Fig. 7A–18). The order of potencies for alpha-adrenergic agonists and antagonists for presynaptic receptors is different from that for classic postsynaptic receptors. For this reason, receptors with pharmacologic properties of the postsynaptic receptor have been termed *alpha$_1$*, whereas those with properties of the presynaptic receptor have been designated *alpha$_2$*. There is evidence that alpha$_2$ receptors are also located postsynaptically in some vascular beds and in the brain. Thus, the classification is functional rather than anatomic.

Stimulation of a presynaptic beta receptor increases exocytotic release of norepinephrine. It appears that the vascular presynaptic receptor may be beta$_2$ in type, and thus more sensitive to circulating epinephrine than to norepinephrine released from nerves. It is apparent that adrenoreceptors play a large role in homeostasis throughout the sympathetic and central nervous systems.

As previously noted, adrenergic receptors have been divided into alpha and beta types based on their pharmacologic properties (i.e., their relative responsiveness to norepinephrine vs isoproterenol). The alphas have been further subtyped into alpha$_{1A}$, alpha$_{1B}$, alpha$_{1C}$; alpha$_{2A}$, alpha$_{2B}$, alpha$_{2C}$, and alpha$_{2D}$.(12) The alpha$_1$ receptors are found in peripheral vascular smooth muscle of the coronary arteries, skin, intestinal mucosa, and splanchnic beds. They are postsynaptic activators of vascular and intestinal smooth muscle as well as endocrine glands. Their stimulation results in either increased or decreased tone, depending on the effector organ. In resistance and capacitance vessels constriction results, while relaxation occurs in the intestine. The myocardium per se has been thought to have no alpha receptors but alpha$_1$-receptor-mediated effects have been reported (13). The physiologic and

Table 7A–4. Responses of Effector Organs to Autonomic Nerve Impulses

| Effector Organs | Adrenergic Impulses[a] | | Cholinergic Impulses[a] |
	Receptor Type	Responses[b]	Responses[b]
Eye			
Radial muscle, iris	α	Contraction (mydriasis) + +	—
Sphincter muscle, iris		—	Contraction (miosis) + + +
Ciliary muscle	β	Relaxation for far vision +	Contraction for near vision + + +
Heart			
SA node	β_1	Increase in heart rate + +	Decrease in heart rate; vagal arrest + + +
Atria	β_1	Increase in contractility and conduction velocity + +	Decrease in contractility, and (usually) increase in conduction velocity + +
AV node	β_1	Increase in automaticity and conduction velocity + +	Decrease in conduction velocity; AV block + + +
His-Purkinje system	β_1	Increase in automaticity and conduction velocity + + +	Little effect
Ventricles	β_1	Increase in contractility, conduction velocity, automaticity, and rate of idioventricular pacemakers + + +	Slight decrease in contractility claimed by some
Arterioles			
Coronary	α, β_2	Constriction +; dilation[c] + +	Dilation ±
Skin and mucosa	α	Constriction + + +	Dilation[d]
Skeletal muscle	α, β_2	Constriction + +; dilation[c,e] + +	Dilation[f] +
Cerebral	α	Constriction (slight)	Dilation[d]
Pulmonary	α, β_2	Constriction +; dilation[c]	Dilation[d]
Abdominal viscera; renal	α, β_2	Constriction + + +; dilation[e] +	—
Salivary glands	α	Constriction + + +	Dilation + +
Veins (Systemic)	α, β_2	Constriction + +; dilation + +	—
Lung			
Bronchial muscle	β_2	Relaxation +	Contraction + +
Bronchial glands	?	Inhibition (?)	Stimulation + + +
Stomach			
Motility and tone	α_2, β_2	Decrease (usually)[g] +	Increase + + +
Sphincters	α	Contraction (usually) +	Relaxation (usually) +
Secretion		Inhibition (?)	Stimulation + + +
Intestine			
Motility and tone	α_2, β_2	Decrease[g] +	Increase + + +
Sphincters	α	Contraction (usually) +	Relaxation (usually) +
Secretion		Inhibition (?)	Stimulation + +
Gallbladder and Ducts		Relaxation +	Contraction +
Kidney	β_2	Renin secretion + +	—
Urinary Bladder			
Detrusor	β	Relaxation (usually) +	Contraction + + +
Trigone and sphincter	α	Contraction + +	Relaxation + +
Ureter			
Motility and tone	α	Increase (usually)	Increase (?)
Uterus	α, β_2	Pregnant: contraction (α); nonpregnant: relaxation (β)	Variable[h]
Sex Organs, Male	α	Ejaculation + + +	Erection + + +
Skin			
Pilomotor muscles	α	Contraction + +	—
Sweat glands	α	Localized secretion[i] +	Generalized secretion + + +
Spleen Capsule	α, β_2	Contraction + + +; relaxation +	—
Adrenal Medulla		—	Secretion of epinephrine and norepinephrine
Liver	α, β_2	Glycogenolysis, gluconeogenesis[j] + + +	Glycogen synthesis +

Table 7A–4. Responses of Effector Organs to Autonomic Nerve Impulses—cont'd

Effector Organs	Adrenergic Impulses[a]		Cholinergic Impulses[a]
	Receptor Type	Responses[b]	Responses[b]
Pancreas			
Acini	α	Decreased secretion +	Secretion + +
Islets (β cells)	α	Decreased secretion + + +	—
	β_2	Increased secretion +	—
Fat Cells	α, β_1	Lipolysis[j] + + +	—
Salivary Glands	α	Potassium and water secretion +	Potassium and water secretion
	β	Amylase secretion +	+ + +
Lacrimal Glands		—	Secretion + + +
Nasopharyngeal Glands		—	Secretion + +
Pineal Gland	β	Melatonin synthesis	—

[a]A long dash signifies no known functional innervation.

[b]Responses are designated 1+ to 3+ to provide an approximate indication of the importance of adrenergic and cholinergic nerve activity in the control of the various organs and functions listed.

[c]Dilation predominates in situ owing to metabolic autoregulatory phenomena.

[d]Cholinergic vasodilatation at these sites is of questionable physiologic significance.

[e]Over the usual concentration range of physiologically released, circulating epinephrine, β-receptor response (vasodilation) predominates in blood vessels of skeletal muscle and liver; α-receptor response (vasoconstriction), in blood vessels of other abdominal viscera. The renal and mesenteric vessels also contain specific dopaminergic receptors, activation of which causes dilatation, but their physiologic significance has not been established.

[f]Sympathetic cholinergic system causes vasodilation in skeletal muscle, but this is not involved in most physiological responses.

[g]It has been proposed that adrenergic fibers terminate at inhibitor β receptors on smooth muscle fibers, and at inhibitory α receptors on parasympathetic cholinergic (excitatory) ganglion cells of Auerbach's plexus.

[h]Depends on stage of menstrual cycle, amount of circulating estrogen and progesterone, and other factors.

[i]Palms of hands and some other sites ("adrenergic sweating").

[j]There is significant variation among species in the type of receptor that mediates certain metabolic responses.

(From Gilman, A.G., Goodman, L.S., and Gilman, A., eds. The Pharmacological Basis of Therapeutics, 6th ed. Macmillan, New York, 1980.)

clinical significance of myocardial alpha$_1$ receptors remains somewhat of an enigma.

Alpha$_2$ receptors occur both pre- and postsynaptically in peripheral tissues. Alpha$_2$ receptors occur on prejunctional sympathetic nerve terminals and function to decrease the amount of norepinephrine released, thus serving as a negative feedback mechanism (Fig. 7A–18). In addition, prejunctional alpha$_2$ receptors have been identified on cholinergic, serotonergic, and GABAergic neurons, where they are thought to be important in neuromodulation. Stimulation of central alpha$_2$ receptors is associated with sedation, analgesia, decreased sympathoadrenal outflow, anxiolysis, and decreased thermal-induced shivering.(12)

In the arterial vasculature, alpha$_1$ receptors are thought to occur postsynaptically on the neuroeffector junction near the amine uptake pump, while alpha$_2$s are located at a location distant from this site. Thus, it would seem that the alpha$_1$ receptor mediates sympathetically driven neuronally induced vasoconstriction, while alpha$_2$ receptors mediate vasoconstriction induced by circulating catecholamines. This arrangement appears to be reversed in the venous capacitance vessels. There appear to be some differences in how the receptors utilize calcium in mediating vasoconstriction: alpha$_1$ receptors utilize intracellular calcium, while alpha$_2$s utilize extracellular calcium.(12)

There are no known direct effects of alpha$_2$ stimulation on myocardial tissue. However, alpha$_2$ activation indirectly effects cardiac function through centrally mediated decreases in sympathetic tone (CNS postsynaptic receptors), by decreased release of norepinephrine from sympathetic nerve terminals (prejunctional receptors), and by altering coronary blood flow (vascular receptors). In the gastrointestinal tract, alpha$_2$s act pre- and postjunctionally to regulate motility and secretions. Vagally mediated increases in motility and secretions are inhibited at the intramural parasympathetic ganglia and prejunctionally at postganglionic cholinergic neurons. Alpha$_2$ stimulation decreases gastric secretion and increases net fluid absorption. The uterus is richly supplied with alpha$_2$ receptors, and their number increases under the influence of estrogen but no functional role has been identified. In the endothelium, alpha$_2$A receptors have been shown to mediate release of nitric oxide, the endothelium-derived relaxing factor (Chapter 5). Other substances that result in nitric oxide release include acetylcholine, bradykinin and substance P. Alpha$_2$ stimulation has been shown to offset adrenergic vasoconstriction in coronary vessels of dogs.

Renal effects of alpha$_2$ stimulation include diuresis induced by inhibition of release of antidiuretic hormone (ADH), blockade of ADH's action at the renal tubule, increased glomerular filtration rate (GFR), and inhibition of renin release. Endocrine effects include decreased insulin, norepinephrine, ACTH, and cortisol release and enhanced growth hormone (GH) release. Alpha$_2$ receptors located on platelets stimulate aggregation.

As previously mentioned, beta receptors are characterized as beta$_1$ (cardiac), beta$_2$ (noncardiac) and beta$_3$ (atypical). Beta$_1$ receptors are located in the myocardium, SA node, ventricular conduction system, and adipose tissue. Beta$_2$ receptors are located in smooth muscle of blood vessels in the skin, muscles, and mesentery, and in bronchial smooth muscle. Stimulation of beta$_2$ receptors results in vasodilation and bronchial relaxation. Beta$_2$ receptors are much more sensitive to epinephrine than norepinephrine, unlike beta$_1$s, which respond equally to each. It is suggested that beta$_1$ receptors, like alpha$_1$s, are responsive to neurally released norepinephrine, while the beta$_2$s respond to circulating epinephrine.

Dopamine receptors have been identified and have been classified as DA$_1$ and DA$_2$. The DA$_1$ receptor is postsynaptic and mediates splanchnic and renal vasodilation. The DA$_2$ receptor is presynaptic, and like the alpha$_2$ receptor, inhibits subsequent release of norepinephrine and induces vasodilation. There are no known postsynaptic DA$_2$ receptors. Centrally, dopamine receptors are found in the basal ganglia, where they coordinate motor function; in the medullary chemoreceptor trigger zone, to stimulate vomiting; and in the hypothalamus associated with prolactin release. Dopamine receptors are found in the esophagus, stomach, and intestines, where they enhance secretions and diminish motility.

Adrenergic receptors display the phenomena of up and down regulation. That is, the number of receptors is effected by the concentration of agonist to which they are exposed (i.e., there is an inverse relationship between the number of receptors and the ambient concentration of the catecholamines). Extended exposure to the agonist leads to decreased receptor numbers (down regulation). Up regulation, the increase in number of receptors, occurs when blood and tissue catecholamine concentrations are low. The phenomenon is reversible and the same for both alpha and beta receptors. Estrogen and thyroxin increase and progesterone decreases alpha receptor numbers.

Interaction of acetylcholine or norepinephrine (the first messenger) with their receptors alters flux of sodium or potassium ions across ion channels or, most often, activates or inhibits effector enzymes such as adenylate cyclase. The alpha$_2$ receptor is comprised of a single polypeptide chain that weaves back and forth through the cell membrane seven times. The transmembranous portion is very similar to that of other adrenoceptors, suggesting that these are the recognition/binding site for norepinephrine. The cytoplasmic side forms the contact point for the guanine nucleotide binding protein (G protein). G proteins couple the receptor to a discrete effector mechanism which may be a transmembrane ion channel or an intracellular second messenger cascade (Chapter 5). At least four different pertussis toxin–sensitive G proteins can couple to the alpha$_2$ receptor. A common feature of all alpha$_2$-adrenergic receptors is their ability, when activated, to inhibit adenylate cyclase. The resulting decrease in the accumulation of cAMP (the second messenger) attenuates the stimulation of cAMP-dependent protein kinase and hence the phosphorylation of target regulatory proteins.(14) DA$_2$ receptors also inhibit formation of cAMP. Other possible effector mechanisms of alpha$_2$ adrenoceptors include efflux of potassium or suppression of calcium influx. Beta$_1$, beta$_2$, and DA$_1$ adrenergic and cholinergic receptors are also G protein in nature. In the case of the beta$_1$, beta$_2$, and DA$_1$ adrenergic receptors, activation results in stimulation of adenylate cyclase and the formation of the second messenger cAMP. A similar enzyme second messenger system has not been demonstrated for the alpha$_1$ receptor. In general, alpha$_1$ stimulation leads to increased cytosolic calcium released from the internal surface of the plasma membrane adjacent to the alpha$_1$ receptor. This in turn is thought to induce release of calcium from the sarcoplasmic reticulum (Chapter 5). Both alpha- and beta-adrenergic responses are dependent on calcium, calcium being the third messenger for alpha$_2$ and beta responses and serving as both the second and third messenger for alpha$_1$-mediated responses.(15)

Theories of Anesthesia

Despite intensive studies for many years, the exact mechanism of anesthesia at the cellular or subcellular level has not been definitely established. Theories of anesthesia at the molecular and subcellular levels have been proposed.(16-18) They can generally be grouped as follows: (a) lipid theories, (b) aqueous–phase theories, (c) critical–volume theory, (d) protein conformational change theory, (e) microtubule theory, and (f) coacervate theory.

Anesthetic agents differ greatly in structure, as they include hydrocarbons, alcohols, ethers, urethanes, sulfones, amides, steroids, and rare gases. Because general anesthesia is produced by a wide range of compounds with no common chemical structure or activity, it is impossible, except in a series of homologous substances, to show any relationship between anesthetic action and chemical constitution. As a result, many of the theories of narcosis have been based on physical properties of the anesthetics. Anesthesia was presumed to result from physical electrostatic intermolecular forces (Van der Waals forces) rather than intermolecular chemical bonds between atoms and ions.

For many years it has been known that anesthetized animals can be awakened by an environment in which the pressure is increased. The physicochemical approach seeks correlations between anesthetic potency and physical properties of a series of anesthetics.

The Meyer–Overton theory states that anesthetic properties of substances are directly related to their lipid solubility. Pauling and Miller independently proposed that the site of action of anesthetics lies in the aqueous phase of the CNS.(19-20) Pauling proposed the formation of gas hydrates, which increased the impedance of the neural network or occluded pores in membranes. Hydrates also could impair the reactivity of enzymes by trapping protein polar groups. Miller theorized that anesthesia is caused by the ordering that simple solutes induce in nearby water molecules ("iceberg effect"). These "icebergs" were presumed to function in the same manner as Pauling's hydrates. Both theories suffer from lack of evidence.

Biophysical theories involve the site of anesthetic action and the site–anesthetic interaction. In 1954, Mullins proposed that anesthesia commences when a critical volume fraction of an inert substance is attained in membranes.(21) He believed that anesthetics filled holes (free volume) in membranes. Subsequent investigators have not supported free–volume theories, but the critical volume of anesthetic entering the membrane is thought to expand it rather than to fill holes. Thus, sodium or potassium channels, acetylcholine receptors, or enzymes could be modified.

Allison and Nunn believed that general anesthesia results from reversible depolymerization of microtubules in nerve cells.(22) The protein conformational change (PCC) theory proposes that anesthetics directly inactivate lipoproteins and that the site of anesthetic action is protein.(23)

In a spin–probe study of pressure, anesthetics, and membrane structure, Finch and Kiesow proposed that pressure and anesthetics alter the internal hydrophobic effects of cell membranes.(24) They believed that anesthetics decrease membrane polarity by displacing water molecules in the membrane. This proposal differs from other hypotheses concerning the role of water in anesthetic effects on membrane structures, since it involves changes in membrane water penetration rather than water structure.

Ecanow et al. have stated that the cell membrane is a coacervate phase capable of undergoing subtle changes in structuring that correspond to different degrees of anesthesia.(25) This allows the membrane to undergo a continuum of free energy changes from polar to nonpolar properties. The anesthetic state occupies one range on this continuum.

Today, the concept of anesthetic effect has changed from filling of free space to expansion and fluidization of the cell membrane. Evidence is clearly against the aqueous–phase theory of Pauling and Miller. The microtubule theory of Allison and Nunn also has not accumulated supporting evidence.(22)

Although the majority of investigators favor a lipid anesthetic site, the PCC theory remains viable. A hydrophobic protein site of action could cause many of the physical–chemical relationships that point toward the lipid phase. Present evidence supports the assumption that the site of anesthetic action is on the cell membrane. It is believed that anesthetics act chiefly by depressing synaptic transmission. It has also been shown that several general anesthetics hyperpolarize CNS neurons, apparently because of an increase in potassium permeability.(26) This is a nonsynaptic activity that, combined with synaptic depression, can result in decreased neuronal excitability and CNS unresponsiveness. However, the exact mechanism of anesthesia still remains an enigma.

SITES OF ACTION OF GENERAL ANESTHETICS

General anesthesia is the result of reversible changes in neurologic function induced by drugs that alter synaptic transmission. Intravenous agents interfere with membrane protein receptors, and volatile drugs interact with the hydrophobic regions of membrane lipids and proteins. Most discussions of the mechanism of anesthesia are oriented toward the volatile anesthetics and seek a unitary mechanism by which they induce the anesthetic state. Volatile agents probably induce general anesthesia by modifying synaptic transmission from within cell membranes rather than direct binding to receptors as do the intravenous anesthetic drugs. Studies linking anesthetic potency with lipid solubility and those demonstrating pressure reversal implicate the lipid matrix of cell membranes as a principal site for anesthetic activity. Many observations have suggested that volatile anesthetics depress excitatory transmission through their effects on sodium and chloride channels in postsynaptic membranes regardless of the neurotransmitter involved. There has been little evidence to show that volatile anesthetics affect the synthesis, release, or binding of neurotransmitters per se.

Neurotransmitters can be either excitatory or inhibitory. GABA is the primary inhibitory neurotransmitter in the brain, and glycine is the major inhibitory neurotransmitter in the spinal cord. Glutamate is the major excitatory neurotransmitter in the brain. Ketamine has been shown to inhibit glutamate receptors, while neuroleptic drugs such as the butyrophenones and phenothiazines are dopamine antagonists.

Data have accumulated to suggest that modulation of GABA function is responsible for several aspects of anesthesia. GABA modulates motor and autonomic and cardiovascular function. GABA inhibits neural transmission by binding to a postsynaptic receptor causing chloride channels to open. Activation of the GABA-chloride ion channel results in hyperpolarization or an increase in ion conductance that prevents depolarization, thereby decreasing neuronal activity. Benzodiazepines, barbiturates, propofol, steroidal anesthetics, and etomidate have been shown to exert their hypnotic effects by interaction with the GABA receptor. In addition, volatile anesthetics (e.g., isoflurane), similarly activate the GABA chloride channel independent of a generalized membrane bilayer effect.(27)

Opioids and alpha$_2$-adrenergic agonists act by inhibiting presynaptic Ca channels responsible for activating release of neurotransmitter. They also increase presynaptic K^+ conductance, which results in hyperpolarization of the synaptic terminal, reducing Ca entry and neurotransmitter release. GABA receptors and the presynaptic adrenergic muscarinic receptors also can decrease calcium conductance presynaptically. Recently, isoflurane has been shown to depress calcium channel activity.(27)

In the past, it was thought that the stages of anesthesia represented suppression of activity in the nervous system, starting first with the higher centers or those newest phylogenetically. Stage one (analgesia) was thought to be caused by effects on the cerebral cortex; stage two (excitement), by effects on the midbrain that had been released from cerebral control; and stage three (surgical anesthesia) by progressive depression of the midbrain and spinal cord, producing skeletal muscle relaxation. The assumption was made that the medulla, for some reason, was not depressed until the deepest stages of anesthesia were reached. Hence, stage four (toxic), involving respiratory and circulatory arrest, was caused by medullary depression. Larrabee and Posternak were able to demonstrate that pentobarbital, ether, chloroform, and chloretone depressed synaptic transmission in concentrations similar to those existing in the blood during surgical anesthesia, whereas higher concentrations were required to affect conduction along any type of axon.(28) They concluded that this selective action of anesthetics on synapses was caused by either a specific effect on synaptic transmission or by the relatively small "factor of safety" in transsynaptic excitation compared to axonal conduction.

The reticular activating system (RAS) is a multisynaptic structure, which probably accounts for its susceptibility to anesthetics, since anesthetics block synaptic transmission better than nerve trunk conduction. Injection of local anesthetics into the RAS produces general anesthesia, thus supporting the theories that an intact RAS is necessary for conscious perception of impulses and that the RAS is probably the most important site within the central nervous system for anesthetic action.

Nearly 30 years ago it was proposed that pain may be controlled by a presynaptic gating mechanism located in the dorsal horn of the spinal cord.(29) Subsequently, it was demonstrated in cats by Wall that pentobarbital produced progressive "closure of the gate," which prevented cutaneous impulses from ascending to the brain.(30) Cutaneous anesthesia was presumably the result of a selective depression of impulse transmission across the first spinal synapse of the cutaneous sensory pathway located in the dorsal horn. Other early investigators, using halothane as the anesthetic agent, suggested that the hypnotic action of anesthetics may be due to depression of synaptic transmission in the reticular substance, whereas the analgesic action may be due to depression of synaptic transmission in the dorsal horn.(31) Recent findings on the mechanism and site of anesthetic action suggest that the validity of these observations, although general in scope in today's science of anesthesiology, remain to be disproven. Today, the concepts of membrane volume expansion on critical hydrophobic sites, altered fluidity of the lipid matrix of cell membranes, and altered binding to protein sites that interfere with signal transduction are reasonable explanations for the mechanism of generalized altered CNS activity that is defined as general anesthesia.

References

1. Hoerlein BF. Canine neurology: diagnosis and treatment, 3rd ed. Philadelphia: WB Saunders, 1978.
2. Milhorat TH. Choroid plexus and cerebrospinal fluid production. Science 166:1514, 1969.
3. Evans AF, Geddes LA. Vasomotor response to increased cerebrospinal fluid pressure in the spinal animal. Cardiovascular Research Center Bulletin, Baylor College of Medicine 7:100, 1969.
4. deJong RH, Hershey WN, Wagman IH. Nerve conduction velocity during hypothermia in man. Anesthesiology 27:805, 1966.
5. deJong RH, Nace RA. Nerve impulse conduction and cutaneous receptor responses during general anesthesia. Anesthesiology 28:851, 1967.
6. Barchas JD, Akil H, Elliott GR, Holman RB, Watson SJ. Behavioral neurochemistry: neuroregulators and behavioral states. Science 200:964, 1978.
7. Nicoll RA, Iwamoto ET. Action of pentobarbital on sympathetic ganglion cells. J Neurophysiol 41:977, 1978.
8. Goyal RK. Muscarinic receptor subtypes. Physiology and clinical implications. N Engl J Med 321:1022–1028, 1989.
9. Ahlquist RP. A study in the adrenotropic receptors. Am J Physiol 15:586, 1948.
10. Lands AM, Arnold A, McAuliff JB, Luduena FP, Brown TG. Differentiation of receptor systems activated by sympathomimetic amines. Nature 214:597, 1967.
11. Berthelsen S, Pettinger WA. A functional basis for classification of alpha–adrenergic receptors. Life Sci 21:595, 1977.
12. Bloor BC. General pharmacology of alpha-2 adrenoceptors. Anaesth Pharmacol Rev 1:221–232, 1993.
13. Smith NT, Corbascio AN. The use and misuse of pressor agents. Anesthesiology 8:58, 1970.
14. Maze M, Tranquilli W. Alpha-2 adrenoceptor agonists: defining the role in clinical anesthesia. Anesthesiology 74:581–605, 1991.
15. Durrett LR, Lawson NW. Autonomic nervous system physiology and pharmacology. In: Barash PG, Cullen BF, Stoelting RK, eds. Clinical Anesthesia. New York: JB Lippincott, 1989:165–226.
16. Kaufman RD. Biophysical mechanisms of anesthetic action: historical perspective and review of current concepts. Anesthesiology 46:49, 1977.
17. Roth SH. Physical mechanisms of anesthesia. Annu Rev Pharmacol Toxicol 19:159, 1979.
18. Koblin DD, Eger EI, III. Theories of narcosis. N Engl J Med 301:1222, 1979.
19. Pauling L. A molecular theory of general anesthesia. Science 134:3471, 1961.
20. Miller SL. A theory of gaseous anesthetics. Proc Natl Acad Sci 47:515, 1961.
21. Mullins LJ. Some physical mechanisms in narcosis. Chem Rev 54:289, 1954.
22. Allison AC, Nunn JF. Effects of general anaesthetics on microtubules. A possible mechanism of anaesthesia. Lancet 2:1326, 1968.
23. Seeman P. The membrane actions of anesthetics and tranquilizers. Pharmacol Rev 24:583, 1972.
24. Finch ED, Kiesow LA. Pressure, anesthetics, and membrane structure: a spin–probe study. Undersea Biomed Res 6:41, 1979.

25. Ecanow B, Gold BH, Ecanow CS. Unified theory of anesthesia. J Pharm Sci 68:4, 1979.
26. Nicoll RA, Madison DV. General anesthetics hyperpolarize neurons in the vertebrate central nervous system. Science 217:1055, 1982.
27. Study RE. Isoflurane inhibits multiple voltage-gated calcium currents in hippocampal pyramidal neurons. Anesthesiology 81:104–116, 1994.
28. Larrabee MG, Posternak JM. Selection action of anesthetics on synapses and axons in mammalian sympathetic ganglia. J Neurophysiol 15:91, 1952.
29. Melzack R, Wall PD. Pain mechanisms: a new theory. Science 150:971, 1965.
30. Wall PD. The mechanisms of general anesthesia. Anesthesiology 28:46, 1967.
31. deJong RH, Wagman IH. Block of afferent impulses in the dorsal horn of monkey. A possible mechanism of anesthesia. Exp Neurol 20:352, 1968.

chapter **7** B

NERVOUS SYSTEM: EFFECTS OF ANESTHETICS ON CENTRAL NERVOUS SYSTEM FUNCTION

Charles E. Short, Klaus A. Otto

Introduction

While the primary effect of anesthetics and anesthetic adjuncts is to alter central nervous system (CNS) function, detailed studies of their neurophysiologic effects have received comparatively limited attention. Traditionally, subjective evaluation of CNS activity utilizing classic signs of anesthesia has been used because standard electroencephalogram (EEG) recordings required extensive training for interpretation. Michenfelder reviewed the historical and current methodologies of studying the brain during anesthesia and concluded that new experimental models are needed to evaluate EEG, cerebral blood flow (CBF), and cerebral metabolism (CMRO$_2$) in analgesia and anesthesia studies.(1-4)

ELECTROENCEPHALOGRAPHY

Historically, the electric activity of the central nervous system has been used in diagnostics of CNS disorders, especially seizures. The EEG has not gained widespread popularity as a clinical tool for evaluation of analgesia and anesthesia. Standard EEG tracings, frequently utilizing a Grass Polygraph or other recorder, required a degree of subjective interpretation. Over twenty years ago investigators evaluated the effect of preanesthetics and anesthetics on visually evoked potentials.(5, 6) More recently, computer analyses of standard EEG tracings have been used to evaluate the effects of anesthetic adjuncts on neurologic function.(7)

Prior EEG studies, before the development of spectral analysis, could not utilize numeric values. The use of computer-assisted analysis of EEG recordings allows a quantitative comparison of the effects of various anesthetic agents and dosages.(8-15) Spectral edge analysis of the EEG has been correlated to anesthetic depth.(15, 16) Studies have been completed to determine the effects of opioid agonists, including fentanyl, alfentanil, and fentanyl-sufentanil.(17-19) Stone and DiFazio correlated lipid solubility with spectral edge analysis in an effort to explain the anestheticlike action of opiates.(14) Assessing analgesic agents, Szeleny and Nickel were able to determine characteristic EEG frequency responses of flupirtine when compared to clonidine, tramadol, and buprenorphine.(20, 21)

Spontaneous and drug-induced changes in the EEG have been qualitatively and quantitatively characterized by utilizing computer-derived power spectral analysis (CSA). This system converts signals recorded in sequential epochs into numerical values for display of EEG amplitude and frequency distribution. Shifts in the 80% power spectral edge allow the investigator to objectively determine shifts in electric frequencies as influenced by drugs.(8-13, 22) Some investigators have utilized 95% spectral edge for analysis.(14) The spectral edge frequency is defined as that frequency below which a certain percentage (80 or 95%) of the total power (amplitude^2) is located. Concurrent analysis of airway, blood, or tissue drug concentrations, anesthetic depth, and spectral edge frequency provides a method of gauging the correlation of neurologic responses to anesthetics and analgesics.(12, 13)

Computer-assisted spectral analysis of EEG has been adapted to animal anesthetic evaluation.(23) This method has been used to assess the CNS effects of detomidine in horses and medetomidine in dogs.(23-25) The EEG responses can be measured with a computerized spectral analysis system. In addition to the recording of raw electroencephalograms (EEGs), the mean frequencies and amplitudes for delta, theta, alpha, beta$_1$, and beta$_2$ frequency bands can be determined. These frequency bands correspond to below 3.999 Hz, 4.00 to 7.999 Hz, 8.00 to 12.999 Hz, 13.00 to 23.999 Hz, and 24.00 to 31.750 Hz respectively. The summation for all activity is recorded at frequencies up to 31.750 Hz. The response curve for each frequency and the duration of drug effect can be determined at each dosage of anesthetic to assess actions on overall CNS activity. Traditionally, adequacy of anesthesia for major surgery has been based on MAC multiples (quantitative measurement) or absence of patient movement (qualitative measurement). Increases in certain hemodynamic parameters (e.g., blood pressure) during surgical stimulation are due to sympathetic nervous system responses to noxious stimuli and have also been relied upon to assess CNS depression. Details of the use of computerized spectral analysis of the EEG to assess anesthetic depression have been published.(8-15, 22, 23)

CEREBRAL BLOOD FLOW METHODS

Efforts to measure accurately or to control flow of arterial blood to the brain are difficult because of the inaccessibility of the anterior vertebral artery. It does not appear possible to divert all of the cerebral blood supply through an accessible artery so that it can be measured. There is communication between the internal and external carotid with the internal maxillary arteries. As a result, all blood directed toward the brain does not pass through the internal carotid artery. Likewise, it is difficult to achieve 100% accuracy in determining cerebral venous outflow, since there is communication between cerebral sinuses and the azygos system.(2) Efforts by Schmidt prior to 1928 resulted in three methods: (a) measurement of cerebral arterial flow, (b) measurement of cerebral venous flow, and (c) measurement of cerebral perfusion. These early methods made direct measurements of blood flow with a venturi system inserted between vessels supplying or draining the brain and the systemic circulation.(2) Even though the results were not always repeatable, Schmidt was able to determine that systemic blood pressure, vasomotor influences, and chemical influences altered cerebral blood flow. Schmidt, Kety, and Pennes were able to refine the methodology and by 1945 were cannulating the basilar artery of the monkey for cerebral flow measurements and the internal jugular for outflow.(3) Flow was determined using a bubble flow meter and arterial-venous (A-V) oxygen content differences.

Arterial-venous oxygen differences ranged between 6 and 10 volume percent. Another method of measuring CBF is based on the principle that the rate at which the cerebral venous blood content of an inert gas approaches the arterial blood content depends on the volume of blood flowing toward the brain. CBF using this method in humans showed a range of 41 to 78 mL $\cdot$ 100 g^{-1} $\cdot$ min^{-1} and a $CMRO_2$ of 3.0-4.7 mL $\cdot$ 100 g^{-1} $\cdot$ min^{-1}.[4]

One of the more commonly used techniques of determining CBF is measurement of venous outflow. The sagittal sinus is exposed, isolated and cannulated. Measurement of CBF is usually made from the anterior, superior, and lateral portions of both cerebral hemispheres in dogs, representing 54% of the total brain weight.[26-32] Arterial and sagittal sinus blood samples are usually compared for A-V oxygen content difference. Many CBF methods employ radioisotopes and gamma counting technology by comparing tissue versus reference values from blood samples. These methods include the administration of 300,000 to 500,000 radiolabeled 15-m-diameter microspheres by injection [33-36], and xenon [37], or hydrogen clearance.[38-40] Antipyrine ^{14}C as an inert tracer has also been distributed in cerebral tissue based on water content and measured by gamma counting techniques and autoradiography.[41-43]

CEREBRAL PERFUSION AND METABOLISM

Cerebral perfusion and metabolism are influenced by many factors. However, under normal conditions they are autoregulated to maintain cerebral homeostasis. The primary requirements for evaluating perfusion and metabolism are CBF and the A-V oxygen difference.[4, 44] Cerebral metabolic rate for oxygen ($CMRO_2$) is the product of CBF and A-V oxygen content difference expressed as mL $\cdot$ 100 g^{-1} $\cdot$ min^{-1}.[30, 45] Cerebral metabolic rate for glucose (CMR gluc) may also be determined. The product of CBF and A-V glucose difference is expressed as mg $\cdot$ 100 g^{-1} $\cdot$ min^{-1}. To assess global CNS O_2 and glucose requirements, three factors need to be determined: cerebral blood flow by direct flow or radioisotope methodology, A-V O_2 or A-V glucose differences and brain weight. $CMRO_2$ is most frequently used as an index of global cerebral metabolism.

CEREBRAL OXYGEN AND METABOLIC REQUIREMENTS

Cerebral metabolism is characterized by remarkable stability in the normal awake brain. In the normal awake brain, depletion of most of the energy stores occurs within 2 to 4 minutes after oxygen delivery is abruptly discontinued. During the same time period a three- to fivefold increase in the brain lactate concentration occurs depending on the initial blood glucose levels. The primary energy-consuming processes of the brain are divided into those of function and maintenance of integrity. The oxygen requirement in the awake normal canine brain is 5.5 mL $\cdot$ 100 g^{-1} $\cdot$ min^{-1}, with 60% needed for function and 40% for maintenance

of brain cell integrity.[1] Normal EEG function is expected with a PaO_2 of approximately 100 mm Hg, PvO_2 of 35 mm Hg, and CBF of 50 mL $\cdot$ 100 g^{-1} $\cdot$ min^{-1}. Irreversible cerebral tissue damage is likely when PaO_2 drops below 20 to 23 mm Hg and CBF below 10 mL $\cdot$ 100 g^{-1} $\cdot$ min^{-1}.[1]

The mature brain in the nonfasting state relies only on glucose as a substrate for conversion to energy. Under normal conditions 95% of the glucose is metabolized by oxidative phosphorylation. The remaining 5% is metabolized by anaerobic pathways to lactate. Inadequate or marginal oxygen delivery to the brain will result in an increase in anaerobic metabolism reflected by increases in glucose consumption and lactate production. This decrease in the ratio of O_2 to glucose utilized may be reported as the oxygen-glucose index (OGI) and the increase in lactate produced to glucose consumed as the lactate-glucose index (LGI).[1] Oxygen availability, CBF, and $CMRO_2$ may vary by species, age, physical condition, and the influence of drugs.

In man, normal function of the awake brain requires approximately 3.5 mL O_2 $\cdot$ 100 g $\cdot$ min^{-1}, or a total of about 50 mL $\cdot$ min^{-1} extracted from an average normal cerebral blood flow of 57 mL $\cdot$ 100 g $\cdot$min^{-1}. Within clinically accepted dose levels, most general anesthetic and cerebral depressants reduce oxygen consumption of the brain.[46] Complete oxidation of glucose to carbon dioxide and water by cerebral tissue appears to be the principal source of energy metabolism. Approximately 70 mg $\cdot$ min^{-1} of glucose are required for metabolism in the adult human brain (27.8 nmol $\cdot$ 100 g^{-1} brain $\cdot$ min^{-1}). Metabolism utilizes 5.5 mmol of oxygen for each mmol of glucose. The effects of analgesics and anesthetics on cerebral metabolism, CBF, and $CMRO_2$ are critical factors in producing safe depression of the CNS.

Barbiturate Anesthetics

Established methods for determining CBF and $CMRO_2$ have demonstrated the responses of the central nervous system of animals to anesthetics and related medications. Pentobarbital depresses CBF and $CMRO_2$ during the first 3 hours in dogs. After 3 hours a tolerance to deep pentobarbital anesthesia develops and $CMRO_2$ significantly increases, even at similar levels of EEG suppression.[47] Ultra-short-acting anesthetics are frequently used for anesthetic induction. Thiopental effects cerebral metabolism only when it alters cerebral electric function. At temperatures below 18° C with absence of electric function, barbiturates have no effects on $CMRO_2$, whereas further reduction in body temperature continues to have an effect.[48]

Extensive study of the effects of thiopental on regulatory mechanisms of brain energy metabolism demonstrate that glucose-6-phosphate concentration increases in the early stages of thiopental anesthesia, coinciding with depression of EEG beta activity, and decreases with the return of EEG activity.[49] Glucose levels increased during the second stage. Phosphofructokinase activity appears to be inhibited only during the early stages of thiopental anesthesia.

During hypoxia, thiopental does not reduce cerebral function enough to provide cerebral protection nor does it uncouple oxidative phosphorylation in vivo.(50) After massive doses of thiopental, $CMRO_2$ decreased from 3.99 to 2.22 mL $\cdot$ 100 g^{-1} $\cdot$ min^{-1}, CMRgluc decreased from 4.7 to 2.6 mg $\cdot$ 100 g^{-1} $\cdot$ min^{-1}, and CBF decreased from 40 to 18 mL $\cdot$ 100 g^{-1} $\cdot$ min^{-1}.

Inhalant Anesthetics

Halothane has a profound effect on brain function and CBF. Cerebral blood flow has been shown to increase progressively during the first 30 minutes of halothane anesthesia and then decrease to preinduction levels by 150 minutes.(51) Cerebral metabolism ($CMRO_2$) and cerebral vascular resistance decrease significantly during induction and for 30 minutes, after which they increase to baseline values. Halothane anesthesia can produce increases in intracranial pressure.(52) It has been shown that halothane produces significant increases in CBF at 1.0 MAC and impairs autoregulation. Similarly, CBF in cats at 0.5, 1.0, and 1.5 MAC halothane increases by 10 to 25% above control values. Regional CBF in both intact and ischemic brain preparations in dogs increases with increasing halothane concentrations.(53) Because of this effect it is thought that halothane is more likely to cause intracranial compromise than isoflurane. Halothane and CO_2 increase regional cerebral blood flow (rCBF) in both ischemic and normal brain tissues. Carbon dioxide is a potent cerebral vasodilator.

In contrast to similar hemispheric CBF during halothane and isoflurane anesthesia in rats, neocortical CBF is greater with halothane. Some of the differences in cerebral response to halothane versus isoflurane may result from altered rCBF differences. Isoflurane causes cerebral vasodilation and an increase in cerebral perfusion.(54-55) There is a time-related reduction in CBF during long periods of isoflurane-N_2O anesthesia.(56) Over time, CBF changes are similar for the total cerebral cortex, corpus callosum, caudate nuclei, cerebellum, and brain stem.

It would be advantageous to couple measurement of CBF and CMRgluc for assessment of cerebral protection during anesthesia. Autoregulation, with normal blood pressure and ventilation, can be expected to compensate for anesthetic-induced changes. In most instances CBF can change significantly without significantly changing CMRgluc. During high concentrations of isoflurane, the lowest CBF/CMRgluc ratios are found in the hippocampal dentate region.(57) Using the sagittal sinus cannulation technique for CBF, no significant change between control (58.8 $\pm$ 4.8 mL $\cdot$ 100 g^{-1} $\cdot$ min^{-1}) and 1% isoflurane values occur.(58) $CMRO_2$ control values of 4.49 $\pm$ 0.10 mL $\cdot$ 100 g^{-1} $\cdot$ min^{-1} did not change significantly during the subsequent 4 hours of isoflurane anesthesia.

Cerebral metabolic measurements during isoflurane anesthesia suggest a degree of protection similar to that of barbiturates induced by depression of cortical electric activity and cerebral metabolism. In hypotensive dogs cerebral energy stores of ATP and phosphocreatine were sustained at higher levels and cerebral lactate levels were significantly lower during isoflurane versus nitrous oxide administration.(59) The effects of increasing isoflurane concentrations on cerebral metabolism have been evaluated by $CMRO_2$ and CMRgluc methods.(59)

It is conceivable that some variation in results reported between halothane and isoflurane may be due to species differences and the presence of other drugs administered in a specific study. For example, it is clear that CNS responses are related to the actions of both barbiturates and halothane when administered concomitantly.(60) It should be noted that cerebral responses can also be influenced by physiologic factors such as blood pressure, cardiac output, carbon dioxide content, and pH.

The dose-related effects of increasing concentrations of isoflurane on cerebral metabolism and blood flow are predictable (Table 7B–1). Eventually, there is profound suppression of cortical electrical activity reflected by an isoelectric EEG.(61) In one study, this occurred at 3% isoflurane when mean $CMRO_2$ was 2.02 mL $\cdot$ 100 g^{-1} $\cdot$ min^{-1} and CBF was 64 mL $\cdot$ 100 g^{-1} $\cdot$ min^{-1}. Thereafter, increasing isoflurane concentration to 6% had no effect on $CMRO_2$ or CBF. Isoflurane (0.5 and 1.0 MAC) provides brain protection during incomplete ischemia with depression of $CMRO_2$, whereas the addition of N_2O reverses cerebral metabolic depression. N_2O alone or combined with low-dose isoflurane may worsen neuronal injury when cerebral ischemia is present.(62) Isoflurane cannot be expected to provide protection against cerebral ischemia from other causes.(63)

Administration of 50% N_2O during normocapnia has been associated with an 11% increase in rCBF.(64-65) In hypocapnic dogs, there was no significant change. Isoflurane (2%) administration induced a 31% increase in CBF during normocapnic conditions but only a 15% increase during hypocapnia. Table 7B-2 lists CBF, $CMRO_2$, and CMRgluc values derived from animals administered various inhalant and injectable anesthetics and analgesics.(66)

Table 7B–1. Effect of Changing End Expired Concentration of Isoflurane on Parameters of Cerebral Metabolism

	Isoflurane Concentration		
	<0.1%	1.4%	2.4%
$CMRO_2$ ml $\cdot$ 100 g^{-1} $\cdot$ min^{-1}	5.10	3.90	3.58
CMRgluc mg^{-1} $\cdot$ 100 g^{-1} $\cdot$ min^{-1}	6.49	4.95	4.97
CBF ml $\cdot$ 100 g^{-1} $\cdot$ min^{-1}	49.3	65.1	77.8

(Adapted from Newberg, L.A., and Michenfelder, J.D. Cerebral Protection by Isoflurane During Hypoxemia or Ischemia. Anesthesiology 59:29–35, 1983.)

Table 7B–2. Cerebral Responses to Various Inhalation and Injectable Anesthetics in the Dog

Inhalant Anesthetic	CBF $mL \cdot 100\ g^{-1} \cdot min^{-1}$	$CMRo_2$ $mL \cdot 100\ g^{-1} \cdot min^{-1}$	CMRgluc $mg \cdot 100\ g^{-1} \cdot min^{-1}$	Conditions	Reference
Halothane				Ventilated	1
0.3%	63	4.9		MAP 110	
0.8%	60	3.9		MAP 84	
Halothane					
Control	65	3.84		Ventilated	51
Isoflurane + N$_2$O				Time	55
1.3 MAC + N$_2$O (70%)	(Considered 0.8% = 1.3 MAC)			(Radioactive	
2 hour	122	5.6		microspheres,	
3 hour	85	4.9		sagittal	
4 hour	78	4.0		sinus)	
Isoflurane without N$_2$O					
Control	59	4.49		Ventilated	58
1 hour 1%	59	4.54		Time	
2 hour 1%	56	4.41		(Direct blood	
3 hour 1%	56	4.39		flow, sagittal	
4 hour 1%	56	4.40		sinus)	
Isoflurane with changing blood pressure					
1%	59	4.49		107 mm Hg MAP	58
3%	94	2.32		93 mm Hg MAP	1
Isoflurane with other medications				Ventilated	
Control	52	3.17		1% isoflurane	1
Flumazenil (benzodiazepine antagonist)				2 mg	
+5 min	53	3.41			
Methoxyflurane at changing concentrations					
<0.10%	45	5.67	8.9	Ventilated	1
0.25%	61	5.11	8.1		
0.44%	52	4.37	7.7		
Enflurane at changing concentrations					
<0.1%	70	5.54	7.09	Ventilated	50
2.2%	77	3.64	5.33		
4.2%	93	3.69	5.23		
Desflurane at changing concentrations					
1.5 MAC	78	2.5		Ventilated	66
2.0 MAC	52	2.5			
2.0 MAC	87			Phenylephrine MAP 52–72 (3.2 μg/kg/min)	
Injectable Anesthetics					
Pentobarbital					
20–30 mg/kg	22	1.8–2.0		Ventilated	47
Thiopental with changing temperatures					
Control	56	4.95		Ventilated 37° C	48
Control	25	0.45		Ventilated 18° C	
Thiopental (40 mg/kg)	34	0.54		Ventilated 18° C	
	29	2.70		Ventilated 37° C	
Thiopental at contrasting levels					
Control	67	4.3		Ventilated	1
Unconscious	37	2.5		Burst suppression	
Deep anesthesia	28	2.7			
Etomidate					
Control	145	5.52		Ventilated	1
0.1 mg/kg/min	36	3.62			

Table 7B–2.   **Cerebral Responses to Various Inhalation and Injectable Anesthetics in the Dog—cont'd**

Injectable Analgesics	CBF $mL \cdot 100\ g^{-1} \cdot min^{-1}$	CMRo$_2$ $mL \cdot 100\ g^{-1} \cdot min^{-1}$	CMRgluc $mg \cdot 100\ g^{-1} \cdot min^{-1}$	Conditions	Reference
Morphine with varying dosages					
Control	87	5.75		Ventilated	1
1.2 mg/kg	40	4.97			
3.0 mg/kg	35	4.78			
Nalorphine					
Control	70	6.06			
0.3 mg/kg	51	5.71			
Sufentanil with time change					
Control	83	4.05		Ventilated	32
10–50 µg/kg					
+2 min.	119	4.51			
+35 min	85	3.76			
+55 min	72	3.66			
Alfentanil					
Control	30	2.28		Pentobarbitone	30
30 mg/kg	29	2.37		Ventilated	
Fentanyl with time changes					
Control	79	4.40		Ventilated	66
50–100 µg/kg					
+5 min	90	4.09			
+20 min	79	4.16			

Models for Neurologic Evaluations

Chronic models have been developed for evaluation of sedatives, analgesics, and anesthetics on various CNS physiologic parameters. Comparative biochemical and neurologic evaluations have been completed to determine effects of anesthetics and anesthetic adjuncts on CMRO$_2$, CBF, and the EEG. In these models, chronically implanted arterial blood flow probes provide continual data on changes in cerebral blood flow induced by various drugs and over time (Figs. 7B–1 and 7B–2).(67)

As was previously discussed, traditional EEG evaluations are subjective and are based on the degree of burst suppression for determination of the isoelectric point. Quantitative assessment of total activity, spectral edge analysis, and shifts of activity in the frequency spectrum of the EEG are now being used to study more discrete CNS responses to sedatives, analgesics, and anesthetics.(23-25, 66)

EVALUATION OF ALPHA$_2$ AGONISTS

Although studies of the effects of sedative-analgesics on cerebral responses are not commonly performed (68), recently, three studies recording cerebral responses to alpha$_2$-agonists and inhalant anesthesia have been completed.(66, 69, 70) In two of these experiments, the sagittal sinus was exposed, isolated, and cannulated for direct measurements of CBF and collection of blood samples for blood gas analysis. Electromagnetic flow probes continuously recorded blood flow from the sagittal catheter or at timed intervals.(69, 70) EEGs were recorded from bilateral frontal-occipital electrodes. Halothane and isoflurane baseline values were determined prior to alpha$_2$-agonist (dexmedetomidine) administration to determine its effects on cerebral function.(69, 70) In another study medetomidine (30 µg/kg IV) was administered to chronically instrumented dogs followed by halothane or isoflurane administration to determine the effects of these drugs on the frequency distribution of the EEG (Fig. 7B–3).(66)

Dexmedetomidine (10 µg/kg) reportedly reduces halothane MAC in dogs by 90%.(70) In halothane- and isoflurane-anesthetized dogs cerebral blood flow decreases after dexmedetomidine administration while CMRO$_2$ remains unchanged.(69) It was concluded that cerebral vasoconstriction via activation of alpha$_2$-adrenergic receptors was responsible for the decrease in CBF.(69) Despite the large reduction in the CBF, there was no global evidence of cerebral ischemia.(69) Dexmedetomidine was believed to be acting on specific brain regions with dense populations of vascular alpha$_2$ receptors as opposed to producing generalized cerebral vasoconstriction.

The biochemical and cerebral responses to medetomidine and halothane or isoflurane as determined by CMRO$_2$, EEG, and CBF data are similar to those observed for dexmedetomidine. CBF and CMRO$_2$ values are comparable in spite of a difference in potency between dexmedetomidine and medetomidine (Table 7B–3). Together these studies document changes in neurologic function and metabolism produced by alpha$_2$ + inhalant anesthesia.

The relation between CBF and CMRO$_2$ has been evaluated for medetomidine alone, medetomidine with inhalant anesthetics, and medetomidine reversed with atipamezole.(66) The primary factor influencing CBF was the dose of alpha$_2$-agonist administered. The CMRO$_2$ was unchanged in each of the treatment groups regardless of the dose, although decreasing values were observed with the higher doses of medetomidine that corresponded with the lowest cerebral blood flow and oxygen content values.(25, 66)

EVALUATION OF EPIDURAL ANALGESICS

In contrast to traditional intravenous administration of analgesics, recent efforts have concentrated on regional nerve blocks or epidurally administered analgesics to reduce CNS responses evoked by noxious stimuli. EEG

arousal reactions have been used to identify alterations of anesthetic depth and for detection of noxious stimuli applied during general anesthesia. Reports comparing EEG and hemodynamic responses to noxious stimuli in humans and animals provide inconsistent results. Nociceptive input results either in simultaneous changes in quantitated EEG and cardiovascular variables or uncoupled electroencephalographic and hemodynamic responses.

The applicability of various cardiovascular and quantitated EEG variables for early detection of the antinociceptive effects of a fixed dose of xylazine administered epidurally in dogs anesthetized with isoflurane has been performed.(71) The application of a noxious somatic stimulus prior to epidural administration of xylazine resulted in significant increases in both MAP and HR, and a significant decrease in EEG total power (TP), whereas responses in beta:delta ratio, SEF 80, and median power frequency as the fiftieth percentile (MED) were not significant. Because changes in TP

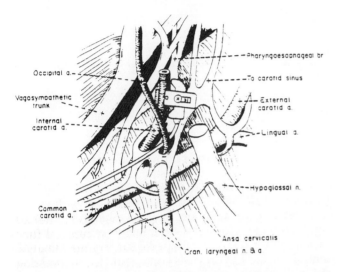

Fig. 7B–1. Nerves and vessels include the internal carotid with placement of the arterial blood flow probe. (Artwork by Lucy Gagliardo.)

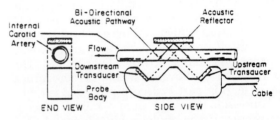

Fig. 7B–2. Schematic views of the perivascular Transonic ultrasonic volume flow sensor. Two transducers pass ultrasonic signals back and forth, alternately intersecting the flowing liquid in upstream and downstream direction. The difference in travel time of the upstream and downstream signals is a measure of volume flow.

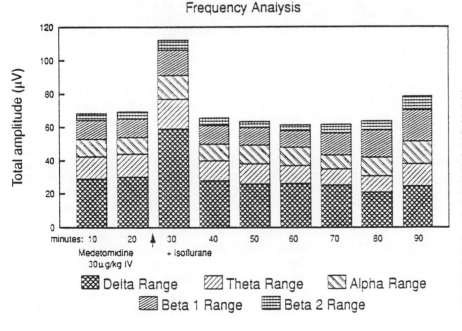

Fig. 7B–3 Frequency distribution of EEG during medetomidine 30 μg/kg followed by isoflurane anesthesia. Note the stability of EEG frequencies except at the onset of isoflurane. The increase in total amplitude and significant increase in delta waves occurred after intubation and the first reaction to inhaling isoflurane. Unconsciousness was demonstrated 10 minutes later by failure to have movement response to strong stimuli and failure to show EEG changes during stimuli. The final increase occurs as medetomidine is no longer effective and isoflurane concentrations are not increased.

Table 7B–3. Alpha₂-Agonist/Anesthetic Cerebral Responses in Dogs

Agents	EEG (μv)	CMRO₂ $ml \cdot 100\ g^{-1} \cdot min^{-1}$	CBF $ml \cdot 100\ g^{-1} \cdot min^{-1}$	Investigator
Medetomidine 30 µg/kg IV	85	2.5–3.3	41	25
Halothane 1 MAC	60	3.8	88	70
Halothane 1 MAC +10 µg/kg IV dexmedetomidine	–	4.4	58	70
Halothane 0.5 MAC +30 µg/kg IV medetomidine	74	2.0–2.7	44	25
Isoflurane 0.5 MAC	–	2.8	90	69
Isoflurane 0.5 MAC +10 µg/kg IV dexmedetomidine	–	2.4	40	69
Isoflurane 0.5 MAC +30 µg/kg medetomidine	65	2.9–3.5	49	25

recorded during stimulation occurred in the same or even higher magnitude during control measurements, it is questionable whether the significant decrease in TP resulted from a nociceptive response. Thus, noxious stimulation caused pronounced changes in cardiovascular variables unaccompanied by EEG changes. This diversion between cardiovascular and cerebrocortical responses, at least in part, reflects a profound cerebrocortical suppression resulting from a mixed effect of isoflurane, acepromazine, and possibly thiopental. Consequently, quantitated EEG variables may not be appropriate predictors of antinociception. On the other hand, if electroencephalography already indicates profound cerebrocortical suppression, increasing anesthetic concentrations (e.g., isoflurane) in order to eliminate cardiovascular nociceptive responses may be inappropriate. Hence, the old dictum that "if the patient has increased cardiovascular responsiveness to a surgical stimulus, increase anesthetic depth" may have to be revised. Pronounced hemodynamic responses to noxious stimuli in the face of adequate cerebrocortical depression may be better treated by administration of specific analgesic drugs or epidural and regional analgesia rather than by increasing concentrations of inhalant anesthetics. Epidurally administered xylazine with its sympatholytic action likely further attenuates hemodynamic responses to noxious stimuli during inhalant anesthesia. This effect may last up to 4 hours without producing serious hemodynamic alterations.

EVALUATION OF PERIOPERATIVE ANALGESIA

The EEG as a noninvasive technique delivers continuous information on the CNS effects of anesthetic agents and thus may become a powerful instrument in establishing pharmacokinetic and pharmacodynamic models for intravenous and inhalation anesthetics. EEG analysis of awake horses compared to anesthetized horses undergoing surgical procedures has been performed.(72) The mean total amplitudes in surgical

groups range from 127 to 169 µV, while nonsurgical groups range from 107 to 115 µV.

When halothane is compared to isoflurane during equine orthopedic surgery, the total amplitude of the EEG during halothane anesthesia is less than with isoflurane. However, the beta:delta power ratio is greater for halothane. During surgical intervention, the beta:delta power ratio and spectral edge increase during halothane but not isoflurane anesthesia. When anesthesia for painful orthopedic surgery is evaluated, analysis of the EEG reveals consistent CNS depression of the amplitude of electric activity with halothane or isoflurane. A significantly greater magnitude of depression is observed when halothane is used in conjunction with xylazine or ketamine. Change in total amplitude is not observed during stimulation of evoked potential by orthopedic surgery during anesthesia. However, there is a shift in the beta:delta ratio during orthopedic manipulation during halothane anesthesia. This shift is not evident during skin incision, is maximum by 30 minutes into the arthroscopic manipulations, and continues during the entire orthopedic procedure.

Observation of frequency shifts in the EEG is of value in assessing neurologic function in human anesthesia and surgery. During arousal from sedation or anesthesia, increases in total amplitude occur. The brain wave activity response to increasing depth of halothane anesthesia in dogs and horses has been described as a predominance of delta and theta activity in the EEG, and a shift from high frequency and low amplitude to lower frequency and higher amplitude. An isoelectric (flat-line) EEG is not expected in the clinical halothane dosage range. Halothane is considered nonseizurogenic. In studies of light anesthesia in man, the EEG activity increased in frequency with some increase in amplitude. Slowing of brain wave activity and burst suppression begins to occur when anesthesia nears surgical planes. In horses using compressed spectral analysis, increasing depth of halothane anesthesia is accompanied by a pronounced shift in EEG activity from beta to theta and delta frequency bands, a decrease in 80% SEF, reduction in beta:delta frequency ratio, and a minor increase in total amplitude.

Anesthesia-mediated stress responses have been studied in halothane-anesthetized horses without surgery. Biochemical changes have also been reported during halothane general anesthesia and arthroscopy. Among the changes reported were decreases in plasma insulin and norepinephrine during surgery and increases in beta-endorphin (transient) and cortisol. Studies in horses undergoing superficial surgery demonstrate that induction affects the stress response as measured by hormonal and metabolic changes. Shifts in EEG frequency may be indicative of a stress response initiated early in the surgical procedure.

Total EEG amplitude is lower during halothane than isoflurane anesthesia at clinically similar depths. This suggests that halothane produces more generalized depression of the CNS than isoflurane. However, the greater values for beta:delta ratio suggest that the CNS is more responsive during halothane anesthesia. This theory is supported by an increase in beta:delta ratio, which is seen during surgical stimulation. The timing of this increase coincides with intense surgical stimulation caused by broaching of the joint cartilage.(23)

Early reports recommend that volatile anesthetic agents should be avoided during measurement of intraoperative somatosensory evoked potentials (SEP) because many patients' SEPs were unrecordable. It was later shown that isoflurane administration results in dose-dependent decreases in the amplitude of cortical wave forms. There is no change in the EEG during isoflurane anesthesia at 1.2 MAC, but a beta:delta shift in the EEG occurs during 1.5 to 1.6 MAC halothane despite significantly lower total EEG amplitude. These results may indicate that halothane suppresses nociception less than isoflurane in horses.(72)

Factors that influence EEG responses besides intrinsic brain activity and anesthetics include hypercarbia, hypercapnia, changes in cerebral blood flow (CBF), arterial hypotension, and hypoxemia. Anesthesia induces ventilatory depression and decreases systemic arterial pressure with increasing MAC multiples. Many anesthetics increase CBF by cerebral arterial dilation and decrease the cerebral metabolic rate of oxygen consumption. Intracranial pressure (ICP) may increase during anesthesia, but can be attenuated by prior hyperventilation and hypocapnia.

The EEG responses mediated in horses sedated with alpha$_2$ agents include significant decreases in total power following doses of detomidine (10 to 60 µg/kg IV). The decrease in power is dose dependent up to about 20 µg/kg, while doses over 10 µg/kg influence duration of depression. The elimination half-life following 80 µg/kg detomidine given intravenously to horses was reported to be 1.19 ± 0.27 hours. Assuming a similar elimination in the anesthetized horses, loss of detomidine's CNS effect is likely to cause changes in the EEG after 1 to 2 hours of anesthesia.

In horses premedicated with xylazine, EEG activity following ketamine administration is characterized as having increasingly high voltage and slower activity. In man, ketamine increases CBF, mainly because of cerebral vasodilation, without significantly changing CMRO$_2$ and cerebral lactate or glucose concentrations. In most species, ketamine increases intracranial pressure and CBF, with little effect on metabolism. Seizures may occur following ketamine administration but are not always obvious on surface EEG recordings. Duration of recumbency following detomidine-ketamine anesthesia in horses ranges from 15 to 30 minutes. Effects of ketamine on EEG 30 minutes or more after its administration are thus assumed to be negligible.

It may be difficult to eliminate all surgical stress responses during inhalation anesthesia in orthopedic patients unless regional nerve blocks are utilized. Extradural and intraarticular opioid agonists and local anesthetics reduce plasma glucose and cortisol responses in surgical patients. The use of CSA of the EEG provides a neurologic measurement that, coupled with standard clinical anesthetic evaluations, contributes to a better understanding of perioperative analgesia. Absence of significant changes in EEG amplitude associated with surgery, insignificant changes in hemodynamics, lack of movement, and stability of measurable parameters in both the nonsurgical and surgical phases of the anesthesia, indicates that adequate analgesia is present.

Summary

At present, EEG brain mapping in dogs given anesthetics and anesthetic adjuncts are in progress (Chapter 23). Documentation of anesthetic effects and cerebral responses are now possible. The effects of anesthetics on CNS responsiveness to major surgical stimulus (i.e., joint surgery) have been demonstrated. Changes in compressed spectral analysis that accompany joint invasion and manipulation are measurable and repeatable. The use of computerized analysis of the EEG provides the opportunity to convert brain wave activity recordings into quantitative values. This is the basis for future analysis of CNS function associated with anesthetic and anesthetic adjunct administration.

Undoubtedly, physiologic mechanisms that protect brain function can be altered by sedatives, analgesics, and anesthetics. Within reasonable limits, autoregulation and coupling of EEG, CBF, and CMRO$_2$ protect brain cells against irreversible damage. Some parameters are well established at normal body temperatures. It is known that 60% of metabolism as measured by CMRO$_2$ supports cell function, while 40% supports cell integrity. Cerebral blood flows of less than 20 mL · 100 g^{-1} · min^{-1} are detrimental to all function and possible integrity. CNS stimulants increase cell requirements, metabolism, and blood flow, just as depressants do the opposite.

As considerations are made for selection of anesthetics, the primary objectives of providing analgesia and avoiding distress should be coupled to the necessity of adequate cerebral perfusion and metabolism. It should be appreciated that prolonged recovery is not always the result of lingering anesthetic action but may, in a small percentage of patients, result from cerebral dysfunction. Reports of postanesthetic seizures in dogs and horses following ketamine, prolonged CNS depression in animals following low oxygen availability or low cardiac output, postanesthetic blindness or deafness, and other possible CNS dysfunction manifested as incoordination or ataxia suggest adverse CNS sequela. Proper selection of anesthetics and techniques, maintenance of needed ventilation and perfusion, and the continuing quest for a better understanding of the effects of anesthetics on CNS physiology will undoubtedly improve anesthetic outcome.

References

1. Michenfelder JD. Anesthesia and the brain. New York: Churchill Livingstone, 1988.
2. Schmidt CF. The influence of cerebral blood-flow on respiration. Am J Physiol 84:202–259, 1928.
3. Schmidt CF, Kety SS, Pennes HH. The gaseous metabolism of the brain of the monkey. Am J Physiol 143:33–52, 1945.
4. Kety SS, Schmidt CF. The determination of cerebral blood flow in man by use of nitrous oxide in low concentrations. Am J Physiol 143:53, 1945.
5. Domino EF, Corssen G, Sweet RB. Effects of various general anesthetics in the visually evoked response in man. Anesth Analg 42:735, 1963.
6. Domino EF. Effects of preanesthetic and anesthetic drugs in visually evoked responses. Anesthesiology 28(1):184–191, 1967.
7. Pastal RH, Fernstrom JD. The effects of clonidine on EEG wavebands associated with sleep in the rat. Brain Res 300:243–255, 1984.
8. Gehrmann JE, Killam KF. Assessment of CNS drug activity in rhesus monkeys by analysis of the EEG. Fed Proc Fed Am Soc Exp Biol 35:2258–2263, 1976.
9. Young GA, Steinfels GF, Khozan N, Glaser EM. Cortical EEG power spectra associated with sleep-awake behavior in the rat. Pharmacol Biochem Behav 8:89–91, 1978.
10. Steinfels GF, Young GA, Khazan N. Opioid self-administration and REM sleep EEG power spectra. Neuropharmacology 19:69–74, 1979.
11. Kareti S, Moreton JE, Khaza N. Effects of buprenorphine, a new narcotic agonist-antagonist analgesic on the EEG power spectrum on behavior of the rat. Neuropharmacology 19:195–201, 1980.
12. Scott JC, Ponganis KV, Stanski DR. EEG quantitation of narcotic effect: The comparative pharmacodynamics of fentanyl and alfentanil. Anesthesiology 62:234–241, 1985.
13. Rampil IJ, Weiskopf RB, Brown JG, Eger EI III, Johnson BH, Holmes MA, Donegan JH. 1653 and isoflurane produce similar dose-related changes in the electroencephalogram of pigs. Anesthesiology 69:298–302, 1988.
14. Stone DJ, DiFazio CA. Anesthetic action of opiates: correlations of lipid solubility and spectral edge. Anesth Analg 67:663–666, 1988.
15. Rampil IJ, Sasse FJ, Smith NT, Hoff BH, Flemming DC. Spectral edge frequency–a new correlation of anesthetic depth. Anesthesiology 73:152, 1990.
16. Smith NT. Personal communication, 1980.
17. Bovill JG, Sebel PS, Wauquier A, Rog P. Electroencephalographic effects of sufentanil anesthesia in man. Br J Anesthet 54:45–52, 1982.
18. Bovill JG, Sebel PS, Wauquier A, Rog P, Schuyt HC. Influence of high dose alfentanil anesthesia on the electroencephalogram:
19. Smith NT, Dec-Silver H, Sanford TJ, Westover, Quinn ML, Klein F, Davis DA. EEG during high-dose fentanyl-sufentanil, or morphine oxygen anesthesia. Anesth Analg 63:386–393, 1984.
20. Nickel B. The antinociceptive activity of flupirtine: A structurally new analgesic. Postgrad Med J 63:19–28, 1987.
21. Szelenyi I, Nickel B. Putatine site(s) and mechanism(s) of action of flupirtine, a novel analgesic compound. Postgrad Med J 63:57–60, 1987.
22. Mathia A, Moreton JE. Electroencephalographic EEG, EEG power spectra, and behavioral correlates in rats given phencyclidine. Neuropharmacology 25(7):763–769, 1986.
23. Otto K, Short CE. EEG power spectrum analysis as a monitor of anesthetic depth in horses. Vet Surg 20(5):362–371, 1991.
24. Short CE, Otto K, Gilbert M, Maylin GA. The responses to detomidine usage as a sole agent or in combination in the horse. Proc Am Assoc Equine Pract 153–166, 1989.
25. Short CE, Kallfelz FA, Otto K, Otto B, Wallace R. The effects of α_2-adrenoceptor agonist analgesia on the central nervous system in an equine model. In: Short CE, Van Poznak A, eds. Animal pain. New York: Churchill Livingstone, 1991.
26. Lassen NA, Ingvar DH. Blood flow of the cerebral cortex determined by radioactive krypton 85. Experientia 17:42, 1961.
27. Rapela CE, Green HD. Autoregulation of canine cerebral blood flow. Circ Res 14:1205–1211, 1964.
28. Michenfelder JD, Messick JM, Theye RA. Simultaneous cerebral blood flow by direct and indirect methods. J Surg Res 8:476–481, 1968.
29. Traystman RJ, Rapela CE. Effect of sympathetic nerve stimulation on cerebral and cephalic blood flow in dogs. Circ Res 36:620–630, 1975.
30. McPherson RW, Traystman RJ. Fentanyl and cerebral vascular responsivity in dogs. Anesthesiology 60:180–186, 1984.
31. Lanier WL, Iaizzo PA, Milde JH. The effects of intravenous succinylcholine on cerebral function and muscle afferent activity following complete ischemia in halothane-anesthetized dogs. Anesthesiology 73:485–490, 1990.
32. Milde LN, Milde JH, Gallagher WJ. Effects of sufentanil in cerebral circulation and metabolism in dogs. Anesth Analg 70:B8–46, 1990.
33. Heymann MA, Payne BD, Hoffman JID, Rudolph AM. Blood flow measurements with radionuclide-labelled particles. Prog Cardiovasc Dis 20:55–76, 1977.
34. Chemtab S, Laudignon N, Beharry K, Rex J, Varma D, Wolfe L, Aranda JV. Effects of prostaglandins and indomethacin on cerebral blood flow and cerebral oxygen consumption in conscious newborn piglets. Div Pharmacol Ther 14(1):1–14, 1990.
35. Hales JRS. Radioactive microsphere techniques for studies of the circulation. Clin Exp Pharm Physiol Suppl 1:31–46, 1974.
36. Monin P, Hascoet JM, Vert P. Autoregulation of cerebral blood flow. Dev Pharmacol Ther 13:120–128, 1989.
37. Hemelrijck JV, Fitch W, Matthussen M, VanAken H, Plets C, Lauwers T. Effect of propofol on cerebral circulation and autoregulation in the baboon. Anesth Analg 71:49–54, 1990.
38. Young W. H_2 clearance measurement of blood flow: a review of technique and polarographic principles. Stroke 11:552–564, 1980.
39. Kaieda K, Todd MM, Warner DS. The effects of anesthetics and $PaCO_2$ on the cerebrovascular, metabolic, and electroencephalographic responses to nitrous oxide in the rabbit. Anesth Analg 68:135–143, 1989.
40. Scheller MS, Todd MM, Drummond JC. Isoflurane, halothane and regional cerebral blood flow at various levels of $PaCO_2$ in rabbits. Anesthesiology 64:598–604, 1986.
41. Schuier FJ, Jones SC, Fedora T, Reivich M. iodoantipyrine and microsphere blood flow estimates in cat brain. Am J Physiol 253:H1289–H1297, 1987.
42. Hansen TD, Warner DS, Todd MM, Vust LJ. Effects of nitrous oxide and volatile anesthetics on cerebral blood flow. Br J Anesth 63:290–295, 1989.
43. Cole DJ, Drummond JC, Shapiro HM, Hertzog RE, Brauer FS. The effect of hypervolemic hemodilution with and without hyperten-

sion on cerebral blood flow following middle cerebral artery occlusion in rats anesthetized with isoflurane. Anesthesiology 71:580–585, 1989.

44. Kety SS, Schmidt CF. The nitrous oxide method for the quantitative determination of cerebral blood flow in man: theory, procedure, and normal values. J Clin Invest 27:476, 1948.

45. Szewczykowski J, Meyer JS, Kondo A, Normura F, Teraura T. Effects of ergot-alkaloids (hydergine) on cerebral hemodynamics and oxygen consumption in monkeys. J Neurol Sci 10:25–31, 1970.

46. Fink BR, Haschke RH. Anesthetic effects on cerebral metabolism. Anesthesiology 39(2):199–215, 1973.

47. Gronert GA, Michenfelder JD, Sharbrough FW, Milde JH. Canine cerebral metabolic tolerance during 24 hours deep pentobarbital anesthesia. Anesthesiology 55:110–113, 1981.

48. Steen PA, Newberg L, Milde JH, Michenfelder JD. Hypothermia and barbiturates: individual and combined effects on canine cerebral oxygen consumption. Anesthesiology 58(6):527–532, 1983.

49. Krieglstein J, Sperling G, Twietmeyer G. Effects of thiopental on regulatory mechanisms of brain energy metabolism, Naunyn-Schmiedeberg's. Arch Pharm 318:56–61, 1981.

50. Michenfelder JD. The interdependency of cerebral functional and metabolic effects following massive doses of thiopental in the dog. Anesthesiology 41(3):231–236, 1974.

51. Albrecht RF, Mileletich DJ, Madaea LR. Normalization of cerebral blood flow during prolonged halothane anesthesia. Anesthesiology 58:26–31, 1983.

52. Todd MM, Drummond JC. A comparison of the cerebrovascular and metabolic effects of halothane and isoflurane in the cat. Anesthesiology 60:276–282, 1984.

53. Smith AL, Larson CP, Hoff JT. Effects of halothane on regional cerebral blood flow in experimental focal ischemia. Anesthesiology 39(4):377–381, 1973.

54. Manohar M, Gustafson R, Goetz TE, Naganwa D. Systemic distribution of blood flow in ponies during 1.45%, 1.96% and 2.39% end-tidal isoflurane-O_2 anesthesia. Am J Vet Res 48(10): 1504–1511, 1987.

55. Manohar M, Goetz TE. Cerebral, renal, adrenal, intestinal and pancreatic circulation in conscious ponies and during 1.0, 1.5 and 2.0 minimal alveolar concentrations of halothane-O_2 anesthesia. Am J Vet Res 46:2492–2497, 1985.

56. Turner DM, Kassell NF, Sasaki T, Comair YG, Boarini DJ, Beck DO. Time dependent change in cerebral and cardiovascular parameters in isoflurane-nitrous oxide anesthetized dogs. Neurosurgery 14(2):135–141, 1984.

57. Maekawa T, Tommasino C, Shapiro HM, Keifer-Goodman J, Kohlenberger RW. Local cerebral blood flow and glucose utilization during isoflurane anesthesia in the rat. Anesthesiology 65:144–151, 1986.

58. Roald OK, Fosman M, Steen PA. The effects of prolonged isoflurane anesthesia on the cerebral blood flow and metabolism in the dog. Acta Anesthesiol Scand 33:210–213, 1989.

59. Newberg LA, Michenfelder JD. Cerebral protection by isoflurane during hypoxemia or ischemia. Anesthesiology 59:29–35, 1983.

60. Anderson RE, Michenfelder JD, Sundt TM Jr. Brain intracellular pH, blood flow, and blood-brain barrier differences with barbiturate and halothane anesthesia in the cat. Anesthesiology 52:201–206, 1980.

61. Newberg LA, Milde JH, Michenfelder JD. The cerebral metabolic effects of isoflurane at and above concentrations that suppress cortical electrical activity. Anesthesiology 59:23–28, 1983.

62. Baughman VL, Hoffman WE, Chinnamma T, Albrecht RF, Miletech DJ. The interaction of nitrous oxide and isoflurane with incomplete cerebral ischemia in the rat. Anesthesiology 70:767–774, 1989.

63. Warner DS, Deshpande JK, Wielock T. The effect of isoflurane on neuronal necrosis following near-complete forebrain ischemia in the rat. Anesthesiology 64:19–23, 1986.

64. Phelps ME, Mazziotta JC, Huang S-C. Study of cerebral function with positron computed tomography. J Cereb Blood Flow Metab 2:113–162, 1982.

65. Archer DP, Labrecque P, Tyler JL, Meyer E, Evans AC, Villemure JG, Casey WF, Diksic M, Hakim AM, Trop D. Measurement of cerebral blood flow and volume with positron emission tomography during isoflurane administration in the hypocapnic baboon. Anesthesiology 72:1031–1037, 1990.

66. Short CE. The effects of selective α_2-adrenoreceptor agonists on cardiovascular functions and brain wave activity in horses and dogs [Dissertation]. Santa Barbara, CA: Veterinary Practice Publishing Company, 1992.

67. Welch KMA, Spira PJ, Knowles L, Lance JW. Effects of prostaglandins on the internal and external carotid blood flow in the monkey. Neurology 24:705–710, 1974.

68. Shapiro HM. Anesthesia effects upon cerebral blood flow, cerebral metabolism, electroencephalogram and evoked potentials. In: Miller RD, ed. Anesthesia, 2nd ed. New York: Churchill Livingstone, 1986:1276.

69. Zornow MH, Fleischer JE, Scheller MS, Nakakimura K, Drummond JC. Dexmedetomidine, an α_2-adrenergic agonist, decreases cerebral blood flow in the isoflurane-anesthetized dog. Anesth Analg 70:624–630, 1990.

70. Karlsson BR, Forsman M, Roald OK, Heier MS, Steen PA. Effect of dexmedetomidine, a selective and potent α_2-agonist, in cerebral blood flow and oxygen consumption during halothane anesthesia in dogs. Anesth Analg 71:125–129, 1990.

71. Otto KA, Rektor AE, Voight RS, Piepenbock S, Short CE. Symposium report: animal pain and its control. Adelaide, Australia, April 1994.

72. Short CE, Ekström PM, Miller SM. Symposium report: animal pain and its control. Adelaide, Australia, April 1994.

PHARMACOLOGY

chapter 8

PREANESTHETICS AND ANESTHETIC ADJUNCTS

Introduction

Preanesthetic drugs are used to prepare the patient for induction and contribute to maintenance and smooth recovery from anesthesia. Specifically, these drugs are chosen to

1. Calm the patient
2. Induce sedation
3. Provide analgesia and muscle relaxation
4. Decrease airway secretion and salivation
5. Obtund autonomic reflex responses

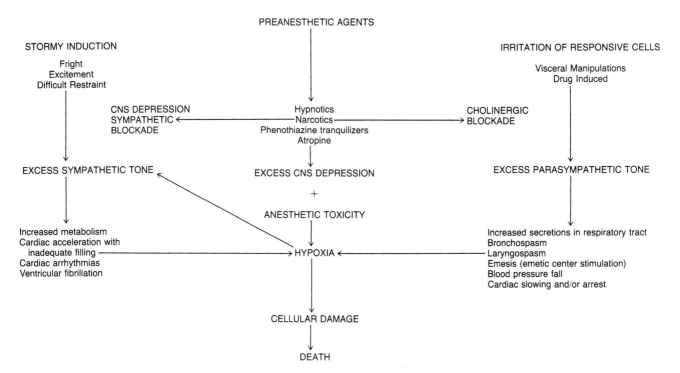

Fig. 8–1. Actions of preanesthetic agents. Adverse effects of stormy induction and/or irritation of responsive cells can be blocked by proper use of preanesthetic agents. Conversely, preanesthetic agents can produce excessive central nervous system depression, which, combined with anesthetic depression, may prove fatal.

6. Decrease gastric fluid volume and acidity
7. Suppress or prevent vomiting or regurgitation
8. Decrease anesthetic requirements
9. Promote smooth induction and recovery from anesthesia

A diagram outlining actions of preanesthetics is given in Figure 8–1. There is no preanesthetic drug or combination of drugs that can be safely and routinely administered to all patients. Preanesthetic drugs should be selected according to patient needs rather than routine administration. Some patients, for example, should not be given tranquilizers that are hypovolemic or hypotensive. The following should be considered in selecting a preanesthetic drug regimen: patient's age, physical status, disposition, species; surgical procedure and duration; inpatient or outpatient; elective or emergency surgery; and your experience with the drugs. Drugs used as preanesthetics include anticholinergics, tranquilizers, sedatives, opioids, and tranquilizer-opioid drug combinations.

Anticholinergics

ATROPINE SULFATE

Atropine blocks acetylcholine at the postganglionic terminations of cholinergic fibers in the autonomic nervous system. Oral, pharyngeal, and respiratory tract secretions are decreased, and the bronchi are dilated. Atropine increases both anatomic and physiologic respiratory dead space and may accentuate postopera-

tive hypoxemia caused by ventilation-perfusion impairment.(1) Motor and secretory activity in the gastrointestinal tract are decreased, and vagal influence on the heart is suppressed. In therapeutic doses, atropine alters arterial blood pressure minimally. It blocks the cholinergic fibers of the short ciliary nerves and relaxes the sphincter muscle of the iris, dilating the pupil. It does not dilate the pupils of birds because their irides are composed of striated muscle (Chapter 24).(2) Atropine sulfate decreases tear formation in both awake and anesthetized dogs.(3, 4) It also suppresses the muscarinic action of anticholinesterases used to reverse nondepolarizing muscle relaxants.

Atropine may be given subcutaneously, intramuscularly, or intravenously. When given intravenously, atropine may initially increase vagal tone both centrally and peripherally. The classic parasympatholytic action of atropine occurs secondarily.(5) Atropine is contraindicated in animals with preexisting tachycardia as may be seen in patients with fever or thyrotoxicosis.

In mature cattle, the dose of atropine is 0.04 mg/kg to 0.06 mg/kg. The dose of atropine for swine is 0.06 to 0.08 mg/kg. Sheep and goats require larger doses, 0.7 mg/kg prior to anesthesia. Even at this dose salivation is not completely obtunded. The effective dose of atropine in the dog is 0.04 mg/kg. At the rate of 0.5 mg/kg administered intravenously, atropine causes excitement but decreases thiopental requirement by 25% and doubles the period of anesthesia in dogs.(6) Atropine given intravenously to dogs recovering from thiopental anesthesia causes reanesthetization, and duration of sleep increases. Using a smaller dose (0.044 mg/kg SQ), Klide et al. reported similar results.(7)

Atropine increases the incidence of cardiac dysrhythmias and sinus tachycardia in dogs. Second-degree atrioventricular block is the most frequent dysrhythmia prior to anesthesia in dogs treated with atropine. Most dysrhythmias are observed during anesthetic induction and early maintenance. The most common dysrhythmias during these periods are unifocal ventricular premature depolarizations and ventricular bigeminy. Indiscriminate use of atropine prior to every anesthesia is not warranted.(8) In ponies, intravenous doses of 0.044 mg/kg and 0.176 mg/kg of atropine sulfate stop intestinal motility and induce colic in 30% of ponies respectively.(9) The response is similar in horses with high doses of atropine.

Metabolism and elimination of atropine vary among species. The cat, rat, and rabbit can destroy large quantities of atropine because they have atropine esterase in the liver.(10, 11) In the dog, atropine is cleared from the blood quickly, being excreted in the urine unchanged or as tropine. Routine administration of atropine as a preanesthetic has decreased, although use with specific drugs is still recommended (e.g., Innovar-Vet).

GLYCOPYRROLATE (ROBINUL-V)

Glycopyrrolate is a synthetic quaternary ammonium anticholinergic. It may be given intravenously, intramuscularly, or subcutaneously to dogs at a dose of 0.011 mg/kg. Glycopyrrolate inhibits the action of acetylcholine on structures innervated by postganglionic cholinergic nerves and on smooth muscles that respond to acetylcholine and lack cholinergic innervation. It decreases the volume and acidity of gastric secretions, intestinal motility, and pharyngeal, tracheal, and bronchial secretions. Its duration of action is reportedly longer than that of atropine.

In anesthetized dogs, intravenous doses of 0.005 to 0.01 mg/kg moderately decrease the amplitude of intestinal contraction. At this dose, respiration, arterial blood pressure, and heart rate are essentially unaffected. Bradycardia, hypertension, and intestinal hyperactivity of vagal origin are decreased. Because glycopyrrolate is a large polar molecule, diffusion across lipid membranes such as the blood-brain barrier and placenta is limited.

After subcutaneous or intramuscular administration, peak effect occurs in 30 to 45 minutes. Its action is evident within 1 minute following intravenous injection. Vagal inhibition lasts for 2 to 3 hours, and the antisialagogue effect may persist for up to 7 hours.

Glycopyrrolate is used to decrease salivary, tracheobronchial, and pharyngeal secretions and the volume and acidity of gastric secretions. Because of the increased pH of gastric secretions and decreased intestinal motility, the likelihood of regurgitation is decreased.

Glycopyrrolate blocks vagal reflexes during induction of anesthesia and intubation.

Tranquilizers

Tranquilizers commonly used by veterinarians include the phenothiazines, butyrophenones, and benzodiazepines. Their primary use is to relieve anxiety. In addition they may be used to quiet a patient for physical examination or transport; prevent animals from licking wounds or chewing bandages and splints; and as an antiemetic (e.g., prevention of car sickness).

When used as a preanesthetic, tranquilizers can be administered intravenously, intramuscularly, or orally. Response to oral administration is slow and unpredictable. Intravenous injection should precede induction of anesthesia by at least 15 to 30 minutes. This permits the full onset of action prior to induction of anesthesia.

Following phenothiazine-induced tranquilization, the animal relaxes and hangs its head; the ears may droop. Some animals may lie down, the eyes may appear glazed, and the membrana nictitans often protrudes. In cattle and horses, the penis relaxes and protrudes from the sheath. Occasionally, acute toxic reactions occur, particularly in horses. Among these are extreme depression, hypotension, tremors, dyspnea, muscle spasticity, hyperirritability, convulsions, ataxia, and death. Occasionally an animal may become aggressive or may show other evidence of central nervous stimulation.

Phenothiazine tranquilizers may potentiate the toxicity of organophosphates and the activity of procaine hydrochloride. These tranquilizers cause a decrease in arterial blood pressure as a result of depression of vasomotor reflexes mediated by the hypothalamus or brain stem, peripheral alpha-adrenergic blockade, a direct relaxing effect on vascular smooth muscle, and direct cardiac depression. Aggressive intravenous fluid therapy with a balanced electrolyte solution is the primary treatment of phenothiazine-induced hypotension. Epinephrine is contraindicated. Norepinephrine, phenylephrine, and ephedrine are indicated because they have minimal beta$_2$ activity, acting primarily at alpha$_1$-receptor sites. Accidental intra-carotid artery injection of a phenothiazine will most often result in convulsions, which can be controlled with guaifenesin and a barbiturate or diazepam given to effect. However, cerebral tissue necrosis and death may occur in spite of treatment. Phenothiazines induce hypothermia by affecting the hypothalamus and decrease the seizure threshold. In stallions, persistent or permanent penile paralysis may occur.

When a tranquilizer is given as a preanesthetic, induction of anesthesia is easier, the dose of anesthetics required is decreased, the incidence of vomiting is decreased, and recovery from anesthesia is usually smoother and free from struggling and vocalization. Further, phenothiazines decrease the incidence of epinephrine-induced dysrhythmias.

Most phenothiazine derivatives—including chlorpromazine hydrochloride (Thorazine), promazine hydrochloride (Sparine), propiopromazine (Tranvet), piperacetazine (Psymod), and Ethyl Isobutrazine (Diquel)—are used infrequently in veterinary medicine today. For a more complete review of their pharmacology and clinical use in veterinary medicine, see the second edition of this book. Acepromazine maleate continues to be widely used.

ACEPROMAZINE MALEATE

Acepromazine, a phenothiazine derivative, is a potent neuroleptic agent with relatively low toxicity. This drug is particularly valuable in dogs, horses, and cats, and has been given to a wide variety of wild animals. The recommended oral dose for dogs and cats is 1 to 3 mg/kg. The following doses are recommended for intravenous, intramuscular, or subcutaneous injection:

Dogs: 0.03 to 0.1 mg/kg, not to exceed a total dose of 3 mg
Cats: 0.03 to 0.1 mg/kg
Horses: 0.02 to 0.05 mg/kg

The LD_{50} in mice is 61.37 mg/kg intravenously, 130.5 mg/kg subcutaneously, and 256.8 mg/kg orally. Acepromazine induces tranquilization, muscle relaxation, and a decrease in spontaneous activity. At high doses, sedation occurs. Preanesthetic administration decreases the amount of general anesthetic required. Acepromazine possesses antiemetic, anticonvulsant, antispasmodic, hypotensive, and hypothermic properties.[12] Nevertheless, acepromazine lowers the convulsive seizure threshold and is contraindicated in treating selected drug-induced seizures (e.g., picrotoxin) and in epileptics. Acepromazine will prevent or decrease severity of the malignant hyperthermia syndrome in susceptible pigs exposed to halothane.[13]

In horses, acepromazine is highly protein-bound with an elimination half-life of 184.8 minutes and is detectable in plasma for up to 8 hours.[14] Penile prolapse occurs with intravenous doses of 0.01 mg/kg to 0.4 mg/kg and is dose related. Acepromazine decreases the packed cell volume and depresses respiration. Locomotor and behavioral responses are decreased.

When given in high doses (0.4 to 1.0 mg/kg) prior to epinephrine administration, acepromazine effectively prevents cardiac dysrhythmias and ventricular fibrillation in dogs during barbiturate, methoxyflurane, and halothane anesthesia.[15-17]

DROPERIDOL

Droperidol is a butyrophenone tranquilizer. In the dog, it induces quiescence with decreased motor activity and tranquilization similar to that induced by acepromazine. Tremors, muscle spasticity, and hyperirritability occur when high doses are administered intravenously (5 to 10 mg/lb). When the drug is given to hyperthermia-susceptible pigs, 20 mg/kg prolongs the reaction time to halothane.[13]

Droperidol inhibits learned responses and antagonizes the CNS-stimulating effects of amphetamine and vomiting produced by apomorphine. Like acepromazine, droperidol is an alpha-adrenergic antagonist and may prevent epinephrine-induced dysrhythmias. Droperidol potentiates the actions of barbiturates and decreases the anesthetic dose. The principal use of droperidol has been as a component of Innovar-Vet, in a mixture with fentanyl. It is especially advantageous in this mixture because of its sedative effects and antiemetic action, which is 1000 times greater than that of chlorpromazine.

DIAZEPAM (VALIUM)

Diazepam, a benzodiazepine, has calming, muscle-relaxant, and anticonvulsant effects. It is used as a preanesthetic for relief of skeletal muscle spasm and as an anticonvulsant.[18] Diazepam is indicated in animals with a history of seizure disorders. It is frequently administered prior to ketamine to prevent seizures and muscle hypertonus.

Diazepam acts on specific benzodiazepine receptor sites located on postsynaptic nerve endings located within the CNS. The greatest concentration of these receptors is located in the cerebral cortex. These receptor sites are found in decreasing density in the hypothalamus, cerebellum, midbrain, hippocampus, medulla, and spinal cord.[19] The anxiolytic and skeletal muscle relaxing effects are a result of increased availability of the inhibitory neurotransmitter glycine. This occurs at the spinal level, resulting in enhanced presynaptic activity, and at supraspinal sites, probably in the brain-stem reticular formation.[20] Diazepam enhances blockade induced by myoneural blocking agents and other central-acting muscle relaxants.[21] The effects of diazepam occur at neuronal pathways in which gamma-aminobutyric acid (GABA) is the primary neurotransmitter.[22] Sedation and anticonvulsant activity are mediated by GABA in the cerebral cortex and motor centers respectively. Pentobarbital has been shown to increase the affinity of diazepam for the benzodiazepine receptor.[23]

Diazepam rapidly passes the blood-brain and placental barriers. Ninety-six percent of the drug is protein-bound.[24] Diazepam is metabolized by demethylation and hydroxylation in people, dogs and rats to N-desmethyldiazepam, 3-hydroxydiazepam, and oxazepam. These metabolites are pharmacologically active.[20] Approximately 70% of diazepam is excreted in urine as conjugated metabolites and 10% in feces.

Diazepam solution should be injected slowly to decrease the incidence of venous thrombosis, and extreme care should be taken to avoid intraarterial administration. Although it is not recommended, diazepam has been administered intramuscularly. Clinical doses cause only minimal respiratory and cardiac depression. High intravenous doses cause a slight decrease in respiration, blood pressure, and left ventricular stroke work. An increase in heart rate and decrease in cardiac output can also occur. In horses, cardiopulmonary dynamics were unchanged with doses of 0.05 to 0.4 mg/kg IV. However, doses exceeding 0.2 mg/kg frequently produced recumbency. Smaller doses resulted in muscular fasciculations, weakness, and ataxia. Diazepam half-life values ranged from 6.94 to 21.6 hours.(25)

The toxicity of diazepam is relatively low, no acute hepatotoxic or nephrotoxic effects being apparent. In rabbits the LD_{50} for intravenous diazepam is 60 mg/kg. Overdoses should be treated with the benzodiazepine antagonist flumazenil and supportive measures including intravenous fluids and an adequate airway.(26) Hypotension may be alleviated by the use of levarterenol or metaraminol. Physostigmine (0.25 to 1.50 mg/kg IV or IP) has been reported as an antidote in rats, rabbits, and cats.(27) Glycopyrrolate may be given to decrease parasympathetic stimulation without altering the antidotal effect. Withdrawal symptoms occur in baboons after as few as 7 days of diazepam treatment.(28) Dosages commonly used in a variety of species are presented in Table 8–1.

MIDAZOLAM (VERSED)

Midazolam is a water-soluble benzodiazepine with a pH of 3.5. At pH values above 4.0 the chemical configuration of midazolam changes such that it becomes lipid soluble. While time to complete recovery is no shorter than with diazepam, it does have a shorter duration of action, with a rapid elimination half-life and total body clearance. In humans, subanesthetic doses induce sedation and heavy hypnosis. These effects are not as evident in dogs and cats. Nevertheless, low doses of midazolam are often combined with a dissociative or opioid to prevent muscle hypertonus and enhance sedation. In small animals, midazolam can be administered by either the intramuscular or intravenous route. It is most frequently given intravenously with ketamine or a thiobarbiturate to induce anesthesia. Midazolam and ketamine induce effects similar to those of either diazepam-ketamine or the proprietary mixture of tiletamine-zolazepam (Telazol). A dose of 0.1 to 0.2 mg/kg of midazolam has been recommended for induction with ketamine or a thiobarbiturate in dogs and cats.(29, 30) Midazolam is nonirritating and well absorbed following intramuscular injection. As with diazepam, midazolam can induce behavioral changes in dogs and cats. Cats may become restless and difficult to

Table 8–1. Tranquilizing Dose of Diazepam in Several Species

Species	Route	Dose mg/kg
Dog and cat	IV	0.1–0.5
	IM	0.3–1.0
Horse	IV	0.05–0.2
Cattle	IM	0.5–1.0
Sheep	IM	0.5–1.0
Pig	IM	0.5–1.0
Chicken	IM	5.0–10
Turkey	IM	5.0–10
Deer	Oral	5
Beaver	Oral	5
Porcupine	Oral	5

approach, and often pace and vocalize. Food consumption may also increase in cats after midazolam administration. In summary, midazolam is a good alternative to diazepam when used in combination with a dissociative (ketamine) or a potent opioid such as oxymorphone or fentanyl to induce or maintain short periods of anesthesia.(29)

Recently it has been reported that midazolam administration with or after erythromycin medication in people results in prolonged and enhanced sedation. Similar prolongation and intensification of midazolam's effects in veterinary patients may occur as well.(31)

FLUMAZENIL (ROMAZICON)

The CNS action of the benzodiazepines can be effectively antagonized by the administration of flumazenil. This drug has a high affinity for benzodiazepine receptors. It reverses all agonist actions of benzodiazepines. Flumazenil's action is rapid, occurring in approximately 2 to 4 minutes. Reversal is not accompanied by anxiety, tachycardia, hypertension, or other responses characterizing stress. Antagonism is achieved in dogs with a dose of 1 part flumazenil to 13 parts diazepam or midazolam.(26) The dose in people ranges from 8 to 15 μg/kg IV. The antagonistic dose of flumazenil is relatively short, lasting approximately 60 minutes. Thus, redosing may be required when attempting to antagonize a large dose of benzodiazepine.(32) Aminophylline and physostigmine have been used to reverse benzodiazepine-induced sedation in people. Aminophylline acts by antagonizing the sedative effect of adenosine accumulating in the CNS in response to benzodiazepine actions. These drugs are no longer used for this purpose, being replaced by the more specific antagonist flumazenil.

Opioids

The term *opioid* is used to refer to all exogenous and synthetic compounds that bind to specific subpopulations of opioid receptors. All these drugs induce some degree of morphinelike agonist action. Their analgesic action is not accompanied by loss of proprioception or consciousness unless excessive doses are given. The opioids are conveniently classified as agonists, agonist-antagonists, and antagonists (Table 8–2). Three sites of action appear to be involved: (a) inhibition of pain transmission in the dorsal horn, (b) inhibition of somatosensory afferents at supraspinal levels, and (c) activation of descending inhibitory pathways.(33)

Studies have led to the recognition of multiple types of opioid receptors with differing physiologic actions.(34, 35) In explaining opioid agonist effects, the most important of these have historically been those produced by sigma-, kappa-, and mu-opioid receptors.(36, 37) Receptor activity of several opioid agonists, antagonists, and agonist-antagonists on specific receptors are shown in Table 8–3. Recent speculation suggests that sigma receptors may not in fact be opioid receptors but are better classified as nonopioid or phencyclidine receptors and that delta opioid receptors

Table 8–2.   Opioid Agonists, Agonist-Antagonists and Antagonists

Agonists	Agonist-Antagonists	Antagonists
Morphine	Pentazocine	Naloxone
Meperidine	Butorphanol	Naltrexone
Fentanyl	Buprenorphine	Nalmefene
Sufentanil	Nalbuphine	
Alfentanil	Nalorphine	
Phenoperidine	Bremazocine	
Codeine	Dezocine	
Dextromethorphan		
Hydromorphone		
Oxymorphone		
Methadone		
Heroin		

play a larger role in altering nociception. Delta receptors appear to mediate antinociception and, because of their selectivity by endogenous opioid peptides, may play a minimal role in mediating the effects of exogenously administered opioids. On the other hand, some opioid drugs do bind to delta receptors, and there is evidence that mu and delta receptors form a molecular complex and interact.

While the actions mediated by the sigma receptor are not entirely understood, studies suggest that it does not mediate the psychomimetic effects produced by agonist-antagonist opioids as originally thought. The sigma receptor shows preference for dextrorotatory compounds and is not sensitive to naloxone, which is levorotatory. Because the psychomimetic effects of agonist-antagonist opioids are mediated by levorotatory enantiomers and can be antagonized by naloxone, it appears that neither sigma nor phencyclidine receptors are involved. Presumably, opioid psychomimetic effects are mediated by kappa receptors or by other, yet-unknown mechanisms.

MORPHINE SULFATE

Morphine is the prototype opioid agonist. Its major pharmacologic effect is analgesia. Morphine induces a rapid and marked increase in serotonin (5-HT) synthesis, which correlates with its analgesic effect.(38) The site of action is probably the nucleus raphe magnus-spinal system. Subarachnoid injection of morphine produces prolonged increases in the pain thresholds of rats, rabbits, cats, and primates without affecting motor function.(39) Morphine depresses the medullary respiratory, cough, and vasomotor centers, while the vomiting center is stimulated. With therapeutic doses, there is a decrease in the basal metabolic rate, resulting in a decrease in body temperature of 1 to 3° F.

Depression of the respiratory centers results in decreased respiratory minute volume and increased alveolar carbon dioxide tension. Both hypercarbia and hypocarbia appear to increase morphine concentrations

and prolong its half-life in the brain over those values found during normocarbia.(40, 41) In most species, morphine does not significantly depress the myocardium: Rate and rhythm are usually unaltered, and there is no significant effect on cardiac output. Morphine can cause histamine release, peripheral vasodilation, bradycardia, and increases in antidiuretic hormone.

Morphine directly stimulates the vomiting center. The sphincters of the gastrointestinal tract are stimulated, causing an overall action that is constipating; increased intestinal peristalsis tends to combat this effect. Dogs given large doses of parenteral morphine usually vomit and defecate soon after its administration.

The reflex centers of the spinal cord are stimulated. Therefore, morphine is contraindicated in strychnine poisoning.(43) Morphine produces an irregular effect on the brain depending upon the species in which it is administered. Because of this, the use of morphine as a preanesthetic agent is confined almost entirely to the dog. The response is variable even within a species. Excitement can occur in the cat, horse, and mouse, and is dose related. In the cat morphine at a dose of 0.1 mg/kg given subcutaneously causes no excitement and analgesia lasts for over 4 hours (44), whereas at 1.0 mg/kg, mydriasis, salivation, and anxiety are evident (Chapter 4).

Table 8–3.   Summary of Receptor Activity of Prototypical Agonists, Antagonists, and Agonist-Antagonists at Hypothetical Opioid Receptor Subtypes

	Mu	Kappa	Phencyclidine or Sigma
Morphine	Ag	Ag	Ag?
*Naloxone	Ant	Ant	—
Nalbuphine	pAg	pAg	—
Pentazocine	Ant	Ag	Ag?
Nalorphine	Ant	pAg	Ag?
Butorphanol	pAg?	pAg	—
Buprenorphine	pAg	Ant?	—
Dezocine	pAg	pAg?	—
Phencyclidine	—	—	Ag

The mu_1- and mu_2- receptors are thought to mediate supraspinal analgesia, respiratory depression, euphoria, and physical dependence; the kappa receptor: spinal analgesia, miosis, and sedation and dysphoria; the sigma receptor: psychomimetic activity, hallucinations, and respiratory and vasomotor stimulation, whereas the delta receptor primarily modifies mu receptor activity.

Ag, agonist; Ant, competitive antagonist; pAg, partial agonist, the absence of an entry means that the compound has not yet been fully studied; −, no significant action.

*Naloxone antagonizes the effects of mu and kappa agonists but not sigma agonists and is thought to have the highest affinity for the mu receptor.

(Modified from Jaffee, J. H. and Martin, W. R. Opioid Analgesics and Antagonists. In: Gilman A.G., Goodman L.G., Gilman A. The Pharmacological Basis of Therapeutics, 6th ed. New York: Macmillan, 1980.

Use of morphine in horses is limited because it produces excitement that can be dangerous to the animal and its handlers. In ponies, morphine (0.66 mg/kg IM) produces good analgesia for superficial pain (2 hours) but has only a slight effect on visceral pain. In horses morphine increases heart rate and systolic, diastolic, and mean blood pressures. Central venous pressure is increased slightly. Cardiac dysrhythmias are not evident. Significant increases in respiratory rate are also evident. Shivering or tremors and restlessness are produced, which may be due to dopamine release.(45) Morphine (0.75 mg/kg) and xylazine (1.2 mg/kg) administered intravenously to horses produces restraint and analgesia considered to be superior to that of xylazine alone. However, sweating, tremors, and cutaneous wheals have been observed following morphine administration.(46)

In most species, morphine is metabolized by the liver to morphine 3–0-glucuronide, which is eliminated in the urine. Morphine stimulates secretion of antidiuretic hormone, with urine production being decreased by as much as 90%. Thus, morphine may be contraindicated in uremic patients.

Historically morphine has been used as a preanesthetic in combination with atropine in dogs. Morphine is a relatively inexpensive opioid preanesthetic. Low doses of morphine (0.1-0.2 mg/kg) can be combined with low doses of xylazine (0.1-0.2 mg/kg) and an anticholinergic administered intramuscularly as a preanesthetic mixture in healthy dogs.

Morphine has been used as the sole analgesic and narcotic agent for cesarean section in the bitch. When it is used for this purpose at a dose of 8.8 mg/kg, maternal and fetal respiration are depressed. The bitch is often ataxic for a long period (18 hours) and may not care for the puppies. When this technique is used, an opioid antagonist is required to speed recovery of the mother and puppies. The use of high doses of morphine to produce profound sedation in dogs is no longer commonly practiced.

MEPERIDINE HYDROCHLORIDE (DEMEROL, PETHIDINE)

The analgesic effect of meperidine is one tenth that of morphine, and it is rapidly excreted. It has a spasmolytic effect similar to atropine and reduces salivary and respiratory secretions. When meperidine is used as a preanesthetic, it decreases the amount of general anesthetic needed and decreases intra- and postoperative pain. It does not cause vomiting and defecation in most patients. Rapid intravenous injection can cause histamine release, hypotension excitement, and convulsions, and is not recommended The preanesthetic subcutaneous dose of meperidine in the dog is 5 to 10 mg/kg. Meperidine should be given 30 minutes prior to induction of anesthesia. The sedative-analgesic actions of meperidine can be reversed by any narcotic antagonists.

In the cat, the effective subcutaneous dose of meperidine is 5 to 10 mg/kg.(47) Cats so treated are tractable and easier to handle, although sedation is not marked.

When 11 mg/kg was given intramuscularly, the onset of analgesia occurred in 30 minutes and lasted approximately 2 hours.(44) The preanesthetic dose of meperidine in the horse is 1.0 to 4.0 mg/kg. Although it does not have a marked sedative effect, its analgesic and spasmolytic actions may be helpful in horses suffering from colic.

METHADONE HYDROCHLORIDE (METHADONE, DOLOPHINE)

Methadone hydrochloride is a synthetic opioid unrelated to morphine. It is active orally and parenterally. Any opioid antagonist will reverse its action. Both clinical and experimental studies indicate that methadone stimulates respiration rate. In dogs, intravenous methadone induces relaxation with partial to complete loss of postural control, generalized depression, copious salivation, and frequently defecation.(48) Analgesia lasts 2 to 6 hours. Even though depressed, the dog will respond to high-pitched noises. The dose of methadone for dogs is 1 mg/kg intravenously or subcutaneously half an hour before induction of anesthesia. Methadone decreases the barbiturate induction dose by approximately one half. When given at a dose of 1 to 1.5 mg/kg, methadone alone will provide sufficient analgesia and restraint for many minor surgeries.

OXYMORPHONE HYDROCHLORIDE (NUMORPHAN)

Oxymorphone hydrochloride is a semisynthetic opioid with a potency approximately 10 times that of morphine.(49) In dogs, oxymorphone appears to induce more sedation and less hypnosis than morphine.(50) Respiratory depression is not marked, and there is little depression of the cough reflex. The anesthetic dose of barbiturates is decreased by one third to two thirds. When combined with a tranquilizer (e.g., acepromazine), neuroleptanalgesia can be induced. The exact degree of sedation and analgesia depends upon the tranquilizer and dose of the two drugs. When combined with 0.1 to 0.2 mg/kg of acepromazine, oxymorphone (0.20 mg/kg) is a safe induction agent in both dogs and cats. When arousal is desired, an opioid antagonist can be administered. The reversal dose of naloxone is 0.4 mg/1.5 mg of oxymorphone and can be given by any parenteral route.

Oxymorphone can be administered intravenously intraoperatively, or epidurally to enhance analgesia during surgery and the postoperative period. A dose of 0.1 mg/kg of oxymorphone or morphine added to 0.22 mL/kg (1 mL/10 lb) sterile isotonic saline injected into the epidural space can provide several hours of analgesia following caudal invasive orthopedic and soft tissue procedures. Advantages of opioid epidural administration include lack of motor nerve blockade, minimal dose requirement, and fewer side effects. Opioids have also been administered in combination with local anesthetics to provide spinal analgesia of several hours' duration.

FENTANYL CITRATE (SUBLIMAZE)

Fentanyl is approximately 250 times more potent than morphine. Its onset of action is rapid following intravenous or intramuscular injection, with analgesia, sedation, ataxia, respiratory depression and exaggerated response to loud noises developing in 3 to 8 minutes. It has a short duration of action, with the peak effect lasting less than 30 minutes. The actions of fentanyl can be reversed by an opioid antagonist.

The respiratory effects range from depression with occasional apnea to panting. Peak respiratory depression is usually noted 5 to 15 minutes after injection. Although fentanyl is short-acting, respiratory depression may persist for several hours after administration. Fentanyl is a highly lipophilic drug that equilibrates rapidly between plasma and CSF.(51) The concentration of fentanyl in plasma and CSF correlates closely with the intensity of respiratory depression. Repeated injections of fentanyl lead to accumulation with increased ventilatory depression. Fentanyl is a basic drug such that an increase in plasma pH shifts the equilibrium to favor the un-ionized moiety. This increases the proportion of fentanyl available for diffusion across the blood-brain barrier. Furthermore, it increases nonspecific brain tissue binding. The reverse is true with respiratory acidosis.(52)

Intravenous or intramuscular injection of fentanyl causes vagal-mediated bradycardia. Prior administration of atropine or glycopyrrolate prevents bradycardia. There is little effect upon cardiac output or blood pressure with normal clinical doses.(53) In dogs anesthetized with barbiturates, intravenous fentanyl (0.04 mg/kg) transiently decreases blood pressure. This occurs in both vagotomized and nonvagotomized dogs, indicating that hypotension is not a function of changing heart rate. Histamine release rarely occurs. Extreme care should be exercised if fentanyl is administered to animals that have already received anesthetizing doses of barbiturates. Bradycardia, hypotension, and respiratory depression may occur and may be difficult to reverse. Nevertheless, low intravenous doses of fentanyl during inhalation anesthesia to enhance analgesia has proven to be both effective and safe with proper monitoring. Fentanyl, unlike morphine, usually does not induce vomiting in dogs; however, the anal sphincter relaxes, and frequently defecation occurs.

Fentanyl has been used in ponies and horses, but has not proved to be particularly effective as an analgesic unless combined with xylazine. Fentanyl (0.055 mg/kg) and xylazine (1.1 mg/kg) in combination are significantly better than xylazine alone in obtunding visceral pain.(54) When fentanyl is used alone, a dose of 0.2 mg/kg produces recumbency in ponies but not surgical anesthesia. A dose of 0.1 mg/kg is not particularly effective in controlling superficial, deep, or visceral pain.

Fentanyl combined with droperidol is marketed as Innovar-Vet. It has been combined with fluanisone in rabbits, rats, swine, primates, dogs, mice, hamsters, and guinea pigs. It has also been used in conjunction with xylazine, metomidate, and short-acting barbiturates.(53)

CARFENTANIL CITRATE (WILDNIL)

Carfentanil, a congener of fentanyl, is approximately 10,000 times more potent than morphine and has been referred to as *superfentanyl*. Because of its potency, it can be administered by swabbing or spraying the buccal or nasal mucosa.(55, 56) It is now available in 10-mL multiple-use vials. Each mL contains 3 mg of drug. Carfentanil is a schedule II controlled substance requiring DEA registration. It has been used almost exclusively for capture of wild and feral animals. Carfentanil is approved for immobilization of free-ranging or confined members of the cervidae family. The usual dose ranges from 0.005 to 0.02 mg/kg IM. Immobilization is usually achieved in 2 to 10 minutes. The upper dose range is suggested for excited animals following extensive pursuit. Its action can be reversed by opioid antagonists, diprenorphine (M5050) probably being the most effective. In free-ranging wild animals carfentanil's potency when compared to etorphine and fentanyl is approximately 20:15:1, respectively.(57) Potent opioids should not be used unless an adequate amount of a similarly potent opioid antagonist is immediately at hand.

SUFENTANIL AND ALFENTANIL (SUFENTA AND ALFENTA)

Sufentanil is a thienyl analog of fentanyl. The analgesic potency of sufentanil is 5 to 10 times that of fentanyl, although the seizure threshold is a 160-fold greater in animals. The elimination half-life of sufentanil is 2 to 2½ hours. Sufentanil rapidly penetrates the blood-brain barrier, and rapid distribution is responsible for its termination of effects following small doses. It is extensively protein-bound in comparison to fentanyl. In people, a single dose of sufentanil induces a longer period of analgesia than does a comparable dose of fentanyl. Bradycardia may be induced, and delayed depression of ventilation has been described. Similar to fentanyl, even large doses of sufentanil induce only minimal hemodynamic effects in patients with strong left ventricular function.(58)

In dogs, sufentanil alone induces unpredictable anesthesia, bradycardia, hypoventilation, and poor muscle relaxation. However, when combined with a potent tranquilizer such as lenperone (0.44 mg/kg IV) and glycopyrrolate, sufentanil, at a dose of 5 micrograms/kg administered IV as a loading dose followed by a continuous infusion at a rate of 0.1 $\mu g \cdot kg^{-1} \cdot min^{-1}$, induces neuroleptanesthesia characterized by good muscle relaxation and good analgesia.(59) Minor muscle twitching occurs sporadically, but chest rigidity (woody chest syndrome) does not develop. Hemodynamic alterations induced by this lenperone-sufentanil combination are negligible when compared with inhalation anesthesia.

In contrast to sufentanil, alfentanil is one fifth to one tenth as potent as fentanyl, and its duration of action is one third that of fentanyl. Its onset of action, however, is much more rapid than fentanyl or sufentanil. Alfentanil and sufentanil have not been used extensively to maintain anesthesia in veterinary patients.

ETORPHINE HYDROCHLORIDE (M–99)

Etorphine hydrochloride is an oripavine derivative that has been used extensively to restrain wild animals. It is chemically related to morphine, and its purchase requires a narcotic license. When given subcutaneously, etorphine is 80 to 1000 times more potent than morphine depending upon test methodology. Etorphine should be administered intramuscularly with either a hand-held syringe or a syringe dart. There is considerable species variation in response. Among the more sensitive species are the elephant, hippopotamus, rhinoceros, tapir, bear, and primates. With medium doses, most animals remain on their feet but can be approached safely.(60) Drugs that have been used in combination with etorphine include acepromazine, scopolamine, promazine, methotrimeprazine, xylazine, and phencyclidine. In ungulates, etorphine produces tachycardia, increased blood pressure, depression of respiration and the cough center, suppression of rumen movements, analgesia, loss of reflexes without loss of consciousness, depression of body temperature, and loss of visual accommodation.

The actions of etorphine resemble those of morphine in rodents, cats, dogs, and monkeys, producing analgesia, catatonia, respiratory depression, antidiuresis, reduced gastrointestinal motility, and blockade of conditioned reflexes. In mice and rats it causes excitement; in rats, dogs, cats, and monkeys, bradycardia and hypotension occur. It does not cause excitement or vomiting in the dog.(61) Etorphine (7.5 μg/kg) combined with methotrimeprazine (6.0 mg/kg) has been used as a neuroleptanalgesic in dogs, pigs, calves, rats, guinea pigs, rabbits, and mice. In all these species, cardiac dysrhythmias and respiratory depression were greater than with equianalgesic doses of fentanyl-fluanisone.(53)

The effects of etorphine can be antagonized with nalorphine or diprenorphine. The dose of the former is in a ratio (etorphine/nalorphine) of 1:10 to 1:20, or 1:1 to 1:2 for diprenorphine.(62) Higher doses of antagonists are not advantageous and may produce protracted recovery times. The antagonist should be given intravenously. Reversal usually occurs within 10 minutes after administration, although 6 to 8 hours may be required.(63) Relapse after reversal has been reported.(64) The extreme potency of etorphine makes it dangerous to handle. Should accidental self-administration occur, death can result if the antidote is not readily available.

AGONIST-ANTAGONIST OPIOIDS

The agonist-antagonist terminology was originally applied to nalorphine and similar drugs. These drugs were believed to be mu-antagonists and kappa-agonists, and thus the hyphenated term *agonist-antagonist* was logical and descriptive; the term *nalorphinelike* was often used interchangeably with *agonist-antagonist*. The drugs most frequently classified as being nalorphinelike included nalorphine, pentazocine, nalbuphine, and butorphanol.

The terms *agonist-antagonist* and *nalorphinelike* have become somewhat vague and unsatisfactory as knowledge of opioid molecular pharmacology has grown. The classification of opioid drugs will probably continue to change as the molecular pharmacology of opioid receptors evolves. A functional definition of agonist-antagonist drugs is needed that reflects current understanding of the opioid receptor system. Perhaps a practical and broadly applicable definition of an agonist-antagonist opioid would include the following requirements:

1. agonist or partial agonist activity at one or more types of opioid receptors; and
2. the ability to antagonize the effects of a full agonist at one or more types of opioid receptors.

As described earlier, antagonist actions of an agonist-antagonist drug can result from partial agonist activity as well as true antagonist activity. Many of the agonist-antagonist drugs appear to be partial agonists at more than one type of receptor, rather than being a full agonist at one type of receptor and a complete antagonist at another.

Classification of agonist-antagonist opioids is further complicated because some of the drugs have significant pharmacologic actions that are not mediated by opioid receptors.

BUTORPHANOL TARTRATE (TORBUTROL, TORBUGESIC)

Butorphanol is a synthetic opioid analgesic that has both agonist and antagonist properties. Its analgesic potency is 3 to 5 times that of morphine. Its opioid antagonist activity is about equipotent with nalorphine, or about 50 times less potent than naloxone.(65) The dose of naloxone required to reverse butorphanol's actions is higher than that required to antagonize complete opioid agonists such as morphine because of butorphanol's greater opioid receptor affinity.

The respiratory depressant effects of butorphanol are less than those of morphine. Respiratory depression appears to reach a "ceiling" beyond which higher doses do not produce an appreciably greater depression. In rats, butorphanol given subcutaneously produces a small increase in $PaCO_2$ and a decrease in the pHa. With doses ranging from 2.5 to 10 mg/kg, no appreciable change in these parameters is evident. In anesthetized dogs, approximately equianalgesic intravenous doses of butorphanol (0.75 mg/kg) and morphine (3 mg/kg) rapidly decrease mean arterial blood pressure, but morphine produce a more marked decrease (77% vs 21% at 1 to 2 minutes after injection).(66) In anesthetized dogs, butorphanol (0.025 mg/kg) and morphine (0.1 mg/kg) have spasmogenic effects, increasing duodenal activity. The maximum effect obtained with butorphanol, however, is only about 13% that of morphine.(67) Butorphanol does not produce any significant changes in bile flow, whereas morphine produces a dose-related significant decrease. When injected intravenously (0.5 mg/kg), butorphanol produces mild sedation in dogs and no changes in blood histamine concentrations.(65) In guinea pigs and dogs, butorphanol is 115 times more effective than codeine or dextromethorphan in suppressing electrically stimulated or pathologic cough.(68) High doses of butorphanol (5 to 30 mg/kg subcutaneously) produce a dose-related diuretic response associated with decreased urinary excretion of antidiuretic hormone.(69)

The analgesic effects of intravenous and intramuscular butorphanol in horses using a colic and superficial pain model have been investigated.(45, 70) Good analgesia for visceral pain was afforded by 0.22 mg/kg IM for 4 hours, and by 0.10 mg/kg IV for 30 minutes. The optimal intravenous dose was believed to be between 0.10 and 0.20 mg/kg. Motor activity in the horses was increased. A combination of butorphanol (0.1 mg/kg IV) plus xylazine (1.1 mg/kg IV) will allow standing surgical procedures in horses for approximately 30 minutes.(71) Butorphanol (0.1 mg/kg IV) can also be combined with xylazine and ketamine to enhance analgesia in horses undergoing short surgical procedures.(72) When the drugs are combined, the analgesic effects of xylazine will wane before those of butorphanol.

In dogs, 0.1 to 0.3 mg/kg of butorphanol decreases enflurane minimum alveolar concentration (MAC) in a dose-dependent fashion. Additional doses do not result in a further reduction of MAC, indicating that an analgesic "ceiling" is also present.(73)

Distribution of butorphanol is mainly to excretory organs and highly perfused tissues, and the drug readily passes into the fetus. Butorphanol is extensively metabolized in humans, approximately 90% to hydroxybutorphanol and 10% to norbutorphanol, neither of which appears to have analgesic activity. Excretion occurs primarily in the urine (70%), with some biliary elimination (11% to 14%).

The LD_{50} of mice given butorphanol intravenously, subcutaneously, and orally is 40 to 57 mg/kg, 299 to 432 mg/kg, and 395 to 527 mg/kg, respectively. Corresponding figures for rats are 17 to 20 mg/kg, 622 to 852 mg/kg, and 570 to 756 mg/kg. In dogs, the LD_{50} following intravenous, intramuscular, or oral administration is 10 to 50 mg/kg, 17 to 29 mg/kg, and greater than 50 mg/kg respectively. The oral LD_{50} in monkeys is more than 50 mg/kg.

Butorphanol is an excellent analgesic to combine with xylazine or detomidine. For example, adult 400- to 500-kg cattle moving in the restraint chute but not necessarily in response to surgical stimulation after a paralumbar block will often stand perfectly still after receiving 8 to 10 mg of butorphanol combined with 8 to 10 mg of xylazine intravenously. In horses, dysphoria may be seen in high-strung individuals when butorphanol is given in high doses or when it is not preceded by a strong sedative (e.g., xylazine).(72, 74)

Butorphanol will antagonize the sedative effects of high doses of a complete opioid agonist (e.g., morphine or oxymorphone).(75) It is interesting that a recent report suggests that the antinociceptive effect of a combination of butorphanol and oxymorphone in cats is greater than additive.(76) These results suggest that the most appropriate method of providing postoperative analgesia while reversing sedation following oxymorphone administration in cats is to administer an appropriate dose of butorphanol rather than an opioid antagonist such as naloxone.

BUPRENORPHINE (BUPRENEX, TEMGESIC)

Buprenorphine is a partial mu-opioid agonist-antagonist derived from thebaine (Table 8–3). Its agonist properties are approximately 30 times that of morphine. Onset of action is relatively slow, requiring 20 to 30 minutes to reach full effect. Its analgesic action may last as long as 8 to 12 hours. It causes respiratory depression that can be reversed with naloxone or naltrexone. Either of these drugs will reverse buprenorphine-induced analgesia. In horses, buprenorphine is best used with a tranquilizer (acepromazine) or with an alpha$_2$-agonist. Because xylazine is much shorter in action than buprenorphine, either detomidine or acepromazine are better choices for prolonged neuroleptanalgesia. A reasonable dose of buprenorphine in the horse is 0.004 to 0.006 mg/kg IV after either xylazine (0.6-0.8 mg/kg IV) or acepromazine (0.04-0.05 mg/kg IV) administration.

In dogs and cats the dose of buprenorphine varies from (0.006-0.010 mg/kg). When administered by the intramuscular or intravenous route to provide postoperative analgesia, the drug appears to act for 6 to 8 hours. When buprenorphine is administered epidurally to provide postoperative analgesia for rear limb orthopedic procedures, the duration of analgesia may be as much as 18 to 24 hours.(77) When it is placed in the epidural space, the high lipid solubility and affinity of buprenorphine for mu receptors limit its cephalad spread and the likelihood of respiratory depression.(58)

PENTAZOCINE LACTATE (TALWIN)

Pentazocine is an opioid analgesic having agonist-antagonist properties (Table 8–3). In people it is one third as potent as morphine. Because of pentazocine's abuse potential it is a controlled substance. Pentazocine has minimal effects on the cardiovascular system and is a mild respiratory depressant. It has been found to be an effective analgesic in horses, dogs, pigs, primates, rabbits, and rats. The doses for horses are 0.5 to 3.0 mg/kg IV and 0.5 to 6.0 mg/kg IM, for pigs 2.0 mg/kg IM, and for dogs 2.0 mg/kg IM. Effects are observed within 15 minutes and last up to 2 hours.(53)

Roughly 80% of a 1 mg/kg dose of pentazocine is excreted in 24 hours in rats and monkeys. About 70% is found in urine and 10% in feces. Intramuscular doses of up to 4 mg/kg four times a day are tolerated by dogs with some sedation and loss of postural reflexes. Higher doses produce moderate salivation, tremors, and mydriasis, whereas toxic doses (20 mg/kg) cause tremors and convulsions. Monkeys and cats exhibit similar symptoms.

In horses suffering from colic, the intravenous injection of 0.55 to 4.4 mg/kg of pentazocine produces analgesia for 15 to 30 minutes. Intramuscular injections of 0.55 to 6.6 mg/kg produce dose-dependent analgesia ranging from 5 to 160 minutes. Doses greater than 4.4 mg/kg result in ataxia and muscle tremors.(78) Naloxone hydrochloride is a good antagonist for pentazocine.(79)

Alpha₂-Adrenergic Agonists

The alpha₂ adrenoceptor is a distinct subclassification of the alpha-adrenergic receptor family. These receptors and their agonists and antagonists hold promise for the anesthetist because they can mediate analgesia, anxiolysis, sedation, sympatholysis, and control of hypertension. They do not profoundly inhibit respiration and are not addictive. Selective antagonists readily reverse all of the actions produced by alpha₂-agonists. The alpha₂ adrenoceptor can be subdivided into several subtypes. Presently alpha$_{2A}$, alpha$_{2B}$, alpha$_{2C}$ and alpha$_{2D}$ have been described via differentiation by radiolabeled antagonists. Alpha$_{2A}$, alpha$_{2B}$ and alpha$_{2C}$ have been cloned in several species. Table 8–4 lists examples of alpha-adrenergic agonists under investigation for their pharmacologic actions.

MECHANISM OF ACTION WITHIN THE CNS

In mammals, a variety of functions are mediated by activation of alpha₂ adrenoceptors. They serve as prejunctional inhibitory receptors (autoreceptors) within the sympathetic nervous system (Chapter 5). They induce vascular smooth-muscle-mediated vasoconstriction and endothelial-dependent mediated vasodilation. They can be found within the GI tract, uterus, kidney, and platelets, and produce a variety of effects within these systems and tissues. Within the CNS alpha₂ adrenoceptors induce both analgesia and sedation not unlike that produced by opioid receptor activation.

There are two reasons for the similar effects of these compounds. First, the alpha₂ and opioid receptors are found in similar regions of the brain and even on some of the same neurons. These receptors share common molecular machinery beyond the receptor. Binding of either alpha₂-adrenergic or mu-opioid receptor agonists to their receptors results in the activation of the same signal transduction system (i.e., membrane-associated G proteins). These proteins induce a chain of events that open potassium channels in the neuronal membrane (i.e., the effector mechanisms). Activation of potassium channels in the postsynaptic neuron causes the cell to lose potassium, becoming more negatively charged (hyperpolarized) as positive ions move to the extracellular space. This action makes the cell unresponsive to excitatory input. The pathway is effectively severed. Consequently alpha₂-agonists and mu-opioid agonists can produce the same pharmacodynamic event because (a) the receptors, although different, may be found in the same location of the brain and even on the same neurons; (b) these receptor types are coupled to the same signal transducer; and (c) the signal transduction mechanism is linked to the same effector mechanism (i.e., the potassium channel). Hence, the functional CNS effects are quite similar between these two receptor systems and their agonists.

The CNS actions of alpha₂ adrenoceptors that may be of clinical utility include sedation, muscle relaxation or inhibition of spasticity, analgesia, anxiolysis, amelioration of opioid withdrawal, and anticonvulsant effects.

Sedation. The locus ceruleus is believed to be the major site of action for the sedative effects of alpha₂-adrenoceptor agonists (Chapter 4). In man, sedation has been the major clinical side effect of clonidine when used as an antihypertensive medication. Xylazine is a

Table 8–4. Examples of Alpha-adrenergic Agonists in Clinical Use or Under Investigation

Nonselective Alpha-Adrenoceptor Agonists	Alpha₁ Adrenoceptor Agonists	Alpha₂ Adrenoceptor Agonists
Norepinephrine	Phenylephrine	Clonidine
Epinephrine	Methoxamine	Guanfacine
	Cirazoline	Guanabenz
	(−) Dobutamine	Xylazine
		Medetomidine
		Detomidine
		Dexmedetomidine
		Romifidine
		Azepexole
		Milvazerol
		Oxymetazoline
		alpha-Methylnorepinephrine

mixed alpha$_1$/alpha$_2$-agonist but has been used for years as a sedative-analgesic in animals. Even the mixed alpha$_1$/alpha$_2$-agonist epinephrine when perfused into brain can produce sedation ranging from sleep to surgical anesthesia.

Muscle Relaxation. The muscle relaxant effects of xylazine, detomidine, and medetomidine that accompany sedation are a well-known and highly utilized property of the alpha$_2$-agonists in veterinary medicine. In man a new alpha$_2$-agonist, tizanidine, has been found to be an effective treatment for muscle spasticity resulting from stroke, cerebral trauma, and multiple sclerosis. Tizanidine has also been proven very effective in treating lower back pain.

Analgesia. Alpha$_2$-adrenoceptor agonists are as efficacious as the opioids in many circumstances and pain syndromes. They are not potent respiratory depressants, however, nor are they addictive, even though the opioids and alpha$_2$-agonists share a common transduction pathway and effector system. Systemic, epidural, and even transdermal routes have been used for administration. It should be appreciated that other compounds also operate via activation of G-protein and potassium channels. Some of the many other drugs utilizing this effector system include adenosine (A$_1$), acetylcholine (M$_2$), GABA$_B$, dopamine (D$_2$), histamine (H$_2$), serotonin (5-HT$_{1A}$), galanin, and somatostatin receptor agonists. Hence, drugs activating these receptors may also prove useful sedative-analgesics. The animal models presently undergoing scrutiny to determine the antinociceptive properties of GABA$_B$-, D$_2$-, galanin-, 5HT$_{1A}$-, H$_2$-, and A$_1$-receptor agonists have demonstrated great promise. The diversity of receptors capable of producing analgesia provides an abundance of sites for new therapeutic agents.

Anxiolysis. Multiple studies have reported the anxiolytic effects of alpha$_2$-agonists perioperatively and during opiate and nicotine withdrawal. Clonidine suppresses the noradrenergic response provoked by immobilization stress. Dexmedetomidine and clonidine have been shown to reduce anxiety associated with the elevated-maze test. These studies demonstrate that alpha$_2$-agonists can provide anxiolytic actions independent of sedation.

Opioid Withdrawal. Alpha$_2$-adrenoceptors and mu-opioid receptors are linked by the same signal transduction mechanism (G-protein) and ion channel (K$^+$) modification. Therefore, these two receptors can modulate the same CNS actions if located in the same areas of the brain. Alpha$_2$-adrenoceptors and mu-opioid receptors are both located within the locus ceruleus (LC) and the C area of the ventrolateral medulla (Chapter 4). Activation of either receptor inhibits the actions of these neurons. The C area responsible for sympathetic outflow projects to the intramedial lateral area of the spinal cord, where it synapses with the sympathetic preganglionic nerves as well as the LC. The LC contains pathways associated with vigilance and is the major site for the hypnotic action of the alpha$_2$-agonists.

During chronic activation of mu-opioid receptors, down regulation of this system occurs. During withdrawal, hyperactivity results. The alpha$_2$-adrenoceptors in this area may invoke the needed inhibitory action that is missing owing to the down regulation of the mu-opioid receptors during the time of withdrawal, giving the mu-opioid system a chance to normalize without hyperactivity.

Anticonvulsant Effects. Clonidine, guanfacine, and other alpha$_2$-adrenoceptor agonists have been tested for anticonvulsant activity. Low doses of clonidine blunt phenothiazine-induced seizures, whereas higher doses reverse any inhibitory effects. The anticonvulsant activity of clonidine is blocked by yohimbine, suggesting an alpha$_2$ mechanism. High-dose effects can be reversed by prazosin suggesting an alpha$_1$- adrenoceptor-mediated mechanism. This is consistent with clonidine's effect on alpha$_1$- and alpha$_2$-adrenoceptors. Low doses can activate alpha$_2$-adrenoceptors, whereas high doses result in alpha$_1$-adrenoceptor stimulation and excitation of the CNS. This may also explain the phenomenon of xylazine CNS stimulation observed in horses following inadvertent intracarotid injection. The "window of sedation" achievable with low doses of a mixed agonist like xylazine is lost when alpha$_1$-adrenoceptors are activated with higher CNS concentrations.

XYLAZINE HYDROCHLORIDE (ANASED, ROMPUN)

Although not identified as such at the time of its introduction into clinical practice, xylazine was the first reported alpha$_2$-agonist to be used as a sedative and analgesic by veterinarians. It was synthesized in Germany in 1962 for use as an antihypertensive but was found to have potent sedative effects in animals. Initially it was used as a sedative in cattle and other ruminants in Europe. In the early 1970s, reports of xylazine's utility as an anesthetic adjunct began appearing in American and European veterinary literature.(80-88) These reports documented the effectiveness of xylazine in eliminating muscular hypertonicity in dogs and cats given ketamine (80, 82, 83), and in producing rapid, predictable sedative, analgesic, and muscle-relaxant actions in horses and cattle following intravenous administration.(81, 84-89) It was also evident that large dose variations in how much xylazine was necessary to produce equivalent levels of sedation and analgesia existed among species. Not until 1981 were xylazine's sedative and analgesic actions definitively linked to the stimulation of central alpha$_2$ adrenoceptors.(90, 91)

Sedative and analgesic activity are related to CNS depression mediated by stimulation of alpha$_2$ receptors.(90) Muscle relaxation is caused by inhibition of intraneural transmission within the CNS. Xylazine is the most commonly administered sedative-analgesic in horses and cattle. In these species it has also proven a safe anesthetic adjunct when coadministered with ketamine to induce short periods of surgical anesthesia.

Xylazine-ketamine anesthetic regimens have been used in dogs (92, 93), cats (94), horses (95), cattle (96, 97), sheep (98, 99), goats (100), most laboratory animal species (101-104), primates (105-107), and many wild and exotic mammalian species.(108-115) Dissociative anesthetics induce minimal muscle relaxation and visceral analgesia, and often cause excitatory phenomena upon emergence.(98) When alpha$_2$-agonists are combined with ketamine, muscle relaxation and visceral analgesia are improved, and emergence is smooth. In one survey conducted over a 7-year period, the same xylazine-ketamine anesthetic combination supplemented with thiamylal was administered to over 2000 dogs with no fatalities or untoward effects encountered.(93) In recent years, butorphanol has been combined with xylazine and other more selective alpha$_2$-agonists to improve analgesia and sedation. Xylazine-butorphanol combinations are employed for sedation and analgesia in the horse, ruminants, dogs, cats, and lab animals.(116-120) Central-acting muscle relaxants such as guaifenesin and the benzodiazepines have also been combined with dissociatives and alpha$_2$-agonists to improve and prolong muscle relaxation for minor surgical procedures and for smoothing emergence.(121-127)

Xylazine is currently approved for use in dogs, cats, horses, deer, and elk in the United States. Doses for several species are listed in Table 8-5. When xylazine is used as a preanesthetic, the dose of barbiturate is decreased by one third to one half. Xylazine decreases the halothane requirement (MAC) for anesthesia by nearly 40%.(128)

Major effects develop in approximately 10 to 15 minutes after intramuscular injection, and within 3 to 5 minutes following intravenous administration. After intramuscular injection, peak plasma concentrations are reached in horses, cattle, sheep, and dogs within 12 to 14 minutes. After intravenous administration, the systemic half-life is 23 minutes for sheep, 30 minutes for dogs, 36 minutes for cattle, and 50 minutes for horses.(129) A dose-dependent sleeplike state is usually maintained for 1 to 2 hours, but the duration of analgesia is only 15 to 30 minutes.(130)

Table 8–5. Xylazine Dosages for Several Species (mg/kg)

	Intravenous	Intramuscular
Horse	0.4–1.1	1.0–2.0
Cattle	0.03–0.1	0.1–0.2
Llama	0.1–0.2	0.2–0.4
Sheep	0.025–0.1	0.1–0.3
Goat	0.05–0.1	0.1–0.3
Pig	1.0–2.0	2.0–4.0
Dog	0.25–0.5	0.5–1.0
Cat	0.25–0.5	0.5–1.0
Bird	—	5.0–10.0

Cardiopulmonary Effects. Concerns over the cardiodepressant and arrhythmogenic effects of xylazine, whether given alone or in combination with ketamine (16, 127, 131-133), have prevented some veterinarians from embracing its use. When injected intravenously as a bolus, xylazine induces bradycardia and a brief period of hypertension (5–10 minutes), followed by a longer-lasting decrease in cardiac output and blood pressure.(134) It is not uncommon for cardiac output to decrease by one third to one half and blood pressure to decrease by one quarter to one third. These effects are observed in nearly all species. Initial hypertension is caused by xylazine's action at peripheral postsynaptic adrenergic receptors, which produces vascular smooth muscle contraction and vasoconstriction. Pretreatment with a calcium channel blocker such as nifedipine results in a dampening of xylazine's initial hypertensive action.(135) Intravenous xylazine administration has also been associated with decreased splenic weight in dogs, suggesting a decrease in systemic vascular capacity.(136) Eventual reductions in blood pressure are due to decreased sympathetic tone resulting from xylazine's activation of central and presynaptic sympathetic neuronal alpha$_2$ adrenoceptors. At this time central alpha$_2$ adrenoceptor effects predominate over the earlier peripheral effects.(137) Additionally, xylazine significantly decreases heart rate by enhancing vagal tone.(138) Except in horses and large ruminants, anticholinergics are routinely recommended prior to xylazine or other alpha$_2$-agonist administration. Nevertheless, controversy over the necessity of anticholinergic administration in small animal species still exists. Pronounced acute bradycardia following intravenous xylazine can usually be prevented by the use of minimal doses and slow administration.

In contrast to the hemodynamic effects observed following intravenous injection, intramuscular administration of xylazine is not associated with as dramatic an increase in blood pressure and vascular resistance.(83, 89, 132) This decreased pressor response is likely caused by reduced peak blood concentrations of the drug. In cats, decreased heart rate and a sustained increase in blood pressure (instead of an increase followed by a decrease) have been reported following the intramuscular administration of xylazine.(127) The mechanism for a sustained hypertensive effect was not determined in this study, although the relevance of this data is questionable, since the dose used (4.4 mg/kg) was approximately four times the recommended clinical dose.(80, 94)

Xylazine-induced decreases in heart rate and cardiac output are moderated by ketamine's sympathomimetic action, while blood pressure and systemic vascular resistance are increased.(131, 139) These acute hemodynamic changes following intravenous xylazine-ketamine administration, coupled with moderate decreases in venous PO$_2$ and oxygen content, have prompted several investigators to conclude that this regimen should not be used in patients with myocardial disease or reduced cardiopulmonary reserve.(131, 139, 140)

The most commonly encountered arrhythmogenic effects of xylazine include sinoatrial block, atrioventricular block, bradycardia, first- and second-degree heart block, AV dissociation, and sinus arrhythmia.(113, 141) Several studies in dogs have assessed the ventricular arrhythmogenic actions of xylazine alone or in combination with other anesthetic agents. This is usually accomplished by measuring the amount of epinephrine required to induce premature ventricular depolarization and is commonly termed the *arrhythmogenic dose of epinephrine* (ADE).(16, 142-145) Muir et al. observed that the epinephrine fibrillation threshold (a more severe test) in thiamylal-halothane-anesthetized dogs decreased with xylazine but increased after acetylpromazine premedication.(16) In a more recent study, ketamine alone reportedly decreased the ADE more than did xylazine.(145) It is interesting that when xylazine and ketamine were combined, they were more arrhythmogenic than when either agent was given alone.(145) Extrapolation of results from ADE studies designed to assess xylazine's arrhythmogenic effects in specific anesthetic protocols (e.g., thiamylal plus halothane anesthesia in dogs) (16) to other anesthetic regimens, different doses or routes of administration, various disease states, different species with both widely varying sensitivities to the anesthetic actions of alpha$_2$-agonists and varying degrees of prevailing autonomic tone (e.g., dog vs horse), and other alpha$_2$-agonists with different receptor specificities and alpha$_2$/alpha$_1$ selectivity ratios is likely fraught with misinterpretation and should be discouraged. For example, in contrast to the numerous reports in the veterinary literature of enhanced arrhythmogenicity after xylazine administration, the selective alpha$_2$-agonist dexmedetomidine has recently been observed to have antiarrhythmogenic effects.(146) This antiarrhythmogenic action was attributed to the stimulation of central alpha$_2$ adrenoceptors, which mediate a sympatholytic action. Recent studies utilizing a saline-controlled ADE model to reduce experimental error associated with repeated epinephrine administration demonstrated no change in arrhythmogenicity after low-dose xylazine or medetomidine preanesthetic administration in halothane- and isoflurane-anesthetized dogs.(147, 148) From the results of these studies it is clear that when anesthetic catecholamine-induced arrhythmogenicity is of concern, the selection of the inhalation anesthetic (halothane vs isoflurane) is more critical in preventing myocardial sensitization than is the preanesthetic administration of an alpha$_2$-agonist.(148)

Although respiratory rate decreases with the administration of clinically recommended doses of xylazine, arterial pH, PaO$_2$, and PaCO$_2$ values remain virtually unchanged in dogs (132, 139) and cats (127), and are only minimally altered in horses (Chapter 6).(81, 87, 95)

Decreased respiration rate is accompanied by increased tidal volume to maintain alveolar ventilation.(139, 149) In horses suffering from recurrent obstructive pulmonary disease (heaves), xylazine administration may be therapeutic by decreasing pulmonary resistance while increasing dynamic compliance.(150) In contrast, when a large dose of xylazine (1.0 mg/kg IV) was given to healthy dogs, decreases in minute ventilation, physiologic dead space, oxygen transport, venous PaO$_2$ and oxygen content, and oxygen consumption were observed along with increases in the tidal volume.(139) Xylazine-induced increases in airway resistance and resonant frequency have been observed in calves.(151) In halothane-anesthetized horses (0.5 to 1.0 mg/kg IV) and sheep (0.02–0.05 mg/kg IV), xylazine administration also increased airway pressure while PaO$_2$ values decreased.(152-153) Similarly, PaO$_2$ values have been observed to decrease after xylazine administration to conscious sheep (0.05–0.3 mg/kg IV).(154-156) Investigators attributed these observations to peripherally located alpha$_2$ adrenoceptors and a perfusion-related imbalance in ventilation and pulmonary circulation (Chapter 6). Thus, although the bulk of evidence would indicate minimal detrimental effect on respiratory function in most domestic animals, caution is advised when administering xylazine or other alpha$_2$-agonists to small ruminants, when administering high singular or cumulative doses to any species, or when combining alpha$_2$-agonists with cardiorespiratory depressant anesthetics.(139)

Specific Species Effects. Sedative doses of xylazine cause heart rate and cardiac output to decrease significantly in dogs while blood pressure and peripheral vascular resistance initially increase. At doses of 1.1 mg/kg intravenously or 2.2 mg/kg intramuscularly, pHa, PaO$_2$ and PaCO$_2$ are unaffected.(132) An initial positive inotropic response after administration of a 1.1-mg/kg intravenous dose to dogs has been observed.(157)

In horses, xylazine induces maximal sedation in about 3 to 5 minutes that lasts for 30 to 40 minutes when given intravenously at a dose of 1.1 mg/kg.(88) When xylazine was compared with several opioids, it was significantly more effective in obtunding deep pain in ponies.(45, 54) Xylazine (1.1 mg/kg) combined with fentanyl (0.055 mg/kg) was significantly better for control of visceral pain than xylazine alone (2.2 mg/kg IV) or xylazine combined with meperidine or oxymorphone.(54)

The recumbent dose of xylazine for beef cows and calves is 0.11 mg/kg intravenously or 0.22 mg/kg intramuscularly. In large bulls, the dose should be decreased by one fourth to one third. When used to supplement local or regional anesthesia for standing surgery, a total dose of 5 to 10 mg given intravenously provides light sedation in adult cattle. Analgesia may be further enhanced with a total dose of 8 to 10 mg of butorphanol given intravenously.

In calves, the hemodynamic effects of sedative doses of xylazine (0.22 mg/kg IM) are characterized by a decrease in heart rate, cardiac output, arterial blood pressure, and left ventricular maximum *dp/dt*.(158) Stroke volume initially decreases and then returns within 15 minutes to baseline values. Total peripheral resistance, end-diastolic left ventricular pressure and volume, and left ventricular residual fraction increase. These changes are indicative of myocardial depression. Only small doses of xylazine are required for sedation of most ruminants when compared to other domestic species (e.g., 0.05 mg/kg in calves vs 0.5 mg/kg in horses).

Pigs are resistant to xylazine's sedative effects, requiring 20 to 30 times the low ruminant dose (Table 8–5). Because of its poor efficacy, it is seldom used alone in swine.

Other Effects of Xylazine. Xylazine has a wide margin of safety. Increasing the dose does not in general increase the degree of sedation but rather the duration of effect. Ten times the recommended dose is tolerated by dogs, cats, and horses; however, this amount results in muscle tremors, bradycardia with partial or complete atrioventricular block, and a decrease in respiratory rate. In some species movement in response to sharp auditory stimuli may also be observed.(132)

Alterations in gastrointestinal function following xylazine administration have been reported in several species. Drooling, likely due to decreased swallowing, is commonly observed in ruminants.(113) Decreased gastroesophageal sphincter pressure in dogs has been reported and may increase the likelihood of gastric reflux.(159) Subcutaneous and to a lesser degree intramuscular administration induces vomiting in both dogs and cats during the early onset of sedation. Xylazine-induced emesis has been linked to central alpha$_2$-adrenoceptor activation as yohimbine (but not cholinergic, dopaminergic, histaminergic, serotonergic, or opioid-receptor antagonists) prevents emesis.(160)

It has been reported that Xylazine prolongs gastrointestinal (GI) transit time in mice (161), dogs (162), sheep (163), bears (164), and tigers.(164) A dose-dependent increase in oesophageal transit time has also been reported in horses following detomidine administration.(165) In cattle, depression of cyclical reticuloruminal motor function can be induced with xylazine, detomidine, or clonidine administration. Ruminants may become tympanitic under xylazine's effects when unfasted. As expected, tolazoline or yohimbine (alpha$_2$-antagonists) can be used to effectively antagonize these actions.(166, 167)

In contrast to xylazine's minimal effects on small intestine function in horses, motor responses in the large bowel (cecum and colon) are inhibited by xylazine, xylazine-butorphanol, and detomidine.(168) A slow return to normal bowel myoelectric activity has been observed after xylazine-ketamine administration.(169) Relaxation of the large intestine coupled with alpha$_2$-mediated analgesia may result in the alleviation of visceral pain.(170) Indeed, xylazine has proven more efficacious than opioids or antiprostaglandins in relieving visceral pain in ponies and horses.(45, 171) In

addition to increasing the visceral pain threshold, xylazine effectively sedates and calms the painful horse. These actions have proven extremely valuable to the veterinarian wanting to restrain and control an equine patient in order to prevent self-induced trauma. However, desirable behavior modifications may be accompanied by a reduction in large bowel motility and blood flow. Reductions in gut blood flow may exceed xylazine-induced decreases in cardiac output, suggesting alpha$_2$-adrenoceptor-mediated vasoconstriction of the gut vasculature.(172) Recent reports of yohimbine's attenuation of equine endoxemia-mediated ileus and hypoperfusion provides further evidence of the important role alpha$_2$ adrenoceptors play in the homeostasis of gastrointestinal function.(173)

Emesis may occur in dogs and frequently in cats soon after xylazine is administered by either the intramuscular or the subcutaneous route. Acute abdominal distension occasionally occurs in large dogs (25 kg or greater) given xylazine intravenously or intramuscularly.(174) Abdominal distension may be caused by aerophagia or may be related to a drug-induced parasympatholytic action, causing gastrointestinal atony with accumulation of gas. This may make xylazine sedation undesirable for upper GI radiographs, because it promotes filling of the stomach with gas and makes interpretation less certain.

Increased urine output following xylazine administration has been reported in cattle (175), horses (176), ponies (177), and cats.(178) Decreases in urine specific gravity and osmolality have been observed in horses and ponies.(176, 177) Although decreased urethral closure pressure has been noted in both female and male dogs given xylazine, normal micturition reflexes are maintained.(179) Decreased urethral closure pressure has been coupled to a reduction in electromyographic activity of the urethral sphincter.(180) However, xylazine administration does not appear to alter the detrusor reflex in dogs.(181)

Transient hypoinsulinemia and hyperglycemia have been observed in several species sedated with xylazine or anesthetized with an anesthetic regimen incorporating xylazine.(182–188) The magnitude and duration of these actions appear to be dose dependent. Hyperglycemia results from inhibition of insulin secretion. Inhibition of insulin release is mediated by alpha$_2$-receptors in pancreatic beta cells.(185) It has been suggested that xylazine should be avoided in animals undergoing a glucose tolerance test.(189) Other hormonal changes induced by xylazine include transient alterations in growth hormone, testosterone, prolactin, antidiuretic hormone, and FSH levels.

Increased myometrial tone and intrauterine pressure have been observed following xylazine administration in cows.(190) In pregnant sheep, myometrial activity doubled for 60 minutes following xylazine administration, while fetal diaphragmatic activity was reduced.(191) Clinically, alpha$_2$-agonists have been administered during all stages of pregnancy in several domestic species but have not been definitively associated with an increased incidence of obstetrical complications.(113) Nevertheless, there have been anecdotal reports of premature labor or even abortion as a result of their use. The indiscriminate use of alpha$_2$-agonists in pregnant animals is not advised.

Mydriasis is commonly observed after xylazine administration. This effect is caused by central inhibition of parasympathetic tone to the iris and/or a direct sympathetic stimulation of alpha$_2$ adrenoceptors located in the iris and CNS.(192) Xylazine lowers intraocular pressure in rabbits, cats, and monkeys by suppressing sympathetic neuronal function and decreasing aqueous flow.(193) Similarly, the topical administration of the more selective alpha$_2$-agonist medetomidine readily induces mydriasis and decreases intraocular pressure (Chapter 24).(194, 195)

Untoward Reactions. Failure to achieve optimum sedation with alpha$_2$-agonists may be owing to preexisting stress, fear, excitement, or pain, as all of these conditions can increase endogenous catecholamine levels that interfere with alpha$_2$-agonist-induced reductions in excitatory neurotransmitter release. Sedation is consistently achieved when xylazine or other alpha$_2$-agonists are given to calm patients in quiet surroundings with minimal environmental stimuli. Experimental and clinical evidence indicates that analgesia is not present throughout the period of sedation. Following a sedative dose, painful procedures should be restricted to the first 10 to 15 minutes after onset of sedation. Continued painful manipulations will shorten the period of sedation and hasten recovery. Extremely apprehensive patients may prove refractory to the sedative actions of alpha$_2$-agonists and are good candidates for untoward reactions. Increasing the dose of xylazine with additional administrations in excited horses often does not improve sedation but results in unwanted side effects, including acute pulmonary hypertension and edema.(196)

Sudden deaths in horses following xylazine administration have been reported.(197, 198) Violent seizures followed by collapse may occur after inadvertent injection into the carotid artery or when an overdose is given intravenously. Presumably, the immediate seizure activity observed with xylazine intracarotid administration in horses is mediated by the activation of central alpha$_1$ adrenoceptors.(199) Cortical concentrations following an intracarotid injection or massive intravenous overdose of a mixed alpha-agonist such as xylazine may extend pharmacodynamic effects beyond the "window of sedation" typically achieved with recommended doses and lower brain concentrations mediating alpha$_2$-adrenoceptor depression. Seizurelike reactions have not been reported after inadvertent carotid arterial injection of the more selective alpha$_2$-agonists detomidine or medetomidine. Excessive CNS stimulation following inadvertent carotid artery injection in the horse can be controlled by an immediate bolus injection of a short acting barbiturate such as thiopental (1–2

gm/500 kg) or infusion of a guaifenesin-thiopental mixture.

Xylazine and other alpha$_2$-agonists should be handled with care in order to avoid accidental self-administration. If absorbed through wounds or mucous membranes serious CNS disturbance may result.

Epidural Administration. Xylazine has a significant local anesthetic effect. This effect is characterized by blockade of action potential and conducting velocity.(200) The iontophoretic application of xylazine to rat cortical neurons suppressed the spontaneous firing of 134 of 137 neurons tested.(201) This effect was not blocked by an alpha$_2$-antagonist, suggesting that the action of locally applied xylazine is caused in part by a membrane stabilizing action.(201)

When comparing xylazine and lidocaine at equal dose and volume in ponies, xylazine induces more profound and longer-lasting epidural analgesia.(202) Xylazine-induced epidural analgesia is not accompanied by the same potential for motor nerve paralysis as is that achieved by local anesthetic injection.(203) Duration of epidural analgesia in horses can be significantly lengthened by coadministering lidocaine and xylazine. The epidural administration of xylazine in horses has not been associated with changes in ECG, blood pressure, blood gases, or enhanced neurotoxicity.(204)

In cattle, epidurally administered xylazine produces a longer duration of increased avoidance threshold than does lidocaine or intramuscularly administered xylazine.(205) The cardiopulmonary depressant effects of epidural xylazine (2% solution at 0.05 mg/kg), which include bradycardia, hypotension, respiratory acidosis, hypoxemia, and ruminal hypomotility, have been reported.(206) These effects were rapidly antagonized with a 0.3-mg/kg IV dose of tolazoline, while sedation and regional analgesia were not.(206) Similar results have been reported in conscious sheep, where intrathecally applied xylazine or clonidine-produced dose-dependent analgesia of the forelimbs when measured by a mechanical pressure device.(207) In these studies, analgesia was abolished by intrathecal administration of idazoxan (an alpha$_2$-antagonist). In addition to its membrane-stabilizing effects, these results indicate that xylazine produces a portion of its analgesic action through the activation of spinal cord alpha$_2$ adrenoceptors. This mechanism of analgesic action is further substantiated by the prolongation of epidural opioid analgesia with the coadministration of selective alpha$_2$-agonists such as clonidine or medetomidine.(208)

DETOMIDINE (DORMOSEDAN)

Detomidine was developed for use as a sedative-analgesic in horses and cattle (Table 8–6). It is a weakly basic, lipophilic imidazole derivative.(209, 210) Compared to xylazine, detomidine has higher potency and greater specificity at central alpha$_2$-adrenoceptor sites.(211) Nevertheless, in very high concentrations,

Table 8-6. Dosage Ranges of Alpha$_2$ Agonists in Several Domestic Species

Domestic Species	Alpha$_2$-Agonists			
	Xylazine ($\mu g/kg$)*	Detomidine ($\mu g/kg$)*	Medetomidine (μ/kg)*	Romifidine ($\mu g/kg$)*
Cat	200–2000	NA	40–80	NA
Dog	200–2000	5–20	10–40	NA
Horse	200–2000	10–40	10–30	30–80
Cattle	20–200	10–40	20–50	NA
Pig	2000–4000	NA	30–80	NA

*Lower doses IV; higher doses IM.
NA, Not available.

detomidine, like xylazine, activates alpha$_1$-adrenoceptors.(212)

Detomidine induces cardiovascular effects similar to those observed with xylazine administration. Decreased contractility, bradycardia, and a biphasic blood pressure response are observed following intravenous injection.(213) Bradycardia may be profound with high dosages. In addition, first- and second-degree AV block commonly occur. These actions can be alleviated by anticholinergic administration or the induction of anesthesia with ketamine.(214)

With the exception of a greater early hypertensive response, detomidine (10–40 $\mu g/kg$ IV) produces cardiovascular alterations in horses nearly identical to those of xylazine (1.1 mg/kg IV).(215) Detomidine-induced sedation and analgesia, however, are of longer duration than that provided by equivalent doses of xylazine.(216, 217) For example, in a cecal balloon colic model, detomidine (20 $\mu g/kg$ IV) provided 45 minutes of analgesia and sedation, whereas the equianalgesic dose (1.1 mg/kg IV) of xylazine was effective for only 20 minutes.(218) Following an IV dose of 40 $\mu g/kg$, it is not uncommon to observe sedation for 90 to 120 minutes and relief of pain for 75 to 80 minutes. For this reason detomidine has become the analgesic of choice for relieving the symptoms of equine colic pain. This allows the veterinarian to undertake further diagnostic procedures as needed. Rarely, alpha$_2$-agonists may relieve intestinal spasm and potentially treat the cause of equine colic. Reductions in intestinal motility also introduce the risk of inducing ileus or impaction, however. It should be understood that "masking" of pain symptoms does not prevent ongoing colic-induced biochemical and tissue deterioration, which typically require aggressive medical and surgical intervention.

Detomidine is often used as a preanesthetic in horses and cattle or is combined with ketamine to induce short periods of anesthesia.(217, 219) Recent studies have also assessed the combined anesthetic actions of detomidine followed by the dissociative tiletamine and the benzodiazepine zolazepam (Telazol). This combination has proven quite effective in both ponies and horses, and incorporates an alpha$_2$-agonist with both a dissociative anesthetic and a benzodiazepine sedative.(220, 221) Although not yet

quantitated in most species, the analgesic and muscle relaxant effects of detomidine undoubtedly reduce the dose requirement of monoanesthetics. Recovery from inhalation anesthesia in horses premedicated with detomidine is usually uneventful and free from excitement phenomena. If necessary, the additional administration of low doses of detomidine (2.5-5 $\mu g/kg$) can be helpful in smoothing emergence during the recovery period. As with xylazine, increased urine output and hyperglycemia commonly result following detomidine administration.

Detomidine is commonly combined with opioids to enhance sedation and analgesia. When given alone to horses, opioids can induce excitation. This response is either greatly diminished or eliminated when opioids are preceded by alpha$_2$-agonist administration. When detomidine is combined with methadone, morphine, meperidine, or butorphanol, opioid stimulatory effects are not observed.(222) In horses, detomidine and butorphanol may be the most effective combination for enhancing sedation and analgesia while minimizing cardiopulmonary depression.(222, 223) This sedative-analgesic combination has proven to be a reliable method of achieving chemical restraint for many diagnostic (e.g., endoscopy) and minor surgical procedures (e.g., dentistry). Detomidine (10-15 $\mu g/kg$ IV) usually precedes butorphanol (20-30 $\mu g/kg$ IV) injection. The full sedative effect should be present before initiating the procedure. Heavy sedation is often accompanied by ataxia, slight tremor of the face and lips, and a tendency to head press and lean forward.

Romifidine is the newest alpha$_2$-agonist to be assessed as a sedative-analgesic in the horse (Table 8–6).(224) At a dose of 80 $\mu g/kg$, romifidine produces sedation similar to both xylazine (1 mg/kg) and detomidine (20 $\mu g/kg$). When compared with romifidine, xylazine and detomidine produce greater ataxia, and their sedative effects are of shorter duration.(224)

MEDETOMIDINE (DORMITOR)

Medetomidine is the newest alpha$_2$-agonist to be approved for veterinary use.(225) It is lipophilic, is rapidly eliminated, and possesses more potency and efficacy than other alpha$_2$-agonists. Its alpha$_2$/alpha$_1$-receptor selectivity binding ratio is 1620 compared to

260, 220, and 160 for detomidine, clonidine, and xylazine, respectively.(226)

In dogs and cats, medetomidine induces dose-dependent sedative-analgesic actions within recommended dose ranges (Table 8–6).(227) As with xylazine and detomidine, higher doses do not result in more sedation but increase the duration of effect. In dogs not premedicated with atropine, blood pressure and respiration rate are decreased in a dose-dependent manner from 10 to 60 μg/kg IM.(228) When compared with 1 MAC (1.38%) isoflurane anesthesia in dogs, a 20-μg/kg IV infusion of medetomidine resulted in less depression of the hypercapnic response curve than did isoflurane.(229) End-tidal CO_2 and $PaCO_2$ values were significantly lower in dogs given medetomidine than those anesthetized with isoflurane. Atropine or glycopyrrolate premedication prevents bradycardia but may increase the initial hypertensive actions during the onset of sedation.(227, 228) Following subcutaneous or intramuscular administration, vomiting may occur with the earliest signs of sedation.(226) Diuresis is observed even with doses as low as 10 μg/kg. Large volumes of dilute urine are produced.(230)

Medetomidine is commonly used as a preanesthetic prior to ketamine, barbiturate, or mask induction with an inhalation anesthetic.(227, 228, 231) The optimal intramuscular preanesthetic dose in dogs is between 10 and 40 μg/kg. Some dogs may not become sedate when given 10 μg/kg. Following a 40-μg/kg dose, bradycardia (atropine responsive) and profound sedation are consistently achieved.(231, 232) Preemptive anticholinergic administration may be more effective at preventing bradycardia than trying to reverse it after its occurrence.(233)

When assessing sedation and analgesia in dogs an intramuscular medetomidine dose of 30 μg/kg is equivalent to a 2.2-mg/kg dose of xylazine. Following medetomidine premedication (20-40 μg/kg IM), propofol (2 mg/kg loading dose; 165 μg · kg^{-1} · min^{-1}), etomidate (0.5 mg/kg loading dose; 50 μg · kg^{-1} · min^{-1}) or ketamine (4 mg/kg IV) provide good surgical anesthesia in dogs.(234-236) A 40-μg/kg dose of medetomidine combined with 5.0 mg/kg of ketamine produces a period of anesthetic action in dogs comparable to that achieved with 1 mg/kg of xylazine and 15 mg/kg of ketamine.(237)

It has been reported that duration of sedation in cats is dose dependent, whereas bradycardia is not.(238) In cats, as in other species, when ketamine is combined with medetomidine, the sympathomimetic properties of ketamine offset the bradycardic actions of medetomidine.(239) When compared to the simultaneous intramuscular administration of acepromazine-ketamine, xylazine-ketamine, or zolazepam-tiletamine, a medetomidine (80 μg/kg)-ketamine (5 mg/kg) regimen produced better visceral analgesia and muscle relaxation.(239)

In horses, medetomidine has a pharmacodynamic profile similar to other alpha₂-agonists but produces more ataxia and disorientation at equal sedative-analgesic doses than does either xylazine or detomidine. These observations indicate that detomidine may be the preferred alpha₂-agonist for use in horses.(240, 241)

In horses, when detomidine or medetomidine were experimentally antagonized with 10 times the agonist dose of atipamezole (a very selective alpha₂-antagonist), mydriasis and analgesia were completely abolished, whereas bradycardia and sedation were only transiently influenced.(240) In horses, atipamezole alone produces consistent dose-related changes in behavioral and autonomic variables, causing mild sedation and cardiac depression unaccompanied by analgesia. Atipamezole-induced sedation has not been reported in the dog or cat.

Medetomidine produces sedation in pigs at dosages ranging from 30 to 80 μg/kg. Higher doses do not increase the level of sedation. Nevertheless, it appears that in swine sedation and analgesia are more predictably achieved with medetomidine than can be achieved with xylazine.(242) Seemingly, variation in potency and/or efficacy among domesticated species is minimal for medetomidine when compared to the less selective alpha₂-agonists such as xylazine (Table 8–6).

In summary, medetomidine produces a reliable degree of sedation, muscle relaxation, and analgesia in a variety of domesticated species. The intramuscular dose recommendations for minor surgical interventions are 30 to 40 μg/kg in dogs and 80 to 110 μg/kg in cats.(243) At these dosages bradycardia is common and vomiting and occasional muscle jerking have been reported.(243) As a preanesthetic much lower doses are commonly used. Medetomidine-ketamine combinations have been effective in providing short periods of anesthesia and immobilization in dogs, cats, and many lab and zoo animal species.(243-248) The coadministration of an opioid or benzodiazepine with medetomidine, as with other alpha₂-agonists, appears quite useful in enhancing sedation and analgesia beyond that achieved with the singular administration of either class of drug alone.(249, 250)

Alpha₂-Adrenergic Antagonists

One of the more significant advances in veterinary anesthesiology during the last decade has been the utilization of antagonists for the reversal of injectable anesthetic regimens. Most notable in this area of investigation has been the clinical application of alpha₂-antagonists such as yohimbine, tolazoline, idazoxan, and atipamezole for reversal of the sedative-muscle relaxant actions induced by xylazine and other alpha₂-agonists (Table 8–7). Alpha₂-antagonists have become valuable tools in the anesthetic management of large domestic and wild species.

YOHIMBINE (YOBINE)

Numerous studies have demonstrated yohimbine's effectiveness in antagonizing alpha₂-agonist-induced sedation and analgesia in laboratory animals, dogs, and cats.(251, 255) Beginning in 1982, a series of studies explored the anesthetic reversal of several injectable drug combinations. Reversal was achieved by combining yohimbine with 4-aminopyridine to antagonize the sedative actions of xylazine in dogs (256) and cattle (257), the complete immobility produced by xylazine-atropine in dogs (258), ketamine anesthesia in cats (259), acepromazine-xylazine sedation in dogs (260), xylazine-ketamine anesthesia in horses (261), the combined anesthetic actions of xylazine-pentobarbital in dogs (262), and the combined anesthetic actions of xylazine-pentobarbital in cats.(263) Emergence from sedation and anesthesia was rapid and permanent in each of these species for each of the anesthetic regimens antagonized. These two drugs were combined because 4-aminopyridine releases acetylcholine and other neurotransmitters from CNS presynaptic nerve endings (264-266) whereas yohimbine antagonizes alpha$_2$-adrenoceptor-mediated depression and enhances the release of norepinephrine and other excitatory neurotransmitters. It was concluded that of the numerous anesthetic regimens assessed for reversal with yohimbine and 4-aminopyridine, the combinations incorporating xylazine, whether combined with ketamine, barbiturates, opioids, or other tranquilizers, resulted in the most reliable, safe, and sustained reversal of sedation and/or anesthesia. In many studies and species, yohimbine alone has also proven effective in antagonizing the sedative-immobilizing actions of anesthetic regimens incorporating xylazine (Table 8–7).(267-281)

TOLAZOLINE (PRISCOLINE)

Tolazoline, idazoxan, and atipamezole have also been used in a number of species to reverse xylazine sedation or partially reverse the depressant effects achieved with anesthetic combinations incorporating alpha$_2$-agonists.(269, 282-300) The effectiveness of the less selective alpha$_2$-antagonists in reversing alpha$_2$-mediated CNS depression does not extend to other classes of anesthetic adjuncts. For example, tolazoline was shown to have no effect on anesthesia induced by tiletamine and zolazepam.(301) Tolazoline possesses the least specificity for alpha$_2$ adrenoceptors of all the alpha$_2$-antagonists commonly used by veterinarians. It induces potent H$_2$-receptor-agonist actions and has been associated with gastrointestinal bleeding following chronic administration in man. Tolazoline has also been implicated in production of abdominal pain, nausea, diarrhea, and exacerbation of peptic ulcer.(302)

ATIPAMEZOLE (ANTISEDAN)

The alpha$_2$/alpha$_1$ selectivity ratio of atipamezole is 200 to 300 times higher than either idazoxan or yohimbine.(296) Atipamezole's specificity for alpha$_2$ adrenoceptors is superior to other clinically available compounds and is devoid of activity at beta, histaminergic, serotonergic, muscarinic, dopaminergic, GABAergic, opioid, and benzodiazepine receptors.(296) The dosage recommendations for atipamezole varies among species and for various alpha$_2$-agonists.(303-306) For instance, a 30-μg/kg dose of atipamezole is effective in reversing a

Table 8–7. Dosage Ranges of Alpha$_2$-Antagonists in Several Domestic Species

Domestic Species and Alpha$_2$-Agonist	Alpha$_2$-Antagonists			
	Yohimbine (μg/kg)	Tolazoline (μg/kg)	Idazoxan (μg/kg)	Atipamezole (μg/kg)
Cat				
Xylazine	100–200	2000	NA	200
Medetomidine	500	NA	NA	200–400 (2–4× M dose)
Dog				
Xylazine	100–150	500–1000	NA	200
Medetomidine	NA	NA	NA	160–240 (4–6× M dose)
Horse				
Xylazine	75–150	4000	NA	150 μg (ponies)
Detomidine	NA	NA	NA	200–400 (10× D dose)
Cattle				
Xylazine	100–200	2000–3000	30–100	10–30 (1/10 the X dose)
Detomidine or Medetomidine	NA	400–1000	30–100	100–200 (5× the M dose)
Pig				
Xylazine	50	2000	NA	NA
Detomidine	NA	NA	NA	NA

NA, Not available; M, Medetomidine; D, Detomidine.

0.3-mg/kg dose of xylazine in calves, (303) whereas four to six times (160 to 240 µg/kg) the medetomidine dose (40 µg/kg) is apparently required for reversal in dogs (Table 8–7).(304)

Administration of an alpha$_2$-antagonist for the reversal of sedation is not completely without risk. Some animals have died following the rapid intravenous administration of high doses of yohimbine and tolazoline.(269) Severe hypotension and tachycardia can occur following rapid intravenous injection. These undesirable effects can be prevented by slow administration to achieve the desired arousal. Overall, the incidence of unfavorable reactions to alpha$_2$-antagonist administration for reversal of alpha$_2$-agonist-mediated CNS depression is extremely rare when the antagonist is appropriately administered. It can be anticipated that the use of more selective and specific alpha$_2$-antagonists will further lessen the likelihood of inducing untoward reactions.

Many questions remain to be answered before the clinical utility of alpha$_2$-antagonists in veterinary practice is fully realized. Are there species differences in the undesirable responses elicited by specific alpha$_2$-antagonist? It is well documented that ruminants are 20 to 30 times more sensitive to xylazine's depressant actions than swine. What are the implications of variation in species sensitivity to alpha$_2$-agonists with regard to the pharmacokinetic and pharmacodynamic profiles of each alpha$_2$-antagonist? In cattle, tolazoline is reported to be more effective than yohimbine in reversing xylazine's CNS actions.(269) Does tolazoline with less specificity and selectivity for alpha$_2$-adrenoceptors have a more desirable pharmacodynamic profile for antagonism of mixed alpha-agonists (e.g., xylazine)? Our collective clinical experiences indicate this is likely in some species (e.g., ruminants).

SUMMARY

Physiologic alterations induced by xylazine and the more selective alpha$_2$-agonists in any species depend on dose, rate, and route of administration, and are variously influenced by the concomitant administration of other classes of drugs. When these factors are appropriately considered, alpha$_2$-agonists have proven to be safe adjunctive agents in augmenting CNS depression, analgesia, and muscle relaxation in healthy patients. In general, the lowest possible dose necessary to achieve the desired depth and duration of effect for a given procedure should be used. The wisdom of many veterinary anesthesiologists indicates that the best utilization of alpha$_2$-agonists is in low doses as preanesthetics in small and large animal practice, and as adjuncts with opioids or monoanesthetics to induce either a profound sedative-analgesic state or to enhance general anesthesia while reducing anesthetic requirement.

In the veterinarian's experience opioids and benzodiazepines do not produce reliable sedation and analgesia in all species or individuals, whereas alpha$_2$-agonists induce more reliable dose-dependent sedative-analgesic actions. Recently, the coadministration of low doses of alpha$_2$-, opioid, and benzodiazepine agonists has focused attention on the activation of separate CNS receptor populations that result in a synergistic anesthetic response with minimal unwanted side effects.(307, 308) Coupled with the fact that each of these classes of drugs can be reversed with selective antagonists (e.g., atipamezole, naloxone, flumazenil), a new era of achieving anesthesia by the activation of different populations of CNS receptors that in turn can be modified or completely antagonized with one or more receptor antagonists may be at hand.(118, 309, 310) In veterinary anesthesia it appears that alpha$_2$-agonists with their excellent spectrum of anesthetic properties will play an important role in the evolution and development of reliable synergistic receptor-mediated analgesia and anesthesia.

Tranquilizer-Opioid Combinations

FENTANYL CITRATE-DROPERIDOL (INNOVAR-VET)

Innovar-Vet, a combination of fentanyl citrate and droperidol, is used to produce neuroleptanalgesia in dogs. This is a state of sedation with analgesia sufficient for minor surgery. Each milliliter of Innovar-Vet contains 0.4 mg of fentanyl and 20 mg of droperidol. Because it contains fentanyl, it is a controlled substance and records must be kept of its use.

This drug combination induces an intense analgesic action of relatively short duration. Droperidol has a long duration of action that extends beyond the analgesic effects of fentanyl.(311) In dogs, this mixture produces sedation, analgesia, immobilization, respiratory depression and/or panting, alpha-adrenergic blockade, a decrease in blood pressure, and bradycardia. Vomiting is seldom observed, although defecation frequently occurs. Innovar-Vet has wide application for use in painful procedures in dogs. Advantages are ease of administration, wide margin of safety, quiet recovery, and partial reversibility with opioid antagonists. Because the mixture potentiates general anesthetics, the dosage of barbiturates should be decreased by one third to one half. When used as a preanesthetic agent, the recommended dosage is 1 mL/7 to 10 kg intramuscularly or 1 mL/12 to 30 kg intravenously, followed in 10 minutes by induction. With this method, induction of anesthesia is smooth and recovery occurs without excitement. Occasionally, the desired degree of depression is not produced by a standard dose of Innovar-Vet. Aggressiveness during the recovery period and other changes in disposition have been noted in some dogs. A prolonged effect, lasting for several days, has been observed with large doses. Other undesirable effects include defecation, salivation, and bradycardia (which may be prevented by pretreatment with atropine), respiratory depression or panting, and spontaneous movements in response to auditory stimuli. Overdosing produces a high incidence of spontaneous movements or even clonic convulsions with extensor rigidity.

Use of an opioid antagonist results in immediate reversal of the effects of fentanyl, including analgesia. Reversal may be used upon completion of the procedure to hasten arousal. A mixture of 4-aminopyridine (0.5 mg/kg) and naloxone hydrochloride (0.04 mg/kg), administered intravenously, markedly antagonizes the CNS effects of 1 mL/9 kg of droperidol-fentanyl.(312)

Innovar-Vet causes central nervous stimulation in cattle, sheep, cats, and horses and thus is not used in these species. Innovar-Vet has been used in pigs to induce mild sedation and in combination with ketamine to induce anesthesia (Chapter 20).

ETORPHINE-ACEPROMAZINE (IMMOBILON LA) AND ETORPHINE-METHOTRIMEPERAZINE (IMMOBILON SA)

Etorphine has been combined with acepromazine for use in large animals and with methotrimeprazine for small animals. The large animal preparation contains 2.45 mg of etorphine and 10.0 mg of acepromazine/mL. The small animal preparation contains 0.074 mg of etorphine and 18.0 mg of methotrimeprazine/mL. Unfortunately, both preparations have been termed *Immobilon*, thus creating confusion. The large animal preparation is used in horses and in wild and zoo animals.

Etorphine-acepromazine has been used to immobilize horses briefly for surgery (e.g., castration). When the drug is given intravenously, recumbency occurs quickly. When it is given intramuscularly, excitement may occur prior to recumbency. Care should be exercised to prevent injury as the horse goes down. Muscular tremors, rigidity, sweating, mydriasis, reduction in intestinal peristalsis, and respiratory depression may also occur. Initially, the heart rate and blood pressure increase; the latter subsequently decreases as a result of the alpha-adrenergic blocking action of acepromazine.(313) Priapism may occur in horses.(314)

Diprenorphine is the recommended antagonist of etorphine. Horses may sometimes become restless and excited 6 to 8 hours following etorphine reversal; in donkeys this may occur within 2 to 3 hours.(315) The dose of diprenorphine for all species is 0.272 mg/kg IV by slow injection. Etorphine-methotrimeprazine has not been widely accepted. In dogs, it produces neuroleptanalgesia and hyperglycemia. It must not be used in cats.

Naloxone (0.6 to 0.8 mg/kg) reverses etorphine's respiratory and cardiovascular depressing effects, but the duration of action of naloxone is short and renarcotization tends to occur within 10 to 15 minutes.(316) Therefore, diprenorphine is recommended for reversal of etorphine-containing mixtures rather than naloxone.

References

1. Atkinson RS, Rusman GB, Lee JA. A synopsis of anaesthesia, 8th ed. Chicago: Year Book, 1977.
2. Gilman AG, Rall TW, Nies AS, Taylor P. The pharmacological basis of therapeutics, 8th ed. New York: Permagon Press, 1990.
3. Gelatt KN, Peiffer RL Jr, Erickson JL, Gum GG. Evaluation of tear formation in the dog, using a modification of the Schirmer Tear Test. J Am Vet Med Assoc 166:368, 1975.
4. Ludders JW, Heavner JE. Effect of atropine on tear formation in anesthetized dogs. J Am Vet Med Assoc 175:585, 1979.
5. Adriani J. Appraisal of current concepts in anesthesiology. Vol. 2. St. Louis: CV Mosby, 1964.
6. Hatch RC. Restraint, preanesthetic medication, and postanesthetic medication of dogs with chlorpromazine and atropine. J Am Vet Med Assoc 150:27, 1967.
7. Klide AM, Rives C, Peters J. Effect of atropine sulfate on thiopental-induced sleeping time in the dog. J Am Vet Med Assoc 35:1029, 1974.
8. Muir WW. Effects of atropine on cardiac rates and rhythm in dogs. J Am Vet Med Assoc 172:917, 1978.
9. Ducharme NG, Fubini SL. Gastrointestinal complications associated with the use of atropine in horses. J Am Vet Med Assoc 182:229, 1983.
10. Godeaux J, Tonnesen M. Investigations into atropine metabolism in the animal organism. Acta Pharmacol Toxicol 5:95, 1949.
11. Stormont C, Suzuki Y. Atropinesterase and cocainesterase of rabbit sterum: localization of the enzyme activity in isozymes. Science 167:200, 1970.
12. Pugh DM. Acepromazine in veterinary use. Vet Rec 76:439, 1964.
13. McGrath CJ, Rempel WE, Addis PB, Crimi AJ. Prophylactic use of major tranquilizers in prevention of malignant hyperthermia in swine. Vet Anesth 8:28, 1980.
14. Ballard S, Shults T, Kownacki AA, Blake JW, Tobin T. The pharmacokinetics, pharmacological responses and behavioral effects of acepromazine in the horse. J Vet Pharmacol Therap 5:21, 1982.
15. Wiersig DO, Davis RH Jr, Szabuniewicz M. Prevention of induced ventricular fibrillation in dogs anesthetized with ultrashort acting barbiturates and halothan. J Am Vet Med Assoc 165:341, 1974.
16. Muir WW, Werner LL, Hamlin RL. Effects of xylazine and acetylpromazine upon induced ventricular fibrillation in dogs anesthetized with thiamylal and halothane. Am J Vet Res 36:1299, 1975.
17. Szabuniewicz M, Davis RH Jr, Wiersig DO. Prevention of methoxyflurane and thiobarbiturate cardiac sensitization of catecholamines in dogs. Pract Vet 47:12, 1975.
18. Wauquier A, Ashton D, Melis W. Behavioral analysis of amygdaloid kindling in beagle dogs and the effects of clonazepam, diazepam, phenobarbital, diphenylhydantoin, and flunarizine on seizure manifestation. Exp Neurol 64:579, 1979.
19. Mohler H, Okada T. Benzodiazepine receptor: demonstration in the central nervous system. Science 198:849, 1977.
20. Schallek W, Schlosser W, Randall LO. Recent developments in the pharmacology of the benzodiazepines. Adv Pharmacol Chemother 10:119, 1972.
21. Dretchen K, Ghoneim MM, Long JP. The interaction of diazepam with myoneural blocking agents. Anesthesiology 34:463, 1971.
22. Costa E, Giudotti A. Molecular mechanisms in the receptor action of benzodiazepines. Ann Rev Pharmacol Toxicol 19:531, 1979.
23. Skolnick P, Moncada V, Barker JL, Paul SM. Pentobarbital: dual actions to increase brain benzodiazepine receptor affinity. Science 211:1448, 1981.
24. van der Kleijn E, van Rossum JM, Muskens ETJM, Rijntjes NVM. Pharmacokinetics of diazepam in dogs, mice and humans. Acta Pharmacol Toxicol 29:109, 1971.
25. Muir WW, Sams RA, Huffman RH, Noonan JS. Pharmacodynamic and pharmacokinetic properties of diazepam in horses. Am J Vet Res 43:1756, 1982.
26. Tranquilli WJ, Lemke K, Williams LL, Ballard G, Ko JCH, Benson GJ, Thurmon JC. Flumazenil efficacy in reversing diazepam or midazolam overdose in dogs. J Vet Anaesthesia 19:65–68, 1992.
27. Nagy J, Decsi L. Further studies on the site of action of diazepam: anticonvulsant effect in the rabbit. Neuropharmacology 18:39, 1979.

28. Lukas SE, Griffiths RR. Precipitated withdrawal by a benzodiazepine receptor antagonist (Ro 15-1788) after 7 days of diazepam. Science 217:1161, 1982.
29. Ilkiw JE. Other potentially useful new injectable anesthetics agents. In: Haskins SC, Klide AM, eds. Veterinary Clinics of North America: Small Animal Practice, Opinions in Small Animal Anesthesia. Philadelphia: WB Saunders, 1992:281–289.
30. Tranquilli WJ, Graning LM, Thurmon JC, et al. Effect of midazolam preanesthetic administration on thiamylal induction requirements in dogs. Am J Vet Res 52(5):662–664, 1991.
31. Olkkola KT, Aranko K, Luurila K, et al. A potential hazard between erythromycin and midazolam. Clin Pharmacol Ther 53:298–305, 1993.
32. Amend F, Ghouri MD, Manuel A, et al. Effects of flumazenil on recovery after midazolam and propofol sedation. Anesthesiology 8(2):333–339, 1994.
33. Pert A. Neuropharmacology of analgesics. Surg Pract News 10:10, 1981.
34. Chang K-J, Cooper BR, Hazum E, Cuatrecasas P. Multiple opiate receptors: different regional distribution in the brain and differential binding of opiates and opioid peptides. Mol Pharmacol 16:91, 1979.
35. Pasternak GW, Childes SR, Snyder SH. Opiate analgesia: evidence for mediation by a subpopulation of opiate receptors. Science 208:314, 1980.
36. Martin WR, Eades CG, Thompson JA, Huppler RE, Gilbert PE. The effects of morphine and nalorphine-like drugs in the nondependent and morphine-dependent chronic spinal dog. J Pharmacol Exp Ther 197:517, 1976.
37. Gilbert PE, Martin WR. The effects of morphine and nalorphine-like drugs in the nondependent, morphine-dependent and cyclazocine-dependent chronic spinal dog. J Pharmacol Exp Ther 198:66, 1976.
38. Godefroy F, Weil-Fugazza J, Coudert D, Besson JM. Effect of acute administration of morphine on newly synthesized 5-hydroxytryptamine in spinal cord of the rat. Brain Res 199:415, 1980.
39. Yaksh TL, Wilson PR., Kaiko RF, Inturrisi CE. Analgesia produced by a spinal action of morphine and effects upon parturition in the rat. Anesthesiology 51:386, 1979.
40. Finck AD, Berkowitz BA, Hempstead BS, Ngai SH. Pharmacokinetics of morphine: effects of hypercarbia on serum and brain morphine concentrations in the dog. Anesthesiology 47:407, 1977.
41. Nishitateno K, Ngai SH, Finck AD, Berkowitz BA. Pharmacokinetics of morphine: concentrations in the serum and brain of the dog during hyperventilation. Anesthesiology 50:520, 1979.
42. Bidwai AV, Stanley TH, Bloomer HA, Blatnik RA. Effects of anesthetic doses of morphine on renal function in the dog. Anesth Analg 54:357, 1975.
43. Jones LM. Veterinary pharmacology and therapeutics, 2nd ed. Ames, IA: Iowa State College Press, 1957.
44. Davis LE, Donnelly EJ. Analgesic drugs in the cat. J Am Vet Med Assoc 153:1161, 1968.
45. Kalpravidh M, Lumb WV, Wright M, Heath RB. Effects of butorphanol, flunixin, levorphanol, morphine and xylazine in ponies. Am J Vet Res 45:217, 1984.
46. Klein LV, Baetjer C. Preliminary report: xylazine and morphine sedation in horses. Vet Anesth 3:2, 1974.
47. Booth NH, Rankin AD. Evaluation of meperidine hydrochloride in the cat. Vet Med 49:249, 1954.
48. Burroughs HE. Methadone narcosis in dogs. J Small Anim Med 1:301, 1953.
49. Eddy NB, Lee LE Jr. The analgesic equivalence to morphine and relative side action liability of oxymorphine (14-hydroxydihydromorphinone). J Pharm Exp Ther 125:116, 1959.
50. Nytch TF. Clinical observations on the preanesthetic use of oxymorphone and its antagonist, N-allyl-noroxymorphone, in dogs. J Am Vet Med Assoc 145:127, 1964.
51. Hug CC, Murphy MR. Fentanyl disposition in cerebrospinal fluid and plasma and its relationship to ventilatory depression in the dog. Anesthesiology 50:342, 1979.
52. Ainslie SG, Eisele JH Jr, Corkill G. Fentanyl concentrations in brain and serum during respiratory acid-base changes in the dog. Anesthesiology 51:293, 1979.
53. Green CJ. Animal anaesthesia. London: Laboratory Animals Ltd., 1979.
54. Pippi NL, Lumb WV. Objective tests of analgesic drugs in ponies. Am J Vet Res 40:1082, 1979.
55. Port JD, Stanley TH, Steffey EM. Narcotic inhalation anesthesia. Anesthesiology 57:A344, 1982.
56. Port JD, Stanley TH, Steffey EP, Henrickson R. Carfentanil: the primate experience. Proc Sci Meeting, Am Coll Vet Anesthesiol, Atlanta, Georgia, 1983.
57. De Vos V. Immobilisation of free-ranging wild animals using a new drug. Vet Rec 103:64, 1978.
58. Stoelting RK. Pharmacology and physiology in anesthetic practice, 2nd ed. Philadelphia: JB Lippincott, 1991.
59. Benson GJ, Thurmon JC, Tranquilli WJ, Corbin JE. Intravenous administration of lenperone and glycopyrrolate followed by continous infusion of sufentanil in dogs: cardiovascular effects. Am J Vet Res 48:1372–1375, 1987.
60. Harthoorn AM. Restraint of undomesticated animals. J Am Vet Med Assoc 149:875, 1966.
61. Blane GF, Boura ALA, Fitzgerald AE, Lister RE. Actions of etorphine hydrochloride (M-99). A potent morphine-like agent. Br J Pharmacol Chemother 30:11, 1967.
62. Burkhart RL. Evaluation of M-99 (etorphine) and antagonists, nalorphine, and M-285 (cyprenorphine) in wild animals. Research and Development Agricultural Division, American Cyanamid Co., Princeton, NJ, 1967.
63. Gray C. Comments on M-99. Am Assoc Zoo Vet, Washington, DC, March 25, 1968. Personal observations.
64. Van Laun T. Anaesthetizing donkeys. Vet Rec 100:391, 1977.
65. Pircio AW, Gylys JA, Cavanagh RL, Buyniski JP, Bierwagen ME. The pharmacology of butorphanol, a 3,14-dihydroxymorphinan narcotic antagonist analgesic. Arch Int Pharmacodyn Ther 220:231, 1976.
66. Schurig JE, Cavanaugh RL, Buyniski JP. Effect of butorphanol and morphine on pulmonary mechanics, arterial blood pressure and venous plasma histamine in the anesthetized dog. Arch Int Pharmacodyn Ther 233:296, 1978.
67. Roebel LE, Baryla UM, Buyniski JP. The effects of butorphanol and morphine on terminal bile duct and duodenal activity in anesthetized dogs. Pharmacologist 19:241, 1977.
68. Cavanaugh RL, Gylys JA, Bierwagen ME. Antitussive properties of butorphanol. Arch Int Pharmacodyn Ther 220:258, 1976.
69. Miller M. Inhibition of ADH release in the rat by narcotic antagonist. Neuroendocrinology 19:241, 1975.
70. Kalpravidh M, Lumb WV, Wright M, Heath RB. Analgesic effects of butorphanol in horses: dose response studies. Am J Vet Res 45:211, 1984.
71. Robertson JT, Muir WW. A new analgesic drug combination in the horse. Am J Vet Res 44:1667, 1983.
72. Tranquilli WJ, Thurmon JC, Turner TA, et al. Preliminary report on butorphanol tartrate as an adjunct to xylazine-ketamine anesthesia in the horse. Equine Practice 5:26–29, 1983.
73. Murphy MR, Hugg CC Jr. "Ceiling Effect" of butorphanol (Stadol) as an anesthetic supplement [abstract]. Anesthesiology 55:260, 1981.
74. Robertson JT, Muir WW, Sams R. Cardiopulmonary effects of butorphanol tartrate in horses. Am J Vet Res 42:41, 1981.
75. Dyson DH, Doherty T, Anderson GI, et al. Reversal of oxymorphone sedation by naloxone, nalmefene and butorphanol. Vet Surg 19:398–404, 1990.
76. Sawyer D, Briggs S, Paul K. Antinociceptive effect of butorphanol-oxymorphone combination in cats [abstract]. 5th International Congress of Veterinary Anesthesia, Guelph, Ontario, August 21–25, 1994:161.
77. Benson GJ, Tranquilli WJ. Advantages and guidelines for using opioid agonist-antagonist analgesics. Vet Clin North America Opin Small Animal Anesth, 22(2):363–365, 1992.
78. Lowe JE. Pentazocine for the relief of abdominal pain in ponies.

Proc 15th Annu Conv Am Assoc Equine Pract. Houston, Texas, 1969.

79. Kallow T, Smith TC. Naloxone reversal of pentazocine-induced respiratory depression. JAMA 204:932, 1968.

80. Amend JF, Klavano PA, Stone EC. Premedication with xylazine to eliminate muscular hypertonicity in cats during ketamine anesthesia. Vet Med Small Anim Clin 67(12):1305–1307, 1972.

81. Kerr DD, Jones EW, Holbert D, Huggins K. Comparison of the effects of xylazine and acetylpromazine maleate in the horse. Am J Vet Res 33(4):777–784, 1972.

82. Moye RJ, Pailet A, Smith MW Jr. Clinical use of xylazine in dogs and cats. Vet Med Small Anim Clin, 68(3):236–239, 1973.

83. Yate S. Clinical use of xylazine. A new drug for old problems. Vet Med Small Anim Clin 68(5):483–486, 1973.

84. Burns SJ, McMullen WC. Clinical application of Bay Va 1470 in the horse. Vet Med 67:77–79, 1971.

85. Clark KW, Hall LW. Xylazine—a new sedative for horses and cattle. Vet Rec 85:512–517, 1969.

86. DeMoor A, Desmit P. Effect of Rompun on acid-base equilibrium and arterial O_2 pressure in cattle. Vet Med Rev 2/3:163–169, 1971.

87. Garner HE, Amend JF, Rosborough JP. Effects of Bay Va 1470 on cardiovascular parameters of ponies. Vet Med 66:1016–1021, 1971.

88. Hoffman PE. Clinical evaluation of xylazine as a chemical restraining agent, sedative, and analgesic in horses. J Am Vet Med Assoc 164(1):42–45, 1974.

89. McCashin FB, Gabel AA. Evaluation of xylazine as a sedative and preanesthetic agent in horses. Am J Vet Res 36(10):1421–1429, 1975.

90. Hsu WH. Xylazine induced depression and its antagonism by alpha-adrenergic blocking agents. J Pharmacol Exp Ther 218:188–192, 1981.

91. Clough DP, Hutton R. Hypotensive and sedative effects of a adrenoceptor agonists: relationship to α_1 and α_2 adrenoceptor potency. Brit J Pharmacol 73:595–604, 1981.

92. Stephenson JC, Blevins DI, Christie GJ. Safety of Rompun/Ketaset combination in dogs: a two year study. Vet Med Small Anim Clin 73(3):303–306, 1978.

93. Kaplan B. A practitioner's report on the use of ketamine and xylazine with or without thiamylal for general anesthesia in dogs. Vet Med Small Anim Clin 74(9):1267–1268, 1979.

94. Cullen LK, Jones RS. Clinical observations on xylazine/ketamine anesthesia in the cat. Vet Rec 101(6):115–116, 1977.

95. Muir MW, Skarda RT, Milne DW. Evaluation of xylazine and ketamine hydrochloride for anesthesia in horses. Am J Vet Res 38(2):195–201, 1977.

96. Waterman AE. Preliminary observations on the use of a combination of xylazine and ketamine hydrochloride in calves. Vet Rec 109(21):464–467, 1981.

97. Thurmon JC, Benson GJ. Anesthesia in ruminants and swine. In: Howard JC, ed. Current veterinary therapy food animal practice 2. Philadelphia: WB Saunders, 1986:51–71.

98. Wright M. Pharmacologic effects of ketamine and its use in veterinary medicine. J Am Vet Med Assoc 180(2):1462–1471, 1982.

99. Nowrouzian I, Schels HF, Ghodsian I, Karimi H. Evaluation of the anesthetic properties of ketamine and a ketamine/xylazine/atropine combination in sheep. Vet Rec 108(16):354–356, 1981.

100. Kumar A, Thurmon JC, Hardenbrook HJ. Clinical studies of ketamine HCl and xylazine HCl in domestic goats. Vet Med Small Anim Clin 71(12):1703–1707, 1976.

101. Green CJ, Knight J, Precious S, Simpkin S. Ketamine alone and combined with diazepam or xylazine in laboratory animals: a 10 year experience. Lab Anim 15(2):163–170, 1981.

102. White GL, Holmes DD. A comparison of ketamine and the combination ketamine-xylazine for effective surgical anesthesia in the rabbit. Lab Anim Sci 26(5):804–806, 1976.

103. Van Pelt LF. Ketamine and xylazine for surgical anesthesia in rats. J Am Vet Med Assoc 171(9):842–844, 1977.

104. Gilroy BA, Varga JS. Use of ketamine-diazepam and ketamine-xylazine combinations in guinea pigs. Vet Med Small Anim Clin 75(3):508–509, 1980.

105. Naccarato EF, Hunter WS. Anaesthetic effects of various ratios of ketamine and xylazine in rhesus monkeys (Macaca mulatta). Lab Anim 13(4):317–319, 1979.

106. Banknieder AR, Phillips JM, Jackson KT, Vinal SI Jr. Comparison of ketamine with the combination of ketamine and xylazine for effective anesthesia in the rhesus monkey (Macaca mulatta). Lab Anim Sci 28(6):742–745, 1978.

107. April M, Tabor E, Gerety RJ. Combination of ketamine and xylazine for effective anaesthesia of juvenile chimpanzees (Pan troglodytes). Lab Anim 16(2):116–118, 1982.

108. Mulder JB. Anesthesia in the coyote using a combination of ketamine and xylazine. J Wildl Dis 14(4):501–502, 1978.

109. Philo LM. Evaluation of xylazine for chemical restraint of captive arctic wolves. J Am Vet Med Assoc 173(9):1163–1166, 1978.

110. Singh AP, Singh J, Peshin PK, Gahlawat JS, Singh P, Nigam JM. Evaluation of xylazine-ketamine anaesthesia in buffaloes (Bubalus bubalus). Zentralbl Veterinarmed 32(1):54–58, 1985.

111. Riebold TW, Kaneps AJ, Schmotzer WB. Anesthesia of llama. Vet Surg 18(5):400–404, 1989.

112. Allen JL, Welsch B, Jacobson ER, Turner TA, Tabeling H. Medical and surgical management of a fractured tusk in an African elephant. J Am Vet Med Assoc 185(11):1447–1449, 1984.

113. Green SA, Thurmon JC. Xylazine—a review of its pharmacology and use in veterinary medicine. J Vet Pharmacol Ther 11:295–313, 1988.

114. Cornick JL, Jensen J. Anesthetic management of ostriches. J Am Vet Med Assoc 200(11):1661–1666, 1992.

115. Mitchell PJ, Burton HR. Immobilization of southern elephant seals and leopard seals with cyclohexamine anesthetics and xylazine. Vet Rec 129(15):332–336, 1991.

116. Tranquilli WJ, Thurmon JC, Turner TA, Benson GJ, Lock TF. Preliminary report on butorphanol tartrate as an adjunct to xylazine-ketamine anesthesia in the horse. Equine Pract 5(6):26–29, 1983.

117. Faulkner DB, Eurell T, Tranquilli WJ, Ott RS, Ohl MW, Cmarik G, Zinn G. Performance and health of weanling bulls after butorphanol-xylazine administration at castration. J Anim Sci 70(10):2970–2974, 1992.

118. Tranquilli WJ, Benson GJ. Advantages and guidelines for using alpha-2 agonists as anesthetic adjuvants. Vet Clin North Am Small Animal Pract 22(2):289–293, 1992.

119. Tranquilli WJ, Thurmon JC, Benson GJ, Speiser J. Butorphanol preanesthetic administration in cats given acepromazine-ketamine and xylazine-ketamine. Vet Med 8:848–854, 1988.

120. Marini RP, Avison DL, Corning BF, Lipman NS. Ketamine/xylazine/butorphanol: a new anesthetic combination for rabbits. Lab Anim Sci 57–62, 1992.42(1).

121. Mathews NS, Dollars NS, Young DB, Shawley RV. Prolongation of xylazine/ketamine induced recumbency time with temazepam in horses. Equine Vet J 23(1):8–10, 1991.

122. McCarty JE, Trim CM, Ferguson D. Prolongation of anesthesia with xylazine, ketamine, and guaifenesin in horses: 64 cases (1986–1989). J Am Vet Med Assoc 197(12):1646–1650, 1990.

123. Brock N, Hildebrand SV. A comparison of xylazine-diazepam-ketamine and xylazine-guaifenesin-ketamine in equine anesthesia. Vet Surg 19(6):468–474, 1990.

124. Lin HC, Thurmon JC, Tranquilli WJ, Benson GJ, Olson WA. Hemodynamic response of calves to tiletamine-zolazepam-xylazine anesthesia. Am J Vet Res 52(10):1606–1610, 1991.

125. Popilskis SJ, Oz MC, Gorman P, Florestal A, Kohn DF. Comparison of xylazine with tiletamine-zolazepam (telazol) and xylazine-ketamine anesthesia in rabbits. Lab Anim Sci 41(1):51–53, 1991.

126. Brown MJ, McCarthy TJ, Bennett BT. Long term anesthesia using a continuous infusion of guaifenesin, ketamine, and xylazine in cats. Lab Anim Sci 41(1):46–50, 1991.

127. Haskins SC, Peiffer RL Jr, Stowe RM. A clinical comparison of CT1341, ketamine, and xylazine in cats. Am J Vet Res 36(10):1537–1543, 1975.

128. Tranquilli WJ, Thurmon JD, Benson GJ, Corbin JE, Davis LE. Halothane sparing effect of xylazine in dogs and subsequent reversal with tolazoline. J Vet Pharmacol Ther 7:23, 1984.

129. Garcia-Villar R, Toutain PL, Alvinerie M, Ruckebusch Y. The pharmacokinetics of xylazine hydrochloride: an interspecific study. J Vet Pharmacol Ther 4:87, 1981.

130. Mozier J. Personal communication. Animal Health Division, Chemagro Corporation, Stilwell, Kansas, 1972.

131. Kolata RJ, Rawlings CA. Cardiopulmonary effects of intravenous xylazine, ketamine, and atropine in the dog. Am J Vet Res 43(12):2196–2198, 1982.

132. Klide AM, Calderwood HW, Soma LR. Cardiopulmonary effects of xylazine in dogs. Am J Vet Res 36(7):931–935, 1975.

133. Kirkpatrick RM. Use of xylazine and ketamine as a combination anesthetic. Canine Practice 5(3):32–57, 1978.

134. Kroneberg G, Oberoff A, Hoffmeister F, Wirth W. Zur pharmakologie von 2-(2,6-dimethylphenylamino)-4-H-5,6-dihydro-1 3-thiazin (Bayer 1470), eines Hemmstoffes adrenergic und cholinergischer neurone. Arch Exp Pathol Pharmakol 258:257–260, 1967.

135. Tranquilli WJ, Thurmon JC, Paul AJ, Benson GJ. Influence of nifedipine on xylazine-induced acute pressor response in halothane anesthetized dogs. Am J Vet Res 46(9):1892–1895, 1985.

136. Hubble JAE, Muir WW. Effect of xylazine hydrochloride on canine splenic weight: an index of vascular capacity. Am J Vet Res 43(10):2188–2191, 1982.

137. Schmitt H, Fournadjiev G, Schmitt H. Central and peripheral effects of 2-(2,6-dimethylphenylamino)-4-H-5,6-dihydro-1,3-thiazin (Bayer 1470) on the sympathetic system. Eur J Pharmacol 10:230–238, 1970.

138. Antonaccio MJ, Robson RD, Kerwin L. Evidence for increased vagal tone and enhancement of baroreceptor reflex activity after xylazine (2-(2,6-dimethylphenylamino)-4-H-5,6-dihydro-1,3-thiazine) in anesthetized dogs. Eur J Pharmacol 23:311–315, 1973.

139. Haskins SC, Patz JD, Farver TB. Xylazine and xylazine-ketamine in dogs. Am J Vet Res 47(3):636–641, 1986.

140. Reutlinger RA, Karl AA, Neiser MJ. Effects of ketamine HCl-xylazine HCl combination on cardiovascular and pulmonary values of the rhesus macaque (Macaca mulatta). Am J Vet Res 41(9):1453–1457, 1980.

141. Dunkle N, Moise NS, Scarlett Kranz J, Short CE. Echocardiographic evaluation of cardiac performance in the cat sedated with xylazine and xylazine-glycopyrrolate. Am J Vet Res 47: 2212–2216, 1986.

142. Tranquilli WJ, Thurmon JC, Benson GJ, Davis LE. Alteration in the arrhythmogenic dose of epinephrine (ADE) following xylazine administration to halothane-anesthetized dogs. J Vet Pharm Ther 9:198–203, 1986.

143. Tranquilli WJ, Thurmon JC, Benson GJ. Alterations in the arrhythmogenic dose of epinephrine after adrenergic receptor blockade with prazosin, metoprolol, or yohimbine in halothane-xylazine anesthetized dogs. Am J Vet Res 47(1):114–118, 1986.

144. Tranquilli WJ, Thurmon JC, Benson GJ. Alterations in epinephrine-induced arrhythmogenesis after xylazine and subsequent yohimbine administration in isoflurane anesthetized dogs. Am J Vet Res 49(7):1072–1075, 1988.

145. Wright M, Heath RB, Wingfield WE. Effects of xylazine and ketamine on epinephrine induced arrythmia in the dog. Vet Surg 16(5):398–403, 1987.

146. Hayashi Y, Sumikawa K, Maze M, Yamatodani A, Kamibayashi T, Kuro M, Yoshiya I. Dexmedetomidine prevents epinephrine-induced arrhythmias through stimulation of central alpha 2 adrenoceptors in halothane-anesthetized dogs. Anesthesiology 75(1):113–117, 1991.

147. Lemke KA, Tranquilli WJ, Thurmon JC, Benson GJ, Olson WA. Alterations in the arrhythmogenic dose of epinephrine following xylazine or medetomidine administration in halothane-anesthetized dogs. Am J Vet Res 54(12):2132–2138, 1993.

148. Lemke KA, Tranquilli WJ, Thurmon JC, Benson GJ, Olson WA. Alterations in the arrhythmogenic dose of epinephrine following xylazine or medetomidine administration in isoflurane-anesthetized dogs. Am J Vet Res 54(12):2139–2145, 1993.

149. Lavoie JP, Pascoe JR, Kurpershock CJ. Effects of xylazine on ventilation in horses. Am J Vet Res 53(6):916–920, 1992.

150. Broadstone RV, Gray PR, Robinson NE, Derksen FJ. Effects of xylazine on airway function in ponies with recurrent airway obstruction. Am J Vet Res 53(10):1813–1817, 1992.

151. Gustin P, Dhem AR, Lekeux P, Lomba F, Landser FJ, Van de Woestijne KP. Regulation of bronchomotor tone in conscious calves. J Vet Pharmacol Ther 12(1):50–64, 1989.

152. Nolan A, Livingston A, Waterman A. The effects of α_2 adrenoceptor agonists on airway pressure in anesthetized sheep. J Vet Pharmacol Ther 9(2):157–163, 1986.

153. Steffey EP, Kelley AB, Farver TB, Woliner MJ. Cardiovascular and respiratory effects of acetylpromazine and xylazine on halothane-anesthetized horses. J Vet Pharmacol Ther 8:290–302, 1985.

154. Waterman AF, Nolan A, Livingston A. Influence of idazoxan on respiratory blood gas changes induced by α_2 adrenoceptor agonist drugs in sheep. Vet Rec 121(5):105–107, 1987.

155. Doherty TJ, Pascoe PJ, McDonell WN, Monteith G. Cardiopulmonary effects of xylazine and yohimbine in laterally recumbent sheep. Can J Vet Res 50(4):517–521, 1986.

156. Hsu WH, Hanson CE, Hembrough FB, Schaffer DD. Effects of idazoxan, tolazoline, and yohimbine on xylazine-induced respiratory changes and central nervous system depression in ewes. Am J Vet Res 50(9):1570–1573, 1989.

157. Muir WW, Piper FS. The effect of xylazine on indices of myocardial contractility in the dog. Am J Vet Res 38:931, 1977.

158. Campbell KB, Klavano PA, Richardson P, Alexander JE. Hemodynamic effects of xylazine in the calf. Am J Vet Res 40:1777, 1979.

159. Strombeck DR, Harrold D. Effects of atropine acepromazine, meperidine, and xylazine on gastroesophageal sphincter pressure in the dog. Am J Vet Res 46(4):963–965, 1985.

160. Hikasa Y, Ogasawara S, Taskase K. Alpha adrenoceptor subtypes involved in the emetic action of dogs. J Pharmacol Exp Ther 261(2):746–754, 1992.

161. Hsu WH. Xylazine-induced delay of small intestinal transit in mice. Eur J Pharmacol 83(1):55–60, 1982.

162. Hsu WH, McNeel SV. Effect of yohimbine on xylazine-induced prolongation of gastrointestinal transit in dogs. J Am Vet Med Assoc 183(3):297–300, 1983.

163. Seifelnasr E, Saleh M, Soliman FA. In vivo investigations on the effect to Rompun on the rumen motility of sheep. Vet Med Rev 2:158–165, 1974.

164. Cook CS, Kane KK. Apparent suppression of gastrointestinal motility due to xylazine: a comparative study. J Zool Anim Med 11:46–48, 1980.

165. Watson TDG, Sullivan M. Effects of detomidine on equine oesophageal function as studied by contrast radiography. Vet Rec 129(4):67–69, 1991.

166. McNeel SV, Hsu WH. Xylazine induced prolongation of gastrointestinal transit in dogs: reversal by yohimbine and potentiation by doxapram. J Am Vet Med Assoc 185(8):878–881, 1984.

167. Ruckebusch Y, Allal C. Depression of reticulo-ruminal motor functions through the stimulation of alpha 2 adrenoceptors. J Vet Pharmacol Ther 10(1):1–10, 1987.

168. Rutkowski JA, Ross MW, Cullen K. Effects of xylazine and/or butorphanol or neostigmine on myoelectric activity of the cecum and right ventral colon in female ponies. Am J Vet Res 50(7):1096–1101, 1989.

169. Lester GD, Bolton JR, Cullen LK, Thurgate SM. Effects of general anesthesia on myoelectric activity of the intestine in horses. Am J Vet Res 53(9):1553–1557, 1992.

170. Ruckebusch RT. Colonic alpha 2 adrenoceptor-mediated responses in the pony. J Vet Pharmacol Ther 10(4):310–318, 1987.

171. Muir WW, Robertson JT. Visceral analgesia: effect of xylazine, butorphanol, meperidine, and pentazocine in horses. Am J Vet Res 46(10):2081–2084, 1985.

172. Rutkowski JA, Eades SC, Moore JN. Effects of xylazine-butorphanol on cecal arterial blood flow, cecal mechanical activity, and systemic hemodynamics in horses. Am J Vet Res 52(7):1153–1158, 1991.

173. Eades SC, Moore JM. Blockade of endotoxin-induced cecal hypoperfusion and ileus with an α_2 antagonist in horses. Am J Vet Res 54(4):586–590, 1993.

174. Haskins SC. Abdominal distention associated with xylazine use. Mod Vet Pract 60:433, 1979.

175. Thurmon JC, Nelson DR, Hartsfield SM, Rumore CA. Effects of xylazine hydrochloride on urine in cattle. Aust Vet J 54:178–180, 1978.

176. Thurmon JC, Steffey EP, Zinke JG, Woliner M, Howland D Jr. Xylazine causes transient dose related hyperglycemia and increased urine volumes in mares. Am J Vet Res 45:224–227, 1984.

177. Trim CM, Henson RR. Effects of xylazine on renal function and plasma glucose in ponies. Vet Rec 118:65–67, 1986.

178. Hartsfield SM. The effects of acetylpromazine, xylazine, and ketamine on urine production in cats. Proc Am Coll Vet Anesthesiol Annu Meeting, St. Louis, Missouri, 1980.

179. Moreau PM, Lees GE, Gross DR. Simultaneous cystometry and uroflowmetry (micturition study) for evaluation of the caudal part of the urinary tract in dogs: reference values for healthy animals sedated with xylazine. Am J Vet Res 44(9):1774–1781, 1983.

180. Richter KP, Ling GV. Effects of xylazine on the urethral pressure profile of healthy dogs. Am J Vet Res 46(9):1881–1886, 1985.

181. Johnson CA, Beemsterbeer JM, Gray PR, Slusser PG, Goullaud EL. Effects of various sedatives on air cystometry in dogs. Am J Vet Res 49(9):1525–1528, 1988.

182. Thurmon JC, Neff-Davis CA, Davis LE, Stoker RA, Benson GJ, Lock TF. Xylazine hydrochloride-induced hyperglycemia and hypoinsulinemia in Thoroughbred horses. J Vet Pharmacol Ther 5:241–245, 1982.

183. Tranquilli WJ, Thurmon JC, Neff-Davis CA, Benson GJ, Hoffman W, Lock TF. Hyperglycemia and hypoinsulinemia during xylazine-ketamine anesthesia in Thoroughbred horses. Am J Vet Res 45(1):11–14, 1984.

184. Symods HW, Mallinson CB. The effect of xylazine and xylazine followed by insulin on blood glucose and insulin in the dairy cow. Vet Rec 102:27–29, 1978.

185. Hsu WH, Hummel SK. Xylazine-induced hyperglycemia in cattle: a possible involvement of a adrenergic receptors regulating insulin release. Endocrinology 109:825–829, 1981.

186. Benson GJ, Thurmon JC, Neff-Davis CA, et al. Effect of xylazine hydrochloride upon plasma glucose and serum insulin concentrations in adult pointer dogs. J Am Anim Hosp Assoc 20:791–794, 1984.

187. Eichner RD, Prior RL, Kvasnicka WB. Xylazine-induced hyperglycemia in beef cattle. Am J Vet Res 40:127, 1979.

188. Felberg W, Symonds HW. Hyperglycaemic effect of xylazine. J Vet Pharmacol Ther 3:197, 1980.

189. Hsu WH, Hembrough FB. Intravenous glucose tolerance test in cats: influenced by acetylpromazine, ketamine, morphine, thiopental, and xylazine. Am J Vet Res 43:2060–2061, 1982.

190. LeBlanc MM, Hubbell JAE, Smith HC. The effects of xylazine hydrochloride on intrauterine pressure in the cow. Theriogenology 21:681–690, 1984.

191. Jansen CA, Lowe KC, Nathaielsz PW. The effect of xylazine on uterine activity, fetal and maternal oxygenation, cardiovascular function and fetal breathing. Am J Obstet Gynecol 148(4):386–390, 1984.

192. Hsu WH, Lee P, Betts DM. Xylazine-induced mydriasis in rats and its antagonism by alpha-adrenergic blocking agents. J Vet Pharmacol Ther 4(2):97–101, 1981.

193. Burke JA, Potter DE. The ocular effects of xylazine in rabbits, cats, and monkeys. J Ocul Pharmacol 2(1):9–21, 1986.

194. Jin Y, Wilson S, Elko EE, Yorio T. Ocular hypotensive effects of medetomidine and its analogs. J Ocul Pharmacol 7(4):285–296, 1991.

195. Potter DE, Ogidigben MJ. Medetomidine-induced alterations of intraocular pressure and contraction of nictitating membrane. Invest Ophthalmol Vis Sci 32(10):2799–2805, 1991.

196. Tranquilli WJ, Thurmon JC. Personal observations.

197. Clarke KW, Hall LW. "Xylazine"—a new sedative for horses and cattle. Vet Rec 85:512, 1969.

198. Fuentes VO. Sudden death in a stallion after xylazine medication. Vet Rec 102:106, 1978.

199. Monti JM. Catecholamines and the sleep-wake cycle. I. EEG and behavioral arousal. Life Sci 30:1145–1157, 1982.

200. Aziz MA, Martin RJ. Alpha agonist and local anesthetic properties of xylazine. Zentrabl Veterinarmed 25:180–188, 1978.

201. O'Regan MH. Xylazine evoked depression of rat cerebral cortical neurons: a pharmacologic study. Gen Pharmacol 20(4):469–474, 1989.

202. Fikes LW, Lin HC, Thurmon JC. A preliminary comparison of xylazine and lidocaine as epidural analgesics in ponies. Vet Surg 18(1):85–86, 1988.

203. LeBlanc PH, Caron JP, Patterson JS, Brown M, Matta MA. Epidural injection of xylazine for perineal analgesia in horses. J Am Vet Med Assoc 193(11):1405–1408, 1988.

204. LeBlanc PH, Eberhart SW. Cardiopulmonary effects of epidurally administered xylazine in the horse. Equine Vet J 22(6):389–391, 1990.

205. Caron JP, LeBlanc PH. Caudal epidural analgesia in cattle using xylazine. Can J Vet Res 53(4):486–489, 1989.

206. Skarda RT, St Jean G, Muir WW. Influence of tolazoline on caudal epidural administration of xylazine in cattle. Am J Vet Res 51(4):556–560, 1990.

207. Waterman A, Livingston A, Bouchenafa O. Analgesic effects of intrathecally applied alpha 2 agonists in conscious, unrestrained sheep. Neuropharmacology 27(2):213–216, 1988.

208. Branson KR, Ko JCH, Tranquilli WJ, Benson GJ, Thurmon JC. Duration of analgesia induced by epidurally administered morphine and medetomidine in the dog. J Vet Pharmacol Ther 16:369–372, 1993.

209. Virtanen R, Ruskoaho H, Nyman L. Pharmacologic evidence for the involvement of α_2 adrenoceptors in the sedative effect of detomidine, a novel sedative-analgesic. J Vet Pharmacol Ther 8(1):30–37, 1985.

210. Virtanen R. Antinociceptive activity and mechanism of action of detomidine. J Vet Pharmacol Ther 9(3):286–292, 1986.

211. Virtanen R, MacDonald E. Comparison of the effects of detomidine and xylazine on some alpha 2 adrenoceptor-mediated responses in the central and peripheral nervous systems. Eur J Pharmacol 115(2):277–284, 1985.

212. Virtanen R, Nyman L. Evaluation of the alpha 1- and alpha 2-adrenoceptor effects of detomidine, a novel veterinary sedative analgesic. Eur J Pharmacol 108(2):163–169, 1985.

213. Wagner AE, Muir WW, Hinchcliff KW. Cardiovascular effects of xylazine and detomidine in horses. Am J Vet Res 52(5):651–657, 1991.

214. Short CE, Matthews N, Harvey R, Tyner L. Cardiovascular and pulmonary function studies of a new sedative/analgesic (detomidine) for use alone in horses or as a preanesthetic. Acta Vet Scand 82:139–155, 1986.

215. Sarazan RD, Starke WA, Krause GF, Garner HE. Cardiovascular effects of detomidine, a new α_2 adrenoceptor agonist, in the conscious pony. J Vet Pharmacol Ther 12:378–388, 1989.

216. Jochle W, Hamm D. Sedation and analgesia with Domosedan (detomidine hydrochloride) in horses: dose response studies on efficacy and its duration. Acta Vet Scand 82:69–84, 1986.

217. Clarke KW, Taylor PM. Detomidine: a new sedative for horses. Equine Vet J 18(5):366–370, 1986.

218. Lowe JE, Hifiger J. Analgesic and sedative effects of detomidine compared to xylazine in a colic model using IV and IM routes of administration. Acta Vet Scand 82:85–95, 1986.

219. Clarke KW, Taylor PM, Watkins SB. Detomidine/ketamine anesthesia in the horse. Acta Vet Scand 82:167–179, 1986.

220. Wan PY, Trim CM, Mueller PO. Xylazine-ketamine and detomidine-tiletamine-zolazepam anesthesia in horses. Vet Surg 21(4):312–318, 1992.

221. Lin HC, Branson KR, Thurmon JC, Benson GJ, Tranquilli WJ, Olson WA, Vaha Vahe AT. Ketamine, telazol, xylazine, and detomidine. A comparative anesthetic drug combinations study in ponies. Acta Vet Scand 33(2):109–115, 1992.

222. Clarke KW, Paton BS. Combined use of detomidine with opiates in horses. Equine Vet J 20:331–334, 1988.

223. LeBlanc PH. Chemical restraint for surgery in the standing horse. Vet Clin North Am Equine Pract 7(3):521–533, 1991.

224. England GC, Clarke KW, Goossen SL. A comparison of the sedative effects of three alpha 2-adrenoceptor agonists (romifi-

dine, detomidine, xylazine) in horses. J Vet Pharmacol Ther 15(2):194–201, 1992.

225. Scheinin M, MacDonald E. An introduction to the pharmacology of α_2 adrenoceptors in the central nervous system. Acta Vet Scand 85:11–19, 1989.

226. Virtanen R. Pharmacologic profiles of medetomidine and its antagonist atipamezole. Acta Vet Scand 85:29–37, 1989.

227. Vainio O. Introduction to the clinical pharmacology of medetomidine. Acta Vet Scand 85:85–88, 1989.

228. Bergstrom K. Cardiovascular and pulmonary effects of a new sedative/analgesic (medetomidine) as a preanesthetic drug in the dog. Acta Vet Scand 29:109–116, 1988.

229. Bloor BC, Abdul-Rasool I, Temp J, Jenkins S, Valcke C, Ward DS. The effects of medetomidine, an α_2 adrenergic agonist, on ventilatory drive in the dog. Acta Vet Scand 85:65–70, 1989.

230. Crighton M. Diuresis following medetomidine. Vet Rec 126(8): 201, 1990.

231. Raiha MP, Raiha JE, Short CE. A comparison of xylazine, acepromazine, meperidine, and medetomidine as preanesthetics to halothane anesthesia in dogs. Acta Vet Scand 85:97–102, 1989.

232. Vainio O, Palmu L. Cardiovascular and respiratory effects of medetomidine in dogs and influence of anticholinergics. Acta Vet Scand 30(4):401–408, 1989.

233. Short CE. Effects of anticholinergic treatment on the cardiac and respiratory systems in dogs sedated with medetomidine. Vet Rec 129(4):310–313, 1991.

234. Thurmon JC, Ko JCH, Benson GJ, Tranquilli WJ. Clinical appraisal of propofol as an anesthetic in dogs premedicated with medetomine. Canine Pract 20(1):21–25, 1995.

235. Ko JCH, Thurmon JC, Bensen GJ, Tranquilli WJ, Olson WA. Hemodynamic and analgesic effects of etomidate infusion in medetomidine-premedicated dogs. Am J Vet Res 55(6):842–846, 1994.

236. Raiha JE, Raiha MP, Short CE. Medetomidine as a preanesthetic prior to ketamine-HCl and halothane anesthesia in laboratory beagles. Acta Vet Scand 85:103–110, 1989.

237. Moens Y, Fargetton X. A comparative study of medetomidine/ ketamine and xylazine/ketamine anaesthesia in dogs. Vet Rec 127(23):567–571, 1990.

238. Stenberg D. Physiologic role of α_2-adrenoceptors in the regulation of vigilance and pain: effect of medetomidine. Acta Vet Scand 85:21–28, 1989.

239. Verstegen J, Fargetton X, Donnay I, Ectors F. An evaluation of medetomidine/ketamine and other drug combinations for anaesthesia in cats. Vet Rec 128(2):32–35, 1991.

240. Kamerling S, Keowen M, Bagwell C, Jochle W. Pharmacologic profile of medetomidine in the equine. Acta Vet Scand 87:161–162, 1991.

241. Bryant CE, England GC, Clarke KW. Comparison of the effects of medetomidine and xylazine in horses. Vet Rec 129(19):421–423, 1991.

242. Sakaguchi M, Nishimura R, Sasaki N, Ishiguro T, Tamura H, Takeuchi A. Sedative effects of medetomidine in pigs. J Vet Med Sci 54(4):643–647, 1992.

243. Vähä Vahe T. The clinical efficacy of medetomidine. Acta Vet Scand 85:151–153, 1989.

244. Jalanka H. The use of medetomidine, medetomidine-ketamine combinations and atipamezole at Helsinki 200 — a review of 240 cases. Acta Vet Scand 85:193–197, 1989.

245. Nevalainen T, Pyhalal, Voipio HM, Virtanen R. Evaluation of anaesthetic potency of medetomidine-ketamine combinations in rats, guinea-pigs and rabbits. Acta Vet Scand 85:139–143, 1989.

246. Arnemo JM, Soli NE. Immobilization of mink (Mustela vison) with medetomidine-ketamine and remobilization with atipamezole. Vet Res Commun 16(4):281–292, 1992.

247. Jalanka HH. Medetomidine and medetomidine-ketamine-induced immobilization in blue foxes (Alopex lagopus) and its reversal by atipamezole. Acta Vet Scand 31(1):63–71, 1990.

248. Van Heerden J, Keffen RH. A preliminary investigation into the immobilising potential of a tiletamine/zolazepam mixture, metomidate, a medetomidine and azaperone combination and medetomidine in ostriches. J S Afr Vet Assoc 62(3):114–117, 1991.

249. England GCW, Clarke KW. The use of medetomidine/fentanyl combinations in dogs. Acta Vet Scand 85:179–186, 1989.

250. Schmidt-Oechtering GU, Becker K. Old and new alpha 2-adrenoceptor agonists xylazine and medetomidine. Tierarztl Prax 20(5):447–458, 1992.

251. Holmberg G, Gershon J. Autonomic and psychic effects of yohimbine hydrochloride. Psychopharmacology 2:93–106, 1961.

252. Lang WJ, Gershon S. Effects of psychoactive drugs on yohimbine induced responses in conscious dogs. Arch Int Pharmacodyn 142:457–472, 1963.

253. Delbarre B, Schmitt H. Sedative effects of α-sympathomimetic drugs and their antagonism by adrenergic and cholinergic blocking drugs. Eur J Pharmacol 13:356–363, 1971.

254. Delbarre B, Schmitt H. A further attempt to characterize sedative receptors activated by clonidine in chickens and mice. Eur J Pharmacol 22:355–359, 1973.

255. Hsu WH. Antagonism of xylazine-induced CNS depression by yohimbine in cats. Calif Vet 37:19–21, 1983.

256. Hatch RC, Booth NH, Clark JD, et al. Antagonism of xylazine sedation in dogs by 4-aminopyridine and yohimbine. Am J Vet Res 43:1009–1014, 1982.

257. Kitzman JV, Booth NH, Hatch RC, et al. Antagonism of xylazine sedation by 4—aminopyridine and yohimbine in cattle. Am J Vet Res 43:2165–2169, 1982.

258. Wallner BM, Hatch RC, Booth NH, et al. Complete immobility produced in dogs by xylazine-atropine: antagonism by 4—aminopyridine and yohimbine. Am J Vet Res 43:2259–2265, 1982.

259. Hatch RC, Booth NH, Kitzman JV, et al. Antagonism of ketamine anesthesia in cats by 4-aminopyridine and yohimbine. Am J Vet Res 44:417–423, 1983.

260. Cronin MF, Booth NH, Hatch RC, et al. Acepromazine-xylazine combination in dogs: antagonism with 4-aminopyridine and yohimbine. Am J Vet Res 44:2037–2042, 1983.

261. Kitzman JV, Wilson RC, Hatch RC, et al. Antagonism of xylazine and ketamine anesthesia by 4-aminopyridine and yohimbine in geldings. Am J Vet Res 45(5):875–879, 1984.

262. Hatch RC, Clark JD, Booth NH, Kitzman JV. Comparison of five preanesthetic medicaments in pentobarbital-anesthetized dogs: antagonism by 4-aminopyridine, yohimbine, and naloxone. Am J Vet Res 44(12):2312–2319, 1983.

263. Hatch RC, Kitzman JV, Clark JD, Zahner JM, Booth NH. Reversal of pentobarbital anesthesia with 4-aminopyridine and yohimbine in cats pretreated with acepromazine and xylazine. Am J Vet Res 45(12):2586–2590, 1984.

264. Loffelholz K, Weide W. Aminopyridines and the release of acetylcholine. Trends Pharmacol Sci 3:147–149, 1982.

265. Sia RL, Boonstra S, Westra P, et al. An electroencephalographic study of 4-aminopyridine. Anesth Analg 61:354–357, 1982.

266. Glover WE. The aminopyridines. Gen Pharmacol 13:259–285, 1982.

267. Hatch RC, Kitzman JV, Zahner JM, Clark JD, Booth NH. Comparison of five preanesthetic medicaments in thiopental anesthetized cats: antagonism by selected compounds. Am J Vet Res 45(11):2322–2327, 1984.

268. Kreeger TJ, Faggella AM, Seal US, Mech LD, Callahan M, Hall B. Cardiovascular and behavioral responses of gray wolves to ketamine-xylazine immobilization and antagonism by yohimbine. J Wildl Dis 23(3):463–470, 1987.

269. Hsu WH, Schaffer DD, Hanson CE. Effects of tolazoline and yohimbine on xylazine-induced central nervous system depression, bradycardia, and tachypnea in sheep. J Am Vet Med Assoc 190(4):423–426, 1987.

270. Deresienski DT, Rupprecht CE. Yohimbine reversal of ketamine-xylazine immobilization of raccoons (Procyon lotor). J Wildl Dis 25(2):169–174, 1989.

271. Freed D, Baker B. Antagonism of xylazine HCl sedation in raptors by yohimbine HCl. J Wildl Dis 25(1):136–138, 1989.

272. Jessup DA, Clark WE, Jones KR, Lance WR. Immobilization of free ranging desert bighorn sheep, tule elk, and wild horses using carfentanil and xylazine: reversal with naloxone, diprenophine, and yohimbine. J Am Vet Med Assoc 187(11): 1253–1254, 1985.

273. Jessup DA, Jones K, Mohr R, Kucera T. Yohimbine antagonism to xylazine in free ranging mule deer and desert bighorn sheep. J Am Vet Med Assoc 187(11):1251–1253, 1985.
274. Jacobson ER, Allen J, Martin H, Kollias GV. Effects of yohimbine on combined xylazine-ketamine-induced sedation and immobilization in juvenile African elephants. J Am Vet Med Assoc 187(11):1195–1198, 1985.
275. Hsu WH, Shulaw WP. Effect of yohimbine on xylazine-induced immobilization in whitetailed deer. J Am Vet Med Assoc 185(11):1301–1303, 1984.
276. Jessup DA, Clark WE, Gullett PA, Jones KR. Immobilization of mule deer with ketamine and xylazine, and reversal of immobilization with yohimbine. J Am Vet Med Assoc 183(11):1339–1340, 1983.
277. McGruder JP, Hsu WH. Antagonism of xylazine-pentobarbital anesthesia by yohimbine in ponies. Am J Vet Res 46(6):1276–1281, 1985.
278. Hsu WH. Xylazine-pentobarbital anesthesia in dogs and its antagonism by yohimbine. Am J Vet Res 46(4):852–855, 1985.
279. Hsu WH, Bellin SI, Dellmann HD, Hanson LE. Xylazine-ketamine-induced anesthesia in rats and its antagonism by yohimbine. J Am Vet Med Assoc 189(9):1040–1043, 1986.
280. Heaton JT, Brauth SE. Effects of yohimbine as a reversing agent for ketamine-xylazine anesthesia in budgerigars. Lab Anim Sci 42(1):54–56, 1992.
281. Nishimura R, Sakaguchi M, Mochizuki M, Sasaki N, Takahashi H, Tamura H, Takeuchi A. A balanced anesthesia with a combination of xylazine, ketamine, and butorphanol and its antagonism by yohimbine in pigs. J Vet Med Sci 54(4):615–620, 1992.
282. Allen JL, Oosterhuis LE. Effect of tolazoline on xylazine-ketamine- induced anesthesia in turkey vultures. J Am Vet Med Assoc 189(9):1011–1112, 1986.
283. Kreeger TJ, Seal US, Faggella AM. Xylazine HCl-ketamine HCl immobilization of wolves and its antagonism by tolazoline HCl. J Wildl Dis 22(3):397–402, 1986.
284. Kreeger TJ, Del-Giudice GD, Seals US, Karns PD. Immobilization of whitetailed deer with xylazine HCl and ketamine HCl and antagonism by tolazoline HCl. J Wildl Dis 22(3):407–412, 1986.
285. Allen JL. Use of tolazoline as an antagonist to xylazine-ketamine-induced immobilization in African elephants. Am J Vet Res 47(4):781–783, 1986.
286. Tranquilli WJ, Thurmon JC, Corbin JE, Benson GJ, Davis LE. Halothane sparing effect of xylazine in dogs and subsequent reversal with tolazoline. J Vet Pharmacol Ther 7(l):23–28, 1984.
287. Thurmon JC, Lin HC, Tranquilli WJ, Benson GJ, Olson WA. A comparison of yohimbine and tolazoline as antagonists of xylazine sedation in calves. Proc 4th Vet Midwest Anesth Conf, Urbana, Illinois, 1987.
288. Takase K, Hikasa Y, Ogasa-Wara S. Tolazoline as an antagonist of xylazine in cattle. Jpn J Vet Sci 48:859–862, 1986.
289. Hartsfield SM. Comparison of the effects of tolazoline, yohimbine and 4-aminopyridine in cats medicated with xylazine. Proc 2nd Vet Midwest Anesth Conf, Urbana, Illinois, 1985.
290. Doherty T, Ballinger JA, McDonell WW, Pascoe P. Antagonism of xylazine induced sedation by a new α_2 antagonist idazoxan. Can J Vet Res 55:244–248, 1987.
291. Doherty TJ, Tweedie DP. Evaluation of xylazine HCl as the sole immobilization agent in moose and caribou — and its subsequent reversal with idazoxan. J Wildl Dis 25(1):95–98, 1989.
292. Virtanen R, MacDonald E. Reversal of the sedative/analgesic and other effects of detomidine and medetomidine by MVP1248, a novel alpha-2-antagonist. Pharmacol Toxicol 60(SIII):2–5, 1987.
293. Jalanka H. The use of medetomidine, medetomidine-ketamine combinations and atipamezole at Helsinki zoo — A review of 240 cases. Acta Vet Scand 85:193–197, 1989.
294. Jalanka H. Evaluation of medetomidine- and ketamine-induced immobilization in Markhors (Capra falconeri megaceros) and its reversal by atipamezole. J Zoo Med 19(3):95–105, 1988.
295. Clarke KW, England GCW. Medetomidine, a new sedative-analgesic for use in the dog and its reversal with atipamezole. J Small Anim Pract 30:343–348, 1989.
296. Virtanen R, Savola JM, Saano V. Highly selective and specific antagonism of central and peripheral alpha 2-adrenoceptors by atipamezole. Arch Int Pharmacodyn Ther 297:190–204, 1989.
297. Jalanka HH. Medetomidine- and ketamine-induced immobilization of snow leopards (Panthera unica): doses, evaluation, and reversal by atipamezole. J Zoo Wildl Med 20(2):154–162, 1989.
298. Verstegen J, Fargetton X, Zanker S, Donnay I, Ectors F. Antagonistic activities of atipamezole 4-aminopyridine and yohimbine against medetomidine/ketamine induced anesthesia in cats. Vet Rec 128(3):57–60, 1991.
299. Jones RS, Young LE. Medetomidine premedication in dogs and its reversal by atipamezole. Acta Vet Scand 87:165–167, 1991.
300. Vainio O. Reversal of medetomidine-induced cardiovascular and respiratory changes with atipamezole in dogs. Vet Rec 127(18):447–450, 1990.
301. Bednarski RM, Muir WW, Tracy LH. The effects of tolazoline, doxapram, RO15-1788 on the depressant action of telazol. Vet Med 84(9):1016–1022, 1989.
302. Silverman AG, Wilner HI, Okun R. A case of gastrointestinal bleeding following the use of tolazoline. Toxicol Appl Pharmacol 16:318–320, 1970.
303. Thompson JR, Kersting KW, Hsu HW. Antagonistic effect of atipamezole on xylazine-induced sedation, bradycardia and ruminal atony in calves. Am J Vet Res 52(8):1265–1268, 1991.
304. Vaha Vahe AT. The clinical effectiveness of atipamezole as a medetomidine antagonist in the dog. J Vet Pharmacol Therap 132(2):198–205, 1990.
305. Jarvis N, England CG. Reversal of xylazine sedation in dogs. Vet Rec 128(14):323–325, 1991.
306. Luna SP, Beale NJ, Taylor PM. Effects of atipamezole on xylazine sedation in ponies. Vet Rec 130(13):268–271, 1992.
307. Tranquilli WJ, Gross ME, Thurmon JC, Benson GJ. Evaluation of three midazolam-xylazine mixtures: preliminary trials in dogs. Vet Surg 19:168–172, 1990.
308. Gross ME, Tranquilli WJ, Thurmon JC, Benson GJ, Olson WA. Hemodynamic effects of intravenous midazolam-xylazine-butorphanol in dogs. Vet Surg 19:173–180, 1990.
309. Maze M, Tranquilli WJ. Alpha 2 adrenoceptor agonists: defining a role in clinical anesthesia. Anesthesiology 74(3):581–605, 1991.
310. Tranquilli WJ, Maze M. Clinical pharmacology and use of α_2 agonists in veterinary anesthesia. Anaesth Pharmacol Rev 1(3):297–309, 1993.
311. Moore J, Dundee JW. Alterations in response to somatic pain associated with anesthesia. VII. The effects of nine phenothiazine derivatives. Br J Anaesth 33:422, 1961.
312. Booth NH, Hatch RC, Crawford LM. Reversal of the neurolept-analgesic effect of droperidol-fentanyl in the dog by 4-aminopyridine and naloxone. Am J Vet Res 43:1227, 1982.
313. Bogan JA, MacKenzie G, Snow DH. An evaluation of tranquilizers for use with etorphine as neuroleptanalgesic agents in the horse. Vet Rec 103:471, 1978.
314. Pearson H, Weaver BMQ. Priapism after sedation, neuroleptanalgesia and anesthesia in the horse. Equine Vet J 10:85, 1978.
315. Dobbs HE, Ling CM. The use of etorphine/acepromazine in the horse and donkey. Vet Rec 91:40, 1972.
316. Dodman NH, Waterman AE. Clinical observations on the antagonism of immobilon by nalaxone in dogs. Vet Rec 103:334, 1978.

chapter 9

INJECTABLE ANESTHETICS

Introduction

There is no injectable anesthetic that produces all of the components of general anesthesia without depressing some vital organ function. Because the available drugs have rather selective actions within the CNS, combinations of drugs are necessary to provide surgical anesthesia without depressing vital functions. Other than ketamine, intravenous anesthetics generally provide only the mental depression of the anesthetic state. Additional analgesics, inhaled anesthetics, and/or muscle relaxants are required to provide and maintain all of the components of general anesthesia. Thus, drugs discussed in this chapter have been variously described as sedatives, hypnotics, anxiolytics, and incomplete anesthetics. The terms *sleep, hypnosis,* and *unconsciousness* have often been used interchangeably in describing the drug-induced sleep produced by these drugs. Characteristics of the ideal injectable anesthetic are given in Table 9–1.

Injectable drugs are used to induce the unconscious state or are given by repeated injection and infusion to maintain the mental depression necessary for anesthesia. In recent years, more specific and controllable compounds that provide hypnosis, analgesia, and muscle relaxation have been developed (e.g., propofol). Total intravenous anesthesia refers to the production of general anesthesia with injectable drugs only. The advantage of total intravenous anesthesia is its facility

Table 9–1.   Characteristics of an Ideal Injectable Anesthetic

I. Physiochemical and pharmacokinetic
   a. Water soluble
   b. Long shelf life
   c. Stable when exposed to light
   d. Small volume required for induction of anesthesia

II. Pharmacodynamics
   a. Minimal individual variation
   b. Safe therapeutic ratio
   c. Onset, one vein to brain circulation time
   d. Short duration of action
   e. Inactivated to nontoxic metabolites
   d. Smooth emergence
   e. Absence of anaphylaxis
   f. Absence of histamine release

III. Side effects
   a. Absence of local toxicity
   b. No effect on vital organ function, except anesthetically desirable CNS effects

to provide each component of anesthesia with a dose of a specific drug. In contrast, inhalation anesthetics increase or decrease the intensity of all components of anesthesia (CNS depression, analgesia, muscle relaxation) at the same time, including their unwanted side effects. The search for new drugs and combinations with appropriate pharmacokinetic-pharmacodynamic profiles for use in domestic and wild animals is ongoing. In animals, unlike man, a state approaching general anesthesia is not achievable with opioids alone. Consequently, in veterinary anesthesia they have been primarily utilized as analgesics perioperatively and as anesthetic adjuncts to induce a state of neuroleptanesthesia and are not employed alone as intravenous anesthetics. For this reason opioids are included in the chapter on preanesthetics and anesthetic adjuncts (Chapter 8). Because the dissociatives have such a widespread use in domestic, feral, and wild species, and are commonly combined with a variety of other drugs, they are also discussed in a separate chapter (Chapter 10).

STRUCTURE-ACTIVITY RELATIONSHIPS

Structure-activity relationships are descriptions of the way modifications of chemical structure affect pharmacologic activity. The addition, modification, or removal of functional groups on the fundamental structure of a drug lend it physiochemical properties that alter its ability to gain access to its site of action (receptor) and determine the effect it has on the receptor and cellular function (intrinsic activity). The structure activity relationships of anesthetic induction drugs have been reasonably described.

Modification of the structure of barbituric acid converts the inactive compound into a hypnotic. The addition of aliphatic side chains in position 5 and 5' produces hypnotic activity. The length of the side chains influences the duration of action as well as

potency. Replacement of the oxygen atom in position 2 of an active barbiturate with a sulfur atom results in a faster onset and a shorter duration of action (e.g., thiopental or thiamylal). If an active barbiturate is methylated in the 1 position, it produces a drug with a rapid onset and short duration of action at the expense of excitatory side effects (e.g., methohexital). Generally, any modification that increases lipophilicity will increase potency and rate of onset and shorten the duration of action.

Several imidazoles possess hypnotic activity. This activity in such a molecule requires an alkyl branched carbon atom between the aryl moiety and the imidazole nitrogen and an ester moiety. Etomidate is the most widely used imidazole anesthetic derivative. Propofol is a diortho-substituted phenol with strong hypnotic actions. Sleep time increases with side-chain length. Potency increases with the length of the side chain up to a total of seven to eight carbon atoms. Longer chains decrease potency, while induction and recovery times are prolonged. The arylcycloalkylamines, of which ketamine is a derivative, derive their anesthetic activity from a cyclohexane ring geminally substituted with an aromatic ring and a basic nitrogen. The potency of these compounds is influenced by substitution on the nitrogen, while their pharmacologic activity is unaffected.

An often-overlooked aspect of structure-activity relationships is the role of stereoisomerism to biologic activity. Except for the asymmetric centers, the stereoisomers of a given molecule are physically and chemically identical. Nevertheless, activity is predicated on the active stereoisomer of a given neurotransmitter, hormone, or drug interfacing with the chiral active center of a receptor or enzyme. Because side effects are often caused by nonspecific action of drugs, the inactive stereoisomer can contribute to side effects of racemic mixtures. Some isomers may have the opposite effect on a receptor or enzyme than that of the active isomer. Several barbiturates have asymmetric carbon atoms with isomers of varying potency. Nevertheless, all barbiturates are marketed as racemic mixtures. The (+) isomer of etomidate has hypnotic activity and is the only anesthetic to be marketed as a single active isomer. The stereoisomers of ketamine vary in their hypnotic and analgesic potency, with the (+) isomer being three times more potent than the (−) isomer. The (−) isomer produces more untoward emergence reactions. Nevertheless, ketamine is marketed as a racemic mixture. Neither propofol nor the benzodiazepines possess asymmetric carbon atoms.(1)

MECHANISMS OF ACTION

The complexity of the CNS has contributed to the lack of a full understanding of the mechanisms of action of injectable anesthetic drugs. No drug has a single action. Some theories suggest that anesthetics alter cell membranes (Chapter 7). Other theories emphasize interaction with neurotransmitter-receptor-ionophore systems. There is considerable evidence suggesting that most injectable anesthetics alter gamma-aminobutyric acid (GABA)-mediated neurotransmission. GABA is a inhibitory neurotransmitter that activates postsynaptic receptors that in turn increase chloride conductance, thus hyperpolarizing and inhibiting the neuron (Chapter 7). Barbiturates and benzodiazepines activate distinct receptors on the GABA receptor complex. Benzodiazepines increase the frequency of chloride ion channel openings produced by GABA. Barbiturates decrease the rate of dissociation of GABA from its receptors increasing the duration of time chloride ion channels are open. Etomidate and propofol may also induce CNS depression by modulation of GABAergic neurotransmission. In contrast to barbiturates, etomidate appears to increase the number of GABA receptors.(1) It is likely that the anatomic site of action within the CNS differs among barbiturates, benzodiazepines, etomidate, and propofol.(2)

Although the effects on neurotransmission are not as well understood as the effects of barbiturates and benzodiazepines, dissociatives are thought to interact with CNS muscarinic cholinergic receptors as antagonists and opioid receptors as agonists. Recent data also suggests that they interact with N-methyl-D-aspartate (NMDA) receptors as nonselective antagonists. Further discussion on the mechanisms of action of dissociatives can be found in Chapter 10.

Barbiturates

Barbituric acid was first prepared by Conrad and Gutzeit in 1882. In 1903, Fischer and von Mering introduced a derivative, diethyl barbituric acid (veronal, barbital), for use as a hypnotic. Fischer is believed to have named the drug veronal from the Latin *vera*, since he thought it to be the "true" hypnotic.

CHEMICAL STRUCTURE

The barbiturates all contain a pyrimidine nucleus resulting from the condensation of malonic acid and urea (Fig. 9–1). Barbituric acid itself has no hypnotic activity. Substituting alkyl or aryl groups on the R_1 or R_2 positions (Fig. 9–2) produces various compounds with hypnotic activity. Replacement of the oxygen atom in position X by a sulfur atom produces the ultra-short-acting thiobarbiturates.

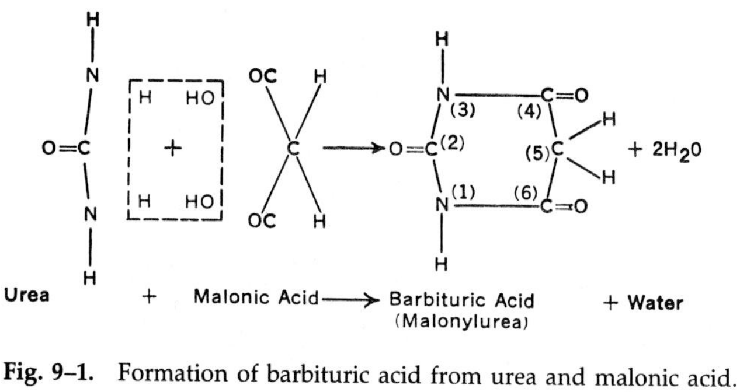

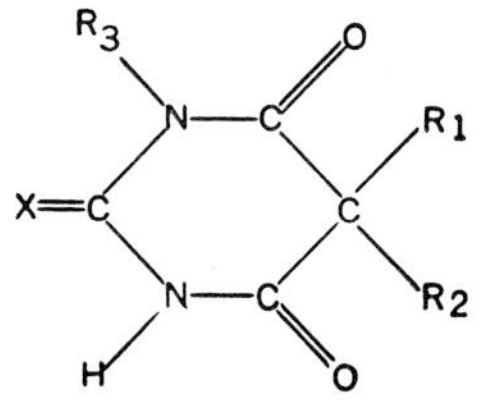

Fig. 9–2. General formula of the barbiturates.

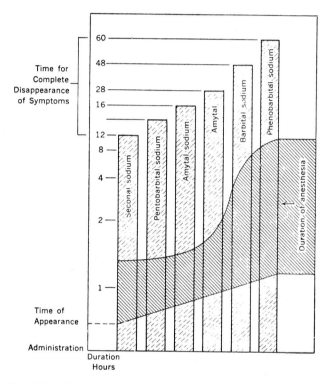

Fig. 9–3. Time of appearance, duration of anesthesia, and time needed for complete disappearance of symptoms after oral administration of equivalent single anesthetic doses in animals. (From Jones, L.M. Veterinary Pharmacology and Therapeutics, 4th ed. Iowa State University Press, Ames, Iowa, 1977.)

Fig. 9–1. Formation of barbituric acid from urea and malonic acid.

Substituted R_1-R_2 derivatives of barbituric acid behave as weak acids and unite with fixed alkalies to form soluble salts. These salts hydrolyze in water to varying degrees and form alkaline solutions. Those commonly employed in veterinary medicine have a pH of 10 or above, and for this reason may cause severe tissue damage and slough if injected perivascularly in any appreciable quantity.

CLASSIFICATION

The barbiturates have been classified into four groups according to duration of action (Fig. 9–3, Tables 9–2, 9–3): long, intermediate, short, and ultrashort. All of those used for clinical anesthesia fall in the short or ultrashort classification, whereas those used for seda-

Table 9–2. Names, Status, Chemical Structures, Duration of Action, and Excretion of the Barbiturates

Barbiturate	Status	Commercial Names or Synonyms	R_1	R_2	R_3	X	Duration of Action	Organ of Degradation and/or Excretion
Allylbarbituric acid	N.F.	Sandoptal	allyl	isobutyl	H	O	Intermediate	III
Amobarbital	U.S.P.	Amytal	ethyl	isoamyl	H	O	Intermediate	III
Aprobarbital	N.F.	Alurate	allyl	isopropyl	H	O	Intermediate	II
Barbital	N.F.	Veronal, Barbitone	ethyl	ethyl	H	O	Long	I
Butabarbital*	N.N.R.	Butisol	ethyl	sec-butyl	H	O	Intermediate	—
Butallylonal*	N.F.	Pernoston	2-bromallyl	sec-butyl	H	O	Intermediate	II
Butethal	N.F.	Neonal	ethyl	n-butyl	H	O	Intermediate	II
Cyclobarbital	N.F.	Phanodorn	ethyl	cyclohexenyl	H	O	Short	II
Cyclopal	–	–	allyl	cyclopentenyl	H	O	Short	II
Diallylbarbituric acid	N.F.	Dial	allyl	allyl	H	O	Long	II
Hexethal*	N.N.R.	Ortal	ethyl	n-hexyl	H	O	Intermediate	III
Hexobarbital†	N.F.	Evipal, Hexobarbitone	methyl	cyclohexenyl	CH$_3$	O	Ultrashort	IV
Kemithal†	–	–	allyl	cyclohexenyl	H	S	Ultrashort	IV
Mephobarbital	N.F.	Mebaral	ethyl	phenyl	CH$_3$	O	Long	II
Pentobarbital	U.S.P.	Nembutal	ethyl	1-methylbutyl	H	O	Short	III
Phenobarbital	U.S.P.	Luminal, Phenobarbitone	ethyl	phenyl	H	O	Long	I
Probarbital*	N.F.	Ipral	ethyl	isopropyl	H	O	Intermediate	III
Propallylonal	–	Nostal	isopropyl	2-bromallyl	H	O	Intermediate	III
Secobarbital*	U.S.P.	Seconal	allyl	1-methylbutyl	H	O	Short	III
Thiamylal†	N.N.R.	Surital	allyl	1-methylbutyl	H	S	Ultrashort	IV
Thiopental†	U.S.P.	Pentothal	ethyl	1-methylbutyl	H	S	Ultrashort	IV
Vinbarbital*	N.F.	Delvinal	ethyl	1-methyl-1-butenyl	H	O	Intermediate	II

*Employed principally as the sodium salt.
†Used for intravenous anesthesia, as sodium salt.
I Mainly excreted by kidney.
II Degraded by liver and excreted by kidney.
III Degraded by liver.
IV Absorbed by body fat, degraded by liver, and excreted by kidney.
(Adapted from Goodman, L.S., and Gilman, A. The Pharmacological Basis of Therapeutics, 2nd ed. Macmillan Publishing Co., New York, 1958.)

Table 9–3. Historical and Clinical Data of the Oxybarbiturates and Thiobarbiturates

Agent (Generic Name)	OXYBARBITURATES		
	Pentobarbital	Secobarbital	Hexobarbital
Trade Name	Nembutal Sodium Registered by Abbott Laboratories	Seconal Sodium Registered by Eli Lilly & Co.	Evipal Sodium Registered by Parke, Davis & Co.
Chemical Name	Sodium 5-ethyl-5(1-methylbutyl)-barbiturate	Sodium 5-allyl-5-(1-methylbutyl)-barbiturate	Sodium 1,5-dimethyl-5-(1-cyclo-hexenyl)-barbiturate
Formula	$C_{11}H_{17}N_2O_3$ Na	$C_{12}H_{17}N_2O_3$ Na	$C_{12}H_{15}N_2O_5$ Na
Discovery of Compound	1930 by Volwiler	1930 by Shonle	1932 by Krepp and Taub
Discovery of Anesthetic or Relaxant Properties	1930 by Volwiler and Tabern	1931 by Swanson	1932 by Weese and Scharpff
Type of Compound	5-substituted barbiturate	5 substituted barbiturate	N-substituted barbiturate
Molecular Weight	248.26	260.27	258.25
Buffer Employed	None	None	None
Preservative or Stabilizing Agent Used	None	Phenol, 0.25% and polyethylene glycol 200, 50%	None
Thermostability	Precipitates on heating	Precipitates on heating	Free acid melts at 146° C
Chemostability	Solution stable indefinitely	Solution stable up to 18 mo in sealed container; decomposes on exposure to air	Solution stable for 48 h if tightly stoppered
Onset of Action Duration of Action	30–60 s 1–2 h	30–60 s 1–2 h	30–60 s 15–30 min
Route and/or Organ of Detoxification or Elimination	Detoxified by the liver	Detoxified by the liver	Detoxified by the liver
Usual Mode of Administration	Intravenous, intrathoracic, intraperitoneal	Intravenous	Intravenous
Specific Pharmacologic Antagonist	Yohimbine plus 4-aminopyridine will partially antagonize pentobarbital and probably other barbiturates. Oxygen administration and artificial respiration recommended in respiratory arrest.		
pH of Solution	6%-pH 10.0–10.3	5%-pH 9.8–10.1	2.5%-pH 8.5–10.5

(Adapted from data compiled by Dr. W.H.L. Dornette and published by the Ohio Chemical and Surgical Equipment Company.)

tion or control of convulsions are of long or intermediate action.

GENERAL PHARMACOLOGY

Racemic mixtures of the barbiturates are used as both hypnotics and general anesthetics. The principal effect of a barbiturate is depression of the central nervous system by interference with passage of impulses to the cerebral cortex. Barbiturates act directly on CNS neurons in a manner similar to that of the inhibitory transmitter GABA. Barbiturate anesthesia is thought to be produced by the combined effect of enhanced inhibition and diminished excitation. Using mouse spinal cord tissue cultures, it has been demonstrated that barbiturate anesthetics and barbiturate anticonvulsants possess qualitative and quantitative differences that explain their different clinical effects.(3) The distinction between an anesthetic and an anticonvulsant barbiturate depends on the concentration at which amino acid modulation and GABA-mimetic activities occur. If both effects are present at similar concentrations, the agent will have anesthetic properties, whereas, if the threshold for modulatory activity is lower, the agent will be an effective anticonvulsant, with sedation only at toxic doses.

Ganglionic transmission is approximately 20 times more sensitive to pentobarbital than is axonal conduction (Chapter 7).(4) The fast excitatory postsynaptic

Methohexital	THIOBARBITURATES		
	Thiamylal	Thiopental	Thialbarbitone
Brevital	Surital Sodium	Pentothal Sodium	Kemithal Sodium
Registered by Eli Lilly & Co.	Registered by Parke, Davis & Co.	Registered by Abbott Laboratories	Registered by Fort Dodge Laboratories
Sodium a-dl-1-methyl-5-allyl-5-(1-methyl-2-pentynyl)-barbiturate	Sodium 5-allyl-5-(1-methylbutyl)-2-thiobarbiturate	Sodium 5-ethyl-5-(1-methylbutyl)-2-thiobarbiturate	Sodium 5-allyl-5-(2-cyclohexenyl)-2-thiobarbiturate
$C_{14}H_{17}N_2O_3$ Na	$C_{12}H_{17}N_2O_2$ SNa	$C_{11}H_{17}N_2O_2$ SNa	$C_{13}H_{15}N_2O_2$ SNa
1955 by Doran	1929 by Dox	1929 by Taburn and Volwiler	1938 by Carrington
1955 by Gibson	1933 by Gruhzit	1933 by Tatum	1946 by Carrington and Raventos
N-5-substituted barbiturate	5-substituted thiobarbiturate	5-substituted thiobarbiturate	5-substituted thiobarbiturate
284.0	276.33	264.23	286.3
Sodium carbonate	6% Sodium carbonate	6% Sodium carbonate	None
None	None	None	None
Deteriorates when boiled	Precipitates when boiled	Precipitates when boiled	Thermolabile
Solution stable at room temperature for 6 mo	Solution stable for 48–72 h if tightly stoppered	Solution stable for 48–72 h if tightly stoppered	Solution stable 7 days; indefinitely if frozen
10–30 s 5–15 min	20–30 s 10–15 min	20–30 s 10–15 min	20–30 s 15–45 min
Detoxified by the liver	Absorbed by fat and detoxified by the liver	Absorbed by fat and detoxified by the liver	Absorbed by fat and detoxified by the liver
Intravenous	Intravenous	Intravenous	Intravenous, intrathoracic, intraperitoneal
Yohimbine plus 4-aminopyridine will partially antagonize pentobarbital and probably other barbiturates. Oxygen administration and artificial respiration recommended in respiratory arrest.			
5%-pH 10.4–11.4	2.5%-pH 10.5–11	2.5%-pH 10.5–11	10%-pH 10.6

potential (EPSP) is approximately 10 times more sensitive to pentobarbital than are the slow potentials (slow EPSP and slow IPSP). Phenobarbital also exerts some degree of selectivity toward the fast EPSP. Anesthetic concentrations of pentobarbital selectively block the fast EPSP. A selective postsynaptic block of the nicotinic action of acetylcholine also occurs and may account for the anesthetic depressant effects of pentobarbital on ganglionic transmission. This selective depression on the nicotinic action of acetylcholine could occur by various molecular mechanisms, for example, by altering the binding of acetylcholine. Barbiturates might also be acting at some step after receptor activation by decreasing ion-channel conduction.

In hypnotic doses, the barbiturates have little effect upon respiration, whereas in anesthetic doses, respiration is depressed. Overdose produces respiratory paralysis and death. With anesthetic doses, there is cardiovascular depression, both centrally and peripherally, with a fall in blood pressure. In hypotic doses, barbiturates have little effect on the basal metabolic rate. With anesthetic doses, basal metabolism is depressed, resulting in lowered body temperature.

Following barbiturate administration leukocyte counts decrease in normal and splenectomized dogs.(5) Packed cell volume also decreases in nonsplenectomized dogs, presumably owing to splenic sequestration of red blood cells. There is no significant change in the differential counts (Tables 9–4 and 9–5).

The oxidation of pentobarbital, hexobarbital, and amobarbital is noncompetitively inhibited by halothane, methoxyflurane, and diethyl ether.(6) Saturation of the enzyme system by the anesthetic appears responsible. Chloramphenicol, a microsomal inhibitor, can markedly prolong recovery from barbiturate anesthesia.

Barbiturates administered during the prenatal period can produce permanent alterations in sexual maturity of hamsters and rats (7, 8), and perhaps an increased incidence of congenital malformations in humans.(9, 10)

DISTRIBUTION OF BARBITURATES

Barbiturates diffuse throughout the body, penetrating cell walls and crossing the placenta. The extent of ionization, lipid solubility (partition coefficient), and protein binding are the three most important factors in distribution and elimination of barbiturates.

Barbiturates are sodium salts of barbituric acid derivatives. When dissolved in water, they ionize. The degree of ionization is determined by the pH of the solution and the dissociation constant (pKa) of the agent. This dissociation constant is the pH at which the compound exists in equal quantities in the dissociated (ionized or polar) and undissociated (un-ionized or nonpolar) forms (Fig. 9–4). For a barbiturate to penetrate the lipoid of cell membranes, it must be in the undissociated or nonpolar form (Fig. 9–5). The more acidic the solution containing the drug, the more undissociated form that exists and the greater the amount that can penetrate cell membranes to produce deeper anesthesia. The reverse is also true; the more alkaline the solution, the greater the dissociation and the less the cell penetration that occurs.

At a blood pH of 7.4, a barbiturate assumes a "normal" distribution within the cells of the central nervous system and produces the desired degree of anesthesia. A change in blood pH, however, may lead to a change in the depth of anesthesia. An increase in acidity, such as commonly occurs with respiratory or metabolic acidosis, increases the depth. An increase

in alkalinity, caused by hyperventilation or administration of alkalinizing agents, increases dissociation. As a result, barbiturate migrates outward from the cells to the plasma, and anesthesia will lighten.(11) Alkalinization of the urine also decreases tubular reabsorption.

The undissociated form has a high affinity for nonpolar solvents. This varies between compounds as shown in Table 9–6. The highly lipid-soluble agents have a rapid onset and are short-acting. They are rapidly metabolized and also easily reabsorbed by the kidney tubules.

A reversible bond develops to plasma proteins, chiefly albumin, the degree of which agrees roughly with the partition coefficient. Because cerebrospinal fluid is practically protein-free, it contains less barbiturate than plasma (Table 9–7). Organ tissues contain a slightly higher level of barbiturate, while fat contains very high concentrations. Highly lipid-soluble compounds penetrate brain tissue quite rapidly, reaching equilibrium with two or three circulations of blood. Gray matter of the brain is penetrated rapidly, with white matter being slower to reach equilibrium (Table 9–8).

Termination of barbiturate anesthesia is produced by physical redistribution, metabolic degradation, and renal excretion. Again, the solubility coefficient dictates the chief route of elimination. Short-acting agents with a high solubility coefficient are largely reabsorbed from the kidney tubules. Their action ceases when they are metabolically transformed into inactive substances, principally in the liver. Long-acting agents with low lipid solubility are chiefly excreted through the kidneys. As much as 85% of barbital and phenobarbital may be recovered from the urine over several days following administration.(12) The short-acting barbiturates (pentobarbital, amobarbital, and secobarbital) are destroyed principally by the liver. Their rapid destruction in the body accounts for their shorter action. With anesthetic-inducing doses ultra-short-acting barbiturates are quickly redistributed, accounting for their short duration of action. Thiobarbiturates are not metabolized more rapidly than the oxybarbiturates.

Table 9–4. Leukocyte Counts and Packed-Cell Volumes in 12 Dogs Following Barbiturate Anesthesia

Time in minutes	Pentobarbital Leukocytes × 10³	PCV, %	Thiopental Leukocytes × 10³	PCV, %	Thiamylal Leukocytes × 10³	PCV, %	Methohexital Leukocytes × 10³	PCV, %
−30	13.7 ± 1.5*	50 ± 1.2	12.4 ± 1.0	49 ± 1.2	12.5 ± 1.1	48.5 ± 1.5	13.4 ± 1.4	50 ± 1.4
Anesthesia 0	13.6 ± 1.5	48 ± 1.5	12.2 ± 0.9	47 ± 1.0	12.7 ± 1.0	48 ± 1.2	13.5 ± 1.4	49 ± 1.1
+30	10.8 ± 1.3	40 ± 1.2	10.8 ± 1.0	40 ± 1.4	10.8 ± 1.0	41 ± 1.2	10.9 ± 1.2	42 ± 0.7
+60	10.9 ± 1.3	40 ± 1.5	10.7 ± 0.9	40 ± 1.6	10.1 ± 1.0	41 ± 1.4	11.0 ± 1.4	42 ± 1.0
+120	10.7 ± 1.4	40 ± 1.4	10.9 ± 1.1	42 ± 1.6	10.3 ± 1.1	43 ± 1.2	11.1 ± 1.2	44 ± 1.0
+180	10.8 ± 1.3	41 ± 1.0	11.3 ± 1.2	42 ± 1.3	10.7 ± 1.1	43 ± 1.2	10.9 ± 1.4	44 ± 1.1

*Mean ± standard deviation.

(From Usenik, E.A., and Cronkite, E.P. Effects of Barbiturate Anesthetics on Leukocytes in Normal and Splenectomized Dogs. Anesth Analg 44:167, 1965.)

Table 9–5. Leukocyte Counts and Packed Cell Volumes in 6 Splenectomized Dogs (2 Trials/Dog) Following Pentobarbital Anesthesia

Time in Minutes	Leukocytes × 10³	PCV, %
−30	14.2 ± 1.0*	46.5 ± 1.6
Anesthesia 0	13.9 ± 1.0	46 ± 1.9
+30	11.6 ± 1.1	45 ± 1.8
+60	11.2 ± 1.0	45 ± 1.8
+120	11.0 ± 1.1	45 ± 1.8
+180	11.0 ± 1.0	45 ± 1.9

*Mean ± standard deviation.
(From Usenik, E.A., and Cronkite, E.P. Effects of Barbiturate Anesthetics on Leukocytes in Normal and Splenectomized Dogs. Anesth Analg 44:167, 1965.)

THE "GLUCOSE EFFECT"?

A unique reanesthetizing action, termed the *glucose effect*, has been observed in animals recovering from barbiturate anesthesia that were subsequently given glucose. A species variation in susceptibility to this effect has been demonstrated; guinea pigs, chickens, pigeons, rabbits, and hamsters are susceptible; dogs are intermediate; and mice, rats, goldfish, and tadpoles are refractory or negative. Intermediates in the glycolysis of glucose and in the Krebs cycle have been shown to have the same effect. The *glucose effect* presumably occurs with most barbiturates and thiobarbiturates, but not with inhalation or other anesthetics. Glucose causes a decrease in activity of the components of the microsomal electron chain, resulting in decreased microsomal metabolism.(13) A study on the *glucose effect* on respiration and EEG in dogs following pentobarbital administration found no evidence of significant deepening of anesthesia as judged by cortical depression, decreasing rate or depth of respiration, or a decrease in minute volume.(14)

Epinephrine given intravenously to dogs or mice also causes a return of sleep on awakening from hexobarbital or chloral hydrate anesthesia. Norepinephrine is less effective in producing this effect.(15) This phenomenon presumably is caused by increased glucose levels in the blood and should be remembered when the use of epinephrine is considered in barbiturate-anesthetized dogs. The effect of glucose, sodium lactate, and epinephrine on thiopental anesthesia in dogs has also been studied (Table 9–9). It does not appear that the *glucose effect* is of practical concern as long as these drugs are used in therapeutic doses.(16)

THERAPEUTIC USES OF BARBITURATES

Barbiturates are used to induce sedation and hypnosis, as anticonvulsants, and as anesthetics. Their use as sedatives and hypnotics in low doses has been supplanted,

pK_a = dissociation constant
or
pH at which equal amount of drug is in ionized and unionized forms.

$$HA \rightleftarrows H^+ + A^-$$

Barbiturate	pK_a
Thiopental	7.4
Secobarbital	7.9
Pentobarbital	8.0

Fig. 9–4. Dissociation of barbiturates.

in most instances, by tranquilizers. The ability of barbiturates to depress the motor cortex has been utilized to treat convulsions associated with poisoning, particularly strychnine, "running fits," distemper encephalitis, and overdosage of local anesthetics. In modern veterinary medicine, the thiobarbiturates are primarily used as induction agents or short-acting anesthetics, whereas pentobarbital is now used sparingly because of its propensity to cause prolonged, rough recoveries when administered in anesthetic doses.

ADDICTION TO BARBITURATES

Although barbiturate addiction can be produced in animals, it is by its very nature self-limiting; however, in man repeated oral use of barbiturates as soporifics or sedatives may become habit-forming. For this reason, legislation in many countries prohibits use of these drugs without a prescription. Veterinarians should be acquainted with applicable laws regarding their use and sale to avoid infraction and to prevent liability.

OXYBARBITURATES

Phenobarbital Sodium, U. S. P. (Phenobarbital). Phenobarbital was synthesized in 1912 in Germany and marketed under the trade name Luminal. It is a long-acting barbiturate, and advantage has been taken of its prolonged action in treating various convulsive disorders (Fig. 9–3). In control of convulsions due to distemper encephalitis, it appears to be as effective as any of the newer drugs and considerably cheaper. Because it is excreted slowly in the urine, it tends to be cumulative. An oral "loading dose" should be administered first, followed by a daily maintenance dose. In the average dog (10 kg), this would be 60 mg initially followed by 15 mg three times a day. Loss of motor coordination results from overdose; when this occurs, the dose should be reduced. Serial assays on serum, saliva, and cerebrospinal fluid (CSF) have shown considerable daily fluctuation of phenobarbital levels, even after several weeks of therapy. A gradually increasing phenobarbital concentration occurs in the three fluids up to doses of 9.0 mg/kg. Serum or saliva assays can accurately indicate the phenobarbital concentration in CSF.(17)

In animals suffering from strychnine poisoning, phenobarbital solution may be given intravenously "to effect" in the same manner as one would administer pentobarbital sodium. Phenobarbital is a hepatic microsomal enzyme inducer. Concomitant administration of phenobarbital and digoxin can shorten the biologic half-life of the latter by approximately 30%.(18)

Pentobarbital Sodium, U. S. P. (Nembutal). Pentobarbital sodium came into general use as an anesthetic agent for dogs and cats in the early 1930s and slowly supplanted ether administered by open mask methods as the anesthetic of choice. By 1940 its use was widespread. Today, it has largely been replaced by inhalation and balanced anesthetic techniques.

Commercial preparations of pentobarbital are racemic mixtures. Administration of subanesthetic doses is often associated with stimulation of the central nervous system and preanesthetic excitation. The (+) isomer of pentobarbital causes a transient period of hyperexcitability before depressing the CNS, whereas the (−) isomer produces relatively smooth and progressively deeper hypnosis.(19)

Studies of the cellular mechanisms underlying this phenomenon have revealed that the drug depresses neuronal excitability in various ways.(20) Two depressant effects appear to be caused primarily by the (−) isomer of the drug. One of these involves an increase in Cl^- conductance. It is likely that the effects of the (−) isomer of pentobarbital are mediated through activation of GABA receptors. Pentobarbital opens GABA-activated channels that remain open for longer periods than when activated by GABA alone.

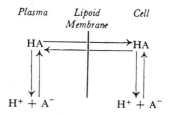

Fig. 9–5. Barbiturate dissociation. Cell membrane is permeable only to undissociated (un-ionized) barbiturate.

Pentobarbital sodium occurs as a white powder or crystalline granules. It is freely soluble in water or alcohol. It forms a clear, colorless solution that is marketed under several trade names. Aqueous solutions have an alkaline pH and may precipitate on standing, but the drug can be redissolved by addition of alkali such as sodium hydroxide. The calculated dose for dogs and cats is 30 mg per kg of body weight; however, it should be emphasized that pentobarbital is given "to effect." Following a single intravenous dose of pentobarbital, there is a decrease in arterial blood pressure. The heart rate increases for 10 to 20 minutes and then stabilizes or decreases. Cardiac output is variable, while peripheral vascular resistance increases (Fig. 9–6).

The cardiovascular effects of prolonged pentobarbital (2½ hours) anesthesia in dogs has been assessed. Systolic blood pressure, initial ventricular impulse, stroke volume, pulse pressure, central venous pressure, PaO_2, pH, and body temperature are all decreased following anesthetic doses of pentobarbital. Heart rate, $PaCO_2$, and peripheral resistance increased after 1½ hours. Cardiac output eventually decreases. Mean arterial pressure significantly decreases during induction, but usually returns to awake values in approximately 30 minutes (Table 9–10).(21) Intravenous pentobarbital administration alters myocardial function and distribution of blood flow. In dogs, it was found that intravenous pentobarbital decreases contractile force by 17.4%, arterial blood pressure by 4.8%, and renal blood flow by 8.4%, while increasing cardiac output by 4.8% and superior mesenteric artery flow by 14.1%. The decreased arterial blood pressure was believed to be due to vasodilation of major vascular beds, and the increased cardiac output due to increased venous return.(22) Respiration is initially depressed and gradually increases during recovery (23).

Light pentobarbital anesthesia has little influence on renal hemodynamics. Deep anesthesia depresses renal

Table 9–6.   **Barbiturates: Relation Between Physicochemical Factors, Distribution, and Fate**

Barbiturate	Partition Coefficient[a]	Plasma Protein Binding[b]	Brain Protein Binding[c]	Delay in Onset of Activity[d]	Excreted by Kidney[e]	Degradation by Liver Slices[f]	pKa[g]
Barbital	1	0.05	0.06	22	65–90	−	7.8
Phenobarbital	3	0.20	0.19	12	30	−	7.3
Pentobarbital	39	0.35	0.29	0.1	−	0.21	8.0
Secobarbital	52	0.44	0.39	0.1	−	0.28	7.9
Thiopental	580	0.65	0.50	−	−	0.38	7.4

[a](Concentration in methylene chloride):(concentration in aqueous phase) of the nonionized form at approximately 25° C.
[b]Binding of 0.001 M barbituric acid by 1% bovine serum albumin in M/15 phosphate buffer at pH 7.4; fraction bound.
[c]Fraction of barbiturate bound by rabbit brain homogenates.
[d]Minutes until anesthesia after intravenous injection in mice.
[e]Approximate percentage of total dose excreted unchanged in urine of man.
[f]Fraction degraded in vitro by liver slices in 3 hours.
[g]Ionization exponent at 25° C.
(From Goodman, L.S., and Gilman, A., eds. The Pharmacological Basis of Therapeutics, 4th ed. Macmillan, New York, 1970.)

Table 9–7. Rates of Passage of Drugs from Bloodstream into CSF of Dogs and Degrees of Ionization of Drugs at pH 7.4

Drug	Percent Un-ionized at pH 7.4	Permeability Coefficient*	Heptane-Water Partition Coefficient of Un-ionized Form of Drug
Barbital	55.7	0.026	0.002
Thiopental	61.3	0.50	3.3
Pentobarbital	83.4	0.17	0.05

*The higher the permeability coefficient, the more rapid the rate of entry into the CSF.
(From Shanker, L.S. Penetration of Drugs into the Central Nervous System. In: Uptake and Distribution of Anesthetic Agents. Edited by E.M. Papper and R.J. Kitz. McGraw-Hill, New York, 1963.)

Table 9–8. Influence of Carbon Dioxide on Penetration of Brain by Drugs

Area	Concentration in Brain		Relative Penetration
	Hypercapnic Acidosis	Hypocapnic Alkalosis	
	Urea (1 hr)		
Gray	0.40	0.16	2.50
White	0.12	0.05	2.40
	Phenobarbital (½ hr)		
Gray	1.20	0.72	1.67
White	1.08	0.40	2.70
	Salicylic Acid (1 hr)		
Gray	0.44	0.11	4.00
White	0.38	0.04	9.50

Concentration in brain is expressed as a fraction of levels in plasma (relative penetration: brain fractions under conditions of hypercapnia to brain fraction under conditions of hypocapnia). Note the disproportionate increase in penetration of white matter by salicylic acid under conditions of hypercapnia. Gray: cerebral cortex; white: cerebral white matter.
(From Roth, L.J., and Barlow, C.F. Drugs in the Brain. Science 134:22, 1961. Copyright 1961 by the American Association for Advancement of Science.)

Table 9–9. Relative Ability of Glucose, Sodium Lactate, and Epinephrine to Cause Anesthetic Rebound* in Dogs Recovering from Thiopental Anesthesia

Drug and Dosage	Dogs Given Injections (No.)	Dogs Rebounded (No.)	(%)	Average Increase in Sleep Time (%)
Glucose, 600.0 mg/kg	18	2	11.1	47.9
Sodium lactate, 60.0 mg/kg	18	7	38.9	48.9
Epinephrine, 0.1 mg/kg	13	11	84.6	38.8
Saline solution, 1.0 ml/kg	12	0	0	0

*Apparent reanesthetization as indicated by loss of voluntary and involuntary movements and possible loss of pedal reflexes.
(From Hatch, R.C. The Effect of Glucose, Sodium Lactate and Epinephrine on Thiopental Anesthesia in Dogs. J Am Vet Med Assoc, 148:135, 1966.)

function, both blood and urine flow, by circulatory depression and also by reflex vasoconstriction. Pentobarbital inhibits water diuresis by stimulating release of antidiuretic hormone (24).

Leukopenia is found in dogs anesthetized with pentobarbital (25). Leukocyte counts drop to 20% of control values (Fig. 9–7). Although the absolute differential white count decreases, there is a relative lymphocytosis that reaches its peak at 90 minutes and then returns to normal. Red cell numbers decrease also. Hemoglobin and hematocrit values show corresponding changes. Pentobarbital, amobarbital, and thiopental produce dilation of the spleen, which presumably accounts for the decrease in erythrocytes (26). Maximum dilation usually occurs 20 to 30 minutes after injection of the anesthetic. Sedimentation rate and coagulation time are both increased, while prothrombin time is decreased. Oral administration of pentobarbital sodium in sedative doses does not affect the blood constituents in the same fashion.

In some animals, the effect produced by high doses of pentobarbital is difficult to differentiate from shock. The size of the dose and method of its administration are the major factors in variation of response to pentobarbital. Individual variations undoubtedly exist. Roughly one of four animals given a dose of 30 mg/kg develops side effects that mimic some phase of shock.(27)

On intraperitoneal administration, the peak concentration in the blood is reached more slowly than with intravenous injection, and the portion of drug absorbed into the portal system is subjected to early destruction in the liver. When a 2.5% aqueous solution is given intraperitoneally in a dose of 30 mg/kg of body weight, anesthesia is not accompanied by impaired renal function and arterial blood pressure increases.(28) When given radiolabeled pentobarbital orally, dogs excrete about 60% of the total dose in the urine during the first 24 hours.(29) Over 92% is excreted as metabolic products derived from the drug, and only 3% is in the form of pentobarbital. Elimination of pentobarbital from the blood of both intact and bilaterally nephrectomized

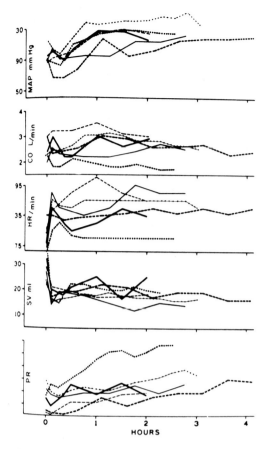

Fig. 9–6. Long-term changes from pentobarbital in 6 dogs. MAP, mean arterial pressure; CO, cardiac output; HR, heart rate; SV, stroke volume; and PR, peripheral resistance. Note large and abrupt increase in heart rate and decrease in stroke volume at the onset of the experiments. (From Olmsted, F., and Page, I.H. Hemodynamic Changes in Dogs Caused by Sodium Pentobarbital Anesthesia. Am J Physiol 210:817, 1966.)

dogs is similar because elimination is totally dependent upon biotransformation of pentobarbital by the liver (30). The absence of renal function per se does not seem to alter the pharmacokinetics of pentobarbital; however, the sensitivity of a patient to the action of barbiturates may be increased by uremia. This phenomenon is probably caused by the decreased capacity of plasma protein to bind acidic drugs.

Pentobarbital freely crosses the placental barrier and enters the fetus. For this reason, its use as a monoanesthetic (high dose) for cesarean section results in high mortality in the newborn. Neonates can be viable at birth but usually do not recover from anesthesia and are unable to nurse.

The duration of surgical analgesia with anesthetizing doses of pentobarbital varies widely with individual animals, averaging about 30 minutes. Complete recovery usually occurs in 6 to 18 hours. Occasional animals, particularly cats, may not rouse for as long as 24 to 72 hours.

Pentobarbital is no longer used in North America to produce anesthesia in cattle and horses, owing to the prolonged recovery period and marked respiratory depression. It has been administered by slow intravenous injection (15 to 30 mg/kg) in foals and young cattle. Because of prolonged recovery, pentobarbital should not be administered to animals under 1 month of age. In adult cattle, anesthesia has been induced with 14 mg/kg intravenously; half of the dose is injected rapidly, the animal is positioned on its sternum, and the remainder is injected slowly to effect.(31) Pentobarbital has also been administered with chloral hydrate or thiopental sodium to induce anesthesia in adult horses (32) and in goats before administration of inhalant anesthetics.(33)

The intravenous anesthetic dose in adult goats is 30 mg/kg, which maintains anesthesia for approximately 20 minutes. Anesthesia can be maintained by doses of 6 to 36 mg · kg^{-1} · h^{-1} of pentobarbital. The induction and intubation dose ranges from 10 to 42 mg/kg. A similar technique for intravenous pentobarbital in sheep has been described.(34) Like goats, sheep rapidly metabolize pentobarbital, and additional doses are required to maintain anesthesia for periods longer than 20 to 30 minutes. The anesthetic dose of pentobarbital sodium is approximately 25 mg/kg in adult sheep. In all ruminants, immediate intubation to prevent aspiration of regurgitated rumen contents is essential.

In swine, a 10- to 30-mg/kg dose of pentobarbital given intravenously provides anesthesia for 15 to 45 minutes. If anesthesia is induced until reflex response to surgical stimulation is abolished, respiratory depression is often severe, and apnea may occur.

Animals awakening from pentobarbital anesthesia tend to exhibit the same signs as when they are anesthetized, except in reverse order. These include crying, shivering, involuntary running movements, thrashing, increased respiratory movements followed by recovery of the righting reflex, and later, ability to stand with a staggering gait. Because recovery is slow, without preanesthetic medication these actions may become so exaggerated that the animal injures itself through contact with the cage or stall or causes wound disruption. Greyhounds are notable for this effect. Show animals have been known to break teeth, much to the embarrassment of the veterinarian. Administration of a narcotic or a tranquilizer is always indicated in cases of emergence excitement. Yohimbine plus 4-aminopyridine will incompletely antagonize pentobarbital-induced CNS depression in dogs preanesthetized with atropine-xylazine or atropine-acepromazine.(35)

Methohexital Sodium (Brevital). Methohexital sodium is an ultra-short-acting barbiturate that is unique in that it contains no sulfur atom. Its short duration is owing more to redistribution than to rapid metabolism. Blood concentrations necessary to produce anesthesia are approximately one half of those required with thiopental or thiamylal. According to the manufacturer, a

Table 9–10. Cardiovascular Responses to Pentobarbital Anesthesia in 12 Dogs

Parameters	Control	Time After Pentobarbital					
		0 h[a]	½ h	1 h	1½ h	2 h	2½ h
Systolic blood pressure (mm Hg)	142 ± 3	116 ± 5[c]	123 ± 4[c]	121 ± 3[c]	122 ± 3[c]	124 ± 3[c]	130 ± 3[c]
	100%[b]	82 ± 3	87 ± 3	86 ± 3	86 ± 2	88 ± 2	92 ± 2
Mean blood pressure (mm Hg)	108 ± 4	95 ± 4[c]	104 ± 4	106 ± 3	108 ± 2	111 ± 3	117 ± 3
	100%	89 ± 4	97 ± 4	99 ± 4	101 ± 3	104 ± 4	109 ± 4
Diastolic blood pressure (mm Hg)	83 ± 3	80 ± 4	89 ± 4	93 ± 3[c]	95 ± 2[c]	90 ± 3[c]	105 ± 3[c]
	100%	98 ± 5	109 ± 5	115 ± 6	117 ± 5	122 ± 6	127 ± 6
Pulse pressure (mm Hg)	59 ± 2.6	36 ± 2.4[c]	34 ± 1.9[c]	28 ± 2.2[c]	27 ± 1.9[c]	26 ± 1.3[c]	25 ± 1.4[c]
Central venous pressure (mm Hg)	+1.44 ± 0.7	+0.14 ± 0.4[c]	−0.4 ± 0.4[c]	−1.00 ± 0.5[c]	−1.25 ± 0.5[c]	−1.08 ± 0.5[c]	−1.55 ± 0.6[c]
Heart rate (beats/min)	96 ± 5	157 ± 5[c]	153 ± 7[c]	157 ± 8[c]	141 ± 7[c]	135 ± 7[c]	146 ± 10[c]
	100%	167 ± 9	165 ± 11	168 ± 9	155 ± 10	146 ± 11	157 ± 12
Initial ventricular impulse (angle in °)	7 ± 0.4	9 ± 0.4[c]	9.8 ± 0.5[c]	10.1 ± 1[c]	12.5 ± 0.9[c]	13.8 ± 1[c]	14.7 ± 0.9[c]
	100%	130 ± 6	142 ± 8	147 ± 15	180 ± 11	193 ± 11	212 ± 11
Cardiac output (L/min)	1.734 ± 0.15	1.834 ± 0.14	1.811 ± 0.09	1.502 ± 0.11[c]	1.324 ± 0.12[c]	1.195 ± 0.10[c]	1.172 ± 0.09[c]
	100%	111 ± 8	111 ± 8	90 ± 5	79 ± 6	71 ± 5	70 ± 5
Stroke volume (ml/beat)	18.6 ± 2	11.8 ± 1[c]	12.3 ± 1[c]	10.1 ± 1[c]	9.5 ± 1[c]	9.4 ± 1[c]	8.9 ± 1[c]
	100%	66 ± 4	68 ± 3	54 ± 2	51 ± 1	50 ± 3	47 ± 4
Total peripheral resistance (dynes-sec/cm⁵)	5287 ± 558	4574 ± 385	4819 ± 419	6200 ± 551	7370 ± 696[c]	8535 ± 942[c]	8864 ± 1928[c]
	100%	91 ± 7	95 ± 6	124 ± 11	142 ± 8	163 ± 10	168 ± 8
P_aO_2 (mm Hg)	93.5 ± 3	60 ± 5[c]	70 ± 3[c]	73.5 ± 6[c]	70 ± 6[c]	77 ± 4[c]	75 ± 5[c]
	100%	61 ± 5	72 ± 4	75 ± 7	80 ± 6	79 ± 5	76 ± 6
P_aCO_2 (mm Hg)	30.9 ± 0.8	40.9 ± 3[c]	44 ± 2[c]	41 ± 3[c]	38 ± 3[c]	38 ± 3[c]	38 ± 3[c]
	100%	132 ± 9	141 ± 5	133 ± 8	121 ± 7	123 ± 9	123 ± 7
pH arterial	7.38 ± 0.01	7.27 ± 0.03[c]	7.27 ± 0.03[c]	7.29 ± 0.03[c]	7.30 ± 0.02[c]	7.30 ± 0.03[c]	7.32 ± 0.03[c]
Temperature (°C)	38.8 ± 0.2	38.7 ± 0.2[c]	38.5 ± 0.2[c]	38.1 ± 0.2[c]	37.9 ± 0.2[c]	37.6 ± 0.2[c]	37.4 ± 0.2[c]

[a]0, time values taken 3 to 5 min after pentobarbital IV.
[b]Each value indicates mean ± S.E. with % of control ± S.E. below.
[c]Denotes statistically significant changes with P < .05.
(From Priano, L.L., Traber, D.L., and Wilson, R.D. Barbiturate Anesthesia: An Abnormal Physiologic Situation. J Pharmacol Exp Ther 165:126, 1969.)

double dose rapidly administered intravenously causes temporary apnea. The lethal dose is said to be approximately 2.5 times greater than the median anesthetic dose. Animals die because of respiratory failure. Methohexital sodium is supplied as 500 mg of dry powder in glass vials. It is diluted with water or normal saline to form a 2.5% solution for injection. Solutions are said to

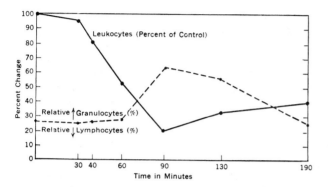

Fig. 9–7. The relative percent change in white cell counts with intravenous pentobarbital sodium anesthesia in 12 dogs as compared to control levels in unanesthetized dogs. The relative percent distribution of lymphocytes and granulocytes is shown on the same scale. (From Graca, J.G., and Garst, E.L. Early Blood Changes in Dogs Following Intravenous Pentobarbital Anesthesia. Anesthesiology 18:461, 1957.)

be stable for as long as 6 months at room temperature. The dose for the dog or cat is 6 to 10 mg/kg of body weight. Half of the estimated dose is injected intravenously at a rapid rate, following which administration is continued to effect. Surgical anesthesia for 5 to 15 minutes is obtained by an initial injection. More prolonged anesthesia can be maintained by intermittent administration or continuous drip. Recovery is quick and may be accompanied by muscular tremors and violent excitement, which detract from the usefulness of the drug. Dogs are usually ambulatory 30 minutes after administration ceases.

Methohexital has been used alone and with several preanesthetics in horses (Table 9–11). Even with preanesthetic sedation, the recovery period is characterized by muscle tremors and struggling.(36) For this reason, the anesthesia produced is undesirable except when followed by administration of an inhalant anesthetic. Under these circumstances, it proves to be a good drug for induction, since its effects are short-lasting. One injection provides just sufficient time for intubation and administration of the inhalant before its effect ceases, leaving the horse anesthetized with only the inhalant. The induction dose in the horse is approximately 6 mg/kg. It must be given rapidly or anesthesia will not be achieved.

Methohexital has been used to induce anesthesia in calves at the rate of 3 to 5 mg/kg. A smooth, rapid induction allowing endotracheal intubation is pro-

Table 9–11. Effect of Methohexital Sodium on the Horse Following Premedication with Morphine, Meperidine, or Promazine (Using 4 Horses per Treatment)

Premedication	Induction Time (sec)		Duration (min)		Time to Stand (min)		Number of Horses and Type of Recovery*
	Mean	Range	Mean	Range	Mean	Range	
Nil	26	23–32	4	3–5.5	21	15–29	4+++
Meperidine†	18	10–25	6	3–16	18	11–30	2+++ 2++
Morphine†	16	10–20	5	2–9	19	10–27	2+++ 1++ 1+
Meperidine Morphine	20	20–21	5	2–7	17	10–34	2+++ 1++ 1+
Promazine†	32	25–35	9	7–10	12	9–16	4+++
Promazine Meperidine	21	13–30	10	7–13	18	9–26	1++ 3+
Promazine Morphine	24	20–30	7	4–9	27	22–30	1++ 3+
Promazine Meperidine Morphine	27	21–35	8	6–11	17	5–30	1++ 3+

*+ Hyperesthesia; ++ mild paddling; +++ severe paddling.

†The dose rates used in this trial were: meperidine 1 mg/lb body weight subcutaneously; morphine sulphate 20 mg/100 lb body weight; promazine 0.25 mg/lb body weight; methohexital sodium 1 g/300 to 400 lb body weight.

(From Grono, L.R. Methohexital Sodium Anaesthesia in the Horse. Aust Vet J 42:398, 1966.)

duced.(37) In adult cattle, the dose for induction is 6 mg/kg.(38)

A high percentage of the metabolites of methohexital is excreted in the bile of dogs and rats. Following administration of ^{14}C-labeled methohexital to dogs and rats, 30.1 and 82.7% of the radioactivity is found in the feces, respectively. In the dog, 21.7% is excreted in bile and urine in the first hour and 52.4% in 8 hours.(39)

THIOBARBITURATES

Thiopental Sodium, U. S. P. (Pentothal). Thiopental was the first thiobarbiturate to gain popularity as an anesthetic agent for animals. It is the thio analogue of pentobarbital sodium, and only differs in that the number 2 carbon has a sulfur atom attached to it instead of an oxygen atom. Thiopental sodium is a yellow crystalline powder that is unstable in aqueous solution or when it is exposed to atmospheric air. For this reason, it is dispensed in sealed containers as a powder buffered with sodium carbonate. It is usually mixed with sterile water or saline to form 2.5%, 5.0%, or 10% solutions. Thiopental solutions should be stored in a refrigerator at 5 to 6° C (41 to 42° F) to retard deterioration. As solutions age, they become turbid and crystals precipitate. This results in progressive loss of activity but does not increase toxicity of the drug. Because the potency is decreased, larger quantities of solution must be used to produce the desired effect.(40)

The metabolism of thiopental is exceedingly complex. Following injection with thiopental containing radioactive sulfur (^{35}S), monkeys produce at least 12 different metabolic products that are excreted in the urine. About 86% is found in the urine within 4 days after intravenous injection; small amounts are also found in the tissues and feces.(41)

The initial toxic effect produced by thiopental is a marked depression of the respiratory centers. Both rate and amplitude are affected. Five minutes after administration of thiopental, heart rate, aortic pressure, peripheral vascular resistance, and left ventricular systolic and end-diastolic pressures increase.(42) Bigeminy is common. Cardiac arrhythmias associated with thiobarbiturate anesthesia can be accentuated by xylazine, halothane, methoxyflurane, and epinephrine.(43-46) These arrhythmias include sinus tachycardia, bigeminy, extrasystoles, ventricular tachycardia, multifocal ventricular tachycardia, and ventricular fibrillation. Administration of a lidocaine bolus concurrently with thiopental (11 mg/kg) reduces the cardiopulmonary depressive effects of the latter and has been advocated for anesthetic induction of patients predisposed to cardiac arrhythmias.(42)

During prolonged thiopental anesthesia, there is a pronounced hyperglycemia, increased lactic acid and amino acids in blood, and decreased liver glycogen.(47) Insulin either prevents a decrease or favors increased storage of liver glycogen. Animals on a high-protein diet or high-carbohydrate diet require more thiopental for surgical anesthesia than animals maintained on a "normal diet." Repeated doses of thiopental have a cumulative effect, as shown in Figure 9–8. Prolonged periods of anesthesia may result from this effect if numerous doses are administered.

Thiopental has an ultrashort action because it is rapidly redistributed (e.g., muscle tissue) and becomes localized in body fat.(48) As concentrations in the plasma, muscle, and viscera fall, thiopental concentration in fat continues to rise. On the other hand, an appreciable amount is metabolized by the liver, and this contributes to the early rapid reduction of arterial thiopental concentration.(49) The same effect occurs after a fatty meal. A high chylomicron level in the blood produces a significant reduction in sleeping time because thiopental is in more intimate contact with chylomicrons and a smaller diffusion distance is present. Blood fat is more potent than depot fat in decreasing thiopental sleeping time.(50) Leukopenia, hyperglycemia, elevated arterial PCO_2, and decreased arterial PO_2 have been observed in thiopental-anesthetized horses (Table 9–12), and are comparable to changes observed with other barbiturates and in other species.

For small animals, 1.25%, 2.5%, and 5.0% solutions of thiopental are used, depending upon the animal's size. Whenever convenient, the more dilute solutions should be used, since overdosing is less likely and irritation is less in the event of accidental perivascular injection. As in other species, thiopental may be used in the dog and cat as the sole anesthetic or for induction prior to inhalation anesthesia. For rapid induction of anesthesia of short duration, the dose is 10 to 12 mg/kg. Should 10 to 20 minutes of surgical anesthesia be required, the dose range is 20 to 30 mg/kg. One third of the estimated

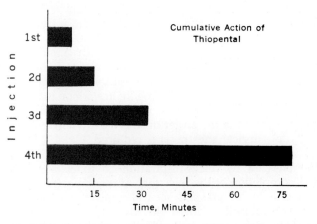

Fig. 9–8. The average duration of anesthesia after successive hourly intravenous injections of equal doses of thiopental to dogs. (From Wyngaarden, J.N., Woods, L.A., Ridley, R., and Seevers, M.H. Anesthetic Properties of Sodium-5-allyl-5-(1-methylbutyl)-2-thiobarbiturate (Surital) and Certain Other Thiobarbiturates in Dogs. J Pharmacol Exp Ther 95:322, 1949.)

Table 9–12. Mean Values of the Parameters Listed Below Following a Single Intravenous Anesthetic Dosage of Thiopental Sodium in 8 Horses*

	Preanesthetic Value	Minutes after Administering Anesthesia			Statistical Differences
		5	15	25	
Leukocyte count cell/mm^3	9700	7800	7500	6100	I
Packed-cell volume (vol %)	32	31	30.5	31	
Blood glucose (mg %)	82.1	85.0	91.2	103.1	I
Heart rate† (per min)	61	85	95	81	I
Blood pressure‡ (mm Hg) Systolic/diastolic	158/117	188/153	173/141	176/140	I
Respiratory rate‡ (per min)	29	8	14	21	I
O$_2$ content of arterial blood (vol %)	19.2	19.0	18.2	18.4	II
O$_2$ content of venous blood (vol %)	14.3	13.5	13.0	12.8	II
CO$_2$ content of arterial blood (vol %)	43.3	44.2	49.9	49.2	I
Arterial blood (pH)	7.39	7.31	7.21	7.22	I
Plasma level of thiopental Na (mg/L)	–	49.3	37.1	35.8	I

*To produce surgical anesthesia, 9 to 17 mg/kg were required.
†Mean values in 6 horses because of equipment failure.
‡Mean values in 5 horses because of equipment failure.
I Statistically significant difference at the 1% level before and after administration of thiopental sodium.
II Statistically significant difference at the 5% level before and after administration of thiopental sodium.
(From Tyagi, R.P.S., Arnold, J.P., Usenik, E.A., and Fletchers, T.P. Effects of Thiopental Sodium (Pentothal Sodium) Anesthesia on the Horse. Cornell Vet 54:584, 1964.)

dose is injected rapidly within 15 seconds, and the remainder is administered slowly to effect. Additional doses may be administered to prolong anesthesia when required. Following large dose administration recovery (to standing) usually requires 1 to 1½ hours. Large doses will saturate the tissues and cause a prolonged emergence. When induction is preceded by preanesthetic sedation, a dose range of 8 to 15 mg/kg is used. As in other species, too large a dose prior to inhalation anesthesia depresses respirations and impairs the uptake of inhaled gases. The use of thiopental is contraindicated in the neonate and in feline porphyria.

Thiopental was commonly used for rapid induction of anesthesia in the horse during the 1950s and early 1960s. After preanesthetic sedation with a suitable tranquilizer (e.g., xylazine, acepromazine), 6 to 10 mg/kg of thiopental are injected intravenously. If injected as rapidly as possible, 6.0 to 9.0 mg/kg are adequate. The smaller dose is used prior to the use of inhalant anesthetics, while the larger dose is used when a short period of surgical anesthesia is required.

The response to thiopental induction in horses is characterized by deep inspiration 20 to 30 seconds after completion of the injection. At this time, the head rope should be grasped securely and the head extended and pulled down slightly. This usually prevents the horse from falling backward. By pulling on both the head and tail at the time of induction, one can usually dictate the side on which the horse falls. Since the horse may occasionally fall heavily, animals with full stomachs should not be induced in this

manner, for gastric rupture may result. In the event that a longer duration of anesthesia is required, larger doses are used, half being injected rapidly and the remainder slowly after the horse is recumbent. Anesthesia may also be prolonged by combination of the thiopental with glyceryl guaiacolate. Occasionally an induction dose of thiopental is injected in the horse without apparent effect. This usually results from perivascular injection, inadequate dosage, or too slow an injection. Since the margin of safety is large, the procedure may be repeated without ill effect, although recovery may be prolonged. If preanesthetic sedation is inadequate, emergence struggling and floundering may occur. The recovery period (to standing) is prolonged if limb movement is restricted by bandages, splints, or casts.

To facilitate subsequent intubation, an induction dose of thiopental may be immediately followed, before the animal falls, by intravenous injection of 0.15 mg/kg of succinylcholine chloride. This has the same disadvantage as the use of succinylcholine alone, namely tachycardia, cardiac arrhythmia, and apnea. Rapid induction with thiopental alone, on the other hand, induces a moderate tachycardia, a slight reduction in mean arterial blood pressure, and a short period of respiratory depression.(51) Rapid intravenous injection of thiopental is usually followed by slow irregular respirations and sometimes a brief period of apnea (up to 1 or 2 minutes). Should apnea occur, a sharp slap on the thoracic wall usually initiates spontaneous respiration. Because recovery may be unduly prolonged, the use of thiopental is contraindicated in the newborn foal.

This rapid injection technique is also contraindicated in animals in shock or in those with uncompensated cardiovascular disease.

Similar doses of thiopental alone (4–6 mg/kg) or with 5% guaifenesin in 5% dextrose in water may be given to induce anesthesia in the horse and cow. Once anesthesia is induced in cattle, endotracheal intubation to prevent possible aspiration of rumen contents is essential. The possibility of this is reduced by positioning the animal so that the anterior thoracic and caudal cervical region is higher than any other part of the body. As in the newborn foal, use of thiopental is contraindicated in the neonatal calf. Thiopental is also used in doses of 8 to 15 mg/kg in small ruminants. Rapid intravenous induction can be achieved with 8 to 12 mg/kg, whereas larger doses are given by slow intravenous injection to effect. The latter technique provides 10 to 20 minutes of surgical anesthesia.

The dose of thiopental required to induce anesthesia in swine is variable. The minimal dose required ranges from 4.0 mg to 8.0 mg/kg. Half the dose is injected rapidly, and the remainder more slowly over the next several minutes. Even during light anesthesia, respiratory depression, irregular breathing, and apnea commonly occur in swine.

Thiamylal Sodium (Surital). Thiamylal sodium is the thio analogue of the barbiturate, secobarbital sodium. It differs from thiopental sodium in that the ethyl radical of the latter (on R_1) is replaced by an allyl radical.(52) Thiamylal sodium was marketed as a mixture with sodium carbonate, the mixture being prepared by adding thiamylal sodium and sodium carbonate to just enough sodium hydroxide solution to dissolve the salts. The pH is adjusted to between 10.7 and 10.9. The solution is made to volume with water, filtered, sterilized, and lyophilized. The finished product consists of pale yellow, hygroscopic, agglutinated masses of crystals with no pronounced odor. On addition of distilled water, it readily dissolves forming a clear yellow solution with a pH of 10.3 (in 2.5% solution). Solutions have a pungent odor that has been described as that of sulfur or garlic. Reduction in pH of the solution results in precipitation of the drug; a few drops of alkali redissolve precipitated material. Normal saline has been suggested as the preferred diluent.(53) Solutions of thiamylal and saline have been kept for as long as 14 days without loss of potency or change in appearance. In dogs the anesthetic potency of thiamylal is 1.5 times that of thiopental.(54) Thiamylal was found to be less cumulative than thiopental as shown in Figure 9–9.

Tolerance does not develop following repeated administration of thiamylal every other day for 4 weeks.(52) Significant increases in heart rate, arterial blood pressure, and myocardial oxygen consumption are produced by 8.0 mg/kg of thiamylal administered intravenously.(55) Even more commonly than after thiopental, intravenous injection of thiamylal sodium will result in the genesis of ventricular bigeminy (ventricular premature depolarization coupled to the

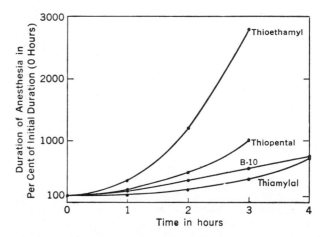

Fig. 9–9. Cumulative action of hourly injections of four thiobarbiturates. Time values on the abscissa represent the hour on which injections were administered. (From Wyngaarden, J.B., Woods, L.A., Ridley, R., and Seevers, M.H. Anesthetic Properties of Sodium-5-allyl-5-(1-methylbutyl)-2-thiobarbiturate (Surital) and Certain Other Thiobarbiturates in Dogs. J Pharmacol Exp Ther 95:326, 1949.)

preceding sinus beat). This appears to originate in the ventricle distal to the bundle of His.(43) Most investigators have found thiamylal to be more arrhythmogenic than thiopental. Because of its arrhythmogenic effect, it has been suggested that thiamylal is contraindicated in any dog with impaired cardiac function.(56)

With a dose of 8.0 mg/kg, respiratory rate is not significantly changed although the tidal volume and minute volume are decreased. This results in significant increases in arterial $PaCO_2$ with decreases in pH and PaO_2.(55) Depression of respiration is pronounced on rapid intravenous injection. When dogs are given excessive doses of thiamylal or thiopental by continuous injection, the respiratory rate and amplitude progressively decrease, but blood pressure does not drop significantly until respiratory arrest occurs (57). Dogs artificially ventilated will tolerate 1½ to 3½ times the dose of thiamylal tolerated with spontaneous respiration. Artificially ventilated animals show a gradual decline in blood pressure. With overdose, hypoxia secondary to respiratory failure is the cause of death.

The effect of dog collars containing dichlorovos on thiamylal anesthesia in dogs has been investigated.(58) After wearing collars for 7 days, dogs had significant decrease in plasma cholinesterase but not in red blood cell cholinesterase. When the dog was anesthetized, PaO_2 was slightly but not significantly reduced and $PaCO_2$ was increased. It was concluded that no significant synergism occurred between the two agents.

Since thiamylal sodium is similar in its action to thiopental, it is used in a like manner. In small animals it is usually prepared as a 4% or weaker solution by adding sterile water or saline to 1 g of powder. A dose of 17.5 mg/kg intravenously produces surgical anesthesia in dogs for approximately 15 minutes, with complete recovery in about 3 hours. If anesthesia of longer duration is desired, repeated increments can be administered. It has been used with a wide variety of preanesthetic agents and muscle relaxants with excellent results. After tranquilization, thiamylal alone (3–4 mg/kg) or in combination with guaifenesin is commonly used for induction prior to inhalation anesthesia in horses and cattle. In unsedated animals the intravenous dose for rapid induction is 4.0 to 8.0 mg/kg. The animal usually relaxes within 15 to 20 seconds and remains recumbent for 20 to 40 minutes. Provision should be made for artificial respiration when thiamylal is used to maintain anesthesia, since apnea may be produced. Nevertheless, because of its low toxicity, thiamylal has been used in young, aged, and poor-risk patients. It has won universal acclaim for its safety and was probably the most widely used thiobarbiturate in small animal and equine practice before manufacturers discontinued production in 1993.

ADMINISTRATION OF BARBITURATES

Intravenous Injection. Barbiturates are administered by several routes, depending upon the patient and the effect desired. For anesthesia, the intravenous route is preferable, since the anesthetic can be given "to effect." Because of wide variation in patient response, this type of dose control is desirable. Intraperitoneal and intramuscular administration is not widely employed. The oral route is slow and unpredictable, and therefore is used chiefly when sedation is sought.

Care should be taken in selection of needles and syringes for administration. In large species of animals, 12- to 18-gauge 1½- to 2-inch needles are used, depending upon the quantity of anesthetic that must be injected rapidly to carry the patient through the excitement stage. When large quantities are to be injected, a vascular catheter is preferred. In smaller animals, 20- to 24-gauge needles aid in venipuncture and help slow the rate of injection. There is a careless tendency to use large syringes on very small animals. This is dangerous because the dose cannot be accurately controlled. A syringe size commensurate with the dose should always be employed; use of large syringes with small doses is an invitation to disaster.

In many practices, an indwelling venous catheter is inserted prior to anesthetic administration. This is used for anesthetic injection and subsequent fluid administration during operation. It also helps ensure that inadvertent perivascular injection does not occur when animals are transported. In small animals (less than 5 kg), it is advisable to dilute the anesthetic with sterile water. By making a 100% dilution, or larger, more accurate dose control is achieved.

When intravenous injection is to be made, hair over the vein may be removed with clippers and the skin prepared by swabbing with a suitable antiseptic. The latter procedure, in addition to cleaning the area, tends to distend the vein. For intravenous anesthesia, the cephalic vein on the anterior aspect of the forelimb is most commonly used in small animals. In dogs, the second choice is generally the saphenous vein on the lateral surface of the hind limb just proximal to the hock. In cats, the saphenous or femoral vein on the inner surface of the thigh is a good second choice. Other veins less frequently used are the jugular and the marginal vein of the ear. In large dogs already anesthetized, the lingual veins on the ventral surface of the tongue are easily accessible. These veins tend to bleed rather profusely, however. In horses, cattle, and sheep, the jugular vein is used almost exclusively. In swine, the marginal vein of the ear or the anterior vena cava is most commonly employed.

In the dog, if injection is to be made into the cephalic vein of the right foreleg, the assistant stands by the animal's left side with the left arm circling the neck and the right arm extended over the dog's back. The right hand grasps the right foreleg just below the elbow. The right index finger is extended over the dorsal surface of the limb, the thumb is held around the ventral surface of the leg, and, by compressing thumb and forefinger, the vein is occluded, causing it to distend with blood. The wrist is turned slightly so that the skin covering the dorsal aspect of the foreleg and the cephalic vein is rotated outward. The veterinarian grasps the paw of the right foot with the left hand and, if the vein is not easily seen, by rapidly squeezing the paw several times, pumps blood from the paw to distend the vein. If the carpus is flexed acutely, the vein is stretched tightly over the underlying muscles and rolling is prevented. Good technique demands that the needle used for injection be threaded into the vein so that the hub is at the site of venipuncture. The leg and syringe are both held in the left hand during injection so they will move as a unit if the animal moves. This prevents accidental retraction of the needle from the vein.

Persons experienced with administration of barbiturates to dogs and cats usually estimate the weight of the animal and draw an excess of solution into a syringe. The first one third to one half of the dose is rapidly injected while watching the animal's facial expression closely. As injection is made, the animal often licks its lips as though tasting the drug. Frequently, dogs move the head from side to side as the anesthetic effect begins. These movements are seen early in the course of administration and indicate more drug must be given. The eyes begin to lose their alert expression, and the animal then relaxes. As injection is continued, the veterinarian can, with thumb and forefinger placed behind the canine teeth, open the animal's jaw. If in a light state of anesthesia, the patient will further open the jaw, curl the tongue, and simulate a yawn. At this point, the cornea and pedal reflexes are still present and the animal is not in a state of surgical anesthesia. Administration of anesthetic should be continued cautiously and in small amounts, with careful attention paid to respiration and reflexes. Surgical anesthesia is reached when the pedal reflex is abolished. At this point, further administration of drug is not necessary.

One should constantly bear in mind that anesthesia is most safely accomplished when the final portion is administered quite slowly. In many small animal practices, it is routine procedure to anesthetize the animal lightly, and then to tape the syringe containing the agent to the limb. A short piece of tape is applied parallel to the barrel and plunger of the syringe to prevent venous back-pressure from pushing the plunger out of the barrel. At this point the animal is clipped, scrubbed, and prepared for surgery. Then the final dose of anesthetic is administered. The syringe is left in position throughout the operation so that small increments can be given as needed.

Intraperitoneal Injection. Intraperitoneal injection has been employed extensively in the past but has the disadvantage that the dose cannot be as accurately controlled as it can by intravenous administration. Usually with this method, the animal is restrained in a vertical position against the assistant's body with the abdomen facing outward. An area just lateral to the umbilicus is clipped and a suitable antiseptic applied. The needle is passed through the abdominal wall and the injection made. The dose for intraperitoneal administration is calculated in the same manner as the intravenous dose. The peak concentration in the blood is reached more slowly, and drug absorbed into the portal system is subject to early metabolism.(28) This technique is not recommended in the clinical practice of veterinary anesthesia.

Intramuscular and Intrathoracic Injection. Under unusual circumstances, such as when wild animals are anesthetized, intramuscular or subcutaneous injection of barbiturates may be indicated. Because of their high alkalinity, there is a tendency for tissue necrosis to develop following this procedure. For moderate anesthesia, 30 mg/kg, and for surgical anesthesia of 1 to 2 hours, 40 mg/kg of pentobarbital can be administered. Induction requires about 15 minutes, and anesthesia reaches its peak effect about 30 minutes following injection.

Although pentobarbital has been given intrathoracically using the same dose as for intravenous anesthesia, veterinarians should strongly oppose intrathoracic administration of anesthetic, as there is risk of puncture to the heart, pericardium, and lung, while the barbiturates are irritating to the serosal surfaces. The latter fact can be confirmed on necropsy of animals destroyed with intrathoracic barbiturates. Pleural thickening, bronchitis, and coagulative necrosis of the lung has been observed on examination of experimentally injected cats.

In general, thiobarbiturates produce more respiratory depression on induction than oxybarbiturates; often one third of the calculated dose causes the patient to collapse and respiration to stop. This transient apnea is alarming to those not aware of this reaction. When it occurs, injection of anesthetic should be suspended until spontaneous rhythmic respirations resume. This usually occurs as soon as the blood carbon dioxide level rises to stimulate respiration and rapid redistribution decreases CNS concentration.

BARBITURATE SLOUGH

Occasionally, an animal may struggle during induction of barbiturate anesthesia and some of the drug may be administered perivascularly. This should be avoided if at all possible because a tissue slough may develop. Experienced anesthetists prevent barbiturate slough by threading the needle into the vein. This procedure makes it unlikely that the needle will come out of the vein if the syringe is jarred or the animal moves. Sloughs caused by anesthesia require 2 to 4 weeks to heal and leave an unsightly scar. Nothing can infuriate an owner more than development of a slough in his animal.

If it is suspected that barbiturate solution has been injected perivascularly, the area should be infiltrated with 1 or 2 mL of 2% procaine solution.(59) Lidocaine can also be used for this purpose. Local anesthetics are effective for two reasons. First, they are vasodilators and prevent vasospasm in the area, and thus aid in dilution and absorption of the barbiturate. Second, they are broken down in an alkaline medium and this reaction neutralizes the alkali (barbiturate). Injection of a corticosteroid or nonsteroidal antiinflammatory drug, and/or the use of hot packs or hydrotherapy may be beneficial, as is infiltration of the area with saline to further dilute the barbiturate.

Nonbarbiturate Drugs

Although the barbiturates have been the most commonly used short-acting anesthetics, many other injectable drugs have been used to induce and maintain unconsciousness. Chloral hydrate alone and in combination with magnesium sulfate and pentobarbital sodium has been used for induction and maintenance of anesthesia in large domestic animals (i.e., the horse and cow). Many drugs have been used to depress the CNS and immobilize laboratory animals but do not find application in routine small animal clinical use. Among them are chloral hydrate, chloralose, urethan, metomidate, and magnesium sulfate. Newer drugs, such as etomidate and propofol, have been developed to provide short periods of unconsciousness from which recovery is rapid. These hypnotic drugs are most effective when given in combination with preanesthetics and analgesics to achieve a state of anesthesia. Several of these combinations have recently been developed and assessed for use in animal anesthesia and are presented in this and various chapters within Sections 3, 7, and 8.

ALTHESIN (SAFFAN)

Althesin is a combination of two steroids: alphaxalone and alphadolone acetate. The solubility of alphaxalone (9 mg/mL) is increased by alphadolone acetate (3 mg/mL) and by 20% w/v polyoxyethylated castor oil (Cremophor EL). The combination of the two steroids

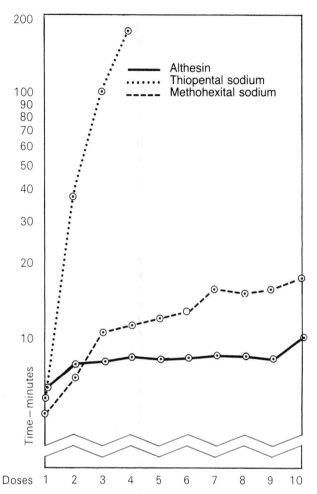

Fig. 9–10. Duration of loss of righting reflex in mice given repeated intravenous doses of althesin and other anesthetics. Second and subsequent doses given 30 seconds after return of the righting reflex. Five mice per group. (After Child, K.J., Currie, J.P., Davis, B., Dodds, M.G., Pearce, D.R., and Twissell, D.J. The Pharmacological Properties in Animals of CT 1341 – A New Steroid Anaesthetic. Br J Anaesth 43:2, 1971.)

has an exceptionally high therapeutic index (30.6). It has little cumulative effect (Fig. 9–10); the duration of anesthesia varies with species (Fig. 9–11). Administration of the combination before or after barbiturates is not advised, although adverse effects when used with other anesthetic drugs have not been reported.

In the cat, a dose of 9 mg/kg is recommended for intravenous administration and 12 to 18 mg/kg for intramuscular administration. Intravenous injection produces relaxation in approximately 9 seconds and surgical anesthesia in about 25 seconds. Intramuscular administration produces variable results but may be useful in fractious animals. The onset after intramuscular injection occurs in 6 to 12 minutes and lasts for approximately 15 minutes. A quiet area for induction is desirable. In the fractious cat, where drugs must be administered intramuscularly, ketamine is the drug of

choice, since althesin is less reliable by this route (Chapter 10).(60)

Althesin has a neutral pH and does not produce pain or inflammation when injected perivascularly or intramuscularly. Additional doses can be given to prolong anesthesia without cumulative effects, and recovery is rapid. In contrast to ketamine, althesin produces good muscular relaxation. Althesin has a slightly protective effect against epinephrine-induced arrhythmias in the cat.(61) Urination, defecation, muscle tremors, paddling, salivation, and hyperesthesia have been reported as side effects. Edema of the feet, ears, and muzzle occur in approximately 25% of cats injected, but is usually transient and disappears within 2 hours. This condition apparently occurs in females more often than in males. Antihistamine administration reduces this occurrence.

In the dog and some other canidae, polyoxyethylene derivatives of hexitol anhydride partial fatty acid esters produce an allergic response.(62) This response is manifested by a prolonged fall in blood pressure and a positive skin wheal if the drug is injected intradermally. Urticaria and erythema are believed to be the result of release of histamine or histaminelike substances. Cremophor EL, a nonionic polyoxyethylated emulsifying agent used as the vehicle in althesin, elicits

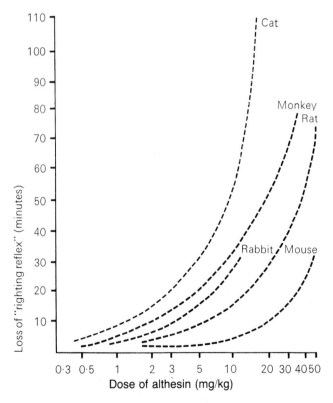

Fig. 9–11. Anesthetic activity of althesin in different species. (After Child, K.J., Currie, J.P., Davis, B., Dodds, M.G., Pearce, D.R., and Twissell, D.J. The Pharmacological Properties in Animals of CT 1341 – A New Steroid Anaesthetic. Br J Anaesth 43:2, 1971.)

the same response. Apparently allergic reactions can occur caused by the vehicle (polyoxyethylated castor oil) or either of the two steroids. The reaction can be of the true hypersensitivity type, which requires previous exposure to the drug, or of the complement activation type, which requires no previous sensitization.(63)

Horses anesthetized with althesin developed violent paddling and galloping movements during recovery, which can be eliminated by prior administration of xylazine (1 mg/kg).(64) The minimum dose of althesin for induction of anesthesia is approximately 1.2 to 1.34 mg/kg in the unpremedicated horse. Although xylazine administration increases the recovery time, its administration would appear prudent.

The dose of althesin for sheep is approximately 2.2 mg/kg intravenously. This produces light surgical anesthesia for 8 to 15 minutes. The average maintenance dose to produce surgical anesthesia for a 3-hour period is $0.23 \text{ mg} \cdot \text{kg}^{-1} \cdot \text{min}^{-1}$. Sheep given althesin develop bradycardia with a decrease in systolic and diastolic pressures of 20 to 35% of preinjection levels. Left ventricular end-diastolic pressure elevates, and cardiac output decreases. These parameters return to normal within 6 to 8 minutes of injection. Myocardial depression measured as a decrease in maximum dp/dt is produced.(64) Althesin has also been used to induce anesthesia prior to administering inhalants to maintain anesthesia in ruminants (goats, sheep, young calves).(65) The dose of althesin for pigs is approximately 6 mg/kg to produce 10 to 15 minutes of anesthesia. In pigs known to develop malignant hyperthermia under anesthesia, althesin does not induce this reaction, and it has been used safely in animals known to be susceptible to this condition.(64)

Althesin decreases cerebral blood flow accompanied by a fall in intracranial pressure in baboons.(66) Neither of the two steroids is extensively protein-bound by the serum of the rat, cat, horse, or man. Approximately 60 to 70% of a radioactive dose of alphaxalone or alphadolone acetate is excreted as metabolic products in the feces during the 5 days following intravenous injection; the other 20 to 30% appears in the urine within the same period.(67)

CHLORAL HYDRATE, U. S. P.

Liebrich, who introduced chloral hydrate as a hypnotic in 1869, thought that because it released chloroform in vitro it would do the same in vivo. This has subsequently been proved a misconception. Chloral hydrate occurs as colorless translucent crystals that volatilize on exposure to air with an aromatic, penetrating odor. It has a bitter, caustic taste. One gram of the crystals dissolves in 0.25 mL of water. It may be administered orally, or solutions may be injected intravenously or intraperitoneally. It irritates the gastric mucosa and may cause vomiting if not diluted in water but is readily absorbed from the gastrointestinal tract. A small amount of chloral hydrate is excreted unchanged in the urine.

The greater portion is reduced to trichloroethyl alcohol, a less potent hypnotic, and this in turn is conjugated with glycuronic acid to form urochloralic (trichloroethylglycuronic) acid, which has no hypnotic property. The latter is excreted in the urine. In animals with liver damage, chloral hydrate may be found in larger quantities and urochloralic acid in smaller quantities in the urine.

Chloral hydrate depresses the cerebrum with loss of reflex excitability. In subanesthetic doses, motor and sensory nerves are not affected. Chloral hydrate is a good hypnotic but a poor anesthetic; the amount needed to produce anesthesia approaches the minimal lethal dose, and it produces deep sleep that lasts for several hours. It has weak analgesic action. In hypnotic doses, the medullary centers are not affected. Anesthetic doses of chloral hydrate depress the vasomotor center severely, resulting in a fall in blood pressure. Hypnotic doses depress respiration, and anesthetic doses markedly depress the respiratory center. Death from chloral hydrate administration is caused by progressive depression of the respiratory center. The margin of safety is such that it is not a satisfactory surgical anesthetic.

Chloral hydrate is not used for small animal anesthesia and has lost most of its popularity as a general anesthetic in large animals. Its continued use in large animals depends on the simplicity of administration and on the duration of effect of the induction dose—an interval adequate for many routine procedures. It is relatively inexpensive and may be combined with barbiturates. It is an irritant when inadvertently injected outside the vein. Use of a vascular catheter obviates this hazard. The concentration of the chloral hydrate solution should not be too high: 7 to 12% w/v aqueous solutions are generally used.

Doses reported for intravenous chloral hydrate vary extensively, probably owing to the rate of administration and to varying interpretations of the depth of resulting anesthesia. The recommended intravenous dose for chloral hydrate in the horse varies from 2 to 3 g/45 kg as a sedative and up to 10 g/45 kg when used alone for general anesthesia. When the drug is used to enhance xylazine or xylazine-butorphanol sedation, a dose of 0.6-1.2 g/45 kg is usually effective. A dose of 1.8 g/45 kg may be necessary. This mixture of drugs can be used to provide effective standing restraint during low epidural analgesia achieved with a local anesthetic in the horse undergoing surgical correction of a rectovaginal fistula.

Chloral hydrate solution was once commonly administered at 15 to 30 g/min and was given until the horse was about to fall, at which time the intravenous tubing was disconnected and the animal restrained until recumbent. If necessary, additional solution was administered slowly until the desired degree of sedation or anesthesia was achieved. Because of conversion to trichloroethanol and slow passage across the blood-

PHARMACOLOGY

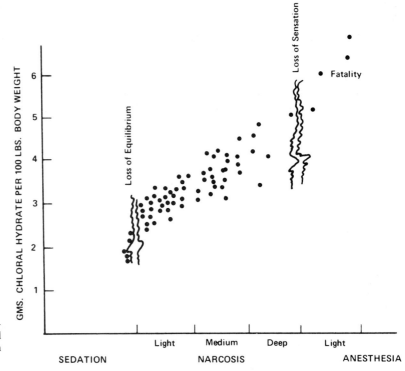

Fig. 9–12. Chloral hydrate and magnesium sulfate anesthesia (2:1) in the horse. Dose of chloral hydrate used and degree of anesthesia obtained in clinical cases.

brain barrier, anesthetic depression increases for several minutes after initial induction. Therefore, additional doses should not be administered immediately. The chief disadvantage with chloral hydrate is that the dose required to induce general anesthesia causes prolonged recovery. For this reason, in modern practice, chloral hydrate is primarily used to induce a degree of narcosis or sedation, and analgesia is produced by means of local or regional anesthesia. Premedication with tranquilizers reduces the amount of chloral hydrate required, facilitates induction, and minimizes struggling during recovery.(68)

The time required for horses to stand after cessation of administration of anesthetic doses varies from 1 to 4 hours and is similar in duration to that observed after chloral hydrate and magnesium sulfate administration. If anesthesia is maintained for a long period, recovery may also be prolonged. The nature of the recovery period can vary; if left undisturbed, the horse often passes quietly into a hypnotic state, remaining thus until it is ready to stand. Excitement and struggling during recovery are not uncommon and can be minimized by use of tranquilizers.

Chloral hydrate is also occasionally used to induce narcosis or anesthesia in cattle and swine. In the former, it has been largely replaced with xylazine. The chloral hydrate dose required is similar to that for horses. In cattle, premedication with atropine sulfate and early intubation are indicated. Chloral hydrate may also be administered to horses and cattle by stomach tube to induce varying degrees of sedation or narcosis (3 to 6 g/45 kg body weight).

Chloral hydrate has been combined with magnesium sulfate or with magnesium sulfate and pentobarbital sodium for anesthesia in horses and cattle (Fig. 9–12). Investigators claimed that these drug combinations resulted in a more rapid and excitement-free induction, increased anesthetic depth, smoother emergence, a wider margin of safety, and less irritation than anesthesia achieved with chloral hydrate alone. Nevertheless, with the advent of rapid-onset, short-acting, and safer drugs, there seems to be little merit in the use of chloral hydrate alone or in combination with other drugs to induce and maintain anesthesia.

CHLORALOSE

Chloralose is prepared by heating anhydrous glucose and trichloroacetaldehyde (anhydrous chloral) in a water bath. Both alpha- and beta-chloralose are formed, with the alpha form being active. Chloralose has been advocated for use in cardiovascular studies because it produces minimal depression and maintains more active reflexes than other anesthetics.(69)

Chloralose is usually prepared as a 1.0% aqueous solution. Heat is necessary to dissolve the drug, but solutions should not be boiled. The intravenous anesthetic dose of alpha-chloralose is approximately 110 mg/kg in dogs and 80 mg/kg for adult cats.(70) Alpha-chloralose appears to depress neuronal function of the cortex and routes of afferent input less than pentobarbital. Many investigators still consider chloralose a valuable drug for maintenance of unconsciousness for long, nonsurvival, surgical experiments (71).

URETHAN, N. F.

Urethan is prepared by heating urea with alcohol under pressure or by warming urea nitrate with alcohol and sodium nitrite. The drug is marketed in the crystalline state. One gram dissolves in 0.5 mL of water, the aqueous solution being neutral. It is most often used as an anesthetic in laboratory animals and fish. The lethal intravenous dose for rabbits is 2.0 g/kg. The dose for dogs and cats is 0.6 to 2.0 g/kg. Up to 0.5 g/kg may be used as a hypnotic dose.

Urethan is mutagenic, carcinostatic, and carcinogenic.(72) Mice given urethan develop an exceptionally high incidence of lung tumors, regardless of the route of administration. Tumors also develop in treated rats and rabbits. Concern over the health of individuals in prolonged contact with urethan or its solutions is justified.(73) For this reason urethan is no longer commonly used in any species.

MAGNESIUM SULFATE

A saturated solution of magnesium sulfate has been used for euthanasia. However, it should only be administered after animals have been rendered unconscious with a barbiturate or another rapid-acting anesthetic. In small animals, anesthesia has been achieved with dilute solutions of magnesium sulfate; however, the CNS is globally depressed and respiratory arrest often occurs at anesthetic doses. Animals will become excited just prior to collapse. Respiratory arrest likely results from complete neuromuscular block and paralysis of the muscles of respiration rather than a consequence of CNS depression. Therefore, one cannot be assured that magnesium sulfate administered alone is a humane method for achieving anesthesia or euthanasia.

METOMIDATE (HYPNODIL)

Metomidate hydrochloride is a hypnotic with muscle relaxant properties. Its hypnotic effect is exerted on mammals, birds, reptiles, and fish. Given alone, it induces sleep without analgesia. General anesthesia can be produced by combining it with neuroleptics or analgesics. It is available in powdered form, which dissolves readily in water to make 1% or 5% solutions. These solutions have a pH of 2.9 and 2.4, respectively. Combined with the butyrophenone tranquilizer azaperone, metomidate produces anesthesia in swine for approximately 2 hours. Respiration slows and deepens. With rapid intravenous injection, apnea may occur. The cardiovascular system remains stable. When metomidate is used for cesarean section in sows, the piglets are usually alert at delivery.(74)

ETOMIDATE (AMIDATE)

Etomidate is an imidazole derivative synthesized in 1965 and was first used for induction of anesthesia in people in 1975. It is a congener of metomidate and contains 2 mg/mL of the drug in 35% ethylene glycol. It should be refrigerated at 2 to 8° C until used, and should not be frozen or exposed to extreme heat. The brainstem reticular formation appears to be the site of hypnotic activity. It is not a good analgesic. Single injections produce relatively brief hypnosis. In dogs, doses of 1.5 and 3.0 mg/kg last 8 ± 5 and 21 ± 9 minutes, respectively.(55) The duration of hypnosis is dose related. Etomidate is rapidly hydrolyzed in the liver and excreted in the urine. The pharmacokinetics of a 3-mg/kg intravenous dose of etomidate in cats is best described as a three-compartment open model similar to those determined in people and rats. Induction and recovery are rapid, with a brief period of myoclonus occurring early in the recovery period.(75)

Etomidate in powder and injectable forms has been used as an anesthetic for exotic species of animals. It was introduced in the United States as an induction agent for poor-risk human patients because it does not depress the cardiovascular and respiratory systems or release histamine. When used alone in dogs it produces no change in heart rate, blood pressure, or myocardial performance.(55) Neonates born to mothers anesthetized with etomidate have minimal respiratory depression. Etomidate does not trigger malignant hyperthermia in susceptible swine.(76) Etomidate qualifies as a good induction drug for neurosurgical procedures. It decreases cerebral metabolic rate of oxygen consumption ($CMRO_2$) and has anticonvulsant properties. It may have brain-protective properties following episodes of global ischemia associated with cardiac arrest.

Etomidate inhibits adrenal steroidogenesis in dogs, suppressing the usual increase in plasma cortisol observed during surgery. A single induction dose of etomidate may depress adrenal function for up to 3 hours. However, the lack of a "stress response" to surgery does not have deleterious effects, and it has been argued that attenuation of metabolic and endocrine responses to surgery actually reduces morbidity and may make this unique action of etomidate beneficial to overall patient outcome. Attention has been given to the development of addisonian crisis resulting from etomidate-induced blockade of corticosteroid production during prolonged infusion to maintain sedation in intensive care patients. Consequently, long-term infusion is not recommended.(77, 78) Etomidate (2 mg/kg) can cause acute hemolysis. The mechanism of hemolysis appears to be due to propylene glycol, which causes a rapid increase in osmolality resulting in red cell rupture.(79)

Etomidate is compatible with other common preanesthetic agents. Venous pain is common on injection in humans, and myoclonia may occur without administration of premedication. Nausea and vomiting are troublesome, especially after the use of multiple doses and can occur at recovery as well as induction. For the most part, these side effects can be prevented by adequate preanesthetic sedation. In summary, etomidate may be one of the better induction drugs in traumatized patients and those with severe myocardial disease, cardiovascular instability, cirrhosis, or intracranial lesions, or ones requiring cesarean section surgery (Chapters 20, 23, 24).(76)

PROPOFOL (RAPINOVET, DIPRIVAN)

Propofol (2,6-diisopropylphenol) is unrelated to barbiturates, euganols, or steroid anesthetics. It is only slightly soluble in water and is marketed as an aqueous emulsion containing 10 mg of propofol, 100 mg of soybean oil, 22.5 mg of glycerol, and 12 mg of egg lecithin per mL. Sodium hydroxide is added to adjust the pH. It is available in sterile glass ampules and contains no preservatives. Propofol emulsion is capable of supporting microbial growth and endotoxin production.(80) Because of the potential for iatrogenic sepsis, unused propofol remaining in an open ampule should be discarded and not be kept overnight for use the next day.

The pharmacokinetics of propofol in dogs fits a two-compartment open model. Rapid onset of action is caused by rapid uptake into the CNS. The short duration of action and rapid smooth emergence results from rapid redistribution from the brain to other tissues and efficient elimination from plasma by metabolism.(81) Propofol has a large volume of distribution as would be expected from its lipophilic nature. It is metabolized primarily by conjugation, but propofol's rapid disappearance from plasma is greater than hepatic blood flow, suggesting extra hepatic sites of metabolism.(82) The pharmacokinetics of propofol has not been reported in cats, but its anesthetic action is similar to that in dogs.(83) In general, after a single bolus injection, propofol induces a rapid, smooth induction followed by a short period of unconsciousness.(84) In people, recovery is rapid and free of emergence excitement after constant infusion or repeated bolus administration.(2) In dogs, recoveries may be prolonged following continuous infusion of propofol exceeding 30 minutes.(85)

Propofol is usually injected as a single bolus for induction of general anesthesia in dogs and cats to allow intubation and initiation of inhalation anesthesia.(84) It should be remembered that propofol is a sedative-hypnotic and has only minimal analgesic action at a subanesthetic dose. Even when an animal is rendered unconscious with propofol, it will respond to painful stimuli unless analgesic drugs such as the opioids or alpha$_2$-agonists are administered concurrently. If administration is preceded by a preanesthetic such as morphine or medetomidine, the induction dose of propofol can be decreased substantially. The dose for induction of anesthesia in unpremedicated dogs ranges from 6 to 8 mg/kg IV, whereas the dose in sedated animals may be as low as 2 to 4 mg/kg IV.(85, 86) Following a single dose of 6 mg/kg IV, recovery in dogs is complete in approximately 20 minutes. A similar dose given to cats provides about 30 minutes of anesthesia to

complete recovery. The incidence of postanesthetic side effects, such as vomiting, sneezing or pawing is about 15% but can be decreased with acepromazine or alpha$_2$ premedication. When the patient is premedicated with 0.02 to 0.04 mg/kg of acepromazine, the induction dose of propofol is decreased by approximately 30 to 40%. Propofol can be used for maintenance of anesthesia either by intermittent bolus or continual infusion.(86, 87) The rate of administration depends on the adjunctive drugs administered and the degree of surgical stimulation.(87) The continual infusion rate ranges from 0.15 to 0.4 mg $\cdot$ kg^{-1} $\cdot$ min^{-1}. When using an intermittent bolus technique, doses of 0.5 to 2 mg/kg are administered as needed.

Propofol induces depression by enhancing the effects of the inhibitory neurotransmitter GABA and decreasing the brain's metabolic activity.(88) It decreases intracranial and cerebral perfusion pressures. Propofol transiently depresses arterial pressure and myocardial contractility similar to that observed with the ultra-short-acting thiobarbiturates. Hypotension is primarily the result of arterial and venous vasodilation.(89) Propofol enhances the arrhythmogenic effects of epinephrine but is not inherently arrhythmogenic.(2)

Propofol is a phenolic compound, and as such it can induce oxidative injury to feline red blood cells when administered repeatedly over several days. This toxicity is likely the result of the cat's reduced ability to conjugate phenol. Heinz body formation occurs, and clinical signs of anorexia, diarrhea, and malaise can result.(90) Apnea of short duration may occur after induction with propofol. In animals breathing spontaneously, hypercapnia may occur for a short period of time following rapid bolus injection.(91) Propofol is excreted primarily by the kidney. However, renal insufficiency has little or no affect on the dog's clinical response to propofol. Propofol has been used for cesarean section surgery with generally good results.(84, 92) Because puppies have good conjugation enzyme activity, there is minimal fetal depression in neonates delivered from mothers anesthetized with propofol.

Complaints of pain on intravenous injection of propofol are common in people. This likely occurs in small animals, but the prevalence appears to be much less. Pain can be minimized by premedication with an opioid or alpha$_2$-agonist and/or injection into larger vessels. Propofol, unlike barbiturates, does not cause tissue damage when injected perivascularly or intraarterially. When combined with an opioid, acepromazine, or an alpha$_2$-agonist, propofol provides dependable anesthesia of short duration for procedures such as castrations, ear flushes, exploration for foxtails, ultrasound examinations, biopsies, and suturing of small lacerations. Additionally, the advantage of rapid smooth recovery is beneficial in patients with chronic respiratory disease or those undergoing bronchoscopy or transtracheal aspiration procedures. Light propofol anesthesia has been advocated for patients undergoing upper airway examination.(93) At the present time, induction of anesthesia with propofol in a 20-kg dog costs approximately $5.00. Maintenance of anesthesia for 1 hour costs approximately $20.00. This is in comparison to a cost of approximately $1.00 for 1 hour of halothane anesthesia and $4.00 for isoflurane anesthesia. For this reason, the use of propofol anesthesia has been restricted to small patients undergoing short surgical or diagnostic procedures.

Propofol is as a satisfactory drug for immobilization of neonatal foals when given in combination with 0.5 mg/kg IV of xylazine. Immobilization is induced with 2 mg/kg IV propofol and maintained with 0.33 mg · kg^{-1} · min^{-1} IV. Cardiovascular changes are characterized by decreased pressure and cardiac output, and a decrease in respiration rate. Although further investigation of the use of propofol in large species such as the horse is ongoing, the current cost of propofol prohibits its routine use in larger animals.

The primary disadvantages of propofol are cost, lack of FDA approval, limited shelf life once the ampule is opened and risk of iatrogenic sepsis. Nevertheless, with the recent termination of production and unavailability of thiamylal, the use of propofol for inducing and maintaining short periods of anesthesia has gained popularity in small animal practice.

PROPANIDID (EPONTOL)

The eugenols are derivatives of oil of cloves. Propanidid was the third eugenol to be developed and became available in Europe in 1967. It has an extremely short duration of action, and it is difficult to administer fast enough to maintain anesthesia in adult horses. Violent excitement follows administration of subanesthetic doses. In dogs, severe respiratory depression and hypotension are induced with anesthetic doses and are probably associated with reaction to the cremophor carrier.

TRICAINE METHANESULFONATE (MS-222; FINQUEL)

Tricaine methanesulfonate, a crystalline water-soluble powder, is marketed under the commercial name, MS-222. It is used as an anesthetic to immobilize amphibia, fish, and other cold-blooded animals by complete bathing of small subjects, by gill spraying in large fish, or by injecting larger species. It exerts a prompt, intense action and has a low degree of toxicity, being approximately three times less toxic than procaine and about 10 times less toxic than cocaine. A 1:1000 solution may be autoclaved without loss of narcotic properties or increase in toxicity.

When rapid or moderately rapid anesthesia is required, fish can be immersed in an anesthetic solution of MS-222. Galvanized or brass containers should not be used because dissolution of zinc is possible. The fish should not be overcrowded in the container. Anesthetic solution should be discarded when loss in potency is suspected or the solution has been fouled with mucus

or excrement. Fish are anesthetized to loss of reflex and positioned so that the gills can be bathed in a sedating concentration during surgery. Large fish such as sharks and rays can be anesthetized in minutes by spraying the gills with a 1-g/L solution of MS-222 with a water pistol or bulb syringe. The action of MS-222 is slowed at cooler temperatures, in extremely soft water, and in larger fish. A preliminary test of the anesthetic solution can be made with a small number of fish to determine the rate of anesthesia and required exposure times under the prevailing conditions. The concentration necessary to induce rapid anesthesia varies among species of fish. For example, salmonidae require 80 to 135 mg/L whereas centrarchidae (blue gill and bass) require a concentration of 260 to 330 mg/L to induce rapid anesthesia within 5 minutes. Excessive exposure can be avoided by carefully observing sensory and motor responses of the fish. Sedation is characterized by decreased reactivity to visual and vibrational stimuli and decreased opercular activity. Deep anesthesia is characterized by loss of equilibrium, with the fish turning over and locomotion ceasing. Prior to use, MS-222 may be weighed out into 2-g units. Two grams of MS-222 dissolved in 5 gallons of water yields a concentration of about 100 mg/L. For rougher approximations, one level teaspoon full of MS-222 contains 2.2 to 2.5 g and when placed in 5 gallons of water provides a concentration of about 120 mg/L. The anesthetic solution should be well oxygenated, and its temperature should be similar to the water from which the fish were taken. As long as opercular activity is still present, the anesthetic action of MS-222 is readily reversed by transferring the fish to fresh water.

Other Methods of Producing Anesthesia

Hypothermia has been limited to use in veterinary teaching hospitals, primarily in cardiac surgery. Electronarcosis and immobilization have not proven to be effective clinical modalities for producing general anesthesia. Acupuncture has gained some popularity, chiefly for chronic pain relief rather than for surgical anesthesia. These techniques will be briefly reviewed.

HYPOTHERMIA

As the body temperature of a warm-blooded animal falls, metabolism is reduced, and therefore the need for oxygen is diminished. Oxygen uptake in dogs is reduced by approximately 50% at 30° C and 65% at 25° C.(94) The metabolic rate of isolated slices of rat heart is reduced 90% by lowering the temperature to 10° C.(95) The potassium-arrested heart at 37° C utilized four times as much glycogen and produced three times as much lactic acid as the heart at 17° C.(96) Thus, the heart, brain, liver, or other vital organs can survive at a low temperature for a considerably increased period when deprived of all or a portion of their blood supply. Hypothermia may be artificially produced in the entire body, or in only a portion such as the heart or head. It

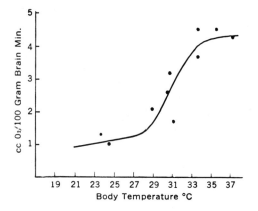

Fig. 9–13. Relation of oxygen uptake by the brain to temperature. (From Bering, E.A., Jr., Taren, J.A., McMurray, J.D., and Bernhard, W.F. Surg Gynecol Obstet 102:134, 1956.)

has found its greatest usefulness in surgery of the heart and central nervous system.(97)

The colder an animal becomes, the less oxygen is required by a given organ. It has been shown, however, that the reduction of oxygen consumption varies for different organs. For example, the work done by the heart at 26 to 27° C is little less than that at normal temperature, and while the general oxygen uptake by the body at this temperature is reduced to 40% of normal, that of the heart is still 50%. In monkeys, little change in cerebral oxygen uptake occurs until a temperature of 31° C is reached.(98) At this point it falls sharply, and through the next 4° C there is a drop of about 25%. Below 27° C oxygen consumption continues to fall but at a much slower rate. The relationship of cerebral oxygen consumption to temperature is sigmoid rather than linear (Fig. 9–13).

Several species of warm-blooded animals have been subjected to drastic hypothermia. It is possible to cool small laboratory animals to 0° C, and even lower, followed by recovery. Recovery in rats after cooling to temperatures just above the freezing point with cardiac and respiratory arrest for 1 hour was between 80 and 100%.(99) Golden hamsters have been kept "on ice" with circulatory arrest for up to 7 hours. These animals even survived supercooling to −5 or −6° C.(100) When the circulation is maintained with a pump-oxygenator, dogs have survived cooling to 1.5° C.(101)

In order to induce the hypothermic state as quickly as possible, it is necessary to control shivering, since it is an important mechanism in protection against cold. Shivering is induced by an increased temperature gradient between cold receptors in the skin and centers in the hypothalamus.(102) Even without visible shivering, there is general hypertonicity of the skeletal muscles, which results in increased metabolic, heart, and respiratory rates. Shivering can be prevented by deep anesthesia, or light anesthesia with curarization or

tranquilization with a phenothiazine. The latter drugs exert their effect through a peripheral action on muscle fibers and on the hypothalamic temperature control center.

Moderate hypothermia produces a rectilinear decrease in anesthetic requirements (MAC) for cyclopropane, diethyl ether, fluroxene, halothane, and methoxyflurane (Fig. 9–14).(103) Moderate hypothermia also reduces the concentration of anesthetic required to produce apnea. There is little difference between halothane, pentobarbital, and chloralose in their effects on whole-body oxygen consumption during surface cooling in dogs (Fig. 9–15).(104)

Three methods of whole-body cooling have been utilized: (a) surface, (b) body cavity, and (a) extracorporeal. Surface cooling is usually accomplished by directly immersing the unprotected body in ice water or by placing the body on a mattress through which ice water is circulated. Hyperventilation is maintained throughout the procedure to keep the blood pH on the alkaline side of normal. This has been shown to reduce cardiac arrhythmias and fibrillation. Below 28° C (82.4° F) no anesthetic is needed, and the patient is maintained on artificial ventilation alone. Active cooling is stopped when approximately two thirds of the desired temperature fall has been accomplished. Otherwise, the temperature continues to drop once the desired degree of hypothermia has been reached.

Body cavity cooling is accomplished by pouring cold saline solution into the open thoracic cavity.(105) This method has the disadvantage of being slow and requiring large volumes of saline solution. Extracorporeal cooling can be accomplished by running blood from

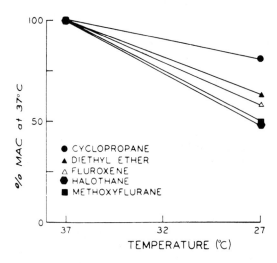

Fig. 9–14. The percentage decline between 37 and 27° C of the minimum alveolar concentration (MAC) required for anesthesia. Cyclopropane, the least oil-soluble agent, declines least, and halothane and methoxyflurane, the most soluble, decline most. (From Regan, M.J., and Eger, E.I.: Effect of Hypothermia in Dogs on Anesthetizing Apneic Doses of Inhalation Agents. Anesthesiology, 23:689, 1967.)

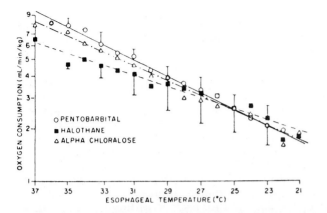

Fig. 9–15. Whole-body oxygen consumption vs esophageal temperature during surface cooling in dogs. The least-squares best-fit lines are shown for three anesthetics: pentobarbital, halothane, and alpha-chloralose. Each point represents the mean, each bar 1 SD. (From Westenskow, D.R., Wong, K.C., Johnson, C.C. and Wilde, C.S.: Physiologic Effects of Deep Hypothermia and Microwave Rewarming: Possible Application for Neonatal Cardiac Surgery. Anesth. Analg., 58:397, 1979.)

a cannulated artery through a heat exchanger using cold tap water as the cooling medium. A pump is required to force the blood through the system. Thrombosis is prevented by administration of heparin. Extracorporeal cooling has been used to lower the brain temperature below that of the general body temperature. Extracorporeal cooling carries with it the dangers of hemolysis and interference with the blood coagulation mechanism. It also presents the hazard of thrombosis. The most obvious advantage is that it provides the best control over body temperature and rewarming can be carried out quickly and efficiently by running warm water through the heat exchanger. Warming also may be accomplished by covering the patient with electric blankets or by using warm water baths. Microwave rewarming has been used experimentally.(104)

Since hypothermia is a form of general anesthesia, it carries the risks of profound CNS and vital organ depression. In addition, it has its own hazards for the circulatory system, skin and internal organs, and metabolism. Blood pressure falls during hypothermia, owing to decreased cardiac output, whereas peripheral vascular resistance increases. Occasionally, severe drops in blood pressure may occur. The fall in heart rate seen with hypothermia is due to depression of the SA node and bundle of His. These conduction changes are manifested by a prolonging of the PR interval, spreading of the QRS complex, and lengthening of the ST interval. In dogs, a cardiac crisis occurs between 23 and 15° C. This is characterized by cessation of sinus rhythm, intense bradycardia, ventricular extrasystoles, and ventricular fibrillation or standstill. As expected, atropine does not relieve the bradycardia. Ventricular fibrillation has been shown to occur most often when the temperature of the heart muscle is below 28° C and when the

heart is manipulated. Fibrillation rapidly depletes cardiac muscle energy stores. It occurs less frequently in young animals than in adults. Hypercapnia with acidemia, hyperkalemia, and myocardial hypoxia also appears to cause fibrillation. The incidence of spontaneous ventricular fibrillation has been shown to vary with the anesthetic used to initiate hypothermia. For example, pentobarbital results in a higher incidence than does thiopental or ether.(106)

Several cardioplegic solutions have been used to stop the heart and to prevent fibrillation. Hypothermia plus cardioplegia is more protective of cardiac tissue than hypothermia alone.(107, 108) Combined with deep hypothermia, cardioplegia allows 30 minutes of cardiac arrest without heart-lung bypass.

During hypothermia there is a prolongation of clotting time. In addition, there is a decrease in platelets, hemoconcentration with sludging, and a reduction in eosinophil and leukocyte counts with a fall in the mean corpuscular hemoglobin concentration.

Prolonged periods of hypothermia have detrimental effects on the patient.(109-111) In dogs held at 29° C for 24 hours, cardiac output and whole-body oxygen consumption decreased progressively to 7% and 28% of control, respectively. Cerebral blood flow and cerebral oxygen consumption responded similarly. On rewarming, cardiovascular collapse with severe tissue hypoxia and metabolic acidosis occurs. Cerebral blood flow becomes grossly inadequate, with depletion of brain energy stores. Hypothermia causes severe damage to the liver, kidneys, and adrenal glands in dogs when temperatures of around 25° C are maintained for several hours.(112) Shorter periods of cooling, however, do not appear to cause demonstrable damage.

Hypothermia has been used for surgery of the heart and great vessels, brain, and spinal cord, and in some other surgical procedures. It also has been advocated in treatment of shock, stroke, cerebral, and spinal contusion, and in prevention of brain damage following a severe hypoxic episode. The chief factor limiting its use alone in heart surgery is the danger of hypoxic brain damage. For this reason older patients and those with cardiac defects requiring extensive repair should be managed with heart-lung bypass. Hypothermia has also been used in dogs for removal of heartworms and repair of cardiac anomalies, but its use is not widespread. This is probably because many veterinarians are not aware of the simplicity of the technique and do not appreciate its potential.

INDUCTION OF HYPOTHERMIA

To produce hypothermia in the dog, a phenothiazine tranquilizer may be given intravenously as a preanesthetic agent. A thiobarbiturate is injected for general anesthesia, following which an endotracheal catheter is inserted and an inhalant anesthetic is used for maintenance. A slow intravenous drip of Ringer's lactate or 5% dextrose is started, and a muscle relaxant is given in the drip tubing to abolish respirations. Controlled ventilation is then initiated. Unless a cooling mattress is available, the animal is positioned in a sink, bathtub, or other container, with its head above water. Electronic thermometer probes are placed in the esophagus at heart level and in the rectum, and electrodes of an ECG machine are attached to the feet. From this point, constant monitoring of the ECG on an oscilloscope is desirable, since cardiac fibrillation may occur at any time during the cooling period and requires immediate corrective measures.

Ice water is used for rapid cooling. It should be constantly agitated by hand or with a pump. The dog should be removed from the bath before the desired body temperature is reached, as temperature will continue to decline even after removal from the water.

After removal, the dog should be dried with towels and placed on an inactive heating pad during the operative period. Rewarming can then be started as soon as closure of the surgical wound is begun. As anesthesia is discontinued and shivering commences, the body temperature quickly begins to rise. If the operation is short, rewarming in a water bath may be necessary along with administration of atropine and neostigmine to reverse the muscle relaxant.

ELECTRONARCOSIS AND IMMOBILIZATION

Electric stimulation of the brain can activate either opioid or nonopioid pain control pathways or both (Chapter 7).(113) Passage of electricity through the brain to produce anesthesia has been investigated for many years. In the veterinary field, clinical trials were conducted by Sir Frederic Hobday in England as early as 1932. Despite extensive research, much remains to be learned about this technique. Early work documented the occurrence of respiratory depression, hyperthermia, convulsions, and fatalities. Electronarcosis may be of

greatest use in situations where prolonged anesthesia is required for experimental purposes.

Most instruments deliver the current through needle electrodes applied to the head. Direct, pulsating direct, and alternating current have been used to produce electronarcosis. Alternating current of 700 cycles, 35 to 50 milliamperes, and approximately 40 volts has been employed.(114) Others have used combined direct and alternating current, modified to produce a rectangular wave of 1.0 to 1.4 ms duration, with a frequency of 100 waves per second.(115) Continuous electrode contact is important to maintain electronarcosis anesthesia. Individual variation among animals requires that the current be adjusted for each according to the response observed.

Electronarcosis is characterized by convulsions on induction unless a muscle relaxant is first administered. An exception to this is the method employing direct current for induction and then both direct and alternating current.(115) Profuse salivation develops on induction and continues throughout. This can be counteracted by using atropine. Endotracheal intubation should always be performed. Hyperthermia, probably caused by disturbance of the thermoregulatory center in the hypothalamus, is commonly seen. The EEG immediately following anesthesia is decreased in amplitude and increased in frequency, but returns to normal within 30 minutes. Brain lesions have been found following electronarcosis (116), and skin burns from the electrodes have been reported.(117)

Electronarcosis appears to produce severe stress, as evidenced by an increased plasma level of hydroxycorticoids, epinephrine, and norepinephrine (Fig. 9–16). The blood pressure rises sharply and then gradually falls to near normal levels (Fig. 9–17). The clotting time, sedimentation rate, hemoglobin, hematocrit, and total and differential white blood cell counts

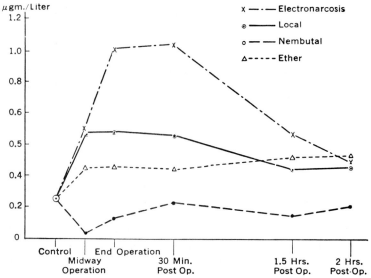

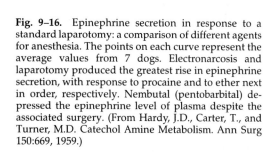

Fig. 9–16. Epinephrine secretion in response to a standard laparotomy: a comparison of different agents for anesthesia. The points on each curve represent the average values from 7 dogs. Electronarcosis and laparotomy produced the greatest rise in epinephrine secretion, with response to procaine and to ether next in order, respectively. Nembutal (pentobarbital) depressed the epinephrine level of plasma despite the associated surgery. (From Hardy, J.D., Carter, T., and Turner, M.D. Catechol Amine Metabolism. Ann Surg 150:669, 1959.)

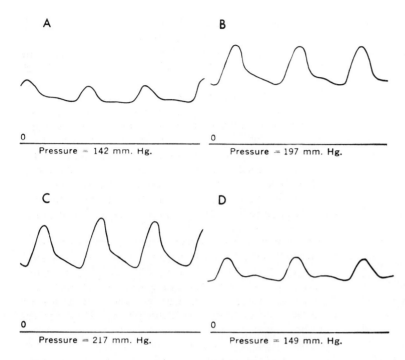

A

0

Pressure = 142 mm. Hg.

B

0

Pressure = 197 mm. Hg.

C

0

Pressure = 217 mm. Hg.

D

0

Pressure = 149 mm. Hg.

Fig. 9–17. Mean femoral artery blood pressure in a dog under electronarcosis: A, preinduction; B, induction; C, beginning surgical anesthesia; and D, 15 minutes after onset of surgical anesthesia. (Courtesy of Dr. R.A. Herin, Colorado State University, Fort Collins, Colorado.)

do not differ from preinduction values.(118) There is little effect on arterial oxygen partial pressure; carbon dioxide content and pH are lowered while blood glucose rises. It was originally thought that electronarcosis, which produces an uninhibited response of the adrenal medullary and cortical systems, may be more desirable than drug-induced anesthesia, which usually depresses this response.(119) This is in contrast to the modern concept of anesthesia, which endeavors to minimize sympathetic nervous system response associated with the production of general anesthesia. Consequently, there has been a loss of interest in electronarcosis and immobilization as humane alternatives for producing general anesthesia.

In addition to questionable humaneness, it is difficult to assess the depth of unconsciousness achieved by electronarcosis. Muscle relaxation varies from adequate to poor. Pain induced by surgery may cause body movements in animals that appear unconscious. The photomotor reflex is probably the best means of determining the depth of anesthesia if a large dose of atropine has not been used. Early investigators indicated that analgesia persists for several minutes following removal of the current and the animal often appears hypnotized. A slight stimulus may then cause complete arousal, and the patient resumes all normal activities.

In the mid-1980s, electroimmobilization was advocated and used by sheep and cattle producers and some veterinarians for restraint and processing of food animals. This technique was recommended for minor surgery although strong evidence exists that electroimmobilization is aversive and does not eliminate pain. Amnesia and unconsciousness are not achieved with the manufacturer's recommended electrode placement and electric current application, and this technique may induce pain and dysphoria. Consequently, electroimmobilization is no longer widely used nor can it be recommended as a humane method of animal restraint.(120)

ACUPUNCTURE

Acupuncture has been advocated for providing analgesia during the operative and postoperative periods, to treat chronic pain, and to even treat selected disease states. Charts for humans and farm animals (horses, cattle, and pigs) can be commonly found in the Oriental literature. Acupuncture points can be stimulated in many different ways, including needling, injection of saline, electric stimulation, or metal implantation. It has been shown that electroacupuncture minimally decreases halothane MAC in dogs. Although the mechanism of action of acupuncture has been suggested to be the activation of the endogenous opioid neurotransmitter system, the administration of opioid antagonists does not reverse acupuncture-induced decreases in halothane MAC. Some investigators have indicated that acupuncture induces surgical analgesia. However, there appear to be three reasons why acupuncture should not be solely relied upon for surgical anesthesia; lack of restraint, inadequate analgesia, and lack of adequate information on acupuncture points to be used for specific surgical sites. These factors — along with the disadvantages of unfamiliarity, time-consuming methods of application, and inconsistent effects — have made acupuncture an unreliable and nonviable method of producing general anesthesia. Acupuncture may be best used for treatment of chronic pain in animals. Treatment of laminitis and chronic back pain in horses has reportedly been effective.(121)

PHYSIOLOGIC HYPNOSIS

Certain species of animals are highly susceptible to hypnosis (immobility reflex). These include arthropods, amphibians, reptiles, birds, guinea pigs, and rabbits. This modality is seldom used in animal anesthesia because of a lack of analgesia associated with the state of physiologic hypnosis. Hypnosis should be viewed as a legitimate method of producing immobilization, not anesthesia.

REFERENCES

1. Fragen RJ, and Avram MJ. Nonopioid intravenous anesthetics. In: Barash PG, Cullen BF, and Stoelting RK, eds. Clinical Anesthesia. Philadelphia: JB Lippincott, 1989:227–253.
2. Branson KE, and Gross ME. Propofol in veterinary medicine. J Am Vet Med Assoc 204(12):1888–1890, 1994.
3. MacDonald RL, and Barker JL. Different actions of anticonvulsant and anesthetic barbiturates revealed by use of cultured mammalian neurons. Science 200:775, 1978.
4. Nicoll RA, and Iwamoto ET. Action of pentobarbital sympathetic ganglion cells. J Neurophysiol 41:977, 1978.
5. Usenik EA, and Cronkite EP. Effects of barbiturate anesthetics on leukocytes in normal and splenectomized dogs. Anesth Analg 44:167, 1965.
6. Brown BR, and Vandam LD. A review of current advances in metabolism of inhalation anesthetics. Ann N Y Acad Sci 179:235, 1971.
7. Clemens LG, Popham RV, and Ruppert PH. Neonatal treatment of hamsters with barbiturate alters adult sexual behavior. Dev Psychobiol 12:49, 1979.
8. Gupta C, Sonawane BR, and Yaffe SJ. Phenobarbital exposure in utero: alterations in female reproductive function in rats. Science 208:508, 1980.
9. Aase JM. Anticonvulsant drugs and congenital abnormalities. Am J Dis Child 127:758, 1974.
10. Barr M Jr, Poznanski AK, and Schmikel RD. Digital hypoplasia and anticonvulsants during gestation: A teratogenic syndrome? J Pediatr 84:254, 1974.
11. Waddell WJ, and Butler TC. The distribution and excretion of phenobarbital. J Clin Invest 36:1217, 1957.
12. Maynert EW, and Van Dyke HB. The absence of localization of barbital in divisions of the central nervous system. J Pharmacol Exp Ther 98:184, 1950.
13. Peters M, and Strother A. A study of some possible mechanisms by which glucose inhibits drug metabolism in vivo and in vitro. J Pharmacol Exp Ther 180:151, 1972.
14. Hamlin RL, Redding RW, Rieger JE, Smith RC, and Prynn B. Insignificance of the "glucose effect" in dogs anesthetized with pentobarbital. J Am Vet Med Assoc 146:238, 1965.
15. Lamson PD, Greig ME, and Williams L. Potentiation by epinephrine of the anesthetic effect in chloral and barbiturate anesthesia. J Pharmacol Exp Ther 106:219, 1952.
16. Hatch RC. The effect of glucose, sodium lactate, and epinephrine on thiopental anesthesia in dogs. J Am Vet Med Assoc 148:135, 1966.
17. Skinner SF, Robertson LT, Artero M, and Gerding RK. Longitudinal study of phenobarbital in serum, cerebrospinal fluid, and saliva in the dog. Am J Vet Res 41:600, 1980.
18. Breznock EM. Effects of phenobarbital on digitoxin and digoxin elimination in the dog. Am J Vet Res 364:371, 1975.
19. Huang LYM, and Barker JL. Pentobarbital: Stereospecific actions of (+) and (−) isomers revealed on cultured mammalian neurons. Science 207:195, 1980.
20. Mathers DA, and Barker JL. (−) Pentobarbital opens ion channels of long duration in cultured mouse spinal neurons. Science 209:507, 1980.
21. Priano LL, Traber DL, and Wilson RD. Barbiturate anesthesia: An abnormal physiologic situation. J Pharmacol Exp Ther 165:126, 1969.
22. MacConnell HL. The effect of barbiturates on regional blood flows. Can Anaesth Soc J 16:1, 1969.
23. Hamlin RL, and Smith CR. Characteristics of respiration in healthy dogs anesthetized with sodium pentobarbital. Am J Vet Res 28:173, 1967.
24. Blake WD. Some effects of pentobarbital and anesthesia on renal hemodynamics. Water and electrolyte excretion in the dog. Am J Physiol 191:393, 1957.
25. Graca JG, and Garst EL. Early blood changes in dogs following intravenous pentobarbital anesthesia. Anesthesiology 18:461, 1957.
26. Hausner E, Essex HE, and Mann FC. Roentgenologic observations of the spleen of the dog under ether, sodium amytal, pentobarbital sodium and pentothal sodium anesthesia. Am J Physiol 121:387, 1938.
27. Mylon E, Winternitz MC, and De Suto-Nagy GJ. Studies on therapy in traumatic shock. Am J Physiol 139:313, 1943.
28. Corcoran AC, and Page IH. Effects of anesthetic dosage of pentobarbital sodium on renal function and blood pressure in dogs. Am J Physiol 140:234, 1943.
29. Van Dyke HB, Scudi JV, and Tabern DL. The excretion of N^{15} in the urine of dogs after the administration of labeled pentobarbital. J Pharmacol Exp Ther 90:364, 1947.
30. Davis LE, Baggot JD, Davis CAN, and Powers TE. Elimination kinetics of pentobarbital in nephrectomized dogs. Am J Vet Res 34:231, 1973.
31. Toosey MB. The uses of concentrated pentobarbitone sodium solution in bovine practice. Vet Rec 71:24, 1959.
32. Jones EW, Johnson L, and Heinze CD. Thiopental sodium anesthesia in the horse: A rapid induction technique. J Am Vet Med Assoc 137:119, 1960.
33. Linzell JL. Some observations on general and regional anesthesia in goats. In: Small animal anaesthesia. 2nd ed. London: Pergamon Press, 1964.
34. Harrison FA. The anaesthesia of sheep using pentobarbitone sodium and cyclopropane. In: Small animal anaesthesia. 2nd ed. London: Pergamon Press, 1964.
35. Hatch RC, Clark JD, Booth NH, and Kitzman JV. Comparison of five preanesthetic medicaments in pentobarbital-anesthetized dogs: Antagonism by 4-aminopyridine, yohimbine, and naloxone. Am J Vet Res 44:2312, 1983.
36. Grono LR. Methohexital sodium anaesthesia in the horse. Aust Vet J 42:398, 1966.
37. Robertshaw D. Methohexital sodium anaesthesia in calves, Vet Rec 76:357, 1964.
38. Monahan CM. The use of methohexitone for induction of anaesthesia in large animals. Vet Rec 76:1333, 1964.
39. Welles JS, McMahon RE, and Doran WJ. The metabolism and excretion of methohexital in the rat and dog. J Pharmacol Exp Ther 139:166, 1963.
40. Robinson MH. Deterioration of solutions of pentothal sodium. Anesthesiology 8:166, 1947.
41. Taylor JD, Richards RK, and Tabern DL. Metabolism of S^{35} thiopental (pentothal). J Pharmacol Exp Ther 104:93, 1952.
42. Rawlings CA, and Kolata RJ. Cardiopulmonary effects of thiopental/lidocaine combination during anesthetic induction in the dog. Am J Vet Res 44:144, 1983.
43. Muir WW. Electrocardiographic interpretation of thiobarbiturate-induced dysrhythmias in dogs. J Am Vet Med Assoc 170:1419, 1977.
44. Wiersig DO, Davis RH, and Szabuniewicz M. Prevention of induced ventricular fibrillation in dogs anesthetized with ultrashort acting barbiturates and halothane. J Am Vet Med Assoc 165:341, 1974.
45. Szabuniewicz M, Davis RH, and Wiersig DO. Prevention of methoxyflurane and thiobarbiturate cardiac sensitization to catecholamines in dogs. Practicing Vet 47:12, 1975.
46. Muir WW, Werner LL, and Hamlin RL. Effect of xylazine and acetylpromazine upon induced ventricular fibrillation in dogs anesthetized with thiamylal and halothane. Am J Vet Res 36:1299, 1975.
47. Booker WM, Maloney AH, Tureman JR, and Ratliff C. Some

metabolic factors influencing the course of thiopental anesthesia in dogs. Am J Physiol 170:168, 1952.

48. Brodie BB, Bernstein E, and Mark LC. The role of body fat in limiting the duration of action of thiopental. J Pharmacol Exp Ther 105:424, 1952.

49. Saidman LJ, and Eger EI. The effect of thiopental metabolism on duration of anesthesia. Anesthesiology 27:118, 1966.

50. Anderson EG, and Magee DF. A study of the mechanism of the effect of dietary fat in decreasing thiopental sleeping time. J Pharmacol Exp Ther 117:281, 1956.

51. Tavernor WD, and Lees P. The influence of thiopentone and suxamethonium on cardiovascular and respiratory function in the horse. Res Vet Sci 11:45, 1970.

52. Swanson EE. Sodium 5-allyl-5-(1-methylbutyl)-2-thiobarbiturate, a short acting anaesthetic. J Pharm Pharmacol 3:112, 1951.

53. Helrich M, Papper EM, and Rovenstine EA. Surital sodium: A new anesthetic agent for intravenous use. Preliminary clinical evaluation. Anesthesiology 11:33, 1950.

54. Wyngaarden JB, Woods LA, and Seevers MH. The cumulative action of certain thiobarbiturates in dogs. Fed Proc 6:388, 1947.

55. Nagel ML, Muir WW, and Nguyen K. Comparison of the cardiopulmonary effects of etomidate and thiamylal in dogs. Am J Vet Res 40:193, 1979.

56. Musselman EE. Arrhythmogenic properties of thiamylal sodium in the dog. J Am Vet Med Assoc 168:145, 1976.

57. Woods LA, Wyngaarden JB, Rennick B, and Seevers MH. Cardiovascular toxicity of thiobarbiturates: Comparison of thiopental and 5-allyl-5-(1-methylbutyl)-2-thiobarbiturate (surital) in dogs. J Pharmacol Exp Ther 95:328, 1949.

58. Ritter C, Hughes R, Snyder G, and Weaver L. Dichlorovos-containing dog collars and thiamylal anesthesia. Am J Vet Res 31:2025, 1970.

59. Elder CK, and Harrison EM. Pentothal sodium slough: Prevention by procaine hydrochloride. JAMA 125:116, 1944.

60. Jones RS. Injectable anaesthetic agents in the cat: A review. J Small Anim Pract 20:345, 1979.

61. Dodds MG, and Twissell DJ. Effect of althesin (CT 1341 on circulatory responses to adrenaline and on halothane-adrenaline cardiac dysrhythmias in the cat. Postgrad Med J 48(suppl 2):17, 1972.

62. Child KJ, Currie JP, Davis B, Dodds MG, Pearce DR, and Twissell DJ. The pharmacological properties in animals of CT 1341—a new steroid anaesthetic agent. Br J Anaesth 43:2, 1971.

63. Watkins J, and Clark RSJ. Report of a symposium: Adverse responses to intravenous agents. Br J Anaesth 50:1159, 1978.

64. Hall LW. Althesin in the larger animal. Postgrad Med J 48(suppl 2):55, 1972.

65. Camburn MA. Use of alphaxalone-alphadolone in ruminants. Vet Rec 111:166, 1982.

66. Pickerodt V, McDowall DG, Coroneos NJ, and Keaney N P. Effect of althesin on carotid blood flow and intracranial pressure in the anaesthetized baboon: Preliminary communication. Postgrad Med J 48(suppl 2):58, 1972.

67. Child KJ, Harnby G, Gibson W, and Hart JW. Metabolism and excretion of althesin (CT 1341) in the rat. Postgrad Med J 48(suppl. 2):37, 1972.

68. Stopiglia AV. Contribuicao para o estudo da anestesia genal de equideos. Fac de Med Vet, Universidad de Sao Paulo, Brasil, 1962.

69. Brown RV, and Hilton JG. The effectiveness of the baroreceptor reflexes under different anesthetics. J Pharmacol Exp Ther 118:198, 1956.

70. King EE, and Unna KR. The action of mephenesin and other interneuron depressants on the brain stem. J Pharmacol Exp Ther 111:293, 1954.

71. Harding GW, Stogsdill RM, and Towe AL. Relative effects of pentobarbital and chloralose on the responsiveness of neurons in sensorimotor cerebral cortex of the domestic cat. Neuroscience 4:369, 1979.

72. Auerbach C. The chemical production of mutations. Science 158:1141, 1967.

73. Wood EM. Urethane as a carcinogen. Progressive Fish Culturist 18:135, 1956.

74. Dimigen J, and Reetz I. Versuche zur schmerzausschaltung beim schwein mit neuroleptikum azaperon und dem hypnotikum metomidat. DTW Dtsch Tierarztl Wochenschr 77:470., 1970.

75. Wertz EM, Benson GJ, Thurmon JC, Tranquilli WJ. Pharmacokinetics of etomidate in cats. Am J Vet Res 51(2):281–285, 1990.

76. Robertson S. Advantages of etomidate as an anesthetic agent. Vet Clin North Am Small Anim Pract Opin Small Anim Anesth 22(2):277–280, 1992.

77. Kruse-Elliott KT, Swanson CR, Aucion, D. P. Effects of etomidate function on canine surgical patients. Am J Vet Res 48:1098–1100, 1987.

78. Muir WW, and Mason DE. Side effects of etomidate in dogs. J Am Vet Med Assoc 194:1430–1434, 1989.

79. Ko JCH, Thurmon JC, Benson GJ, Tranquilli WJ, and Hoffmann WE. Acute hemolysis associated with etomidate-propylene glycol infusion in dogs. J Vet Anesth 20:92–94, 1993.

80. Arduino MJ, Bland LA, McAllister SK, et al. Microbial growth and endotoxin production in the intravenous anesthetic propofol. Infect Control Hosp Epidm 12:535–539, 1991.

81. Zoran DL, Riedesel DH, and Dyer DC. Pharmacokinetics of propofol in mixed breed dogs and greyhounds. Am J Vet Res 54:755–760, 1993.

82. Langley MS, and Heel RC. Propofol: A review of its pharmacodynamic and pharmacokinetic properties and use as an intravenous anaesthetic. Drugs 35:334–372, 1988.

83. Weaver BM, Raptopoulos D. Induction of anaesthesia in dogs and cats with propofol. Vet Rec 126:617–620, 1990.

84. Morgan DWT, Legge K. Clinical evaluation of propofol as an intravenous anaesthetic agent in cats and dogs. Vet Rec 124:31–33, 1989.

85. Robertson SA, Johnston S, Beemsterboer, J. Cardiopulmonary, anesthetic, and postanesthetic effects of intravenous infusions of propofol in greyhounds and non-greyhounds. Am J Vet Res 53:1027–1032, 1992.

86. Thurmon JC, Ko JCH, Benson GJ, Tranquilli WJ, Olson WA. Hemodynamic and analgesic effects of propofol infusion in medetomidine-premedicated dogs. Am J Vet Res 55(3):363–367, 1994.

87. Smith JA, Gaynor JS, Bednarski RM, et al. Adverse effects of administration of propofol with various preanesthetic regimens in dogs. JAMA 202:1111–1115, 1993.

88. Concas A, Santoro G, Serra M, et al. Neurochemical action of the general anaesthetic propofol on the chloride ion channel coupled with GABA receptors. Brain Research 542:225–232, 1991.

89. Ilkiw JE, Pascow PJ, Haskins SC, et al. Cardiovascular and respiratory effects of propofol administration in hypovolemic dogs. Am J Vet Res 53:2323–2327, 1992.

90. Day TK, Andress DG, Day DG. Effects of consecutive day propofol anesthesia on feline red blood cells [abstract]. Proc Annu Mtg Am Coll Vet Anesthesiol, Washington, DC, 1993:15.

91. Smith I, White PF, Nathanson M, and Gouldson R. Propofol, an update on its clinical use. Anesthesiology 81(4):1005–1043, 1994.

92. Dailland P, Cockshott ID, Litzin JD, et al. Intravenous propofol during cesarean section: Placental transfer, concentrations in breast milk, and neonatal effects. A preliminary study. Anesthesiology 71:827–834, 1989.

93. Ilkiw JE. Other potentially useful new injectable anesthetic agents. Vet Clin North Am Small Anim Prac Opin Small Anim Anesth 22(2):281–288, 1992.

94. Bigelow WG, Lindsay WK, Harrison RC, Gordon RA, and Greenwood WF. Oxygen transport and utilization in dogs at low body temperatures. Am J Physiol 160:125, 1950.

95. Fuhrman GJ, Fuhrman FA, and Field J. Metabolism of rat heart slices, with special reference to effects of temperature and anoxia. Am J Physiol 163:642, 1950.

96. Gott VL, Bartlett M, Long DM, Lillehei CW, and Johnson JA. Myocardial energy substances in the dog heart during potassium and hypothermic arrest. J Appl Physiol 17:815, 1962.

97. Swan H, Zeavin I, Holmes JH, and Montgomery V. Cessation of circulation in general hypothermia. Ann Surg 138:360, 1953.

98. Bering EA Jr, Taren JA, McMurray JD, and Bernhard W F. Studies on hypothermia in monkeys. II. The effect of hypothermia on the

general physiology and cerebral metabolism of monkeys in the hypothermic state. Surg Gynecol Obstet 102:134, 1956.

99. Andjus RK, and Lovelock JE. Reanimation of rats from body temperatures between 0 and 1° C by microwave diathermy. J Physiol 128:541, 1955.

100. Smith AU. Resuscitation of hypothermic, supercooled and frozen mammals. Proc R Soc Med 49:357, 1956.

101. Gollan F, Tysinger DS Jr, Grace JT, Kory RC, and Meneely GR. Hypothermia of 1.5 degrees C in dogs followed by survival. Am J Physiol 181:297, 1955.

102. Davis TRA, and Mayer J. Nature of the physiological stimulus for shivering. Am J Physiol 181:669, 1955.

103. Regan MJ, and Eger EI. Effect of hypothermia in dogs on anesthetizing and apneic doses of inhalation agents. Anesthesiology 23:689, 1967.

104. Westenskow DR, Wong KC, Johnson CC, and Wilde CS. Physiologic effects of deep hypothermia and microwave rewarming: Possible application for neonatal cardiac surgery. Anesth Analg 58:397, 1979.

105. Blades B, and Pierpont HC. A simple method for inducing hypothermia. Ann Surg 140:557, 1954.

106. Covino BG, Charleson DA, and D'Amato HE. Ventricular fibrillation in the hypothermic dog. Am J Physiol 178:148, 1954.

107. Hess ML, Krause SM, and Greenfield LJ. Assessment of hypothermic, cardioplegic protection of the global ischemic canine myocardium. J Thorac Cardiovasc Surg 80:293, 1980.

108. Rosenfeldt FL, Hearse DJ, Cankovic-Darracott S, and Braimbridge MV. The additive protective effects of hypothermia and chemical cardioplegia during ischemic cardiac arrest in the dog. J Thorac Cardiovasc Surg 79:29, 1980.

109. Michenfelder JD, and Milde JH. Failure of prolonged hypocapnia, hypothermia or hypertension to favorably alter stroke in primates. Stroke 8:87, 1977.

110. Steen PA, Soule EH, and Michenfelder JD. The detrimental effect of prolonged hypothermia in cats and monkeys with and without regional cerebral ischemia. Stroke 10:522, 1979.

111. Steen PA, Milde JH, and Michenfelder JD. The detrimental effects of prolonged hypothermia and rewarming in the dog. Anesthesiology 52:224, 1980.

112. Knocker P. Effects of experimental hypothermia on vital organs. Lancet 2:837, 1955.

113. Watkins LR, and Mayer DJ. Organization of endogenous opiate and nonopiate pain control systems. Science 216:1185, 1982.

114. Hardy JD, Turner MD, and McNeil CD. Electrical anesthesia. III. Development of a method and laboratory observations. J Surg Res 1:152, 1961.

115. Smith RH, Goodwin C, Fowler E, Smith GW, and Volpitto PP. Electronarcosis produced by a combination of direct and alternating current. A preliminary study. Anesthesiology 22:163, 1961.

116. Herin RA. Electroanesthesia: A review of the literature (1819–1965). Act Nerv Super 10:439, 1968.

117. Smith RH, Gramling ZW, Smith GW, and Volpitto PP. Electronarcosis by combination of direct and alternating current and effects on dog brain as shown by EEG and microscopic study. Anesthesiology 22:970, 1961b.

118. Herin RA. Electrical anesthesia in the dog. J Am Vet Med Assoc 142:865, 1963.

119. McNeil CD, and Hardy JD. Electrical anesthesia: Some metabolic observations and comparisons. Surg Forum 9:394, 1959.

120. Thurmon JC. Injectable anesthetic agents and techniques in ruminants and swine. Vet Clin North Am Food Anim Pract Anesth 2(3):567–591, 1986.

121. Klide AM. Acupuncture analgesia. Vet Clin North Am Small Anim Pract Opin Small Anim Anesth 374–379, 1992.

chapter 10

DISSOCIATIVE ANESTHETICS

Hui Chu Lin

Introduction

The term *dissociative anesthesia* is used to describe an anesthetic state induced by drugs that interrupt ascending transmission from the unconscious to conscious parts of the brain, rather than by generalized depression of all brain centers.(1) There is electroencephalographic (EEG) evidence of dissociation between the thalamus and limbic system. Phencyclidine, ketamine, and tiletamine are used to induce taming and immobilization as well as general anesthesia.(2, 3) Dissociative anesthesia is characterized by a cataleptoid state in which the eyes

remain open with a slow nystagmic gaze.(4) Varying degrees of hypertonus and purposeful or reflexive skeletal muscle movements often occur unrelated to surgical stimulation. Although analgesia is intense, it is of short duration. In most respects the pharmacodynamics of tiletamine are similar to those induced by ketamine, but its potency and duration of action are intermediate between phencyclidine, the most potent, and ketamine, the least potent. Phencyclidine was the first dissociative used for animal anesthesia, but it is no longer available

241

to the practicing veterinarian. Ketamine is the most commonly used dissociative for animal anesthesia. Tiletamine is only approved for use in combination with a benzodiazepine derivative, zolazepam. In a 1:1 ratio this drug combination is marketed as Telazol.

Ketamine (Vetalar, Ketaset, Ketalar, Ketaject)

Ketamine, chemically designated as [2-(O-chlorophenyl)-2-methylaminocyclohexanone], has a molecular weight of 238, is water soluble and has a lipid solubility 5 to 10 times that of thiopental.(5-7) The ketamine molecule exists as two optical isomers. This racemic mixture is currently used clinically; however, in animals the (+) isomer induces hypnosis lasting nearly twice as long as the (−) isomer.(8, 9) The mixture is intermediate in effect. Analgesia with the (+) isomer is more profound, and there is less locomotor activity during recovery.(10) After bolus intravenous (IV) injection, ketamine rapidly crosses the blood-brain barrier, quickly entering the brain, and the brain/plasma concentration ratio becomes constant in less than 1 minute.(11) Tissue irritation occurs after intramuscular (IM) injection because the pH of the aqueous preparation of ketamine is 3.5.(12)

PHARMACOLOGY

Effects on the Central Nervous System. Ketamine produces dose-related unconsciousness and analgesia. Doses of 0.1, 1, 1.5, and 2 mg/kg IV induce a duration of unconsciousness from 1.5 to 10 minutes. Because of its small molecular weight, a pKa near the physiologic pH (7.5), and high lipid solubility, ketamine has a rapid onset of action, with maximal effect occurring in approximately 1 minute. Termination of effect after a single bolus of ketamine is caused by rapid redistribution of the drug from brain to other tissues.(11)

The primary site of central nervous system (CNS) action of ketamine appears to be the thalamoneocortical projection system. It selectively depresses neuronal function of the neocorticothalamic axis and the central nucleus of the thalamus while it stimulates parts of the limbic system, including the hippocampus (Chapter 7).(13, 14) Evidence indicates that ketamine also depresses nociceptive cells in the medial medullary reticular formation and activity of laminae I and V of the feline dorsal horn.(15, 16) Ketamine administration to people with a history of seizures does not induce seizure activity in spite of the presence of thalamic and limbic epileptiform EEG patterns.(17, 18) In fact, low doses of ketamine may have anticonvulsant properties through antagonism of N-methyl-D-aspartate (NMDA) receptors.(19-22) Nevertheless, ketamine-induced seizure has been reported in some dogs and cats known to be epileptic.(23-26) In general, use of ketamine in animals with a history of epilepsy, should be avoided.

Intense analgesia produced by ketamine occurs at subanesthetic doses with elevated pain threshold correlated with plasma level of 0.1 µg/mL or greater.(27) The degree of analgesia appears to be greater for somatic pain than for visceral pain.(28) Proposed mechanisms responsible for the analgesic actions of ketamine include blockade of spinoreticular tracts(29, 30), depression of nuclei of the medial medullary reticular formation(15), suppression of lamina of the spinal cord(16, 31, 32), interaction with CNS and spinal cord opiate receptors(33-36), and NMDA receptor antagonism. In cats visceral analgesia induced by ketamine (2, 4, and 8 mg/kg IV) is similar to that produced by butorphanol (0.1 mg/kg IV). With increasing doses of ketamine, or when ketamine and butorphanol were administered simultaneously, there is no increase in visceral analgesia.(37) However, even at the highest dose of ketamine (8 mg/kg), when cats appeared anesthetized they still responded to colonic nociceptor stimulation. Therefore, ketamine alone is not recommended to relieve visceral pain associated with abdominal or thoracic procedures lasting more than 30 minutes. Ketamine appears to be more effective for minor surgery and postoperative analgesia involving skeletal/integumentary structures and extremities.(37, 38)

Epidural administration of ketamine produces dose-dependent selective analgesia.(39, 40) In rats, a dose of 6 mg/kg induced motor function blockade for 5 to 15 minutes, while only sensory blockade occurred with 4 mg/kg.(41) Similar to systemic administration, epidural ketamine produces profound somatic but poor visceral analgesia. Simultaneous administration of a local anesthetic and ketamine improves visceral analgesia.(42) Subarachnoid administration of ketamine (1–2 mg/kg) between L1 and L2 of dogs produces analgesia of the hind limbs.(43) Subarachnoid injection of ketamine between T18 and L1 allowed performance of abdominal surgery in the standing horse.(44) The actual mechanism of epidural and subarachnoid ketamine-induced analgesia is not clear, though several mechanisms have been suggested, including interaction with opiate receptors(35, 45), lamina selective suppression of dorsal horn unit activity(16), local anesthetic effect of ketamine(46), and blockade of alpha-adrenoceptor pathways(47).

Ketamine induces significant increase in cerebral blood flow (CBF), intracranial pressure (ICP), and cerebrospinal fluid (CSF) pressure as a result of cerebral vasodilation and elevated systemic blood pressure.(48-54) The mechanism of ketamine-induced elevated ICP remains controversial. Ketamine increases CBF and ICP in awake goats when $PaCO_2$ is allowed to rise but has no effect on CBF and ICP when $PaCO_2$ is maintained at a preketamine level.(55, 56) In piglets with increased ICP, ketamine induced a further increase in ICP, paralleling a rise in $PaCO_2$. When ventilation was controlled, no increase in ICP was observed in piglets with normal or elevated ICP.(56) Increased skeletal, thoracic, and abdominal muscle tone can impede venous return from the head, increasing intracranial blood volume and pressure.(56, 57) Administration of a nondepolarizing muscle relaxant (e.g., pancuronium) may normalize ICP in patients with increased ICP.(56) Diazepam or thiopental attenuates ketamine-induced cerebral vasodilation and the increase in CSF pressure.(53, 58-60) Similarly, midazolam and fentanyl attenuate ketamine-induced increases in ICP in dogs.(60) Regardless of the mechanism, if controlled ventilation is used to maintain $PaCO_2$ between 25 and 30 mm Hg, further increases in ICP can be prevented.(60) Based on these studies, ketamine should be avoided in spontaneously breathing patients with increased CSF pressure or head injury.

Hallucinatory behavior, which may progress to delirium, may occur during emergence from ketamine anesthesia. Ketamine-induced depression of the inferior colliculus and medial geniculate nucleus leading to misperception of auditory and visual stimuli may be responsible for this reaction.(5) In cats, emergence reactions are characterized by ataxia, increased motor activity, hyperreflexia, sensitivity to touch, avoidance behavior of an invisible object, and sometimes violent recovery.(22, 61, 62) These reactions usually disappear within several hours without recurrence. Premedication or concurrent administration of xylazine (63, 64), acetylpromazine,(65) or a benzodiazepine derivative (e.g., diazepam or midazolam)(66-68) decreases the incidence of adverse emergence reactions (Chapter 20).

Effects on the Cardiovascular System. The cardiovascular action of ketamine is characterized by indirect cardiovascular stimulation. Various effects on target organs include (a) sympathomimetic effects mediated within CNS (69); (b) inhibition of neuronal uptake of catecholamines by sympathetic nerve endings(70); (c) direct vasodilation of vascular smooth muscle(71); and (d) an inotropic effect on the myocardium(72). Heart rate and arterial blood pressure increase as a result of direct stimulation of the CNS, leading to increased sympathetic outflow.(73) Plasma concentrations of epinephrine and norepinephrine increase within 2 minutes after intravenous administration of ketamine and return to control levels 15 minutes later.(74) In dogs and cats anesthetized with ketamine, mean arterial pressure, heart rate, and cardiac output increases while peripheral vascular resistance remains unchanged.(28, 75-80) Increased myocardial stimulation is associated with increased cardiac work and myocardial O_2 consumption. Increases in myocardial O_2 supply result from increased cardiac output and a decrease in coronary vascular resistance such that increases in coronary blood flow parallel the increase in O_2 consumption.(81, 82) However, some studies indicate that ketamine-induced increases in coronary blood flow may be insufficient to meet myocardial O_2 demand.(83, 84) The cardiovascular stimulating effects induced by ketamine are blunted or prevented by prior administration of a benzodiazepine(85, 86), droperidol(87), acetylpromazine, alpha$_2$-agonists, or the concomitant administration of inhalation anesthetics, including nitrous oxide.(88, 89)

The effect of ketamine on the myocardium remains controversial. A positive inotropic effect has been demonstrated in patients whose heart rates were kept constant by atrial pacing(72) and in isolated mammalian papillary muscle.(90-93) In denervated hearts, ketamine induces direct myocardial depression in vivo(94, 95) and in vitro.(93, 96-98) Cook et al. suggested that the predominant inotropic mechanism of ketamine is inhibition of catecholamine uptake at the neuroeffector junction, leading to activation of beta-adrenoceptors.(93) The importance of an intact and normally functioning CNS in stimulating cardiovascular function is underscored when ketamine is administered in the presence of other anesthetics. For example, when administered to dogs anesthetized with pentobarbital, ketamine induces a biphasic response in blood pressure(96), whereas in conscious dogs it only induces a pressor response.(75) Likewise, in pentobarbital-anesthetized rats, ketamine induces myocardial depression.(99) A negative inotropic effect of ketamine has been clearly demonstrated in isolated perfused rabbit hearts(96) and in left ventricular trabeculae carneae preparations of rats.(100) In right heart bypass, ketamine repeatedly depresses myocardial performance.(101) In rabbits anesthetized with pentobarbital, intravenous injection of ketamine depresses preganglionic sympathetic activity and arterial pressure, but heart rate is not altered significantly.(102) In anesthetic doses, ketamine may inhibit catecholamine uptake and enhance beta-adrenergic activity, negating a direct depressant effect upon the heart.(103)

An antiarrhythmic action based on ketamine's ability to reverse epinephrine-induced ventricular arrhythmias in dogs anesthetized with halothane has been reported.(96) In another study in dogs, ketamine increased the ventricular arrhythmogenic dose of epinephrine (ADE) during halothane anesthesia.(104) Results from more recent studies in which ketamine has been shown to sensitize the myocardium to catecholamines conflict with the earlier reports.(105) In halothane-anesthetized cats, ketamine infusion significantly decreases ventricular ADE.(106) In cats, the arrhythmogenic action of ketamine is greater during halothane than during isoflurane anesthesia.(107)

The survival rate of animals in shock is reportedly greater when they are anesthetized with ketamine versus halothane.(108) Ketamine has been recommended for anesthesia of critically ill patients in which there is a risk of cardiac depression and hypotension. However, when ketamine was used in patients with valvular heart disease, the workload of the heart increased, as evidenced by increasing pulmonary vascular resistance, pulmonary arterial and capillary and capillary wedge pressures, mean arterial pressure, and central venous pressure.(82, 109) While blood pressure may be better maintained with ketamine, arterial lactate concentrations increase more than in animals with lower blood pressure anesthetized with a volatile anesthetic.(110) Critically ill patients occasionally respond to ketamine with an unexpected decrease in blood pressure and cardiac output.(95) This likely results from depletion of catecholamine stores and an uncovering of ketamine's direct myocardial depressant effects.(111)

Effects on the Respiratory System. Ketamine differs from most other anesthetics in that it does not depress ventilatory responses to hypoxia.(12) Skeletal muscle tone is maintained or even increased; thus, arterial oxygenation and functional residual capacity are usually well maintained during ketamine anesthesia.(112-115) In dogs, when compared to halothane, a continuous infusion of ketamine induces a consistently lower shunt fraction and higher PaO_2 values during one-lung anesthesia.(116) Computed tomography reveals that during ketamine anesthesia and spontaneous breathing only occasional development of atelectasis occurs and gas exchange is minimally affected.

In dogs anesthetized with ketamine, respiratory rate and minute volume decrease initially, but both return to baseline values within 15 minutes.(118) In cats and sheep, ketamine induces a transient decrease in PaO_2 in the presence of decreased or increased respiratory rate.(28, 119-123) The transient apnea induced by ketamine appears to be dose dependent. At higher doses, respiration is characterized by an apneustic, shallow, and irregular pattern.(2, 25, 80) Severe respiratory depression or arrest with overdosage has been reported in human patients and cats.(80, 124-126)

Ketamine often causes increased salivation and secretion of respiratory track mucus, which can easily be controlled by administration of an anticholinergic. Laryngeal and pharyngeal reflexes usually are well maintained during ketamine anesthesia. Nevertheless, swallowing reflexes may be somewhat obtunded because most species can be intubated when anesthetized with ketamine.(62) Careful airway management and/or endotracheal intubation should always be performed to prevent aspiration.

Effects on the Hepatic, Renal, and Reproductive Systems. A significant increase in serum concentrations of liver enzymes has been observed in humans anesthetized with a ketamine infusion.(127) Dogs given higher intramuscular doses (40 mg/kg daily, for 6 weeks) of ketamine also have a transient increase in liver enzymes.(1) Nevertheless, hepatic dysfunction is not evident in either humans or dogs.(1, 127) In rats, ketamine induces hepatic microsomal enzymes similar to phenobarbital-associated induction but to a lesser extent.(128)

Ketamine undergoes extensive hepatic metabolism in the dog, horse, and human. Very little hepatic metabolism occurs in the cat, and the majority of the injected ketamine is eliminated unchanged via the kidney.(129) Rapid recovery following ketamine administration is caused by rapid redistribution of ketamine from the CNS to all body tissues, primarily body fat, lung, liver, and kidney.(130) Clinically, animals with hepatic dysfunction do not metabolize ketamine as rapidly as normal animals. Animals with renal dysfunction or obstruction to urine flow also have prolonged sleep times.(121) Ketamine should be given cautiously in animals with hepatic or renal dysfunction.

Just as the administration of chloramphenicol and acetoxycycloheximide prolongs the sleep time of subsequent administrations of pentobarbital, the use of chloramphenicol also increases ketamine sleep time in cats.(131)

Pregnant ewes have been successfully anesthetized for up to 2 hours with intravenous ketamine (2 mg/kg) followed by continuous infusion of ketamine (0.2% ketamine in 5% glucose) at a rate of 4 mL/min.(132) Levinson et al. reported that ketamine increased uterine blood flow and did not produce deleterious effects on fetal cardiovascular or acid-base status.(133) When given intramuscularly or intravenously to pregnant goats, ketamine rapidly traverses the placental membrane and increases in both fetal heart rate and blood pressure occur. Fetal pHa and PaO_2 decrease while $PaCO_2$ increases during ketamine anesthesia. These effects are greater with intravenous than intramuscular administration.(134) When used for induction, ketamine reportedly increases basal uterine tone and the intensity of contractions in both pregnant and nonpregnant women. Nevertheless, human fetal mortality is less with ketamine than with other anesthetics.(135)

Effects on Intraocular Pressure. In people a slight but statistically significant increase in intraocular pressure (IOP) independent of changes in blood pressure occurs with ketamine anesthesia.(136, 137) Conflicting results have been reported, however. Intravenous or intramuscular administration of 2 mg/kg or 8 mg/kg of ketamine did not produce a significant effect on IOP.(138, 139) In dogs, IOP increases during xylazine and ketamine anesthesia while in horses it tends to decrease.(41, 140) Increases in extraocular muscle tone induced by ketamine may be responsible for the increase in IOP.(142) With this in mind, ketamine should be used with caution in patients with corneal injuries where increased IOP may result in expulsion of intraocular contents (Chapter 24).

CLINICAL USE

Dogs. Ketamine, when used alone, induces extreme muscle tone, exuberant spontaneous movement, violent recovery, and occasional convulsions in dogs.(62, 118) Clinically, ketamine is used in combinations with or after a tranquilizer or sedative to eliminate many of the side effects cited in Table 10–1. Benzodiazepines induce a central muscle relaxant effect that decreases muscle hypertonus associated with ketamine.(143) Midazolam maleate, a water-soluble benzodiazepine, has a potency three times that of diazepam. Midazolam (0.5 mg/kg IV) and ketamine (10 mg/kg IV) induce a significant increase in heart rate and mild respiratory depression as evidenced by increased $PaCO_2$. Duration of anesthesia induced by this combination is approximately 12 to 15 minutes.(144) In a comparative study, both midazolam/ketamine and diazepam/ketamine combinations induced minimal cardiovascular and respiratory effects in greyhounds. Time to intubation was significantly shorter with midazolam/ketamine, but recovery seemed to be smoother with diazepam/ketamine.(145) Intrave-

Table 10–1. Use of Ketamine or Ketamine Combinations in Dogs

Drug(s)	Dose and Route (mg/kg)	Duration (min)	Comment	Reference
Ketamine	10, IV	15 ± 8	↑ Muscle tone Short duration Anesthesia inadequate for surgery	118
Ketamine	1 or 2, intrathecal	—	Analgesia of the hindlimbs	43
Acepromazine Ketamine Thiamylal	0.55, IM 11–22, IM To effect, IV	20–90	Occasional seizures	23
Acepromazine Ketamine	0.22 IM 11–18, IM	—	Restraint for aggressive dogs Spastic movements Prolonged recovery	146
Acepromazine Ketamine	0.5, IV 10, IM	—	Good restraint	298
Acepromazine Ketamine	0.2, IV 10, IV	39 ± 8	Less muscle rigidity Useful for clinical anesthesia Not suitable for patients with hypotension or respiratory depression	299
Xylazine Ketamine	0.55–1.1, IM 22, IV; to effect	—	Excellent surgical anesthesia Good muscle relaxation and analgesia for abdominal surgery	148
Xylazine Ketamine	2.2, IM 11, IM	—	Occasional seizures	300
Xylazine Ketamine	2.2, IM 11, IM	25–50	Occasional seizures	147
Xylazine Ketamine	2.2, IM 5.5, IM	30	Occasional seizures	301
Xylazine Ketamine Thiamylal	1.1, IM 11–22, IM To effect, IV	25–60	Occasional seizures	302
Xylazine Ketamine	0.22, IM 10, IM	28–36	—	303
Atropine Xylazine Ketamine	0.04, IV 1.1, IV 11, IV	—	—	304
Atropine Xylazine Ketamine	0.044, IM 1.1, IM 22, IM	22 (17–35)	↑ Risk in dogs with cardiopulmonary disease	305
Guaifenesin Xylazine Ketamine	50 mg/mL 0.25 mg/mL 1 mg/mL Induction 0.55 mL/kg, IV Maintenance 2.2 mL/kg/h, IV	120	Stable anesthesia	150
Xylazine Ketamine	1, IV 10, IM	32 ± 6	Better muscle relaxation than ketamine alone	306
Xylazine Ketamine Medetomidine Ketamine Medetomidine Ketamine	1, IM 15, IM 0.04, IM 2.5, IM 0.04, IM 5, IM	24 ± 5.5 7 ± 0.9 30 ± 4.9	— — Longer duration of muscle relaxation and recovery than xylazine/ketamine Prolonged recovery	154

Table 10–1.   Use of Ketamine or Ketamine Combinations in Dogs (continued)

Drug(s)	Dose and Route (mg/kg)	Duration (min)	Comment	Reference
Medetomidine Ketamine	0.04, IM 7.5, IM	51 ± 8	—	154
Medetomidine Ketamine	0.04, IM 5, IM	>75	Significant cardiovascular changes	155
Diazepam Ketamine	0.28, IV 5.5, IV	—	Suitable induction for greyhound	145
Midazolam Ketamine	0.28, IV 5.5, IV	—	More myoclonic movements Shorter time to intubation Suitable induction for greyhound	
Midazolam Ketamine	0.5, IV 10, IV	13.3 ± 3.1	↑ Heart rate Mild respiratory depression Better muscle relaxation	144

nous administration of acepromazine (0.11 mg/kg) and ketamine (11 mg/kg) induces anesthesia for 10 to 35 minutes with good muscle relaxation and smooth recovery.(62) This combination can be administered intramuscularly for restraint of aggressive dogs when intravenous injection is difficult.(146) Kaplan suggested that administering an intravenous dose of 0.5 to 3 mL of 2.5% thiamylal following acepromazine and ketamine induces more predictable anesthesia.(23)

Xylazine (1.1 mg/kg IM) is often used with ketamine (11 mg/kg IM) for short-term anesthesia of 25 to 40 minutes. The dose of ketamine can be adjusted (4-22 mg/kg) according to the duration for surgery.(118, 147) In "high-strung" small breed dogs, small ketamine doses produce insufficient anesthesia and have greater tendency to cause seizure. Excessive salivation may occur during ketamine anesthesia, but this can be controlled with atropine. Xylazine-induced bradycardia and second-degree AV block may be minimized by ketamine's cardiovascular stimulating effect. However, atropine should be given if xylazine-induced cardiac effects are severe. The use of xylazine-ketamine for cesarean section in the dog has been evaluated.(148) The authors indicated that xylazine (0.55 mg/kg IM) and ketamine (22 mg/kg IV, to effect) produced surgical anesthesia with analgesia and muscle relaxation that were more than adequate for abdominal surgery. Some puppies were depressed after delivery, and the depression was believed to be caused by the combined factors of dystocia and anesthetic effects.(148) An advantage of xylazine-ketamine combination is the reversibility of xylazine-induced CNS and cardiopulmonary depression. Antagonism should not be initiated for at least 20 minutes after administration of ketamine. Earlier antagonism of xylazine in xylazine-ketamine-anesthetized dogs may result in ketamine-induced hyperexcitability and seizures.(149)

Guaifenesin has been added to a xylazine-ketamine combination to enhance muscle relaxation. The mixture for use in dogs is prepared by adding 1 g of ketamine and 250 mg of xylazine to 1 L of 5% guaifenesin. The final concentration is 1 mg/mL, 0.25 mg/mL, and 50 mg/mL for ketamine, xylazine, and guaifenesin, respectively. The intravenous dose used to induce anesthesia is 0.55 mL/kg and for maintenance is 2.2 mL/kg/h. Significant decreases in cardiac index and hypoventilation have been observed when using this mixture for anesthetic maintenance.(150)

Medetomidine is an new alpha$_2$-agonist, similar to xylazine, with a higher alpha$_2$/alpha$_1$ selectivity (1620) than that of xylazine (160).(151) It has been used with ketamine to induce short-term anesthesia in dogs.(152, 153) Medetomidine (40 μg/kg IM) and ketamine (5 mg/kg IM) induce anesthesia (duration of 20 to 35 minutes) comparable to that of xylazine (1 mg/kg IM) and ketamine (15 mg/kg IM). Duration of muscle relaxation and recovery are longer with the medetomidine/ketamine combination. Both xylazine/ketamine and medetomidine/ketamine combinations induce significant decreases in heart rate and respiration rate, but the decrease is more profound and longer lasting with medetomidine/ketamine.(154) In another study medetomidine/ketamine did not induce significant effects on respiratory function, but significant cardiovascular depression occurred as evidenced by a decrease in heart rate, cardiac output, stroke volume, and left and right ventricular stroke index.(155)

Cats. In cats, ketamine produces a profound anesthesia with doses ranging from 11 to 44 mg/kg intramuscularly. Depending upon the dose, cats become recumbent within 1 to 8 minutes after injection with peak plasma levels at 10 minutes. Duration of anesthesia is approximately 30 to 45 minutes.(156, 157) Repeat doses of ketamine can be given to cats to prolong anesthesia. However, large doses to prolong anesthesia are not recommended.(156) Rapid induction and faster recovery with a short duration of anesthesia (10 to 15 minutes) occur when ketamine (2 to 6 mg/kg) is administered intravenously. Cardiac arrest or apnea may occur when a large intravenous dose is rapidly injected. Therefore, intravenous ketamine should be administered slowly and to effect.(157)

Diazepam (0.3 mg/kg) has been mixed in the same syringe with ketamine (5.5 mg/kg) and given slowly intravenously for short-term anesthesia. This has proven to be a safe combination in cats with compromised cardiovascular function. Diazepam (0.22 mg/kg IV or 0.44 mg/kg IM) followed by a total dose of 1 to 5 mg/kg of ketamine has also been used successfully in geriatric cats.(157) Administration of butorphanol prior to diazepam-ketamine may increase analgesia and permit diagnostic or surgical procedures to be performed when endotracheal intubation and delivery of an inhalant anesthetic is not feasible.(149) When various doses of midazolam (0.05, 0.5, 1.0, 2.0, or 5 mg/kg IV) are combined with ketamine (3 mg/kg IV), the duration of anesthesia increases slightly. However, increasing the dose (5 mg/kg) prolongs objectionable behavioral signs (restlessness, vocalization, and changes in ability to approach and restrain).(158) Phenothiazine tranquilizers such as acepromazine, promazine, and triflupromazine have been combined with ketamine for better muscle relaxation and a smoother recovery. However, phenothiazine derivatives are alpha-adrenoceptor antagonists, and hypotension, prolonged recovery, and hypothermia may occur if they are used at high doses. Hartsfield suggests that doses of 0.1 to 0.6 mg/kg (IV, IM, or SQ) of acepromazine not to exceed a total dose of 3 mg is effective in decreasing the undesirable effects of ketamine anesthesia.(157)

In clinical practice, xylazine and ketamine is a popular anesthetic combination for use in cats. Xylazine (0.5–1.1 mg/kg IM), with or without atropine, is administered 20 minutes before ketamine (11–22 mg/kg IM).(64, 159) Emesis is a common side effect of xylazine in cats, and this should be allowed to occur prior to ketamine administration to prevent aspiration of stomach contents.(62) When compared to acepromazine-ketamine (acepromazine 0.11 mg/kg and ketamine 4.6 mg/kg, IM), the simultaneous administration of xylazine-ketamine (xylazine 0.23 mg/kg and ketamine 4.6 mg/kg, IM) produces a longer duration of action. Xylazine-ketamine is accompanied by cardiopulmonary depression that is more profound and of longer duration.(160)

Medetomidine (80 µg/kg IM) has been combined with several different doses of ketamine (2.5, 5, 7.5, and 10 mg/kg IM) in cats undergoing ovariohysterectomy. The higher doses of ketamine will not prolong the duration of anesthesia. Apnea may occur when the ketamine dose approaches 10 mg/kg. A dose of 5 mg/kg with medetomidine (80 µg/kg) produces anesthesia of approximately 1 hour. Good muscle relaxation and profound analgesia are comparable to that achieved with xylazine (1 mg/kg IM) and ketamine (10 mg/kg IM). Duration of anesthesia is longer than that achieved with acepromazine (1 mg/kg IM) and ketamine (10 mg/kg IM).(161, 162) Specific alpha$_2$-antagonists such as atipamezole and yohimbine and CNS stimulants such as 4-aminopyridine have been used to reverse medetomidine/ketamine anesthesia.

Atipamezole (0.2 mg/kg IM) and yohimbine (0.5 mg/kg IM) have been effective in antagonizing the anesthetic effects of medetomidine/ketamine.(163, 164)

A continuous infusion of guaifenesin, ketamine, and xylazine has been used to maintain anesthesia for up to 6 hours in laboratory cats. This combination is prepared by adding 1 g of ketamine and 250 mg of xylazine to 1 L of 5% guaifenesin. Fifty milliliters of this mixture is added to 200 mL of saline to make the final concentration 0.2 mg/mL, 0.05 mg/mL, and 10 mg/mL of ketamine, xylazine, and guaifenesin, respectively. Cats premedicated with 3 to 4 mg/kg of ketamine intramuscularly can be induced with approximately 1 to 1.5 mL of this mixture injected slowly intravenously to effect. Anesthesia has been maintained for approximately 6 hours with this mixture. Heart rate, respiratory rate, PvO$_2$, and PvCO$_2$ did not change significantly from baseline values. Only venous pH decreased slightly during the study period. Cats were in sternal recumbency within 2 hours after discontinuation of infusion.(165)

Oxymorphone, morphine, meperidine, and butorphanol have been used in combination with ketamine in the cat.(38, 166, 167) When administered at oxymorphone's peak effect, the ketamine requirement is decreased by 2.5 to 10%.(166) Administration of morphine or meperidine neither improves nor complicates the anesthetic effects of ketamine.(167) Adding butorphanol (0.1 mg/kg IV) to ketamine (8 mg/kg IV) appears to increase the intensity and duration of analgesia for a variety of procedures. The most effective dose of butorphanol ranges from 0.05 to 0.2 mg/kg intravenously. Some clinicians' experiences suggest that doses below and above this range provide less analgesia. It is important to realize that butorphanol is an opioid agonist-antagonist that possesses a "ceiling effect" on analgesia as well as undesirable opioid actions (e.g., respiratory depression). Doses above 0.2 mg/kg may result in increased CNS stimulation that is unaccompanied by an increased analgesic action. Table 10–2 summarizes the use of ketamine in cats.

Horses. Ketamine should not be used as a monoanesthetic in horses. Preanesthetic sedation and tranquilization must be present before ketamine is administered. Xylazine is most commonly used for this purpose. Xylazine (1.1 mg/kg IV), followed in 5 to 10 minutes by ketamine (2.2–3.0 mg/kg IV), induces a short period of safe and effective anesthesia in all breeds of horses. Higher doses of ketamine (2.75–3.0 mg/kg IV) are required for ponies, young "high-strung" Arabians, Hackneys, and Thoroughbreds.(168) Ketamine should not be administered if xylazine fails to produce adequate sedation, and an alternative anesthetic technique (e.g., guaifenesin-thiobarbiturate mixture) should be considered.(168) It is not uncommon for heart rate and respiratory rate to decrease by one third after xylazine administration.(169) After ketamine injection, heart rate may remain decreased while respiratory rate returns to prexylazine values.(169) Cardiac output, systemic arterial, pulmonary and central venous pres-

Table 10–2. Use of Ketamine or Ketamine Combinations in Cats

Drug(s)	Dose and Route (mg/kg)	Duration (min)	Comment	Reference
Ketamine	<22, IM	20–40	Chemical restraint	26
Ketamine	22–44, IM	—	Cataleptoid anesthesia Lack of muscle relaxation	
Ketamine	11–44, IM	20–45	—	307
Ketamine	22 IM	—	Castration, onychectomy, restraint	
Ketamine	33, IM	—	Ovariohysterectomy, cesarean section, laparotomy, orthopedic procedures	
Ketamine	4–30, IM	—	—	308
Ketamine	5–20, IM	—	—	
Ketamine	4, IM	—	Incomplete immobilization	
Ketamine	10, IM	—	Chemical restraint Little analgesia	
Ketamine	20, IM	—	Better muscle relaxation Minor surgical procedures	
Ketamine	33, IM	77	Little analgesia Respiratory depression Occasional apnea	28
Oxymorphone	0.16, SQ, IM, IV	10–20	Light anesthesia	166
Triflupromazine	1.1, SQ, IM, IV			
Ketamine	1.1–2.2, SQ, IM, IV			
Xylazine	1.1, IM	25–40	—	309
Ketamine	15.4–22, IM			
Xylazine	1.1, IM	30	Vomiting	159
Ketamine	22, IM			
Xylazine	2.2, IM	118	Vomiting	63
Ketamine	11, IM			
Xylazine	0.23, IM	120	Vomiting	310
Ketamine	4.6, IM			
Acepromazine	0.11, IM	35–45	—	
Ketamine	4.6, IM			
Xylazine	0.23, IM	100 ± 15	Longer duration than acepromazine/ketamine	160
Ketamine	4.6, IM			
Acepromazine	0.11, IM	37 ± 10	Better maintained heart rate than xylazine/ketamine	
Ketamine	4.6, IM			
Xylazine	2.2, IM	60	—	311
Ketamine	6.6, IM			
Xylazine	4.4, IM	100	—	
Ketamine	6.6, IM			
Atropine	0.3, IM	20	Satisfactory anesthesia	312
Xylazine	1.1, IM			
Ketamine	22, IM			
Guaifenesin	10 mg/mL	360	Easy administration	165
Xylazine	0.05 mg/mL		Stable anesthetic depth	
Ketamine	0.2 mg/mL		Rapid recovery compared to other anesthetics	
	Induction 1.32 ± 0.33 ml/kg, IV		Reversible with yohimbine or tolazoline	
	Maintenance 10 mL/kg/h, IV			
Acepromazine	1, IM	20 ± 14.8	Poor muscle relaxation and analgesia	162
Ketamine	10, IM			
Xylazine	1, IM	46 ± 22.6	Satisfactory anesthesia Depression of cardiovascular system	
Ketamine	10, IM			
Medetomidine	0.08, IM	36.2 ± 11.5	Better muscle relaxation	
Ketamine	2.5, IM		Satisfactory anesthesia	

Table 10–2. Use of Ketamine or Ketamine Combinations in Cats (continued)

Drug(s)	Dose and Route (mg/kg)	Duration (min)	Comment	Reference
Medetomidine	0.08, IM	59 ± 6.4	Better muscle relaxation	162
Ketamine	5, IM		Satisfactory anesthesia	
Medetomidine	0.08, IM	65.6 ± 22.9	Better muscle relaxation	
Ketamine	7.5, IM		Satisfactory anesthesia	
Medetomidine	0.08, IM	99.7 ± 26.7	Better muscle relaxation	
Ketamine	10, IM		Satisfactory anesthesia	
			Occasional apnea	
Ketamine	2, IV	105	Visceral analgesia	37 38
Ketamine	4, IV	110	Visceral analgesia	
Ketamine	8, IV	115	Visceral analgesia	
Diazepam	0.2, IV	20	Visceral analgesia	
Ketamine	2, IV			
Diazepam	0.2, IV	60	Visceral analgesia	
Ketamine	4, IV			
Diazepam	0.2, IV	100	Visceral analgesia	
Ketamine	8, IV			
Acepromazine	0.1, IV	65	Visceral analgesia	
Ketamine	2, IV			
Acepromazine	0.1, IV	80	Visceral analgesia	
Ketamine	4, IV			
Acepromazine	0.1, IV	125 ± 22	Visceral analgesia	
Ketamine	8, IV			
Butorphanol	0.1, IV	280	Visceral analgesia	
Ketamine	2, IV			
Butorphanol	0.1, IV	325	Visceral analgesia	
Ketamine	4, IV			
Butorphanol	0.1, IV	360	Visceral analgesia	
Ketamine	8, IV			
Medetomidine	0.08, IM	46 ± 15	Vomiting	163
Ketamine	7, IM		Surgical anesthesia	
			Good muscle relaxation	
Medetomidine	0.08, IM	50.2	—	164
Ketamine	5, IM			
Ketamine	3, IV	—	↑ Muscle tone	158
			Immobilization	
Midazolam	0.05, IV	—	↓ Muscle tone	
Ketamine	3, IV		Dose-related behavioral signs	
			Suitable for clinical use	
Midazolam	0.5, IV	5 ± 1.1	Muscle relaxation	
Ketamine	3, IV		Suitable for clinical use	
Midazolam	1, IV	—	Suitable for clinical use	
Ketamine	3, IV			
Midazolam	2, IV	—	—	
Ketamine	3, IV			
Midazolam	5, IV	6.2 ± 1.62	Prominent and long-lasting behavioral signs	
Ketamine	5, IV			

sures remain within normal ranges during xylazine-ketamine anesthesia.(169) Duration of anesthesia (15–20 minutes) is related to redistribution of ketamine to other body tissues and hepatic metabolism. In horses, approximately 60% of ketamine is metabolized by the liver, with the remainder excreted unchanged in the urine.(170) Anesthesia can be extended by redosing with one third to one half of the original dose of each drug.

Xylazine (1.1 mg/kg IV) does not always produce adequate sedation in mules. Butorphanol (0.04 mg/kg IV) has been combined with xylazine and ketamine to enhance analgesia, improve muscle relaxation, and prolong duration of recumbency in mules.(171) Tranquilli et al. reported that the addition of butorphanol (0.11 or 0.22 mg/kg) enhances muscle relaxation and analgesia when using a xylazine-ketamine combination. Behavioral changes caused by butorphanol may be breed dependent. Central nervous system stimulation characterized by hyperresponsiveness and spasmodic lip movements has been reported in high-strung individuals after butorphanol administration, whereas deep sedation and ataxia were observed in a Belgian stallion.(172) For extremely painful procedures, methadone with and without acepromazine has been administered to enhance analgesia during xylazine-ketamine anesthesia.(173, 174)

Ketamine (2 mg/mL) can be added directly to a 5% solution of guaifenesin and the mixture administered as a rapid infusion, or it can be administered as a bolus (1.5–2.2 mg/kg IV) after administration of enough guaifenesin to produce limb weakness. Less cardiovascular depression occurs with this combination, as compared to thiopental- or thiamylal-guaifenesin.(168) When premedicated with xylazine (1 mg/kg IV) and atropine (1 mg/100 kg), ketamine plus guaifenesin rapidly induces anesthesia with good muscle relaxation and analgesia followed by a smooth recovery in foals.(175) In these foals the mean induction and maintenance doses of ketamine were 2.3 mg/kg and 12.1 $mg \cdot kg^{-1} \cdot h^{-1}$, respectively. Heart rate, arterial blood pressure, and respiratory rate remained within the normal range.(175) Only slight respiratory acidosis, as evidenced by changes in blood gas and pH, was observed 5 minutes after induction.(175) Marked respiratory depression did not occur during anesthesia.(175)

Continuous infusion of a guaifenesin-ketamine-xylazine combination is safe and effective for extending anesthesia in adult horses following xylazine (1.1 mg/kg IV) and ketamine (2.2–3.0 mg/kg IV) induction. This drug combination is prepared by adding 500 mg of xylazine and 2.0 g of ketamine to 1 L of 5% guaifenesin in dextrose.(176, 177) In ponies anesthetized for 2 hours with this mixture, arterial blood pressure and left ventricular stroke work index were transiently decreased for the first 15 to 30 minutes after induction.(176) Cardiac index and arterial pH were also decreased for 15 minutes after induction.(176) Hypoventilation with mild hypercapnia was noted throughout the study.(176) These changes are transient and comparable to those reported for other injectable anesthetic drugs or drug combinations.(176) In untranquilized ponies and foals, anesthesia can be induced with a rapid intravenous injection of 1.1 mL/kg of the guaifenesin-ketamine-xylazine mixture. Anesthesia may be maintained by continuous intravenous infusion of 2 to 4 $mL \cdot kg^{-1} \cdot h^{-1}$ depending upon anesthetic requirement. Standing recovery usually occurs within 25 to 30 minutes.(168, 176, 177) An alpha$_2$-antagonist such as yohimbine (0.125 mg/kg) or tolazoline (2 to 4 mg/kg) can be administered intravenously to hasten recovery.(168, 177) In 1993, Young et al. reported his experiences with guaifenesin (100 mg/mL), ketamine (2 mg/mL), and xylazine (1 mg/mL) anesthesia in horses undergoing various orthopedic and soft tissue surgeries.(178) The average anesthetic infusion rate was 1.1 $mL \cdot kg^{-1} \cdot h^{-1}$. Anesthesia was characterized by active palpebral re-

flexes, variable degrees of nystagmus, occasional swallowing, and ear movement. Swallowing was considered undesirable in horses undergoing laryngeal surgery, but the infusion produced satisfactory anesthesia for all other procedures. When compared to halothane anesthesia, arterial blood pressure was better maintained (mean pressure at 70–110 mm Hg) in horses anesthetized with a continuous infusion of this mixture. Heart rate was significantly lower during infusion anesthesia than during halothane anesthesia. This may be attributed to a maintenance of blood pressure and the bradycardic effect of xylazine.(179) In Youngs et al.'s study, PaCO$_2$ was lower and PaO$_2$ higher with infusion anesthesia than during halothane anesthesia.(178) This indicated to the authors that infusion of guaifenesin-ketamine-xylazine caused less respiratory depression than halothane. Recovery of infusion anesthesia was judged good in the majority of horses, with sternal recumbency and standing occurring in 24 and 38 minutes, respectively.(178)

Detomidine is approved for use in horses in the United States as a sedative/analgesic for colic. Short-term anesthesia in horses can be achieved with detomidine (20 µg/kg IV) followed in 6 to 8 minutes by ketamine (2.2 mg/kg IV). Mean arterial blood pressure increases after detomidine/ketamine injection.(180, 181) When compared with xylazine and ketamine, detomidine and ketamine induce better muscle relaxation. Recovery can be somewhat unpredictable. Occasionally, horses and ponies experience a rough recovery. This is thought to be caused by the longer duration of sedation and muscle relaxation associated with detomidine.(180, 181) Adding butorphanol (0.04 mg/kg IV) to the detomidine and ketamine combination may improve the quality of recovery but also increases the duration of recumbency.(181) A combination of guaifenesin (50 mg/mL), ketamine (2 mg/mL), and detomidine (5 µg/mL) has been used for castrating ponies. Ponies were premedicated with 22 µg/kg of detomidine administered intramuscularly. Fifteen minutes later, anesthesia was induced with 0.67 to 1.1 mL/kg of the mixture and maintained at an infusion rate of 2.2 $mL \cdot kg^{-1} \cdot h^{-1}$. This combination produces good muscle relaxation and analgesia with minimal cardiopulmonary effects during surgery. Standing recovery occurs 25 to 40 minutes after termination of infusion.(182)

When diazepam (0.1 mg/kg) is combined with xylazine (0.3 mg/kg) and ketamine (2 mg/kg), muscle relaxation is improved. Diazepam provides practical advantages in commercial preparation, small volume, and ease of administration over guaifenesin.(183) Similarly, temazepam (0.044 mg/kg IV), another benzodiazepine derivative, has been used to prolong the duration of anesthesia induced by xylazine and ketamine.(184) Luna et al. used an intravenous infusion of methotrimeprazine (0.5 mg/kg), midazolam (0.1 mg/kg), and 10% guaifenesin (100 mg/kg), with or without ketamine (1.6 mg/kg), to induce recumbency in 15 horses. Anesthesia was maintained with halothane in 100% O$_2$. Horses receiving ketamine required lower halothane concentrations to maintain surgical anesthesia. Subsequently, standing recovery of these horses occurred more rapidly than for those not receiving ketamine.(185) Table 10–3 summarizes the use of ketamine combinations in horses.

Ruminants. A bolus injection of ketamine (2 mg/kg IV) followed by continuous intravenous infusion of 0.2% ketamine in physiologic saline at a rate of 10 mL/min induces dissociative anesthesia for major and minor surgeries (toe amputation, laparotomy, etc.) in cows.(186) Presently, xylazine (0.1 to 0.2 mg/kg IV) is commonly administered prior to or concomitantly with ketamine (2.2–3 mg/kg IV) for short-term anesthesia of ruminants. Tracheal intubation is easily achieved in cattle anesthetized with this combination.(187) Anesthesia may be safely prolonged by administration of 1 to 2 mg/kg of ketamine given slowly to effect. Alternatively, anesthesia can be maintained with a continuous infusion of ketamine in saline or 5% dextrose solution (2 mg/mL) at a rate of 10 mL/min.(188) Clinical experience shows that guaifenesin-ketamine-xylazine mixture is an effective anesthetic combination in ruminants. The concentration of each drug in the mixture is 50 mg/mL, 2 mg/mL, and 0.1 mg/mL for guaifenesin, ketamine, and xylazine, respectively. Anesthesia can be induced with 0.55–1.1 mL/kg initially and maintained with $2.2 \text{ mL} \cdot \text{kg}^{-1} \cdot \text{h}^{-1}$ in adult cattle and $1.65 \text{ mL} \cdot \text{kg}^{-1} \cdot \text{h}^{-1}$ in calves, kids, and lambs. Onset of anesthesia is gradual but smooth. Muscle relaxation is excellent, easily allowing tracheal intubation. Supplementation with O_2 (5 to 10 L/min) during prolonged procedures may help prevent hypoxemia. Mild hypoventilation is induced by the anesthetic mixture. Surgical procedures that can be performed in cattle anesthetized with guaifenesin-ketamine-xylazine include femoral fracture plating and pinning, penile surgery, umbilical hernia repair, cesarean section, and celiotomy.(188)

In calves anesthetized with xylazine-ketamine, decreases in heart rate induced by xylazine are reversed by subsequent administration of ketamine. When xylazine and ketamine are administered simultaneously, no significant changes in heart rate, cardiac output, and arterial blood pressure are observed.(189, 190) Thus, it appears that the simultaneous administration of xylazine and ketamine offers the advantage of minimizing the decrease in cardiac output and stroke volume induced by xylazine alone.(191) Respiratory rate often increases after xylazine-ketamine administration but is usually accompanied by a decrease in PaO_2 and an increase in $PaCO_2$.(192, 193) Arterial pH decreases slightly as a result of accumulation of CO_2. Only minor changes in base excess and standard bicarbonate are observed.(192)

When compared to pentobarbital and saffan, the intravenous administration of ketamine in sheep induces anesthesia of shorter duration than pentobarbital but longer than saffan. Transient respiratory depression is reflected in changes in PaO_2 and $PaCO_2$ 10 to 15 minutes following ketamine and saffan administration. In contrast, respiratory depression persists with pentobarbital anesthesia.(122) Premedication with xylazine (0.2 mg/kg IM) prior to ketamine (2.2 mg/kg IV) administration prolongs the duration of anesthesia (67.0 ± 21.6 minutes) and eliminates some of the undesirable effects of ketamine, including muscle rigidity, insufficient suppression of reflexes, and tachycardia.(194) However, increased salivation, urination, and regurgitation associated with xylazine and/or ketamine administration occur.(194) It has been reported that the addition of atropine to xylazine-ketamine decreases salivation, urination, and regurgitation.(194) In sheep, the administration of either diazepam (0.375 mg/kg IV)-ketamine (7.5 mg/kg IV) or xylazine (0.1 mg/kg IV)-ketamine (7.5 mg/kg IV) reportedly decreases cardiac output.(195)

When a mixture of guaifenesin (50 mg/mL), ketamine (1 mg/mL), and xylazine (0.1 mg/mL) in 5% dextrose was used to induce and maintain anesthesia for 1 hour in spontaneously breathing sheep, a significant decrease in PaO_2 and a significant increase in respiratory rate were observed. These changes were attributed to lateral recumbency and anesthetic-induced respiratory depression. Supplementation with 100% O_2 and repositioning to sternal recumbency greatly improved arterial oxygenation. This mixture induced minimal cardiovascular depression. Induction and recovery from anesthesia was smooth.(196) In goats, atropine, acetylpromazine, diazepam, or xylazine has been used prior to ketamine anesthesia. The duration of anesthesia is longest (45.2 minutes) in goats anesthetized with atropine (0.44 mg/kg IM), xylazine (0.22 mg/kg IM), and ketamine (11 mg/kg IM). An increase in $PaCO_2$ and a decrease in PaO_2 occurred with all combinations. Xylazine and ketamine caused the largest increase in $PaCO_2$ and decrease in PaO_2.(197) This drug combination has been used successfully to maintain anesthesia for a variety of surgical procedures including laparotomy, abomasotomy, enucleation, and amputation of claw. Surgical anesthesia can be maintained for 2.5 to 3 hours by supplemental increments of ketamine (6 mg/kg IM) or a mixture of xylazine (0.045 mg/kg IM) and ketamine (2.45 mg/kg IM). Full recovery occurs more rapidly in goats in which anesthesia was supplemented with ketamine alone than in those in which anesthesia was prolonged with the xylazine-ketamine mixture.(198)

In llamas, xylazine (0.25 mg/kg IM) followed in 15 minutes by ketamine (5 mg/kg IM) induces 30 to 60 minutes of anesthesia and restraint sufficient for minor procedures such as suturing lacerations, abscess drainage, or cast application.(199) If tracheal intubation is desired, intravenous xylazine (0.25 mg/kg IV) and ketamine (2.5 mg/kg IV) can be used. Changes in heart rate and blood pressure are similar to those observed in other species.(200) Ketamine (1 mg/mL) in 5% guaifenesin can be given to effect (1.5–2.2 mL/kg IV) to induce and maintain anesthesia.(201) Table 10–4 summarizes the use of ketamine combinations in cattle.

Table 10–3.   Use of Ketamine or Ketamine Combinations in Horses

Drug(s)	Dose and Route (mg/kg)	Duration (min)	Comment	Reference
Xylazine	1.1, IV	16.1 ± 7.3	Excellent analgesia	169
	wait 3–5 min		Light anesthesia	
Ketamine	2.2, IV			
Xylazine	1.1, IV	—	Excitement following	
Ketamine	2.2, IV		induction	
	simultaneously			
Xylazine	1.1, IV	12.1 ± 3.2	Muscle twitching	
	wait 3–5 min		Rapid nystagmus	
Ketamine	6.6, IV		Prolonged and rough recovery	
Xylazine	1.1, IV	Arabian: 18.25	Behavioral changes	172
Butorphanol	0.1 or 0.2, IV	Belgian: 52.5	Enhanced muscle relaxation and	
Ketamine	2.2, IV	Appaloosa: 56.5	analgesia	
		Mean: 38.25 ± 6.64		
Xylazine	1.1, IV	—	Satisfactory anesthesia	173
Ketamine	2.2, IV			
Methadone	0.1, IV			
Acepromazine	0.1, IV	—	—	
Ketamine	2.2, IV			
Methadone	0.1, IV			
Methadone	0.1, IV	—	Inadequate anesthesia	
Acepromazine	0.15, IV			
Xylazine	1.1, IV			
Ketamine	2.2, IV			
Acepromazine	0.04, IV	10.2	Muscle tremor lasted < 1 min	174
Methadone	0.04, IV	(3–18)	after induction	
Ketamine	2–2.5, IV			
Xylazine	1.1, IV	24	Inadequate muscle relaxation	181
Ketamine	2.2, IV			
Xylazine	1.1, IV	37	Adequate muscle relaxation	
Butorphanol	0.044, IV		Good analgesia	
Ketamine	2.2, IV			
Guaifenesin	50 mg/mL	49 ± 3	Surgical anesthesia	177
Xylazine	0.5 mg/mL			
Ketamine	1 mg/mL			
	Induction 1.1 mL/kg, IV			
	Maintenance 4.5 mL/kg/h, IV			
Guaifenesin	50 mg/mL	44 ± 2	Better muscle relaxation and	
Xylazine	0.5 mg/mL		analgesia	
Ketamine	2 mg/mL		Surgical anesthesia	
	Induction 1.1 mL/kg, IV			
	Maintenance 4.3 mL/kg/h, IV			
Guaifenesin	50 mg/mL	120	↓ Blood pressure initially	176
Xylazine	0.5 mg/mL		Hypoventilation	
Ketamine	1 mg/mL			
	Induction 1.1 mL/kg, IV			
	Maintenance 2.75 mL/kg/h, IV			
Guaifenesin	100 mg/mL	51–95	Presence of swallowing reflex, not	178
Xylazine	1 mg/mL		suitable for laryngeal surgery	
Ketamine	2 mg/mL		Surgical anesthesia	
	Maintenance 1.1 mL/kg/h, IV		Smooth recovery	
Xylazine	0.3, IV	—	Supplemental ketamine 200–500 mg	183
Diazepam	0.05, IV			
Ketamine	2, IV		Maintain with halothane	
Xylazine	1.1, IV	—	Supplemental ketamine 200–750 mg	
Diazepam	0.1, IV			
Ketamine	2, IV		Maintain with halothane	
			Good muscle relaxation	

Table 10–3. Use of Ketamine or Ketamine Combinations in Horses (continued)

Drug(s)	Dose and Route (mg/kg)	Duration (min)	Comment	Reference
Xylazine Guaifenesin Ketamine	1.1, IV 100, IV 2, IV	—	Supplemental ketamine 200–1000 mg Maintain with halothane Good muscle relaxation	183
Xylazine Temazepam Ketamine	1.1, IV 0.044, IV 2.2, IV	—	Longer duration of recumbency	184
Methotrimeprazine Midazolam Guaifenesin Ketamine	0.5, IV 0.1, IV 100, IV 1.6, IV	—	Induction of anesthesia Smooth recovery	185
Detomidine Ketamine	0.02, IV 2.2, IV	—	Second dose of ketamine (1.4 mg/kg) given 15 min after first dose Improve anesthesia	173
Xylazine Ketamine	1.1, IV 2.2, IV	12–35	Smooth induction and recovery	180
Detomidine Ketamine	0.02, IV 2.2, IV	10–43	Required more time than xylazine and ketamine to assume recumbency Occasional poor recovery Longer lasting hypertension	
Detomidine Ketamine	0.02, IV 2.2, IV	26.8 (14–42)	Smooth induction Occasional rough recovery	181
Detomidine Butorphanol Ketamine	0.02, IV 0.04, IV 2.2, IV	36.2 (18–67)	Smooth induction Smoother recovery Muscle relaxation	
Guaifenesin Detomidine Ketamine	50 mg/mL 5 μg/mL 2 mg/mL Induction 0.67–1.1 mL/kg, IV Maintenance 2.2 mL/kg/h, IV	—	Good muscle relaxation and analgesia Minimal cardiovascular effects	182
Ketamine	5–6 mg/100 kg, injected into subarachnoid space	—	Effective spinal block	44
Ketamine	10–12 mg/100 kg, injected into subarachnoid space	—	Blockade of T13 to L3 Effective surgical analgesia	

Swine. Ketamine has been used extensively in pigs premedicated with atropine (0.04 mg/kg IM) for minor surgical and diagnostic procedures. At intramuscular doses of 11 to 20 mg/kg, muscle relaxation is poor and analgesia is brief.(2) Green et al. reported that pigs react violently to intramuscular injections of ketamine and then exhibit muscle tremor, extensor rigidity, panting respiration, and erythema.(202) These shortcomings can be minimized by combining diazepam (1 mg/kg IM) or xylazine (2 mg/kg IM) with ketamine (10–20 mg/kg IM). Deep sedation and good muscle relaxation occurs with these drug combinations, but pigs may still respond to noxious stimuli such as incision of the abdominal wall.(202, 203) Supplemental dosing with half of the original dose of xylazine and ketamine can be given for tracheal intubation.(203) In our clinical experience, simultaneous xylazine (2.2 mg/kg IV) and ketamine (2.2 mg/kg IV) administration induces a short period of anesthesia. Alternatively, a combination of oxymorphone (0.075 mg/kg), xylazine (2 mg/kg), and ketamine (2 mg/kg) mixed in the same syringe and given intravenously induces surgical anesthesia. When given intramuscularly, satisfactory response can be achieved by doubling the dose of each drug.(187, 204)

Xylazine (1–2 mg/kg) and ketamine (3–5 mg/kg) have been injected into the testicles to induce immobilization for castration of mature boars. Half the calculated dose is injected into each testicle. Surgical removal of the testicle removes drug not yet absorbed, which hastens recovery.(187)

Table 10–4. Use of Ketamine or Ketamine Combinations in Ruminants

Species	Drug(s)	Dose and Route (mg/kg)	Duration (min)	Comment	Reference
Cattle	Ketamine	2 mg/mL in saline, given at 10 mL/min, IV	—	—	186
Cattle	Xylazine Ketamine	0.1, IV 2, IV *Suppl. 2% ketamine in saline	—	Recovery in 45 minutes	313
Cattle	Ketamine Xylazine Ketamine	1.5–4.6, IV 0.22, IM, IV 1.8–4.6, IV	— —	— Muscle relaxation adequate for tracheal intubation	314
Cattle	Xylazine Ketamine	0.22, IM 11, IM	40–55	Good muscle relaxation Surgical anesthesia	315
Cattle	Ketamine Xylazine Ketamine	11, IV 0.14, IM 2.8, IV	— —	Dose repeated every 30 minutes for a duration of 3–4 hours Better muscle relaxation	316
Cattle	Xylazine Ketamine Xylazine Ketamine Xylazine Ketamine	0.2, IM 5, IV Given separately 0.2, IM 10, IM Given separately 0.2, IM 10, IM Simultaneously	20 23.5 ± 1.8 37 ± 3.4	Rapid onset of action Easy tracheal intubation Transient respiratory depression Rapid breathing Easy tracheal intubation Good muscle relaxation Good muscle relaxation Good analgesia	189
Cattle	Xylazine Ketamine	0.088, IM 4.4, IM	55.7 ± 10.4	Good muscle relaxation Good analgesia	190
Cattle	Diazepam Guaifenesin Ketamine	1.16 ± 0.05, IV 115.23 ± 5.13, IV 5.49 ± 0.6, IV	22.2 ± 3.2	Surgical anesthesia	317
Cattle	Diazepam Ketamine	1.18 ± 0.04, IV 10.63 ± 0.56, IV	36 ± 3.67	Smooth induction and recovery	318
Sheep	Ketamine Xylazine Ketamine Atropine Xylazine Ketamine	22, IV 0.2, IM 22, IV 0.2, IM 0.2, IM 22, IV	23 ± 12.05 67 ± 21.6 34 ± 5.5	Marked muscle rigidity Mild salivation Salivation Regurgitation ↓ Muscle rigidity Prolonged anesthesia ↓ Salivation Urination Regurgitation Tachycardia	194
Sheep	Diazepam Ketamine Xylazine Ketamine	0.375, IV 7.5, IV 0.1, IV 7.5, IV	15 25	↓ Cardiac output ↑ Systemic vascular resistance ↓ Cardiac output, systemic vascular resistance and mean arterial pressure Avoid in compromised heart function	195
Sheep	Medetomidine Ketamine	0.025, IM 1, IM	—	Good muscle relaxation Tachypnea	319
Sheep	Diazepam Ketamine	0.375, IV 7.5, IV Maintenance D; 0.188, IV K; 3.75, IV every 15 min	120	Satisfactory anesthesia Hypotension Respiratory acidosis ↑ Systemic and pulmonary vascular resistance	320

*Suppl.: Supplemental dose

Table 10–4. Use of Ketamine or Ketamine Combinations in Ruminants (continued)

Species	Drug(s)	Dose and Route (mg/kg)	Duration (min)	Comment	Reference
Sheep	Guaifenesin Xylazine Ketamine	50 mg/mL 0.1 mg/mL 1 mg/mL Induction 0.67–1.1 mL/kg, IV Maintenance 2.2 mL/kg, IV	60	Surgical anesthesia ↑ Respiratory rate, ↓ Pa_{O_2} Supplemental 100% O_2	196
Goats	Atropine Xylazine Ketamine	0.44, IM 0.22, IM 11, IM	40–45	Good muscle relaxation	198
Goats	Ketamine	3, IV	—	Adequate for tracheal intubation	321
Goats	Ketamine Atropine Ketamine	22, IM 0.44, IM 22, IM	10.3 10.2	Apneustic breathing ↓ Salivation	197
	Atropine Acepromazine Ketamine	0.44, IM 0.88, IM 22, IM	22.2	↑ Duration and degree of analgesia and muscle relaxation	
	Atropine Diazepam Ketamine	0.44, IM 0.88, IM 22, IM	22.4	↑ Duration and degree of analgesia and muscle relaxation	
	Atropine Xylazine Ketamine	0.44, IM 0.22, IM 11, IM	45.2	↑ Duration and degree of analgesia and muscle relaxation	
Llamas	Xylazine Ketamine	0.35, IM 0.25, IV 5–8, IM 3–5, IV	30–60	Restraint Anesthesia	201
	Guaifenesin Ketamine	80, IV 1.6, IV	15–20	Good muscle relaxation Little analgesia	
Llamas	Xylazine Ketamine	0.35, IM 0.25, IV 5–8, IM 3–5, IV	30–60	Restraint Anesthesia	322
	Diazepam Ketamine	0.2–0.3, IM 0.1–0.2, IV 5–8, IM 3–5, IV	—	Anesthesia	

As in horses and ruminants, the combination of guaifenesin (50 mg/mL), xylazine (1 mg/mL), and ketamine (1 mg/mL) is a very useful anesthetic regimen for pigs of all ages. It should be recognized that the concentration of xylazine in this mixture is twice that used in horses and ten times that used in ruminants. Anesthesia is induced with rapid administration of the mixture at a dose of 0.5 to 1 mL/kg via a catheterized central auricular vein. For prolonged procedures, anesthesia is maintained by continuous infusion at a rate of 2.2 $mL \cdot kg^{-1} \cdot h^{-1}$.(188) Mean arterial pressure and systemic vascular resistance increase in pigs anesthetized with guaifenesin-ketamine-xylazine. Heart rate decreases but remains within an acceptable range. The $PaCO_2$ decreases while PaO_2 remains unaltered. In summary, the continuous infusion of guaifenesin, ketamine, and xylazine induces minimal cardiopulmonary changes similar to those observed in swine anesthetized with inhalation anesthetics. This mixture has been used to induce satisfactory anesthesia in healthy swine for up to 2 hours.(205)

In miniature swine, a combination of acepromazine (0.39 mg/kg IM) and ketamine (15 mg/kg IM) induces anesthesia for 65 to 80 minutes.(206) When used with droperidol-fentanyl (Innovar-Vet, 1 mL/15 kg IM), ketamine (12 to 16 mg/kg IM) induces 30 to 40 minutes of surgical anesthesia. Prolongation of anesthesia can be achieved with supplemental ketamine (2.2 mg/kg IV or 6.6 mg/kg IM).(207) A xylazine (2 mg/kg IM), ketamine (5 mg/kg IM), and butorphanol (0.1 mg/kg IM) regimen has been used successfully to induce light anesthesia in Vietnamese potbellied pigs for the purpose of electroejaculation and artificial insemination.(208) Ketamine has also been combined with diazepam (0.5–1 mg/kg IM) or midazolam (0.2–0.4 mg/kg IM) for inducing anesthesia for short procedures.(209–211) Table 10–5 summarizes the use of ketamine combinations in swine.

Table 10–5.   Use of Ketamine or Ketamine Combinations in Swine

Drug(s)	Dose and Route (mg/kg)	Duration (min)	Comment	Reference
Atropine	0.044, IM	10–30	Poor muscle relaxation and analgesia	2
Ketamine	20, IM			
Xylazine	2, IM	—	Required supplemental dose for intubation	203
Ketamine	20, IM			
Innovar-Vet	1 mL/13.6 kg, IM	41.75	Good muscle relaxation	323
Ketamine	11, IM			
Acepromazine	0.5, IM	18.25	Strong, muscle activity	
Ketamine	15, IM			
Xylazine	0.2, IM	24.5	Strong, muscle activity	
Ketamine	11, IM			
Ketamine	10–20, IM	—	Violent reaction, muscle tremor, extensor rigidity, ↑ heart rate and respiratory rate, panting respiration, erythema	202
Diazepam	1, IM	40	Deep sedation, respond to incision	
Ketamine	10, IM		Good muscle relaxation	
Xylazine	2, IM	40	Deep sedation	
Ketamine	15, IM		Good analgesia	
			Excellent muscle relaxation	
Xylazine	2, IV	20–30	Good analgesia and muscle relaxation	187
Ketamine	2, IV		Smooth recovery, can be shortened by naloxone	204
Oxymorphone	0.075, IV			
Xylazine	1, IV	25	Good analgesia	324
Ketamine	10, IV			
Guaifenesin	50 mg/mL	120	Good muscle relaxation and analgesia	188
Xylazine	1 mg/mL		Minimal cardiovascular changes	
Ketamine	1 mg/mL			
	Induction 0.67–1.1 mL/kg, IV			
	Maintenance 2.2 mL/kg/h, IV			
Meperidine	2.2, IM	60.6 ± 18.6	Surgical anesthesia	325
Azaperone	2.2, IM		Rapid & smooth recovery	
Ketamine	22, IM		Anesthesia can be prolonged by supplemental ketamine and morphine	
Morphine	1.7, IM			
Miniature pigs				
Xylazine	2, IM	—	Light anesthesia	208
Ketamine	5, IM			
Butorphanol	0.1, IM			
Xylazine	2.2, IM	—	Induction of anesthesia	210
Ketamine	11–17.6, IM		Short procedures	
Diazepam	1.1, IM	—	—	
Ketamine	11–17.6, IM			
Diazepam	0.05–0.1, IM	20–30	Deep sedation	211
Ketamine	10–30, IM			
Midazolam	0.2–0.4, IM	20–30	Deep sedation	
Ketamine	10–30, IM			
Xylazine	4, IM	20–30	Deep sedation	
Ketamine	5–10, IM			
Innovar-Vet	1 mL/20 kg, IM	20–30	Deep sedation	
Ketamine	10–20, IM			
Atropine	0.04, IM	—	Anesthesia can be prolonged with supplemental ketamine, 2–4 mg/kg IV	209
Xylazine	2.2, IM			
Ketamine	12–20, IM			
Diazepam	1–2, IM	—	—	
Ketamine	12–20, IM			
Butorphanol	0.22, IM	—	Enhanced analgesia	
Xylazine	2, IM		Satisfactory anesthesia for abdominal surgery	
Ketamine	11, IM			

Nondomestic Animals. Ketamine has been used extensively for immobilization of wild animals. However, its use has been somewhat limited owing to its lack of potency coupled with the high volume required to dose larger species. In 1973, freeze-dried ketamine was prepared and used at a concentration of 200 mg/mL when combined with various concentrations of xylazine to capture wild carnivores.(212-214) Duration of anesthesia is highly dose dependent. In free-ranging ungulates, prolonged recovery and ataxia have been reported following the use of ketamine.(215) In zoo animals, where predation is not a problem, the use of ketamine/xylazine combinations for immobilization is satisfactory.(216) Tables 10–6 and 10–7 present a brief summary on the use of ketamine in nondomesticated mammals and birds.

Telazol

Telazol (CI-744), is a nonopioid, nonbarbiturate injectable anesthetic. It consists of a 1:1 (wt:wt) combination of tiletamine and zolazepam. Tiletamine (CI-634), a dissociative anesthetic agent, has a longer duration of action and greater analgesic effect than does ketamine. Zolazepam (CI-716), a benzodiazepine tranquilizer, was combined with tiletamine because of its effectiveness as an anticonvulsant and muscle relaxant.

PHARMACOLOGY

Tiletamine Hydrochloride (CI-634). The basic descriptive pharmacology of tiletamine [2-(ethylamino)-2-(2-thienyl) cyclohexanone hydrochloride] was first reported in 1969.(217) In most respects the pharmacodynamics of tiletamine are similar to those of ketamine, but its potency and duration of action is intermediate between phencyclidine, the most potent, and ketamine, the least potent of the dissociatives.

Effects on the Central Nervous System

The CNS effects induced by tiletamine are highly species specific. In rats and mice tiletamine causes excitation and ataxia even at small doses. This effect is not as marked in other species. Catalepsy occurs in all species when tiletamine is given in moderate doses.(217) With large doses, analgesia and general anesthesia occur in mice, rats, pigeons, cats, and monkeys, and only minimal depression is produced in guinea pigs and rabbits. Similar to phencyclidine, tiletamine is more effective in producing general anesthesia in cats and primates. However, at extremely large doses (approaching the lethal dose: 150 mg/kg IM in cats and 50 mg/kg IV in monkeys), brief and mild clonic seizures occur in these two species. A dose of 20 mg/kg intravenously in dogs induces inconsistent responses (i.e., light surgical anesthesia and analgesia occur in some dogs, while clonic convulsions are induced in others). It is interesting that CNS intraventricular injection of a very low dose of tiletamine (0.001 μmol) antagonized N-methyl-D-aspartate (NMDA)- and quinolinate-induced convulsions and decreased spinal flexor reflexes. However, tiletamine at

higher doses (0.0297 μmol) induced convulsions. It was suggested that the anticonvulsant and reflex suppressant effects of tiletamine are caused by antagonism of NMDA receptor-mediated excitation, while the convulsant action is caused by an interaction with non-NMDA receptors.(218) Similar antagonism of NMDA-induced neuronal excitation in the spinal cord has been demonstrated with phencyclidine and ketamine.(21)

In general, the CNS effects induced by tiletamine seem to be dose related, inducing progressive loss of sensory perception and consciousness without producing a deep sleep-like condition. The eyes remain open, and the corneal reflex remains intact. Muscle relaxation and analgesia are insufficient for painful visceral surgery but can be easily augmented by supplementation with other drugs.

The EEG activity of tiletamine has been studied in monkeys (219) and cats (14). In monkeys, tiletamine produces a fairly consistent depth and duration of anesthesia. The EEG tracings and the electrocardiogram (ECG) recordings were consistent with stable clinical anesthesia. Bradycardia is variable, and the respiratory rate is well maintained. Minimal movement of extremities occurs. Some reflexes remain intact and recovery is rapid.(219) The EEG recorded from cats given 20 mg/kg of tiletamine intramuscularly revealed an anoxic pattern, characterized by extreme pulsatory action (i.e., convulsive activity). This EEG pattern, when accompanied by peripheral clonic rhythmic motor seizures, could be life threatening. However, cats usually recover uneventfully.(14)

Effects on the Cardiovascular System

The cardiorespiratory effects of 11 mg/kg of tiletamine given intravenously to cats have been studied.(220) Heart rate and arterial blood pressure decrease from 5 to 30 minutes postinjection, gradually returning to baseline, but these changes are not significant. In four cats, intravenous injection of tiletamine produced a consistently increased heart rate and blood pressure with coincidental arrhythmias characterized by premature ventricular beats of short duration shortly after injection. When a combination of tiletamine (IM) and chloral hydrate (IV) is given to rabbits, blood pressure remains unchanged for 1.5 hours. After an additional dose of both tiletamine and chloral hydrate, blood pressure decreases markedly. Hypotension seems to be caused by the second dose of chloral hydrate.(221) In unanesthetized dogs, 2 mg/kg of tiletamine given intravenously results in an increase in blood pressure and heart rate. In pentobarbital-anesthetized dogs, increased blood pressure occurs after intravenous injection of 0.5 to 2 mg/kg of tiletamine, whereas a dose of 4 to 8 mg/kg decreases blood pressure. Intraarterial (IA) injection of 0.4 to 1.6 mg of tiletamine into the autoperfused hindquarters of the dog does not change the perfusion pressure. However, increasing the dose to 3.2 to 6.4 mg did decrease perfusion pressure. In contrast, IA injection of 0.1 to 0.8 mg of phencyclidine increases

Table 10–6. Use of Ketamine or Ketamine Combinations in Exotic and Wildlife Animals

Common Names (Genus and Species)	Drug(s)	Dose and Route (mg/kg)	Duration (min)	Comment	Reference
Order Artiodactyla, Family Bovidae					
Buffalo Calves (*Bubalus bubalis*)	Ketamine	2, IV	4.45 ± 0.34 (3–5.5) range	—	326
	Ketamine Chlorpromazine	2, IV 2, IM	11.17 ± 0.77 (6–14) range	Prolong analgesia, recovery time, and degree of muscle relaxation	
Buffalo Calves (*Bubalus bubalis*)	Ketamine	Induction 2, IV Maintenance 0.2% infusion to effect	60	Abdominal muscle relaxation	327
Alpine Goat (*Capra hircus*)	Xylazine	0.35, IM (0.1–0.62) range	—	—	328
	Ketamine	2.92, IM (1.65–6.2) range			
Goat (*Capra hircus*)	Ketamine	10–20, IM	—	—	329
Bighorn Sheep (*Ovis canadensis*)	Xylazine	• Male: 70–300 mg, IM • Female: 70–250 mg, IM • Lambs: 80–90 mg, IM	—	—	330
	Ketamine	• 200 mg, IM			
Alpine Ipex (*Capra ibex*)	Medetomidine Ketamine	0.08–0.1, IM 1.5–2, IM	—	Complete immobilization	331
Barbary Sheep (*Ammotragus lervia*)	Medetomidine Ketamine	0.08–0.1, IM 1.5–2, IM	—	Satisfactory immobilization Supplemental IV medetomidine (20–25% of first dose) induced complete immobilization	332
Markhor (*Capra falconerii megaceros*)	Medetomidine Ketamine	0.069, IM 1.6, IM	—	Immobilization Good muscle relaxation	332
Mouflon Sheep (*Ovis musimon*)	Medetomidine Ketamine	0.125, IM 2.5, IM	—	Complete immobilization	331
Zebu (*Bos indicus*)	Ketamine	5–20, IM	—	—	329
Order Artiodactyla, Family Cervidae					
Chital deer (*Axis axis*)	Xylazine/Ketamine mix (1:1) Xyl: 100 mg/mL Ket: 100 mg/mL	Stags (90–100 kg) • 1.5–2 mL, IM	—	—	333
Fallow Deer (*Dama dama*)	Xylazine/Ketamine mix (1:1) Xyl: 100 mg/mL Ket: 100 mg/mL	Yearlings (30–50 kg) • 1 mL, IM Young buck (50–75 kg) • 1.5 mL, IM Large buck (>75 kg) • 2 mL, IM Large buck (>90 kg) • 2.5 mL, IM	— — — —	— — — —	333
Fallow Deer (*Dama dama*)	Xylazine Ketamine	4, IM 3, IM	—	—	334
Fallow Deer (*Dama dama*)	Medetomidine Ketamine	0.08–0.12, IM 1–2, IM	—	Complete immobilization	331

• Total dose

Table 10–6. Use of Ketamine or Ketamine Combinations in Exotic and Wildlife Animals (continued)

Common Names (Genus and Species)	Drug(s)	Dose and Route (mg/kg)	Duration (min)	Comment	Reference
Order Artiodactyla, Family Cervidae—cont'd					
Red Deer (*Cervus elaphus*)	Xylazine/Ketamine mix (1:1) Xyl: 100 mg/mL Ket: 100 mg/mL	Mature stags • 2 mL, IM Yearlings • 1.5 mL, IM	— —	— —	333
Red Deer (*Cervus elaphus*)	Xylazine Ketamine	1.2, IM 1, IM	—	—	334
Domestic Reindeer	Medetomidine Ketamine	0.025, IM 0.5, IM	—	Complete immobilization	331
Forest Reindeer (*Rangifer tarandus fennicus*)	Medetomidine Ketamine Medetomidine Ketamine	0.059 ± 0.013, IM (0.04–0.08) range 0.9 ± 0.3, IM (0.4–1.9) range 0.05, IM 1.1, IM	— —	Immobilization Complete immobilization	335 332
Forest Reindeer (*Rangifer tarandus fennicus*)	Medetomidine Ketamine	0.06, IM 0.6, IM	—	Complete immobilization	331
White-tailed Deer (*Odocoileus virginianus*)	Xylazine Ketamine	0.5–1.9, IM 3.7–14.7, IM	—	Immobilization	336
White-tailed Deer (*Odocoileus virginianus*)	Xylazine Ketamine	100 mg total, IM 300 mg total, IM	—	—	337
White-tailed Deer (*Odocoileus virginianus*)	Xylazine Ketamine	0.35, IM (0.1–0.6) range 2.92, IM (1.6–6.2) range	—	—	328
White-tailed Deer (*Odocoileus virginianus*)	Medetomidine Ketamine Medetomidine Ketamine	0.06, IM 1.7, IM 0.06, IM 1.7, IM	— —	Complete immobilization Complete immobilization	331 332
Formosan Sika Deer	Medetomidine Ketamine	0.23 ± 0.06, IM (0.16–0.36) range 2.3 ± 0.6, IM (1.69–3.63) range	—	Immobilization	331
Elk (*Cervus canadensis*)	Xylazine Ketamine	600 mg total, IM 1200 mg, total, IM	—	Immobilization	338
Order Carnivora, Family Canidae					
Coyote (*Canis latrans*)	Ketamine Xylazine Ketamine	12.3, IM 1.8–2.9, IM 9.2–14.7, IM	52 —	Immobilization Extensive salivation Rigidity Chemical restraint	339
Coyote (*Canis latrans*)	Xylazine Ketamine	2, IM 4, IM	—	—	340
Cape Hunting Dogs (*Lycaon pictus*)	Medetomidine Ketamine	0.04–0.12, IM 2.6–3, IM	—	Partial or complete immo- bilization Bradycardia ↓ Respiration rate	341
Arctic Fox (*Alopex lagopus*)	Medetomidine Ketamine	0.05, IM 2.5, IM	—	Complete immobilization	331

• Total dose

Table 10–6. Use of Ketamine or Ketamine Combinations in Exotic and Wildlife Animals (continued)

Common Names (Genus and Species)	Drug(s)	Dose and Route (mg/kg)	Duration (min)	Comment	Reference
Order Carnivora, Family Canidae—cont'd					
Blue Fox (Alopex lagopus)	Medetomidine Ketamine	0.05, IM 2.5, IM	—	Immobilization	342
Grey Fox (Urocyon cinereoargenteus)	Xylazine Ketamine	6.6–11, IM 11–17.6, IM	—	Chemical restraint	339
Kit Fox (Vulpes macrotis)	Xylazine Ketamine	6.6–11, IM 11–17.6, IM	—	Chemical restraint	339
Red Fox (Vulpes fulva)	Xylazine Ketamine	6.6–11, IM 22–33, IM	—	Chemical restraint	339
Grey Wolf (Canis lupus)	Xylazine Ketamine	2.2, IM 6.6, IM	—	Significant bradycardia	343
Wolf (Canis lupus L.)	Xylazine Ketamine	30 mg total, IM 400 mg total, IM	148 ± 52.7	—	344
Wolf (Canis lupus L.)	Xylazine Ketamine	2–3, IM 5–6, IM	35–40	—	345
Order Carnivora, Family Felidae					
Bobcat (Lynx rufus)	Acepromazine Ketamine Ketamine	0.66–1.1, IM 17.6, IM (11.9–34.9) range 33.4, IM (22.4–60.3) range	— —	Immobilization —	339
California Bobcat (Felis rufus californieus)	Ketamine	5.5–17, IM	—	—	346
Fishing Cat (Felis viverrina)	Ketamine	19–25, IM	—	—	347
Flat-headed Cat (Felis planiceps)	Ketamine	8, IM	—	—	347
Jungle Cat	Medetomidine Ketamine	0.1, IM 2.5, IM	—	Immobilization	331
Leopard Cat (Felis bengalensis)	Ketamine	8–25, IM	—	—	348
Cheetah (Acinonyx jubatus)	Ketamine	8–12, IM	—	—	348
Cheetah (Acinonyx jubatus)	Ketamine	10, IM	—	—	347
Cheetah (Acinonyx jubatus)	Medetomidine Ketamine	0.06–0.07, IM 2.5–3, IM	—	Immobilization	331
Jaguar (Panthera onca)	Ketamine	13–18, IM	—	—	348
Jaguar (Panthera onca)	Medetomidine Ketamine	0.05, IM 1.5–2, IM	—	Immobilization	331
Leopard (Panthera pardus)	Medetomidine Ketamine	0.07–0.08, IM 2.5–3, IM	—	Immobilization	331
Black Leopard (Panthera pardus)	Ketamine	15, IM	—	Occasional convulsion Inadequate muscle relaxation	348
Black Leopard (Panthera pardus)	Ketamine Ketamine Ketamine	11, IM (5.5–17) range 7.5, IM 10–15, IM	— — —	— — —	346 349 329

Table 10–6. Use of Ketamine or Ketamine Combinations in Exotic and Wildlife Animals (continued)

Common Names (Genus and Species)	Drug(s)	Dose and Route (mg/kg)	Duration (min)	Comment	Reference
		Order Carnivora, Family Felidae—cont'd			
Chinese Leopard (*Panthera pardus Japonensis*)	Ketamine	15, IM	—	Occasional convulsion Inadequate muscle relaxation	348
Clouded Leopard (*Neofelis nebulosa*)	Ketamine	8.6, IM	—	Occasional convulsion Inadequate muscle relaxation	348
	Ketamine	7, IM	—	—	347
Snow Leopard (*Panthera uncia*)	Ketamine	10, IM 10–12, IM	—	—	347
Snow Leopard (*Panthera uncia*)	Medetomidine Ketamine	0.06–0.08, IM 2.5–3, IM	—	Complete immobilization	331
	Medetomidine	0.067 ± 0.016, IM (0.038–0.107) range	45	Complete immobilization Allowed tracheal intubation	332
	Ketamine	2.7 ± 0.8, IM (1.3–5.7) range			
Snow Leopard (*Panthera uncia*)	Xylazine	2.2 ± 0.2, IM (1.9–2.6) range	30–45	Immobilization Moderate to good muscle relaxation	350
	Ketamine	10.9 ± 1, IM (9.6–12.8) range			
	Medetomidine	0.067 ± 0.014, IM (0.038–0.109) range	30–60	Immobilization Shorter recovery compared to xylazine-ketamine	
	Ketamine	2.9 ± 0.8, IM (1.6–5.7) range		Good to excellent muscle relaxation	
Lion (*Panthera leo*)	Medetomidine Ketamine	0.03, IM 1–1.5, IM	—	Immobilization	331
Lion (*Panthera leo*)	Ketamine	10–20, IM	—	Rapid immobilization	348
	Ketamine	5–7, IM	—	—	351
	Ketamine	5–7.5, IM	—	—	349
	Xylazine Ketamine	110 total, IM 450 total, IM	240	Immobilization	329
	Xylazine Ketamine	3.2, IM 8, IM	—	—	352
Mountain Lion (*Felis concolor*)	Xylazine Ketamine	0.88–0.99, IM 7.3–7.7, IM *Suppl. 4.4–8.8, IM	—	Immobilization	339
Mountain Lion, Puma (*Felis concolor*)	Ketamine Xylazine Ketamine	11–25, IM 1.8, IM 11, IM	— —	— —	348 353
Margay (*Felis wiedii*)	Ketamine	15, IM	—	Occasional convulsion Inadequate muscle relaxation	348
Tiger (*Panthera tigris*)	Ketamine	7–14, IM	—	—	348
Tiger (*Panthera tigris*)	Medetomidine Ketamine	0.03, IM 1–1.5, IM	—	Immobilization	331
		Order Carnivora, Family Mustelidae			
Badger (*Taxidea taxus*)	Ketamine	11–33, IM	—	Immobilization	339

*Suppl.: Supplemental dose

Table 10–6. Use of Ketamine or Ketamine Combinations in Exotic and Wildlife Animals (continued)

Common Names (Genus and Species)	Drug(s)	Dose and Route (mg/kg)	Duration (min)	Comment	Reference
		Order Carnivora, Family Mustelidae—cont'd			
Beaver (*Castor canadensis*)	Ketamine	22, IM	—	Immobilization	354
	Acepromazine	0.22, IM	—	Immobilization	339
	Ketamine	11, IM			
Beaver (*Castor canadensis*)	Diazepam	0.1, IM	—	Smooth induction	355
	Ketamine	25, IM			
Ferret (*Mustela putorius*)	Ketamine	20–25, IM	—	—	356
	Xylazine	2, IM	80 ± 11.4	—	357
	Ketamine	25, IM			
	Ketamine	60, IM	—	Muscle rigidity Incomplete analgesia	358
	Diazepam	3, IM	—	Muscle rigidity Incomplete analgesia	
	Ketamine	35, IM			
	Xylazine	2, IM	—	Acceptable analgesia	
	Ketamine	25, IM		Muscle relaxation	
Ferret (*Mustela putorius furo*)	Ketamine	25, IM	—	Excessive salivation Muscle tremor Paddling motions	359
	Xylazine	2, IM	—	Good muscle relaxation	
	Ketamine	25, IM			
Fisher (*Martes pennati*)	Ketamine or with	7.5, IM (11–24.2) range	—	Immobilization	339
	Acepromazine	1.1, IM			
Mink (*Mustela vision*)	Ketamine	5–20, IM	—	—	356
	Ketamine	10–15, IM	—	Suitable for electroejaculation	
	Ketamine	100, IM	—	Surgical anesthesia	
Mink (*Mustela vision*)	Ketamine	15.4–22, IM	—	Immobilization	339
Pine Marten (*Marten americana*)	Ketamine	11–22, IM	—	Immobilization	339
European Otter (*Lutra lutra*)	Diazepam	0.5, IM	—	Good muscle relaxation Smooth recovery	360
	Ketamine	18, IM			
Asian Small-clawed Otter (*Aonyx cinerea*)	Medetomidine	0.1–0.12, IM	—	Good muscle relaxation Immobilization	361
	Ketamine	4–5, IM			
River Otter (*Lutra canadensis*)	Ketamine	22, IM	—	—	339
Sea Otter (*Enhydra lutris*)	Ketamine	1, IM	—	Immobilization	339
Australian Skink and Bobtail Skink (*Tiliqua rugosa*) King's Skink (*Egernia kingii*)	Ketamine	170–230 mg total, IM	—	Good muscle relaxation	362
Common Skunk (*Spilogale putoris*)	Ketamine	10–20, IM	—	—	363
Spotted Skunk (*Spilogale gracilis*)	Ketamine	30.1, IM	—	Immobilization	339
Striped Skunk (*Mephitis mephitis*)	Ketamine	4.5–60	—	Immobilization	364
Striped Skunk (*Mephitis mephitis*)	Ketamine	27, IM	44	Immobilization	339

Table 10–6. Use of Ketamine or Ketamine Combinations in Exotic and Wildlife Animals (continued)

Common Names (Genus and Species)	Drug(s)	Dose and Route (mg/kg)	Duration (min)	Comment	Reference
	*Order Carnivora, Family Mustelidae—cont'd*				
Weasel (*Mustela frenata*)	Ketamine	15.4–22, IM	–	Immobilization	339
	*Order Carnivora, Family Ursidae*				
American Black Bear (*Ursus americana*)	Medetomidine Ketamine	0.03–0.04, IM 1–1.5, IM	–	Immobilization	331
American Black Bear (*Ursus americana*)	Xylazine Ketamine	2–4.5, IM 5–9, IM	–	Good chemical restraint	212
	Xylazine Ketamine	1.9–9.25, IM 1.9–9.25, IM	45–100	–	213
	Xylazine Ketamine	3.6–10.5, IM 3.6–10.5, IM	–	Immobilization	365
Brown Bear (*Ursus arctos horribilis*)	Medetomidine Ketamine	zoo: 0.02–0.03, IM wild: 0.06–0.08, IM zoo: 0.5–1, IM wild: 1–1.6, IM	–	Immobilization	331
Grizzly Bear (*Ursus arctos*)	Xylazine Ketamine	11.1, IM (6.3–14) range 11.1, IM (6.3–14) range	–	–	365
Himalayan Bear (*Selnarctos thibetanus*)	Medetomidine Ketamine	0.03–0.04, IM 1–1.5, IM	–	–	331
Polar Bear (*Ursus maritimus*)	Medetomidine Ketamine	0.03, IM 1–1.5, IM	–	Immobilization	331
Polar Bear (*Ursus maritimus*)	Xylazine Ketamine	6.8, IM 6.8, IM	–	Immobilization Good muscle relaxation	214
Sloth Bear (*Melursus ursinus*)	Xylazine Ketamine	1.4–2.44, IM 5.8–9.75, IM	–	Immobilization	366
	*Miscellaneous Species*				
Camel (*Camelus bactrianus*)	Xylazine Ketamine Xylazine Ketamine	0.25, IM 5.5, IM 0.15, IM 2.5, IM	– –	Good muscle relaxation Good analgesia Good muscle relaxation Good analgesia	367
African Elephant (*Loxodonta africana*)	1st dose Xylazine Ketamine 2nd dose Xylazine Ketamine or Ketamine	1st dose 0.14 ± 0.03, IM 1.14 ± 0.21, IM 2nd dose 0.08 ± 0.03, IM 0.61 ± 0.19, IM 0.47, IV	11.6 ± 6.9 (7–31) range 27 ± 8.9 (13–50) range	Deep sedation to immobilization –	368
African Elephant (*Loxodonta africana*)	Xylazine Ketamine	0.2, IM 1–1.5, IM	–	–	369
African Elephant (*Loxodonta africana*)	Xylazine Ketamine	0.1 ± 0.04, IM 0.6 ± 0.13, IM	–	Chemical restraint	370
Spotted Hyena (*Crocuta crocuta*)	Xylazine Ketamine	6.3, IM 13.2, IM	100	Immobilization	371
Collared Peccaries (*Tayassu tajacu*)	Ketamine	14.7–24.6, IM	71.7	Smooth recovery	372
Rabbit (*Sylvilagus floridanus*)	Xylazine Ketamine	5, IM 70, IM	–	–	373

Table 10–6. Use of Ketamine or Ketamine Combinations in Exotic and Wildlife Animals (continued)

Common Names (Genus and Species)	Drug(s)	Dose and Route (mg/kg)	Duration (min)	Comment	Reference
		Miscellaneous Species—cont'd			
Rabbit (*Sylvilagus floridanus*)	Ketamine †EMTU	35, IM 25–45.5, IV	18.75 (15–60)	Lack of consistency in induction of surgical anesthesia	374
	Xylazine Acepromazine Ketamine	5, SQ 0.75, IM 35, IM	95.25 (58–177)	Respiratory depression Hypothermia Surgical anesthesia	
	Ketamine Chloral hydrate	20, IM 250, IV	15 (0–30)	Lack of consistency in induction of surgical anesthesia	
	Xylazine Ketamine	5, IM 35, IM	46.5 (15–83)	Lack of consistency in induction of surgical anesthesia	
Rabbit (*Sylvilagus floridanus*)	Xylazine Ketamine	5, IM 35, IM	—	—	375
	Xylazine Butorphanol Ketamine	5, IM 0.1, IM 35, IM	68 ± 2	—	
New Zealand White Rabbit	Xylazine Ketamine	5, IM 35, IM	35 ± 6	Surgical anesthesia	287
New Zealand White Rabbit	Xylazine Ketamine	5, IV 25, IV	—	—	376
New Zealand White Rabbit	Xylazine Ketamine	5, IM 35, IM	77 ± 5	—	377
	Xylazine Acepromazine Ketamine	5, IM 0.75, IM 35, IM	99 ± 20	—	
New Zealand White Rabbit	Guaifenesin Ketamine	200, IV 50, IM	30	Surgical anesthesia	378
Raccoon (*Procyon lotor*)	Ketamine	10–14, IM	—	Inadequate jaw muscle relaxation	379
	Ketamine	20–29, IM	180 (150–270)	Adequate jaw relaxation (30–100 minutes) Immobilization	
Raccoon (*Procyon lotor*)	Ketamine Xylazine Ketamine	16.7, IM 2.2–3.3, IM 11–16.5, IM	— —	Chemical restraint Incomplete restraint with low dose of ketamine	339
	Acepromazine Ketamine	1.25, IM 13.6, IM	—	—	
Feral Pig	Xylazine Ketamine	9.8–19.6, IM 9.8–19.6, IM	47.9 ± 12.7	Immobilization	380
Ringtail (*Bassariscus astutus*)	Ketamine	15, IM	—	Immobilization	339
Gopher Snake (*Pituophis melanoleucus catenifer*)	Ketamine	75, IM	43.6 ± 8.1 (11–63)	Sedation to surgical anesthesia	381

†EMTU: ethyl-(1-methyl-propyl) malonyl-thio-urea

Table 10–6. Use of Ketamine or Ketamine Combinations in Exotic and Wildlife Animals (continued)

Common Names (Genus and Species)	Drug(s)	Dose and Route (mg/kg)	Duration (min)	Comment	Reference
Miscellaneous Species—cont'd					
Richardson's Ground Squirrel (*Spermophilus richardsonii*)	Xylazine Ketamine	10.6 ± 0.5, IM 85.5 ± 3.4, IM or	16 ± 3	Surgical anesthesia	382
		10.7 ± 0.7, SQ 85.6 ± 4, SQ	19 ± 9	—	
	Ketamine	86 ± 7, IM	12 ± 10	Did not induce surgical anesthesia	
Bennett Wallabies (*Protemnodon rufogrisea*)	Xylazine Ketamine	187.5, IM 150, IM	—	Rapid immobilization	383
	Xylazine Ketamine	80, IM 160, IM	—	Rapid immobilization	
Marine Animals					
Crabeater Seal (*Lobodon carcinophagus*)	Diazepam Ketamine	0.2, IM 6, IM	20–40	—	384
Northern Elephant Seal (*Mirounga angustirostris*)	Ketamine	1.4–6.9, IM	—	Immobilization	385
Fur Seals (*Arctocephalus galapagoensis*)	Xylazine Ketamine	0–1.16, IM 3.1–18.7, IM	—	Satisfactory immobilization	386
Gray Seal (*Halischoerus grypus*)	Xylazine Ketamine	5.15, IM 4.96, IM	—	—	387
	Diazepam Ketamine	0.3, IM 6, IM	—	Immobilization	388
	Diazepam Ketamine	0.03–0.1, IM 1–3, IM	—	—	389
Harbor Seal (*Phoca vitulina*)	Ketamine Diazepam Ketamine	3–3.2, IM 0.04–0.06, IM 1.4–1.9, IM	— —	— —	389
	Diazepam Ketamine	0.05, IM, IV 1.5, IM, IV	45	Immobilization	390
	Ketamine	4.5, IM	<70	Smooth induction and recovery	
Ringed Seal (*Pusa hispida*)	Ketamine	4.5–11, IM	—	Sedation to surgical anesthesia	390
Southern Elephant Seal (*Miroubga leonina*)	Diazepam Ketamine	0.3, IM 6, IM	—	Immobilization	388
Weddell Seal (*Leptonychotes weddellii*)	Diazepam Ketamine	0.05 ± 0.01, IM 7.99 ± 1.99, IM	12.7 ± 20.7	Immobilization	391
California Sea Lion (*Zalophus californianus*)	Ketamine	4.5–5, IM	<65	Avoid use in ill patients	390
Galapagos Sea Lion (*Zalophus californianus wollebaeki*)	Xylazine Ketamine	0.3–1.43, IM 2.1–7.1, IM	—	—	386

Table 10–7.   Use of Ketamine or Ketamine Combinations in Birds

Species (Genus and Species)	Drug(s)	Dose and Route (mg/kg)	Duration (min)	Comment	Reference
Accipiters	Diazepam Ketamine	1, IM 30, IM	—	—	392
Bald Eagle (*Haliaeetus leucocephalus*)	Diazepam Ketamine	1, IM 10–30, IM	—	—	392
Budgerigar (*Melopsittacus undulatus*)	Xylazine Ketamine	10, IM 40, IM	—	—	393
Double Wattled Cassowary (*Casuarius casuarius*)	Etorphine Ketamine	10–12 total, IM 200–300 total, IM	—	Immobilization suitable for minor procedures	394
Chicken (*Gallus gallus*)	Ketamine	14, IV	15	Muscle tremor LD$_{50}$: 67.5 mg/kg	395
Columbiformes and Corvids	Diazepam Ketamine	2–5, IM 20–40, IM	—	—	392
Ducks and Geese	Diazepam Ketamine	2–4, IM 20–60, IM	—	—	392
Pekin Duck (*Anas platyrhyncos*)	Ketamine Xylazine Ketamine	20, IV 1, IV 20, IV	— — —	— Respiratory depression	396
Emu (*Dromiceius novaehollandiae*)	Ketamine	25, IM initially 5–8, IV additionally	—	Anesthesia	397
Emu (*Dromiceius novaehollandiae*)	Ketamine	25 initially, IM 5, *Suppl. IV	—	Short-term immobilization	397
Leghorn	Xylazine Ketamine	2, IM 2, IM	—	—	398
Red-tailed Hawk (*Buteo jamaicensis*)	Xylazine Ketamine	2.2, IV 4.4, IV	—	—	399
Herons	Diazepam Ketamine	1–2, IM 20, IM	—	—	392
Ostrich (*Struthio camelus*)	Diazepam Ketamine Diazepam Ketamine Xylazine Diazepam Ketamine Xylazine Xylazine Ketamine	0.22, IV 4.4, IV 0.33, IV 6.6, IV 0.44, IM 0.15, IV 2.8, IV 0.9, IM 0.03, IV 4.8, IV	— — — — —	Good induction and recovery Poor induction Good recovery Poor induction Good recovery Fair induction Poor recovery	400
Blue Necked Ostrich (*Struthio camelus austrealis*)	Etorphine Ketamine	10–12 total, IM 200–300 total, IM	—	Immobilization suitable for minor procedure	394
Barred, Long-eared, and Short-eared Owls	Diazepam Ketamine	1, IM 10, IM	—	—	392
Great horned and Screech Owls	Diazepam Ketamine	1, IM 25, IM	—	—	392

*Suppl.: Supplemental dose

Table 10–7.   Use of Ketamine or Ketamine Combinations in Birds—cont'd

Species (Genus and Species)	Drug(s)	Dose and Route (mg/kg)	Duration (min)	Comment	Reference
Parakeets	Ketamine	1 total, IM	—	Sedation	401
	Ketamine	2 total, IM	—	Surgical anesthesia	
	Ketamine	3 total, IM	—	Surgical antesthesia	
Pigeon (Columbia livia)	Ketamine	1 total, IM	—	Respiratory depression	401
	Ketamine	2 total, IM	—	—	
	Ketamine	3 total, IM	—	—	
Cape Vulture (Gyps coprotheres)	Ketamine	7.5–28.8, IM	—	Immobilization	402
Turkey Vulture (Cathartes aura)	Xylazine	1, IM	19.8 ± 25.4	Good muscle relaxation	403
	Ketamine	10, IM		Consistent level of anesthesia	

perfusion pressure.(217) It appears phencyclidine induces direct vasoconstriction at the lower IA doses, while tiletamine does not.

Tiletamine directly depresses the denervated myocardium, whereas it increases cardiac performance following injection in animals with intact cardiac innervation. No inotropic or chronotropic effects were observed when 0.05 to 5.0 mg of tiletamine was injected into the coronary circulation of an isolated rabbit heart preparation. The authors suggested that the increase in blood pressure and heart rate produced by tiletamine in intact animals might be caused, in part, by its influence on the central cardiovascular regulatory mechanisms.(217) This is further supported by the report of White et al., who concluded that ketamine produces its primary sympathomimetic action by direct stimulation of the CNS, which results in increased circulating plasma catecholamines.(5)

Effects on the Respiratory System

Tiletamine does not cause respiratory depression when given in cataleptic doses to cats, but signs of overdose are characterized by hypoventilation and apnea.(222) A moderate decrease in respiration rate 5 minutes after tiletamine injection that returns to normal by 6 hours has been reported.(14) An irregular respiration rate, apneusis, an increase in $PaCO_2$, and a decrease in pHa and PaO_2 have been reported in cats. Apneustic breathing can be decreased or even converted to a normal respiratory pattern by the intravenous injection of either a phenothiazine (e.g., acepromazine) or a benzodiazepine (e.g., diazepam) tranquilizer. This results from a decrease in hypertonicity of the antigravity muscles.(220) Tiletamine has not been used in humans. Ketamine is preferred because it does not produce significant respiratory depression except when given as a rapid intravenous infusion.(5)

Metabolic Disposition and Effect on Urine Output

Plasma half-life ($t_{1/2}$) of tiletamine in cats is 2 to 4 hours. Only 5 to 10% of the dose is detected in urine, none appears in the feces, and some drug is found in

bile.(223) In dogs, monkeys, and rats, plasma $t_{1/2}$ was 1.2 hours, 1 to 1.5 hours, and 30 to 40 minutes, respectively. Tissue $t_{1/2}$ was considerably longer than plasma $t_{1/2}$ in the cat and rat. Three metabolites, 2-(ethylamino)-2-(2-thienyl) cyclohexanol , 2-amino-2-(2-thienyl) cyclohexanol (metabolite 1), and 2-amino-2-(2-thienyl) cyclohexanone (metabolite 3) have been isolated from cat urine, while only metabolites 1 and 2 were isolated in monkey urine.(223)

Tiletamine, at 4, 8, and 16 mg/kg, increases urine excretion for 2 hours in water loaded rats. The increase in urine output lasted for 3 hours when tiletamine was given at total doses of 32 and 64 mg.(217)

Zolazepam Hydrochloride (CI-716). Zolazepam is a benzodiazepine derivative that has taming effects in animals. The advantageous pharmacologic characteristics of benzodiazepines (e.g., chlordiazepoxide, diazepam, midazolam, and zolazepam) have been described as (a) production of amnesia, (b) minimal depression of cardiorespiratory function, (c) strong anticonvulsant action, (d) relative safety even if overdosed, and (e) rare development of significant tolerance or physical dependence. Benzodiazepines have a rapid onset and short duration of action but lack analgesic effects.(224) Although the benzodiazepines are not approved for use alone in animals, diazepam is being used with increasing frequency in veterinary patients. Zolazepam was first investigated for use in humans and is the only benzodiazepine approved by the FDA for use in animals when combined with tiletamine (i.e., Telazol).

Effects on the Central Nervous System

In cats, zolazepam does not induce anesthesia or tranquilization when administered either intramuscularly or intravenously.(14) After intraperitoneal injection in mice, it induces a delayed increase in random motor activity. When compared with chlordiazepoxide and diazepam, zolazepam is the least apt to cause CNS depression. This observation played a major role in the selection of zolazepam as the benzodiazepine of choice to be combined with tiletamine in the development of Telazol. The objective was to develop an anesthetic free from the undesirable sedative-hypnotic-respiratory depressant effects seen with the commonly approved injectable anesthetics. From the results of rat behavioral studies, zolazepam was reported to produce significant anxiolytic effects at doses ranging from 0.63 mg/kg to 10 mg/kg. However, doses of 0.08, 0.16, 0.31, 20, and even 40 mg/kg did not produce significant anxiolytic effects. It seems that zolazepam only produces anxiolytic activity in a rather precise dose. At lower doses, the effects are not prominent enough, and at higher doses, the depressant side effects became too prominent for the anxiolytic effect to be observed.(225) When a dose of 10 mg/kg of zolazepam was given intramuscularly to cats, a "fear reaction," extreme continuous territorial exploration, or a hysterical jumping-climbing behavior occurred that was not unlike that often observed with high doses of midazolam administration.(14) The fear reaction was characterized by a cowering behavior and seeking dark corners, cabinets, chairs, and tables. Territorial exploration was characterized by mouthing objects on the floor and continuous movement. Jumping-climbing behavior was characterized by seeking anything high off the floor and attempting repeatedly to jump on top of it. These behaviors continued for 15 minutes after drug injection, gradually decreasing in frequency. Calm behavior gradually returned, with the cats appearing normal in 24 hours. Concurrently with the development of changing behaviors, EEG recordings revealed a pattern with extremely high amplitude and high frequency. This high amplitude and frequency activity occurred within 2 minutes of zolazepam injection, reaching a maximum at 5 minutes. Decreased frequency and amplitude were present at 24 hours but returned to preinjection or baseline levels at 48 hours.(14)

Effects on the Cardiovascular System

The effect of diazepam on cardiovascular action is mild even in doses of 15 mg/kg given intravenously.(226) In dogs, 2.5 mg/kg of diazepam given intravenously does not significantly alter heart rate and mean arterial pressure.(227) When given in a dose of 10 mg/kg intramuscularly, zolazepam produced an increase in heart rate in cats.(14) In pentobarbital-anesthetized dogs, zolazepam is reportedly free of untoward action on cardiovascular function even when given in massive intravenous doses (cumulative dose of 61 mg/kg). In chronically instrumentated, nonanesthetized adult beagles, 2 mg/kg IV of zolazepam induces no discernible changes in cardiovascular function, while 10 mg/kg and 50 mg/kg induces a decrease in systemic vascular resistance with an associated decrease in systemic blood pressure. A reflex tachycardia with a decrease in stroke volume and an increase in ventricular contractility occurs in response to systemic hypotension.(225)

Effects on the Respiratory System

Zolazepam (10 mg/kg IM) has only minimal effects on the respiration rate in cats.(14) Diazepam (0.3 mg/kg IV)

and midazolam (0.15 mg/kg IV) decrease ventilatory and mouth occlusion pressure in response to CO_2 as a result of respiratory depression in healthy human volunteers.(228) When diazepam is given at doses of 5 to 10 mg intravenously to human patients with heart disease for treatment of anxiety during cardiac catheterization, hypoventilation occurs, which appears to be in response to a decrease in tidal volume.(229) However, the changes in ventilation are not severe and do not require mechanical support. Information on the effect of zolazepam in animals is limited.

Effects on Other Systems

Zolazepam is free of alpha-adrenergic blocking activity, ganglionic activity, and anticholinergic effects.(14) Zolazepam has little or no measurable effect on stomach secretory activity in pylorus-ligated rats when compared with the effect produced by a potent anticholinergic drug such as atropine. The dose of zolazepam required to decrease the mean volume of gastric secretion by 50% when injected subcutaneously is 34 mg/kg, whereas the dose for atropine is 1 mg/kg.(221) In mice, oral zolazepam significantly delays stomach emptying time at a dose of 30 mg/kg. Fecal output is not significantly decreased by 50 mg/kg of oral zolazepam. Zolazepam does not appear to adversely affect normal gastrointestinal function when given in clinically effective doses.(225)

Zolazepam has no discernible effect on mating behavior, gonadotrophin secretion, or ovarian function in adult rats even at doses up to eight times the therapeutic dose. In immature intact and immune hypophysectomized rats treated with exogenous gonadotrophins, zolazepam at antianxiety doses (0.63–10 mg/kg) or higher significantly decreases the number of eggs ovulated per rat without altering the percentage of rats ovulating. It appears that zolazepam acts either directly or indirectly on the immature ovary to decrease the number of ova released. Ovarian and uterine weight are not affected.(225)

Metabolic Disposition

Plasma $t_{1/2}$ of zolazepam in dogs, cats, rats, and monkeys is 4 to 5 hours, 4.5 hours, 3 hours, and 1 hour, respectively. In beagle dogs, about 2.9 to 8.7% of the dose of zolazepam is detected in the urine and 1% is recovered in the feces. The major metabolite isolated from cat urine is 8-dimethyl-1,6-hydroxy-zolazepam [metabolite 5]. Two other metabolites, 8-dimethyl-zolazepam [metabolite 1] and 1,8-dimethyl-zolazepam [metabolite 3] are also found in cat urine after a single dose, but the concentration decreases with repeated dosing. In beagle dogs, 1-dimethyl-zolazepam [metabolite 2] and a hydroxylated derivative of metabolite 2 [metabolite 6] are found in urine. Six-hydroxy-zolazepam [metabolite 4] is found in both male and female rats, whereas metabolite 2 is found in female rats only.(230)

Telazol (CI-744). Several combinations of tiletamine and zolazepam were investigated in the early stage of Telazol development. Massopust et al. reported that 20 mg/kg of tiletamine and 10 mg/kg of zolazepam in cats prolonged surgical anesthesia for 1.5 hours, twice the anesthetic time produced by tiletamine alone.(14) The muscular clonus, body rigidity, and convulsive movements produced by tiletamine alone were absent when combined with zolazepam. The bizarre behavior (fear reaction, territorial exploration and jumping-climbing behaviors) induced by zolazepam alone was also absent when cats awoke from tiletamine-zolazepam anesthesia. Palpebral and corneal reflexes, flexion of limbs, and body extension to back pinch were either absent or decreased. The pharyngeal-tracheal reflexes remain intact.(14) Studies in dogs and primates also demonstrate that the effectiveness of tiletamine was greatly enhanced by combining it with zolazepam (also referred to as *flupyrazapon*) in a 2:1 ratio. This combination of drugs resulted in general anesthesia, excellent muscle relaxation, no nystagmus or athetoid movement, and smooth recovery in dogs and monkeys.(231, 232) The combination of zolazepam at the dose used did not completely suppress, but did attenuate the side effects of tiletamine. This suggested that tiletamine could be used in combination with zolazepam for animal anesthesia and adjustment of drug ratio might even lessen the side effects.(14) Subsequently, tiletamine and zolazepam were combined in a 1:1 ratio by weight of base and marketed. Telazol is supplied in a sterile vial as a lyophilized powder containing 250 mg of tiletamine and 250 mg of zolazepam. It is recommended that the drug be reconstituted with 5 mL of sterile water, resulting in a combination of 50 mg of tiletamine and 50 mg of zolazepam per mL. Telazol has a wide margin of safety, and reactions to intramuscular injection are minimal. Induction of anesthesia is rapid and smooth, as is recovery in most species. The swallowing and eructation/vomiting reflex are retained. Muscle relaxation and general lack of response to external stimuli add to Telazol's usefulness.

Effects on the Central Nervous System

Telazol induces analgesia from interruption of sensory input into the brain, which usually persists after the anesthetic effect has subsided. The patient's eyes remain open, even during surgical anesthesia. Protective reflexes such as coughing, swallowing, and corneal and pedal reflexes are maintained. Increased salivation is a common occurrence in most animals given Telazol. This can be easily prevented by administration of atropine or glycopyrrolate.

After intravenous injection of Telazol (4 mg/kg) in calves, the EEG moves toward electric silence. Suppression is followed by a short period of high-amplitude-slow-frequency activity.(233) Similar EEG patterns have been observed after tiletamine (20 mg/kg IM)-zolazepam (10 mg/kg IM) administration to cats.(14) Changes in EEG activity in animals under general anesthesia have been shown to be characterized by a waveform pattern of slow frequency and high amplitude or voltage.(1)

Effects on the Cardiovascular System

In cats and llamas, Telazol causes no significant changes in heart rate.(234, 235) In conflict with these observations are the results of a study that reported an increase in heart rate after Telazol (12.8 mg/kg, IV or IM) administration to cats.(236) Increased heart rate has also been observed in dogs given Telazol (2 to 19.8 mg/kg) with no premedication.(236-238) When dogs are premedicated with acepromazine, the magnitude of heart rate increase is decreased. (238) In calves, Telazol (4 mg/kg IV) induces a transient decrease followed by an increase in heart rate. The mechanism of the transient decrease in heart rate is believed to be caused by the negative inotropic and chronotropic effects of the tiletamine.(233) The direct depressant effect of tiletamine has been clearly demonstrated in denervated myocardium.(225) A decreased amplitude of myocardial contraction has been observed when tiletamine (0.5 to 5 mg) was administered into the coronary circulation of an isolated rabbit heart preparation.(217) The subsequent increase in heart rate is attributed to direct CNS stimulation leading to increased sympathetic tone and perhaps decreased vagal tone.(239) In monkeys, the heart rate decreases 5% in animals given 1.5 mg/kg (IM) and 7% in those given 3.0 mg/kg (IM). Decreased left ventricular *dp/dt*, *V*max, and left ventricular end-diastolic pressure indicates that Telazol produces a transient decrease in myocardial contractility.(240)

Changes in arterial blood pressure and systemic vascular resistance induced by Telazol are characterized by a decrease followed by an increase after intravenous injection in cats, dogs, and calves.(233, 234, 237) Tiletamine may play a major role in the unique biphasic hemodynamic changes occurring after Telazol injection.(233) Because tiletamine (3.2 mg/kg to 6.4 mg/kg) has been observed to decrease perfusion pressure when administered intraarterially into the hindquarters of the dog, it may be responsible for the initial hypotension of the biphasic response.(217) Subsequent hypertension is likely caused by direct CNS stimulation accompanied by increased sympathetic tone, a releasing of catecholamine from peripheral storage sites, prevention of uptake of catecholamine back into the postganglionic nerve endings, and inhibition of vagal baroreceptor reflex activity.(62, 241-244)

In calves, the biphasic response in arterial blood pressure induced by Telazol (4 mg/kg IV) is reversed when combined with xylazine (0.1 mg/kg IV). The hemodynamic effects of Telazol are offset by the initial vasoconstrictive and delayed sympatholytic and parasympathomimetic effects of intravenous xylazine.(245) In horses, blood pressure increases initially following injection of xylazine but returns to baseline value after Telazol injection. Xylazine typically induces a biphasic increase followed by a decrease in arterial blood pressure after intravenous injection in horses.(246) The injection of Telazol may attenuate the hypotensive response of xylazine via tiletamine's ability to increase sympathetic activity.(247) In sheep, butorphanol (0.5 mg/kg IV) preanesthetic administration does not influence the decrease in mean systemic and pulmonary arterial pressures induced by Telazol (12 mg/kg IV). Heart rate does not change significantly when butorphanol is given simultaneously or prior to Telazol, although increased systemic vascular resistance is observed.(248)

In calves, left ventricular stroke work index and rate pressure product follow a similar biphasic response as seen with blood pressure and systemic vascular resistance after Telazol injection.(233) Cardiac output remains unchanged in calves and llamas,(233, 235) and only decreases briefly in cats, 1 minute after intravenous injection with doses of 15.8 and 23.7 mg/kg of Telazol.(234) In dogs, Telazol injection induces either an increase or no change in cardiac output. The increase is attributed to an increase in heart rate.(237) Decreased cardiac output is observed in horses given xylazine-Telazol and in sheep given butorphanol-Telazol.(247, 248) In calves given xylazine-Telazol, cardiac output decreases transiently and is associated with an increase in afterload and a decrease in heart rate.(245)

The cardiovascular effects induced by Telazol vary markedly between species.(249) In cats, dogs, and calves, Telazol produces generalized cardiovascular stimulation, while depression has generally been observed in monkeys. Phencyclidine(250, 251) and ketamine(252, 253) also cause cardiovascular effects that are species dependent.

Effects on the Respiratory System

Respiration rate increases in most species following Telazol injection. In calves, low doses of Telazol (4 to 8 mg/kg, IV or IM) increase respiration rate for 30 to 60 minutes. Apnea may occur with larger doses (10 mg/kg IM), but spontaneous breathing usually resumes shortly with minimal respiratory support.

Respiratory rate in cats generally decreases and is characterized by an apneustic breathing pattern after intramuscular or intravenous injection. A normal breathing pattern returns within 10 to 15 minutes.(236) Respiratory depression in cats appears to be dose dependent, with higher doses causing an increase in $PaCO_2$ and a decrease in pHa.(234) Respiration rate is increased in most dogs when doses ranging from 6.6 to 19.8 mg/kg are given intramuscularly. However, minute ventilation and tidal volume decrease when larger doses are given.(237) When a dose of 2 to 4 mg/kg is given intravenously to dogs without premedication, the ventilatory pattern is characterized by a short period of apnea (1 min) followed by irregular, slow, shallow breathing. This is accompanied by slight hypoxemia, but the $PaCO_2$ remains near normal.(238) In sheep,

although respiration rate remains unchanged, apneustic breathing and decreased inspired minute ventilation and tidal volume are observed after Telazol administration (12 or 24 mg/kg IV).(254) In llamas, mild respiratory depression accompanied by hypoxemia is also evident.(235) In nonhuman primates, low doses of Telazol (1.5 mg/kg or 3.0 mg/kg IM) induce respiratory depression, with the peak effect occurring within 10 minutes after injection. Respiratory rate gradually returns to preinjection values.(240)

CLINICAL USE

In general, Telazol induces an increase in heart rate in most species. Tachycardia and hypertension may occur during surgical manipulations. With high doses, apneustic breathing, apnea, decreased tidal volume, and other forms of respiratory depression have been observed. Low but clinically effective doses have only minimal effect on respiration. Complete skeletal muscle relaxation of selected muscle groups (e.g., anterior temporal, posterior temporal, anterior border of the superficial head of the masseter, orbicularis musculature) has been described in monkeys and has been demonstrated in the electromyogram following Telazol (3 mg/kg IM). Slight muscle hyperactivity has been observed during the recovery period.(255) Hypothermia may occur after Telazol injection as a result of profound muscle relaxation. Body temperature should be monitored, as supplemental heat may be required, particularly in small patients. Telazol can be used concurrently with other anesthetics (e.g., ultra-short-acting barbiturates and inhalation anesthetics). Excessive salivation following Telazol injection can be controlled with an anticholinergic (e.g., atropine or glycopyrrolate). Telazol's duration of action varies widely among species for reasons not fully understood.(256)

Although only approved for use in dogs and cats, Telazol has proven to be a very useful drug for restraint and induction of anesthesia in a wide variety of wild (257) and domestic species.(233, 235, 247)

Dogs. Onset of surgical anesthesia occurs within 7 to 8 minutes following intramuscular injection of Telazol and within 30 to 60 seconds after intravenous injection. Recommended doses and duration of surgical anesthesia for dogs are given in Table 10–8. Dogs usually are fully recovered within 4 hours after a single intramuscular injection. The duration of surgical anesthesia can be prolonged by increasing the dose or administering supplemental doses.

Tachycardia and transient hypotension occur after intramuscular injection of 10 or 20 mg/kg Telazol.(258) Hellyer et al. reported that intravenous injection of 6.6, 13.2, and 19.8 mg/kg caused an increase in heart rate.(237) The two larger doses caused an increase in cardiac output. All doses caused a biphasic blood pressure response. Blood pressure first decreased then increased. The initial decrease could be caused in large part by the rate of injection. Depression of minute ventilation occurred and appeared to be dose depen-

Table 10–8. Use of Telazol or Telazol Combinations in Dogs

Drug(s)	Dose and Route (mg/kg)	Duration (min)	Comment	Reference
Telazol	9.9, IM	21 ± 10.9	Unsatisfactory recovery in two dogs	236
Telazol	9.9, IV	20.1 ± 6.38	—	
Telazol	6.6, IV	17.5 ± 11.7	Smooth recovery	237
Telazol	13.2, IV	37 ± 18.1	Rougher recovery	
Telazol	19.8, IV	50.8 ± 27.27	Rougher recovery	
Telazol	6.6–9.9, IM	30	Diagnostic examinations Restraint	256
Telazol	2–4, IV	15–20	Diagnostic examinations Restraint	
Telazol	9.9–13.2, IM	30–90	Minor surgical procedures (mild to moderate analgesia)	
Telazol	4–9.9, IV	20–80	—	
Telazol	2, IV	11.9 ± 6.6	Minor procedures requires no intubation Easy intubation	238
Telazol	4, IV	22.7 ± 7.3	—	
Telazol	15.4, IM	40	Anesthesia	259
Telazol	6.6, IV or IM	20–25	Light surgical anesthesia	
Telazol	5.7, IM (4–8.6) range	41.5 (15–77) range	Satisfactory anesthesia	268
Telazol	9.7, IM (8.8–13)	56.6 (33–106) range	Satisfactory anesthesia	
Telazol	17.8, IM (13–22) range	79.7 (37–124) range	Satisfactory anesthesia	
Telazol	4, IV	—	Satisfactory restraint from intradermal skin testing	404 405
Telazol	5, IV	38.5 ± 23	Injection of flumazenil shorten recovery	266
Telazol	6–12, IM	—	—	232
Telazol	4–100, IM	—	—	268
Telazol Xylazine Butorphanol	8.8, IM 1.1, IM 0.22, IM	100	Anesthesia Good muscle relaxation Good analgesia	260

dent. When given intramuscularly at the recommended doses, Telazol provides a broad margin of safety. Dogs survived without any lasting effects when doses of 29.9 mg/kg were given daily for 8 consecutive days.(256) In dogs, plasma $t_{1/2}$ of tiletamine is 1.2 hours as compared to 1 hour for zolazepam.(223) When dogs recover from Telazol anesthesia, the tranquilizing effects of zolazepam appear to wane before those of tiletamine. Therefore, the characteristic rough recovery seen with dissociative drugs alone is often seen following Telazol anesthesia in dogs. Adverse responses during recovery may also be influenced by dose and route of Telazol administration and the procedure performed. The higher the dose, the more likely dogs will have a rough, prolonged recovery. Muscle rigidity is common, and some seizurelike activity may be observed.(259) In one study, a dog was given 0.1 mg/kg of diazepam intravenously to reduce muscle activity as it began to recover from Telazol anesthesia. Smoothness of recovery reportedly improved after diazepam injection.(238) Premedication with acepromazine, opioids (morphine or

butorphanol), or xylazine has proven to enhance smoothness of recovery.(259) A combination of Telazol-xylazine-butorphanol has been used successfully in dogs for ovariohysterectomy. Duration of surgical anesthesia was 100 minutes, and recovery occurred in 130 minutes.(260)

In pentobarbital-anesthetized dogs, concurrent injection of chloramphenicol prolongs anesthesia sleep time by protein-synthesis inhibition(261,262), whereas chloramphenicol (213.8 mg/kg, orally) administration does not prolong Telazol (11 mg/kg IM) anesthesia.(263)

Telazol (20 mg/kg IM) does not sensitize the heart to epinephrine-induced ectopic ventricular tachycardia or fibrillation.(264) When administered prior to or after halothane anesthesia, the ventricular arrhythmogenic dose of epinephrine did not change significantly (6.7 ± 2.8 μg/kg) from that in dogs anesthetized with halothane alone (8.9 ± 4.3 μg/kg).(265)

Tolazoline (5 mg/kg IV), doxapram (5 mg/kg IV) and flumazenil (5 mg/kg IV; a benzodiazepine antagonist) have been investigated as antagonists to Telazol's depressant effects. Only flumazenil significantly shortened recovery, but continuous paddling and whining were observed in these dogs. Apparently, flumazenil reversed the effect of zolazepam, unmasking the excitatory effects of tiletamine.(266) In another study, Hatch et al. suggested that doxapram (5.5 mg/kg IV) may be the optimal drug for reversal of Telazol overdose (30 mg/kg IM)(267), although it is a generalized CNS stimulant and not a drug that acts on specific receptor sites.

Cats. The onset of surgical anesthesia in cats occurs in 1.5 to 6 minutes after intravenous or intramuscular injection of Telazol. Recommended doses and duration of surgical anesthesia for cats are given in Table 10–9. Cats react painfully to intramuscular injection of Telazol. The margin of safety of Telazol in cats is 4.5 times

the recommended dose.(256) For anesthesia, it has been suggested that Telazol is superior to ketamine because of fewer undesirable side effects.(166, 268)

In cats, Telazol causes a slight decrease in blood pressure when doses of 10 to 20 mg/kg are given intramuscularly.(269) After intravenous injection arterial blood pressure decreases initially, then increases.(234) Heart rate may increase after both intravenous and intramuscular injection, but tachycardia occurs more often in dogs than in cats.(236) Telazol has been reported to cause no significant change in heart rate after intravenous injection in cats.(234) Respiratory rate usually decreases and is dose dependent.(234, 236) The plasma $t_{1/2}$ of tiletamine and zolazepam in cats is 2.5 and 4.5 hours, respectively. Thus, as the cat recovers

Table 10–9. Use of Telazol or Telazol Combinations in Cats

Drug(s)	Dose and Route (mg/kg)	Duration (min)	Comment	Reference
Telazol	6–40, IM	—	—	268
Telazol	6–12, IM	—	Anesthesia	289
Telazol	12.8, IM	52.6 ± 22.0	Salivation Apneustic breathing Salivation	236
Telazol	12.8, IV	52.8 ± 17.3	Salivation Apneustic breathing Salivation	
Telazol	7.5, IM	49.9 ± 12.7	Surgical anesthesia Mild muscle relaxation Rough recovery	161 162
Telazol	9.7–11.9, IM	30	Diagnostic examinations Dentistry	256
Telazol	9.9, IV	25	Diagnostic examinations Dentistry	
Telazol	10.6–12.5, IM	60	Minor procedure (mild to moderate analgesia)	
Telazol	4.5, IM	30–60	Ovariohysterectomy	
Telazol	4.5, IM		Onychectomy	
Telazol	14.3–15.8, IM	60–135	—	
Telazol	10.4, IM (6–16) range	64.6 (32–135) range	Satisfactory surgical anesthesia Salivation	268
Telazol	9.7, IV	60	—	234
Telazol	15.8, IV	>90	Respiratory depression	
Telazol	23.7, IV	>90	Respiratory depression	
Telazol	3.1 ± 0.99, IM	—	Inadequate analgesia for castration	406
Telazol	2.7 ± 1.0, IV			
Acepromazine	0.1, IM	—	Adequate anesthesia for castration	
Telazol	3.4 ± 1.09, IM 2.7 ± 0.97, IV			
Telazol	4.5 ± 0.9, IM	—	Adequate anesthesia for castration	
Telazol	4.5 ± 0.9, IV	—	—	
Telazol	5, IV	20.2 ± 10.3	Injection of doxapram and flumazenil shorten recovery	266
Telazol*	3.3, IM	43.4 ± 9.1	Smooth induction and recovery	272
Ketamine	2.64, IM		Excellent muscle relaxation	
Xylazine	0.66, IM		Good analgesia	

*Reconstitute with 4 mL of ketamine and 1 mL of 10% xylazine.

from Telazol anesthesia there is a prolongation of tranquilization as a result of the long plasma $t_{1/2}$ of zolazepam. Because of this longer plasma $t_{1/2}$, the recovery time for cats is twice as long as that of dogs.(223) Tolazoline (5 mg/kg IV), doxapram (5 mg/kg IV), and flumazenil (5 mg/kg IV) have been used to antagonize Telazol's depressant effects (5 mg/kg IV) in cats. Doxapram and flumazenil promoted a more rapid arousal.(266) Prior administration of chloramphenicol (204.2 mg/kg, orally) causes an increase in duration of surgical anesthesia and time to return of righting reflex in cats given Telazol.(270)

Epinephrine-induced cardiac fibrillation is not enhanced in cats anesthetized with clinical doses of Telazol (20 mg/kg IM).(264) Likewise, in halothane-anesthetized cats, injection of Telazol (3 mg/kg, IV or IM) did not alter the ventricular arrhythmogenic dose of epinephrine.(265)

Telazol or ketamine-acepromazine have been combined with either butorphanol or oxymorphone and analgesia assessed using circulating catecholamine concentration as an indicator of analgesic response during onychectomy (declaw). Telazol alone or the Telazol combinations with opioids appear to depress catecholamine plasma concentrations during pre- and postoperative periods.(271)

A combination of Telazol, ketamine, and xylazine has been recommended as an alternative anesthetic regimen for onychectomy and castration of cats. Four milliliters of 10% ketamine and 1 mL of 10% xylazine are used to reconstitute 500 mg of Telazol. Each mL of the resulting solution contains 50 mg of tiletamine, 50 mg of zolazepam, 80 mg of ketamine, and 20 mg of xylazine. The final concentration of dissociative (i.e., tiletamine and ketamine) in this combination is 130 mg/mL. Intramuscular injection of 0.15 mL/4.5 kg of this combination produces approximately 40 to 45 minutes of surgical anesthesia adequate for onychectomy and castration. The advantages of this combination include small injection volume, rapid onset of action with smooth induction, excellent muscle relaxation with analgesia, and smooth recovery.(272)

Horses. When used alone in horses, Telazol causes hyperresponsiveness. Muscle spasm, rapid eye movement, or movement of the limbs occur during anesthesia. In horses, Telazol is recommended only in combination with a tranquilizer or sedative to reduce excitement and improve muscle relaxation.(273) Different doses of Telazol have been used in combination with xylazine and detomidine in horses(181, 247, 273-275), ponies(276), mules(277), and donkeys.(278) When combined with xylazine (1.1 mg/kg IV), Telazol (1.1, 1.65, 2.2 mg/kg IV) rapidly induces safe short-term anesthesia ($\geq$ 20 minutes) and smooth recovery.(247, 273) When xylazine (2.2 mg/kg) is given intramuscularly, some horses have a rough recovery.(247) When butorphanol (0.04 mg/kg IV) is added to xylazine-Telazol, duration of recumbency is prolonged (41.3 minutes), and emergence is usually smoother.(181)

With xylazine premedication, heart rate decreases but gradually returns to baseline following Telazol, while cardiac output remains decreased.(247) Respiration rate decreases and is accompanied by decreased pHa and PaO_2 and increased $PaCO_2$.(247) Ventilation is characterized by a short period of apneustic breathing following Telazol injection.(247, 273) Xylazine (1.1 mg/kg IV)-Telazol (0.55, 1.1, or 1.6 mg/kg IV) can be used to safely induce anesthesia, permitting tracheal intubation for maintenance with an inhalant.(279)

When mules are anesthetized with xylazine (1.1 mg/kg IV) and Telazol (1.1 mg/kg IV) under field conditions, recoveries are frequently rough.(277) In donkeys, xylazine (1.1 mg/kg IV) – Telazol (1.1 mg/kg IV) induced safe and satisfactory anesthesia with a duration of action and good muscle relaxation for approximately three quarters of an hour. Nevertheless, recoveries were prolonged and rough.(278) In ponies, Telazol (2 or 3 mg/kg IV) has also been used with detomidine (0.02, 0.04, or 0.06 mg/kg IV). These combinations produce rapid induction, profound analgesia and good muscle relaxation. Higher doses increase the duration of anesthesia and the roughness of recovery. Doses of 2 mg/kg of Telazol (IV) and 0.04 mg/kg of detomidine (IV) induce rapid recumbency, good analgesia, and smooth recovery. With this combination the duration of anesthesia is twice (30 – 40 minutes) that of intravenous xylazine-ketamine.(276) Arterial blood pressure in horses increases significantly after detomidine and Telazol administration. Heart rate decreases after detomidine but returns toward baseline after Telazol administration. Respiratory rate increases but is accompanied by lower PaO_2 values when compared to horses anesthetized with xylazine/ketamine.(274) A summary of doses, routes of injection, and duration of action of Telazol for horses is presented in Table 10–10.

Ruminants. In calves, Telazol induces rapid immobilization when administered in doses of 4 to 12 mg/kg intramuscularly. At a dose of 10 mg/kg or greater, apnea may occur. Muscle relaxation is profound, but analgesia is minimal. The overall response is characteristic of general anesthesia. A combination of xylazine (0.1 mg/kg IV) and Telazol (4 mg/kg IV) appears to increase muscle relaxation and analgesia and have a longer duration of action than that of Telazol (4 mg/kg IV) alone.(245, 280)

Telazol (8 to 20 mg/kg IV) has been used successfully to anesthetize sheep undergoing surgical procedures. Induction is rapid and exceptionally smooth, and duration of surgical anesthesia ranges from 40 minutes to 3.7 hours. Excessive salivation can be controlled by administration of 0.066 mg/kg of atropine sulfate.(268) Intravenous doses of 12 or 24 mg/kg of Telazol cause a significant decrease in minute ventilation and respiratory airflow that is characterized by an apneustic breathing pattern.(254) Intramuscular administration of 12 mg/kg of Telazol appears to be the optimal dose, with surgical anesthesia lasting approximately 30 minutes. The analgesic effect was found to be most profound

Table 10–10. Use of Telazol or Telazol Combinations in Horses

Species	Drug(s)	Dose and Route (mg/kg)	Duration (min)	Comment	Reference
Horse	Xylazine Telazol	1.1, IV 1.65, IV	—	Anesthesia Smooth recovery	247
Horse	Xylazine Telazol	1.1, IV 0.5, IV	26.25	Adequate anesthesia Easy intubation Hyperresponsiveness during recovery	273
	Xylazine Telazol	1.1, IV 0.75, IV	29.25	Adequate anesthesia Easy intubation Hyperresponsiveness during recovery	
	Xylazine Telazol	1.1, IV 2.2, IV	34.33	Adequate anesthesia Easy intubation Smooth recovery	
Horse	Xylazine Telazol	1.1, IV 1.65, IV	32.8 ± 2.8	Good muscle relaxation Smooth recovery[b]	276
	Detomidine Telazol	0.02, IV 2, IV	38.5 ± 9	Balanced anesthesia Smooth recovery[b]	
	Detomidine Telazol	0.04, IV 2, IV	66.5 ± 10.3	Balanced anesthesia Excellent recovery[a]	
	Detomidine Telazol	0.06, IV 3, IV	91.5 ± 18	Balanced anesthesia Prolonged duration Rough recovery[c]	
Horse	Detomidine Telazol	0.015, IV 2, IV	25.5 ± 3	Satisfactory induction and recovery	275
Horse	Xylazine Telazol Xylazine Butorphanol Telazol	1.1, IV 1.1, IV 1.1, IV 0.04, IV 1.1, IV	30.7 (24–35) range 41.3 (33–66)	Good muscle relaxation Smooth recovery[b] Good muscle relaxation Prolonged analgesia Smooth recovery[b]	181
Horse	Detomidine Telazol	0.02, IV 1.1, IV	26 ± 4	Good muscle relaxation Prolonged analgesia Hypoxemia	274
	Detomidine Telazol	0.04, IV 1.4, IV	39 ± 11	Good muscle relaxation Prolonged analgesia Hypoxemia	
Mules	Xylazine Telazol	1.1, IV 1.1, IV	21.1	Smooth recovery[b]	277
Donkeys	Xylazine Telazol	1.1, IV 1.1, IV	46	Satisfactory anesthesia Good muscle relaxation Smooth recovery[b]	278

[a]Animals stood at first attempt.
[b]Animals stood requiring less than three attempts.
[c]Animals stood requiring greater than five attempts.

around the head, neck, and the trunk, whereas poor analgesia was found in the distal portion of the limb and perineal area.(281) When Telazol (12 mg/kg IV) is combined with butorphanol (0.5 mg/kg IV) in sheep, heart rate remains unchanged when butorphanol is given simultaneously or prior to Telazol. Analgesia lasts 25 to 50 minutes.(248) Xylazine (0.11 mg/kg IV) has also been combined with Telazol (13.2 mg/kg IV) to induce anesthesia in sheep. Compared to Telazol (13.2 mg/kg IV) alone, xylazine/Telazol produces a longer duration of analgesia (101.7 vs 41.6 minutes); however, some sheep may become apneic requiring assisted ventilation immediately after intravenous injection. Apnea is short lived, with spontaneous breathing returning within 2 minutes.(282)

In llamas, Telazol (4.4 mg/kg IM) provides good chemical restraint, but muscle relaxation and analgesia are not sufficient for surgery.(235) Table 10–11 summarizes the use of Telazol and Telazol combinations in ruminants.

Swine. Telazol alone in pigs (doses range from 4.4 to 22 mg/kg) induces rapid immobilization but does not

Table 10–11. Use of Telazol or Telazol Combinations in Domestic Ruminants

Species	Drug(s)	Dose and Route (mg/kg)	Duration (min)	Comment	Reference
Calves	Telazol	4, IV	50–60	Anesthesia	233
Calves	Xylazine Telazol	0.1, IV 4, IV	66	Anesthesia	245 280
Cattle	Telazol	2–6, IV	–	–	363
Sheep	Telazol Butorphanol	12, IV 0.5, IV	31 (25–45) range	Adequate anesthesia	248
Sheep	Telazol	11.9 ± 2.7, IV (8.1–16.8) range *Suppl.: 5.7, IV	150 (48–222) range 210 (48–318) range	Cataleptoid anesthesia Excellent muscle relaxation Muscle relaxation not as good as single dose.	407
Sheep	Telazol	14.4, IV (12–22) range	41.5 (25–65) range	Satisfactory anesthesia for neuro- surgical procedures	268
Sheep	Telazol	2.2–4.4, IM	–	Immobilization	289
Sheep	Telazol	8–22, IM	–	–	268
Sheep	Telazol Telazol	12, IV 24, IV	39 ± 5 40 ± 14	Smooth induction Gradual but unremarkable recovery Apneustic breathing Smooth induction Gradual but unremarkable recovery Apneustic breathing	254
Sheep	No Atropine: Telazol Telazol Telazol With Atropine: Telazol Telazol Telazol	 9, IM 12, IM 15, IM 0.04, IM 9, IM 12, IM 15, IM	 14 35 51 13 28 42	 Variable anesthetic response Surgical anesthesia Prolonged anesthetic duration – – –	281
Sheep	Atropine Telazol Xylazine Telazol	0.03, IM 13.2, IV 0.01, IM 13.2, IV	41.6 ± 15 101.7 ± 26	– Better muscle relaxation Larger anesthetic duration Apnea	282
Llama	Telazol	4.4, IM	25–50	Chemical restraint	235

*Suppl.: Supplemental dose

produce adequate muscle relaxation and analgesia sufficient for surgery. Hyperresponsive reflexes characterized by exaggerated limb withdrawal are common and often persist during the course of immobilization. Similar responses have been described in swine receiving ketamine alone.(2) Ganter and Ruppert reported that 10 mg/kg of Telazol given intramuscularly induced rapid immobilization with an average duration of 33.7 ± 15 minutes.(283) Although muscle relaxation was described as good, analgesia was poor. During recovery the pigs were excited and salivated excessively. It appears that zolazepam in pigs does not induce the same degree of muscle relaxation or suppress hyperresponsiveness as effectively as in other species.(231, 234, 257, 268) However, when xylazine (1.1 or 2.2 mg/kg IM) is combined with Telazol (6 mg/kg IM), this combination induces effective and safe anesthesia with good muscle relaxation.(284) Pigs become recumbent within 60 to 120 seconds following xylazine-Telazol injection. Heart rate increases initially and gradually decreases below baseline values at 45 minutes. Respiratory rate also increases initially but returns to baseline values in 15 minutes. Duration of analgesia is prolonged with the larger xylazine dose (68 minutes vs 47 minutes).(284) This combination can be used for induction (xylazine: 2.2 mg/kg IV; Telazol: 2.2 mg/kg IV), where anesthesia is to be maintained with an inhalant, or alone for short-elective surgical procedures.

Prolonged recoveries associated with Telazol anesthesia in swine seem to be related to the zolazepam fraction of Telazol. When using Telazol alone, it is impossible to increase the concentration of tiletamine without increasing the concentration of zolazepam. In a recent study, 2.5 mL of ketamine and 2.5 mL of 10% xylazine were used to reconstitute Telazol powder. The resulting solution contains 50 mg each of tiletamine, ketamine, zolazepam, and xylazine per mL, and the final dissociative concentration (i.e., ketamine and tiletamine) is 100 mg/mL, providing a 2:1 ratio of dissociative to either zolazepam or xylazine. The addition of ketamine and xylazine to this combination increases the anesthetic action and dissociative concentration relative to the concentration of zolazepam. The dose volume necessary to produce anesthesia is decreased, as is the dosage component of zolazepam. Consequently, the prolonged recovery observed with Telazol alone in swine, thought to be caused by zolazepam, is shortened.(187, 209, 285, 286) The response induced by this combination is dose dependent. In potbellied pigs, the intramuscular dose required to induce sedation and immobilization for a duration of 35 to 40 minutes is 0.007 to 0.013 mL/kg. Doses of 0.02 to 0.026 mL/kg induce adequate muscle relaxation for tracheal intubation and surgical anesthesia for 25 to 35 minutes.(187, 285) Anesthesia can be safely extended by supplemental intravenous dose of 0.006 mL/kg given slowly over 60 seconds.(187) When this combination is used to induce anesthesia, the maintenance requirement for inhalation anesthetic is decreased by approximately 40 to 50%.(285) The use of this combination in market swine to induce anesthesia revealed a 50 to 75% increase in dosage requirement. However, this increase in dosage requirement is associated with longer recoveries in older swine (breeding boars and sows). Table 10–12 summarizes the use of Telazol in swine.

Nondomestic Animals. Telazol (15 mg/kg IM)—xylazine (5 mg/kg IM) anesthesia has been compared to ketamine (35 mg/kg IM)—xylazine (5 mg/kg IM) in rabbits. The Telazol-xylazine combination produces effective surgical anesthesia for 72 ± 8 minutes, which was significantly longer than that of ketamine-xylazine mixture (35 ± 6 minutes). The Telazol-xylazine combination induces profound muscle relaxation and visceral analgesia. Decreased arterial pressure and PaO_2 with increased $PaCO_2$ are observed, but respiration rate and PaO_2 are higher with the ketamine-xylazine combination.(287)

In ferrets, Telazol (22 mg/kg IM) produces excellent immobilization, variable muscle relaxation, and smooth induction and recovery, and analgesia is sufficient for minor surgical procedures of short duration (Table 10–13).(288)

Telazol has been used extensively in a wide variety of exotic and wild animals species.(257, 289-291) The small volume required, ease of administration, wide safety margin, and dose-related effects (from immobilization to anesthetization) has made Telazol a popular immobilizing drug for use in many wild and exotic species.

A combination of detomidine (66 µg/kg IM) and Telazol (2.2 mg/kg IV) has been administered to anesthetize a tame ("home raised") zebra. Anesthesia was induced safely and rapidly within 60 to 90 seconds. The amount of halothane required to maintain anesthesia was decreased markedly.(292) In lesser pandas, the anesthetic effect of Telazol (1.8–6.3 mg/kg IM) has been compared to that of ketamine (12.6–15.3 mg/kg IM). Telazol, at a mean dose of 4.1 mg/kg, produced rapid induction, short-term immobilization (25–40 minutes), and smooth recovery. Muscle relaxation was sufficient for the procedures performed, whereas with ketamine muscle relaxation was poor and tremors and convulsions were observed in two pandas.(293) When used in Alaskan moose, Telazol (2.4–5.3 mg/kg IM) alone does not induce predictable immobilization and prolonged

Table 10–12. Use of Telazol or Telazol Combinations in Swine

Drug(s)	Dose and Route (mg/kg)	Duration (min)	Comment	Reference
Xylazine Telazol	1.1, IM 6, IM	47 ± 11	Satisfactory anesthesia Easy administration	284
Xylazine Telazol	2.2, IM 6, IM	67.5 ± 9	Longer duration of analgesia	
Telazol	10, IM	33.7 ± 15	Good muscle relaxation Poor analgesia Excited recovery	283
Telazol	2–4, IM 4–8.8, IM	—	Immobilization Anesthesia	289
Telazol* Ketamine Xylazine	0.007–0.013 mL/kg, IM 0.02–0.026 mL/kg, IM	35–40 25–35	Sedation and Immobilization Surgical anesthesia	188 209 285 286

*Reconstitute Telazol with 2.5 mL of ketamine and 2.5 mL of 10% xylazine.

Table 10–13. Use of Telazol or Telazol Combinations in Exotic and Wildlife Animals

Common Name (Genus and species)	Drug(s)	Dose and Route (mg/kg)	Duration (min)	Comment	Reference
Order Artiodactyla, Family Bovidae					
Aoudad (*Ammotagus lervia*)	Telazol	3.5–8.6, IM	—	Immobilization	257
Bison (*Bison bison*)	Telazol	2.2–4.4, IM	—	Good immobilization	289
White-tailed Gnu (*Connochaeters gnou*)	Telazol	37, IM	—	Immobilization	289
African Pygmy Goat (*Capra hircus*)	Telazol Telazol	2.2, IM 4.4–27.6, IM	— —	Immobilization —	289 257
Mexican Goat (*Capra species*)	Telazol	5.5–9.5, IM	—	Immobilization	289
Mouflon Sheep (*Ovis musimon*)	Telazol	5.5–7.5, IM	—	Immobilization	289
Rocky Mountain Bighorn Sheep (*Ovis canadensis*)	Telazol	4.4–5.5, IM	—	Immobilization	289
Tahr (*Hemitragus jemiahicus*)	Telazol	3.3–4.4, IM	—	Immobilization	289
Order Artiodactyla, Family Cervidae					
Pronghorn Antelope (*Antilocapra americana*)	Telazol	4.6, IM	—	Good chemical restraint	289
Sable Antelope (*Hippotragus niger*)	Telazol	22–23.8, IM	—	—	257
Sitatunga Antelope (*Tragelaphus spekii*)	Telazol Telazol	8.3–20.7, IM 1.7–4.25, IM	— —	— —	257 290
Suni Antelope (*Neotragus moschatus*)	Telazol	6.6–30, IM	—	—	257
Blesbuck (*Damaliscus dorcus*)	Telazol	3.09–11, IM	—	—	257
Bushbuck (*Tragelaphus scriptus*)	Telazol	8.5–12.7, IM	—	—	257
Black-tailed Deer	Telazol	2.5–20, IM	—	—	333
White-tailed Deer (*Odocoilleus virginianus*)	Telazol Telazol Telazol	4.4, IM (1.1–8.8) range 5, IM 8.9, IM	30–60 (3–186) range 21 —	— Good immobilization Immobilization	289 408 409
White-tailed Deer (*Odoceus virginianus*)	Telazol	1.5–10, IM	—	—	333
Fallow Deer (*Dama dama*)	Telazol	33, IM	—	Immobilization	289
Luzon Samber Deer (*Cervus meriannus meriannus*)	Telazol	6.6, IM	—	Immobilization	289
Mule Deer (*Odocoileus hemionus*)	Telazol	14.6–22, IM	—	Immobilization	289
Mule Deer (*Odocoileus hemionus*)	Telazol	14–20, IM	—	—	333

Table 10–13.   Use of Telazol or Telazol Combinations in Exotic and Wildlife Animals (continued)

Common Name (Genus and species)	Drug(s)	Dose and Route (mg/kg)	Duration (min)	Comment	Reference
Order Artiodactyla, Family Cervidae — cont'd					
Sika Deer (*Cervus nippon pseudaxis*)	Telazol	4.4, IM	—	Immobilization	289
Crowned Duiker (*Sylvicapra grimmia coronata*)	Telazol	4.4–11, IM	—	—	257
Maxwell Duiler (*Cephalophus maxwelli*)	Telazol	2.2–13.2	—	—	257
Common Eland Cape Eland (*Taurotragus oryx*)	Telazol	11.5, IM	—	—	257
Dorcas Gazelle (*Gazella dorcas*)	Telazol	2.6–16.5, IM	—	Supplemented with inhalation anesthesia	289
	Telazol	4.4–22, IM	—	Good restraint for minor surgery	
Grant's Gazelle (*Gazella granti*)	Telazol	4.8–13.2, IM	—	Immobilization	289
	Telazol	7.3–15.4, IM	—	—	257
Persian Gazelle (*Gazella subqutturosa*)	Telazol	6.6, IM	—	Immobilization	289
Slender-horned Gazelle (*Gazella leptoceros*)	Telazol	6.6–11.4, IM	—	Immobilization	289
	Telazol	4.8–15.4, IM	—	—	257
Soemmering's Gazelle (*Gazella soemmeringi*)	Telazol	11, IM	—	—	257
Thomson's Gazelle (*Gazella thomsoni*)	Telazol Acepromazine	8.8, IM 5 mg, IM	—	Immobilization	289
	Telazol	4.4–14.1, IM	—	—	257
Gemsbok (*Oryx gazella*)	Telazol	31, IM	—	Immobilization	289
	Telazol	5.5, IM	—	—	257
Blue-bearded Gnu (*Connochaetes taurinus taurinus*)	Telazol	6.6, IM	—	—	257
Brindled Gnu (*Connochaettes taurinus*)	Telazol	4.4, IM	—	—	257
Impala (*Aepyceros melampus*)	Telazol	4.85, IM	—	—	257
Greater Kudu (*Tragelaphus strepsiceros*)	Telazol	6.1, IM	—	—	257
Alaskan Moose (*Alces alces gigas*)	Telazol	4.4–7.9, IM	—	Chemical restraint Lower dose produces ataxia	289
	Telazol	2.4–5.3, IM	0–103	Unpredictable response Prolonged ataxia during recovery	215
Nyala (*Tragelaphus angasi*)	Telazol	6.6–11, IM	—	—	257
Siberia Reindeer (*Rangifer tarandus*)	Telazol	4.4–5.3, IM	—	Immobilization	289
Springbok (*Antidorcas marsupialis*)	Telazol	10.6, IM	—	—	257

Table 10–13. Use of Telazol or Telazol Combinations in Exotic and Wildlife Animals (continued)

Common Name (Genus and species)	Drug(s)	Dose and Route (mg/kg)	Duration (min)	Comment	Reference
Order Artiodactyla, Family Cervidae—cont'd					
Wapiti (*Cervus canadensis*)	Telazol	9.2, IM	—	Immobilization	289
Zebu (*Bos indicus*)	Telazol	3.6, IM	—	—	257
Order Carnivora, Family Canidae					
Cacomistle (*Bassariscus astutus*)	Telazol	3.3–16.5, IM	—	Desirable immobilization	289
Coyote (*Canis latrans*)	Telazol	11, IM	—	Desirable immobilization	289
Cape Hunting Dogs (*Lycaon pictus*)	Telazol	8.8–10, IM	—	Desirable immobilization	289
Racoon Dog (*Nyctereutes procyonoides*)	Telazol	6.6, IM	—	Desirable immobilization	289
Red Fox (*Vulpes vulpes*)	Telazol	10, IM	25.1 ± 2.5	Good cardiovascular and respiratory support	410
	Telazol	8.8, IM	—	Desirable immobilization	289
	Telazol	4, IM	34	Excellent immobilization	290
Fennec Fox (*Fennecus zerda*)	Telazol	13 (12–16) range	53 (32–65) range	Excellent immobilization	290
Gray Wolf (*Urocyon cinereoargenteus*)	Telazol	5.3 (2.6–14.1) range	63 (12–135) range	Surgical anesthesia	290
	Telazol	8.8, IM	—	Desirable immobilization	289
Iranian Wolf	Telazol	3.6 (2.1–5.5) range	34 (15–78) range	Excellent immobilization	290
Timber Wolf (*Canis lupis*)	Telazol	2.2–6.6, IM	—	Needed physical restraint	289
Order Carnivora, Family Felidae					
Carcal (*Felis caracal*)	Telazol	3.3–5.5, IM	—	Needed some restraint	289
	Telazol	6.6–7.3, IM	—	—	257
African Wild Cat (*Felis libyca*)	Telazol	4.4, IM	—	Desirable immobilization	289
Bobcat (*Lynx rufus*)	Telazol	13.3, IM	99	Additional dose for maintenance	290
Dusky Jungle Cat (*Felis chaus*)	Telazol	1.1–5.5, IM	—	Desirable immobilization	289
Geoffrey Cat (*Felis geoffreyi*)	Telazol	4, IM	—	Desirable immobilization	289
Golden Cat (*Felis temnincki*)	Telazol	4, IM (4–4.1) range	31 (26–37) range	Excellent immobilization	290
	Telazol	2–4.4, IM	—	Desirable immobilization	289
	Telazol	4–4.1, IM	—	—	290
Fishing Cat (*Felis viverrina*)	Telazol	2.2–4.4, IM	—	Desirable immobilization	289
Jungle Cat (*Felis chaus*)	Telazol	4.2, IM	58	Surgical anesthesia	290
	Telazol	1.1–5.5, IM	—	—	289
Leopard Cat (*Felis begalensis*)	Telazol	7, IM (5–10) range	61 (25–87) range	Excellent immobilization	290
	Telazol	2.2–6.6, IM	—	Desirable immobilization	289

Table 10–13. Use of Telazol or Telazol Combinations in Exotic and Wildlife Animals (continued)

Common Name (Genus and species)	Drug(s)	Dose and Route (mg/kg)	Duration (min)	Comment	Reference
		Order Carnivora, Family Felidae—cont'd			
Pampes Cat (*Felis manul*)	Telazol	2.2–5.5, IM	—	Desirable immobilization	289
Cheetah (*Acinonyx jubatus*)	Telazol	1.6–3.5, IM	60–90	Light anesthesia Moderate muscle relaxation Muscle rigidity and voluntary movement with low dose	411
	Telazol	4.6, IM (2.9–9.2) range	117 (39–395) range	Surgical anesthesia Salivation	290
	Telazol	2.2–2.75, IM	—	Desirable immobilization	289
	Telazol	2.2–8.8, IM	—	—	257
Jaguar (*Panthera onca*)	Telazol	4.2, IM (3.5–4.4) range	60 (40–115) range	Excellent immobilization	290
	Telazol	2–4, IM	—	Desirable immobilization	289
Jaguarondi (*Felis jaguarondi*)	Telazol	6.6, IM	—	Desirable immobilization	289
Black Leopard (African Spotted Leopard) (*Panthera pardus*)	Telazol	5–6.25, IM	<180	Desirable immobilization	412
	Telazol	6.6, IM (1.4–11.5) range	141 (23–228) range	Surgical anesthesia at higher dose Lowest dose did not produce immobilization	290
	Telazol	3.4–11, IM	—	—	257
	Telazol	3.6–6, IM	—	—	413
	Telazol	4–5, IM	—	—	289
Clouded Leopard (*Panthera nebulosa*)	Telazol	4.7, IM (1.5–8.3) range	121 (23–293) range	Excellent immobilization	290
Snow Leopard (*Panthera uncia*)	Telazol	4, IM (3.9–4) range	65 (56–75) range	Good immobilization	290
Lion (*Panthera leo*)	Telazol	3.76 ± 0.48, IM	—	Rapid induction time Good muscle relaxation Freedom from convulsion	295
	Telazol	1.6–2.9, IM	—	Sufficient muscle relaxation Licking movement	289
	Telazol	2.2–3, IM	—	Desirable immobilization	
	Telazol	2.2–8.4, IM	—	—	257
African Lion (*Panthera leo*)	Telazol	5, IM (3.2–8.9) range	69 (21–139) range	Good immobilization	290
	Telazol	<2.2, IM	—	Desirable immobilization	289
Mountain Lion, Puma (*Felis concolor*)	Telazol	8.2, IM (2.7–16) range	96 (20–280) range	Poor muscle relaxation at lower dose Repeated doses for root canal and tooth-capping	290
	Telazol	2.2–3.3, IM	—	Need a little restraint	289
Ocelot (*Felis pardalis*)	Telazol	8.3, IM (4.5–12.2) range	42 (30–55) range	Surgical anesthesia	290
	Telazol	4.4, IM	—	—	257
Serval (*Felis serval*)	Telazol	4.4–5.5, IM	—	Desirable immobilization	289
	Telazol	2.2–12.2, IM	—	—	257

Table 10–13.   Use of Telazol or Telazol Combinations in Exotic and Wildlife Animals (continued)

Common Name (Genus and species)	Drug(s)	Dose and Route (mg/kg)	Duration (min)	Comment	Reference
		Order Carnivora, Family Felidae—cont'd			
Tiger (Panthera tigris)	Telazol	2–2.8, IM	—	Slight physical restraint needed	289
	Telazol	4, IM	—	Anesthesia	
	Telazol	3.5–4, IM	180–300	Desirable immobilization	412
	Telazol	2.3–11.7, IM	—	Minimum dose of 4.6 mg/kg for female and 4 mg/kg for male	414
	Telazol	4.4–19.3, IM	—	—	257
		Order Carnivora, Family Ursidae			
American Black Bear (Ursus americana)	Telazol	4.7 ± 0.8, IM	—	—	294
	Telazol	0.6–0.73, IM	—	—	257
	Telazol	3.3–7, IM	—	—	
Asiatic Bear (Selenarctos thibetanus)	Telazol	2.8–4.4, IM	—	—	257
Brown Bear (Ursus arctos syriacus)	Telazol	3.5 ± 1.8, IM	—	—	294
Grizzly Bear (Ursus arctos horribilis)	Telazol	7–9, IM	45–75	Rapid induction Predictable recovery Wide safety margin Few adverse side effects	415
	Telazol	2.4–6.3, IM	—	—	257
Kamchacka Bear (Ursus arctos beringianus)	Telazol	4.3, IM (3.1–5.2) range	41 (26–75) range	Surgical anesthesia Additional dose can be given for prolonged procedures	290
Kodiak Bear (Ursus arctos middendorffi)	Telazol	5.5, IM	20	Good anesthesia	289
Polar Bear (Thalarctos maritimus)	Telazol	4.9, IM (3.5–7) range	83 (15–230) range	Surgical anesthesia Additional IM or IV dose may be necessary to maintain anesthesia Immobilization	290
	Telazol	5, IM	—	Inadequate analgesia	416
Polar Bear (Thalarctos maritimus)	Telazol	8–9, IM	—	Immobilization Satisfactory analgesia Fast recovery	417
	Telazol	3.5–7, IM	—	—	290
Sloth Bear (Melursus ursinus)	Telazol	5.5–6.6, IM	—	—	257
Spectacled Bear (Tremartos ornatus)	Telazol	5.7, IM (3.2–11.1) range	35 (23–45) range	Excellent immobilization	290
	Telazol	2.8 ± 0.5, IM	—	—	294
Sun Bear (Helarctos malaynus)	Telazol	4–5.5, IM	—	—	290
	Telazol	2.8–4.7, IM *Suppl. 29–75% of original dose	15–180	Adequate immobilization Rapid induction Smooth recovery Free of convulsion	294
	Telazol	4.8, IM (4–5.5) range	35 (30–45) range	Surgical anesthesia	290

*Suppl.: Supplemental dose.

Table 10–13. Use of Telazol or Telazol Combinations in Exotic and Wildlife Animals (continued)

Common Name (Genus and species)	Drug(s)	Dose and Route (mg/kg)	Duration (min)	Comment	Reference
Order Carnivora, Family Viverridae					
Binturong (*Arctictis binturong*)	Telazol	1.1, IM	—		289
African Palm Civet (*Nandinia binotata*)	Telazol	5.5–8.8, IM	—	Needed higher dose	289
Banded Palm Civet (*Hemigalus derbyanus*)	Telazol	6.6, IM	—	Desirable immobilization	289
Formosan Masked Civet (*Paguma larvata*)	Telazol	<2–4, IM	—	Manual restraint needed	289
Palm Civet (*Paradoxurus hermaphroditus*)	Telazol	2.2–4.9, IM	—	Needed some restraint	289
Lesser Oriental Civet (*Viverricula indica*)	Telazol	4.4, IM	—	Desirable immobilization	289
Fanaloka (*Cryptoprocta fosse*)	Telazol	2–8, IM	—	Needed some physical restraint	289
Genet (*Genetta tigrina*)	Telazol	2.2, IM	—	Desirable immobilization	289
Linsand (*Prionodon linsang*)	Telazol	4.4, IM	—	Desirable immobilization	289
African Water Mongoose (*Atilax paludinosus*)	Telazol	5.5, IM	—	Desirable immobilization	289
Ring Tail Mongoose (*Gallidia elegans*)	Telazol	4.4, IM	—	Desirable immobilization	289
Black-footed Mongoose (*Bdeogale species*)	Telazol	4.4, IM	—	Desirable immobilization	289
Ratel (*Mellivora capnsis*)	Telazol	2.2, IM	—	Woke up fast	289
Miscellaneous Species					
Acouchi (*Myoprocta pratti*)	Telazol	4.4–6.6, IM	—	—	289
Badger (*Taxidea taxus*)	Telazol	4.4, IM	—	Surgical anesthesia	290
Chimpanzee (*Pan troglodytes*)	Telazol	16, orally *Suppl. 2.5, IM	40 >40	Immobilization Analgesia	418
Chinchilla (*Chinchilla villidera laniger*)	Telazol Telazol Telazol	11–44, IM 4.4, IM 5.5–44, IM	115–431 — —	Surgical anesthesia — —	419 257 289
African Elephant (*Loxodonta africana*)	Telazol	3, IM	—	—	289
Ferrets (*Mustela putorius*)	Telazol Telazol Telazol Telazol	12, IM 22, IM 19.8, IM 5.8, IM (1.5–10) range	31 (15–51) range 73 (45–165) range — 32 (17–58) range	Poor analgesia Immobilization Immobilization Good muscle relaxation Adequate analgesia — Excellent immobilization Halothane can be used for prolonged anesthesia	288 257 290

*Suppl.: Supplemental dose.

Table 10–13. Use of Telazol or Telazol Combinations in Exotic and Wildlife Animals (continued)

Common Name (Genus and species)	Drug(s)	Dose and Route (mg/kg)	Duration (min)	Comment	Reference
		Miscellaneous species—cont'd			
Gerbils (*Meriones Unguiculatus*)	Telazol	60, IM	Male 5.7 ± 0.37 Female 4.3 ± 1.18	Surgical anesthesia	297
	Telazol	20–40, IM	1.58–4.03	Immobilization	
Guinea pig (*Cavia porcellus*)	Telazol	52, IM	122 (70–163) range	Unsatisfactory anesthesia Useful for procedures requiring prolonged recumbency without manipulation	268
Hamster (*Outbred syrian*)	Telazol	20–80, IP	7–27	Immobilization Inadequate analgesia	296
	Telazol	60–80, IM	19–32	Immobilization Inadequate analgesia	
European Hedgehog (*Erinaceus europaeus*)	Telazol	0.75–10, IM	—	—	257
Feral Horse (*Equus equus*)	Telazol Butorphanol Xylazine	3.5, IM 0.07, IM 3, IM	88 (16–210) range	Immobilization	420
Hutia (*Plagiodontia aedium*)	Telazol	6.6, IM	—	—	289
Spotted Hyena (*Croctuta crocuta*)	Telazol	1.8, IM	—	Desirable immobilization	289
Long-nose Rat Kangaroo (*Potorous tridactylus*)	Telazol	14.7, IM	—	—	421
Red Kangaroo (*Mactropus rufus*)	Telazol	4.1, IM (2.8–6.9) range	107 (30–217) range	Desirable anesthesia Salivation	422
	Telazol	<4, IM	—	Poor muscle relaxation	
	Telazol	>4, IM	—	Good muscle relaxation	
	Telazol	6–8, IM	20–30	Prolonged procedures	
	Telazol	1.8–6.2 *Suppl. 25–60% of original dose	60–120	Sufficient anesthesia	421
Tree Kangaroo (*Dendrolagus matschiei*)	Telazol	1.6–4.9, IM	20	Minor muscle rigidity Adequate immobilization	421
Kinkajou (*Potos flavus*)	Telazol	0.7–7.7, IM	—	Desirable immobilization Higher dose may be necessary for surgery	289
Koala (*Phascolarctos cinereus*)	Telazol	7, IM (5–7.7) range *Suppl. 2.5, IM	30–45 90	Anesthesia Mild salivation	423
Koala (*Phascolarctos cinereus*)	Telazol	6.9, IM	86.3 ± 1.1 (80–98) range	Surgical anesthesia	424
Mice (*Outbred or inbred*)	Telazol	100–160, IP or IM	4–119	Respiratory depression	296
Mink (*Mustela vison*)	Telazol	30, IM	27	Surgical anesthesia	290
	Telazol	1.2–2.6, IM	—	Good immobilization	289
	Telazol	3.6–7.5, IM	5–35	Surgical anesthesia	
	Telazol	12–16, IM	36–57	Surgical anesthesia	

*Suppl.: Supplemental dose.

Table 10–13.   Use of Telazol or Telazol Combinations in Exotic and Wildlife Animals (continued)

Common Name (Genus and species)	Drug(s)	Dose and Route (mg/kg)	Duration (min)	Comment	Reference
		Miscellaneous species—cont'd			
Monkeys	Telazol	5–10, IM	30–55	Excellent muscle relaxation Absence of ocular move- ment Gradual emergence	425
Red Howler Monkey (*Alouatta seniculus*)	Telazol	23.3, IM (13–37.5) range	45	Good muscle relaxation Immobilization	426
Otter (*Lutra cunadeasis*)	Telazol	5.4, IM (4.1–6.7) range	38 (20–57) range	Surgical anesthesia	290
River Otter (*Lutra canadensis*)	Telazol Telazol Telazol	2.2, IM 4.1–6.7, IM 0.66–11, IM	10 — —	Chemical restraint — —	289 290 257
Sea Otter (*Enhydra lutris*)	Telazol Telazol Telazol Telazol	1.2, IM 1.4–2.9, IM 9.3, IM 1–2, IM	40 25–45 360 —	Unable to resist handling Surgical anesthesia Surgical anesthesia Apnea Immobilization	427 339
Pacarana (*Dinomys branickii*)	Telazol	4.4, IM	—	—	289
Lesser Pandas (*Ailurus fulgens*)	Telazol	4.1, IM (1.8–6.3) range	25–40	Moderate muscle relaxation Mild salivation Increased salivation Muscle tremors	293
Collard Peccary (*Tayassu tajacu sonoriensis*)	Telazol Telazol	4.6–32.3, IM >19, IM	— —	Good immobilization Surgical anesthesia	289
Phalanger (*Trichosurus vulpecula*)	Telazol	7.7–11.5, IM	—	—	421
Nonhuman Primates	Telazol Telazol	0.6–10, IM 2–22, IM	— —	Chemical immobilization Surgical anesthesia	428
Rabbits (*Sylvilagus floridanus*)	Telazol Xylazine	15, IM 5, IM	72 ± 8	Surgical anesthesia Profound visceral analgesia	287
Rabbits (*Sylvilagus floridanus*)	Telazol	23.6, IM (13–40) range	68 (20–120) range	Unsatisfactory surgical anesthesia Immobilization	268
Rabbits (*Sylvilagus floridanus*)	Telazol	8.8–23.4, IM	—	—	257
Raccoon (*Procyon lotor*)	Telazol Telazol Telazol Telazol	11.8, IM (4.3–225) range 5.9–13.7, IM 0.8–7, IM 6.6–14.8, IM	45 (17–65) range — — —	Surgical anesthesia with higher dose Poor muscle relaxation with lower dose Desrable immobilization Lower dose given IV —	290 289 257
Rat (Sprague-Dawley)	Telazol	20–30, IP	68 (41–110) range	Satisfactory anesthesia Good muscle relaxation	268
Rat (Outbred or inbred)	Telazol	20–40, IP or IM	6–300+	Satisfactory anesthesia	296
Rhesus (*Macaca mulatta*)	Telazol	3–5, IM	—	—	231
Hoffman's Sloth (*Choloepus hoffmanni*)	Telazol	2.2–4.4, IM	—	—	289

Table 10–13.   Use of Telazol or Telazol Combinations in Exotic and Wildlife Animals (continued)

Common Name (Genus and species)	Drug(s)	Dose and Route (mg/kg)	Duration (min)	Comment	Reference
Miscellaneous species—cont'd					
Striped Skunk (*Mephitis mephitis*)	Telazol	9.3, IM (3–14) range	42 (10–102) range	Surgical anesthesia	290
	Telazol	5.5–11, IM	—	—	289
	Telazol	17.6–54.2, IM	—	—	257
Grey Squirrel (*Scirus carolinensis*)	Telazol	4.4–6.6, IM	—	—	257
Formosan Tree Squirrel (*Callosciurus erythraeus*)	Telazol	8.3–17, IM	—	—	289
Striped Skunk (*Mephitis mephitis*)	Telazol	5.5–11, IM	—	Desirable immobilization	289
Tayra (*Eira barbara*)	Telazol	3.3, IM	—	—	289
Mainland Wombat (*Phascolomis hirsutus*)	Telazol	2–2.2, IM	—	—	421
Grey Seal (*Halischoerus grypus*)	Telazol	1, IM	—	—	429
Elephant Seal (*Mirounga anqustirostris*)	Telazol	0.7–1.6, IM	—	Lower dose not sufficient for good restraint	289
	Telazol	1–2, IM	—	Satisfactory immobilization	
Southern Elephant Seal (*Miroubna leonina*)	Telazol	1, IM	—	—	429
Tasmanian Devil (*Sarcophilus harrisi*)	Telazol	2.8–5.5, IM	— —	Higher dose may be necessary	289
Northern Sea Lion (*Eumetopias jubatus*)	Telazol	1.8–2.5, IM	—	Smooth recovery	430
Tapir (*Tapirus terrestris*)	Telazol	2.8, IM	—	Immobilization	289

Table 10–14.   Use of Telazol or Telazol Combinations in Reptiles

Common Name (Genus & species)	Drug(s)	Dose and Route (mg/kg)	Duration (min)	Comment	Reference
Order Reptilia					
Alligator (*Alligator mississippiensis*)	Telazol	15, IM	183.8 ± 33.8	Long induction time Painful on injection Incomplete loss of response	431
Boa Constrictor (*Boa constrictor*)	Telazol	15–29, IM	—	Adequate for minor procedures	289
Crocodiles (*Crocodylus noloticus*)	Telazol Acepromazine	5–10, IM 1, IM	—	Sedation	432
Common Iguana (*Iguana iguana*)	Telazol Telazol	10, IM 26.5, IM	— —	Desirable immobilization —	289 257
Indian Python (*Python molurus*)	Telazol	15.4, IM	—	—	257
Rattlesnake (*Crotalus atrox*)	Telazol	35–210, IM	—	Long duration of sedation	289
Timer Rattlesnake (*Crotalus horridus*)	Telazol	75, IM	—	Prolonged recovery	289
Tortoise (*Testudo species*)	Telazol	1.1–22, IM	—	—	257

Table 10–15. Use of Telazol or Telazol Combinations in Birds

Common Name (Genus and species)	Drug(s)	Dose and Route (mg/kg)	Duration (min)	Comment	Reference
Mynah Bird (Acridotheres tristis)	Telazol	26.5, IM	—	—	257
Sulfur-crested Cockatoo (Cacatua galerita)	Telazol	2.64–25.2, IM	—	—	257
Ring-necked Dove (Streptopelia risoria)	Telazol	50–75, IM	—	—	289
Rock Dove (Columba livia)	Telazol	10–70, IM	—	—	268
Muscovy Duck (Cairina moschate)	Telazol	5.9–15.6, IM	—	5.9 and 8.4 mg/kg did not produce sufficient analgesia	289
	Telazol	13.2–22, IM	—	—	257
Bald Eagle (Haliaetus leucocephalus)	Telazol	13.2–22, IM	—	—	257
Emu (Dromaius novaehollandiae)	Telazol	15, IM	—	Needed some physical restraint	257
	Telazol	22, IM	—	—	
Flamingo (Phoenicopteri species)	Telazol	22, IM	—	—	257
Chilean Flamingo (Phoenicopterus ruber chilensis)	Telazol	6.6, IM	—	Desirable immobilization	289
Egyptian Goose (Alopochen aegyptiacus)	Telazol	22–24.5, IM	—	—	257
Lesser Magelian Goose (Choephaga picta)	Telazol	6.6–8.8, IM	—	Desirable immobilization	289
White Fronted Goose (Anser aibiforms frontalis)	Telazol	2.7, IM	—	Desirable immobilization	289
Roadside Hawk (Buteo magnirostris)	Telazol	16–33, IM	—	Desirable immobilization	289
Pea Hen (Pavo cristatus)	Telazol	11.3, IM	—	—	257
Green Heron (Butorides virescens)	Telazol	75, IM	—	Excellent anesthesia	289
Rhinoceros Hornbill (Buceros rhinoceros)	Telazol	28.7, IM	—	—	257
Blue Gold Macaw (Ara alarauna)	Telazol	12.1–22, IM	—	—	257
Scarlet Macaw (Ara macao)	Telazol	4.4–11, IM	—	—	289
	Telazol	5.5–19.8, IM	—	—	257
Mallard (Anas platyrhynchos)	Telazol	44.1–55.1, IM	—	—	257
Osprey (Pardion haliaetus)	Telazol	9.26–17.6, IM	—	—	257
Ostrich (Sruthio camelus)	Telazol	4–5, IM	—	Desirable immobilization	289
	Telazol	3.7, IV	—	Good induction Poor recovery	400
Barn Owl (Tyto alba)	Telazol	8.8–30.2, IM	—	—	257
African Ring-neck Parakeet (Psittacula krameri)	Telazol	26, IM	—	Desirable immobilization	289

Table 10–15.   Use of Telazol or Telazol Combinations in Birds (continued)

Common Name (Genus and species)	Drug(s)	Dose and Route (mg/kg)	Duration (min)	Comment	Reference
Parakeet (Melopsittacus undulatus)	Telazol	20–22, IM	—	—	257
Patagonian Parrot (Cyrsolophus patagonus)	Telazol	11, IM	—	Excellent immobilization	289
Crested Green Wood Partridge (Rollulus roulroul)	Telazol	10, IM	—	Good immobilization	289
Pigeon (Columbia livia)	Telazol	30.6, IM (20–48) range	41.4 (25–70) range	Immobilization Poor relaxation	268
Pigeon (Columbia livia)	Telazol	40–60, IM	—	Good anesthesia	289
Plover (Charadriidae species)	Telazol	17.6, IM	—	—	257
Rhea (Rhea americana)	Telazol	2–5, IM	—	Tranquilized, resisted handling	289
Greater Rhea (Rhea americana)	Telazol Telazol	2–22, IM 35.8	— —	— —	289 257
Yellow-bellied Sapsucker (Sphyrapicus varius)	Telazol	33–100, IM	—	Good immobilization	289
Black Swan (Cygnus atratus)	Telazol	6.6, IM	—	—	289
Black Neck Swan (Cygnus malanocoryphus)	Telazol	4.4–6.6, IM	—	Some physical restraint needed	289
Wood Stork (Mycteria americana)	Telazol	11, IM	—	—	257
Blue Wing Teal (Anas discors)	Telazol	22–35, IM	—	Prolonged recovery with higher dose	289
Green Wing Teal (Anas crecca carolinensis)	Telazol	35, IM	—	Prolonged recovery with higher dose	289
Woodcock (Philohela minor)	Telazol	44, IM	—	Desirable immobilization	289

ataxia occurs during recovery. The uncertainty associated with establishing optimum dosages for many wild species may be responsible for much of the variability in response.(215) Rough recoveries in many larger species may be caused by the muscle-relaxing effects of zolazepam, which seem to affect the rear quarters more profoundly.

When compared to a phencyclidine (1.4–1.8 mg/kg IM)-promazine (1.4–2.0 mg/kg IM) combination, Telazol (2.8–4.7 mg/kg IM) produces immobilization that is free of the convulsive activity usually observed in phencyclidine-promazine immobilized bears.(294) In lions immobilized with ketamine-phencyclidine-promazine, xylazine-phencyclidine-promazine, and xylazine-ketamine-phencyclidine-promazine, convulsive episodes often occur, whereas Telazol provides rapid induction, free of convulsions, and sufficient muscle relaxation for electroejaculation, blood collection, and electrocardiography.(295) Differences in con-

vulsive activity following phencyclidine and Telazol administration are likely caused by the CNS inhibition produced by zolazepam.

Size, age, temperament and condition of each animal should be considered before using Telazol. Males and females of some species apparently respond to Telazol differently.(291, 296, 297) The use of Telazol alone and in combination with other drugs in wild mammals, reptiles, and birds is summarized in Tables 10-13 through 10-15.

References

1. Corssen G, Miyasaka M, Domino EF. Changing concepts in pain control during surgery: Dissociative anesthesia with CI-581, a progress report. Anesth Analg 47:746, 1968.
2. Thurmon JC, Nelson DR, Christie GJ. Ketamine anesthesia in swine. J Am Vet Med Assoc 160:1325, 1972.
3. Chen G, Ensor C. 2–(Ethylamino)-2–(2–Thienyl) Cyclohexanone · HCl (CI-634): A taming, incapacitating, and anesthetic agent for the cat. Am J Vet Res 29:863, 1968.

4. Winters WD, Ferrer-Allado T, Guzman-Flores C. The cataleptic state induced by ketamine: A review of the neuropharmacology of anesthesia. Neuropharmacology 11:303, 1972.

5. White PF, Way WL, Trevor AJ. Ketamine — Its pharmacology and therapeutic uses. Anesthesiology 56:119, 1982.

6. Corssen G, Reves JG, Stanley TH. Dissociative anesthesia. In: Intravenous Anesthesia and Analgesia. Philadelphia: Lea & Febiger, 1988:99.

7. Cohen ML, Trevor AJ. On the cerebral accumulation of ketamine and the relationship between metabolism of the drug and its pharmacological effects. J Pharmacol Exp Ther 189:351, 1974.

8. Marietta MP, Way WL, Castognoli N Jr, Trevor AJ. On the pharmacology of the ketamine enantiomorphs in the rat. J Pharmacol Exp Ther 202:157, 1977.

9. Ryder S, Way WL, Trevor AJ. Comparative pharmacology of the optical isomers of ketamine in mice. Eur J Pharmacol 49:15, 1978.

10. White PF, Ham J, Way WL, Trevor AJ. Pharmacology of ketamine isomer in surgical patients. Anesthesiology 52:231, 1980.

11. Cohen ML, Chan SL, Way WL, Trevor AJ. Distribution in the brain and metabolism of ketamine in the rat after intravenous administration. Anesthesiology 39:370, 1973.

12. Booth NH. Intravenous and other parenteral anesthetics. In: Veterinary Pharmacology and Therapeutics, ed. by Booth, N.H., and McDonald, L.E. Ames, IA: Iowa State University Press, 1988:212.

13. Miyasaka M, Domino EF. Neuronal mechanisms of ketamine-induced anesthesia. Int J Neuropharmacol 7:557, 1968.

14. Massopust LC, Wolin LR, Albin MS. The effect of a new phencyclidine derivative on the electroencephalographic and behavioral responses in the cat. T.-I.-T. J Life Sci 3:1–10, 1973.

15. Ohtani M, Kikuchi H, Kitahata LM, Taub A, Toyooka H, Hannaoka K, Dohi S. Effects of ketamine on nociceptive cells in the medial medullary reticular formation of the cat. Anesthesiology 51:414, 1979.

16. Kitahata LM, Taub A, Kosaka Y. Lamina-specific suppression of dorsal-horn unit activity by ketamine hydrochloride. Anesthesiology 38:4, 1973.

17. Corssen G, Little SG, Tavakoli M. Ketamine and epilepsy. Anesth Analg 53:319, 1974.

18. Ferrer-Allado T, Brechner VL, Dymond A, Cozen H, Crandall P. Ketamine-induced electroconvulsive phenomena in the human limbic and thalamic regions. Anesthesiology 38:333, 1973.

19. Reder BS, Trapp LD, Troutman KG. Ketamine suppression of chemically induced convulsions in the two-day-old white leghorn cockerel. Anesth Analg 59:406, 1980.

20. Church J. The anticonvulsant activity of ketamine and other phencyclidine receptor ligands, with particular reference to N-methyl-D-aspartate receptor mediated events. In: Status of Ketamine in Anesthesiology, ed. by Domino, E.F. Ann Arbor, MI: NPP Books, 1990:521.

21. Anis NA, Bery SC, Burton NR, Lodge D. The dissociative anesthetics, ketamine and phencyclidine, selectively reduce excitation of central mammalian neurons by N-methyl-D-aspartate. Br J Pharmacol 79:565, 1983.

22. Velíšek L, Mareš P. Anticonvulsant action of ketamine in laboratory animals. In: Status of Ketamine in Anesthesiology, ed. by Domino, E.F. Ann Arbor, MI: NPP Books, 1990:541.

23. Kaplan B. Ketamine HCl anesthesia in dogs: Observation of 3 cases. Vet Med Small Anim Clin 67:631, 1972.

24. Humphrey WJ. Ketamine HCl as a general anesthetic in dogs. Mod. Vet Pract. 52:38, 1971.

25. Evans AT, Krahwinkel DJ, Sawyer DC. Dissociative anesthesia in the cat. J Am Vet Med Assoc 8:371, 1972.

26. Beck CC. Evaluation of Vetalar (ketamine HCl): A unique feline anesthetic. Vet Med Small Anim Clin 66:993, 1971.

27. Nimmo WS, Clements JA. Ketamine. In: Pharmacokinetics of Anesthesia, ed. by Prys-Roberts, C., and Hug, C.C. Boston: Blackwell Scientific Publications, 1984:235.

28. Haskins SC, Peiffer RL, Stowe CM. A clinical comparison of CT-1341, ketamine, and xylazine in cats. Am J Vet Res 36:1537, 1975.

29. Sparks DL, Corssen G, Sides J, Black J, Kholeif A. Ketamine-induced anesthesia: Neural mechanisms in the rhesus monkey. Anesth Analg 52:288, 1973.

30. Sparks DL, Corssen G, Aizenman B, Black J. Further studies of the neural mechanisms of ketamine-induced anesthesia in the rhesus monkey. Anesth Analg 54:189, 1975.

31. Conseiller C, Benoist JM, Hamann KF, Maillard MC, Besson JM. Effects of ketamine (CI 581) on cell responses to cutaneous stimulations in laminae IV and V in the cat's dorsal horn. Eur J Pharmacol 18:346, 1972.

32. Tang AH, Schroeder LA. Spinal cord depressant effects of ketamine and etoxadrol in the cat and the rat. Anesthesiology 39:37, 1973.

33. Vincent JP, Cavey D, Kamenka JM, Geneste P, Lazdunski M. Interaction of phencyclidines with the muscarinic and opiate receptors in the central nervous system. Brain Res 152:176, 1978.

34. Finck AD, Ngai SH. Opiate receptor mediation of ketamine analgesia. Anesthesiology 56:291, 1982.

35. Smith DJ, Pokoe GM, Monroe PJ, Martin LL, Cabral MEY, Crisp T. Ketamine analgesia in rats may be mediated by an interaction with opiate receptors. In: Status of Ketamine in Anesthesiology, ed. by Domino, E.F. Ann Arbor, MI: NPP Books, 1990:199.

36. Hanaoka K, Tagami M, Nagase M, Ide Y, Yamamura H. Spinal analgesia mechanisms of ketamine: Antagonism by naloxone. In: Status of Ketamine in Anesthesiology, ed. by Domino, E.F. Ann Arbor, MI: NPP Books, 1990:229.

37. Sawyer DC, Rech RH, Durham RA. Effects of ketamine and combination with acetylpromazine, diazepam, or butorphanol on visceral nociception in the cat. In: Status of Ketamine in Anesthesiology, ed. by Domino, E.F. Ann Arbor, MI: NPP Books, 1990:247.

38. Sawyer DC, Rech RH, Durham RA. Does ketamine provide adequate visceral analgesia when used alone or in combination with acepromazine, diazepam, or butorphanol in cats? J Am Anim Hosp Assoc 29:257, 1993.

39. El-Khateeb OE, Ragab A, Metwalli M, Hassan HA. Assessment of epidural ketamine for relief of pain following vaginal and lower abdominal surgery. In: Status of Ketamine in Anesthesiology, ed. by Domino, E.F. Ann Arbor, MI: NPP Books, 1990:403.

40. El-Khateeb OE. Caudal ketamine for relief of pain following anorectal surgery. In: Status of Ketamine in Anesthesiology, ed. by Domino, E.F. Ann Arbor, MI: NPP Books, 1990:411.

41. Guinto-Enriquez G, Enriquez RY, Reyes de Castro L. Epidural injection of ketamine hydrochloride: An experimental study in rats. In: Status of Ketamine in Anesthesiology, ed. by Domino, E.F. Ann Arbor, MI: NPP Books, 1990:381.

42. Shulman SM, Peng ATC, Blancato LS, Cutrone F, Nyunt K. Studies with epidural ketamine and local anesthetic combinations for obstetrical analgesia and anesthesia. In: Status of Ketamine in Anesthesiology, ed. by Domino, E.F. Ann Arbor, MI: NPP Books, 1990:395.

43. Baha F, Malbert CH. Effect of ketamine given by the intrathecal route in dogs. Rev Med Vet 142:283, 1991.

44. Bolte S, Igna C, Padurean D, Draghici H. Alternative anesthesia (segmental subarachnoid analgesia with ketamine) in abdominal surgery in horses in the standing position. Zooteh Med Vet 40:28, 1990.

45. Smith DJ, Pekoe GM, Martin LL, Colgate B. The interaction of ketamine with opiate receptor. Life Sci 26:789, 1980.

46. Kawana Y, Sato H, Shimade H, Fujita N, Ueda Y, Hayashi A, Araki Y. Epidural ketamine for postoperative pain relief after gynecological operations: A double-blind study and comparison with epidural morphine. Anesth Analg 66:735, 1987.

47. Gordh TJ. Alpha-adrenergic and cholinergic mechanisms of analgesia. Acta Anaesthesiol Scand 86:31, 1987.

48. Evans J, Rosen M, Weeks RD, Wise C. Ketamine in neurosurgical procedures. Lancet 1:40, 1971.

49. Gardner AE, Olson BE, Lichtiger M. Cerebrospinal fluid pressure during associative anesthesia with ketamine. Anesthesiology 35:226, 1971.

50. Shapiro HM, Wyte SR, Harris AB. Ketamine anesthesia in patients with intracranial pathology. Br J Anaesth 44:1200, 1972.

51. Takeshita H, Okuda Y, Sari A. The effects of ketamine on

cerebral circulation and metabolism in man. Anesthesiology 36:69, 1972.

52. List WF, Crumrine RS, Cascorbi HF, Weiss MH. Increased cerebrospinal fluid pressure after ketamine. Anesthesiology 36:98, 1972.

53. Wyte SR, Shapiro HM, Turner P, Harris AB. Ketamine-induced intracranial hypertension. Anesthesiology 36:174, 1972.

54. Schulte am Esch J, Pfeifer G, Thiemig I, Entzian W. The influence of intravenous anaesthetic agents on primarily increased intracranial pressure. Acta Neurochir (Wien) 51:560, 1979.

55. Schwedler M, Miletich DJ, Albrecht RF. Cerebral blood flow and metabolism following ketamine administration. Can Anaesth Soc J 29:222, 1982.

56. Pfenninger E, Reith A. Ketamine and intracranial pressure. In: Status of Ketamine in Anesthesiology, ed. by Domino, E.F. Ann Arbor, MI: NPP Books, 1990:109.

57. Lassen NA. Cerebral and spinal cord blood flow. In: Anesthesia and Neurosurgery, ed. by Cottrell, J.E., and Turndoff, H. St. Louis: CV Mosby, 1986:1.

58. Albin MS, Gonzalez-Abola E, Chang JL, Helsel P, Bunegin L. Attenuation of intracranial hypertension after ketamine by diazepam pretreatment. Fifth European Congress of Anesthesiology, Expcerpta Medica, Amsterdam, 1978:213.

59. Thorsen T, Gran L. Ketamine/diazepam infusion anaesthesia with special attention to the effect on the cerebrospinal fluid pressure and arterial blood pressure. Acta Anaesthesiol Scand 24:1, 1980.

60. Artru AA. Hypocapnia or diazepam reverse, and midazolam or fentanyl attenuates ketamine induced increase of cerebral blood volume and/or CSF pressure. In: Status of Ketamine in Anesthesiology, ed. by Domino, E.F. Ann Arbor, MI: NPP Books, 1990:119.

61. Beck CC. Vetalar (ketamine hydrochloride): A unique cataleptoid anesthetic agent for multispecies usage. J Zoo Anim Med 7:11, 1976.

62. Wright M. Pharmacologic effects of ketamine and its use in veterinary medicine. J Am Vet Med Assoc 180:1462, 1982.

63. Faulk RH. Xylazine and ketamine synergism for ultrashort anesthesia in cats. Feline Pract 8:15, 1978.

64. Amend JF, Klavano PA, Stone EC. Premedication with xylazine to eliminate muscular hypertonicity in cats during ketamine anesthesia. Vet Med Small Anim Clin 67:1305, 1972.

65. Manziano CF, Manziano JR. The combination of ketamine HCl and acepromazine maleate as a general anesthetic in dogs. Vet Med Small Anim Clin 73:727, 1978.

66. Kothary SP, Zsigmond EK. A double-blind study of the effective antihallucinatory doses of diazepam prior to ketamine anesthesia. Clin Pharmacol Ther 21:108, 1977.

67. Cartwright PD, Pingel SM. Midazolam and diazepam in ketamine anesthesia. Anaesthesia 59:439, 1984.

68. Toft P, Romer U. Comparison of midazolam and diazepam to supplement total intravenous anaesthesia with ketamine for endoscopy. Can J Anaesth 34:466, 1987.

69. Ivankovitch AD, Miletich DJ, Reinmann C, Albrecht RF, Zahed B. Cardiovascular effects of centrally administered ketamine in goats. Anesth Analg 53:924, 1974.

70. Salt PJ, Barnes PK, Beswick FJ. Inhibition of neuronal and extraneuronal uptake of noradrenaline by ketamine in the isolated perfused rat heart. Br J Anaesth. 51:835, 1979.

71. Altura BM, Altura BT, Carella A. Effects of ketamine on vascular smooth muscle function. Br J Pharmacol 70:257, 1980.

72. Tweed WA, Minuck M, Nymin D. Circulatory responses to ketamine anesthesia. Anesthesiology 37:613, 1972.

73. Wong DHW, Jenkins LC. An experimental study of the mechanism of action of ketamine on the central nervous system. Can Anaesth Soc J 21:57, 1974.

74. Baraka A, Harrison T, Kachachi T. Catecholamine levels after ketamine anesthesia in man. Anesth Analg 52:198, 1973.

75. Traber DL, Wilson RD, Priano LL. A detailed study of the cardiopulmonary response to ketamine and its blockade by atropine. South Med J 63:1077, 1970.

76. McCarthy DA, Chen G, Kaump DH, Ensor C. General anesthesia and other pharmacological properties of 2–(O-chlorophenyl)-2–

77. methylamino cyclohexanone HCl (CI-581). J New Drugs 5:21, 1965.

77. Traber DL, Wilson RD, Priano LL. Blockade of the hypertensive response to ketamine. Anesth Analg 49:420, 1970.

78. Traber DL, Wilson RD, Priano LL. The effect of alpha-adrenergic blockade on the cardiopulmonary response to ketamine. Anesth Analg 50:737, 1971.

79. Nakajima T, Azumi T, Yatabe Y. Mechanism of positive chronotropic response of the canine SA node to selective administration of ketamine. Arch Int Pharmacodyn Ther 234:247, 1978.

80. Child KJ, Davis B, Dodds MG, Twissell DJ. Anaesthetic, cardiovascular and respiratory effects of a new steroidal agent CT 1341: A comparison with other intravenous anaesthetic drugs in the unrestrained cat. Br J Pharmacol 46:189, 1972.

81. Sonntag H, Heiss HW, Knoll D, Regensburger D, Schenk HD, Bretschneider HJ. Myocardial perfusion and myocardial oxygen consumption in patients during induction of anesthesia with droperidol/fentanyl or ketamine. Z Kreislaufforsch 61:1092, 1972.

82. Smith G, Thorburn J, Vance JP, Brown DM. The effect of ketamine on the canine coronary circulation. Anaesthesia 34:555, 1979.

83. Folts JD, Afonso S, Rowe GG. Systemic and coronary hemodynamic effects of ketamine in intact anaesthetized and unanaesthetized dogs. Br J Anaesth 47:686, 1975.

84. Kaukinen S. The combined effects of antihypertensive drugs and anaesthetics (halothane and ketamine) on the isolated heart. Acta Anaesthesiol Scand 22:649, 1978.

85. Zsigmond EK, Kothary SP, Matsuki A, Kelsch RC, Martinez O. Diazepam for prevention of the rise in plasma catecholamines caused by ketamine. Clin Pharmacol Ther 15:223, 1974.

86. Jackson APF, Dhadphale PR, Callaghan ML. Haemodynamic studies during induction of anaesthesia for open-heart surgery using diazepam and ketamine. Br J Anaesth 50:375, 1978.

87. Båfors E, Häggmark S, Nyhman H, Rydvall A, Reiz S. Droperidol inhibits the effects intravenous ketamine on central hemodynamics and myocardial O_2 consumption in patients with generalized atherosclerotic disease. Anesth Analg 62:193, 1983.

88. Bidwai AV, Stanley TH, Graves CL, Sentker CR. The effects of ketamine on cardiovascular dynamics during halothane and enflurane anesthesia. Anesth Analg 54:588, 1975.

89. Reich DL, Silvay G. Ketamine: An update on the first twenty-five years of clinical experience. Can J Anaesth 36:186, 1989.

90. Barrigin S, De Miguel B, Tamargo J, Tejerina T. The mechanism of the positive inotropic effect of ketamine on isolated atria of the rat. Br J Pharmacol 76:85, 1982.

91. Riou B, Lecarpentier Y, Viars P. Inotropic effect of ketamine on rat cardiac papillary muscle. Anesthesiology 71:116, 1989.

92. Riou B, Viars P, Lecarpentier Y. Effects of ketamine on the cardiac papillary muscle of normal hamsters and those with cardiomyopathy. Anesthesiology 73:910, 1990.

93. Cook DJ, Carton EG, Housemans PR. Mechanism of the positive inotropic effect of ketamine in isolated ferret ventricular papillary muscle. Anesthesiology 74:880, 1991.

94. Schwartz DA, Horwitz LD. Effects of ketamine on left ventricular performance. J Pharmacol Exp Ther, 194:410, 1975.

95. Waxman K, Shoemaker WC, Lippmann M. Cardiovascular effects of anesthetic induction with ketamine. Anesth Analg 59:355, 1980.

96. Dowdy EG, Kaya K. Studies of the mechanism of cardiovascular responses to CI-581. Anesthesiology 29:931, 1968.

97. Urthaler F, Walker AA, James TN. Comparison of the inotropic action of morphine and ketamine studied in canine cardiac muscle. J Thorac Cardiovasc Surg 72:142, 1976.

98. Rusy BF, Amuzu JK, Bosscher HA, Redon D, Komai H. Negative inotropic effect of ketamine in rabbit ventricular muscle. Anesth Analg 71:275, 1990.

99. Chang P, Chan KE, Ganendran A. Cardiovascular effects of 2–(O-chlorophenyl)-2–methylamine cyclohexanone (CI-581) in rats. Br J Anaesth 41:391, 1969.

100. Goldberg AH, Keane PW, Phear WPC. Effects of ketamine on contractile performance and excitability of isolated heart muscle. J Pharmacol Exp Ther 175:388, 1970.

101. Diaz FA, Bianco JA, Bello A, Beer N, Velarde H, Izquierdo JP, Jaen R. Effects of ketamine on canine cardiovascular function. Br J Anaesth 48:941, 1976.

102. McGrath JC, Mackenzie JE, Miller RA. Effects of ketamine on central sympathetic discharge, circulation and baroreceptor responses. Br J Anaesth. 47:634, 1975.

103. Roberts JG. Intravenous anesthetic agents. In: Circulation in Anesthesia, ed. by Prys-Roberts, C. Oxford: Blackwell, 1980:459.

104. Koehntop DE, Liao J, Van Bergen FH. Effects of pharmacologic alterations of adrenergic mechanisms by cocaine, tropolone, aminophylline, and ketamine on epinephrine-induced arrhythmias during halothane-nitrous oxide anesthesia. Anesthesiology 46:89, 1977.

105. Hamilton JT, Bryson JS. The effect of ketamine on transmembrane potentials of Purkinje fibers of the pig heart. Br J Anaesth 46:636, 1974.

106. Bednarski RM, Sams RA, Majors LJ, Ashcraft S. Reduction of the ventricular arrhythmogenic dose of epinephrine by ketamine administration in halothane-anesthetized cats. Am J Vet Res 49:350, 1988.

107. Bednarski RM, Majors LJ. Ketamine and the arrhythmogenic dose of epinephrine in cats anesthetized with halothane and isoflurane. Am J Vet Res 47:2122, 1986.

108. Longnecker DE, Sturgill BC. Influence of anesthetic agents on survival following hemorrhage. Anesthesiology 45:516, 1976.

109. Spotoft H, Korshin JD, Sørensen MB, Skovsted P. The cardiovascular effects of ketamine used for induction of anesthesia in patients with valvular heart disease. Can Anaesth Soc J 26:463, 1979.

110. Weiskopf RB, Townley MI, Riordan KK, Baysinger M, Mahoney E. Comparison of cardiopulmonary responses to graded hemorrhage during enflurane, halothane, isoflurane, and ketamine anesthesia. Anesth Analg 60:481, 1981.

111. Stoelting RK. Nonbarbiturate induction drugs. In: Pharmacology and Physiology in Anesthetic Practice, Philadelphia: JB Lippincott, 1991:134.

112. Domino EF, Chodoff P, Corssen G. Pharmacologic effects of CI-581, a new dissociative anesthetic in man. Clin Pharmacol Ther 6:279, 1965.

113. Gooding JM, Dimick AR, Tavakoli M, Corssen G. A physiological analysis of cardiopulmonary responses to ketamine anesthesia in noncardiac patients. Anesth Analg 27:205, 1977.

114. Shulman D, Beardsmore CS, Aronson HB, Godfrey S. The effects of ketamine on the functional residual capacity in young children. Anesthesiology 62:551, 1985.

115. Mankikian B, Cantineau JP, Sartene R, Clergue F, Viars P. Ventilatory pattern and chest wall mechanics during ketamine anesthesia in humans. Anesthesiology 65:492, 1986.

116. Lumb PD, Silvay G, Weinreich AI, Shiang H. A comparison of the effects of continuous ketamine infusion and halothane on oxygenation during one-lung anesthesia in dogs. Can Anaesth Soc J 26:394, 1979.

117. Tokics L. Gas exchange and atelectasis during ketamine and halothane anesthesia. In: Status of Ketamine in Anesthesiology, ed. by Domino, E.F. Ann Arbor, MI: NPP Books, 1990:133.

118. Haskins SC, Farver TB, Patz JD. Ketamine in dogs. Am J Vet Res 46:1855, 1985.

119. Hatch RC. Prevention of ketamine catalepsy and enhancement of ketamine anesthesia in cats pretreated with methiothepin. Pharmacol Res Commun 5:311, 1973.

120. Hatch RC, Ruch T. Experiments on antagonism of ketamine anesthesia in cats given adrenergic, serotonergic, and cholinergic stimulants alone and in combination. Am J Vet Res 35:35, 1974.

121. Short CE. Dissociative anesthesia. In: Principles and Practice of Veterinary Anesthesia. Baltimore: Williams & Wilkins, 1987:158.

122. Waterman A, Livingston A. Some physiological effects of ketamine in sheep. Res Vet Sci 25:225, 1978.

123. Thurmon JC, Kumar A, Link RP. Evaluation of ketamine hydrochloride as an anesthetic in sheep. J Am Vet Med Assoc 162:293, 1973.

124. Sears BE. Complications of ketamine. Anesthesiology 35:231, 1971.

125. Lofty AO. Anesthesia with ketamine: Indications, advantages, and shortcomings. Anesth Analg 49:969, 1970.

126. Szappanyas G, Gemperle M, Isard A. Utilization of ketamine (Ketalar) as an anesthetic in veterinary surgery. Bull Soc Sci Vet Med Comp 72:149, 1970.

127. Dundee JW, Fee JPH, Moore J, McIlroy PD, Wilson DB. Liver function studies after ketamine infusions. Br J Clin Pharmacol 6:450, 1978.

128. Marietta MP, Vore ME, Way WL, Trevor AJ. Characterization of ketamine induction of hepatic microsomal drug metabolism. Biochem Pharmacol 26:2451, 1977.

129. Paddleford RR. General anesthesia. In: Manual of Small Animal Anesthesia. New York: Churchill Livingstone, 1988:31.

130. Lanning CF, Harmel MH. Ketamine anesthesia. Annu Rev Med 26:137, 1975.

131. Bree MM, Park JS, Short CE. Responses of cats to ketamine-antibiotic combinations. Vet Med Small Anim Clin 70:1309, 1975.

132. Taylor P, Hopkins L, Young M, McFadyen IR. Ketamine anesthesia in the pregnant sheep. Vet Rec 90:35, 1972.

133. Levinson G, Shnider SM, Gildea JE, DeLorimier AA. Maternal and foetal cardiovascular and acid-base changes during ketamine anesthesia in pregnant ewes. Br J Anaesth 45:1111, 1973.

134. Kumar A, Thurmon JC, Nelson DR, Link RD. Effects of ketamine hydrochloride on maternal and fetal arterial pressure and acid-base status in goats. Vet Anesthesiol 5:28, 1978.

135. White PF. Ketamine update: Its clinical uses in anesthesia. In: Status of Ketamine in Anesthesiology, ed. by Domino, E.F. Ann Arbor, MI: NPP Books, 1990:343.

136. Yoshikawa K, Murai Y. Effect of ketamine on intraocular pressure in children. Anesth Analg 50:199, 1971.

137. Corssen G, Hoy JE. A new parenteral anesthetic–CI 581: Its effect on intraocular pressure. J Pediatr Ophthalmol 4:20, 1967.

138. Peuler M, Glass DD, Arens JF. Ketamine and intraocular pressure. Anesthesiology 43:575, 1975.

139. Ausinsch B, Rayburn RL, Munson ES, Levy NS. Ketamine and intraocular pressure in children. Anesth Analg 55:773, 1976.

140. Gelatt KN, Peiffer RL, Gum GG, Gwin RM, Erickson JL. Evaluation of applanation tonometers for the dog eye. Invest Ophthalmol Vis Sci 16:963, 1977.

141. Trim CM, Colbern GT, Martin CL. Effect of xylazine and ketamine on intraocular pressure in horses. Vet Rec 117:442, 1985.

142. Wilson RP. Complications associated with local and general ophthalmic anesthesia. In: Complications of Ocular Surgery, ed. by Smolin, G., and Friedlaender, M.H. Int Ophthalmol Clin 32:1, 1992.

143. Rucker MC. Panel report: Combining anesthesia in dogs. Mod Vet Pract 57:320, 1976.

144. Jacobson JD, Hartsfield SM. Cardiorespiratory effects of intravenous administration and infusion of ketamine-midazolam in dogs. Am J Vet Res 54:1710, 1993.

145. Hellyer PW, Freeman L, Hubbell JAE. Induction of anesthesia with diazepam-ketamine and midazolam-ketamine in greyhounds. Vet Surg 20:143, 1991.

146. Werner RE. Panel report: Combining anesthesia in dogs. Mod Vet Pract 57:320, 1976.

147. Kirkpatrick RM. Use of xylazine and ketamine as a combination anesthetic. Canine Pract 5:53, 1978.

148. Navarro JA, Friedman JR. A clinical evaluation of xylazine and ketamine HCl for cesarean section in the dog. Vet Med Small Anim Clin 70:1075, 1975.

149. Hartsfield SM. Advantages and guidelines for using ketamine for induction of anesthesia. Vet Clin North Am Opin Small Anim Anesth 22(2):268, 1992.

150. Benson GJ, Thurmon JC, Tranquilli WJ, Smith CW. Cardiopulmonary effects of an intravenous infusion of guaifenesin, ketamine, and xylazine in dogs. Am J Vet Res 46:1896, 1985.

151. Virtanen R. Pharmacological profiles of medetomidine and its antagonist, atipamezole. Acta Vet Scand 85:29, 1989.

152. Räihä JE, Räihä MP, Short CE. Medetomidine as a preanesthetic prior to ketamine-HCL and halothane anesthesia in laboratory beagles. Acta Vet Scand 85:103, 1989.

153. Jalanka H, Skutnabb K, Damstén Y. Preliminary results on the use of medetomidine-ketamine combinations in the dogs. Acta Vet Scand 85:125, 1989.
154. Moens Y, Fargetton X. A comparative study of medetomidine/ketamine and xylazine/ketamine anaesthesia in dogs. Vet Rec 127:567, 1990.
155. Serteyn D, Coppens P, Jones R, Verstegen J, Philippart C, Lamy M. Circulatory and respiratory effects of the combination medetomidine-ketamine in beagles. J Vet Pharmacol Ther 16:199, 1993.
156. Lumb WV, Jones EW. Other methods for producing general anesthesia. In: Veterinary Anesthesia, 2nd ed. Philadelphia: Lea & Febiger, 1984:307.
157. Hartsfield SM. Injectable drugs and drug combinations for feline premedication, sedation, anesthesia and analgesia. Proc 54th Annu Mtg (Feline medicine), AAHA, Phoenix, Ariz. 1987:277.
158. Ilkiw JE, Suter C, McNeal D, Steffey EP. Effect of intravenous administration of variable-dose midazolam following fixed-dose ketamine in healthy awake cats. Proc Annu Mtg Am Coll Vet Anesthesiol, Las Vegas, Nevada, 1990:18.
159. Cullen LK, Jones RS. Clinical observations on xylazine/ketamine anesthesia in the cat. Vet Rec 101:115, 1977.
160. Colby ED, Sanford TD. Feline anesthesia with mixed solutions of ketamine/xylazine and ketamine/acepromazine. Feline Pract 12:14, 1982.
161. Verstegen J, Fargetton X, Ectors F. Medetomidine/ketamine anesthesia in cats. Acta Vet Scand 85:117, 1989.
162. Verstegen J, Fargetton X, Donnay I, Ectors F. An evaluation of medetomidine/ketamine and other drug combinations for anaesthesia in cats. Vet Rec 128:32, 1991.
163. Young LE, Jones RS. Clinical observations on medetomidine/ketamine anesthesia and its antagonism by atipamezole in the cat. J Small Anim Pract 31:221, 1990.
164. Verstegen J, Fargetton X, Zanker S, Donnay I, Ectors F. Antagonistic activities of atipamezole 4-aminopyridine and yohimbine against medetomidine/ketamine-induced anesthesia in cats. Vet Rec 128:57, 1991.
165. Brown MJ, McCarthy TJ, Bennett BT. Long term anesthesia using a continuous infusion of guaifenesin, ketamine, and xylazine in cats. Lab Anim Sci 41:46, 1991.
166. Reid JS, Frank RJ. Prevention of undesirable side reactions of ketamine anesthetic in cats. J Am Anim Hosp Assoc 8:115, 1972.
167. Hatch RC. Effects of ketamine when used in conjunction with peridine or morphine in cats. J Am Vet Med Assoc 162:964, 1973.
168. Benson GJ, Thurmon JC. Intravenous anesthesia. In: Principles and Techniques of Equine Anesthesia, ed. by Riebold, T.W., Philadelphia: W.B. Saunders, Vet Clin North Am 6(3):513, 1990.
169. Muir WW, Skarda RT, Milne DW. Evaluation of xylazine and ketamine hydrochloride for anesthesia in horses. Am J Vet Res 38:195, 1977.
170. Heath RB, Hubbell JAE, Muir WW. Intravenous anesthesia. In: Equine Medicine and Surgery, 3rd ed., ed. by Mansmann, R.A., McAllister, E.S., and Pratt, P.W. Santa Barbara, CA: American Veterinary Publications, 1982:257.
171. Matthews NS, Taylor T. Sedation and anesthesia of mules and donkeys. In: Current Therapy in Equine Medicine, vol. 3, ed. by Robinson, N.E. Philadelphia: WB Saunders, 1992:101.
172. Tranquilli WJ, Thurmon JC, Turner TA, Benson GJ, Lock TF. Butorphanol tartrate as an adjunct to xylazine-ketamine anesthesia in the horse. Equine Pract 5:26, 1983.
173. Fisher RJ. A field trial of ketamine anaesthesia in the horse. Equine Vet J 16:176, 1984.
174. Parsons LE, Walmsley JP. Field use of an acetylpromazine/methadone/ketamine combination for anaesthesia in the horse and donkey. Vet Rec 111:395, 1982.
175. Hikasa Y, Takase K, Kakuta T, Ogasawara S. Clinical application of 0.2% ketamine micro-drip infusion anesthesia in foals. Bull Equine Res Inst Jpn 26:31, 1989.
176. Greene SA, Thurmon JC, Tranquilli WJ, Benson GJ. Cardiopulmonary effects of continuous intravenous infusion of guaifenesin, ketamine, and xylazine in ponies. Am J Vet Res 47:2364, 1986.

177. Lin HC, Thurmon JC, Benson GJ, Tranquilli WJ, Olson WA. Guaifenesin-ketamine-xylazine anesthesia for castration in ponies: A comparative study with two different doses of ketamine. J Equine Vet Sci 13:29, 1993.
178. Young LE, Bartram DH, Diamond MJ, Gregg AS, Jones RS. Clinical evaluation of an infusion of xylazine, guaifenesin and ketamine for maintenance of anaesthesia in horses. Equine Vet J 25:115, 1993.
179. Kerr DD, Jones EW, Huggins K, Edwards WC. Sedative and other effects of xylazine given intravenously to horses. Am J Vet Res 33:525, 1972.
180. Clarke KW, Taylor PM, Watkins SB. Detomidine/ketamine anesthesia in the horse. Acta Vet Scand 82:167, 1986.
181. Matthews NS, Hartsfield SM, Cornick JL, Williams JD, Beasley A. A comparison of injectable anesthetic combinations in horses. Vet Surg 20:268, 1991.
182. Thurmon JC, Ko JCH, Benson GJ, Tranquilli WJ, Olson WA. Guaifenesin-ketamine-detomidine anesthesia for castration of ponies: A preliminary report. Fourth International Congress of Veterinary Anesthesia, Utrecht, The Netherlands. 48, 1991.
183. Brock N, Hildebrand SV. Xylazine-diazepam ketamine compared with xylazine-guaifenesin ketamine in equine anesthesia. Vet Surg 19:468, 1990.
184. Matthews NS, Dollars NS, Young DB, Shawley RV. Prolongation of xylazine/ketamine induced recumbency time with temazepam in horses. Equine Vet J 23:8, 1991.
185. Luna SPL, Massone F, Castro GB, Fantoni DT, Hussni CA, Aguiar AJA. A combination of methotrimeprazine, midazolam and guaiphenesin, with and without ketamine, in an anaesthetic procedure for horses. Vet Rec 131:33, 1992.
186. Fuentes VO, Tellez E. Ketamine dissociative analgesia in cattle. Vet Rec 94:482, 1974.
187. Thurmon JC, Benson GJ. Anesthesia in ruminants and swine. In: Current Veterinary Therapy, Food Animal Practice, ed. by Howard, J.L. Philadelphia: WB Saunders, 1993:58.
188. Thurmon JC. Injectable anesthetic agents and techniques in ruminants and swine. In: Anesthesia, ed. by Thurmon, J.C. Philadelphia: WB Saunders, Vet Clin North Am Food Anim Pract 2(3):567, 1986.
189. Waterman AE. Preliminary observations on the use of a combination of xylazine and ketamine hydrochloride in calves. Vet Rec 109:464, 1981.
190. Rings DM, Muir WW. Cardiopulmonary effects of intramuscular xylazine-ketamine in calves. Can J Comp Med 46:386, 1982.
191. Campbell KB, Klavano PA, Richardson P, Alexander JE. Hemodynamic effects of xylazine in the calf. Am J Vet Res 40:1777, 1979.
192. Waterman AE. Effects of a combination of ketamine and xylazine on respiratory gas tensions and acid-base status in calves. Vet Rec 113:517, 1983.
193. Blaze CA, Holland RE, Grant AL. Gas exchange during xylazine-ketamine anesthesia in neonatal calves. Vet Surg 17:155, 1988.
194. Nowrouzian I, Schels HF, Ghodsian I, Karimi H. Evaluation of the anaesthetic properties of ketamine and a ketamine/xylazine/atropine combination in sheep. Vet Rec 108:354, 1981.
195. Coulson NM, Januszkiewicz AJ, Dodd KT, Ripple GR. The cardiorespiratory effects of diazepam-ketamine and xylazine-ketamine anesthetic combinations in sheep. Lab Anim Sci 39:591, 1989.
196. Lin HC, Tyler JW, Welles EG, Spano JS, Thurmon JC, Wolfe DF. Effects of anesthesia induced and maintained by continuous intravenous administration of guaifenesin, ketamine, and xylazine in spontaneously breathing sheep. Am J Vet Res 54:1913, 1993.
197. Kumar A, Thurmon JC, Nelson DR, Benson GJ, Tranquilli WJ. Response of goats to ketamine hydrochloride with and without premedication of atropine, acetylpromazine, diazepam, or xylazine. Vet Med Small Anim Clin 78:955, 1983.
198. Kumar A, Thurmon JC, Hardenbrook HJ. Clinical studies of ketamine HCl and xylazine HCl in domestic goats. Vet Med Small Anim Clin 71:1707, 1976.
199. Koch MD. Canine tooth extraction and pulpotomy in the adult male llama. J Am Vet Med Assoc 185:1304, 1984.

200. Gavier D, Kittleson MA, Fowler ME, Johnson LE, Hall G, Nearenberg D. Evaluation of a combination of xylazine, ketamine, and halothane for anesthesia in llamas. Am J Vet Res 49:2047, 1988.

201. Riebold TW, Kaneps AJ, Schmotzer WB. Anesthesia in the llama. Vet Surg 18:400, 1989.

202. Green CJ, Knight J, Precious S, Simpkin S. Ketamine alone and combined with diazepam or xylazine in laboratory animals: A 10 years experience. Lab Anim 15:163, 1981.

203. Kyle OC, Novak S, Bolooki H. General anesthesia in pigs. Lab Anim Sci 29:123, 1979.

204. Breese CE, Dodman NH. Xylazine-ketamine-oxymorphone: An injectable anesthetic combination in swine. J Am Vet Med Assoc 184:182, 1984.

205. Thurmon JC, Tranquilli WJ, Benson GJ. Cardiopulmonary responses of swine to intravenous infusion of guaifenesin, ketamine, and xylazine. Am J Vet Res 47:2138, 1986.

206. Gray KN, Raulston GL, Flow BL, Jardine JH, Huchton JI. Repeated immobilization of miniature swine with an acepromazine-ketamine combination. Southwest Vet 31:27, 1978.

207. Benson GJ, Thurmon JC. Anesthesia of swine under field conditions. J Am Vet Med Assoc 174:594, 1979.

208. Evens LE, Ko JCH. Electroejaculation and artificial insemination in Vietnamese potbellied miniature pigs. J Am Vet Med Assoc 197:1366, 1990.

209. Braun W. Anesthetic and surgical techniques useful in the potbellied pig. Vet Med 88:441, 1993.

210. Matthews NS. Anesthesia of small ruminants, llamas, and miniature pigs in small animal practice. North American Veterinary Conference, Orlando, Fla. 17, 1992.

211. Williams LL. The Vietnamese pot-bellied pig: Anesthetic friend or foe? In: Symp Am Coll Vet Surg, ed. by Greene, S.A. 1992:222.

212. Addison EM, Kolensky GB. Use of ketamine hydrochloride, xylazine hydrochloride to immobilize black bears. J Wildl Dis 15:253, 1977.

213. Haigh JC. Freeze-dried ketamine and Rompun for use in exotic species. Proc Am Assoc Zoo Vet, 1978:21.

214. Lee J, Schweinsburg R, Kernan F, Haigh J. Immobilization of polar bears (Ursus maritimus, Phipps) with ketamine hydrochloride and xylazine hydrochloride. J Wildl Dis 17:331, 1981.

215. Franzmann AW, Arneson PD. Immobilization of Alaskan moose. J Zoo Anim Med 5:26, 1974.

216. Weisner H. Zur Neuroleptanalgesie bei Zootesen und Gatterwild unter Anwendung des Tele-inject systems. Kleintier Praxis 20:18, 1975.

217. Chen G, Ensor CR, Bohner B. The pharmacology of 2-(Ethylamino)-2-(2-Thienyl)-Cyclohexamine · HCl (CI-634). J Pharmacol Exp Ther 168:171, 1969.

218. Klockgether T, Lechoslaw T, Schwarz M, Sontag KH, Lehmann J. Paradoxical convulsant action of a novel non-competitive N-methyl-D-aspartate (NMDA) antagonist, tiletamine. Brain Res 461:343, 1988.

219. Hinko PJ, Wendt W, Wollin LR, Massopust LC. Neurophysiologic and behavioral effects of certain anesthetics administered intramuscularly in the rhesus monkey (Macaca mulatta). Am J Vet Res 31:1661, 1970.

220. Calderwood HW, Klide AM, Cohn BB, Soma LR. Cardiorespiratory effects of tiletamine in cats. Am J Vet Res 32:1511, 1971.

221. Chen G, Bohner B. Surgical anesthesia in the rabbit with 2-(Ethylamino)-2-(2-Thienyl)Cyclohexanone · HCl (CI-634) and chloral hydrate. Am J Vet Res 29:869, 1968.

222. Bennet RR. The clinical use of 2-(Ethylamino)-2-(2-Thienyl)-Cyclohexanone · HCl (CI-634) as an anesthetic for the cat. Am J Vet Res 30:1469, 1969.

223. Baukema J, Glazko AJ. Metabolic disposition of CI-744 in cats and dogs. Data on file. Ann Arbor, Michigan: Parke-Davis & Co., 1975.

224. Stoelting RK. Benzodiazepine. In: Pharmacology and Physiology in Anesthetic Practice, Philadelphia: JB Lippincott, 1987:117.

225. Parke-Davis & Co. Pharmacology of CI-716. Detroit, MI: December 1, 1974.

226. Randall LO, Heise GA, Schallek W, Bagdon RE, Ranziger R, Boris A, Moe RA, Abrams WB. Pharmacological and clinical studies on valium, a new psychotherapeutic agent of the benzodiazepine class. Current Ther Res Clin Exp 3:405, 1961.

227. Jones DJ, Stehling LC, Zauder HL. Cardiovascular responses to diazepam and midazolam maleate in the dog. Anesthesiology 51:430, 1979.

228. Forster A, Gardaz JP, Suter PM, Gemperle M. Respiratory depression by midazolam and diazepam. Anesthesiology 53:494, 1980.

229. Dalen JE, Evans GL, Banas JS, Brooks HL, Paraskos JA, Dexter L. The hemodynamic and respiratory effects of diazepam (Valium®). Anesthesiology 30:259, 1969.

230. Baukema J, Overholm RA, Glazko AT. Metabolism of Flupyrazopon (CI-716) in laboratory animals. Paper presented to American Society of Pharmacology and Experimental Therapeutics, August, 1973.

231. Bree MM. Dissociative anesthesia in Macaca mulatta: Clinical evaluation of CI 744. J Med Primatol 1:256, 1972.

232. Bree MM, Cohen BJ, Rowe SE. Dissociative anesthesia in dogs and primates: Clinical evaluation of CI-744. Lab Anim Sci 22:878, 1972.

233. Lin HC, Thurmon JC, Benson GJ, Tranquilli WJ, Olson WA. The hemodynamic responses of calves to tiletamine-zolazepam anesthesia. Vet Surg 18:328, 1989.

234. Hellyer P, Muir WW, Hubbell JAE, Sally J. Cardiorespiratory effects of the intravenous administration of tiletamine-zolazepam to cats. Vet Surg 18:105, 1988.

235. Klein L, Tomasic M, Olson K. Evaluation of Telazol in llamas. Proc Annu Mtg Am Coll Vet Anesthesiol, New Orleans, Louisiana, 1989:23.

236. Tracy CH, Short CE, Clark BC. Comparing the effects of intravenous and intramuscular administration of Telazol. Vet Med 83:104, 1988.

237. Hellyer P, Muir WW, Hubbell JAE, Sally J. Cardiorespiratory effects of the intravenous administration of tiletamine-zolazepam to dogs. Vet Surg 18:160, 1989.

238. Donaldson LL, McGrath CJ, Tracy CH. Testing low doses of intravenous Telazol in canine practice. Vet Med 84:1202, 1989.

239. McGrath JC, MacKenzie JE, Miller RA. Effects of ketamine on central sympathetic discharge and baroreceptor reflex during mechanical ventilation. Br J Anaesth 47:1141, 1975.

240. Booker JL, Erickson HH, Fitzpatrick EL. Cardiodynamics in the rhesus macaque during dissociative anesthesia. Am J Vet Res 43:671, 1982.

241. McGrath JC, MacKenzie JE, Miller RA. Effects of ketamine on central sympathetic discharge, circulatory and baroreceptor responses. Br J Anaesth 47:634, 1975.

242. Millar RA. On the mechanism and occurrence of cardiovascular stimulation by ketamine. Br J Anaesth 48:268, 1976.

243. Nedergaard OE. Cocaine-like effect of ketamine on vascular adrenergic neurons. Eur J Pharmacol 23:153, 1973.

244. Tanaka K, Pettinger WA. Renin release and ketamine-induced cardiovascular stimulation in the rat. J Pharmacol Exp Ther 188:229, 1974.

245. Lin HC, Thurmon JC, Benson GJ, Tranquilli WJ, Olson WA. Hemodynamic responses of calves to tiletamine-zolazepam-xylazine anesthesia. Am J Vet Res 52:1606, 1991.

246. Kerr DD, Jones EW, Holbert D, Huggins K. Comparison of the effects of xylazine and acetylpromazine maleate in the horse. Am J Vet Res 33:777, 1972.

247. Hubbell JAE, Bednarski RM, Muir WW. Xylazine and tiletamine-zolazepam anesthesia in horses. Am J Vet Res 50:737, 1989.

248. Howard BW, Lagutchik MS, Januszkiewicz AJ, Martin DG. The cardiovascular response of sheep to tiletamine-zolazepam and butorphanol tartrate anesthesia. Vet Surg 19:461, 1990.

249. Chen G. Sympathomimetic anesthetics. Can Anesth Soc J 20:180, 1973.

250. Chen G, Ensor CR, Russel D, Bohner B. The pharmacology of 1-(1-phenylcyclohexyl) piperidine HCl. J Pharmacol Exp Ther 127:241, 1959.

251. Popovic NA, Mullane JF, Vick JA, Kobrine A. Effects of phencyclidine hydrochloride on certain cardiorespiratory values of rhesus monkey (Macaca mulatta). Am J Vet Res 33:1649, 1972.

252. Traber DJ, Wilson RD, and Priano LL. Differentiation of the cardiovascular effects of CI-581. Anesth Analg 47:769, 1968.
253. Ochsner AJ. Cardiovascular and respiratory responses to ketamine hydrochloride in the rhesus monkey (*Macaca mulatta*). Lab Anim Sci 27:69, 1977.
254. Lagutchik MS, Januszkiewicz AJ, Dodd KT, Martin DG. Cardiopulmonary effects of tiletamine-zolazepam combination in sheep. Am J Vet Res 52:1441, 1991.
255. McNamara JA, Sly DL, Cohen BJ. Effect of CI 744 on skeletal muscle activity in monkeys (*Macaca mulatta*). Am J Vet Res 35:1089, 1974.
256. Short CE, Tracy CH. Technical discussion about Telazol. Vet Med 83:8, 1988.
257. Schobert E. Telazol use in wild and exotic animals. Vet Med 82:1080, 1987.
258. Potoczak R, Corey R. The effects of CI-744 upon cardiovascular function in the dog. Fed Proc 34:771, 1975.
259. Short CE. Talking about Telazol: Roundtable. Vet Med 84:1, 1989.
260. Benson GJ, Wheaton LG, Thurmon JC, Tranquilli WJ, Olson WA. Effects of Telazol-xylazine-butorphanol anesthesia for ovariohysterectomy of dogs. Proc Am Coll Vet Anesthesiol, New Orleans, Louisiana, 1989:12.
261. Dunbar RW, Knapp DE, Morrow DH. The effect of protein-synthesis inhibitors on anesthetic action. Anesth Analg 48:778, 1969.
262. Adams RH, Dixit BN. Prolongation of pentobarbital anesthesia by chloramphenicol in dogs and cats. J Am Vet Med Assoc 156:902, 1970.
263. Bree MM, Park JS, Beck CC, Moser JH. Effects of chloramphenicol on Telazol (CI-744) anesthesia in dogs. Vet Med Small Anim Clin 71:1243, 1976.
264. Smith RD, Pettway CE. Absence of sensitization to epinephrine-induced cardiac arrhythmia and fibrillation in dogs and cats anesthetized with CI-744. Am J Vet Res 36:695, 1975.
265. Bednarski RM, Muir WW. Ventricular arrhythmogenic dose of epinephrine in dogs and cats anesthetized with tiletamine/zolazepam and halothane. Am J Vet Res 51:1468, 1990.
266. Bednarski RM, Muir WW, Tracy CH. The effects of tolazoline, doxapram, and RO15-1788 on the depressant action of Telazol. Vet Med 84:1016, 1989.
267. Hatch RC, Clark JD, Jernigan AD, Tracy CH. Searching for a safe, effective antagonist to Telazol overdose. Vet Med 83:112, 1988.
268. Ward GS, Johnson DO, Roberts CR. The use of CI-744 as an anesthetic for laboratory animals. Lab Anim Sci 24:737, 1974.
269. Parke-Davis & Co. Effects of CI-744 on cardiovascular and respiratory function. Data on file. Ann Arbor, Michigan, 1976.
270. Bree MM, Park JS, Short CE, Beck CC, Moser JH. Effects of chloramphenicol on Telazol (CI-744) anesthesia in cats. Vet Med Small Anim Clin 71:764, 1976.
271. Lin HC, Benson GJ, Thurmon JC, Tranquilli WJ, Olson WA. Influence of anesthetic regimens on the perioperative catecholamine response associated with onychectomy in cats. Am J Vet Res 54:1721, 1993.
272. Ko JCH, Thurmon JC, Benson GJ, Tranquilli WJ. An alternative drug combination for use in declawing and castrating cats. Vet Med 88:1061, 1993.
273. Short CE, Tracy CH, Sanders E. Investigating xylazine's utility when used with Telazol in equine anesthesia. Vet Med 8:228, 1989.
274. Wan PY, Trim CM, Mueller POE. Xylazine-ketamine and detomidine-tiletamine-zolazepam anesthesia in horses. Vet Surg 21:312, 1992.
275. Marsico F, Tendillo FJ, Segura G, Criado A. The tiletamine-zolazepam-detomidine combination in horses: Preliminary results. J Vet Anaesth. 20:33, 1993.
276. Lin HC, Branson KR, Thurmon JC, Benson GJ, Tranquilli WJ, Olson WA. Ketamine, Telazol, xylazine and detomidine: A comparative study of anesthetic drug combinations in ponies. Acta Vet Scand 33:109, 1992.
277. Matthews NS, Taylor TS, Hartsfield SM. A comparison of injectable anesthetic regimens in mules. Proc Am Coll Vet Anesthesiol, New Orleans, Louisiana, 1989:15.
278. Matthews NS, Taylor TS, Hartsfield SM. A comparison of injectable anesthetic combinations in donkeys. Proc Am Coll Vet Anesthesiol, Las Vegas, Nevada, 1990:13.
279. Abrahamsen EJ, Hubbell JAE, Bednarski RM, Muir WW, Macioce BA. Xylazine and tiletamine-zolazepam for induction of anesthesia maintained with halothane in 19 horses. Equine Vet J 23:224, 1991.
280. Thurmon JC, Lin HC, Benson GJ, Tranquilli WJ, Olson WA. Telazol-xylazine: An anesthetic drug combination for calves. Vet Med 84:824, 1989.
281. Taylor JH, Botha CJ, Swan GE, Mülders MSG, Grobler MJ. Tiletamine hydrochloride in combination with zolazepam hydrochloride as an anesthetic agent in sheep. J S Afr Vet Assoc. 63:63, 1992.
282. Lin HC, Tyler JW, Wallace SS, Thurmon JC, Wolfe DF. Telazol and xylazine anesthesia in sheep. Cornell Vet 83:117, 1993.
283. Ganter M, Ruppert K. The effect of the anesthetic Tilest in swine. Dtsch Tierarztl Wochensch 97:360, 1990.
284. Thurmon JC, Benson GJ, Tranquilli WJ, Olson WA, Tracy CH. The anesthetic and analgesic effects of Telazol and xylazine in pigs: Evaluating clinical trials. Vet Med 83:841, 1988.
285. Ko JCH, Thurmon JC, Tranquilli WJ, Benson GJ, Olson WA. Problems encountered when anesthetizing potbellied pigs. Vet Med 88:435, 1993.
286. Ko JCH, Thurmon JC, Benson GJ, Tranquilli WJ, Olson WA. A new drug combination for use in porcine cesarean sections. Vet Med 88:466, 1993.
287. Popilskis SJ, Oz MC, Gorman P, Florestal A, Kohn DF. Comparison of xylazine with tiletamine-zolazepam (Telazol) and xylazine-ketamine anesthesia in rabbits. Lab Anim Sci 41:51, 1991.
288. Payton AJ, Pick JR. Evaluation of a combination of tiletamine and zolazepam as an anesthetic for ferrets. Lab Anim Sci 39:243, 1989.
289. Gray CW, Bush M, Beck CC. Clinical experience using CI-744 in chemical restraint and anesthesia of exotic specimens. J Zoo Anim Med 5:12, 1974.
290. Boever WJ, Holden J, Kane KK. Use of Telazol (CI-744) for chemical restraint and anesthesia in wild and exotic carnivores. Vet Med Small Anim Clin 72:1722, 1977.
291. King JM, Bertram BCR, Hamilton PH. Tiletamine and zolazepam for immobilization of wild lions and leopards. J Am Vet Med Assoc 171:894, 1977.
292. Lin HC, Thurmon JC, Benson GJ, Tranquilli WJ. Immobilization and anesthesia of hand-reared zebras. J Am Vet Med Assoc 202:988, 1993.
293. Custer RW, Bush M, Smeller JM, Smith EE. Clinical experience with dissociative anesthetics in lesser pandas (*Ailurus fulgens*): Hematology and blood chemistry values. J Zoo Anim Med 9:22, 1978.
294. Bush M, Custer RS, Smith EE. Use of dissociative anesthetics for the immobilization of captive bears: Blood gas, hematology and biochemistry values. J Wildl Dis 16:481, 1980.
295. Bush M, Custer R, Smeller J, Bush LM, Seal US, Barton R. The acid-base status of lions, *Panthera leo*, immobilized with four drug combinations. J Wildl Dis 14:102, 1978.
296. Silverman J, Huhndorf M, Balk M, Slater G. Evaluation of a combination of tiletamine and zolazepam as an anesthetic for laboratory rodents. Lab Anim Sci 33:457, 1983.
297. Hrapkiewicz KL, Stein S, Smiler KL. A new anesthetic agent for use in the gerbil. Lab Anim Sci 39:338, 1989.
298. Gelatt KN, Henderson JD, Steffen GR. Fluorescein angiography of the normal and diseased ocular fundi of the laboratory dogs. J Am Vet Med Assoc 169:980, 1976.
299. Farver TB, Haskins SC, Patz JD. Cardiopulmonary effects of acepromazine and of the subsequent administration of ketamine in the dog. Am J Vet Res 47:631, 1986.
300. Billar RR. Panel report: Combining anesthesia in dogs. Mod Vet Pract 57:319, 1976.
301. Stephenson JC, Blevins I, Christie GJ. Safety of rompun/ketaset combination in dogs: A two-year study. Vet Med Small Anim Clin 73:303, 1978.

302. Kaplan B. A practitioner's report on the use of ketamine and xylazine with or without thiamylal for general anesthesia in dogs. Vet Med Small Anim Clin 74:1267, 1979.
303. Kumar A, Pandiya SC, Singh H. Canine anesthesia with a combination of ketamine and xylazine in experimental and clinical cases. Indian J Anim Health 18:39, 1979.
304. Kolata RJ, Rawlings CA. Cardiopulmonary effects of xylazine, ketamine, and atropine in the dog. Am J Vet Res 43:2196, 1982.
305. Clark DM, Martin RA, Short CE. Cardiopulmonary responses to xylazine/ketamine anesthesia in the dog. J Am Anim Hosp Assoc 18:815, 1982.
306. Haskins SC, Patz JD, Farver TB. Xylazine and xylazine-ketamine in dogs. Am J Vet Res 47:636, 1986.
307. DeYoung DW, Paddleford RR, Short CE. Dissociative anesthetics in the cat and dog. J Am Vet Med Assoc 161:1442, 1972.
308. Glen JB. The use of ketamine (CI-581) in feline anesthetic practice. Vet Rec 92:65, 1973.
309. Amend JF. Rompun (Bay Va 1470), an effective premedication for ketamine anesthesia in the cat. Vet Med Rev 2:142, 1973.
310. Colby ED, Sanford TD. Blood pressure and heart and respiratory rates of cats under ketamine/xylazine, ketamine/acepromazine anesthesia. Feline Pract 11:19, 1981.
311. Hsu WH, Lu ZX. Effect of yohimbine on xylazine-ketamine anesthesia in cats. J Am Vet Med Assoc 185:886, 1984.
312. Duke T, Hale GJ, Jones RS. Clinical observations on the simultaneous administration of xylazine and ketamine for anesthesia in the cat. Companion Anim Pract 2:3, 1988.
313. Fuentes VO, Tellez E. Midline caesarian section in a cow using ketamine anesthesia. Vet Rec 99:338, 1976.
314. Tadmor A, Narcus S, Eting E. The use of ketamine hydrochloride for endotracheal intubation in cattle. Aust Vet J 55:537, 1979.
315. Kumar A, Singh H. Ketamine and xylazine anesthesia in bovine paediatric surgery. Indian Vet J 56:219, 1979.
316. Aouad JI, Wright EM, Shaner TW. Anesthesia evaluation of ketamine and xylazine in calves. Bovine Pract 2:22, 1981.
317. Khushpalinder S, Sharma SN, Sobti VK. Clinical evaluation of diazepam-glycerylguaiacolate-ketamine anesthesia for bone surgery in calves. Indian J Vet Surg 11:1, 1990.
318. Singh KI, Sharma SN, Mirakhur KK, Singh S. Clinical and biochemical effects of diazepam-ketamine combination anaesthesia in calves. Indian Vet J 68:253, 1991.
319. Laitinen DM. Clinical observations on medetomidine/ketamine anaesthesia in sheep and its reversal by atipamezole. J Assoc Vet Anesth Gr Br Ir 17:17, 1990.
320. Coulson NM, Januszkiewicz AJ, Ripple GR. Physiological responses of sheep to two hours anesthesia with diazepam-ketamine. Vet Rec 129:329., 1991.
321. Tadmor A, Zukerman I. The use of ketamine hydrochloride for endotracheal intubation in goats. Aust Vet J 57:303, 1981.
322. Fowler ME. Anesthesia. In: Medicine and Surgery of South American Camelids. Ames, IA: Iowa State University Press, 1989:51
323. Cantor GH, Brunson DB, Riebold TW. A comparison of four short-acting anesthetic combinations for swine. Vet Med Small Anim Clin 76:715, 1981.
324. Trim CM, Gilroy BA. Cardiopulmonary effects of a xylazine and ketamine combination in pigs. Res Vet Sci 38:30, 1985.
325. Hoyt RF, Hayre MD, Dodd KT, Phillips YY. Long-acting intramuscular anesthetic regimen for swine. Lab Anim Sci 36:413, 1986.
326. Pathak SC, Nigam JM, Peshin PK, Singh AP. Anesthetic and hemodynamic effects of ketamine hydrochloride in buffalo calves (Bubalus bubalis). Am J Vet Res 43:875, 1982.
327. Ramakrishna O, Murphy DK, Nigam JM. Ketamine anesthesia in buffalo calves. Indian Vet J 58:503, 1981.
328. Dew TL. Use of tolazoline hydrochloride to reverse multiple anesthetic episodes induced with xylazine hydrochloride and ketamine hydrochloride in white-tailed deer and goats. J Zoo Anim Med 19:8, 1988.
329. Langrehr D, Muller R. Significance of CI-581 for anesthesiology in veterinary medicine with special attention to zoo animals. Proc 9th Int Symp Dis Zoo Anim, Prague, Akademie. Verlag, Berlin, 1967.
330. Festa-Bianchet M, Jorgenson JT. Use of xylazine-ketamine to immobilize bighorn sheep in Alberta. J Wildl Dis 49:162, 1985.
331. Barnett JEF, Lewis JCM. Medetomidine and ketamine anesthesia in zoo animals and its reversal with atipamezole: A review and update with specific reference to work in British zoos. Proc Am Zoo Vet, South Padre Island, Tex. 1990:207.
332. Jalanka H. The use of medetomidine, medetomidine-ketamine combinations and atipamezole at Helsinki Zoo: A review of 240 cases. Acta Vet Scand 85:193, 1989
333. English AW. Chemical restraint of deer. Deer Refresher Course: Proc Refresher Course for Veterinarians. Sydney, Australia: The University of Sydney. 72:325–72:350, 1984.
334. Keep JM. The sedation and immobilization of deer. Deer Refresher Course: Proc Refresher Course for Veterinarians, Sydney, Australia: The University of Sydney. 49:21–49:28, 1984.
335. Jalanka HH. Medetomidine- and ketamine-induced immobilization in Forest Reindeer (Rangifer tarandus fennicus) and its reversal by atipamezole. Proc Am Zoo Vet, Greensboro, NC. 1989:1.
336. Mech LD, Giudice GDD, Karns PD, Seal US. Yohimbine hydrochloride as an antagonist to xylazine hydrochloride immobilization of white-tailed deer. J Wildl Dis 21:405, 1985.
337. Kreeger TJ, Giudice GDD, Seal US, Karns PD. Immobilization of white-tailed deer with xylazine hydrochloride and ketamine hydrochloride and antagonism by tolazoline hydrochloride. J Wildl Dis 22:407, 1986.
338. Golightly RT, Hofstra TD. Immobilization of elk with a ketamine-xylazine mix and rapid reversal with yohimbine hydrochloride. Wildl Soc Bull 17:53, 1989.
339. Jessup DA. Restraint and chemical immobilization of carnivores and furbearers. In: Chemical Immobilization of North American Wildlife, ed. by Nielsen, L., Haigh, J.C., and Fowler, M.E. Milwaukee, WI: Wisconsin Humane Society, 1982:227.
340. Kreeger TJ, Seal US. Immobilization of Coyotes with xylazine hydrochloride-ketamine hydrochloride and antagonism by yohimbine hydrochloride. J Wildl Dis 22:604, 1986.
341. Heerden JV, Swan GE, Dauth J, Burroughs REJ, Dreyer MJ. Sedation and immobilization of wild dogs (Lycaon pictus) using medetomidine or a medetomidine-ketamine combination. S Afr J Wildl Res 21:88, 1991.
342. Jalanka HH. Medetomidine- and medetomidine-ketamine-induced immobilization in blue foxes (Alopex lagopus) and its reversal by atipamezole. Acta Vet Scand 31:63, 1990.
343. Kreeger TJ, Faggella AM, Seal US, Mech LD, Callahan M, Hall B. Cardiovascular and behavioral responses of gray wolves to ketamine-xylazine immobilization and antagonism by yohimbine. J Wildl Dis 23:463, 1987.
344. Kreeger TJ, Seal US, Faggella AM. Xylazine hydrochloride-ketamine hydrochloride immobilization of wolves and its antagonism by tolazoline hydrochloride. J Wildl Dis 22:397, 1986.
345. Fuller TK, Kuehn DW. Immobilization of wolves using ketamine in combination with xylazine or promazine. J Wildl Dis, 19:69, 1983.
346. Mathews M. The use of ketamine to immobilize a black leopard. J Zoo Anim Med 2:25, 1971.
347. Dolensek EP. Reports to Parke-Davis, 1971.
348. Hime JM. Use of ketamine hydrochloride in non-domesticated cats. Vet Rec 95:193, 1974.
349. Parke-Davis. Reports on file, 1965–1971.
350. Jalanka HH. Evaluation and comparison of two ketamine-based immobilization techniques in snow leopards (Panthera uncia). J Zoo Wildl Med 20:163, 1989.
351. Herbst LH, Packer C, Seal US. Immobilization of free-ranging African lions (Panthera leo) with a combination of xylazine hydrochloride and ketamine hydrochloride. J Wildl Dis 21:401, 1985.
352. Wyk TCV, Berry HH. Tolazoline as an antagonist in free-ranging lions immobilized with a ketamine-xylazine combination. J S Afr Vet Assoc 57:221, 1986.
353. Logan KA, Thorne ET, Irwin LL, Skinner R. Immobilizing wild mountain lions (Felis concolor) with ketamine hydrochloride and xylazine hydrochloride. J Wildl Dis 22:97, 1986.

354. Melquist WE, Hornocker MG. Methods and techniques for studying and censusing river otter populations. University of Idaho Technical Report B, Moscow, Idaho. 1979:17.

355. Greene SA, Keegan RD, Gallagher LV, Alexander JE, Harari J. Cardiovascular effects of halothane anesthesia after diazepam and ketamine administration in beavers (Castor canadensis) during spontaneous or controlled ventilation. Am J Vet Res 52:665, 1991.

356. Aulerich RJ. Reports to Parke-Davis, 1971.

357. Sylvina TJ, Berman NG, Fox JG. Effects of yohimbine on bradycardia and duration of recumbency in ketamine/xylazine anesthetized ferrets. Lab Anim Sci 40:178, 1990.

358. Moreland AF, Glaser C. Evaluation of ketamine, ketamine-xylazine and ketamine-diazepam anesthesia in the ferret. Lab Anim Sci 35:287, 1985.

359. Bone L, Battles AH, Goldfarb RD, Lombard CW, Moreland AF. Electrocardiographic values from clinically normal, anesthetized ferrets (Mustela putorius furo). Am J Vet Res 49:1884, 1988.

360. Kuiken T. Anesthesia in the European otter (Lutra lutra). Vet Rec 123:59, 1988.

361. Lewis JCM. Reversible immobilization of Asian small-clawed otters with medetomidine and ketamine. Vet Rec 128:86, 1991.

362. Arena PC, Richardson KC, Cullen LK. Anaesthesia in two species of large Australian skunk. Vet Rec 123:155, 1988.

363. Beck CC. Chemical restraint of exotic species. J Zoo Anim Med 3:3, 1972.

364. Rosatte RC, Hobson DP. Ketamine hydrochloride as an immobilizing agent for striped skunk. Can Vet J 24:134, 1983.

365. Lynch GM, Hall W, Pelchat B, Hanson JA. Chemical immobilization of black bear with special reference to the use of ketamine-xylazine. In: Chemical Immobilization of North American Wildlife, ed. by Nielsen, L., Haigh, J.C., and Fowler, M.E. Milwaukee, WI: Wisconsin Humane Society, 245, 1982.

366. Page CD. Sloth bear immobilization with a ketamine-xylazine combination: Reversal with yohimbine. J Am Vet Med Assoc 189:1050, 1986.

367. White RJ, Bali S, Bark H. Xylazine and ketamine anaesthesia in the dromedary camel under field condition. Vet Rec 120:110, 1987.

368. Jacobson ER, Allen J, Martin H, Kollins GV. Effects of yohimbine on combined xylazine-ketamine-induced sedation and immobilization in juvenile african elephants. J Am Vet Med Assoc 187:1195, 1985.

369. Allen JL. Use of tolazoline as an antagonist to xylazine-ketamine-induced immobilization in African elephants. Am J Vet Res 47:781, 1986.

370. Heard DJ, Kollias GV, Webb AI, Jacobson ER, Brock KA. Use of halothane to maintain anesthesia induced with etorphine in juvenile African elephants. J Am Vet Med Assoc 193:254, 1988.

371. Stander PE, Gasaway WC. Spotted hyenas immobilized with ketamine/xylazine and antagonized with tolazoline. Afr J Ecology 29:168, 1991.

372. Gallagher JF, Lochmiller RL, Grant WE. Immobilization of collared peccaries with ketamine hydrochloride. J Wildl Manag 49:356, 1985.

373. Mills TM, Copland JA. Effects of ketamine-xylazine anesthesia on blood levels of luteinizing hormone and follicle stimulating hormone in rabbits. Lab Anim Sci 32:619, 1982.

374. Hobbs BA, Ralhall TG, Sprenkel TL, Anthony KL. Comparison of several combinations for anesthesia in rabbits. Am J Vet Res 52:669, 1991.

375. Marini RP, Avison DL, Corning BF, Lipman NS. Ketamine/xylazine/butorphanol: A new anesthetic combination for rabbits. Lab Anim Sci 42:57, 1992.

376. Borkowski GL, Danneman PJ, Russell GB, Lang CM. An evaluation of three intravenous anesthetic regimens in New Zealand rabbits. Lab Anim Sci 40:270, 1990.

377. Lipman NS, Marini RP, Erdman SE. A comparison of ketamine/xylazine and ketamine/xylazine/acepromazine anesthesia in the rabbit. Lab Anim Sci 40:395, 1990.

378. Olson ME, McCabe K, Walker RL. Guaifenesin alone or in combination with ketamine or sodium pentobarbital as an anesthetic in rabbits. Can J Vet Res 51:383, 1987.

379. Gregg DA, Olson LD. The use of ketamine hydrochloride as an anesthetic for raccoons. J Wildl Dis 11:335, 1975.

380. Baber DW, Coblentz BE. Immobilization of feral pigs with a combination of ketamine and xylazine. J Wildl Manag 46:557, 1982.

381. Custer RS, Bush M. Physiologic and acid-base measures of Gopher snakes during ketamine or halothane-nitrous oxide anesthesia. J Am Vet Med Assoc 177:870, 1980.

382. Olson ME, McCabe K. Anesthesia in the Richardson's ground squirrel: Comparison of ketamine, ketamine and xylazine, droperidol and fentanyl, and sodium pentobarbital. J Am Vet Med Assoc 189:1035, 1986.

383. England GCW, Kock RA. The use of two mixtures of ketamine and xylazine to immobilize free ranging Bennett Wallabies. Vet Rec 122:11, 1988.

384. Shaughnessy PD. Immobilization of crabeater seals, Lobodon carcinophagus, with ketamine and diazepam. Wildl Res 18:165, 1991.

385. Briggs GD, Henrickson RV, Boeuf JL. Ketamine immobilization of Northern elephant seals. J Am Vet Med Assoc 167:546, 1975.

386. Trillmich F. Ketamine/xylazine combination for the immobilization of Galapagos sea lions and fur seals. Vet Rec 112:279, 1983.

387. Baker JR, Gatesman TJ. Use of carfentanil and a ketamine-xylazine mixture to immobilise wild grey seals (Halichoerus grypus). Vet Rec 116:208, 1985.

388. Baker JR, Anderson SS, Fedak MA. The usetamine-diazepam mixture to immobilise wild grey seals (Halichoerus grypus) and Southern elephant seals (Mirounga leonina). Vet Rec 123:287, 1988.

389. Geraci JR, Skirnisson K, St. Aubin DJ. A safe method for repeated immobilizing seals. J Am Vet Med Assoc 179:1192, 1981.

390. Geraci JR. An appraisal of ketamine as an immobilizing agent in wild and captive pinnipeds. J Am Vet Med Assoc 163:574, 1973.

391. Gales NJ, Burton HR. Use of emetics and anaesthesia for dietary assessment of weddell seals. Aust Wildl Res 15:423, 1988.

392. Evans RH. Anesthesia for orthopedics. Vet Tech 6:44, 1985.

393. Heaton JT, Brauth SE. Effects of yohimbine as a reversing agent for ketamine-xylazine anesthesia in budgerigars. Lab Anim Sci 42:54, 1992.

394. Stoskopf MJ, Beall FB, Ensley PK, Neely E. Immobilization of large ratites: Blue necked ostrich (Struthio Camelus austrealis) and double wattled cassowary (Casuarius casuarius) with hematologic and serum chemistry data. J Zoo Anim Med 13:160, 1982.

395. McGrath CJ, Lee TC, Campbell VL. Dose-response anesthetic effects of ketamine in the chicken. Am J Vet Res 45:531, 1984.

396. Ludders JW, Rode J, Mitchell GS, Nordheim EV. Effect of ketamine, xylazine, and a combination of ketamine and xylazine in Pekin ducks. Am J Vet Res 50:245, 1989.

397. Grubb B. Use of ketamine to restrain and anesthetize emus. Vet Med Small Anim Clin 78:247, 1983.

398. Harvey RB, Kubena LF, Lovering SL, Phillips TD. Ketamine/xylazine anesthesia for chickens. Avian/Exotic Pract 2:6, 1985.

399. Degernes LA, Kreeger TJ, Mandsager R, Redig PT. Ketamine-xylazine anesthesia in red-tailed hawks with antagonism by yohimbine. J Wildl Dis 24:322, 1988.

400. Cornick JL, Jensen J. Anesthetic management of ostriches. J Am Vet Med Assoc 200:1661, 1992.

401. Stunkard JA, Miller JC. An outline guide to general anesthesia in exotic species. Vet Med Small Anim Clin 69:1181, 1974.

402. Heerden JV, Komen J, Myer E. The use of ketamine hydrochloride in the immobilization of the cape vulture (Gyps coprotheres). J S Afr Vet Assoc 58:143, 1987.

403. Allen JL, Oosterhuis JE. Effect of tolazoline on xylazine-ketamine-induced anesthesia in turkey vultures. J Am Vet Med Assoc 189:1011, 1986.

404. Codner EC, McGrath CJ. The effect of tiletamine-zolazepam anesthesia on the response to intradermally injected histamine. J Am Anim Hosp Assoc 27:189, 1991.

405. Codner EC, Lessard P, McGrath CJ. Effect of tiletamine/

zolazepam sedation on intradermal allergy testing in atopic dogs. J Am Vet Med Assoc 201:1857, 1992.

406. McGrath CJ, Donaldson LL, Richey MT. Use of combined intramuscular and intravenous tiletamine-zolazepam in cats for elective castration. Proc Am Coll Vet Anesthesiol, New Orleans, Louisiana, 1989:14.

407. Conner GH, Coppock RW, Beck CC. Laboratory use of CI-744, a cataleptoid anesthetic, in sheep. Vet Med Small Anim Clin 69:479, 1974.

408. Lindzey and Griel: Laboratory study of CI-744 as an anesthetic agent in deer. Pennsylvania State University, State College, August, 1972.

409. Mautz WW, Seal US, Boardman CB. Blood serum analyses of chemically and physically restrained white-tailed deer. J Wildl Manag. 44:343, 1980.

410. Kreeger TJ, Seal US, Tester JR. Chemical Immobilization of red foxes (Vulpes vulpes). J Wildl Dis 26:95, 1990.

411. Smeller J, Bush M. A physiological study of immobilized Cheetahs (Acinonyx jubatus). J Zoo Anim Med 7:5, 1976.

412. Seidensticker J, Tamang KM, Gray CW. The use of CI-744 to immobilize free-ranging tigers and leopards. J Zoo Anim Med 5:22, 1974.

413. Bertram BCR, King JM. Lion and leopard immobilization using CI-744. East Afr Wildl J 14:237, 1976.

414. Smith JLD, Sunquist ME, Tamang KM, Rai PB A technique for capturing and immobilizing tigers. J Wildl Manag 47:255, 1983.

415. Taylor WP, Reynolds HV, Ballard WB. Immobilization of grizzly bears with tiletamine hydrochloride and zolazepam hydrochloride. J Wildl Manag 53:978, 1989.

416. Haigh JC, Stirling I, Broughton E. Clinical experiences with Telazol for polar bear (Ursus maritimus, Phipps) immobilization. Am Assoc Zoo Vet 130:1984.

417. Stirling I, Spencer C, Andriashek D. Immobilization of polar bears (Ursus maritimus) with Telazol in the Canadian Arctic. J Wildl Dis 25:159, 1989.

418. Knottenbelt MK, Knottenbelt DC. Use of oral sedative for immobilization of a chimpanzee (Pan troglodytes). Vet Rec 126:404, 1990.

419. Schultz TA, Fowler ME. The clinical effects of CI-744 in Chinchillas, Chinchilla villidera (Laniger). Lab Anim Sci 24:810, 1974.

420. Matthews NS, Myers MM. The use of tiletamine-zolazepam for darting feral horses. J Equin Vet Sci 13:264, 1993.

421. Smeller JM, Bush M, Custer RW. The immobilization of marsupials. J Zoo Anim Med 8:16, 1977.

422. Boever WJ, Stuppy D, Kane KK. Clinical experience with Telazol (CI-744) as a new agent for chemical restraint and anesthesia in the red kangaroo (Macropus rufus). J Zoo Anim Med 8:14, 1977.

423. Bush M, Graves J, O'Brian SJ, Wildt DE. Dissociative anesthesia in free-ranging male koalas and selected marsupials in captivity. Aust Vet J 67:449, 1990.

424. Wildt DE, O'Brian SJ, Graves JAE, Murray ND, Hurlbut S, Bush M. Anesthesia and reproductive characteristics of free-ranging male koalas (Phascolarctos cinereus). Am Assoc Zoo Vet 109, 1988.

425. Kaufman L, Hahnenberger R. CI-744 anesthesia for ophthalmological examination and surgery in monkeys. Invest Ophalthalmol 14:788, 1975.

426. Crissey SD, Edwards MS. Telazol immobilization of red howlers (Alouatta seniculus) under free-ranging conditions. Am Assoc Zoo Vet 207, 1989.

427. Williams TD, Kocher FH. Comparison of anesthetic agents in the sea otter. J Am Vet Med Assoc 173:1127, 1978.

428. Eads FE Telazol (CI-744): A new agent for chemical restraint and anesthesia in nonhuman primates. Vet Med Small Anim Clin 71:648, 1976.

429. Baker JR, Fedak MA, Anderson SS, Arnbom T, Baker R. Use of tiletamine-zolazepam mixture to immobilize wild grey seals and southern elephant seals. Vet Rec 126:75, 1990.

430. Loughlin TR, Spraker T. Use of Telazol to immobilize female northern sea lions (Eumetopias jubatus) in Alaska. J Wildl Dis 25:353, 1989.

431. Clyde VL, Cardeilhac P, Jacobson E. Chemical restraint of american alligator (Alligator Mississippiensis) with atracurium and tiletamine-zolazepam. Proc Am Assoc Zoo Vet, South Padre Island, Tx. 1990:288.

432. Bonath KH, Haller RD, Bonath I, Amelang D. Tiletamine-zolazepam-acepromazine-sedation in Crocodylus niloticus with regard to respiratory and cardiovascular system. Proc 4th International Congress of Vet Anaesthesia. 78, 1991.

chapter 11

INHALATION ANESTHETICS

Eugene P. Steffey

Introduction

Inhalation anesthetics are used widely for the anesthetic management of animals. They are unique among the anesthetic drugs because they are administered, and in large part removed from the body, via the lungs. Their popularity arises in part because their pharmacokinetic characteristics favor predictable and rapid adjustment of anesthetic depth. In addition, a special apparatus is usually used to deliver the inhaled agents. This apparatus includes a source of oxygen (O_2) and a patient breathing circuit that in turn usually includes an endotracheal tube or face mask, a means of eliminating carbon dioxide (CO_2), and a compliant gas reservoir. These components help minimize patient morbidity or mortality because they facilitate lung ventilation and improved arterial oxygenation. In addition, inhalation anesthetics in gas samples can now be readily and affordably measured almost instantaneously. Measurement of inhalation anesthetic concentration enhances the precision and safety of anesthetic management beyond the extent commonly possible with injectable anesthetic agents.

Over the nearly 150 years that inhalation anesthesia has been used in clinical practice, less than 20 agents have actually been introduced and approved for general use with patients (Fig. 11–1). Less than 10 of these have had any history of widespread clinical use in

Inhalation Anesthetics in Clinical Practice

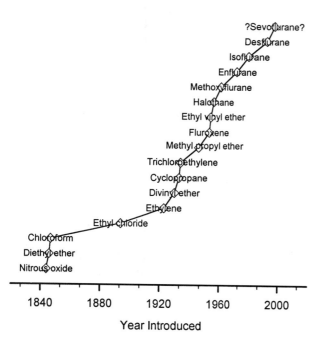

Fig. 11–1. Inhalation anesthetics introduced for widespread clinical use. (Adapted from Eger.) (251)

Table 11–1. Inhalation Anesthetic Agents

Group 1: Agents in current clinical use for animals
Major use
Halothane
Isoflurane
Minor use
Enflurane
Methoxyflurane
Nitrous oxide
Group 2: New agents
Desflurane
Sevoflurane
Group 3: Agents of historical interest
Chloroform
Cyclopropane
Diethyl ether
Fluroxene
Trichlorethylene

veterinary medicine, and only 5 are of current clinical importance in North America. It is this group of anesthetics that are the focus of this chapter (Table 11–1). The first group in the table includes halothane and isoflurane, which together are the most widely used inhaled anesthetics. In addition, nitrous oxide (N_2O), methoxyflurane, and enflurane enjoy varying degrees of popularity.

Since the search for anesthetic agents with ever-greater safety and fewer side effects is ongoing, newer anesthetics will continue to be found. Consequently, a brief discussion of desflurane, which has been recently released in the United States for general clinical use with human patients, and sevoflurane, which is undergoing laboratory and clinical testing, will be presented. Although at this time these agents have no direct impact on the anesthetic management of animals, they have the potential for some use in the anesthetic management of human patients. Such action would likely ultimately influence aspects of anesthetic management of animals, so a review of the characteristics of these anesthetics is considered important.

The third group is comprised of anesthetics that once enjoyed variable popularity for veterinary application (Table 11–1). These agents are no longer broadly used in clinical circumstances, so they will not be discussed beyond brief mention. Data of typical contemporary interest regarding their action in species of clinical importance to veterinary medicine is generally lacking, but readers interested in further information on agents in this group are referred to early editions of veterinary anesthesia textbooks(1-4). This group of anesthetics includes chloroform and cyclopropane. These agents have long been discarded for general use in human and veterinary medical practice because they cause liver failure (chloroform) or are explosive (cyclopropane). Diethyl ether, on the other hand, was widely used for clinical anesthetic management of human patients and a variety of animals up to about 20 years ago.(5) It was

Enflurane
(Ethrane)

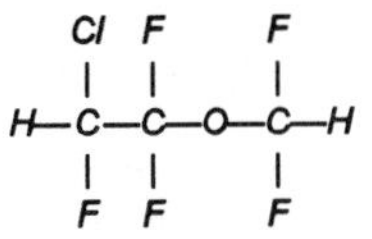

```
      Cl  F   F
      |   |   |
  H—C—C—O—C—H
      |   |   |
      F   F   F
```

Halothane
(Fluothane, Halocarbon)

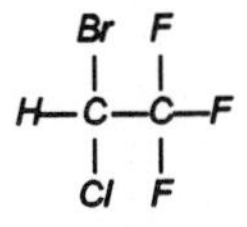

```
      Br  F
      |   |
  H—C—C—F
      |   |
      Cl  F
```

Isoflurane
(Forane, Aerrane)

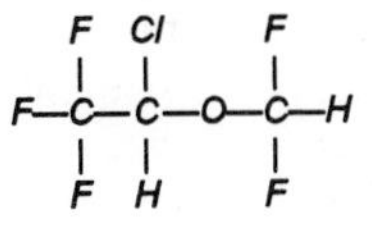

```
      F   Cl  F
      |   |   |
  F—C—C—O—C—H
      |   |   |
      F   H   F
```

Methoxyflurane
(Penthrane, Metofane)

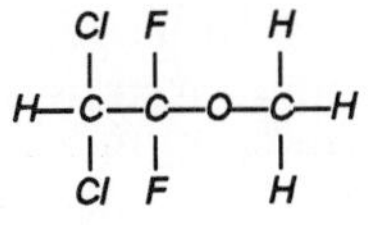

```
      Cl  F   H
      |   |   |
  H—C—C—O—C—H
      |   |   |
      Cl  F   H
```

Nitrous oxide

```
      N
      ‖
  O   |
      N
```

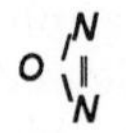

Fig. 11–2. Chemical structure of inhalation anesthetics in current use for animals. Trade names are given in parentheses.

largely replaced by newer anesthetics because of its flammability. This characteristic negated its use in modern operating rooms that include a variety of electric surgical equipment (e.g., electrocautery) and patient monitoring and ventilating devices.

Physiochemical Characteristics

The chemical structure of inhalation anesthetics and their physical properties are important determinants of their actions and safety of administration. An in-depth analysis of the impact of agent chemical structure and physical properties is beyond the scope of this chapter. However, brief discussion of aspects of Figures 11–2 and 11–3, and Tables 11–2 and 11–3 is appropriate because physiochemical characteristics determine and/or influence practical considerations such as how the agents are supplied by the manufacturer (e.g., as a gas or liquid) and the resistance of the anesthetic molecule to degradation by physical factors (e.g., heat, light) and substances it contacts during use (e.g., metal, soda lime). The equipment necessary to safely deliver the agent to the patient (e.g., vaporizer, breathing apparatus) is influenced by some of these properties, as are the agent's uptake, distribution within, and elimination (including potential for metabolic breakdown) from the patient. In summary, a knowledge and understanding

of fundamental properties permits intelligent use of contemporary anesthetics.

CHEMICAL CHARACTERISTICS

All contemporary inhalation anesthetics are organic compounds except N_2O (Fig. 11–2) (cyclopropane is the other notable inorganic anesthetic). Agents of current interest are further classified as either aliphatic (i.e., straight or branch chained) hydrocarbons or ethers (i.e., two organic radicals attached to an atom of oxygen; the general structure is ROR). In the continued search for a less reactive, more potent, nonflammable inhalation anesthetic, focus on halogenation (i.e., addition of fluorine, chlorine, or bromine; iodine is least useful) of these compounds has predominated. Chlorine and bromine especially convert many compounds of low anesthetic potency into more potent drugs. Historically, interest in fluorinated derivatives was delayed until the 1940s because of difficulties in synthesis, and thus quantities available for study were limited. Methods of synthesis, although difficult, have improved considerably and have facilitated new agent discovery (Figs. 11–2 and 11–3). It is interesting that organic fluorinated compounds are a group of extreme contrasts—some are toxic, others are not; some are extremely inert, others are highly reactive. In some anesthetics fluorine is substituted for chlorine or bromine to improve stability, but at the expense of reduced anesthetic potency and solubility.

Halothane (Fig. 11–2) is a halogenated, aliphatic saturated hydrocarbon (ethane). Predictions that halogenated structure would provide nonflammability and molecular stability encouraged the development of halothane in the early 1950s. However, soon after clinical introduction it was observed that the concurrent presence of halothane and catecholamines increased the incidence of cardiac arrhythmias, especially in

Desflurane
(Suprane, 1653)

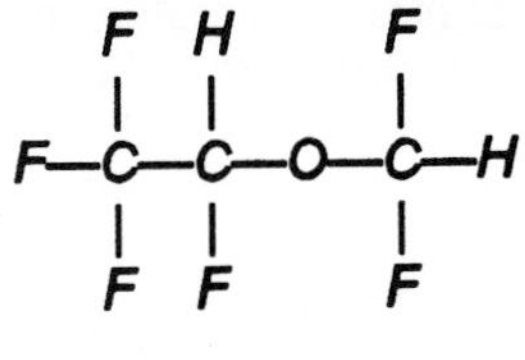

```
      F   H   F
      |   |   |
  F—C—C—O—C—H
      |   |   |
      F   F   F
```

Sevoflurane
(Ultane)

```
              F
              |
      H   F—C—F
      |   |
  F—C—O—C—H
      |   |
      H   F—C—F
              |
              F
```

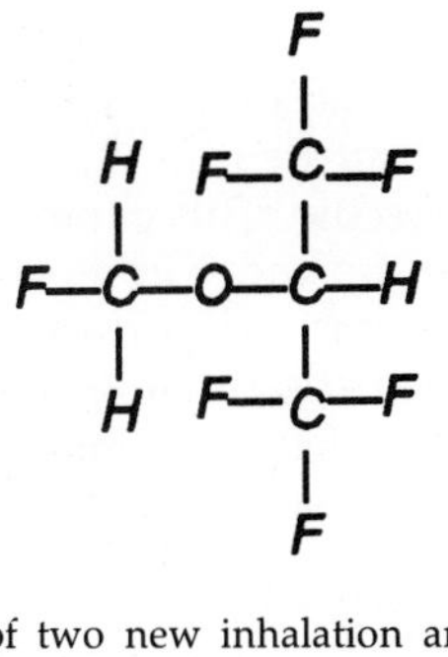

Fig. 11–3. Chemical structure of two new inhalation anesthetics. Trade name is given in parentheses.

Table 11–2. Some Physical and Chemical Properties of Inhalation Anesthetics in Current Clinical Use for Animals (6, 251)

Property	Enflurane	Halothane	Isoflurane	Methoxyflurane	Nitrous Oxide
Molecular weight	185	197	185	165	44
Liquid specific gravity (20° C) (g/mL)	1.52	1.86	1.49	1.42	—
Boiling point (°C)	57	50	49	105	−89
Vapor pressure (mm Hg)					
20° C (68° F)	172	243	240	23	—
24° C (75° F)	207	288	286	28	—
mL vapor/mL liquid @ 20° C	197.5	227	194.7	206.9	—
Preservative	None	Required	None	Required	None
Stability in					
Soda lime	Stable	Decomposes	Stable	Decomposes	Stable
UV light	Stable	Decomposes	Stable	Decomposes	Stable

Table 11–3. Some Physical and Chemical Properties of Two New Inhalation Anesthetics

Property	Desflurane	Sevoflurane
Molecular weight	168[255]	200[255]
Liquid specific gravity @ 20° C (g/mL)	1.47[256]	1.52[256]
Boiling point (° C)	23.5[255]	59[44]
Vapor pressure (mm Hg) @ 20° C (68° F)	664[257]	160[44]
mL of vapor/mL of liquid @ 20° C	209.7	182.7
Preservatives	None	None
Stability in soda lime	Yes	No?

References indicated by superscript.

human patients. An ether linkage in the molecule favors a reduced incidence of cardiac arrhythmias. Consequently, this chemical structure is a predominant characteristic of all agents developed or proposed for clinical use since the introduction of halothane (Figs. 11–2 and 11–3).

Despite many favorable characteristics and improvements over earlier anesthetics (Fig. 11–1) that included improved chemical stability, halothane is susceptible to decomposition. Accordingly, halothane is stored in dark bottles and a very small amount of a preservative, thymol, is added to it to retard breakdown. Thymol is much less volatile than halothane and over time collects within the devices used to control delivery of the volatile anesthetic (i.e., vaporizers) and causes them to malfunction. To accomplish greater molecular stability fluorine is substituted for chlorine or bromine in the anesthetic molecule. This chemical manipulation adds shelf life to the substance and negates the need for additives such as thymol. Unfortunately, the fluorine ion is also toxic to some tissues (e.g., kidneys), which is of substantial concern if the parent compound (e.g., methoxyflurane) is not resistant to metabolism (Fig. 11–2).

PHYSICAL CHARACTERISTICS

There is a constant interchange of respiratory gases (O_2 and CO_2) between cells and the external environment via blood. Inhalation anesthesia involves additional considerations whereby an anesthetic must be transferred under control from a container to sites of action in the central nervous system. Early in this process the agent is diluted to an appropriate amount (concentration) and supplied to the respiratory system in a gas mixture that contains enough O_2 to support life. The chain of events that ensues is influenced by many physical and chemical characteristics that can be quantitatively described (Tables 11–2 to 11–6). The practical clinical applications of these quantitative descriptions are reviewed here. Limited space does not permit in-depth review of all underlying principles, and readers interested in further background information are referred elsewhere.(6, 7)

The physical characteristics of importance to our understanding of the action of inhalation anesthetics can be conveniently divided into two general categories; those that determine the means by which the agents are administered and those that help determine their kinetics in the body. This information is applied in the clinical manipulation of anesthetic induction and recovery and in facilitating changes in anesthetic-induced CNS depression in a timely fashion.

Properties Determining Methods of Administration

A variety of physical/chemical properties determine the means by which inhalation anesthetics are administered. These include characteristics such as molecular weight, boiling point, liquid density (specific gravity) and vapor pressure.

GENERAL PRINCIPLES: A BRIEF REVIEW

Molecules are in a constant state of motion and exhibit a force of mutual attraction. The degree of attraction is evident by the state in which the substance exists (i.e., solid, liquid, or gas). Molecular motion increases as energy (e.g., in the form of heat) is added to the molecular aggregate and decreases as energy is removed. With increased motion there is a reduction in the intermolecular forces; if conditions are extreme enough, a change in physical state may ensue. All substances exist naturally in a particular state but can be

Table 11–4. Partition Coefficients (Solvent/Gas) of Some Inhalation Anesthetics at 37° C

Solvent	Desflurane	Enflurane	Halothane	Isoflurane	Methoxyflurane	Sevoflurane	Nitrous Oxide
Water	–	0.78	0.82	0.62	4.50	0.60	0.47
Blood	0.42	2.00	2.54	1.46	15.00	0.68	0.47
Olive oil	18.70	96.00	224.00	91.00	970.00	47.00	1.40
Brain	1.30	2.70	1.90	1.60	20.00	1.70	0.50
Liver	1.30	3.70	2.10	1.80	29.00	1.80	0.38
Kidney	1.00	1.90	1.00	1.20	11.00	1.20	0.40
Muscle	2.00	2.20	3.40	2.90	16.00	3.10	0.54
Fat	27.00	83.00	51.00	45.00	902.00	48.00	1.08

Tissue samples are derived from human sources.
(Data are from Eger [13, 63, 254, 258], Steward et al. [259], Strum and Eger [260], and Wallin et al [44]).

Table 11–5. Solvent/Gas Partition Coefficients for Halothane at 37° C in a Variety of Species (261)

Solvent	Dog	Horse	Ox	Rabbit
Blood	3.51	1.77	2.40	4.02
Brain	6.03	5.42	4.80	6.22
Liver	6.64	8.51	5.10	9.17
Kidney	4.95	3.21	3.80	6.96
Muscle	5.45	3.55	5.40	3.67

made to exist (at least in theory) in any or all phases by altering conditions. Water, as an example, exists as ice (mutual molecular attraction is great), liquid water, or water vapor (attraction considerably reduced) depending upon conditions.

Gas vs Vapor

Inhalation anesthetics are either gases or vapors. In relation to inhalation anesthetics the term *gas* refers to an agent, such as N_2O (or cyclopropane), that exists in its gaseous form at room temperature and sea level pressure. The term *vapor* indicates the gaseous state of a substance that at ambient temperature and pressure is a liquid. With the exception of N_2O, all the contemporary and new anesthetics fall into this category. Desflurane (Table 11–3) is one of the new volatile liquids that comes close to the transition stage and offers some unique (among the inhalation anesthetics) considerations to be discussed later in this chapter.

Behavior of Gases

Whether inhalation agents are supplied as a gas or volatile liquid under ambient conditions, the same physical principles apply to each agent when it is in the gaseous state. Molecules move about in haphazard fashion at high speeds and collide with each other (more frequently in liquid than in gas) or the walls of the containing vessel. The force of the bombardment is measurable and referred to as pressure. In the case of gases, if the space or volume in which the gas is enclosed is increased, the number of bombardments decreases (i.e., a smaller number of molecular collisions per unit time) and then the pressure decreases. The

behavior of gases is predictably described by various gas laws. Relationships such as those described by Boyle's law (volume vs pressure), Charles's law (volume vs temperature), Gay-Lussac's law (temperature vs pressure), Dalton's Law of Partial Pressure (the total pressure of a mixture of gases is equal to the sum of the partial pressures of all of the gaseous substances present), and others are important to our overall understanding of aspects of respiratory and anesthetic gases and vapors. However, in-depth descriptions of these principles are beyond the scope of this chapter and readers are referred elsewhere for this information.(7)

Methods of Description

Quantities of inhalation anesthetic agent are usually characterized by one of three methods: pressure (e.g., in mm Hg), concentration (in vol %) or mass (in mg or g). The form most familiar to clinicians is that of concentration (e.g., X% of agent A in relation to the whole gas mixture). Modern monitoring equipment samples inspired and expired gases and provides concentration readings for inhalation anesthetics. Precision vaporizers used to control delivery of inhalation anesthetics are calibrated in percentage of agent, and effective doses are almost always reported in percentages.

Pressure is also an important way of describing inhalation anesthetics and is further discussed under the heading of anesthetic potency. A mixture of gases in a closed container will exert a pressure on the walls of the container. The individual pressure of each gas in a mixture of gases is referred to as its *partial pressure*. As noted earlier, this expression of the behavior of a mixture of gases is known as Dalton's law, and its use in understanding inhalation anesthesia is inescapable. Use of the concept of partial pressure is important in understanding inhalation anesthetic action in a multiphase biologic system because, unlike concentration, the partial pressure of an agent is the same in different compartments that are in equilibrium with each other. That is, in contradistinction to concentration or volume percent, an expression of the relative ratio of gas molecules in a mixture, partial pressure is an expression of the absolute value.

Table 11–6. Rubber or Plastic/Gas Partition Coefficients at Room Temperature (63)

Solvent	Enflurane	Halothane	Isoflurane	Methoxyflurane	Nitrous Oxide
Rubber	74	120	62	630	1.2
Polyvinyl chloride	120	190	110	—	—
Polyethylene	~2	26	~2	118	—

a. Isoflurane specific gravity = 1.49 g/ml, therefore:
   1 ml liquid isoflurane = 1 ml × 1.49 g/ml = 1.49 gm
b. Since molecular weight of isoflurane = 185 gm (from Table 3), then:
   1.49 gm ÷ 185 gm = 0.0081 mol of liquid
c. Since 1 mol of gas = 22.4 L, then:
   0.0081 mol × 22400 ml/mol = 181.4 ml of isoflurane vapor at 0°C, 1 atm
d. But vapor is at 20°C not 0°C (i.e., 273°K),
   So 181.4 × 293/273 = 194.7 ml vapor/ml liquid isoflurane at 20°C at sea level pressure
For substantial variation in ambient pressure, the final figure noted above would have to be further "corrected" by a factor of: 760/ambient barometric pressure

Fig. 11–4. Example of calculations to determine the volume of isoflurane vapor at 20° C from one mL of isoflurane liquid.

Molecular weight and agent density are used in many calculations to convert from liquid to vapor volumes and mass. Briefly (and in simplified fashion), Avogadro's principle is that equal volume of all gases under the same conditions of temperature and pressure contain the same number of molecules (6.0226×10^{23} [Avogadro's Number] per gram molecular weight). Furthermore, under standard conditions the number of gas molecules in a gram molecular weight of a substance occupies 22.4 liters. In order to compare properties of different substances of similar state, it is necessary to do so under comparable conditions; with respect to gases and liquids this usually means with reference to pressure and temperature. Unless otherwise indicated, physical scientists have arbitrarily selected *standard conditions* as 0° C (273° K in absolute scale) and 760 mm Hg pressure (1 atmosphere at sea level). If conditions differ, appropriate temperature and/or pressure corrections must be applied to resultant data.

The weight of a given volume of liquid, gas, or vapor may be expressed in terms of its density or specific gravity. The density is an absolute value of mass (usually grams) per unit volume (for liquids, volume = 1 mL; for gases, 1 liter at standard conditions). The specific gravity is a relative value; that is, the ratio of the weight of a unit volume of one substance to a similar volume of water in the case of liquids or air in the case of gases (or vapors) under similar conditions. The value of both air and water is one. At least for clinical purposes the value for density and specific gravity for an inhalation anesthetic is the same. Thus, for example, we can determine the volume of isoflurane gas (vapor) at 20° C from a mL of isoflurane liquid according to the scheme given in Figure 11–4. This type of calculation has practical applications. For example, to determine

a. Total isoflurane vapor delivered over 2 hours (120 min) estimated at:

   3%/100 × 6 LPM = 0.18 LPM × 120 min =
   $\qquad$ 21.60L/120 min = 21,600 ml/120 min

   vs

   3%/100 × 4 LPM = 0.12 LPM × 120 min =
   $\qquad$ 14.4 L/120 min = 14,400 ml/120 min

b. Total vapor volume saved:

   21,600 ml/120 min − 14,400 ml/120 min =
   $\qquad$ 7,200 ml vapor/120 min saved

c. Total liquid isoflurane volume saved/2 hours

   7200 ml vapor ÷ 194.7 ml vapor/ml liquid =
   $\qquad$ 36.98 ml of isoflurane liquid

   (194.7 ml vapor/ml liquid can be calculated as in Fig. 4 or taken from Table 2)
   The economic value of reducing isoflurane consumption can then be determined by calculating the product of the liquid volume saved and the purchase cost/ml of isoflurane liquid.

Fig. 11–5. Problem: Determine the savings in isoflurane liquid afforded by reducing the fresh gas (e.g., O_2) inflow rate from 6 Lpm (liters per minute) to 4 Lpm, given that the average delivered (vaporizer setting) concentration for 2 hours is 3%.

the savings in isoflurane liquid afforded by reducing the fresh gas (e.g., O_2) inflow rate, a series of calculations as presented in Figure 11–5 can be made.

VAPOR PRESSURE

Molecules of liquids are in constant random motion. Some of those in the surface layer gain sufficient velocity to overcome the attractive forces of neighboring molecules and in escaping from the surface enter the vapor phase. The change in state from a liquid to a gas phase is known as *vaporization* or *evaporation*. This process is dynamic and in a closed container that is kept at a constant temperature eventually reaches an equilibrium whereby there is no further net loss of molecules to the gas phase (i.e., the numbers of molecules leaving and returning to the liquid phase are equal). The gas phase at this point is saturated.

Molecules of a vapor exert a force per unit area or pressure in exactly the same manner as do molecules of a gas. The pressure (units of measure are mm Hg) that the vapor molecules exert when the liquid and vapor phases are in equilibrium is known as the *vapor pressure*. Thus, the vapor pressure of an anesthetic is a measure of its ability to evaporate; that is, it is a measure of the tendency for molecules in the liquid state to enter the gaseous (vapor) phase. The vapor pressure of a volatile anesthetic must be at least sufficient to provide enough

Vapor Pressure - Temperature Relationship

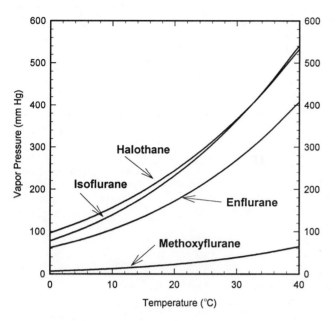

Fig. 11–6. Vapor pressure as a function of temperature for four contemporary volatile anesthetics. Curves are generated from Antoine equations.(252)

molecules of anesthetic in the vapor state to produce anesthesia at ambient conditions. The *saturated vapor pressure* represents a maximum concentration of molecules in the vapor state that can exist for a given liquid at each temperature. Herein lies a practical difference between substances classified as a gas or vapor; a gas can be administered over a range of concentrations from 0 to 100%, whereas the vapor has a ceiling that is dictated by its vapor pressure. The saturated vapor concentration can be easily determined by relating the vapor pressure to the ambient pressure. For example, in the case of halothane (Table 11–2), a maximal concentration of 32% halothane is possible under usual conditions (i.e., [244/760] − 100 = 32%, where 760 mm Hg is the barometric pressure at sea level). With other variables considered constant, the greater the vapor pressure, the greater the concentration of the drug deliverable to the patient. Therefore, again from Table 11–2, halothane, for example, is more volatile than methoxyflurane under similar conditions. The barometric pressure also influences the final concentration of an agent. For example, in locations such as Denver, Colorado, where the altitude is about 5000 feet above sea level and the barometric pressure is only about 635 mm Hg, the saturated vapor concentration of halothane at 20° C is now (243/635) − 100 = 38.3%.

It is important to recognize that the saturated vapor pressure at one atmosphere is unique for each volatile anesthetic agent and depends only on its temperature. In this case the effect of barometric pressure can be neglected over ranges normally encountered in the practice of anesthesia. Thus, for a given agent, the graph

of the saturated vapor pressure vs temperature is a curve as shown in Figure 11–6. From this graph it can be seen that if the temperature of the liquid is increased, more molecules escape the liquid phase and enter the gaseous phase. The greater number of molecules in the vapor phase results in a greater vapor pressure and vapor concentration. Conversely, if the liquid is cooled, the reverse situation occurs and vapor concentration decreases. Liquid cooling may occur not only as a result of ambient conditions but also as a natural consequence of the vaporization process. For example, during vaporization the "fastest" molecules at the surface escape first. With depletion of these "high-energy" molecules, the average kinetic energy of those left behind is reduced and there is a tendency for the temperature of the remaining liquid to fall if this process is not compensated for externally. As the temperature decreases the vapor pressure, and thus the vapor concentration, also decreases.

Special Considerations

BOILING POINT

The boiling point of a liquid is defined as the temperature at which the vapor pressure of the liquid is equal to the atmospheric pressure. Customarily, the boiling temperature is stated at the standard atmospheric pressure of 760 mm Hg. The boiling point decreases with increasing altitude because the vapor pressure does not change but the barometric pressure decreases. The boiling point of N_2O is −89° C (Table 11–2) at one atmosphere pressure at sea level. It is thus a gas under operating room conditions. Because of this, it is distributed for clinical purposes in steel tanks compressed to the liquid state at about 750 psi (pounds per square inch; 750 psi/14.9 psi [one atmosphere] = 50 atmospheres). As the N_2O gas is drawn from the tanks, liquid N_2O is vaporized and the overriding gas pressure remains constant until no further liquid remains in the tank. At that point only N_2O gas remains, and the gas pressure decreases from this point as remaining gas is vented from the tank. Consequently, the weight of the N_2O minus the weight of the tank rather than the gas pressure within the tank is a more accurate guide to the remaining amount of N_2O in the tank.(8)

Desflurane, the newest clinically available volatile anesthetic, also possesses an interesting consideration because its boiling point (Table 11–3) is near room temperature. This characteristic accounted for an interesting engineering challenge in developing an administration device (i.e., a vaporizer) for routine use in the relatively constant environment of the operating room and limits further consideration of its use in all but a narrow range of circumstances commonly encountered in veterinary medical applications. For example, because of its low boiling point, even evaporative cooling has large influences on vapor pressure and thus the vapor concentration of gas mixtures delivered to the patient.

CALCULATION OF ANESTHETIC CONCENTRATION DELIVERED BY A VAPORIZER

The saturated vapor pressure of most volatile anesthetics is of such magnitude that the maximal concentration of anesthetic attainable at usual operating room conditions is above the range of concentrations that are commonly necessary for safe clinical anesthetic management. Therefore, some control of the delivered concentration is necessary and usually provided by a device known as a *vaporizer*. The purpose of the vaporizer is to dilute the vapor generated from the liquid anesthetic with O_2 (or an O_2 and N_2O mixture) to produce a more satisfactory inspired anesthetic concentration. This anesthetic dilution is usually accomplished as indicated in the Figure 11–7 model by diverting the gas entering the vaporizer into two streams, one that

enters the vaporizing chamber (anesthetic chamber volume: V_{anes}) and the other that bypasses the vaporizing chamber (dilution volume or $V_{dilution}$). If the vaporizer is efficient, the carrier gas passing through the vaporizing chamber becomes completely saturated to an anesthetic concentration (%) reflected by (anesthetic agent vapor pressure/atmospheric pressure) × 100, at the vaporizer chamber temperature. The resultant anesthetic concentration then is decreased (diluted) downstream by the second gas stream to a "working" concentration. In modern, precision, agent-specific vaporizers no mental effort is required—just set the dial, the manufacturers have precalibrated the vaporizer for accurate delivery of the dialed concentration. Nevertheless, it is helpful to our overall understanding to know the principles underlying this convenience and

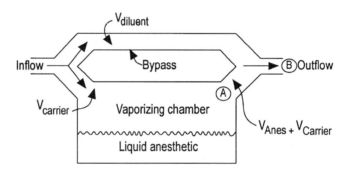

3

Steps:

1. The saturated *concentration* of anesthetic in the anesthetic vaporizing chamber and leaving it (ideally at A above) is calculated knowing the saturated vapor pressure (P_{VP}) (from Table 2) and barometric pressure (P_B).

For example:

$$\text{Halothane\%} = \frac{243}{760} \times 100 = 32.0\% \qquad (a)$$

2. The *volume* of anesthetic leaving the vaporizing chamber is the original volume of the carrier gas (O_2) entering the anesthetic vaporizing chamber ($V_{carrier}$) and the volume of anesthetic (V_{halo}) added to it.

$$\text{Halothane\%} = \frac{V_{halo}}{V_{carrier} + V_{halo}} \times 100 \qquad (b)$$

Halothane% is known from (a) above and $V_{carrier}$ is known from control of a flowmeter (e.g., a measured flow vaporizer) or via the design characteristics of a commercial, agent-specific, vaporizer that automatically "splits" the fresh gas flow from a single flow meter. In the first case, two gas flow controls are necessary, one for $V_{carrier}$ and one for a larger gas dilution flow ($V_{dilution}$). In either the case of manual or automatic fresh gas flow alteration, the equation is then solved for V_{halo} (expressed in ml of halothane vapor).

For example, if $V_{carrier} = 100$ mL O_2, then

$$32\% = \frac{V_{halo}}{100 + V_{halo}} \times 100$$

$$3200 + 32V_{halo} = 100V_{halo}$$

$$3200 = 68V_{halo}$$

$$V_{halo} = 47.1 \text{ mL halothane vapor}$$

3. V_{halo} is then contained in a total gas volume at B of

$$V_{\text{total gas}} = V_{halo} + V_{carrier} + V_{diluent} \qquad (c)$$

Where $V_{diluent}$ is set by the anesthetist using a second gas control (i.e., flowmeter; units here of mL/min) or by the vaporizer design and dial setting.

Then in our example for a $V_{diluent}$ of 1000 mL (in 1 minute)

$$V_{total} = 47.1 + 100 + 1000$$

$$= 1147 \text{ ml (rounded off)}$$

4. So the final halothane vapor concentration is determined by

$$\text{halothane \%} = \frac{V_{halo}}{V_{Total}} \times 100$$

Again, in our example,

$$\text{halothane \%} = \frac{47.1}{1147} = 4.1\%$$

Alternatively, with some basic algebraic work with equations given above, the same numbers can be applied to the resultant formula given below to arrive at the anesthetic concentration. The condensed formula is:

$$\text{Anesthetic concentration (\%)} = \frac{V_{carrier} \cdot P_{VP} \cdot 100}{V_{diluent} \cdot (P_B - P_{VP}) + (V_{carrier} \cdot P_B)}$$

Fig. 11–7. An anesthetic vaporizer model to assist in illustrating the principles associated with the calculation of the vapor concentration of an inhalation anesthetic emerging from a vaporizer. Conditions associated with halothane delivery in San Francisco (i.e., at sea level; barometric pressure = 760 mm Hg) at 20° C are used as an example of general principles.

how to apply these principles in the use of older noncompensated measured flow vaporizers.

To calculate the anesthetic concentration from the vaporizer one must know the vapor pressure of the agent (at the temperature of use), the atmospheric pressure, the fresh gas flow entering the vaporizing chamber, and the diluent gas flow. Then,

% anesthetic = flow of anesthetic from the vaporizing chamber/total gas flow

More detail for interested readers is given in Figure 11–7.

Properties Influencing Drug Kinetics: Solubility

Anesthetic gases and vapors dissolve in liquids and solids. The solubility of an anesthetic is a major characteristic of the agent and has important clinical ramifications. For example, anesthetic solubility in blood and body tissues is a primary factor in the rate of uptake and its distribution within the body. It is therefore a primary determinant of the speed of anesthetic induction and recovery. Solubility in lipid bears a strong relationship to anesthetic potency, and its tendency to dissolve in anesthetic delivery components such as rubber goods influences equipment selection and other aspects of anesthetic management.

SOLUBILITY OF GASES

As previously mentioned, molecules of a gas that overlie a liquid surface are in random motion and some penetrate the liquid surface. After entering the liquid they intermingle with the molecules of the liquid (i.e., the gas dissolves in the liquid). There is a net movement of the gas into the liquid until an equilibrium is established between the dissolved gas in the liquid and the undissolved portion above the liquid. At this time there is no further net gain of gas molecules by the liquid, and the number of gas molecules entering the liquid equals the number leaving. The gas molecules within the liquid exert the same pressure or tension that they exert in the gas phase. If the pressure (i.e., the number of gas molecules overlying the liquid) is increased, more molecules pass into the liquid and the pressure within the liquid is increased. This net inward movement of gas molecules continues until a new equilibrium is established between the pressure of the gas in the liquid and that overlying the liquid. Alternatively, if the pressure of gas overlying the liquid is somehow decreased below that in the liquid, gas molecules escape from the liquid. This net outward movement of gas molecules from the liquid phase continues until equilibrium between the two phases is reestablished.

The amount, that is, the total number of molecules of a given gas dissolving in a solvent, depends on the chemical nature of the gas itself, the partial pressure of the gas, the nature of the solvent and the temperature. This relationship is described by Henry's law,

$$V = S \times P$$

where V is the volume of gas, P is the partial pressure of the gas, and S is the solubility coefficient for the gas in the solvent at a given temperature. Henry's law applies to gases that do not combine chemically with the solvent to form compounds.

Before leaving this basic information, a brief focus on a number of variations may be helpful. First, it is important to recognize that if the atmosphere that overlies the solvent is made up of a mixture of gases, then each gas dissolves in the solvent in proportion to the partial pressure of the individual gases. The total pressure exerted by the molecules of all gases within the solvent equals the total gas pressure lying above the solvent.

Within the body there is a partition of anesthetic gases between blood and body tissues in accordance with Henry's law. This process can be perhaps better understood by visualizing a system composed of three compartments (e.g., gas, water, and oil) contained in a closed container (Fig. 11–8). In such a system the gas overlies the oil, which in turn overlies the water. Because there is a passive gradient from the gas phase to the oil, gas molecules move into the oil compartment. This movement in turn develops a gradient for the gas molecules in oil relative to water. If gas is continually added above the oil, there will be a continual net movement of the gas molecules from the gas phase into both the oil and, in turn, the water. At a given temperature, when no more gas dissolves in the solvent, the solvent is said to be *fully saturated.* At this point the pressure of the gas molecules within the three compartments will be equal but the amount (i.e., the number of molecules or volume of gas) partitioned between the two liquids will vary with the nature of the liquid and gas. Finally, it is important to understand that the amount of gas that goes into solution depends upon the temperature of the solvent. Less gas dissolves in a solvent as temperature increases, and more gas is taken up as solvent temperature decreases. For example, as water is heated air bubbles appear inside the container as a result of the decreasing solubility of the air in water. Conversely, as blood is cooled from a normal body temperature (e.g., hypothermia), gases become more soluble in blood.

SOLUBILITY COEFFICIENTS

The extent to which a gas will dissolve in a given solvent is usually expressed in terms of its solubility coefficient (Table 11–4). With inhalation anesthetics, solubility is most commonly measured and expressed as a partition coefficient (PC). Other measurements of solubility include the Bunson and Ostwald solubility coefficients.(7, 9)

The PC is the concentration ratio of an anesthetic in the solvent and gas phases (e.g., blood and gas, Fig. 11–9) or between two tissue solvents (e.g., brain and

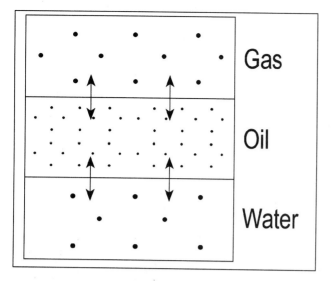

Fig. 11–8. Diagrammatic representation of an anesthetic gas distributing itself among three compartments (gas, oil, water). At equilibrium, the number of anesthetic molecules in the three compartments differ but the pressure exerted by the anesthetic molecules is the same in each compartment.

blood, Table 11–4). It thus describes the capacity of a given solvent to dissolve the anesthetic gas. That is, how the anesthetic will *partition* itself between the gas and the liquid solvent phases after equilibrium has been reached. Remember, anesthetic gas movement occurs because of a partial pressure difference in the gas and liquid solvent phases, so when there is no longer any anesthetic partial pressure difference there is no longer any net movement of anesthetic and equilibrium has been achieved. Solvent/gas PCs are summarized in Table 11–4. Values noted in this table are for human tissues because they are most widely available in the anesthesia literature. Comparative data for halothane with some species of clinical interest in veterinary medicine is given in Table 11–5. Regardless of the species, it is important to emphasize that many factors can alter anesthetic agent solubility.(9-12) Perhaps the most notable after the nature of the solvent is that of temperature.

Of all the PCs that have been described or are of interest, two are of particular importance in the practical understanding of anesthetic action. They are the blood/gas and the oil/gas solubility coefficients.

Blood/Gas Partition Coefficient

Blood/gas solubility coefficients (Tables 11–4 and 11–5) provide a means for predicting the speed of anesthetic induction, recovery, and change of anesthetic depth. Assume, for example, that anesthetic A has a blood/gas PC value of 15. This means that the concentration of the anesthetic in blood will be 15 times greater at equilibrium than that in alveolar gas. Expressed differently, the same volume of blood, say 1 mL, will hold 15 times more of anesthetic A than 1 mL of alveolar gas despite an equal partial pressure. Alternatively, consider anesthetic

B with a PC of 1.4. This PC indicates that at equilibrium, the amount of anesthetic B is only 1.4 times greater in blood than it is in alveolar air. Comparing the PC of anesthetic A with that of anesthetic B indicates that anesthetic A is much more soluble in blood than B (nearly 11 times more soluble: 15/1.4). From this, and assuming other conditions are equal, anesthetic A will require a longer time of administration to attain a partial pressure in the body for a particular end point (say, anesthetic induction) than will anesthetic B. Also, since there is more of anesthetic A contained in blood and other body tissues under similar conditions, elimination (and therefore anesthetic recovery) will be prolonged when compared to anesthetic B.

Oil/Gas Partition Coefficient

The oil/gas PC is another solubility characteristic of clinical importance (Tables 11–4, 11–5). This PC describes the ratio of the concentration of an anesthetic in oil (olive oil is the standard) and gas phases at equilibrium. The oil/gas PC correlates inversely with anesthetic potency (see "Anesthetic Dose: The Minimum Alveolar Concentration (MAC)" in this chapter) and describes the capacity of lipids for anesthetic.

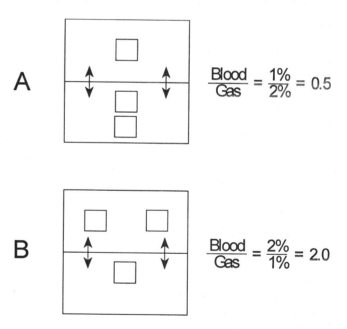

In example A, anesthetic A is introduced into a closed container of equal gas and blood volume. The anesthetic distributes itself between the two phases (gas and blood) until equilibrium is attained (i.e., no anesthetic partial pressure difference between the two phases). At that time, there is no further net transfer of anesthetic into the blood and the equilibrium concentrations of anesthetic A are as shown. The ratio of the final concentration of anesthetic A in blood compared to gas is thus 0.5, i.e., the anesthetic concentration in blood is only ½ that of the gas at equilibrium. In example B, at equilibrium anesthetic B is twice as soluble in blood.

Fig. 11–9. Blood gas partition coefficient illustration. (Adapted from Eger.) (9)

Other Partition Coefficients

Solubility characteristics for various tissues (Tables 11–4 and 11–5) and other media, such as rubber and plastic (Table 11–6), are also important. For example, the solubility of a tissue determines in part the quantity of anesthetic removed from the blood to which it is exposed. The higher the tissue solubility, the longer it will take to saturate the tissue with anesthetic agent. Thus, other things considered equal, anesthetics that are very soluble in tissues will require a longer period for induction and recovery. If the amount of rubber goods in the apparatus used to deliver the anesthetic to the patient is substantial and the anesthetic agent solubility in rubber is large, the amount of uptake of anesthetic agent by the rubber may be of clinical significance.

Pharmacokinetics: Uptake and Elimination of Inhalation Anesthetics

The aim in administering an inhalation anesthetic to a patient is to achieve an adequate partial pressure or tension of anesthetic (P_{anes}) in the brain to cause a desired level of CNS depression commensurate with the definition of general anesthesia. Anesthetic depth varies directly with P_{anes} in brain tissue. The rate of change of anesthetic depth is of obvious clinical importance and is directly dependent upon the rate of change in anesthetic tensions in the various media in which it is contained before reaching the brain. Thus, knowledge of the factors that govern these relationships is of fundamental importance to skillful control of general inhalation anesthesia.

Inhalation anesthetics are unique among the classes of drugs that are used to produce general anesthesia because they are administered via the lungs. The pharmacokinetics of the inhaled anesthetics describes the rate of their uptake by blood from the lungs, distribution in the body, and eventual elimination by the lungs and other routes. Readers seeking more in-depth coverage are directed to reviews by Eger (9, 13) and Mapleson.(14)

Inhalation anesthetics, similar to O_2 and CO_2, move down a series of partial pressure gradients from regions of higher tension to those of lower tension until equilibrium (i.e., equal pressure throughout the apparatus and body tissues) is established. Thus on induction, the P_{anes} at its source in the vaporizer is high, as is dictated by the vapor pressure, and progressively decreases as anesthetic travels from vaporizer to patient breathing circuit, from circuit to lungs, from lungs to arterial blood, and finally, from arterial blood to body tissues (e.g., the brain, Fig. 11–10). Of these the alveolar partial pressure (P_A) of anesthetic is most crucial. The brain has a rich blood supply and the anesthetic in arterial blood (PaAnes) rapidly equilibrates with brain tissue (P_{brain}Anes). Usually gas exchange at the alveolar level is sufficiently efficient that the PaAnes is close to P_AAnes. Thus, the P_{brain}Anes closely follows P_AAnes, and by controlling the P_AAnes

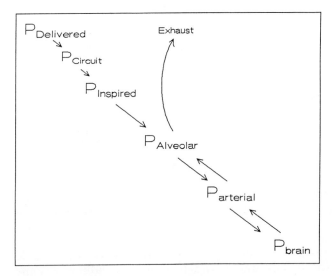

Fig. 11–10. The flow pattern of inhaled anesthetic agents during anesthetic induction and recovery. Inhalation anesthesia may be viewed as the development of a series of partial pressure (tension) gradients. During induction there is a high anesthetic tension in the vaporizer that decreases progressively as the flow of anesthetic gas moves from its source to the brain. Some of these gradients are easily manipulated by the anesthetist; others are not, or are done so with difficulty. (From Steffey with permission of the publishers.) (253)

there is a reliable indirect way for controlling P_{brain}Anes and anesthetic depth.

At this point it may be also helpful to recall that although the partial pressure of anesthetic is of primary importance, we frequently define clinical dose of an inhaled anesthetic in terms of concentration (C; i.e., vol %). As previously noted, this is because it is common practice for the clinician to regulate and/or measure respiratory and anesthetic gases in volume percent. In addition, in the gaseous phase, the relationship between the P_{anes} and the C_{anes} is a simple one:

$$P_{anes} = \text{fractional anesthetic concentration} \times \text{total ambient pressure}$$

The fractional anesthetic concentration is of course $C_{anes}/100$. However, as reviewed in the preceding section, in blood or tissues the actual quantity of anesthetic depends on both the P_{anes} and the anesthetic solubility (as measured by partition coefficient) within the solvent (e.g., blood or oil). Consequently, at equilibrium, the partial pressure of the gas in the alveoli and among tissue compartments will be equal although concentrations will vary within these tissues.

ANESTHETIC UPTAKE: FACTORS THAT DETERMINE THE P_A OF ANESTHETIC

The P_A of anesthetic is a balance between anesthetic input (i.e., delivery to the alveoli) and loss (uptake by blood and body tissues) from the lungs. A rapid rise in the P_A of anesthetic is associated with a rapid anesthetic induction or change in anesthetic depth. Factors that contribute to a rapid change in the P_A of anesthetic are summarized in Table 11–7.

DELIVERY TO THE ALVEOLI

Delivery of anesthetic to the alveoli and therefore the rate of rise of the alveolar concentration or fraction (F_A) toward the inspired concentration or fraction (F_I) depends on the inspired anesthetic concentration itself and the magnitude of alveolar ventilation. Increasing either one of these or both increases the rate of rise of the P_A of anesthetic; that is, with other things considered equal there is an increase in speed of anesthetic induction or change in anesthetic level.

Inspired Concentration. The inspired concentration has a number of variables controlling it. First of all, the upper limit of inspired concentration is dictated by the agent vapor pressure, which in turn is dependent on temperature. This may be especially important considering the breadth of veterinary medical application of inhaled anesthesia and methods of vaporizing volatile anesthetics under widely diverse conditions (some environmental conditions are quite hostile).

Characteristics of the patient breathing system can also be a major factor in generating a suitable inspired concentration under usual operating room conditions. Characteristics of special importance include the volume of the system, the amount of rubber or plastic

Table 11–7. Factors Related to a Rapid Change in Alveolar Anesthetic Tension (P_A)

A. Increased alveolar delivery
  1. Increased inspired anesthetic concentration
    a. Increased vaporization of agent
    b. Increased vaporizer dial setting
    c. Increased fresh gas inflow
    d. Decreased gas volume of patient breathing circuit
  2. Increased alveolar ventilation
    a. Increased minute ventilation
    b. Decreased dead space ventilation
B. Decreased removal from the alveoli
  1. Decreased blood solubility of anesthetic
  2. Decreased cardiac output
  3. Decreased alveolar-venous anesthetic gradient

(Modified from Steffey [253]).

components of the system, the position of the vaporizer relative to the breathing circuit (i.e., within or outside of the circuit), and the fresh gas inflow to the patient breathing circuit. The patient breathing circuit contains a gas volume that must be replaced with gas containing the desired anesthetic concentration. Thus, the volume of the breathing circuit serves as a buffer to delay the rise of anesthetic concentration. In the management of small animals (i.e., animals less than 10 kg), a nonrebreathing patient circuit and/or a relatively high fresh gas inflow into the patient breathing circuit is usually used, so there should *not* be a clinically important difference between the delivered (e.g., vaporizer dial setting) and the inspired concentration. That is, when the vaporizer dial setting is adjusted to the desired concentration setting, the fresh gas plus anesthetic flowing from the vaporizer almost immediately contains the dialed anesthetic vapor concentration. In addition, the total gas flow is high relative to the volume of the delivery circuit, so the anesthetic concentration in the inspired breath is rapidly increased. However, with animals larger than 10 kg, a circle, CO_2 absorber (i.e., rebreathing), patient breathing circuit is most commonly used for inhalation anesthesia. The volume of this breathing circuit may be very large compared to fresh gas inflow. This volume markedly delays the rate of rise of inspired anesthetic concentration because the residual gas volume must be "washed out" and replaced by anesthetic containing fresh gas in order for the inspired concentration to increase to that delivered from the vaporizer (Fig. 11–11). In addition, rebreathing of exhaled gas (minus CO_2) occurs to varying degrees with these circuits. The inspired gas is composed of exhaled and fresh gases. Because the expired gas contains less anesthetic than the fresh gas, the inspired anesthetic gas concentration will be less than that of the fresh gas leaving the vaporizer.

In veterinary applications, the delaying influence of the circle circuit is most notable with anesthetic management of very large animals such as horses (15) and cattle and/or when using a closed circuit fresh-gas flow

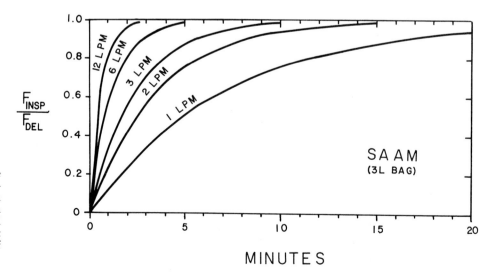

Fig. 11–11. A comparison of the rate of increase of inspired halothane concentration toward a constant delivered concentration F_{insp}/F_{del} in a 7-liter small animal anesthetic breathing circuit (SAAM) at fresh gas flow rates of 1, 3, 6, and 12 Lpm.(15)

Table 11–8. Vaporizer Positioning Within or Outside of a Circle Patient Rebreathing Circuit Influences Inspired Anesthetic Concentration (16)

Factor	Vaporizer Positioning	
	Out of Circuit	In Circuit
Increase ventilation	Decrease	Increase
Increase fresh gas (O_2) in-flow to circuit	Increase	Decrease

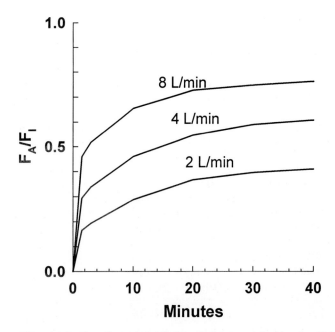

Fig. 11–12. The effect of ventilation on the rise of the alveolar (F_A) concentration of halothane toward the inspired (F_I) concentration. As noted, the F_A/F_I ratio increases more rapidly as ventilation is increased from 2 to 8 L/min. (Redrawn from Eger.) (9)

rate (i.e., where O_2 is the fresh gas and its inflow [plus anesthetic] to the circuit just meets the metabolic needs of the patient). With closed circuit delivery, the fresh gas inflow is very low relative to the circuit volume. (6, 9, 13)

The high solubility of some anesthetics (e.g., methoxyflurane; Table 11–6) in rubber and plastic will also delay development of an appropriate inspired anesthetic concentration. The loss of anesthetic to these equipment "sinks" serves to increase the apparent volume of the anesthetic circuitry and may, in some cases, be clinically important (e.g., the use of rubber hoses and a large rubber rebreathing bag on circuits designed for anesthetic management of horses).

Positioning the vaporizer in relation to the patient breathing circuit will influence inspired anesthetic concentration.(14, 16) For example, with the vaporizer positioned within a circle rebreathing circuit, a decrease in inspired concentration will follow an increase in fresh gas inflow to the circuit, whereas an increase in inspired concentration will result if the vaporizer is positioned outside the circuit (Table 11–8).

Alveolar Ventilation. An increase in alveolar ventilation increases the rate of delivery of inhalation anesthetic to the alveolus (Fig. 11–12). If unopposed by anesthetic tissue uptake, alveolar ventilation would rapidly increase the alveolar concentration of anesthetic so that within minutes the alveolar concentration would equal the inspired concentration. However, in reality the input created by alveolar ventilation is countered by absorption of anesthetic into blood. Predictably, hypoventilation decreases the rate at which the alveolar concentration increases over time compared to the inspired concentration (i.e., anesthetic induction is slowed). Alveolar ventilation is altered by changes in anesthetic depth (increased depth usually means decreased ventilation), mechanical ventilation (usually increased ventilation), and dead space ventilation (i.e., for constant minute ventilation a decrease in dead space ventilation results in an increase in alveolar ventilation) (Chapter 6).

Alveolar ventilation and thus the alveolar anesthetic concentration can also be influenced by administering a potent inhalation anesthetic like halothane in conjunction with N_2O. Very early in the administration of N_2O (during the period of large volume uptake; the first 5–10 minutes of delivery) the rate of rise of the alveolar concentration of the concurrently administered inhalation anesthetic is increased. This is commonly referred to as the *second gas effect,* and this phenomenon can be applied clinically to speed anesthetic induction. (9, 13, 17)

REMOVAL FROM ALVEOLI: UPTAKE BY BLOOD

As noted by Eger (13), anesthetic uptake is the product of three factors: solubility (S, the blood/gas solubility, Table 11–4), cardiac output (CO), and the difference in the anesthetic partial pressure between the alveolus and venous blood returning to the lungs (P_A P_v; expressed in mm Hg): that is,

$$Uptake = S \times CO(P_A - P_v/P_{bar})$$

where P_{bar} = barometric pressure in mm Hg. Note that if any of these three factors equals zero there is no further uptake of anesthetic by blood.

Solubility. As previously discussed the solubility of an inhalation anesthetic in blood and tissues is characterized by its partition coefficient (PC; Tables 11–4 and 11–5). Remember that a PC describes how an inhalation anesthetic distributes itself between two phases or two solvents (e.g., the quantity of agent in blood and alveoli [gas] or blood and muscle, respectively) once equilibrium is established (i.e., when the anesthetic partial pressure is equal). Based on blood/gas PCs, inhalation anesthetics range from highly soluble (methoxyflurane) to poorly soluble (N_2O and desflurane). Agents such as halothane and isoflurane are intermediary.

Compared to an anesthetic with high blood solubility (PC), an agent with low blood solubility is associated with a more rapid equilibration because a smaller amount of anesthetic must be dissolved in the blood before equilibrium is reached with the gas phase. In the

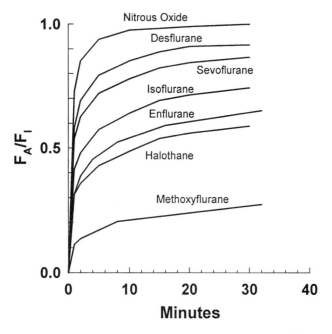

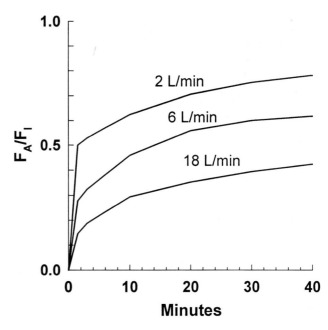

Fig. 11-13. The rise in the alveolar (F_A) anesthetic concentration toward the inspired (F_I) concentration. Note the rise is most rapid with the least soluble anesthetic, N_2O, and slowest with the most soluble anesthetic, methoxyflurane. All data are from studies of humans. (The curves are redrawn from Eger.) (63, 254)

Fig. 11-14. The effect of cardiac output on the rise of the alveolar (F_A) concentration of halothane toward the inspired (F_I) concentration. As noted, the F_A/F_I ratio increases more rapidly as cardiac output is decreased from 18 to 2 L/min. (Redrawn from Eger.) (9)

case of the agent with a high blood/gas PC, the blood acts like a large "sink" into which the anesthetic is poured and accordingly blood is "reluctant" to give up the agent to other tissues (such as the brain). The blood serves as a conduit for drug delivery to the brain and as such can be visualized as a pharmacologically inactive reservoir that is interposed between the lungs and the agent's site of desired pharmacologic activity (i.e., brain). Therefore, an anesthetic agent with a low blood/gas PC is usually more desirable than a highly soluble agent, because it is associated with (a) a more rapid anesthetic induction (i.e., more rapid rate of rise in alveolar concentration during induction; Fig. 11-13); (b) more precise control of anesthetic depth (i.e., alveolar concentration during the anesthetic maintenance); and (c) a more rapid elimination of anesthetic and recovery (i.e., a rapid decrease in alveolar concentration during recovery).

Cardiac output. The amount of blood flowing through the lungs and on to body tissues also influences anesthetic uptake from the lungs. The greater the CO, the more blood passing through the lungs carrying away anesthetic from the alveoli. Thus a large CO, like increased anesthetic agent blood solubility, delays the alveolar rise of P_{anes} (Fig. 11-14). Patient excitement is an example in which a relatively large CO is anticipated. Conversely, a reduced CO should be anticipated with a patient in shock. Such a situation would be associated with an increase in the rate of rise of the P_A of the anesthetic, making anesthetic induction more rapid and risky.

Alveolar to Venous Anesthetic Partial Pressure Difference. The magnitude of difference in anesthetic partial

pressure between the alveoli and venous blood is related to the amount of uptake of anesthetic by tissues. It is not surprising that the largest gradient occurs during induction. Once the tissues no longer absorb anesthetic (i.e., equilibrium is reached), there is no longer any uptake of anesthetic from the lungs because $P_v = P_A$ (i.e., the venous blood returning to the lungs contains as much anesthetic as when it left the lungs). The changes in gradient between the initiation of induction and equilibration result in part from the relative distribution of CO. In this regard it is important to recognize that roughly 70 to 80% of the CO is normally directed to only a small volume of body tissues in a lean individual (Chapter 5).(18, 19) Tissues such as the brain, heart, hepatoportal system, and kidneys represent only about 10% of the body mass but normally receive about 75% of the total blood flow each minute. As a result, these highly perfused tissues equilibrate with arterial anesthetic partial pressure rapidly when compared to other body tissues (actual timing is influenced by agent solubility). Since the venous anesthetic pressure or tension equals that in the tissue within 10 or 15 minutes, about 75% of the blood returning to the lungs is the same as the alveolar tension. This presumes there has been no change in arterial anesthetic partial pressure during this time and thus uptake is reduced. Skin and muscle comprise the major bulk of the body (about 50% in humans) but at rest receive only about 15 to 20% of the CO, so saturation of these tissues takes a few hours to accomplish. Fat is a variable component of body bulk and receives only a small proportion of blood flow. Consequently, anesthetic saturation of this tissue is very slow because all anesthetics are considerably more soluble in fat than other tissue groups (Tables 11–4 and 11–5).

Other factors can influence the magnitude of the alveolar to arterial anesthetic partial pressure gradient. For example, abnormalities of ventilation/perfusion result in an alveolar-arterial gradient proportional to the degree of abnormality.(20) Others include loss of anesthetic via the skin (21-23) and into closed gas spaces (9, 13, 17) and metabolism.(9, 13)

Overview. The rate with which the alveolar anesthetic concentration increases relative to the inspired concentration (i.e., the rate of change in anesthetic level) is often summarized as a plot of the ratio of F_A/F_I versus time. The position of individual curves representing different anesthetics on a plot is related to the solubility characteristics of the anesthetics (Fig. 11–13). The shape of the graph of F_A/F_I versus time is similar for all anesthetics (Fig. 11–13). There is a rapid rise initially that results from the effect of alveolar ventilation bringing anesthetic into the lung. There is then a decrease in the rate of rise of the curve as uptake by the blood occurs. With time the highly perfused tissues of the body equilibrate with incoming blood so that eventually about three quarters of the total blood flow returning to the heart has the same anesthetic partial pressure as it had when it left the lungs. Thus, further uptake from the lung is decreased and the rate of approach of the F_A to F_I over time is further decreased.

ANESTHETIC ELIMINATION

Recovery from inhalation anesthesia results from the elimination of anesthetic from the brain. This requires a decrease in alveolar anesthetic partial pressure (concentration), which in turn fosters a decrease in arterial and then brain anesthetic partial pressure (Fig. 11–10). Prominent factors accounting for recovery are the same as those for anesthetic induction. Therefore, factors such as alveolar ventilation, cardiac output, and especially agent solubility greatly influence recovery from inhalation anesthesia. Indeed, the graphic curves representing the washout of anesthetic from alveoli versus time (Fig. 11–15) are essentially inverses of the wash-in curves. That is, the washout of the less soluble anesthetics is high at first (i.e., rapid washout by ventilation of the lung functional residual capacity), then rapidly declines to a lower output level that continues to decrease but at a slower rate. The washout of more soluble agents is also high at first, but the magnitude of decrease in alveolar anesthetic concentration is less and decreases more gradually with time (Fig. 11–15).

A factor that is important during the washout period is the duration of anesthesia. This effect and a comparison of this effect between three agents spanning a range of blood solubilities is summarized in Figure 11–16.(24) If a patient rebreathing anesthetic circuit (e.g., circle system) is in use and the patient is not disconnected from the circuit at the end of anesthesia, the circuit itself may also reduce the rate of recovery, just as the circuit was shown to decrease the rate of rise of anesthetic during induction. This influence of rebreathing circuits can be reduced by directing high flow rates of anesthetic-free O_2 into the anesthetic circuit.

Other factors that are important to varying degrees to inhalation anesthetic elimination from the body include percutaneous loss, intertissue diffusion of agents, and metabolism. Transcutaneous movement of inhalation agent occurs, but the amount under consideration is small.(21-23, 25) Intertissue diffusion is of theoretical interest, but its clinical importance is limited.(26, 27) Metabolism may also play a small role with some inhalation anesthetics (e.g., methoxyflurane and perhaps even halothane), especially when associated with prolonged anesthesia.(26, 28-30)

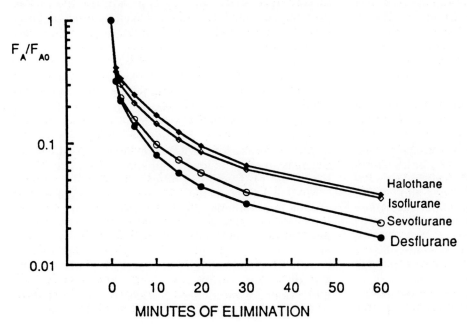

Fig. 11–15. The fall in alveolar (F_A) concentration relative to the alveolar concentration at the end of anesthesia (F_{AO}). Note that the newest, most insoluble, volatile anesthetic, desflurane, is eliminated in humans more rapidly than the other contemporary potent anesthetics. Not shown is information for methoxyflurane. If present, the curve for methoxyflurane would appear above that for halothane. (From Eger with permission.) (254)

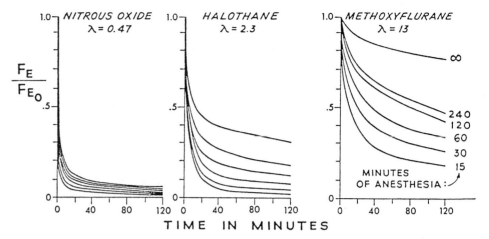

Fig. 11–16. The decrease in the alveolar (F_E) anesthetic concentration from the concentration at the time of breathing circuit disconnect (i.e., the beginning of recovery from anesthesia; F_{EO}) is influenced by both the solubility (λ) of anesthetic and the duration of anesthesia. (From Stoelting and Eger with permission.) (24)

A special consideration associated with recovery following use of N_2O also deserves comment. *Diffusion hypoxia* is a possibility at the end of N_2O administration when the patient breathes air immediately rather than O_2 for at least a brief transition period (i.e., 5–10 minutes).(31-33) In this case a large volume of N_2O enters the lung from the blood. This early rapid inflow of N_2O to the lung displaces other gases within the lung. If at this time the patient is breathing air (only about 21% O_2) rather than 100% O_2, N_2O dilutes alveolar O_2, further reducing O_2 tension from levels found in ambient air. This action may cause life-threatening reductions in arterial oxygenation. Since the major effect is in the first few minutes after discontinuing N_2O, the condition can be prevented by administering pure O_2 at the conclusion of N_2O administration rather than allowing the patient to immediately breathe ambient air.

BIOTRANSFORMATION

Inhalation anesthetics are not chemically inert.(34) They undergo varying degrees of metabolism primarily in the liver, but also to lesser degrees in the lung, kidney, and intestinal tract.(28, 35-38) The importance of this is twofold. First, in a very limited way with older anesthetics, metabolism may facilitate anesthetic recovery. Second and more important is the potential for acute and chronic toxicities by intermediary or end-metabolites of inhalation agents, especially on kidneys, liver, and reproductive organs.(28, 38)

The magnitude of metabolism of inhalation anesthetic agents is determined by a variety of factors including the chemical structure, hepatic enzyme activity (cytochrome P = 450 enzymes located in the endoplasmic reticulum of the hepatocyte), the blood concentration of the anesthetic(39), disease states, and genetic factors (i.e., some species and individuals are more active metabolizers of these drugs than others, e.g., humans vs rats).

An indication of the extent of biotransformation of contemporary inhalation anesthetics is given in Table 11–9. The degradation of sevoflurane occurs in vivo to about the same extent as isoflurane and as indicated by transient postanesthetic increases in blood and urinary

fluoride levels in rats(40-44), dogs(42), and humans.(45) The peak serum fluoride concentrations observed in humans during and following sevoflurane anesthesia are low, and nephrotoxicity is not expected.(45, 46) Desflurane resists degradation in vivo.(47-49) The increase in serum inorganic fluoride is much smaller than that found with isoflurane.(47, 49)

For further information on the biotransformation of inhalation anesthetics in general and for specific details regarding individual anesthetic agents readers are referred to reviews by Baden and Rice (28) and Mazze and Fujinaga.(38)

Anesthetic Dose: the Minimum Alveolar Concentration (MAC)

The term *potency* refers to the quantity of an inhalant anesthetic that must be administered to cause a desired effect (e.g., general anesthesia). In the case of anesthetics there is an obvious clinical need to have an appropriate quantitative expression of central nervous system depression (i.e., general anesthesia) because there are variable influences on vital organ function that accompany the use of general anesthetics. In 1963 Merkel and Eger described what has become the standard index of anesthetic potency for inhalation anesthetics, MAC (Chapter 2).(50) Anesthetic potency of an inhaled anesthetic is inversely related to MAC (i.e., potency = 1/MAC). From information presented earlier, it also follows that MAC is inversely related to the oil/gas PC. Thus, a very potent anesthetic (e.g., methoxyflurane) has a low MAC value and a high oil/gas PC, whereas an agent of low anesthetic potency (e.g., N_2O) has a high MAC and low oil/gas PC.

MAC is defined as the minimum alveolar concentration of an anesthetic at one atmosphere that produces immobility in 50% of subjects exposed to a supramaximal noxious stimulus. Thus MAC corresponds to the effective dose$_{50}$ or ED$_{50}$; half of the subjects are anesthetized and half have not yet reached that "level." The dose that corresponds to the ED$_{95}$ (95% of the individuals are anesthetized), at least in humans, is 20 to 40% greater than MAC.(51)

A number of characteristics of MAC deserve emphasis.(9) MAC is defined in terms of a percent of one atmosphere and therefore represents an anesthetic partial pressure at the anesthetic site of action (i.e., remember $P_x = (C/100) \cdot P_{bar}$, where P_x stands for the partial pressure of the anesthetic in the gas mixture, C is the anesthetic concentration in vol % and P_{bar} is the barometric or total pressure of the gas mixture). Thus, although the concentration at MAC for a given agent may vary depending on ambient pressure conditions (e.g., sea level vs high altitude), the anesthetic partial pressure always remains the same.

Second, the A in MAC represents *alveolar* concentration, not inspired or delivered (as for example, from a vaporizer). This is important because the alveolar concentration is easily monitored with contemporary technology. Also, as we reviewed earlier, after sufficient time for equilibration (minutes) alveolar partial pressure will closely approximate arterial and brain anesthetic partial pressures.

Finally, it is important to note that MAC is determined in healthy animals under laboratory conditions in the *absence* of other drugs and circumstances common to clinical use that may modify the requirements for anesthesia. General techniques for determining MAC in animals are given elsewhere.(9, 52-56)

The MAC values for contemporary inhalation anesthetics for a variety of animals commonly encountered in veterinary medicine are summarized in Table 11-10. Values for humans are also given for comparison. Readers interested in values for agents such as diethyl ether or cyclopropane are referred elsewhere.(9, 52, 53)

In a single species the variability in MAC is generally small and is not substantially influenced by gender, duration of anesthesia, variation of $PaCO_2$ (from 10 to 90 mm Hg), metabolic alkalosis or acidosis, variation in PaO_2 (from 40 to 500 mm Hg), moderate anemia, or moderate hypotension (9, 52, 53) (Table 11-11). Even between species the variability in MAC for a given agent is usually not large. However, there is at least one notable exception (Table 11-10). In humans, the MAC for N_2O is 104%, making it the least potent of the inhalation anesthetics currently used in this species. Its potency in other species is less than half that in humans (i.e., around 200%). Because the N_2O MAC is above

100% it cannot be used by itself at one atmosphere pressure in any species and still provide adequate amounts of O_2. Consequently, and assuming that MAC values for combinations of inhaled anesthetics are additive, N_2O is usually administered with another more potent agent to thereby reduce the concentration of the second agent necessary for anesthesia (Fig. 11-17). However, because of the potency difference between animals and humans the amount of reduction differs in an important way. For example, administration of 60% N_2O with halothane reduces the amount of halothane needed to produce MAC by about 55% in healthy humans (Fig. 11-17) but reduces it only by about 20 to 30% in dogs. As noted in Figure 11-17, the response of other animals most closely resembles the dog. Some factors that are known to influence MAC are given in Table 11-11. Several other factors influencing MAC have been reviewed in Chapter 2.

Equipotent doses (i.e., equivalent concentrations of different anesthetics at MAC) are useful for comparing effects of inhalation anesthetics on vital organs. In this regard anesthetic dose is commonly defined in terms of multiples of MAC (i.e., 1.5 or 2.0 times MAC, or simply 1.5 MAC or 2.0 MAC). From the preceding discussion, therefore, the ED_{50} equals MAC or 1.0 MAC and represents a light level of anesthesia (clearly inadequate in 50% of otherwise unmedicated, healthy animals). The ED_{95} is 1.2 to 1.4 MAC, and 2.0 MAC represents a deep level of anesthesia, in some cases even an anesthetic overdose. The concept of MAC multiples can be used to compare drug effects and contrast doses of a specific drug.

Pharmacodynamics: Actions and Toxicity of the Volatile Inhalation Anesthetics on Body Systems

All contemporary inhalation anesthetic agents in one way or another influence vital organ function. Some actions are inevitable and accompany the use of all agents, whereas other actions are a special or prominent feature of one or a number of the agents. Differences in action, and especially undesirable action, of specific anesthetic agents forms the basis for selecting one agent over another for a particular patient and/or procedure. Undesirable actions also provide primary impetus for development of new agents and/or anesthetic techniques.

Data from healthy animals exposed to equipotent alveolar concentrations of these drugs under controlled circumstances provide foundation information for this review. In other cases, results of studies of human volunteers form the basis of our understanding of some drug actions. Because animals are commonly allowed to breathe spontaneously during general anesthesia (vs controlled mechanical ventilation) it usually is considered baseline. It is important to stress that many variables other than mode of ventilation commonly accompany anesthetic management of animals in both clinical and laboratory settings. These variables influence drug pharmacodynamics and may cause individuals to respond differently than test subjects that were

Table 11-9. Biotransformation of Inhalation Anesthetics in Humans

Anesthetic	Anesthetic Recovered as Metabolites (%)
Methoxyflurane[37]	50
Halothane[36,262]	20-25
Sevoflurane[92]	3.0
Enflurane[263]	2.4
Isoflurane[264]	0.17
Desflurane[92]	0.02
Nitrous oxide[215]	0.004

References indicated by superscript.

Table 11–10.　MAC Values for a Variety of Species

	Methoxyflurane	Halothane	Isoflurane	Enflurane	Sevoflurane	Desflurane	N$_2$O
Cat	0.23[265]	1.14[266] 0.82[268] 1.19[269] 0.99[270]	1.63[105] 1.61[269]	1.20[265] 2.37[269]	2.58[66]	9.79[267]	255.00[266]
Dog	0.23[271] 0.24[276] 0.29[277]	0.86[272] 0.87[266,276] 0.92[278] 0.93[281] 0.89[274]	1.28[105] 1.39[274] 1.30[86]	2.20[273] 2.06[87] 2.25[279] 2.06[279]	2.36[274] 2.10[66]	7.20[275]	188.00[271] 222.00[266] 297.00[280]
Horse	0.28[346]	0.88[54]	1.31[54]	2.12[54]	2.31[282]		205.00[147]
Monkey		0.89[266] 1.15[283]	1.28[283] 1.46[86]	1.84[283] 1.97[284] 2.19[285]			200.00[266]
Mouse		0.96[284] 1.00[285]	1.35[284] 1.41[285]				275.00[285] 150.00[286]
Calf		0.76[287]					223.00[287]
Pig		0.91[288] 1.25[291] 0.94[344]	1.45[289] 2.04[56] 1.51[86] 1.55[293] 1.75[344]		2.66[290] 1.97[292]	10.00[56]	277.00[291] 162.00[293] 195.00[344]
Rabbit		0.82[294] 0.80[297] 1.39[295] 1.56[298]	2.05[295]	2.86[295]	3.70[296]	8.90[275]	
Rat	0.27[299]	1.17[299] 0.81[300] 1.11[304] 1.10[301] 1.13[309,310] 1.03[284] 1.23[306]	1.17[300] 1.38[304] 1.52[284] 1.46[306]	2.17[284]	2.40[301] 2.50[40]	5.72[302] 7.10[305] 6.85[306]	136.00[303] 204.00[110] 155.00[307] 235.00[308] 221.00[308]
Sheep	0.26[311]	0.97[311]	1.58[311]				
Birds							
Chicken		0.85[55]					
Ducks		1.04[312]	1.30[313]				
Cranes			1.34[314]				
Pigeon			1.51[315]				154.00[315]
Hawk			1.45[315]				220.00[315]
Amazon Parrot			1.47[316]				
Cockatoo			1.44[316]				
African Gray Parrot			1.91[316]				
Miscellaneous							
Toad	0.22[317]	0.67[317]					82.20[317]
Goldfish	0.13[318]	0.76[318]					
Human	0.16[319]	0.77[319] 0.73[324] 0.74[326,327]	1.15[320]	1.68[321]	2.05[296] 1.71[325]	6.00[322] 7.25[322]	104.00[323]

References indicated by superscript.

studied under standardized conditions. Such confounding variables include species, duration of anesthesia, noxious (surgical) stimulation, coexisting disease, concurrent medications, and extremes of age as examples.

CENTRAL NERVOUS SYSTEM (CNS)

Inhalation anesthetics induce a reversible generalized CNS depression. The degree of depression is often described as depth of anesthesia (Chapter 7). Cerebral electric activity varies with anesthetic dose. Several

Table 11–11. Some Factors That Influence the Value of MAC (Anesthetic Requirement)

Increase
Hyperthermia (to 42° C)
Hypernatremia
Drugs causing CNS stimulation
  amphetamine
  ephedrine
  morphine (horse[328])
  laudanosine[298]
  physostigmine[329]

No change
Duration of anesthetic
Hyperkalemia, hypokalemia
Gender
$Paco_2$ (15–95 mm Hg)
Pao_2 > 40 mm Hg
Arterial blood pressure > 50 mm Hg[330]
Metabolic acid-base change
Atropine, Glycopyrrolate, Scopolamine (peripheral)[270]

Decrease
Hypothermia
Hyponatremia
Pregnancy
Pao_2 < 40 mm Hg
$Paco_2$ > 95 mm Hg
Arterial blood pressure < 50 mm Hg
Increasing adult age
Drugs causing CNS depression
  other inhalation anesthetics
  • N_2O[17]
  injectable anesthetics
  • ketamine[331]
  • thiopental[332]
  preanesthetic medication
  • xylazine[333,345]
  • medetomidine[334,335]
  • morphine[86]
  • alfentanil[336]
  • fentanyl[337]
  • midazolam[337]
  • diazepam[333,338]
  • acepromazine[333,339]
  • meperidine[333,340]
  other
  • adenosine[341]
  • central anticholinergic[329]
  • 5HT antagonist[342]

Lists of example drugs are intended to be representative, not exhaustive.
(Summarized from Eger [9], Quasha et al., [52] and Cullen [53] except where indicated by superscript reference numbers.)

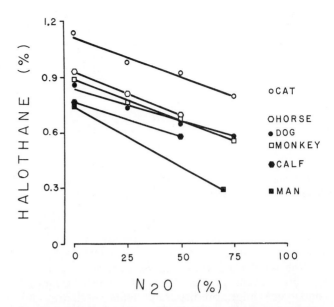

Fig. 11–17. The alveolar concentration of halothane needed to produce MAC decreases when halothane is combined with N_2O. The halothane sparing imposed by N_2O is less in animals compared to humans. (From Steffey and Eger with permission.) (149)

studies have attempted to correlate depth of anesthesia with various EEG parameters.(57-60) In general, as the depth of anesthesia (i.e., concentration of anesthetic) is increased from awake states, the electric activity of the cerebral cortex becomes desynchronized. There is initially an increased frequency of the EEG activity. With further increases in anesthetic concentration, a decrease in frequency and increased amplitude of EEG waves occur (Chapter 7A). Because of these general changes, some studies have attempted to correlate depth of anesthesia with various EEG parameters. However, despite some weak correlations and its usefulness as an indication of changing anesthetic depth, no parameter has had sensitivity and specificity sufficient to justify use of the EEG alone as a reliable index of anesthetic depth.(61)

Several anesthetics in contemporary use have epileptogenic potential, especially in individuals predisposed to seizures. Enflurane is most prominent in this regard among inhalant anesthetics. Seizure activity is of concern because neuronal injury may result if demands for substrate (especially O_2) for maintaining neuronal function are greater than supply. A second concern is trauma to the patient experiencing tonic/clonic muscle twitching, especially in the horse. People assisting in the anesthetic and surgical management of these large patients may become injured. Finally, there is concern that seizures may persist into the postanesthetic period, especially in unpredictable fashion and when they occur in less-well-controlled circumstances.

A systematic study of EEG activity in dogs showed that enflurane was associated with spontaneous or noise-initiated intensified seizures. In addition, enflurane induces seizure activity that is associated with substantial increases in cerebral blood flow and cerebral metabolic use of O_2. In the studies by Joas et al.(62), halothane, methoxyflurane, and isoflurane did not cause the frank epileptoid activity in dogs that was induced by enflurane. Indeed, both halothane and isoflurane have the capacity to produce an isoelectric EEG, with isoflurane doing so at a lower dose.(63)

Table 11–12. Apneic Index in Various Species

	Species									
	Cat		Dog		Rat		Horse		Humans	
Agent	MAC	AI	MAC	AI	MAC	AI	MAC	AI	MAC	AI
Desflurane									7.25[322]	1.8[71]
Enflurane	–	–	2.06	2.57[87]	2.17[284]	1.8[110]	2.12	2.26[54]	1.68[321]	1.6[71]
Halothane	–	–	0.87	2.90[276]	1.11[304]	2.3[111]	0.88	2.60[54]	0.77[319]	2.3[71]
Isoflurane	1.63	2.40[105]	1.28	2.51[105]	1.38[304]	3.1[110]	1.31	2.33[54]	1.15[320]	1.7[71]
Methoxyflurane	0.24	3.4[276]	0.24	3.4[276]	0.27[299]	2.2[110]				

MAC, minimal alveolar concentration in vol %; AI, apneic index = % at apnea/MAC; $\overline{X} \pm SE$
Reference numbers are given as superscripts.

The EEG responses with the two newest anesthetics, desflurane and sevoflurane, are reportedly similar to those of isoflurane(58, 64), but not devoid of CNS actions.(65, 66) Because of the EEG activating property of enflurane it seems prudent to avoid its use in situations when events might predispose patients to seizures and when reasonable anesthetic alternatives exist.

RESPIRATORY SYSTEM

Inhalation anesthetics depress respiratory system function. The volatile agents in particular affect ventilation in a drug-specific and species-specific manner. In general, spontaneous ventilation progressively decreases as inhalation anesthetic dose is increased because at low doses tidal volume decreases more than frequency increases. As anesthetic dose is further increased, respiratory frequency also decreases. In otherwise unmedicated animals respiratory arrest occurs at 2 to 3 MAC (Table 11–12). The overall decrease in minute ventilation and the likely variable increase in dead space ventilation (resulting in an increase in the dead space to tidal volume ratio, V_D/V_t, from a normal of about 0.3 to 0.5 or more) results in a reduction in alveolar ventilation (Chapter 6). Decreases in alveolar ventilation are out of proportion to decreases in CO_2 production (O_2 utilization is decreased by general anesthesia), such that $PaCO_2$ increases (Fig. 11–18). In addition, the normal stimulation to ventilation caused by increased $PaCO_2$ (or decreased PaO_2) is depressed by the inhalation anesthetics; presumably via the action of these agents directly on the medullary and peripheral (aortic and carotid body) chemoreceptors.(63) Changes in perianesthetic PaO_2 other than what might be related to the magnitude of alveolar ventilation are not notably different among the various inhalation anesthetics in a given species.

Bronchospasm is associated with some diseases and other patient conditions and contribute to increased airway resistance. A variety of studies strongly suggest that among anesthetics, halothane is the most effective bronchodilator.(67, 68) It therefore has been the anesthetic agent of choice for patients at risk of bronchospasm. The work of Hirshman and colleagues suggests that isoflurane and perhaps enflurane are as effective in decreasing experimentally produced airway resistance and therefore are good alternatives to halothane.(69, 70)

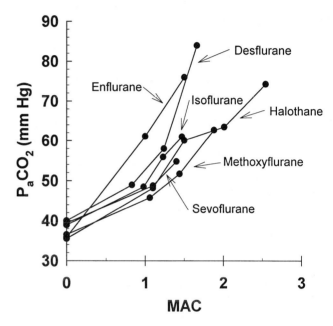

Fig. 11–18. Respiratory response to an increase in the alveolar concentration (expressed in as a multiple of MAC) of inhalation anesthetics in humans. (Data are taken from multiple sources.) (71-76)

Comparable data are not yet available for the two newest agents, desflurane and sevoflurane.

Arterial Carbon Dioxide Tension (PaCO₂). The $PaCO_2$ is the most frequently used index of respiratory system response to general anesthetics. All contemporary inhalation anesthetics depress alveolar ventilation and as a consequence increase $PaCO_2$ in dose-related fashion. Figure 11–18 summarizes the effects of inhalation anesthetics in humans, the species for which data are most complete.(71-76) As Figure 11–18 indicates, enflurane is the agent that is most depressing to ventilation and halothane is the least. Although there is some difference in the rank order of the anesthetics between species, the difference is generally small.

FACTORS INFLUENCING RESPIRATORY EFFECTS

Mode of Ventilation. Ventilation is often assisted or controlled during inhalation anesthesia to compensate for the anesthetic-induced respiratory depression. Controlled mechanical ventilation (i.e., the anesthetist controls both respiratory frequency and tidal volume) is used to predictably maintain a normal PaCO$_2$ during anesthesia (Chapter 17). Assisted ventilation (i.e., the anesthetist augments tidal volume but the animal determines its own breathing frequency) is used to attempt to improve the efficiency of oxygenating arterial blood and reduce the work of breathing but is usually not effective in substantially lowering PaCO$_2$ compared to circumstances associated with spontaneous ventilation (i.e., the animal controls both the rate and depth of breathing).(77-79)

Surgery and Other Noxious Stimulation. Noxious stimulation may result in sufficient central nervous stimulation to lessen the ventilatory depression of the inhalation anesthetic.(80, 81) The effect is diminished with increasing anesthetic depth. In some circumstances respiratory depression, as evidenced by an increasing PaCO$_2$, may increase with anesthetic duration. Changes are most notable in the horse anesthetized with a constant doses of isoflurane.(82, 83)

Concurrent Drugs. In humans the substitution of N$_2$O for an equivalent amount of a concurrently administered, more potent volatile agent such as isoflurane results in a lower PaCO$_2$ than the volatile agent alone.(17) In dogs and monkeys anesthetized with halothane, ventilation was at least as, and sometimes more, depressed when N$_2$O was substituted for a portion of the halothane requirement.(84, 85) The addition of opioid drugs like morphine may increase the respiratory depression produced by an inhalation anesthetic.(81, 86)

CARDIOVASCULAR SYSTEM

All of the volatile inhalation anesthetics cause dose-dependent and drug-specific changes in cardiovascular performance. The magnitude and sometimes direction of change may be influenced by other variables that often accompany general anesthesia (Table 11–13). The mechanisms of cardiovascular effects are diverse but often include direct myocardial depression and a decrease in sympathoadrenal activity.

Cardiac Output (CO). All of the volatile anesthetics decrease CO. The magnitude of change is dose related and dependent upon agent. In general, enflurane is most depressing to CO and isoflurane least.(63, 87-91) As with isoflurane, desflurane and sevoflurane tend to preserve CO at clinically useful concentrations.(90, 92-96) The decrease in CO is largely due to a decrease

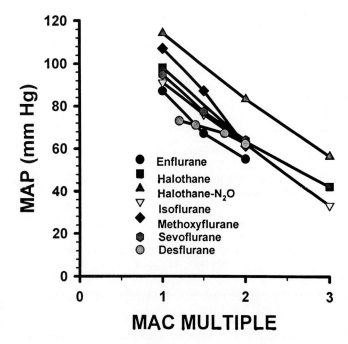

Fig. 11–19. Inhalation anesthetics cause a dose (expressed as multiples of MAC) dependent decrease in mean arterial blood pressure (MAP) in dogs whose ventilation is mechanically controlled to produce eucapnia. Data are from the literature and referenced in the text.

in stroke volume as a result of dose-related depression in myocardial contractility.(63, 96-100)

The effect of inhalation anesthetics on heart rate (HR) is variable and depends on agent and species. For example, in humans HR is not substantially altered with halothane anesthesia but is usually increased by enflurane, isoflurane, desflurane, and sevoflurane.(63, 92, 96, 101) Compared to conditions in awake, calm dogs, HR is increased with all four of the anesthetics listed.(95) The HR usually remains constant over a range of clinically useful alveolar concentrations in the absence of other modifying factors (e.g., noxious stimulation).(63, 87, 88, 90, 95, 102) The distribution of blood flow to organs is altered during inhalation anesthesia. Readers with special interest in these changes are referred elsewhere for further information.(63, 103, 104)

Arterial Blood Pressure. Volatile anesthetics cause a dose-dependent decrease in arterial blood pressure (Fig. 11–19).(87, 89, 93, 105-107) In general, the dose-related decrease in arterial blood pressure is similar regardless of the species studied.(54, 63, 87, 89, 91, 105, 106, 108, 109) The decrease in blood pressure is usually related at least to a decrease in stroke volume regardless of the agent or species studied. In some cases (agent and/or species) a decrease in peripheral vascular resistance may also play an important but lesser role. Indices of anesthetic influence on cardiovascular collapse are given in Table 11–14.(87, 110, 111)

Cardiac Rhythm and Catecholamines. Inhalation anesthetics may increase the automaticity of the myocardium and the likelihood of propagated impulses from

Table 11–13.   Factors That Influence Cardiovascular Effects of Inhalation Anesthetics

Anesthetic dose
Magnitude of PaCO$_2$
Mechanical ventilation
Noxious stimulation
Duration of anesthesia
Concurrent drug therapy
Intravascular fluid volume

Table 11–14. Anesthetic-Induced Cardiovascular Depression as Expressed by Cardiovascular Anesthetc Indices

Agent	Dog[a]	Pig[b]	Rat[c]	Rhesus Monkey[d]
Desflurane-O_2	—	2.45	—	—
Enflurane-O_2	4.10	—	3.3	2.24
Halothane-O_2	4.43	—	3.0	2.38
Halothane–50% N_2O	—	—	3.7	—
Isoflurane-O_2	4.11	3.02	5.7	—
Methoxyflurane-O_2	—	—	3.7	—

[a]The theoretical anesthetic concentration at zero mean arterial pressure related to MAC.(87)
[b]Mean fatal dose (343).
[c]Heart concentration of anesthetic at cardiovascular failure related to heart concentration of anesthetic at establishment of anesthesia (110, 111).
[d]The theoretical anesthetic concentration at zero mean arterial pressure related to MAC.(87)

ectopic sites, especially from within the ventricle (Chapter 5).(112) This effect is exaggerated by adrenergic agonists.(113) The association of cardiac dysrhythmias with adrenergic drugs and anesthetic agents has received extensive study.

Inhalation anesthetics may sensitize the heart to arrhythmogenic effects of catecholamines. Halothane is most notable in this regard, as it markedly reduces the amount of epinephrine necessary to cause ventricular premature contractions.(114) There is some evidence that deeper levels of halothane decrease this incidence(115-117), but this is not a consistent finding.(118) Enflurane and methoxyflurane are less potent in regard to their ability to sensitize the heart to arrhythmogenic effects of epinephrine, and isoflurane, desflurane, and sevoflurane are least arrhythmogenic.(63, 92, 117, 119-123) Such considerations are important in the design of anesthetic plans for patients in which it is desirable/necessary to administer catecholamines, for example, local application to minimize blood oozing from highly vascular surgical sites or in patients in which high blood levels of endogenous catecholamines are anticipated.(124, 125)

FACTORS INFLUENCING CIRCULATORY EFFECTS

A variety of circumstances occasionally or usually associated with the anesthetic management of veterinary patients that may add to or oppose the primary effects of the anesthetic. In most cases the most profound modifications of drug action are on cardiovascular function. They may include mechanical ventilation and alterations in $PaCO_2$, noxious (surgical) stimulation, duration of anesthesia, and coexisting drugs.

Mode of Ventilation and $PaCO_2$. There may be considerable difference in the cardiovascular effects of inhalation anesthetics in animals breathing spontaneously versus when breathing is mechanically controlled (e.g., intermittent positive pressure ventilation or IPPV) to produce and maintain a normal $PaCO_2$. In general, and considering a broad range of circumstances, cardiovascular function is usually depressed during IPPV relative to actions during spontaneous ventilation. Such action results from either the direct

mechanical actions (i.e., intermittent elevation of intrathoracic pressure and resultant decrease in venous return to the heart) or lessening of the indirect pharmacologic action of $PaCO_2$(126) or both. Carbon dioxide has three pharmacologic actions important to these considerations; an increased $PaCO_2$ has direct depressant actions on the heart and smooth muscle of the peripheral blood vessels (i.e., dilation) and indirect (via sympathetic nervous system) stimulation of circulatory function.

In sympathetically intact animals, the stimulatory actions of CO_2 usually predominate, so increased CO and arterial blood pressure usually accompany an increase in $PaCO_2$, becoming lower when $PaCO_2$ is normalized.(77, 89, 91, 108, 109, 127-130)

Noxious Stimulation. Noxious stimulation during anesthesia modifies the circulatory effect of inhalation anesthetics via stimulation of the sympathetic nervous system. An increase in arterial blood pressure and heart rate (cardiac output) commonly accompanies noxious stimulation.(81, 131, 132) The response is anesthetic dose related. For example, Roizen et al. showed that deeper levels of halothane and enflurane decreased or prevented surgically induced increases in serum norepinephrine levels in human patients.(131) Anesthetic doses that block the response are in the range of 1.5 to 2.0 MAC.(131, 132)

Duration of Anesthesia. Some cardiovascular effects of inhalation anesthetics may change with duration of anesthesia. For example in humans, halothane anesthesia lasting 5 to 6 hours is associated with an increase in values of some measures of cardiovascular function such as CO and heart rate.(128, 133) Similarly, varying degrees of time-related changes have been reported with enflurane (75), desflurane (134), and others.(135-138)

Temporal changes in cardiovascular function have also been reported in a variety of animals with halothane (139-142) and isoflurane.(82, 141) Dose of anesthetic (83, 135, 139) and body posture during anesthesia (143, 144) apparently also play a temporal role in some species.

The causes of these changes remain unclear. In vitro, depression of the cat papillary muscle exposed to a constant concentration of halothane does not vary over a 3-hour period.(145) This observation suggests that temporal effects associated with inhalation anesthetics are not the result of improved intrinsic cardiac function. Studies of human volunteers have shown that temporal responses to halothane can be prevented if the subjects are given propranolol before anesthesia, suggesting the mechanism is related to increasing sympathetic nervous system activity.(146)

Usually the temporal changes associated with inhalation anesthetics are of only minor or no concern to the clinician but must be considered in interpreting results of laboratory studies in which these agents are used for anesthetic management.

Concurrent Drugs. Drugs administered immediately before or in conjunction with inhalation anesthetics (preanesthetic medication, injectable anesthetic induction drugs, vasoactive and cardiotonic drugs, etc.) may influence cardiovascular function by altering the anesthetic requirement (i.e., MAC) or by their own specific cardiovascular actions.

For example, N_2O is used on occasion to substitute for a portion of a more potent inhalation anesthetic. In reducing the amount of the potent volatile agent, some cardiovascular sparing usually occurs. Nitrous oxide also may depress the myocardium directly, but these effects are usually counterbalanced by its sympathomimetic effect and indirect stimulation of cardiovascular function. Thus the resultant effect of its use is related to the amount administered and the interaction between N_2O and the basal anesthetic. Overall its use usually promotes slight cardiovascular sparing effect when compared to the use of more potent inhalants alone. The magnitude of N_2O effect is clinically limited and species dependent.(84, 85, 106, 147, 148) A more complete summary of its cardiovascular actions appears elsewhere.(100, 149)

Injectable drugs such as acepromazine, alpha$_2$-agonists, thiobarbiturates, dissociatives (e.g., ketamine), and others are frequently administered to animals as part of their anesthetic management. They confound the primary effects of the inhalation anesthetics and may accentuate cardiovascular depression. On the other hand, sympathomimetic drugs such as ephedrine (150), dopamine, and dobutamine(151, 152) are frequently given to counteract unwanted cardiovascular depressions of the anesthetic.

EFFECTS ON THE KIDNEYS

All present-day potent inhalation anesthetics reduce renal blood flow and glomerular filtration rate in a dose-related manner. This action is a common finding regardless of the species studied. During anesthesia healthy animals produce small volumes of concentrated urine. An increase in serum urea nitrogen, creatinine, and inorganic phosphate may accompany especially prolonged anesthesia.(63, 153-156) The reduction in renal function is highly influenced by the animal's state of hydration and hemodynamics during anesthesia. Accordingly, attendant intravenous fluid therapy and

prevention of a marked reduction in renal blood flow will lessen or counteract the tendency for reduced renal function (Chapter 24). In most cases effects of inhalation anesthesia on renal function are usually rapidly reversed after anesthesia.

Among the inhalation anesthetics, methoxyflurane is the most nephrotoxic. Particularly in humans and some strains of rats, methoxyflurane causes renal failure that is characterized not by oliguria but by a large urine volume unresponsive to vasopressin.(157) This is caused by the biotransformation of methoxyflurane and the release of free fluoride ion that in turn causes direct damage to the renal tubules. Because of this complication, methoxyflurane is no longer used as an anesthetic in human patients. Renal injury has been reported in the dog when methoxyflurane was used in combination with tetracycline antibiotics(158) and flunixin.(159)

With the possible exception of enflurane and sevoflurane, the breakdown of other inhalation anesthetics does not pose a risk of fluoride-induced nephrotoxicity. Biotransformation of enflurane by humans following moderate duration of anesthesia causes serum inorganic fluoride concentrations to increase. However, serum levels are usually lower than 50 μmol/L, which is normally considered the nephrotoxic threshold in humans.(38, 157, 160)

Sevoflurane is degraded by CO_2 absorbents such as soda lime and Baralyme. A nephrotoxic compound, olefin, is produced.(44, 107, 161) The concentration threshold for nephrotoxicity in rats(162, 163) is within the range of concentrations that may be found associated with the anesthetic management of human patients.(92, 160)

EFFECTS ON THE LIVER

Depression of hepatic function and hepatocellular damage may be caused by the action of volatile anesthetics. Effects may be transient or permanent and may be by direct or indirect action. Studies by Reilly et al. (164) suggested that at least halothane (but likely also other potent inhalation anesthetics) substantially inhibits drug metabolizing capacity by the liver. A reduction in intrinsic hepatic clearance of drugs along with anesthetic-induced alteration of other pharmacokinetically important variables (e.g., reduced hepatic blood flow) fosters a delayed drug removal or an increase in plasma drug concentration during anesthesia. Prolonged or increased (relative to conditions in the unanesthetized animal) plasma concentrations of some drugs have important toxic implications, especially in physiologically comprised patients.

Hepatocellular injury (toxicity) is associated with inhalation anesthetics. This may be manifested histologically as centrilobular necrosis. Evidence of injury may vary from slight to moderate increases in serum levels of hepatic derived enzymes (such as transaminases, sorbitol dehydrogenases, etc., depending upon species) to the rare severe, often fatal, case, especially with humans of fulminant hepatic failure (e.g., the halothane hepatitis syndrome).(28, 165, 166) The cause of hepatocellular injury is not known and is a topic of much debate. Numerous animal models have been developed in attempt to define the mechanism(s).(167)

All of the potent inhalation anesthetics are capable of causing hepatocellular injury by reducing liver blood flow and oxygen delivery. However, available data suggest that of the six contemporary volatile anesthetics, isoflurane is most likely to better maintain tissue O_2 supply and thereby is the agent least likely to produce liver injury even when administered for prolonged periods.(63, 168) The two new agents sevoflurane and desflurane are nearly similar to isoflurane, whereas halothane produces the most striking adverse changes.(92, 104, 107, 169-172) Results of investigations indicate that ancillary influences including N_2O(173), concurrent hypoxia(171, 174, 175), prior induction of hepatic drug-metabolizing enzymes, mode of ventilation(176), and positive end-expired pressure(177) may worsen conditions and increase the likelihood of hepatocellular damage.

Localized hypoxia may damage the hepatocyte directly and/or perhaps result in the production of reactive intermediary compounds from agent (most notably halothane) biotransformation. These compounds then act to produce hepatocellular damage via an autoimmune-mediated reaction(178, 179) or some other as-yet-undescribed process.

The principal factor leading to the decreased use of halothane for human patients nearly two decades ago was the rare occurrence of a fulminant form of hepatic necrosis (usually signs of the condition began a few days after halothane anesthesia). The popular view of the cause of this often fatal, more extreme form of anesthetic-related hepatic injury is that products from halothane biotransformation form hapten-protein conjugates that lead to immunologically mediated hepatic necrosis. Current research uses the guinea pig as a model.(180-182) The mechanism may be family related.(183)

EFFECTS ON SKELETAL MUSCLE: MALIGNANT HYPERTHERMIA

Malignant hyperthermia (MH) is a potentially life-threatening pharmacogenetic myopathy that is most commonly reported in susceptible human patients(184, 185) and swine(186) (e.g., Landrace, Pietrain, or Poland China strains) (Chapter 20). However, reports of its occurrence in other species are available.(187-194) Volatile anesthetics can initiate MH, but halothane is the most potent triggering agent relative to other inhalation anesthetics.(185, 195) The syndrome is characterized by a rapid rise in body temperature that if not treated quickly causes death. Monitoring of temperature and CO_2 production is warranted in susceptible/suspected patients. Patients known to be susceptible to MH can be anesthetized safely. Avoidance of triggering agents and prophylactic dantrolene given before anesthesia are effective in blocking the onset of MH.(184, 185)

Further discussions on the clinical phramacology and use of volatile inhalant anesthetics in various species (Chapter 20) and disease conditions (Chapter 23), and for special procedures and patients (Chapter 24) can be found in Sections 7 and 8, which emphasize anesthetic patient management.

The Gaseous Anesthetic: Nitrous Oxide (N_2O)

Nitrous oxide was introduced into clinical practice more than 150 years ago. Since then its use has formed the basis for more general anesthetic techniques of human patients than any other single inhalation agent.(17) Its widespread use resulted from many desirable properties, including low blood solubility (Table 11-4), limited cardiovascular and respiratory system depression, and minimal toxicity.(17) Its use in the anesthetic management of animals became a natural extension of its use for humans.

However, N_2O is not the ideal anesthetic for humans or animals. As discussed earlier in this chapter, N_2O is not a potent anesthetic (Table 11-10) and will not anesthetize a fit, healthy individual. To get important benefits of N_2O, it is usually used in high inspired concentrations. However, as the concentration of N_2O is increased, there is a change in the proportion and partial pressure of the various other constituents of the inspired breath, notably O_2. Consequently, to avoid hypoxemia 75% of the inspired breath is the highest concentration that can be safely administered. Nitrous oxide has less value in the anesthetic management of animals than in that of humans because the anesthetic potency of N_2O in animals is only about half that found for humans (for example, MAC for the dog is about 200% vs about 100% for humans; Table 11-10).(9, 149) Thus, the value of N_2O in veterinary clinical practice is as an anesthetic adjuvant, that is, accompanying other inhaled or injectable drugs. Since the effects of N_2O on vital organ function (including cardiovascular and respiratory) in the absence of hypoxemia are small in most veterinary patients, benefit is afforded by allowing a certain reduction in the amount of the primary, more potent, inhaled or injectable anesthetic agents.

Nitrous oxide's low blood solubility (Table 11-4) is responsible for a rapid onset of action. Although it does not have the potency to produce anesthesia it may be used to speed induction of inhalation anesthesia as a result of its own (albeit limited) central nervous system effects and, as mentioned earlier, also by augmenting the uptake of a concurrently administered more potent volatile anesthetic such as halothane, the "second gas effect."(9, 17, 196, 197) When a high concentration of N_2O is given concurrently in a mixture with an inhalation agent (e.g., N_2O plus halothane), the alveolar concentration of the simultaneously administered anesthetic (halothane), increases more rapidly than when the "second" gas had been administered without N_2O. The second gas effect is the result of an increased inspiratory volume secondary to the large volume of

N_2O taken up (remember N_2O is used at high concentrations) (196) and a concentrating effect on the second gas in a smaller volume (and thus increased gradient for transfer to blood) as a result of the uptake of the large volume of N_2O.(9, 197)

As noted previously, N_2O's effects on cardiovascular and respiratory function (other than reducing the inspired O_2 concentration) are small compared to other inhalation anesthetics. It does depress myocardial function directly, but its sympathetic stimulation properties counteract some of the direct depression (its own as well as that from accompanying volatile anesthetics).(149) As a result of its sympathetic nervous system activation it may contribute to an increased incidence of cardiac arrhythmias.(198, 199) There is evidence to suggest that its use contributes to myocardial ischemia in some circumstances.(200-203) Overall, a conservative outlook regarding N_2O use relative to respiration and circulation is that significant concern is warranted only in patients with initially compromised function.(204, 205) As with any agent, its advantages and disadvantages should be weighed on an individual patient basis.

Nitrous oxide has little or no effect on liver and kidney function.(206-208) Although there is evidence of N_2O-induced interference with production of red and white blood cells by bone marrow, the risk of adverse outcomes to a subject exposed under most clinical veterinary circumstances is little or none.(207, 209) However, prolonged exposure to N_2O causes megaloblastic hematopoiesis and polyneuropathy. Seriously ill patients may have increased sensitivity to these toxicities. Problems result from N_2O-induced inactivation of the vitamin B_{12}–dependent enzyme methionine synthase, an enzyme that controls interrelations between vitamin B_{12} and folic acid metabolism.(210) Although an occasional patient may develop signs suggestive of vitamin B_{12} and folic acid deficiency after an anesthetic technique that included N_2O, this is a rare event in human and animal patients.(207, 211) Prolonged occupational or abusive exposure to N_2O may be equally harmful and should be considered in management plans of veterinary practices.(28, 207, 212, 213) Nitrous oxide is rapidly and mainly eliminated in the exhaled breath. The extent of biotransformation (to molecular N_2) is very small and mainly by intestinal flora (28, 214, 215) (Table 11–9).

TRANSFER OF N₂O TO CLOSED GAS SPACES

Gas spaces exist or may exist in the body under a variety of conditions and to varying degrees. For example, gas is normally found in the stomach and intestines. The gut is a dynamic reservoir; the gas it contains is freely movable into and out of it according to the laws of diffusion. The gas in the gut originates from air swallowing, normal production of bacterial behavior, chemical reactions, and diffusion from the blood. There is marked variability in both composition and volume of stomach and bowel gas (e.g., herbivore vs carnivore). There are other natural air cavities, such as the air sinuses and the middle ear, and then there are circumstances in which air may be electively or inadvertently introduced as part of diagnostic or therapeutic actions (e.g., pneumoencephalogram, pneumocystogram, endoscopy, vascular air emboli, etc.).

Potential problems associated with gas spaces arise when an animal breathing air is given a gas mixture containing N_2O.(9, 17) Nitrogen (N_2) is the major component of air (80%) and of most gas spaces (methane, CO_2, and hydrogen are also found in variable quantities in the gut). When N_2O is introduced into the inspired breath, a reequilibration of gases in the gas space begins with N_2O quickly entering and N_2 slowly leaving. That is, because of its greater blood solubility the volume of N_2O that can be transported to a closed gas space is many times the volume of N_2 that can be carried away.(9) For example, the blood/gas partition coefficient for N_2O is 0.47 (Table 11–4), whereas that for N_2 is about 0.015.(216) Thus, N_2O is more than 30 times more soluble in blood than N_2 (0.47/0.015). The result of the net transfer of gas to the gas space can be manifested as an increase in volume, as with the gut(217, 218), pneumothorax(218), or blood embolus(219, 220), an increase in pressure (e.g., middle ear[221, 222], pneumoencephalogram[223]), or both (as the distending limits of the compliant container are reached). Usually air is used to inflate the cuff of an endotracheal tube. This cuff is another relatively compliant, enclosed air space. Nitrous oxide will similarly expand this gas space and may increase the pressure exerted on the tracheal wall.(224-226)

DIFFUSION HYPOXIA

A further consideration for the differential movement of N_2O and N_2 occurs at the end of anesthesia when N_2O is discontinued. Because of the large volume of N_2O stored in the body during anesthesia and the unequal change of N_2O for N_2, a deficiency in blood oxygenation may occur at the end of anesthesia if air is abruptly substituted for N_2O. As discussed earlier in this chapter, this condition is referred to as *diffusion hypoxia*.(31, 32) The rapid outpouring of N_2O from the blood into the lung results in a transient but marked decrease in alveolar PO_2 with a resultant decrease in PaO_2.

INTERACTION WITH RESPIRATORY GAS MONITORING

Routine monitoring of expired CO_2 is increasingly important and possible in the operating room of veterinary hospitals. Nitrous oxide interferes with the accurate recording of CO_2 with some monitoring devices. This interaction must be considered in decisions regarding the purchasing of equipment and overall anesthetic management plan. A more complete summary of the advantages and disadvantages of N_2O use is available elsewhere.(17) A brief summary of practical consideration of N_2O use in veterinary practice has also recently appeared.(227, 228)

Occupational Exposure: Trace Concentrations of Inhalation Anesthetics

Operating room personnel are often exposed to low concentrations of inhalation anesthetics (Chapters 2 and 14). Contamination of ambient air occurs via vaporizer filling, known and unknown leaks in the patient breathing circuit, and careless spillage of liquid agent. Measurable amounts of anesthetic gases and vapors are present in operating room air under a variety of conditions.(229-241) Personnel inhale and, as shown by studies, retain these agents for some time.(242, 243) The slow rate of elimination of some vapors (e.g., methoxyflurane and halothane) allows accumulation of retained trace anesthetic quantities from one day to the next.

Concern is raised because epidemiologic studies of humans and laboratory studies of animals have suggested that chronic exposure to trace levels of anesthetics may constitute a health hazard. The possibility that chronic exposure to low levels of anesthetic agents constitute a hazard to health science personnel has attracted and maintained worldwide interest since the early 1970s. Of particular concern are reports that inhaled anesthetics possess mutagenic, carcinogenic, or teratogenic potential. Depending on the point in life at which exposure occurs, there is concern that these underlying mechanisms in turn may result in an increased incidence in fetal death, spontaneous abortion, birth defects or cancer in exposed workers.(244-246) However, "to date, no mutagenic effect of long-term or short-term exposure to inhaled anesthetics has been demonstrated in humans" and "the overwhelming conclusion from both animal and human studies is that there is no carcinogenic risk either from working in the operating or dental suite or from exposure to anesthetics."(28)

Although the data to date, especially regarding effects on human reproduction, remain equivocal, a firm cause-and-effect relationship between chronic exposure to trace levels of anesthetics and human health problems does not exist. Although the risk of long-term exposure to trace concentration of anesthetics for those in operating room conditions appears minimal, current evidence is suggestive enough to cause concern and to encourage practices to reduce the contamination by

anesthetics of operating room personnel. Indeed, levels of exposure have been recommended by the government: 2.0 parts per million (ppm) for volatile agents and 25 ppm for N_2O.(247) In this regard, inexpensive methods to reduce and control anesthetic exposure by operating room personnel are available and should be used(248, 249) (Table 11-15).

Frequent monitoring of actual levels of anesthetic gas/vapor is of obvious value and is encouraged in specialized circumstances and/or environments of high use. Likely the greatest impact results from educating personnel about the potential problem of waste anesthetic gases and methods for controlling exposure levels.(249, 250)

References

1. Soma LR. Textbook of Veterinary Anesthesia. Baltimore: Williams & Wilkins, 1971.
2. Hall LW. Wright's Veterinary Anaesthesia and Analgesia, 7th ed. London: Balliere Tindall, 1971.
3. Lumb WV, Jones EW. Veterinary Anesthesia. Philadelphia: Lea & Febiger, 1973.
4. Short CE. Inhalant Anesthetics. In: Principles & Practice of Veterinary Anesthesia. Edited by C.E. Short. Baltimore: Williams & Wilkins, 1987:70–90.
5. Duncalf D. Flammable anesthetics are nearing extinction. Anesthesiology 56:217–218, 1982.
6. Lowe HJ, Ernst EA. The Quantitative Practice of Anesthesia: Use of Closed Circuit. Baltimore: Williams & Wilkins, 1981.
7. Hill DW. Physics Applied to Anaesthesia, 4th ed. London: Butterworth, 1980.
8. Haskins S, Sansome AL. A time-table for exhaustion of nitrous oxide cylinders using cylinder pressure. Vet Anesth 6:6–8, 1979.
9. Eger EI, II. Anesthetic Uptake and Action. Baltimore: Williams & Wilkins, 1974.
10. Mapleson WW, Allott PR, Steward A. The variability of partition coefficients for halothane in the rabbit. Br J Anaesth 44:650, 1972.
11. Eger RR, Eger EI, II. Effect of temperature and age on the solubility of enflurane, halothane, isoflurane, and methoxyflurane in human blood. Anesth Analg 64:640–642, 1985.
12. Lerman J, Schmitt-Bantel BI, Gregory GA, Willis MM, Eger EI, II. Effect of age on the solubility of volatile anesthetics in human tissues. Anesthesiology 65:307–312, 1986.
13. Eger EI, II. Uptake and distribution. In: Anesthesia, 3rd ed. Edited by R.D. Miller. New York: Churchill Livingstone, 1990:85–104.
14. Mapleson WW. Pharmacokinetics of inhalational anaesthetics. In: General Anaesthesia, 5th ed. Edited by J.F. Nunn, J.E. Utting, and B.R. Brown, Jr. London: Butterworth, 1989:44–59.
15. Steffey EP, Howland D, Jr. The rate of change of halothane concentration in a large animal circle anesthetic system. Am J Vet Res 38:1993–1996, 1977.
16. Mapleson WW. The concentration of anaesthetics in closed circuits, with special reference to halothane. I. Theoretical studies. Br J Anaesth 32:298–309, 1960.
17. Eger EI, II. Nitrous Oxide/N_2O. New York: Elsevier, 1985.
18. Webb AI. The effect of species differences in the uptake and distribution of inhalant anesthetic agents. In: Proceedings of the Second International Congress of Veterinary Anesthesia. Edited by J. Grandy, S. Hildebrand, W. McDonell, et. al. Santa Barbara, CA: Veterinary Practice Publishing Co., 1985:27–32.
19. Staddon GE, Weaver BMQ, Webb AI. Distribution of cardiac output in anaesthetized horse. Res Vet Sci 27:38–45, 1979.
20. Eger EI, II. and Severinghaus, J.W. Effect of uneven pulmonary distribution of blood and gas on induction with inhalation anesthetics. Anesthesiology 25:620–626, 1964.
21. Stoelting RK, Eger EI, II. Percutaneous loss of nitrous oxide, cyclopropane, ether and halothane in man. Anesthesiology 30:278–283, 1969.

Table 11–15. Methods to Reduce Occupational Exposure to Inhalation Anesthetics in the Operating Room (249)

1. Use waste gas *scavenger* to collect gas from the pressure relief (pop off) valve of the patient breathing circuit and anesthesia ventilator.
2. Conduct *regular inspection* and *maintenance* to detect and repair leaks in anesthetic machines and patient breathing circuits, piped gas supplies (N_2O), etc.
3. *Alter work practices* (e.g., minimize leaks around face mask, turn off vaporizer/fresh gas flow when patient breathing circuit not attached to patient).
4. Adequate ventilation in operating rooms.
5. Monitor room trace anesthetic gas levels.
6. Personnel education.

22. Fassoulaki A, Lockhart SH, Freire BA, Yasuda N, Eger EI, II, Weiskopf RB, Johnson BH. Percutaneous loss of desflurane, isoflurane, and halothane in humans. Anesthesiology 74:479–483, 1991.

23. Lockhart SL, Yasuda N, Peterson N, Laster MJ, Taheri S, Weiskopf RB, Eger EI, II. Comparison of percutaneous losses of sevoflurane and isoflurane in humans. Anesth Analg 72:212–215, 1991.

24. Stoelting RK, Eger EI, II. The effects of ventilation and anesthetic solubility on recovery from anesthesia: An in vivo and analog analysis before and after equilibration. Anesthesiology 30:290–296, 1969.

25. Cullen BF, Eger EI, II. Diffusion of nitrous oxide, cyclopropane, and halothane through human skin and amniotic membrane. Anesthesiology 36:168–173, 1972.

26. Carpenter RL, Eger EI, II, Johnson BH, Unadkat JD, Sheiner LB. Does the duration of anesthetic administration affect the pharmacokinetics or metabolism of inhaled anesthetics in humans? Anesth Analg 66:1–8, 1987.

27. Carpenter RL, Eger EI, II, Johnson BH, Unadkat JD, Sheiner LB. Pharmacokinetics of inhaled anesthetics in humans: Measurements during and after the simultaneous administration of enflurane, halothane, isoflurane, methoxyflurane, and nitrous oxide. Anesth Analg 65:575–583, 1986.

28. Baden JM, Rice SA. Metabolism and toxicity. In: Anesthesia, 3rd ed. Edited by R.D. Miller. New York: Churchill Livingstone, 1990:135–170.

29. Cahalan MK, Johnson BH, Eger EI, II. Relationship of concentrations of halothane and enflurane to their metabolism and elimination in man. Anesthesiology 54:3–8, 1981.

30. Carpenter RL, Eger EI, II, Johnson BH, Unadkhat JD, Sheiner LB. The extent of metabolism of inhaled anesthetics in humans. Anesthesiology 65:201–206, 1986.

31. Fink BR. Diffusion anoxia. Anesthesiology 16:511–519, 1955.

32. Rackow H, Salanitre E, Frumin MH. Dilution of alveolar gases during nitrous oxide excretion in man. J Appl Physiol 16:723–728, 1961.

33. Sheffer L, Steffenson JL, Birch AA. Nitrous oxide-induced diffusion hypoxia in patients breathing spontaneously. Anesthesiology 37:436–439, 1972.

34. Van Dyke RA, Chenoweth MB, Van Poznak A. Metabolism of volatile anesthetics–I conversion in vivo of several anesthetics to $^{14}CO_2$ and chloride. Biochem Pharmacol 13:1239–1247, 1964.

35. Stier A, Alter H, Hessler O, Rehder K. Urinary excretion of bromide in halothane anesthesia. Anesth Analg 43:723–728, 1964.

36. Rehder K, Forbes J, Alter H, Hessler O, Stier A. Halothane biotransformation in man: A quantitative study. Anesthesiology 28:711–715, 1967.

37. Holaday DA, Rudofsky S, Treuhaft PS. Metabolic degradation of methoxyflurane in man. Anesthesiology 33:579–593, 1970.

38. Mazze RI, Fujinaga M. Biotransformation of inhalational anesthetics. In: General Anaesthesia, 5th ed. Edited by J.F. Nunn, J.E. Utting, and B.R. Brown. London: Butterworth, 1989:73–85.

39. Sawyer DC, Eger EI, II, Bahlman SH, Cullen BF, Impelman D. Concentration dependence of hepatic halothane metabolism. Anesthesiology 34:230–235, 1971.

40. Cook TL, Beppu WJ, Hitt BA, Kosek JC, Mazze RI. Renal effects and metabolism of sevoflurane in Fischer 344 rats: An in-vivo and in-vitro comparison with methoxyflurane. Anesthesiology 43:70–77, 1975.

41. Cook TL, Beppu WJ, Hitt BA, Kosek JC, Mazze RI. Comparison of renal effects and metabolism of sevoflurane and methoxyflurane in enzyme-induced rats. Anesth Analg 54:829–835, 1975.

42. Martis L, Lynch S, Napoli MD, Woods EF. Biotransformation of sevoflurane in dogs and rats. Anesth Analg 60:186–191, 1981.

43. Rice SA, Dooley JR, Mazze RI. Metabolism by rat hepatic microsomes of fluorinated ether anesthetics following ethanol consumption. Anesthesiology 58:237–241, 1983.

44. Wallin RF, Regan BM, Napoli MD, Stern IJ. Sevoflurane: A new inhalational anesthetic agent. Anesth Analg 54:758–766, 1975.

45. Holaday DA, Smith FR. Clinical characteristics and biotransformation of sevoflurane in healthy human volunteers. Anesthesiology 54:100–106, 1981.

46. Frink EJ, Jr, Malan TP, Jr, Brown EA, Morgan S, Brown BR, Jr. Plasma inorganic fluoride levels with sevoflurane anesthesia in morbidly obese and nonobese patients. Anesth Analg 76:1333–1337, 1993.

47. Koblin DD, Eger EI, II, Johnson BH, Konopka K, Waskell L. I-653 resists degradation in rats. Anesth Analg 67:534–539, 1988.

48. Koblin DD, Weiskopf RB, Holmes MA, Konopka K, Rampil IJ, Eger EI, II, Waskell L. Metabolism of I-653 and isoflurane in swine. Anesth Analg 68:147–149, 1989.

49. Sutton TS, Koblin DD, Gruenke LD, Weiskopf RB, Rampil IJ, Waskell L, Eger EI, II. Fluoride metabolites following prolonged exposure of volunteers to desflurane and patients to desflurane. Anesth Analg 73:180–185, 1991.

50. Merkel G, Eger EI, II. A comparative study of halothane and halopropane anesthesia including method for determining equipotency. Anesthesiology 24:346–357, 1963.

51. De Jong RH, Eger EI, II. MAC expanded: AD_{50} and AD_{95} values of common inhalation anesthetics in man. Anesthesiology 42:408–419, 1975.

52. Quasha AL, Eger EI, II, Tinker JH. Determination and applications of MAC. Anesthesiology 53:315–334, 1980.

53. Cullen DJ. Anesthetic depth and MAC. In: Anesthesia, 2nd ed. Edited by R.D. Miller. New York: Churchill Livingstone, 1986: 553–580.

54. Steffey EP, Howland D, Jr, Giri S, Eger EI, II. Enflurane, halothane and isoflurane potency in horses. Am J Vet Res 38:1037–1039, 1977.

55. Ludders JW, Mitchell GS, Schaefer SI. Minimum anesthetic dose and cardiopulmonary response for halothane in chickens. Am J Vet Res 49:929–933, 1988.

56. Eger EI, II, Johnson BH, Weiskopf B, Holmes MA, Yasuda N, Targ A, Rampil IJ. Minimum alveolar concentration of I-653 and isoflurane in pigs: Definition of a supramaximal stimulus. Anesth Analg 67:1174–1177, 1988.

57. Thomsen CE, Christensen KN, Rosenfalck A. Computerized monitoring of depth of anaesthesia with isoflurane. Br J Anaesth 63:36–43, 1989.

58. Rampil IJ, Weiskopf RB, Brown JG, Eger EI, II, Johnson BH, Holmes MA, Donegan JH. I-653 and isoflurane produce similar dose-related changes in the electroencephalogram of pigs. Anesthesiology 69:298–302, 1988.

59. Schwilden H, Stoeckel H. Quantitative EEG analysis during anaesthesia with isoflurane in nitrous oxide at 1.3 and 1.5 MAC. Br J Anaesth 59:738–745, 1987.

60. Rampil IJ, Lockhart SH, Eger EI, II, Yasuda N, Weiskopf RB, Cahalan MK. The electroencephalographic effects of desflurane in humans. Anesthesiology 74:434–439, 1991.

61. Dwyer RC, Rampil IJ, Eger EI, II, Bennett HL. The electroencephalogram does not predict depth of isoflurane anesthesia. Anesthesiology 81:403–409, 1994.

62. Joas TA, Stevens WC, Eger EI, II. Electroencephalographic seizure activity in dogs during anaesthesia: Studies with Ethrane, fluroxene, halothane, chloroform, divinyl ether, diethyl ether, methoxyflurane, cyclopropane and forane. Br J Anaesth 43:739–745, 1971.

63. Eger EI, II. Isoflurane–A compendium and reference, 2nd ed. Madison, WI: Anaquest, 1985.

64. Scheller MS, Tateishi A, Drummond JC, Zornow MH. The effects of sevoflurane on cerebral blood flow, cerebral metabolic rate for oxygen, intracranial pressure, and the electroencephalogram are similar to those of isoflurane in the rabbit. Anesthesiology 68:548–552, 1988.

65. Osawa M, Shingu K, Murakawa M, Adachi T, Kurata J, Seo N, Murayama T, Nakao S, Mori K. Effect of sevoflurane on central nervous system electrical activity in cats. Anesth Analg 79:52–57, 1994.

66. Scheller MS, Nakakimura K, Fleischer JE, Zornow MH. Cerebral effects of sevoflurane in the dog: Comparison with isoflurane and enflurane. Br J Anaesth 65:388–392, 1990.

67. Coon RL, Kampine JP. Hypocapnic bronchoconstriction and inhalation anesthetics. Anesthesiology 43:635–641, 1975.

68. Klide AM, Aviado DM. Mechanism for the reduction in pulmo-

nary resistance induced by halothane. J Pharmacol Exp Ther 158:28–35, 1967.

69. Hirshman CA, Bergman NA. Halothane and enflurane protect against bronchospasm in an asthma dog model. Anesth Analg 57:629–633, 1978.

70. Hirshman CA, Edelstein H, Peetz S, Wayne R, Kownes H. Mechanism of action of inhalational anesthesia on airways. Anesthesiology 56:107–111, 1982.

71. Lockhart SH, Rampil IJ, Yasuda N, Eger EI, II, Weiskopf RB. Depression of ventilation by desflurane in humans. Anesthesiology 74:484–488, 1991.

72. Munson ES, Larson CPJ, Babad AA, Regan MJ, Buechel DR, Eger EI, II. The effects of halothane, fluroxene and cyclopropane on ventilation: A comparative study in man. Anesthesiology 27:716–728, 1966.

73. Larson CP, Jr, Eger EI, II, Muallem M, Buechel DR, Munson ES, Eisele JH. The effects of diethyl ether and methoxyflurane on ventilation: II. A comparative study in man. Anesthesiology 30:174–184, 1969.

74. Doi M, Ikeda K. Respiratory effects of sevoflurane. Anesth Analg 66:241–244, 1987.

75. Calverley RK, Smith NT, Jones CW, Prys-Roberts C, Eger EI, II. Ventilatory and cardiovascular effects of enflurane anesthesia during spontaneous ventilation in man. Anesth Analg 51:610–618, 1978.

76. Fourcade HE, Stevens WC, Larson CPJ, Cromwell TH, Bahlman SH, Hickey RF, Halsey MJ, Eger EI, II. The ventilatory effects of forane, a new inhaled anesthetic. Anesthesiology 35:26–31, 1971.

77. Hodgson DS, Steffey EP, Grandy JL, Woliner MJ. Effects of spontaneous, assisted, and controlled ventilation in halothane-anesthetized geldings. Am J Vet Res 47:992–996, 1986.

78. Steffey EP, Wheat JD, Meagher DM, Norrie RD, McKee J, Brown M, Arnold J. Body position and mode of ventilation influences arterial pH, oxygen and carbon dioxide tensions in halothane-anesthetized horses. Am J Vet Res 38:379–382, 1977.

79. Gronwall R. Effects of fasting on hepatic function in ponies. Am J Vet Res 36:145–148, 1975.

80. France CJ, Plumer HM, Eger EI, II, Wahrenbrock EA. Ventilatory effects of isoflurane (Forane) or halothane when combined with morphine, nitrous oxide and surgery. Br J Anaesth 46:117–120, 1974.

81. Steffey EP, Eisele JH, Baggot JD, Woliner MJ, Jarvis KA, Elliott AR. Influence of inhaled anesthetics on the pharmacokinetics and pharmacodynamics of morphine. Anesth Analg 77:346–351, 1993.

82. Steffey EP, Hodgson DS, Dunlop CI, Miller MF, Woliner MJ, Heath RB, Grandy J. Cardiopulmonary function during 5 hours of constant-dose isoflurane in laterally recumbent, spontaneously breathing horses. J Vet Pharmacol Ther 10:290–297, 1987.

83. Whitehair KJ, Steffey EP, Willits NH, Woliner MJ. Recovery of horses from inhalation anesthesia. Am J Vet Res 54:1693–1702, 1993.

84. Steffey EP, Gillespie JR, Berry JD, Eger EI, II, Rhode EA. Circulatory effects of halothane and halothane-nitrous oxide anesthesia in the dog: Spontaneous ventilation. Am J Vet Res 36:197–200, 1975.

85. Steffey EP, Gillespie JR, Berry JD, Eger EI, II. Cardiovascular effects with the addition of N₂O to halothane in stump-tailed macaques during spontaneous and controlled ventilation. J Am Vet Med Assoc 165:834–837, 1974.

86. Steffey EP, Baggot JD, Eisele JH, Willits N, Woliner MJ, Jarvis KA, Elliott AR, Tagawa M. Morphine-isoflurane interaction in dogs, swine and rhesus monkeys. J Vet Pharmacol Ther 17:202–210, 1994.

87. Steffey EP, Howland D, Jr. Potency of enflurane in dogs: Comparison with halothane and isoflurane. Am J Vet Res 39:673–677, 1978.

88. Klide AM. Cardiovascular effects of enflurane and isoflurane in the dog. Am J Vet Res 37:127–131, 1976.

89. Steffey EP, Farver TB, Woliner MJ. Circulatory and respiratory effects of methoxyflurane in dogs: Comparison of halothane. Am J Vet Res 45:2574–2579, 1984.

90. Sommer R. Preventing endotracheal tube fire during pharyngeal surgery. Anesthesiology 66:439, 1987.

91. Steffey EP, Howland D, Jr. Comparison of circulatory and respiratory effects of isoflurane and halothane anesthesia in horses. Am J Vet Res 40:821–825, 1980.

92. Eger EI, II. New inhaled anesthetics. Anesthesiology 80:906–922, 1994.

93. Merin RG, Bernard JM, Doursout MF, Cohen M, Chelly JE. Comparison of the effects of isoflurane and desflurane on cardiovascular dynamics and regional blood flow in the chronically instrumented dog. Anesthesiology 74:568–574, 1991.

94. Weiskopf RB, Holmes MA, Eger EI, II, Johnson BH, Rampil IJ, Brown JG. Cardiovascular effects of I-653 in swine. Anesthesiology 69:303–309, 1988.

95. Pagel PS, Kampine JP, Schmeling WT, Warltier DC. Comparison of the systemic and coronary hemodynamic actions of desflurane, isoflurane, halothane, and enflurane in the chronically instrumented dog. Anesthesiology 74:539–551, 1991.

96. Warltier DC, Pagel PS. Cardiovascular and respiratory actions of desflurane: Is desflurane different from isoflurane? Anesth Analg 75:S17–S31, 1992.

97. Pagel PS, Kampine JP, Schmeling WT, Warltier DC. Influence of volatile anesthetics on myocardial contractility in vivo–Desflurane versus isoflurane. Anesthesiology 74:900–907, 1991.

98. Pagel PS, Kampine JP, Schmeling WT, Warltier DC. Evaluation of myocardial contractility in the chronically instrumented dog with intact autonomic nervous system function: Effects of desflurane and isoflurane. Acta Anaesthesiol Scand 37:203–210, 1993.

99. Boban M, Stowe DF, Buljubasic N, Bampine JP, Bosnjak ZJ. Direct comparative effects of isoflurane and desflurane in isolated guinea pig hearts. Anesthesiology 76:775–780, 1992.

100. Eisele JH, Jr. Cardiovascular effects of nitrous oxide. In: Nitrous Oxide/N₂O, 1st ed. Edited by E.I. Eger, II. New York: Elsevier, 1985:125–156.

101. Frink EJ, Jr, Malan TP, Atlas M, Dominguez LM, DiNardo JA, Brown BR, Jr. Clinical comparison of sevoflurane and isoflurane in healthy patients. Anesth Analg 74:241–245, 1992.

102. Bernard J, Wouters PF, Doursout M, Florence B, Chelly JE, Merin RG. Effects of sevoflurane and isoflurane on cardiac and coronary dynamics in chronically instrumented dogs. Anesthesiology 72:659–662, 1990.

103. Seyde WC, Longnecker DE. Anesthetic influences on regional hemodynamics in normal and hemorrhaged rats. Anesthesiology 61:686–698, 1984.

104. Bernard JM, Doursout MF, Wouters P, Hartley CJ, Cohen M, Merin MG, Chelly JE. Effects of enflurane and isoflurane on hepatic and renal circulations in chronically instrumented dogs. Anesthesiology 74:298–302, 1991.

105. Steffey EP, Howland D, Jr. Isoflurane potency in the dog and cat. Am J Vet Res 38:1833–1836, 1977.

106. Steffey EP, Gillespie JR, Berry JD, Eger EI, II, Rhode EA. Circulatory effects of halothane and halothane-nitrous oxide anesthesia in the dog: Controlled ventilation. Am J Vet Res 35:1289–1293, 1974.

107. Frink EJ, Jr, Morgan SE, Coetzee A, Conzen P, Brown BR, Jr. The effects of sevoflurane, halothane, enflurane, and isoflurane on hepatic blood flow and oxygenation in chronically instrumented greyhound dogs. Anesthesiology 76:85–90, 1992.

108. Steffey EP, Howland D, Jr. Cardiovascular effects of halothane in the horse. Am J Vet Res 39:611–615, 1978.

109. Steffey EP, Gillespie JR, Berry JD, Eger EI, II, Rhode EA. Cardiovascular effect of halothane in the stump-tailed macaque during spontaneous and controlled ventilation. Am J Vet Res 35:1315–1319, 1974.

110. Wolfson B, Hebrick WD, Lake CL, Silar ES. Anesthetic indices–Further data. Anesthesiology 48:187–190, 1978.

111. Wolfson B, Kielar CM, Lake C, Hebrick WD, Sikes ES. Anesthetic Index–A new approach. Anesthesiology 38:583–586, 1973.

112. Price HL. The significance of catecholamine release during anesthesia. Br J Anaesth 38:705–711, 1966.

113. Katz RL, Epstein RA. The interaction of anesthetic agents and

adrenergic drugs to produce cardiac arrhythmias. Anesthesiology 29:763–784, 1968.

114. Raventos J. The action of fluothane: A new volatile anaesthetic. Br J Pharmacol 11:394–409, 1956.

115. Muir BJ, Hall LW, Littlewort MCG. Cardiac irregularities in cats under halothane anaesthesia. Br J Anaesth 31:488–489, 1959.

116. Purchase IF. Cardiac arrhythmias occurring during halothane anaesthesia in cats. Br J Anaesth 38:13–22, 1966.

117. Joas TA, Stevens WC. Comparison of the arrhythmic doses of epinephrine during forane, halothane, and fluroxene anesthesia in dogs. Anesthesiology 35:48–53, 1971.

118. Muir WW, Hubbell JAE, Flaherty S. Increasing halothane concentrations abolishes anesthesia-associated arrythmias in cats and dogs. J Am Vet Med Assoc 192:1730–1736, 1988.

119. Moore MA, Weiskopf RB, Eger EI, II, Wilson C, Lu G. Arrhythmogenic doses of epinephrine are similar during desflurane or isoflurane anesthesia in humans. Anesthesiology 79:943–947, 1993.

120. Munson ES, Tucker WK. Doses of epinephrine causing arrhythmia during enflurane, methoxyflurane and halothane anesthesia in dogs. Can Anaesth Soc J 22:495–501, 1975.

121. Navarro R, Weiskopf RB, Moore MA, Lockhart S, Eger EI, II, Koblin D, Lu G, Wilson C. Humans anesthetized with sevoflurane or isoflurane have similar arrhythmic response to epinephrine. Anesthesiology 80:545–549, 1994.

122. Weiskopf RB, Eger EI, II, Holmes MA, Rampil IJ, Johnson BH, Brown JG, Yasuda N, Targ AG. Epinephrine-induced premature ventricular contractions and changes in arterial blood pressure and heart rate during I-653, isoflurane, and halothane anesthesia in swine. Anesthesiology 70:293–298, 1989.

123. Johnston RR, Eger EI, II, Wilson C. A comparative interaction of epinephrine with enflurane, isoflurane and halothane in man. Anesth Analg 55:709–712, 1976.

124. Tucker WK, Rackstein AD, Munson ES. Comparison of arrhythmic doses of adrenaline, metaraminol, ephedrine, and phenylephrine during isoflurane and halothane anesthesia in dogs. Br J Anaesth 46:392–396, 1974.

125. Robertson BJ, Clement JL, Knill RL. Enhancement of the arrhythmogenic effect of hypercarbia by surgical stimulation during halothane anaesthesia in man. Can Anaesth Soc J 28:342, 1981.

126. Cullen DJ, Eger EI, II. Cardiovascular effects of carbon dioxide in man. Anesthesiology 41:345–349, 1974.

127. Grandy JL, Hodgson DS, Dunlop CI, Curtis CR, Heath RB. Cardiopulmonary effects of halothane in cats. Am J Vet Res 50:1729–1732, 1989.

128. Bahlman SH, Eger EI, II, Halsey MJ, Stevens WC, Shakespeare TF, Smith NT, Cromwell TH, Fourcade H. The cardiovascular effects of halothane in man during spontaneous ventilation. Anesthesiology 36:494–502, 1972.

129. Cromwell TH, Stevens WC, Eger EI, II, Shakespear TF, Halsey MJ, Bahlman SH, Fourcade HE. The cardiovascular effects of compound 469 (Forane) during spontaneous ventilation and CO$_2$ challenge in man. Anesthesiology 35:17–25, 1971.

130. Cullen LK, Steffey EP, Bailey CS, Kortz G, da Silva Curiel J, Bellhorn RW, Woliner MJ, Elliott AR, Jarvis KA. Effect of high PaCO$_2$ and time on cerebrospinal fluid and intraocular pressure in halothane-anesthetized horses. Am J Vet Res 51:300–304, 1990.

131. Roizen MF, Horrigan RW, Frazer BM. Anesthetic doses blocking adrenergic (stress) and cardiovascular responses to incision– MAC BAR. Anesthesiology 54:390–398, 1981.

132. Yasuda N, Weiskopf RB, Cahalan MK, Ionescu P, Caldwell JE, Eger EI, II, Rampil IJ, Lockhart SH. Does desflurane modify circulatory responses to stimulation in humans? Anesth Analg 73:175–179, 1991.

133. Eger EI, II, Smith NT, Stoelting RK, Cullen DJ, Kadis LB, Whitcher CE. Cardiovascular effects of halothane in man. Anesthesiology 32:396–409, 1970.

134. Weiskopf RB, Cahalan MK, Eger EI, II, Yasuda N, Rampil IJ, Ionescu P, Lockhart SH, Johnson BH, Freire B, Kelley S. Cardiovascular actions of desflurane in normocarbic volunteers. Anesth Analg 73:143–156, 1991.

135. Stevens WC, Cromwell TH, Halsey MJ, Eger EI, II, Shakespear TF, Bahlman SH. The cardiovascular effects of a new inhalation anesthetic, Forane, in human volunteers at constant arterial carbon dioxide tension. Anesthesiology 35:8–16, 1971.

136. Cullen BF, Eger EI, II, Smith NT, Sawyer DC, Gregory GA, Joas TA. Cardiovascular effects of fluroxene in man. Anesthesiology 32:218–230, 1970.

137. Libonati M, Cooperman LH, Price HL. Time-dependent circulatory effects of methoxyflurane in man. Anesthesiology 34:439–444, 1971.

138. Gregory GA, Eger EI, II, Smith NT. The cardiovascular effects of diethyl ether in man. Anesthesiology 34:19–24, 1971.

139. Steffey EP, Farver TB, Woliner MJ. Cardiopulmonary function during 7 h of constant-dose halothane and methoxyflurane. J Appl Physiol 63:1351–1359, 1987.

140. Steffey EP, Kelly AB, Woliner MJ. Time-related responses of spontaneously breathing, laterally recumbent horses to prolonged anesthesia with halothane. Am J Vet Res 48:952–957, 1987.

141. Dunlop CI, Steffey EP, Miller MF, Woliner MJ. Temporal effects of halothane and isoflurane in laterally recumbent ventilated male horses. Am J Vet Res 48:1250–1255, 1987.

142. Steffey EP, Dunlop CI, Cullen LK, Hodgson DS, Giri SN, Willits N, Woliner MJ, Jarvis KA, Smith CM, Elliott AR. Circulatory and respiratory responses of spontaneously breathing, laterally recumbent horses to 12 hours of halothane anesthesia. Am J Vet Res 54:929–936, 1993.

143. Steffey EP, Kelly AB, Hodgson DS, Grandy JL, Woliner MJ, Willits N. Effect of body posture on cardiopulmonary function in horses druing five hours of constant-dose halothane anesthesia. Am J Vet Res 51:11–16, 1990.

144. Steffey EP, Woliner MJ, Dunlop C. Effects of five hours of constant 1.2 MAC halothane in sternally recumbent, spontaneously breathing horses. Equine Vet J 22:433–436, 1990.

145. Shimosato S, Yasuda I. Cardiac performance during prolonged halothane anaesthesia in the cat. Br J Anaesth 50:215–219, 1978.

146. Price HL, Skovsted P, Pauca AL, Cooperman LH. Evidence for β-receptor activation produced by halothane in man. Anesthesiology 32:389–395, 1970.

147. Steffey EP, Howland D, Jr. Potency of halothane-N$_2$O in the horse. Am J Vet Res 39:1141–1146, 1978.

148. Bahlman SH, Eger EI, II, Smith NT, Stevens WC, Shakespear TF, Sawyer DC, Halsey MJ, Cromwell TH. The cardiovascular effects of nitrous oxide-halothane anesthesia in man. Anesthesiology 35:274–255, 1971.

149. Steffey EP, Eger EI, II. Nitrous oxide in veterinary practice and animal research. In: Nitrous Oxide/N$_2$O. Edited by E.I. Eger, II. New York: Elsiever, 1984:305–312.

150. Grandy JL, Hodgson DS, Dunlop CI, Chapman PL, Heath RB. Cardiopulmonary effects of ephedrine in halothane-anesthetized horses. J Vet Pharmacol Ther 12:389–396, 1989.

151. Dyson DH, Pascoe PJ. Influence of preinduction methoxamine, lactated ringer solution, or hypertonic saline solution infusion on postinduction dobutamine infusion on anesthetic-induced hypotension in horses. Am J Vet Res 51:17–21, 1990.

152. Swanson CR, Muir WW, Bednarski RM, et al. Hemodynamic responses in halothane-anesthetized horses given infusions of dopamine or dubutamine. Am J Vet Res 46:365–371, 1985.

153. Steffey EP, Zinkl J, Howland D, Jr. Minimal changes in blood cell counts and biochemical values associated with prolonged isoflurane anesthesia of horses. Am J Vet Res 40:1646–1648, 1979.

154. Steffey EP, Farver T, Zinkl J, Wheat JD, Meagher DM, Brown MP. Alterations in horse blood cell count and biochemical values after halothane anesthesia. Am J Vet Res 41:934–939, 1980.

155. Stover SM, Steffey EP, Dybdal NO, Franti CE. Hematologic and biochemical values associated with multiple halothane anesthesias and minor surgical trauma of horses. Am J Vet Res 49:236–241, 1988.

156. Steffey EP, Giri SN, Dunlop CI, Cullen LK, Hodgson DS, Willits N. Biochemical and haematological changes following prolonged halothane anaesthesia in horses. Res Vet Sci 55:338–345, 1993.

157. Mazze RI. Anesthesia and the renal and genitourinary systems. In: Anesthesia, 3rd ed. Edited by R.D. Miller. New York: Churchill Livingstone, 1990:1791–1808.

158. Pedersoli WM. Blood serum inorganic ionic fluoride tetracycline and methoxyflurane anesthesia in dogs. J Am Anim Hosp Assoc 13:242–246, 1977.
159. Matthews KA, Doherty T, Dyson DH, Wilcock B, Valliant A. Nephrotoxicity in dogs associated with methoxyflurane anesthesia and flunixin meglumine analgesia. Can Vet J 31:766–771, 1990.
160. Frink WJ, Jr, Malan TP, Jr, Isner RJ, Brown EA, Morgan SE, Brown BR, Jr. Renal concentrating function with prolonged sevoflurane or enflurane anesthesia in volunteers. Anesthesiology 80:1019–1025, 1994.
161. Strum DP, Johnson BH, Eger EI, II. Stability of sevoflurane in soda lime. Anesthesiology 67:779–781, 1987.
162. Gonsowski CT, Laster MJ, Eger EI, II, Ferrell LD, Kerschmann RL. Toxicity of compound A in rats: Effect of a 3-hour administration. Anesthesiology 80:556–565, 1994.
163. Gonsowski CT, Laster MJ, Eger EI, II, Ferrell LD, Kerschmann RL. Toxicity of compound A in rats: Effect of increasing duration of administration. Anesthesiology 80:566–573, 1994.
164. Reilly CS, Wood AJJ, Koshakji RP, Wood M. The effect of halothane on drug disposition: Contribution of changes in intrinsic drug metabolizing capacity and hepatic blood flow. Anesthesiology 63:70–76, 1985.
165. Subcommittee of the National Halothane Study of the Committee on Anesthesia. Summary of the national halothane study: Possible association between halothane anesthesia and postoperative hepatic necrosis. JAMA 197:121–134, 1966.
166. Inman WHW, Mushin WW. Jaundice after repeated exposure to halothane: An analysis of reports to the Committee on Safety of Medicines. Br Med J 1:5–10, 1974.
167. Clarke JB, Lind RC, Gandolfi AJ. Mechanisms of anesthetic hepatotoxicity. In: Advances in Anesthesia, 10th ed. Edited by R.K. Stoelting, P.G. Barash, and R.J.Gallagher. St. Louis: Mosby Year Book, 1993:219–246.
168. Gelman S, Fowler KC, Smith LR. Liver circulation and function during isoflurane and halothane anesthesia. Anesthesiology 61:726–731, 1984.
169. Holmes MA, Weiskopf RB, Eger EI, II, Johnson BH, Rampil IJ. Hepatocellular integrity in swine after prolonged desflurane (I-653) and isoflurane anesthesia: Evaluation of plasma alanine aminotransferase activity. Anesth Analg 71:249–253, 1990.
170. Eger EI, II, Johnson BH, Ferrell LD. Comparison of the toxicity of I-653 and isoflurane in rats: A test of the effect of repeated anesthesia and use of dry soda lime. Anesth Analg 66:1230–1233, 1987.
171. Strum DP, Eger EI, II, Johnson BH, Steffey EP, Ferrell LD. Toxicity of sevoflurane in rats. Anesth Analg 66:769–773, 1987.
172. Eger EI, II, Johnson BH, Strum DP, Ferrell LD. Studies of the toxicity of I-653, halothane, and isoflurane in enzyme-induced, hypoxic rats. Anesth Analg 66:1227–1229, 1987.
173. Ross JAS, Monk SJ, Duffy SW. Effect of nitrous oxide on halothane-induced hepatotoxicity in hypoxic, enzyme-induced rats. Br J Anaesth 56:527–533, 1984.
174. Shingu K, Eger EI, II, Johnson BH. Hypoxia per se can produce hepatic damage without death in rats. Anesth Analg 61:820–823, 1982.
175. Shingu K, Eger EI, II, Johnson BH. Hypoxia may be more important than reductive metabolism in halothane-induced hepatic injury. Anesth Analg 61:824–827, 1982.
176. Cooperman LH, Warden JC, Price HL. Splanchnic circulation during nitrous oxide anesthesia and hypocarbia in normal man. Anesthesiology 29:254–258, 1968.
177. Johnson EE, Hedley-Whyte J. Continuous positive-pressure ventilation and choledochoduodenal flow resistance. J Appl Physiol 39:937–942, 1975.
178. Kenna JG, Satoh H, Christ DD, Pohl LR. Metabolic basis for a drug hypersensitivity: Antibodies in sera from patients with halothane hepatitis recognize liver neoantigens that contain the trifluoroacetyl group derived from halothane. J Pharmacol Exp Ther 245:1103–1109, 1988.
179. Klatskin G, Kimberg DV. Recurrent hepatitis attributable to halothane sensitization in an anesthetist. N Engl J Med 280:515–522, 1969.
180. Lind RC, Gandolfi AJ, Hall PD. A model for fatal halothane hepatitis in the guinea pig. Anesthesiology 81:478–487, 1994.
181. Lunam CA, Cousins MJ, Hall PD. Genetic predisposition to liver damage after halothane anesthesia in guinea pigs. Anesth Analg 65:1143–1149, 1986.
182. Lind RC, Gandolfi AJ, Brown BR, Gall PM. Halothane hepatotoxicity in guinea pigs. Anesth Analg 66:222–228, 1987.
183. Farrell G, Prendergast D, Murray M. Halothane hepatitis: Detection of a constitutional susceptibility factor. N Engl J Med 313:1310–1315, 1985.
184. Denborough MA, Forster JFP, Lovell RRH. Anaesthetic deaths in a family. Br J Anaesth 34:395, 1962.
185. Gronert GA, Schulman SR, Mott J. Malignant hyperthermia. In: Anesthesia, 3rd ed. Edited by R.D. Miller. New York: Churchill Livingstone, 1990:935–956.
186. Hall LW, Woolf N, Bradley JWP, Jolly DW. Unusual reaction to suxamethonum chloride. Br Med J 2:1305, 1966.
187. Kirmayer AH, Klide AM, Purvance JE. Malignant hyperthermia in a dog: Case report and review of the syndrome. J Am Vet Med Assoc 185:978–983, 1984.
188. Deuster PA, Bockman EL, Muldoon SM. In vitro responses of cat skeletal muscle to halothane and caffeine. J Appl Physiol 58:521–528, 1985.
189. Bagshaw RJ, Cox RH, Knight DH, Detwiler DK. Malignant hyperthermia in a grayhound. J Am Vet Med Assoc 172:61, 1978.
190. Rosenberg H, Waldron-Maese E. Malignant hyperpyrexia in horses: Anesthetic sensitivity proven by muscle biopsy [Abstract]. Annu Meet Am Soc Anesth, Park Ridge, Ill; 333, 1977.
191. Hildebrand SV, Howitt GA. Succinylcholine infusion associated with hyperthermia in ponies anesthetized with halothane. Am J Vet Res 44:2280–2284, 1983.
192. Short C, Paddleford RR. Malignant hyperthermia in the dog [Letter]. Anesthesiology 39:462–463, 1973.
193. Waldron-Mease E, Klein LV, Rosenberg H, Leitch M. Malignant hyperthermia in a halothane-anesthetized horse. J Am Vet Med Assoc 179:896–898, 1981.
194. De Jong RH, Heavner JE, Amory DW. Malignant hyperpyrexia in the cat. Anesthesiology 41:608–609, 1974.
195. Gronert GA. Malignant hyperthermia. Anesthesiology 53:395–423, 1980.
196. Epstein RM, Rackow H, Salanitre E, Wolf GL. Influence of the concentration effect on the uptake of anesthetic mixtures: The second gas effect. Anesthesiology 25:364–371, 1964.
197. Stoelting RK, Eger EI, II. An additional explanation for the second gas effect: A concentrating effort. Anesthesiology 30:273–277, 1969.
198. Liu WS, Wong KC, Port JD, Aridriano KP. Epinephrine-induced arrhythmia during halothane anesthesia with the addition of nitrous oxide, nitrogen or helium in dogs. Anesth Analg 61:414–417, 1982.
199. Lampe GH, Donegan JH, Rupp SM, Wauk LZ, Whitendale P, Fouts KE, Rose BM, Litt LL, Rampil IJ, Wilson CB, Eger EI, II. Nitrous oxide and epinephrine-induced arrhythmias. Anesth Analg 71:602–605, 1990.
200. Philbin DM, Foex P, Drummond G, Lowenstein E, Ryder WA, Jones LA. Postsystolic shortening of canine left ventricle supplied by a stenotic coronary artery when nitrous oxide is added in the presence of narcotics. Anesthesiology 62:166–174, 1985.
201. Leone BJ, Philbin DM, Lehot JJ, Foex P, Ryder WA. Gradual or abrupt nitrous oxide administration in a canine model of critical coronary stenosis induces regional myocardial dysfunction that is worsened by halothane. Anesth Analg 67:814–822, 1988.
202. Nathan HJ. Nitrous oxide worsens myocardial ischemia in isoflurane-anesthetized dogs. Anesthesiology 68:407–416, 1988.
203. Diedericks J, Leone BJ, Foex P, Sear JW, Ryder WA. Nitrous oxide causes myocardial ischemia when added to propofol in the compromised canine myocardium. Anesth Analg 76:1322–1326, 1993.
204. Saidman LJ, Hamilton WK. We should continue to use nitrous oxide. In: Nitrous Oxide/N$_2$O, 1st ed. Edited by E.I. Eger, II. New York: Elsevier, 1985:345–353.
205. Eger EI, II, Lampe GH, Wauk LZ, Whitendale P, Cahalan MK,

Donegan JH. Clinical pharmacology of nitrous oxide: An argument for its continued use. Anesth Analg 71:575–585, 1990.

206. Lampe GH, Wauk LZ, Whitendale P, Way WL, Murray W, Eger EI, II. Nitrous oxide does not impair hepatic function in young or old surgical patients. Anesth Analg 71:606–609, 1990.

207. Brodsky JB. Toxicity of nitrous oxide. In: Nitrous Oxide/N₂O, 1st ed. Edited by E.I. Eger, II. New York: Elsevier, 1985:259–279.

208. Lampe GH, Wauk LZ, Donegan JH, Pitts LH, Jackler RK, Litt LL, Rampil IJ, Eger EI, II. Effect on outcome of prolonged exposure of patients to nitrous oxide. Anesth Analg 71:586–590, 1990.

209. Waldman FM, Koblin DD, Lampe GH, Wauk LZ, Eger EI, II. Hematologic effects of nitrous oxide in surgical patients. Anesth Analg 71:618–624, 1990.

210. Nunn JF, Chanarin I. Nitrous oxide inactivates methionine synthetase. In: Nitrous Oxide/N₂O, 1st ed. Edited by E.I. Eger, II. New York: Elsevier, 1985:211–233.

211. Koblin DD, Tomerson BW, Waldman FM, Lampe GH, Wauk LZ, Eger EI, II. Effect of nitrous oxide on folate and vitamin B12 metabolism in patients. Anesth Analg 71:610–617, 1990.

212. Layzer RB, Fishman RA, Schafer JA. Neuropathy following abuse of nitrous oxide. Neurology 28:504–506, 1978.

213. Layzer RB. Myeloneuropathy after prolonged exposure to nitrous oxide. Lancet 2:1227–1230, 1978.

214. Hong K, Trudell JR, O'Neil JR, Cohen EN. Biotransformation of nitrous oxide. Anesthesiology 53:354–355, 1980.

215. Hong K, Trudell JR, O'Neil JR, Cohen EN. Metabolism of nitrous oxide by human and rat intestinal contents. Anesthesiology 52:16–19, 1980.

216. Weathersby PK, Homer LD. Solubility of inert gases in biological fluids and tissues: A review. Undersea Biomed Res 7:277–296, 1980.

217. Steffey EP, Johnson BH, Eger EI, II, Howland D, Jr. Nitrous oxide increases the accumulation rate and decreases the uptake of bowel gases. Anesth Analg 58:405–408, 1979.

218. Eger EI, II, Saidman LJ. Hazards of nitrous oxide anesthesia in bowel obstruction and pneumothorax. Anesthesiology 26:61–66, 1965.

219. Steffey EP, Gauger GE, Eger EI II. Cardiovascular effects of venous air embolism during air and oxygen breathing. Anesth Analg 53:599–604, 1974.

220. Munson ES, Merrick HC. Effect of nitrous oxide on venous air embolism. Anesthesiology 27:783–787, 1966.

221. Davis I, Moore JRM, Lahiri SK. Nitrous oxide and the middle ear. Anaesthesia 34:147–151, 1979.

222. Perreault L, Normandin N, Plamondon L, Blain R, Rousseau P, Girard M, Forget G. Middle ear pressure variations during nitrous oxide and oxygen anaesthesia. Can Anaesth Soc J 29:428–434, 1982.

223. Saidman LJ, Eger EI, II. Change in cerebrospinal fluid pressure during pneumoencephalography under nitrous oxide anesthesia. Anesthesiology 26:67–72, 1965.

224. Stanley TH, Kawamura R, Graves C. Effects of N₂O on volume and pressure of endotracheal tube cuffs. Anesthesiology 41:256–262, 1974.

225. Stanley TH. Effects of anesthetic gases on endotracheal tube cuff gas volumes. Anesth Analg 53:480–482, 1974.

226. Stanley TH. Nitrous oxide and pressures and volumes of high- and low-pressure endotracheal-tube cuffs in intubated patients. Anesthesiology 42:637–640, 1975.

227. Bednarski R.M. Advantages and guidelines for using nitrous oxide. Vet Clin North Am Small Anim Pract 22:313–314, 1992.

228. Klide AM, Haskins SC. Precautions when using nitrous oxide. Vet Clin North Am Small Anim Pract 22:314–316, 1992.

229. Linde HW, Bruce DL. Occupational exposure of anesthetists to halothane, nitrous oxide and radiation. Anesthesiology 30:363–368, 1969.

230. Whitcher CE, Cohen EN, Trudell JR. Chronic exposure to anesthetic gases in the operating room. Anesthesiology 35:348–353, 1971.

231. Nikki P, Pfaffli P, Ahlman K. Chronic exposure to anaesthetic gases in the operating theatre and recovery room. Ann Clin Res 4:266–272, 1972.

232. Millard RI, Corbett TH. Nitrous oxide concentrations in the dental operatory. J Oral Surg 32:593–594, 1974.

233. Campbell RL, Hannifan MA, Reist PC, Gregg JM. Exposure to anesthetic waste gas in oral surgery. J Oral Surg 35:625–630, 1977.

234. Cleaton-Jones P, et al. Nitrous oxide contamination in dental surgeries using relative analgesia. Br J Anaesth 50:1019–1024, 1978.

235. Whitcher C, Zimmerman DC, Piziali RL. Control of occupational exposure to nitrous oxide in the oral surgery office. J Oral Surg 36:431–440, 1978.

236. Ward GS, Byland RR. Concentrations of methoxyflurane and nitrous oxide in veterinary operating rooms. Am J Vet Res 43:360–362, 1982.

237. Ward GS, Byland RR. Concentrations of halothane in veterinary operating and treatment rooms. J Am Vet Med Assoc 180:174–177, 1982.

238. Milligan JE, Sablan JL, Short CE. A survey of waste anesthetic gas concentrations in U.S. Airforce veterinary surgeries. J Am Vet Med Assoc 177:1021–1022, 1980.

239. Dreesen DW, Jones GL, Brown J, Rawlings CA. Monitoring for trace anesthetic gases in a veterinary teaching hospital. J Am Vet Med Assoc 179:797–799, 1981.

240. Manley SV, McDonell WF. Recommendations for reduction of anesthetic gas pollution. J Am Vet Med Assoc 176:519–524, 1980.

241. Manley SV, Taloff P, Aberg N, Howitt GA. Occupational exposure to waste anesthetic gases in veterinary practice. Calif Vet 36:14–19, 1982.

242. Pfaffli P, Nikki P, Ahlman K. Halothane and nitrous oxide in end-tidal air and venous blood of surgical personnel. Ann Clin Res 4:273–277, 1972.

243. Corbett TH. Retention of anesthetic agents following occupational exposure. Anesth Analg 52:614–618, 1973.

244. Ad Hoc Committee on the Effect of Trace Anesthetics on the Health of Operating Room Personnel. Occupational disease among operating room personnel: A national study. Anesthesiology 41:321–340, 1974.

245. Cohen EN, Bellville JW, Brown BW. Anesthesia, pregnancy, and miscarriage: A study of operating room nurses and anesthetists. Anesthesiology 35:343–347, 1971.

246. Cohen EN, Brown BW, Jr, Bruce DL, Cascorbi HF, Corbett TH, Jones TW, Whitcher CE. A survey of anesthetic health hazards among dentists. J Am Dent Assoc 90:1291–1296, 1975.

247. Geraci CL, Jr. Operating room pollution: Governmental perspectives and guidelines. Anesth Analg 56:775–777, 1977.

248. Lecky JH. The mechanical aspects of anesthetic pollution control. Anesth Analg 56:769–774, 1977.

249. Ad Hoc Committee on Effects of Trace Anesthetic Agents on Health of Operating Room Personnel. Waste anesthetic gases in operating room air: A suggested program to reduce personnel exposure. Park Ridge, IL: American Society of Anesthesiologists, 1983.

250. Lecky JH. Anesthetic pollution in the operating room: A notice to operating room personnel. Anesthesiology 52:157–159, 1980.

251. Eger EI, II. Isoflurane (Forane). A compendium and reference. Madison, WI: Ohio Medical Products, 1982.

252. Rodgers RC, Hill GE. Equations for vapour pressure versus temperature: Derivation and use of the Antoine equation on a hand-held programmable calculator. Br J Anaesth 50:415–424, 1978.

253. Steffey EP. Inhalation anesthesia. In: Feline Anaesthesia. Edited by L.W. Hall and P. Taylor. London: Balliere Tindall, 1994.

254. Eger EI, II. Desflurane animal and human pharmacology: Aspects of kinetics, safety, and MAC. Anesth Analg 75:S3–S9, 1992.

255. Jones RM. Desflurane and sevoflurane: Inhalation anaesthetics for this decade? Br J Anaesth 65:527–536, 1990.

256. Laster MJ, Fang Z, Eger EI, II. Specific gravities of desflurane, enflurane, halothane, isoflurane, and sevoflurane. Anesth Analg 78:1152–1153, 1994.

257. Miller ED, Jr, Greene NM. Waking up to desflurane: The anesthetic for the 90s? Anesth Analg 70:1–2, 1990.

258. Eger EI, II. Partition coefficients of I-653 in human blood, saline, and olive oil. Anesth Analg 66:971–974, 1987.

259. Steward A, Allott PR, Cowles AL, Mapleson WW. Solubility coefficients for inhaled anaesthetics for water, oil and biological media. Br J Anaesth 45:282–293, 1973.

260. Strum DP, Eger EI, II. Partition coefficients for sevoflurane in human blood, saline, and olive oil. Anesth Analg 66:654–657, 1987.

261. Webb AI, Weaver BMQ. Solubility of halothane in equine tissues at 37°C. Br J Anaesth 53:479–486, 1981.

262. Cascorbi HF, Blake DA, Helrich M. Differences in the biotransformation of halothane in man. Anesthesiology 32:119–123, 1970.

263. Chase RE, Holaday DA, Fiserova-Bergerova V, Saidman LJ, Mack FE. The biotransformation of ethrane in man. Anesthesiology 35:262–267, 1971.

264. Holaday DA, Fiserova-Bergerova V, Latto IP, Zumbiel MA. Resistance of isoflurane to biotransformation in man. Anesthesiology 43:325–332, 1975.

265. Brown BR, Crout JR. A comparative study of the effects of five general anesthetics on myocontractility: I. Isometric conditions. Anesthesiology 34:236–245, 1971.

266. Steffey EP, Gillespie JR, Berry JD, Eger EI, II, Munson ES. Anesthetic potency (MAC) of nitrous oxide in the dog, cat and stumptail monkey. J Appl Physiol 36:530–532, 1974.

267. McMurphy RM, Hodgson DS. The minimum alveolar concentration of desflurane in cats. Vet Surg 1995.

268. Fyhrquist. Clinical pharmacology of the ACE inhibitors. Drugs 32(5):33–39, 1986.

269. Drummond JC, Todd MM, Shapiro HM. Minimal alveolar concentrations for halothane, enflurane, and isoflurane in the cat. J Am Vet Med Assoc 182:1099–1101, 1983.

270. Webb AI, McMurphy RM. Effect of anticholinergic preanesthetic medicaments on the requirements of halothane for anesthesia in the cat. Am J Vet Res 48:1733–1736, 1987.

271. Eger EI, II, Brandstater B, Saidman LJ, Regan MJ, Severinghaus JW, Munson ES. Equipotent alveolar concentrations of methoxyflurane, halothane, diethyl ether, fluroxene, cyclopropane, xenon, and nitrous oxide in the dog. Anesthesiology 26:771–777, 1965.

272. Eger EI, II, Saidman LJ, Brandstater B. Temperature dependence of halothane and cylcopropane anesthesia in dogs: Correlation with some theories of anesthetic action. Anesthesiology 26:764–770, 1965.

273. Eger EI, II, Lundgren C, Miller SL, Stevens WC. Anesthetic potencies of sulfur hexafluoride, carbon tetrafluoride, chloroform and ethrane in dogs: Correlation with the hydrate and lipid theories of anesthetic action. Anesthesiology 30:129–135, 1969.

274. Kazama T, Ikeda K. Comparison of MAC and the rate of rise of alveolar concentration of sevoflurane with halothane and isoflurane in the dog. Anesthesiology 68(3):435–438, 1988.

275. Doorley MB, Waters SJ, Terrell RC, Robinson JL. MAC of I-653 in beagle dogs and New Zealand white rabbits. Anesthesiology 69:89–92, 1988.

276. Regan MJ, Eger EI, II. Effect of hypothermia in dogs on anesthetizing and apneic doses of inhalation agents. Determination of the anesthetic index (apnea/MAC). Anesthesiology 28:689–700, 1967.

277. Steffey EP, Farver TB, Woliner MJ. Circulatory and respiratory effects of methoxyflurane in dogs: comparison of halothane. Am J Vet Res 45:2574–2579, 1984.

278. Steffey EP, Eger EI, II. The effect of hyperthermia on halothane MAC in dogs. Anesthesiology 41:392–396, 1974.

279. Murphy MR, Hug CC, Jr. The anesthetic potency of fentanyl in terms of its reduction of enflurane MAC. Anesthesiology 57:485–488, 1982.

280. DeYoung DJ, Sawyer DC. Anesthetic potency of nitrous oxide during halothane anesthesia in the dog. J Am Anim Hosp Assoc 16:125–128, 1980.

281. Himez RS, Jr, Di Fazio CA, Burmey RC. Effects of lidocaine on the anesthetic requirements of nitrous oxide and halothane. Anesthesiology 47:437–440, 1977.

282. Aida H, Mizuno Y, Hobo S, Yoshida K, Fujinaga T. Determination of the minimum alveolar concentration (MAC) and physical response to sevoflurane inhalation in horses. J Vet Med Sci 56:1161–1165, 1994.

283. Tinker JH, Sharbough FW, Michenfelder TD. Anterior shift of the dominant EEG rhythm during anesthesia in the Java monkey. Anesthesiology 46:252–259, 1977.

284. Mazze RI, Rice SA, Baden JM. Halothane, isoflurane, and enflurane MAC in pregnant and nonpregnant female and male mice and rats. Anesthesiology 62:339–342, 1985.

285. Deady JR, Koblin DD, Eger EI, II, Heavner JE, D'Aoust B. Anesthetic potencies and the unitary theory of narcosis. Anesth Analg 60:380–384, 1981.

286. Miller KW, Paton WDM, Smith EB, Smith RA. Physiochemical approaches to the mode of action of general anesthetics. Anesthesiology 36:339–351, 1972.

287. Steffey EP, Howland D, Jr. Halothane anesthesia in calves. Am J Vet Res 40:372–376, 1979.

288. Tranquilli WJ, Thurmon JC, Benson GJ, Steffey EP. Halothane potency in pigs (Sus scrofa). Am J Vet Res 44:1106–1107, 1983.

289. Lundeen G, Manohar M, Parks C. Systemic distribution of blood flow in swine while awake and during 1.0 and 1.5 MAC isoflurane anesthesia with or without 50% nitrous oxide. Anesth Analg 62:499–512, 1983.

290. Manohar M, Parks CM. Porcine systemic and regional organ blood flow during 1.0 and 1.5 minimum alveolar concentrations of sevoflurane anesthesia without and with 50% nitrous oxide. J Pharmacol Exp Ther 234:640–648, 1984.

291. Weiskopf R, Bogetz MS. Minimum alveolar concentrations (MAC) of halothane and nitrous oxide in swine. Anesth Analg 63:529–532, 1984.

292. Gallagher TM, Burrows FA, Miyasaka K, Volgyesi GA, Lerman J. Sevoflurane in newborn swine: anesthetic requirements (MAC) and circulatory responses (abstract). Anesthesiology 67:A503, 1987.

293. Eisele PH, Talken L, Eisele JH, Jr. Potency of isoflurane and nitrous oxide in conventional swine. Lab Anim Sci 35:76–78, 1985.

294. Davis NL, Nunnally RL, Malinin TI. Determination of the minimum alveolar concentration (MAC) of halothane in the white New Zealand rabbit. Br J Anaesth 47:341–345, 1975.

295. Drummond JC. MAC for halothane, enflurane, and isoflurane in the New Zealand white rabbit and a test for the validity of MAC determinations. Anesthesiology 62:336–339, 1985.

296. Scheller MS, Saidman LJ, Partridge BL. MAC of sevoflurane in humans and the New Zealand white rabbit. Can J Anaesth 35:153–157, 1988.

297. Wear R, Robinson S, Gregory GA. Effect of halothane on baroresponse of adult and baby rabbits. Anesthesiology 56:188–191, 1982.

298. Shi WZ, Fahey MR, Fisher DM, Eger EI, II, Canfill C, Miller RD. Increase in minimum alveolar concentration (MAC) of halothane by laudanosine in rabbits. Anesth Analg 64:282, 1985.

299. Waizer PR, Baez S, Orkin LR. A method for determining minimum alveolar concentration of anesthetic in the rat. Anesthesiology 39:394–397, 1973.

300. Vitez TS, White PF, Eger EI, II. Effects of hypothermia on halothane MAC and isoflurane MAC in the rat. Anesthesiology 41:80–81, 1974.

301. Crawford MW, Lerman J, Saldivia V, Carmichael FJ. Hemodynamic and organ blood flow responses to halothane and sevoflurane anesthesia during spontaneous ventilation. Anesth Analg 75:1000–1006, 1992.

302. Eger EI, II, Johnson BH. MAC of I-653 in rats, including a test of the effect of body temperature and anesthetic duration. Anesth Analg 66:974–977, 1987.

303. DiFazio CA, Brown RE, Ball CG, Heckel CG, Kennedy SS. Additive effects of anesthetics and theories of anesthesia. Anesthesiology 36:57–63, 1972.

304. White PF, Johnston RR, Eger EI, II. Determination of anesthetic requirement in rats. Anesthesiology 40 52–57, 1974.

305. Taheri S, Halsey MJ, Liu J, Eger EI, II, Koblin DD, Laster MJ. What solvent best represents the site of action of inhaled anesthetics in humans, rats, and dogs? Anesth Analg 72:627–634, 1991.

306. Laster MJ, Liu J, Eger EI, II, Taheri S. Electrical stimulation as a substitute for the tail clamp in the determination of minimum alveolar concentration. Anesth Analg 76:1310–1312, 1993.

307. Russell GB, Graybeal JM. Direct measurement of nitrous oxide MAC and neurologic monitoring in rats during anesthesia under hyperbaric conditions. Anesth Analg 75:995–999, 1992.

308. Gonsowski CT, Eger EI, II. Nitrous oxide minimum alveolar anesthetic concentration in rats is greater than previously reported. Anesth Analg 79:710–712, 1994.

309. Strout CD, Nahrwold MC. Halothane requirement during pregnancy and lactation in rats. Anesthesiology 55:322–323, 1981.

310. Roizen MF, White PF, Eger EI, II, Brownstein M. Effects of ablation of serotonin or norepinephrine brain-stem areas on halothane and cyclopropane MACs in rats. Anesthesiology 49:252–255, 1978.

311. Palahniuk RJ, Shnider SM, Eger EI, II. Pregnancy decreases the requirement for inhaled anesthetic agents. Anesthesiology 41: 82–83, 1974.

312. Ludders JW. Minimal anesthetic concentration (MAC) and cardiopulmonary dose-response of halothane in pekin ducks (abstract). Anaesthes. Fourth International Congress of Veterinary Anesthesia (suppl). 131, 1991.

313. Ludders JW, Mitchell GS, Rode J. Minimal anesthetic concentration and cardiopulmonary dose response of isoflurane in ducks. Vet Surg 19:304–307, 1990.

314. Ludders JW, Rode J, Mitchell GS. Isoflurane anesthesia in sandhill cranes (*Grus canadensis*): Minimal anesthetic concentration and cardiopulmonary dose response during spontaneous and controlled breathing. Anesth Analg 68:511–516, 1989.

315. Fitzgerald G, Blais D. Effect of nitrous oxide on the minimal anesthetic dose of isoflurane in pigeons and red-tailed hawks (abst). Proceedings, Fourth International Congress of Veterinary Anaesthesia. 27, 1991.

316. Curro T, Brunson D, Paul-Murphy J. Evaluation of the ED_{50} of isoflurane and the isoflurane-sparing effect of butorphanol and flunixin meglumine in parrots (Psittaciformes) (abstract). Proceedings, Fifth International Congress of Veterinary Anesthesia. 57, 1994.

317. Shim CY, Andersen NB. The effects of oxygen on minimal anesthetic requirements in the toad. Anesthesiology 34:333–337, 1971.

318. Cherkin A, Catchpool JF. Temperature dependence of anesthesia in goldfish. Science 144:1460–1462, 1964.

319. Saidman LJ, Eger EI, II, Munson ES, Babad AA, Muallem M. Minimum alveolar concentrations of methoxyflurane, halothane, ether and cyclopropane in man: Correlation with theories of anesthesia. Anesthesiology 28:994–1002, 1967.

320. Stevens WC, Dolan WM, Gibbons RD, White A, Eger EI, II, Miller RD, De Jong RH, Elashoff RM. Minimum alveolar concentrations (MAC) of isoflurane with and without nitrous oxide in patients of various ages. Anesthesiology 42:197–200, 1975.

321. Gion H, Saidman LJ. The minimum alveolar concentration of enflurane in man. Anesthesiology 35:361–364, 1971.

322. Rampil IJ, Lockhart SH, Zwass MS, Peterson N, Yasuda N, Eger EI, II, Weiskopf RB, Damask MC. Clinical characteristics of desflurane in surgical patients–Minimum alveolar concentration. Anesthesiology 74:429–433, 1991.

323. Hornbein TF, Eger EI, II, Winter PM, Smith G, Wetstone D, Smith KH. The minimum alveolar concentration of nitrous oxide in man. Anesth Analg 61:553–556, 1982.

324. Miller RD, Wahrenbrock EA, Schroeder CF, Knipstein TW, Eger EI, II, Buechel DR. Ethylene-halothane anesthesia: Addition or synergism?. Anesthesiology 31:301–304, 1969.

325. Katoh T, Ikeda K. The minimum alveolar concentration (MAC) of sevoflurane in humans. Anesthesiology 66:301–304, 1987.

326. Saidman LJ, Eger EI, II. Effect of nitrous oxide and of narcotic premedication on the alveolar concentration of halothane required for anesthesia. Anesthesiology 25:302–306, 1964.

327. Bridges BEJ, Eger EI, II. The effect of hypocapnia on the level of halothane anesthesia in man. Anesthesiology 27:634–637, 1966.

328. Steffey EP, Baggot JD, Eisele JH Jr. Morphine-isoflurane interaction in horses (abstract). FASEB J 4:A879, 1990.

329. Zucker J. Central cholinergic depression reduces MAC for isoflurane in rats. Anesth Analg 72:790–795, 1991.

330. Wouters P, Doursout M, Merin RG, Chelly JE. Influence of hypertension on MAC of halothane in rats. Anesthesiology 72:843–845, 1990.

331. White PF, Johnston RR, Pudwill CR. Interaction of ketamine and halothane in rats. Anesthesiology 42:179 1975.

332. Stone DJ, Moscicki JC, DiFazio CA. Thiopental reduces halothane MAC in rats. Anesth Analg 74:542–546, 1992.

333. Steffey EP, Pascoe PJ. Xylazine reduces the isoflurane MAC in horses (abstract). Vet Surg 20:158, 1991.

334. Ewing KK, Mohammed HO, Scarlett JM, Short CE. Reduction of isoflurane anesthetic requirement by medetomidine and its restoration by atipamezole in dogs. Am J Vet Res 54:294–299, 1993.

335. Vainio OM, Bloor BC. Relation between body temperature and dexmedetomidine-induced minimum alveolar concentration and respiratory changes in isoflurane-anesthetized miniature swine. Am J Vet Res 55:1000–1006, 1994.

336. Pascoe PJ, Steffey EP, Black WD, Claxton JM, Jacobs JR, Woliner MJ. Evaluation of the effect of alfentanil on the minimum alveolar concentration on halothane in horses. Am J Vet Res 54:1327–1332, 1993.

337. Murphy MR, Hug CC Jr. The anesthetic potency of fentanyl in terms of its reduction of enflurane MAC. Anesthesiology 57:485–488, 1982.

338. Matthews NS, Dollar NS, Shawley RV. Halothane-sparing effect of benzodiazepines in ponies. Cornell Vet 80:259–265, 1990.

339. Heard DJ, Webb AI, Daniels RT. Effect of acepromazine on the anesthetic requirement of halothane in the dog. Am J Vet Res 47:2113–2116, 1986.

340. Steffey EP, Martucci R, Howland D, Asling JH, Eisele JH. Meperidine-halothane interaction in dogs. Can Anaesth Soc J 24:459–467, 1977.

341. Seitz PA, Terriet M, Rush W, Merrell WJ. Adenosine decreases the minimum alveolar concentration of halothane in dogs. Anesthesiology 73:990–994, 1990.

342. Doherty TJ, McDonell WN, Dyson DH, Black WD, Valliant AE. The effect of a 5-hydroxytryptamine antagonist (R51703) on halothane MAC in the dog. J Vet Pharmacol Ther 18:153–155, 1995.

343. Weiskopf RB, Holmes MA, Rampil IJ, Johnson BH, Yasuda N, Targ AG, Eger EI, II. Cardiovascular safety and actions of high concentrations of I-653 and isoflurane in swine. Anesthesiology 70:793–799, 1989.

344. Tranquilli WJ, Thurmon JC, Benson GJ. Anesthetic potency of nitrous oxide in young swine (*Sus scrofa*). Am J Vet Res 46:58–60, 1985.

345. Muir WW III, Wagner AE, Hinchcliff KW. Cardiorespiratory and MAC-reducing effects of α_2-adrenoreceptor agonists in horses. In: Animal Pain. Short CE, VanPoznak A, eds. New York: Churchill Livingstone, 1992, pp 201–212.

346. Steffey EP, Kelly AB. Methoxyflurane MAC in horses. Unpublished observations, University of California, Davis, 1979.

chapter 12

LOCAL ANESTHETICS

James E. Heavner

Introduction

Local anesthetics are a group of drugs that reversibly block the propagation of action potentials along nerve axons. They are used to anesthetize a region of the body. Muscle paralysis may or may not occur and may or may not be a desirable effect. These drugs are relatively unique in that they are applied directly at the target site. Absorption into and distribution by the systemic circulation is not necessary to achieve the intended application. The primary action of local anesthetics is interference with voltage-gated sodium channels, but they have other effects as well. Some local anesthetics are employed clinically for purposes other than producing anesthesia (e.g., lidocaine is used to treat cardiac ventricular arrhythmias).

History

Cocaine was the first local anesthetic to be discovered. It is an alkaloid present in the leaves of *Erythroxylon coca*, a shrub that grows in the Andes Mountains. Natives in that region chew or suck the leaves to obtain cocaine and experience a sense of well-being that it produces.

Gaedicke extracted erythroxylin from the leaves of the plant in 1855, and Niemann isolated cocaine in 1860. The first use of cocaine as a local anesthetic was described by a Peruvian army surgeon. In 1884 a report by Koeller revealed that instillation of cocaine into the conjunctival sac anesthetized the eye. This led to appreciation of the clinical usefulness of cocaine. Subsequently, cocaine was widely used by ophthalmologists as a topical anesthetic. Halsted administered cocaine to induce peripheral nerve block and Bier used it to produce spinal anesthesia shortly after Koeller's discovery.

Efforts to develop chemicals that were less addictive and toxic than cocaine, yet with local anesthetic activity, led to the synthesis of procaine by Einhorn in 1905. This ester of para-aminobenzoic acid was the prototype for synthesis of other benzoic acid–derived local anesthetics. The next milestone in the development of local anesthetics was the synthesis of lidocaine by Lofgren in 1943. Lidocaine is an amide derivative of diethylaminoacetic acid and the prototype for the synthesis of other amide-linked local anesthetics.

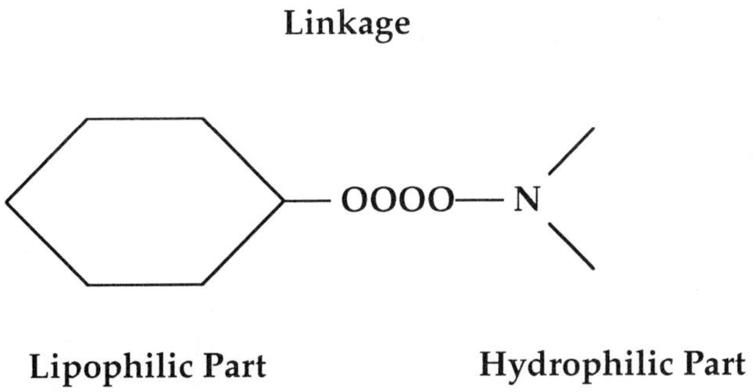

Linkage

Lipophilic Part   Hydrophilic Part

Fig. 12–1. Basic molecular structure of local anesthetics.

Chemistry and Structure-Activity Relationships

Clinically useful local anesthetics have similar physical properties and molecular structures. Most of the drugs are weakly basic tertiary amines (that is, a nitrogen atom with three attached organic groups). A few, such as hexylcaine and prilocaine, are secondary amines. The basic local anesthetic molecule has three parts: a hydrophilic end (imparting water solubility), a lipophilic end (imparting lipid solubility), and an intermediate hydrocarbon chain connecting the hydrophilic and lipophilic ends (Fig. 12–1). The aromatic end (lipophilic) is derived from benzoic acid or aniline. The hydrophilic end is less easily characterized, though amino derivatives of ethyl alcohol or acetic acid are common. Some local anesthetics (for example, benzocaine) lack the hydrophilic tail and are nearly insoluble in water, and thus are not suitable for injection but are satisfactory for topical application to mucosal surfaces and open wounds.

The 6 to 9 Å separation of the lipophilic and hydrophilic components by four or five atoms appears to be critical for a molecule to retain local anesthetic activity. Antihistaminics, anticholinergics, and other classes of compounds have a structure similar to that of local anesthetics and often exhibit weak local anesthetic effects. Further details regarding chemistry and structure-activity relationships of local anesthetics can be found in the review by Courtney and Strichartz.(1)

Grouping Local Anesthetics

Local anesthetics are typically classed as being *ester-linked* or *amide-linked,* depending on the structure of the molecule's intermediate chain. Local anesthetics de-

rived from benzoic acid belong to the ester family, and those derived from aniline belong to the aminoacyl or amide family. The nature of the intermediate chain predetermines the course of biotransformation of local anesthetics. Ester-linked local anesthetics, characterized by procaine (Fig. 12–2), are readily hydrolyzed. Amide-linked local anesthetics, characterized by lidocaine (Fig. 12–3), are generally biotransformed by liver microsomal enzymes.

Time to effect, potency, and duration of action of local anesthetics basically depend upon the physical chemical properties of their molecular structure (Table 12–1). *Lipid solubility* is a major determinant of *intrinsic local anesthetic potency* among drugs. Because axonal membranes are highly lipid in composition, local anesthetics act strongly on these structures. In the ester series of local anesthetics, addition of a butyl group to the lipophilic end of procaine yields the local anesthetic tetracaine, which is considerably more lipid soluble and intrinsically more potent than procaine. In the amide series, the replacement of the methyl group with a butyl group on the lipophilic end of mepivacaine leads to the formation of bupivacaine, which is 15 times more lipid soluble and 4 times more potent than mepivacaine.

Protein binding is believed to be a primary determinant of *local anesthetic duration,* presumably because the site of action of local anesthetics involves the protein within the axonal membrane. The greater the binding affinity to axonal protein, the longer anesthetic activity persists. Tetracaine is 13 times more highly bound to proteins, and its anesthetic duration is 3 to 7 times longer than that of procaine.

The acid dissociation constant (pKa) is generally thought to determine the speed of action of local anesthetics. Local anesthetic agents exist in solution in both the charged cationic (+) and the uncharged base forms. It is generally thought that the base is primarily responsible for onset of action, because the uncharged form diffuses more readily across the nerve sheath.

Mechanism of Action

Local anesthetics prevent the rapid influx of sodium into nerve axons that produces the action potential.(2) Under resting conditions there is a voltage difference

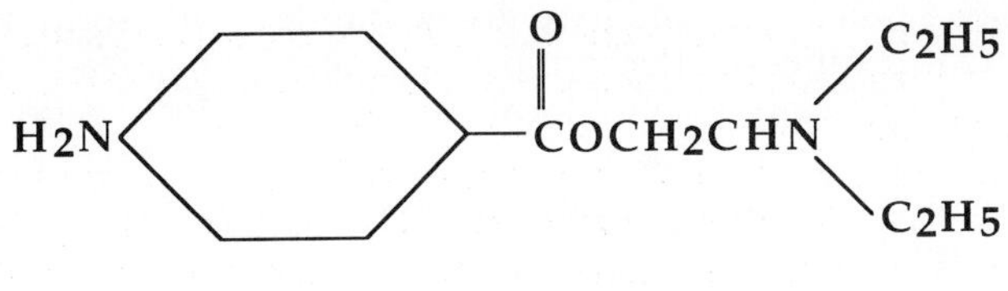

Procaine

Fig. 12–2. Procaine.

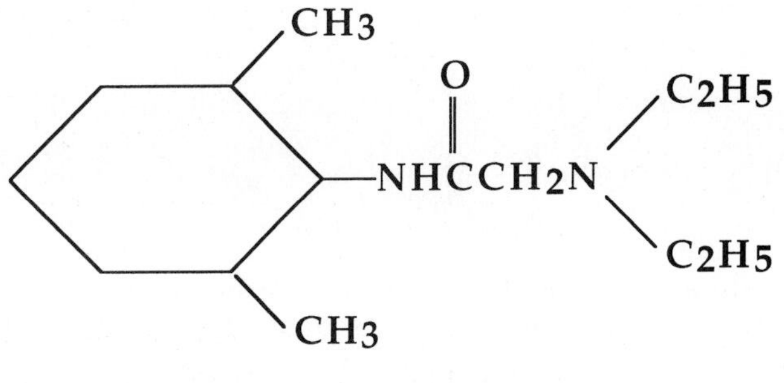

Lidocaine

Fig. 12–3. Lidocaine.

Table 12–1. Physical, Chemical and Biologic Properties of the Commonly Used Local Anesthetic Agents

Agent	Lipid Solubility	Relative Potency	pKa	Onset of Action	Plasma Protein Binding (%)	Duration (min)	Molecular Weight
Low potency, short duration							
Procaine*,†	1	1	8.9	Slow	6	60–90	236
Chloroprocaine†	1	1	9.1	Fast	7	30–60	271
Intermediate potency and duration							
Mepivacaine‡	2	2	7.6	Fast	75	120–240	246
Prilocaine‡	1	2	7.7	Fast	55	120–240	220
Lidocaine‡	3.6	2	7.7	Fast	65	90–200	234
High potency, long duration							
Tetracaine†	80	8	8.6	Slow	80	180–600	264
Bupivacaine‡	30	8	8.1	Intermediate	95	180–600	288
Etidocaine‡	140	6	7.7	Fast	95	180–600	276

*Procaine is the least potent of the local anesthetics in current use; the relative potency given in this chart is relative to procaine.
†ester
‡amide

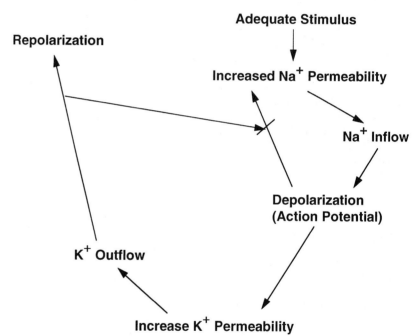

Fig. 12–4. Flow of sodium (Na^+) and potassium (K^+) triggered by an adequate stimulus. (From Heavner, reprinted with permission).(3)

across axonal membranes (the inside being in the range of 70 mV negative with respect to the outside). When the membrane receives an adequate stimulus, it depolarizes, producing an action potential that moves in obligatory fashion along the axon (propagated action potential) (Chapter 7). The depolarization produces a cascade of events as shown in Figure 12–4. The influx of sodium ions into the axon is controlled by sodium channels that exist in various states (Fig. 12–5) depending upon the transmembrane potential.(3)

A number of theories about how local anesthetics prevent the generation of a propagated action potential have been offered. One of the most consistent ones is that local anesthetics, in positively charged form, enter

the sodium channel from inside the axon and "plug" the channel. Another popular theory offered is that local anesthetics, being lipid soluble, nestle in the axon membrane lipids, and in so doing, interfere with sodium channel function. Perhaps best accepted is the idea that most clinically useful local anesthetics block action potential propagation via a combination of actions: channel blocking and indirect interference with sodium channel function.(4)

A recent review of the molecular mechanisms of local anesthetic action suggests that local anesthetics act solely by binding to receptors located on sodium channels (Fig. 12–6).(5) Local anesthetics may differ in their ability to bind to sodium channels depending on

Depolarization

Resting ———► Closed ———► Open ———► Inactivated

Repolarization

Inactivated ———————————► Resting

Fig. 12–5. A very simplified example of the order of sodium "state" changes during membrane depolarization. (From Heavner, reprinted with permission).(3)

channel status. For instance, benzocaine may bind to the channel conformation representing one state, whereas lidocaine may bind to a different conformational state of the sodium channel. There is evidence for this preferential binding among local anesthetics, and clinically observed differences in local anesthetic effects can be explained on this basis. The channel-binding concept does not explain how pressure reversal of benzocaine-induced nerve block is achieved.

It is important to note that there are families of channels (e.g., sodium channels in heart, brain, and axons are not identical) and that a given tissue may contain a variety of different sodium channels.(6) Local anesthetic effects may differ depending on the kind(s) of sodium channels present in the target tissue, and some local anesthetic effects (e.g., CNS toxicity) may be mediated by actions other than interference with sodium channel function.

Differential Nerve Block

Analgesia/anesthesia without loss of motor function frequently is desirable and can be achieved with appropriate use of local anesthetics. This suggests that sensory nerve fibers might be more readily blocked by local anesthetics than are large motor fibers. Human studies as well as in vitro studies have been done to document that such differential sensitivity does indeed exist, to document why, and to rank fibers in order of sensitivity to block. With spinal anesthesia in humans, the level of sympathetic block extends further than does sensory block, which extends further than somatic motor block.(7) This suggests that preganglionic sympathetic nerve fibers (B fibers) are more sensitive to local anesthetics than are small sensory nerve fibers (A-delta), which are more sensitive than larger motor fibers (A-alpha). It has been demonstrated in vitro that cocaine blocks small A-delta fibers more readily than A-alpha fibers.(8) On the other hand, the spectrum of sensitivity of unmyelinated fibers (C fibers) overlaps that of the myelinated fibers.(9)

Studies of differential sensitivity of nerve fibers based on compound action potential analysis have been criticized, and claims have been made that studies of individual axons are more accurate. In the latter case, differential sensitivity has been less clear. However,

such studies have reinforced older ideas regarding differential sensitivity based on a critical length of fiber that must be blocked and/or the rate at which axons discharge. It generally is agreed that spread of local anesthetic in high enough concentration to block three consecutive nodes of Ranvier in myelinated axons is a minimal requirement to stop electric transmission through an axon. Obviously, this does not apply to unmyelinated C fibers and points to this fiber group as standing apart from myelinated fibers with respect to factors influencing local anesthetic block. There is evidence that the frequency with which axons discharge correlates with vulnerability to local anesthetic action. Axons that have a high discharge rate (e.g., C

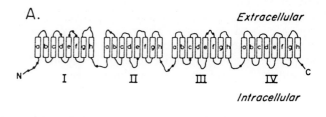

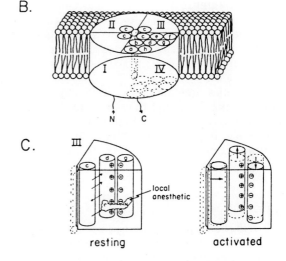

Fig. 12–6. A speculative model for the molecular mechanism of local anesthetic action. (A) The primary sequence of the large subunit of the sodium channel has four repeating domains (I to IV), each containing six to eight sequences of amino acids that probably form α helical structures spanning the nerve membrane, denoted by the rectangles lettered a to h. (B) It has been postulated that these helices pack together in approximately fourfold symmetry, with the polar edges of the four c helices forming the lining of the ion pore and projecting through the center of the complex. For simplicity, only the extracellular (top) and intracellular (bottom, dashed ellipses) edges of the helices are shown. (C) A stripped-down view of quadrant III shows the postulated gating mechanism. Helix d is coupled to the pore-forming helix c and contains a series of basic amino acids that form a strip of positive charges. These charges are stabilized in the low dielectric milieu of the membrane interior by a strip of negative charges counterpoised to them on helix g. Membrane depolarization activates the channel by pulling the g helix in, pushing the d helix out, and thereby moving the c helix to open the channel pore. It is speculated that a local anesthetic binds at a site near or on the gating helices, as drawn on the resting conformation, and prevents these conformational changes. (From Butterworth and Strichartz, permission requested).(5)

and A-delta fibers) are more sensitive to local anesthetics than are fibers with lower discharge rates (e.g., A-beta fibers; frequency-dependent block).(10)

In humans, individual variation in response to local anesthetics exists, but the sensation of pain usually is the first sensory modality to disappear, followed in turn by sensations of cold, warmth, touch, and deep pressure.

Pharmacokinetics of Local Anesthetics

ABSORPTION

With one exception, local anesthetics are not injected intravascularly to induce anesthesia. The exception is when intravenous regional anesthesia (IVRA) is used to anesthetize an anterior or posterior extremity (Chapter 16). Systemic absorption of local anesthetic occurs in the other cases, and the rate of absorption varies directly with the vascularity of the injection site. The faster the absorption rate, the shorter the duration of action of the local anesthetic and the greater the risk of systemic toxicity.

A vasoconstrictor, most commonly epinephrine, is added to local anesthetic solutions to reduce local blood flow, thereby prolonging duration of action and reducing the probability of systemic toxicity. In fact, maximum recommended doses of local anesthetics are increased if a vasoconstrictor is added. Usual concentration of epinephrine is 1:200,000 (5 µg/mL) or 1:400,000 (2.5 µg/mL).

Local anesthetics generally are ineffective when applied to unbroken skin, but they are effective when the skin is broken, when applied to the cornea, or when applied to mucous membranes. Recently a eutectic mixture of prilocaine and lidocaine (EMLA creme) has been marketed that is effective when applied to the skin (Chapter 16).

DISTRIBUTION

Local Distribution. Distribution of local anesthetic at the injection site depends upon the volume of local anesthetic solution injected and how resistant the tissue is to the spread of the local anesthetic. Hyaluronidase is sometimes added to local anesthetic solutions to enhance spread, especially when the local anesthetic is injected into the bony orbit to anesthetize the eye. When a local anesthetic is injected into the subarachnoid space (spinal anesthesia), the specific gravity (baricity) of the solution relative to the specific gravity of cerebrospinal fluid influences distribution. Hyperbaric solutions prepared by adding glucose (10%) combined with patient positioning are used to direct local anesthetic to specific sites.

Systemic Distribution. The liver and lungs are major sites for plasma clearance of local anesthetics. The extraction fraction (amount of local anesthetic extracted from the plasma by an organ) is quite high for the liver for most local anesthetics (e.g., 0.75 for lidocaine). A decrease in liver blood flow can therefore prolong

plasma half-life. The pH of the local anesthetic solution may also affect local distribution. Increasing the pH increases the ratio of uncharged to charged molecules in solution. This speeds the onset of block because the uncharged form readily diffuses to the target site.

ELIMINATION

Local anesthetics undergo biotransformation and are then excreted from the body via the urine or via the bile. The majority of the para-aminobenzoic acid formed after procaine metabolism is excreted unchanged or as a conjugated product in the urine.(11) After intravenous infusion of chloroprocaine in man, approximately 65% of the total dose is recovered over a 90-minute period. Approximately 85% of the metabolite, 2-chloro-4-aminobenzoic acid, is recovered in the form of a conjugate in the urine.(12) The liver plays an important role in the metabolism of local anesthetics. It is a source of plasma cholinesterase that cleaves the ester link or contains the mixed function oxidases that biotransforms amide-linked local anesthetics.

Local Anesthetic Toxicity

Toxic reactions to local anesthetics are easily categorized (Table 12–2), are well characterized, and are generally are not fatal if recognized early and appropriately treated. The most frequent and dramatic reactions observed clinically are acute reactions involving the direct effects of local anesthetics on the cardiovascular system and/or central nervous system. There has been considerable interest in local anesthetic cardiotoxicity alone and relative to the central nervous system toxicity in recent years. This interest stems from cardiac toxicity, induced by bupivacaine, resulting in deaths.(13) Circumstances related to these deaths suggest that bupivacaine affects the heart somewhat differently than do other local anesthetics.

Acute toxicity is usually associated with accidental intravascular injection of local anesthetics. Numerous strategies exist to avoid intoxication via this mechanism including incremental dosing, aspiration before injection, and use of test doses or substances. Studies show that premedication with certain drugs (e.g., diazepam) increases the local anesthetic seizure threshold. Benzodiazepines apparently have value in aborting seizures, as do ultra-short-acting barbiturates (e.g., thiopental). Limited evidence from animal studies show that pro-

Table 12–2. Categories of Local Anesthetic Toxic Reactions

Systemic
Cardiac/Vascular
Central nervous system
Methemoglobinemia
Localized or Systemic
Allergic reactions
Localized
Tissue toxicity

pofol may also be effective in stopping local anesthetic seizures.(14) Cardiac rhythm disturbances and cardiovascular collapse generally are treated symptomatically (e.g., volume expansion, cardiac stimulants, cardioversion, oxygen, sodium bicarbonate).

CNS TOXICITY

Central nervous system symptoms of local anesthetic toxicity usually occur before cardiovascular changes occur. In humans, the first signs of CNS toxicity include drowsiness progressing to numbness of lips, slurring of speech, agitation, tinnitus, diplopia, fine tremors, and then grand mal seizures; large doses produce generalized CNS depression (an isoelectric EEG). Ironically, there is no evidence that epileptics have a heightened susceptibility to the CNS toxicity of these drugs. In fact, local anesthetics have anticonvulsant action and have been used effectively to stop grand mal seizures.(15) Similarly, local anesthetics have been administered intravenously to produce general anesthesia. Conclusive evidence about how local anesthetics produce their effects on the CNS is lacking. Data from human and animal studies indicate that local anesthetic-induced seizures originate in the limbic brain.(16) At the neuronal level, local anesthetics appear to produce CNS symptoms via an effect on sodium conductance, possibly via the same mechanism by which they produce conduction block in axons of the peripheral nervous system. Evidence indicates that some of the cardiotoxic effect of local anesthetics, bupivacaine in particular, may actually result from effects of these drugs on the brain.(17)

CARDIOVASCULAR TOXICITY

Local anesthetics can produce profound cardiovascular changes by direct cardiac and peripheral vascular action, and indirectly by conduction blockade of autonomic fibers. The primary site of action is the myocardium, where decreases in electric excitability, conduction rate, and force of contraction occur.(18) Notable are the cardiac rhythm disturbances associated with local anesthetic cardiotoxicity. High concentrations of local anesthetics dilate blood vessels, but low concentrations may cause vasoconstriction. Inhibition of sodium conductance increase appears to play a major role in the cardiac effects of local anesthetics and probably in the vascular effects as well. However, there is evidence that potassium channel block may also contribute to the cardiotoxicity of local anesthetics.(19)

The direct cardiac depressant effects of local anesthetics have been investigated rather intensively during the last several years. This research was stimulated by the previously mentioned cardiac arrests produced by bupivacaine. Common practice is to compare the effects of bupivacaine and lidocaine. Both drugs can produce a similar pattern of cardiovascular toxicity. However, the profound depression of the cardiac conducting tissue produced by bupivacaine is difficult to treat, whereas prompt treatment of lidocaine depression

usually produces an uneventful recovery.(13) Animal studies show that resuscitation is usually successful if prompt treatment is instituted after bupivacaine overdose.(20)

Recent studies indicate that a host of physiologic changes can affect the cardiotoxicity of local anesthetics (e.g., progesterone [pregnancy], hyponatremia, and diabetes mellitus).(21-23) Even at the height of CNS symptoms, cardiovascular changes may be minimal, with some increase in pulse rate and a corresponding rise in blood pressure.

METHEMOGLOBINEMIA

Most discussions regarding the propensity for local anesthetics to produce methemoglobinemia focus on prilocaine, the only clinically used local anesthetic that is a secondary amine. However, reports implicate prilocaine, benzocaine, lidocaine, and procaine as causative agents.(24) Methemoglobinemia is formed when ferrous iron (Fe^{++}) in hemoglobin is oxidized to the ferric (Fe^{+++}) form. Methemoglobinemia can be induced in sheep by topical administration of benzocaine-containing anesthetic spray.(25)

TISSUE TOXICITY

Tissue toxicity includes irritation and lysis of cells. Muscles and nerves are of primary concern, with skeletal muscle appearing to be the most sensitive. High concentrations of local anesthetics clearly are cytotoxic. This toxic property of local anesthetics became an area of focus following reports of several incidences of prolonged sensory and motor deficits after the accidental intrathecal administration of chloroprocaine.(26) Studies triggered by these reports revealed that a number of factors other than local anesthetics could contribute to or be the primary cause of tissue destruction (e.g., solution pH, preservatives). The potent long-lasting anesthetics with high lipid solubility appear to be more likely to cause tissue damage than are other local anesthetics. Electron microscopy studies indicate that local anesthetics affect the perineurium, Schwann cells, and axons.(27)

ALLERGIC REACTIONS

Allergic reactions to local anesthetics may occur. However, the number of documented reactions is small. Reputedly, allergic reactions are more likely to occur with ester-linked local anesthetics than with amide-linked ones. Methylparaben, a preservative sometimes added to local anesthetic solutions, may cause allergic-type reactions. Cutaneous and respiratory reactions are the most common indicators of anaphylaxis.

There is little information about whether or not toxic responses to local anesthetics are age dependent. Preliminary data from animals suggests that infants may be more resistant to the acute CNS and CV toxic effects of local anesthetics than are adults. This is so despite evidence that plasma clearance of local anesthetics may be slower in infants than in adults. General anesthesia with halothane blocks grand mal seizures but enhances the acute cardiovascular toxicity of bupivacaine in 2-day-old pigs.(28)

Clinical Uses

Local and regional anesthetic techniques and their application in a variety of domestic animals are presented in Chapter 16. The main categories of anesthetics with representative drugs are now given. The number of local anesthetics is so large that it is impractical to list all of them.

Local Anesthetics Suitable for Injection: lidocaine, bupivacaine, ropivacaine, procaine, chloroprocaine, mepivacaine, tetracaine.

Local Anesthetics Largely Restricted to Ophthalmological Use: benoxinate, proparacaine.(29)

Local Anesthetics Used Mainly to Anesthetize Mucous Membranes and Skin: dibucaine, dyclonine, paramoxine, eutectic mixture of prilocaine and lidocaine (skin).

Anesthetics of Low Solubility: benzocaine (very poorly absorbed, applied to wounds and ulcerated surfaces to produce sustained anesthesia).

Local Anesthetics Approved for Veterinary Use per Codified Federal Register (CFR)

Lidocaine injection with epinephrine: cats, cattle, dogs, horses
21 CFR 522.1244 p. 280 4/1/93 edition

Mepivacaine hydrochloride injection: horses
21 CFR 522.1372 p. 281 4/1/93 edition

Proparacaine hydrochloride ophthalmic solution: animal species not specified
21 CFR 524.1883 p. 338 4/1/93 edition

A number of combination products containing local anesthetics plus corticosteroid or antimicrobial agents are also listed in the CFR. The indication for these products generally is to treat surface bacterial infections and/or allergy.

References

1. Courtney KR, Strichartz GR. Structural elements which determine local anesthetic activity. In: Strichartz GR, ed. Handbook of experimental pharmacology, vol. 81. Local anesthetics. Berlin: Springer-Verlag, 1987:53–94.
2. Strichartz GR, Ritchie JM. The action of local anesthetics on ion channels of excitable tissues. In: Strichartz GR, ed. Handbook of experimental pharmacology, vol. 81. Local anesthetics. Berlin: Springer-Verlag, 1987:21–53.
3. Heavner JE. Molecular action of local anesthetics. In: Clinical practice of regional anesthesia. New York: Churchill Livingstone, 1991:67–71.
4. Covino BG, Vassallo HG. Local anesthetics: mechanisms of action and clinical use. New York: Grune & Stratton, 1976.
5. Butterworth JF, Strichartz G. Molecular mechanisms of local anesthesia: a review. Anesthesiology 72:711, 1990.
6. Cattrall WA. Structure and function of voltage-sensitive ion channels. Science 242:50–61, 1988.
7. Greene NM. Area of differential block in spinal anesthesia with hyperbaric tetracaine. Anesthesiology 19:45–50, 1958.
8. Gasser HS, Erlanger J. The role of fiber size in the establishment of a nerve block by pressure or cocaine. Am J Physiol 88:581–591, 1929.
9. Nathan PW, Sears TA. Some factors concerned in differential nerve block by local anaesthetics. J Physiol 157:565–580, 1961.
10. Raymond SA, Strichartz GR. The long and short by differential block. Anesthesiology 70:725–728, 1989.
11. Brodie BB, Lief PA, Poet R. The fate of procaine in man following intravenous administration and methods for the estimation of procaine and diethylaminoethanol. J Pharmacol Exp Ther 94:359–366, 1948.
12. O'Brien JE, Abbey V, Hinsvark O, Perel J, Finster M. Metabolism and measurement of chloroprocaine, an ester-type local anesthetic. J Pharm Sci 68:75–78, 1979.
13. Albright GA. Cardiac arrest following regional anesthesia with etidocaine or bupivacaine. Anesthesiology 51:285–287, 1979.
14. Heavner JE, Arthur J, Zou J, McDaniel K, Tyman-Szram B, Rosenberg PH. Comparison of propofol with thiopentone for treatment of bupivacaine-induced seizures in rats. Br J Anaesthesiol 71:715–719, 1993.
15. Browne T. Paraldehyde, chlormethiazole and lidocaine for treatment of status epilepticus. Adv Neurol 34:509–517, 1983.
16. Wagman JH, de Jong RH, Prince DA. Effects of lidocaine on the central nervous system. Anesthesiology 28:155–172, 1967.
17. Heavner JE. Cardiac dysrhythmias induced by infusing local anesthetics into the lateral cerebral ventricle of cats. Anesth Analog 65:133–138, 1986.
18. Atlee JL, Bosnjak ZJ. Mechanisms for cardiac dysrhythmias during anesthesia. Anesthesiology 72:347–374, 1990.
19. Courtney KR, Kendig JJ. Bupivacaine is an effective potassium channel blocker in heart. Biochem Biophys Acta 939:163–166, 1988.
20. Kasten GW, Martin ST. Bupivacaine cardiovascular toxicity: comparison of treatment with bretylium and lidocaine. Anesth Analg 64911–916, 1985.
21. Moller RA, et al. Progesterone-induced increase in cardiac sensitivity to bupivacaine. Anesthesiology 69:A675, 1988.
22. Imai M, et al. Enhanced myocardial depression from bupivicaine in diabetic rats. Anesthesiology 69:A872, 1988.
23. Betrix L, et al. Effects of hypo- and hypernatremia on the depression of ventricular condition and arrhythmias. Anesthesiology 69:A875, 1988.
24. Anderson ST, Hajduczek J, Barker SJ. Benzocaine-induced methemoglobinemia in an adult: accuracy of pulse oximetry with methemoglobinemia. Anesth Analg 67:1099–1101, 1988.
25. Lagutchik MS, Mundie TG, Martin DG. Methemoglobinemia induced by a benzocaine-based topically administered anesthetic in eight sheep. J Am Vet Med Assoc 201:1407–1410, 1992.
26. Covino BG. Toxicity and systemic effects of local anesthetic agents. In: Strichartz GR, ed. Handbook of experimental pharmacology, vol. 81. Local anesthetics. Berlin: Springer-Verlag, 1987:187–212.
27. Powell HC, Kalichman MW, Garrett RS, Myers RR. Selective vulnerability of unmyelinated fiber Schwann cells in nerves exposed to local anesthetics. Lab Invest 59:271–280, 1988.
28. Badgwell JM, Heavner JE, Kytta J. Bupivacaine toxicity in young pigs is age-dependent and is affected by volatile anesthetics. Anesthesiology 73:297–303, 1990.
29. Durham RA, et al. Topical ocular anesthetics in ocular irritancy testing: a review. Lab Anim Sci 42:535–541, 1992.

chapter 13

MUSCLE RELAXANTS AND NEUROMUSCULAR BLOCK

L. K. Cullen

Development of Muscle Relaxants

The first use of compounds with a known muscle paralyzing action was centuries ago by the South American Indians who used curare on the tips of arrows to immobilize wild animals. Curare is derived from the bark, leaves, and vines of a tropical plant, *Chondodendron tomentosum*. Early in the last century a number of animals in North America and Europe were given curare; to the amazement of onlookers, it was shown that they could be kept alive with artificial ventilation. In 1850 Claude Bernard demonstrated that the paralyzing actions of curare were due to its action at the neuromuscular junction. Much later, in 1914, Dale described the physiologic actions of acetylcholine, which led to the development of the chemical theory of neuromuscular transmission in 1936.(1) King isolated the active substance in curare, d-tubocurarine, in 1935 and determined its chemical structure. In 1912 unpurified curare was used in Leipzig to facilitate surgery, in what was probably its first reported use for this purpose.(2) Thirty years later, in America, Griffith and Johnson introduced a pure and stable preparation of curare (trade name Intocostrin) as an adjunct to anesthesia; better muscle relaxation was provided for surgery. Curare was introduced to Britain in 1945, and in the following year Gray and Halton established its use during human anesthesia.

The first reported use of succinylcholine was in 1906, but its muscle relaxant properties were not recognized because the animals were already curarized or paralyzed. The paralyzing properties of succinylcholine were discovered in 1949, when it was further noted that muscle relaxation was reversible because the drug was hydrolyzed by cholinesterase. Succinylcholine was introduced in 1951 as part of the anesthetic regimen in human patients, and it is now the only depolarizing relaxant used clinically.

One of the first reports of the clinical use of a muscle relaxant in veterinary anesthesia was in 1952 by Hall at the Royal Veterinary College, London.(3) This led to the development of the concept of balanced anesthesia; the three components of the triad are narcosis, analgesia, and muscle relaxation.

The relaxants, d-tubocurarine and succinylcholine, have some undesirable actions on the cardiovascular system; they have actions at autonomic ganglia and cardiac muscarinic receptors, and cause histamine release. Although the rapid onset of relaxation following succinylcholine was desirable for endotracheal intubation in human patients, additional unwanted actions, such as postanesthetic muscle pains and hyperkalemia were produced.

Although d-tubocurarine was introduced into clinical anesthesia, the search continued for synthetic drugs with a similar action. Gallamine triethiodide was developed and used in France in 1948. At the same time decamethonium, a depolarizing relaxant, was described and the paralyzing properties noted. A semisynthetic compound, dimethyltubocurarine or metocurine, was introduced in 1948. Alcuronium was discovered in 1961, and later, in 1968, the steroid relaxant pancuronium was introduced.

Early in the 1980s the effects of two new potent neuromuscular blockers, atracurium and vecuronium, were examined in extensive clinical trials. Both of these compounds have a shorter duration of action than most other nondepolarizing relaxants, and as the adverse actions are few, they have become widely accepted in anesthetic practice.

Pipecuronium, a long-acting nondepolarizing relaxant, was described in about 1980 and is being examined further in human clinical trials. Other nondepolarizing relaxants with minimal cardiovascular effects that are being tested clinically in human patients are doxacurium, mivacurium, and, recently, rocuronium. These compounds may prove useful in veterinary anesthesia. Even with the introduction of these new relaxants, the search continues for other drugs with negligible side effects and a rapid onset of action. Most research into muscle relaxants has concerned humans, for whom they are used very frequently as an adjunct to anesthesia; use of these agents in animals is much less common.

Physiology of the Neuromuscular Junction

Before discussing neuromuscular blockers it is appropriate to present a brief summary of the classical view of the physiology of the neuromuscular junction whereby acetylcholine is released from the nerve ending to trigger receptors on postjunctional muscle membrane, leading to skeletal muscle contraction (Chapter 7). Although neuromuscular transmission has been studied for more than a century and much is known about it, there are still some areas where knowledge is lacking. Further details can be found in recent reviews.(4-8)

A large myelinated nerve from the ventral horn of the spinal cord carries impulses to the skeletal muscle; as it approaches the muscle, the nerve branches extensively. The nerve carries stimuli to a vast number of muscle fibers that must be activated simultaneously for muscle contraction. As the motor nerve approaches the muscle cell, each branch loses its myelin sheath and the minute nerve terminals lie in small grooves on the surface of the muscle fiber under the cover of a Schwann cell. The area where the nerve ending lies in close proximity to the muscle fiber is complex and is known as the *neuromuscular junction* (Fig. 7–13). The muscle fiber membrane forming the groove in which the nerve terminals lie is deeply corrugated vertically; these corrugations are called *secondary clefts*. Deeper to the secondary clefts in the muscle fiber is a region rich in mitochondria that covers the contractile mechanisms of the muscle. The small gap between the nerve terminal and the muscle membrane, which is up to 60 nm wide, is known as the *junctional cleft*. Most skeletal muscle fibers have only one neuromuscular junction; however, extraocular muscle fibers have multiple junctions and all act as a stimulation site.

An impulse traveling down the motor nerve causes depolarization of the nerve terminal, triggering the release of acetylcholine, which crosses the junctional cleft to stimulate nicotinic cholinoceptors on the postsynaptic muscle membrane. Acetylcholine is synthesized in the nerve terminal from choline and acetate in the presence of the enzyme choline acetyltransferase. Transmitter molecules are contained in uniformly sized vesicles or quanta, which are mobilized down the motor nerve fiber to the presynaptic membrane, where they are concentrated in areas called *active zones*. These active zones lie directly opposite high concentrations of cholinoceptors located on the shoulders of the secondary clefts of the postsynaptic muscle membrane. Thus, when the transmitter is released, it travels a minimal distance across the junctional cleft to reach the receptor.

When an impulse travels down the nerve and the nerve terminal is depolarized, a series of events is initiated. Membrane-bound adenylcyclase is activated, converting adenosine triphosphate to cyclic adenosine monophosphate. Calcium channels in the membrane of the nerve terminal open, allowing calcium to enter and combine with the protein calmodulin. Calcium is essential for the transmitter contained within the vesicles to be discharged into the junctional cleft. A nerve action potential releases several hundred vesicles of transmitter into the junctional cleft so that acetylcholine can interact with the postsynaptic cholinoceptors. Interaction between acetylcholine and the receptor triggers an end plate potential (EPP), which is converted to a muscle action potential and then muscle fiber contraction.

After activating the receptors, the transmitter in the junctional cleft is rapidly hydrolyzed by the enzyme acetylcholinesterase to choline and acetate. Some of the choline is taken up by the nerve terminal for acetylcholine resynthesis.

A nerve action potential releases transmitter to activate the postsynaptic receptors, and if the end plate potential that is established in the muscle is of sufficient magnitude, then muscle fiber contraction ensues. Muscle fiber contraction is part of an all–or–none phenomenon. As the intensity of the stimulus increases, more muscle fibers are depolarized and the strength of muscle contraction rises until a peak is reached.

Recording end plate potentials from the postsynaptic muscle membrane, physiologists have demonstrated the presence of miniature end plate potentials (MEPPs). These MEPPs develop as a result of the spontaneous release of very small quantities of transmitter from the nerve terminal into the junctional cleft. The MEPPs occur at a frequency of about two per second, and calculations have indicated that they follow the release of the contents of one vesicle of acetylcholine. The potential established in the muscle membrane from a MEPP is too small for it to propagate a muscle fiber contraction.

POSTSYNAPTIC CHOLINOCEPTORS

The postsynaptic cholinoceptors are concentrated on the shoulders of the secondary clefts directly opposite the acetylcholine active zones of the nerve terminal. In most normal functioning muscle fibers, other than the extraocular muscles, receptors are located at the neuromuscular junction only.(7) Receptors are proteins synthesized in the muscle membrane and are made up of five subunits or protomers, with a molecular weight of about 250,000 daltons. The protomers are arranged in the form of a cylinder, leaving a small pore in the center, and the receptor spans the thickness of the cell membrane from outside to inside. Two of the five subunits are identical and are designated alpha, the others are beta, gamma and delta, though an epsilon subunit replaces the gamma in the adult bovine receptor.(7) When the receptor is in the resting stage, the central pore is closed, preventing any ions from traversing it.

Acetylcholine molecules must react with both alpha subunits of the receptor for it to undergo conformational change and the central pore to open to create what is known as a *channel*. When the pore is open, there is a flow of ions through the channel, sodium and calcium (to a lesser extent) from outside the cell to the inside and potassium from inside the cell to the outside. Cations can pass through the pore, but anions including chloride are excluded from this flow. Sodium influx, which is the major ion to flow, constitutes the end plate current; the amount of current generated is related to the number of channels that open and the influx of sodium ions. Current flow through a membrane changes the potential across it; thus, the end plate potential is produced. When acetylcholine detaches from the alpha subunits of the receptor, the channel in the central pore closes and current flow ceases. The interaction between transmitter and receptor is extremely dynamic, and the receptor ion flow channels open and close in response to acetylcholine. There are millions of postsynaptic receptors at the neuromuscular junction, and many need to be activated for the end plate potential to reach a critical threshold to propagate a muscle action potential and contraction.

There is a considerable safety factor in neuromuscular transmission in both the quantity of acetylcholine released and the number of postsynaptic receptors that need to be triggered to cause muscle contraction.(9) This safety margin varies between muscles; for example, in dogs and cats the margin of safety in the diaphragm is greater than that in the tibialis anterior muscle.(10)

Acetylcholine released from the nerve terminal crosses the junctional cleft and binds with a receptor before being rapidly hydrolyzed by acetylcholinesterase. During normal physiologic function, transmitter destruction is so rapid that acetylcholine does not accumulate from one nerve impulse to another. Although postsynaptic cholinoceptor activity during normal physiologic function is very dynamic, some factors are known to influence it, for example, drugs, temperature, electrolyte balance in surrounding fluids, and changes in fluidity of the surrounding membrane.

Acetylcholinesterase is found in high concentrations at the neuromuscular junction, and a single molecule hydrolyzes a few hundred thousand molecules of acetylcholine per minute. The enzyme is synthesized rapidly by nerve and muscle. The action of acetylcholine is terminated rapidly after interacting with postsynaptic receptors, and the enzyme also protects the nerve terminal from persistent depolarization by large concentrations of transmitter.

PRESYNAPTIC CHOLINOCEPTORS

Over recent years, substantial electrophysiologic and biochemical evidence has demonstrated the presence of nicotinic receptors that bind acetylcholine on the nerve terminal.(11) When acetylcholine is released from the nerve terminal to trigger postsynaptic receptors, it also activates presynaptic receptors. Evidence indicates that presynaptic receptor stimulation facilitates the mobilization of the reserve store of transmitter in the nerve terminal to the presynaptic membrane, thus keeping it available for demand. Activation of the prejunctional receptors is not required for transmitter release.(11) The mechanism by which transmitter is mobilized to the nerve terminal for release after receptor stimulation is still not understood.

PHARMACOLOGIC ACTIONS OF NEUROMUSCULAR BLOCKING DRUGS

The neuromuscular blocking drugs used during general anesthesia are classified as *depolarizing* or *nondepolarizing* according to the effects on the acetylcholine receptor. Succinylcholine is the only depolarizing relaxant used clinically, but there are numerous nondepolarizing relaxants, some of which are still being trialed; these are d-tubocurarine, metocurine, gallamine, alcuronium, pancuronium, atracurium, vecuronium, pipecuronium, doxacurium, mivacurium, and rocuronium. Brief details about the actions of both groups of relaxants on the cholinoceptor follow, but more information is available in reviews.(4, 7, 12,)

Depolarizing Blocking Drugs. The succinylcholine molecule is like two acetylcholine molecules joined back to back, and therefore this compound initially stimulates cholinoceptors at the neuromuscular junction. Although acetylcholine is rapidly destroyed in the junctional cleft, succinylcholine molecules remain present for a much longer period and are available to make multiple contacts with receptors. Pharmacodynamically succinylcholine is similar to that of the neuromuscular transmitter(7), so the relaxant molecules stimulate cholinoceptors to open the central pore or ion channel, allowing the inflow of sodium and calcium ions and outflow of potassium ions. Depolarization occurs at the end plate, which then leads to muscle fiber contraction, seen as fasciculations. In addition, succinylcholine depolarizes the motor nerve terminal, producing repetitive discharge of transmitter, which is another cause of muscle fasciculations. Since succinylcholine molecules persist much longer than acetylcholine, end plate depolarization is prolonged, leading to an area of inexcitability on the muscle membrane. The muscle fibers become flaccid, and relaxation ensues. Succinylcholine can also directly stimulate the cholinergic stretch receptors in the muscle spindles that send impulses to the brain.(12) Extraocular muscles have multiple innervation sites on the muscle membrane, are chemically excitable along the whole surface, and therefore undergo prolonged contracture when succinylcholine is given. In chronically denervated muscle, receptor sites proliferate and there is increased sensitivity to the depolarizing relaxant.

Initially succinylcholine produces a depolarization block. However, with a high dose, many doses, or prolonged action of the drug, the characteristics of the neuromuscular block change slowly. The new phase is the phase II block, which has many similarities to that produced by nondepolarizing neuromuscular blockers. The reason for the change in characteristics is still unclear. It has been suggested that when the phase II block is established, the receptors become desensitized. Receptors become desensitized from the continued presence of the transmitter, acetylcholine, and when in this state they cannot be triggered to undergo conformational change; that is, the ion channels do not open and the muscle membrane is not depolarized. Desensitization has been described in amphibian isolated nerve muscle preparation following succinylcholine administration.(13) As well as postjunctional actions, succinylcholine stimulates prejunctional receptors that may inhibit acetylcholine synthesis and release.(7) Repeated bolus injections or an infusion of succinylcholine causes tachyphylaxis in human patients.(14)

Ion Channel Block. Channel block occurs when the receptor ion channels have been opened by an agonist and the neuromuscular blocker, which is a large molecule, physically plugs the channel to stop ion flow. The extent to which this occurs during clinical use of neuromuscular blockers is not clear; however, ion channel block is likely to be of greater significance when high doses of relaxants, particularly nondepolarizing blockers, are given.

Nondepolarizing Blocking Drugs. The nondepolarizing relaxants recognize the acetylcholine receptor and show affinity for it but do not trigger it. The molecules of the nondepolarizing relaxants are large and prevent acetylcholine from occupying the triggering sites of the receptors. For the receptor to open, acetylcholine needs to bind to both alpha protein subunits to establish a sufficiently large end plate potential and propagate a muscle action potential. The nondepolarizing neuromuscular blocker molecules react dynamically with receptor recognition sites; they predominantly associate and dissociate with the binding sites, so a characteristic of the block of is one of competition. In addition to competing with the transmitter for receptor triggering sites, nondepolarizing blockers are also likely to cause ion channel block.(4) Blockage of the channel reduces the number of receptors that can be activated.

Nondepolarizing blockers have different affinities for prejunctional and postjunctional receptors. Experimental evidence has indicated that pancuronium and alcuronium have a greater affinity for postsynaptic receptors, whereas gallamine and d-tubocurarine have a greater affinity for presynaptic receptors to reduce the amount of acetylcholine released. These differences can be shown by the extent of the train–of–four fade during partial neuromuscular block.(15)

Monitoring Neuromuscular Function

Neuromuscular function should be monitored whenever possible during the administration of muscle relaxants. Monitoring provides details about the quantity of neuromuscular blocker required to produce the desired muscle relaxation for surgery and when to administer an antagonist for reversal of the block. In addition it provides an indication of the muscle function present to permit spontaneous breathing and recovery. Neuromuscular actions of relaxants can be modified by numerous factors such as the presence of other drugs, electrolyte and acid-base disturbances, and ongoing pathologic processes. With monitoring of neuromuscular function during the administration of relaxants, more appropriate dosing can be achieved. During the recovery stage from anesthesia where relaxants are given in human patients, muscle strength can be assessed by voluntary movements to command, a method not available in veterinary anesthesia.

The simplest method for assessing neuromuscular function is to stimulate electrically a peripheral nerve and evaluate the evoked muscle contraction. Under normal conditions and with unimpaired neuromuscular transmission, a single stimulus produces a muscle contraction known as a *twitch*. If strong enough, muscle contraction can be seen. However, evaluation is much more accurate if the muscle response is recorded and measured. Initial attempts to monitor neuromuscular function in human patients were described in 1941.(16)

Contraction of the muscle fiber is an all–or–nothing phenomenon, and as the nerve stimulus intensifies, the strength of contraction of the whole muscle increases until a maximum is reached. Consequently, the intensity of the electric stimulus applied during monitoring should be supramaximal to ensure that all muscle fibers are stimulated and there is maximum muscle contraction. The most appropriate time to commence monitoring neuromuscular function is after the animal has been anesthetized and before the relaxant is administered. Prerelaxant evoked muscle responses in the anesthetized animal should be determined and then compared with those when the animal is paralyzed. To avoid repetitive nerve stimulation and magnified responses, a square stimulus waveform of duration 0.2 ms or less should be applied. Direct muscle stimulation is possible when the duration of stimulus exceeds 0.3 ms.

Many small hand-held nerve stimulators are readily available and are ideal for stimulating a peripheral nerve. An example of a nerve stimulator is shown in Figure 13–1. Depending on the stimulator, it can deliver various patterns of nerve stimulation: single stimulus, tetanic, train–of–four, and double-burst stimulation. In animals needle electrodes are positioned so that the active or negative electrode is placed over the nerve with the positive electrode proximally.(17) In horses needle electrodes are placed on each side of the nerve to be stimulated.

METHODS FOR RECORDING NEUROMUSCULAR FUNCTION

Stimulation of a motor nerve at supramaximal intensity under normal conditions evokes a contraction of the muscles. The evoked muscle response can be recorded in two ways: mechanically, where the tension developed by a muscle is measured with a force displacement transducer, or electromyographically, where the electric response of the muscle action potential is measured. Mechanical measurements are mostly recorded during clinical monitoring. For accurate recording of muscle responses using a force displacement transducer, it

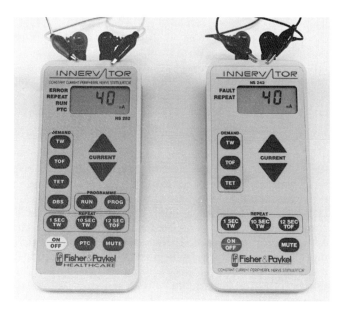

Fig. 13–1. A small nerve stimulator suitable for monitoring neuro-muscular function. These stimulators deliver single-twitch, train–of–four, tetanic, and double–burst stimulation (left stimulator only). The one on the left can be programmed to repeat the stimuli.

should have adequate capacity, the direction of muscle contraction should be applied at right angles to the transducer, and the resting tension on the muscle should be kept constant. Variation in the resting tension when the muscle contracts changes the strength of contraction.(18)

Evoked electromyography measures the compound muscle action potential in those muscles that are contracting. Electromyography uses expensive equipment and requires the insertion of three needle electrodes: The active electrode is inserted into the muscle to be studied, a reference electrode is placed over the tendon of insertion of the muscle, and a ground is positioned between the stimulating and recording electrodes. Consequently, electromyography is usually studied during experimental investigations.

For clinical monitoring of the presence of neuromuscular block in the dog, muscle responses to electric stimulation of the ulnar(19, 20), peroneal(21), tibial(22), and facial(20, 23) nerves have been reported. With the dog in lateral recumbency, the ulnar nerve is stimulated on the medial aspect of the elbow, where it lies subcutaneously, and the strength of contraction of the forepaw is measured. With peroneal nerve stimulation, the nerve is stimulated on the lateral aspect of the stifle and muscle twitch of the hind foot is recorded. Accurate recording of muscle responses is possible with ulnar nerve but not facial nerve stimulation in the dog.(23)

In the anesthetized laterally recumbent horse, the peroneal nerve is stimulated as it crosses the fibula shaft just distal to the head of the fibula.(24) With the hindleg strapped to a frame on the table on which the anesthetized horse lies, mechanical responses of the

digital extensor muscles following peroneal nerve stimulation can be recorded. Alternatively, in the horse, the facial nerve, which is palpated subcutaneously over the masseter muscle ventral to the lateral canthus of the eye, can be stimulated in this region and the evoked muscle contractions of the muzzle recorded.(21, 25) Muscle responses to peroneal nerve stimulation have been recorded in the cow(21) and llama.(26)

The hoof twitch shows greater sensitivity to the effects of relaxants than the facial muscle twitch in horses, ponies, and calves given atracurium and pancuronium.(27-30)

Frequently during clinical anesthesia neuromuscular function is monitored by stimulating a peripheral nerve and observing evoked twitches. Access to a nerve for stimulation is determined by the surgery being performed. Subjective assessment of the muscle twitches, that is, observations of the evoked muscle responses, is not accurate, and muscle responses differ. For example, the facial muscles are more resistant to the effects of relaxants than those muscles served by the ulnar or peroneal nerve. Limb muscle twitches are eliminated before the facial muscle twitch.

PATTERNS OF NERVE STIMULATION

For the monitoring of neuromuscular function, several different nerve stimulation patterns have been developed and muscle responses recorded. The common stimulation patterns are single twitch, train–of–four, tetanic, posttetanic single twitch, and double–burst stimulation. The evoked muscle responses recorded before and after neuromuscular blocker administration correspond to the pattern of nerve stimulation (Fig. 13–2). Partial neuromuscular block with depolarizing or nondepolarizing relaxants modifies the recorded mechanical responses to these stimulation patterns (Table 13–1). Responses can vary according to the onset or recovery from neuromuscular block and the muscle group from where the evoked responses are recorded.(31) The sensitivity of each stimulatory pattern varies.

Single Twitch. The nerve is stimulated at a frequency of 0.1 to 1 Hz, and the muscle response or twitch is recorded. Onset and recovery from neuromuscular block is evident by decreasing or increasing twitch heights respectively. Time for return of twitch height, for example 25 to 75% of control, gives an indication of the duration of return of neuromuscular function. For the recording of single twitch, only about 20 to 25% of the functional acetylcholine receptor pool is necessary–or up to 75 to 80% of receptors require blocking before a single twitch shows depression.(9)

Train of Four. This pattern stimulates the nerve with a train–of–four stimulus over 2 seconds, that is, a frequency of 2 Hz. An interval of 10 seconds usually occurs between each train, and the pattern is applied either continuously or intermittently. Four muscle responses or twitches are measured. In the presence of a partial neuromuscular block with a nondepolarizing

Stimulation Pattern

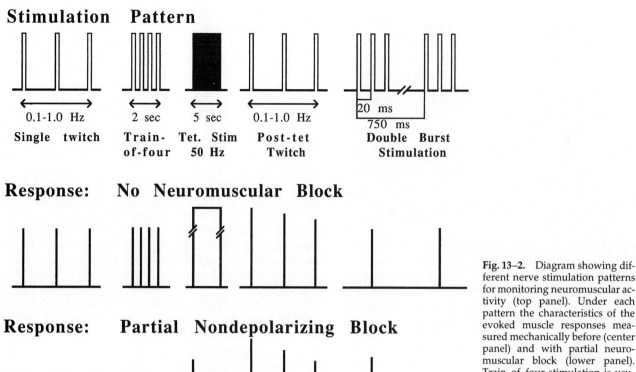

Fig. 13–2. Diagram showing different nerve stimulation patterns for monitoring neuromuscular activity (top panel). Under each pattern the characteristics of the evoked muscle responses measured mechanically before (center panel) and with partial neuromuscular block (lower panel). Train–of–four stimulation is usually repeated at intervals of 10 seconds. See text for further details.

relaxant, a progressive decline in the height of the twitches, from one to four, occurs, the fourth being depressed the greatest (Fig. 13–2). With deepening block twitches are progressively eliminated, the fourth being eliminated initially. During return of neuromuscular function from complete block, twitches reappear; initially the first twitch of the train appears, followed by the second, third, and fourth in that order. Train–of–four nerve stimulation was initially utilized in human patients.(32) Measurements of the four twitch heights are taken, and the ratio of the amplitude of the fourth

to the first twitch in the same train is calculated to give the train–of–four ratio. This ratio is equal to one with no neuromuscular block, and with onset of block the ratio progressively declines until the fourth twitch is eliminated. The ratio describes the extent of block.

The original explanation for the train–of–four fade, that is, a progressive decline in the heights of the four twitches, was a falling reduction in the availability of transmitter for release into the junctional cleft at frequencies of nerve stimulation above 1 Hz. It has recently been shown that fade does not arise from block

Table 13–1. Responses During Partial Neuromuscular Block. **Distinguishing features of depolarizing, nondepolarizing and succinylcholine-induced phase II block. Left column lists the different patterns of nerve stimulation or other characteristic, and in the second, third and fourth columns the respective responses in the presence of partial neuromuscular block**

Criteria	Depolarizing Block	Nondepolarizing Block	Phase II Block
Fasciculation before onset of block	Yes	No	—
Time for onset	Short	Longer	—
Single twitch	Depressed	Depressed	Depressed
Tetanic height	Depressed	Depressed	Depressed
Tetanic fade	Minimal or absent	Present and marked	Present and marked
Train-of-four fade	Minimal or absent	Present and marked	Present and marked
Posttetanic facilitation	Minimal or absent	Present	Present
Response to anti-cholinesterases	Block is prolonged	Block is antagonized	Block is antagonized

of postjunctional cholinoceptors at the muscle end plate, but block of prejunctional receptors.(7, 11) With block of prejunctional receptors by the relaxant, there is inhibition of the triggering mechanism to facilitate the mobilization of transmitter into position for synaptic release. Thus, experimental evidence indicates that the first twitch in a train of four assesses postjunctional receptor block, whereas fade is a prejunctional affect. During clinical monitoring of neuromuscular function the train–of–four ratios can be used to assess neuromuscular transmission without the need for control responses, and this pattern of stimulation does not affect the subsequent recovery from nondepolarizing block as does tetanic stimulation.(33) The train–of–four ratio can be used to assess partial neuromuscular block in dogs without a prerelaxant control twitch height.(34)

Evaluation of mechanical responses to train–of–four stimulation is a more sensitive assessment of neuromuscular function than a single twitch. Due to the margin of safety associated with neuromuscular transmission, the train–of–four ratio decreases when about 70 to 75% of receptors are blocked.(35) For accurate monitoring of clinical cases it is necessary to record and measure the train–of–four ratios to evaluate neuromuscular function; visual observation does not give sufficient accuracy.(36)

Some studies have shown train–of–four stimulation to be more sensitive than single-twitch during monitoring of neuromuscular function(37, 38); however, care is required when comparing responses to both patterns of stimulation. Depressed single-twitch heights have shown signs of recovery before there was evidence of train–of–four ratio increase. Furthermore, different nondepolarizing relaxants have varying ratios at the same stage of block, and during recovery from neuromuscular block fade is usually more pronounced than during onset.(39, 40, 41)

Train–of–four fade is minimal or absent in the presence of depolarizing blockers in human patients (32, 42) and marked with nondepolarizing blockers. Train–of–four fade has been used to characterize succinylcholine neuromuscular block in human patients(42) and dogs;(43) initially, there is minimal fade, indicating the presence of the depolarizing block, but with the prolonged presence of succinylcholine, fade slowly increases to show the presence of a phase II block (Table 13–1).

Tetanic Stimulation. Muscle responses are recorded to short periods of high-frequency nerve stimulation up to 200 Hz. Mostly, nerve stimulation is applied at 50 Hz for 5 seconds, which is considered to be more physiologic (44), with intervals of 5 to 6 minutes between each stimulation. These rates of stimulation may cause arousal in the lightly anesthetized patient. With a partial nondepolarizing block, reduced tetanic height and tetanic fade occur (Fig. 13–2), but tetanic fade is considered to be a prejunctional affect similar to that for train–of–four fade. Responses to tetanic stimulation provide a more accurate assessment of neuromuscular function than train–of–fade.

Posttetanic Twitch. The resumption of single-twitch stimulation about 5 seconds after tetanic stimulation during partial nondepolarizing block produces twitch heights higher than the pretetanic twitches. This effect, which is called *posttetanic facilitation,* is transient and is evident when recordings of evoked muscle responses are measured mechanically (tension) or electromyographically. With intense block, posttetanic facilitation may not be evident. The phenomenon is explained by increased mobilization of transmitter after the tetanic stimulation. In the absence of neuromuscular block, posttetanic twitch stimulation can be demonstrated to a lesser extent when muscle responses are measured mechanically, but not during the recording of electromyographic measurements.(45) The extent of posttetanic facilitation depends on the time interval between the tetanic stimulation and posttetanic twitch, the time interval between each tetanic stimulation, and the frequency and duration of tetanic stimulation. The first clinical indicator of recovery from complete neuromuscular block is posttetanic facilitation.(36, 46)

With intense neuromuscular block, muscle responses to single-twitch or train–of–four stimulation are absent, but a technique has been developed in human patients to indicate approximately when mechanical responses to train–of–four stimulation will become evident during the recovery phase.(46) The technique makes use of the transient posttetanic facilitation response. The twitch height and the number of the twitches seen after tetanic stimulation, called the *posttetanic count,* is determined by the extent of neuromuscular block present; twitches disappear if the block is intense. A relationship between posttetanic count and the return of train–of–four responses has been determined for pancuronium(46), atracurium(47), and vecuronium.(48)

Double–Burst Stimulation. The visual assessment of muscle responses to train–of–four stimulation in human patients is inaccurate; therefore, in the absence of recording equipment, double–burst stimulation is considered to be superior. An initial burst of three impulses to the nerve at a frequency of 50 Hz (one impulse every 20 ms) followed by an interval of 750 ms (Fig. 13–2) allows visualization or manual detection of small amounts of residual neuromuscular block under clinical conditions.(49) In the absence of muscle relaxation, two short muscle contractions of equal strength are produced; in the partially paralyzed muscle the second response is weaker than the first; that is, the responses fade. Absence of fade in response to double-burst stimulation means that clinically significant residual neuromuscular block does not exist.

DISTINGUISHING FEATURES OF NEUROMUSCULAR BLOCK

In the presence of partial neuromuscular block, the mechanical muscle responses to different patterns of nerve stimulation display features characteristic of the type of block present. Responses to single-twitch stimulation show depression of twitch height in all types of block. However, the degree of train–of–four fade, tetanic fade, and posttetanic twitch potentiation differ in the presence of depolarizing and nondepolarizing block (Table 13-1). The evoked muscle responses following initial doses of succinylcholine show characteristics of a depolarizing block, but when high doses are given or its action is prolonged, the characteristics of the block change to resemble those of a nondepolarizing block or phase II block. Spontaneous recovery from the phase II block takes longer than that from the initial depolarizing block.

The train-of-four ratio has been used to characterize the succinylcholine neuromuscular block in human patients (42) and dogs.(43) Initially the depolarizing block is indicated by minimal train–of–four fade; however, the development of the phase II block is indicated by marked fade. The phase II block begins to develop in the dog after a single dose of 0.3 mg/kg of succinylcholine.(43) Tachyphylaxis, defined as "a diminishing paralyzing action in response to an equivalent dose of relaxant," is evident early in the depolarizing phase.(43)

Pharmacology of Neuromuscular Blockers

CHEMISTRY AND METABOLISM

Neuromuscular blocking agents are quaternary ammonium compounds, and the positive charge at these sites in the molecules mimics the quaternary nitrogen atom of the transmitter acetylcholine molecule. Since muscle relaxant molecules are structurally related to acetylcholine, they are attracted to all cholinergic receptors, those at the neuromuscular junction as well as the nicotinic receptors of the autonomic ganglia and muscarinic receptors at postganglionic parasympathetic sites.

Muscle relaxant molecules have positive charges separated by a bridging part and are highly ionized. Their ionization state and hydrophilic nature mean that glomerular filtration is a major route for excretion. Except for pancuronium, vecuronium, pipecuronium, and rocuronium, which have a steroidal chemical structure, neuromuscular blockers rely little on hepatic breakdown.

Being highly water soluble, relaxants are unlikely to cross lipid membranes in high concentrations such as the blood-brain barrier, the placenta, and the renal tubular epithelium to be reabsorbed after being filtered. Muscle relaxants are unable to penetrate the blood-brain barrier effectively and therefore are devoid of sedative, anesthetic, or analgesic properties.

Succinylcholine. Structurally succinylcholine is two acetylcholine molecules joined back to back. This depolarizing relaxant is hydrolyzed by the enzyme pseudocholinesterase (plasma cholinesterase) to choline and succinylmonocholine, which is further hydrolyzed to succinic acid and choline. Succinylmonocholine has very weak neuromuscular blocking actions, about one–twentieth to one–eightieth those of the parent compound. Other minor routes of succinylcholine elimination are alkaline hydrolysis, renal elimination, and redistribution to tissues from where elimination is slower than from plasma.(50) The role of pseudocholinesterase in succinylcholine metabolism was demon-

strated by the increased resistance to paralyzing doses of the relaxant shown by dogs given some of the purified enzyme.(51) Attempts to correlate the duration of action of the relaxant to circulating cholinesterase levels are unreliable in healthy dogs.(52)

Pseudocholinesterase is formed in the liver, and plasma levels of this enzyme are reduced by liver disease, malnutrition, chronic anemia, burns, certain malignancies, cytotoxic drugs, pregnancy, and acetylcholinesterase inhibitors.(53–56) Some specific drug administrations also inhibit cholinesterase activity: lithium(57), echothiopate(54), metoclopramide(58), and neostigmine.(59)

Organophosphate insecticides used as anthelmintics or ectoparasite therapy in animals have a variable effect on succinylcholine activity. In cats with a dichlorvos flea collar fitted for two months, no effect on the duration of succinylcholine paralysis was observed.(60) In horses, however, the anthelmintics dichlorvos and trichlorfon reduce cholinesterase activity and prolong the succinylcholine–induced apnea and the cardiac dysrhythmias associated with this relaxant.(61)

d-Tubocurarine. d-Tubocurarine, or curare, is a naturally occurring substance obtained from an Amazonian vine. d-Tubocurarine is a benzylisoquinoline substance, and it is eliminated predominantly in the urine unchanged. A small proportion is excreted in the bile.

Metocurine. Metocurine (dimethyltubocurarine), a trimethylated derivative of tubocurarine, is a benzylisoquinoline substance. Metocurine relies mostly on renal excretion, with less than 2% being eliminated in human bile.(62)

Gallamine. This synthetic substance is a trisquaternary compound that relies on renal excretion for elimination.

Pancuronium. Pancuronium is a synthetic steroid molecule that relies on the kidney for elimination of more than half of the dose given. The balance of pancuronium is metabolized by the liver to 3-OH-, 17-OH-, and 3,17-OH-pancuronium; all of these metabolites have weaker relaxant properties than the parent compound.(63) Pancuronium neuromuscular block is prolonged in patients with renal failure.(64)

Alcuronium. Alcuronium is a long-acting semisynthetic relaxant that is not available for clinical use in the United States. Excretion is by the kidneys predominantly, eliminating about 80% of the injected portion, and the balance is removed in the bile.

Atracurium. Atracurium is a synthetic bisquaternary isoquinoline compound that is metabolized by esterases and Hofmann elimination. Hofmann elimination spontaneously breaks down atracurium at body pH and temperature to laudanosine (tertiary amine) and a monoquaternary acrylate without renal, hepatic, or enzymatic processes. Additional breakdown is by ester hydrolysis and other metabolic pathways, including some in the liver.(65) A recent in vitro study has shown that approximately 40% of the injected atracurium is eliminated by Hofmann degradation and ester hydrolysis, and the balance is metabolized by other pathways.(66) A decrease in temperature of 5 to 6° C slows the rate of degradation of atracurium to about half that at normal body temperature. Laudanosine at very high concentrations has been shown to cause seizure activity in dogs. However, the concentrations that develop following recommended clinical dose rates of atracurium are unlikely to cause complications.(67)

Atracurium elimination half-life is short and is not altered in patients with renal or hepatic failure.(68) Laudanosine, on the other hand, has a long elimination half-life and is metabolized primarily in the liver and eliminated via the kidney. In human patients with severe renal failure(69) and liver disease(70), laudanosine concentrations are increased for a prolonged period. About 12% of the injected dose of the atracurium metabolite is excreted unchanged in the urine of dogs.(71)

Vecuronium. Vecuronium is the monoquaternary analog of the steroid relaxant pancuronium and was developed to avoid the undesirable actions of pancuronium, namely the ganglion blocking and the indirect sympathomimetic effect. Vecuronium has a potency similar to pancuronium in the cat(72) and is less cumulative.(73) In the rat nearly one half of the injected vecuronium is eliminated in the bile, with very small amounts being excreted via the kidney.(74) Vecuronium is unstable when stored in solution long term and is presented in a lyophilized form that is dissolved in water prior to clinical use. The solution is stable at room temperature for up to 24 hours.

Pipecuronium. Pipecuronium is a long-acting bisquaternary steroid neuromuscular blocker. It is an analog of pancuronium and has a higher potency.(75) Renal elimination of the unchanged molecule accounts for about 77% of the injected drug in the dog, with less than 5% excreted in the bile. More is eliminated in the bile if renal elimination is impaired.(76) In the dog hepatic biliary elimination of pipecuronium is much less important than that of the other two steroidal relaxants pancuronium and vecuronium.

Doxacurium. Doxacurium, a benzylisoquinoline compound, is a new long-acting nondepolarizing relaxant. It is slightly more potent than pipecuronium and much more potent than pancuronium. This compound is predominantly eliminated unchanged in the urine and bile in cats. Human patients with renal or liver failure showed prolonged duration of action of doxacurium.(77)

Mivacurium. Mivacurium, a benzylisoquinoline diester compound, is a new nondepolarizing relaxant with a potency of approximately one third to one half that of atracurium in the monkey. Its short duration of action in human patients is caused by the rapid hydrolysis by pseudocholinesterase. Acetylcholinesterase breakdown and spontaneous hydrolysis appear to be minimal.(78, 79) The breakdown products are pharmacologically inactive. Liver uptake and metabolism and renal elimination have been demonstrated in the cat and dog, though it seems that these routes are of minor significance. Prolonged activity of mivacurium may occur in human patients with low cholinesterase, though this is unlikely to be as significant as with succinylcholine, since other clearance pathways for mivacurium are likely.(79)

Rocuronium. Rocuronium (Org 9426), a steroidal nondepolarizing relaxant, is a derivative of vecuronium and is less potent. It has a rapid onset of action and a duration of effect similar to that for vecuronium in dogs.(80) It is the most recent neuromuscular blocker to undergo clinical trials in human patients.

Nonneuromuscular Blocking Actions of Relaxants

Muscle relaxants act predominantly at the neuromuscular junction, but because of their structure they recognize cholinoceptors elsewhere in the body. Undesirable actions of neuromuscular blockers arise from competing with or mimicking acetylcholine at nicotinic autonomic ganglion receptors and muscarinic receptors, or by weak actions on sympathetic nerve endings. Most of these actions affect the cardiovascular system. Recently, newer drugs (e.g., atracurium and vecuronium) have been developed in an attempt to minimize the undesirable actions associated with the use of the older relaxants. Additional effects on the cardiovascular system arise through the release of histamine by some of the neuromuscular blockers. The adverse actions of neuromuscular blockers have been reviewed recently.(81, 82, 83)

CARDIOVASCULAR ACTION

Muscle relaxants modify cardiovascular variables through their effects on autonomic ganglia, muscarinic receptors, and sympathetic nerve endings. Of the muscle relaxants used clinically, d-tubocurarine has the greatest potential to block transmission at autonomic ganglia. These actions cause a decrease in systemic vascular resistance, hypotension, and a slight rise in heart rate. Ganglion blocking actions of metocurine are low and even less for gallamine and alcuronium.

A vagolytic mechanism to produce tachycardia is variable among nondepolarizing relaxants. Gallamine is the most likely relaxant to have a vagolytic action; other blockers with this potential in decreasing order are d-tubocurarine, pancuronium, alcuronium, metocurine, atracurium, and vecuronium.(81, 84-86) Atracurium and vecuronium cause negligible vagal interference during clinical use.

Pancuronium and, to a lesser extent, gallamine weakly stimulate the release of norepinephrine from adrenergic nerve endings in vitro, mechanisms that increase heart rate and blood pressure. Other contributing actions are inhibition of catecholamine reuptake by sympathetic nerve endings.(87) In dogs pancuronium increases blood pressure, heart rate, and cardiac output.(88, 89) Gallamine increases cardiac output and decreases blood pressure, but has little effect on heart rate.(90) Metocurine and d-tubocurarine decrease blood pressure and slightly increase heart rate.(89, 90) Because vecuronium has no effect on heart rate, arterial pressure, autonomic ganglia, or adrenoceptor or baroreceptor activity in dogs and cats, it has been recommended for patients with myocardial disease.(89, 91, 92)

When anesthetized with halothane, horses have no change in heart rate with gallamine or pancuronium (93, 94), but in ponies, pancuronium increases blood pressure and heart rate.(27) Pancuronium has no effect on the heart rate or blood pressure in halothane–anesthetized calves.(28) Pancuronium in pigs increases blood pressure and heart rate, while vecuronium decreases blood pressure.(95) Atracurium appears to have minimal affect on cardiovascular variables. Heart rate and rhythm and blood pressure changes are not seen in halothane–anesthetized ponies(96), horses(29), and dogs anesthetized with thiopental, nitrous oxide, and oxygen.(97) In halothane–anesthetized sheep, no consistent cardiovascular changes were noted with d-tubocurarine, pancuronium, or vecuronium.(98)

In humans mivacurium and doxacurium have virtually no action at autonomic ganglia or cardiac muscarinic receptors when used in clinical doses.(56) Pipecuronium in dogs and cats has negligible ganglion blocking action and transiently decreases blood pressure at doses in excess of that for neuromuscular block.(75) Profound hypotension has been reported in one dog anesthetized with thiopental and nitrous oxide given pipecuronium.(99) In humans and dogs doxacurium and mivacurium have minimal effects on cardiovascular function, although decreases in the blood pressure and heart rate have been reported.(100–106) Rocuronium in humans and dogs induces minimal cardiovascular side effects.(107)

Succinylcholine can stimulate cholinergic receptors to produce either vagal or sympathetic actions. A decrease in heart rate follows direct stimulation of postganglionic cholinergic receptors in the heart or increased vagal tone caused by carotid body sensory receptor stimulation.(82) Bradycardia is a common finding in human patients given succinylcholine, and this effect can be prevented by pretreatment with atropine. Sympathetic stimulation increases heart rate and blood pressure.

Cardiovascular changes in animals given succinylcholine are variable. Arterial pressure frequently increases in most animals, though a transient decrease may occur occasionally before the increase. Blood pressure changes that accompany the first dose of succinylcholine usually progressively diminish if successive doses are given. Both bradycardia and tachycardia have been observed following succinylcholine injection.(55, 95, 108) Succinylcholine in dogs decreases peripheral resistance and slightly increases cardiac output.(90)

In conscious horses, succinylcholine significantly increases arterial pressure and heart rate(109, 110), and is accompanied by cardiac dysrhythmias and myocardial hemorrhages.(55) These cardiac effects may arise from hyperkalemia, direct cardiac effects, sympathetic stimulation, hypercapnia, or hypoxia. When succinyl-

choline is given to halothane–anesthetized horses, heart rate increases but not blood pressure.(108)

When choosing a neuromuscular blocker, some consideration should be given to the cardiovascular actions of the drugs. Vecuronium and atracurium are nearly free of cardiovascular effects. These are the relaxants of choice if myocardial disease is present, although atracurium has the potential to release histamine.

HISTAMINE RELEASE BY RELAXANTS

Histamine release can accompany the administration of some neuromuscular blockers; of those relaxants that cause histamine release, the higher the dose administered the greater the potential for release. Signs of histamine release in human patients are local skin reactions including erythema, hypotension, and tachycardia. In animals cardiovascular changes occur. Anaphylactic or anaphylactoid reactions are rare. Pretreatment with H_1- and H_2-receptor antagonists are beneficial in avoiding the effects of histamine release.(82) d-Tubocurarine is the most potent liberator of histamine.(81, 82, 111, 112) The potential for relaxants to release histamine in human patients in decreasing order of potency is d-tubocurarine, atracurium, alcuronium, succinylcholine, vecuronium, and pancuronium.(112) Bolus doses of atracurium less than 0.6 mg/kg in humans are unlikely to produce significant histamine release.(82) Gallamine and alcuronium have similar potential to release histamine(82), while metocurine and mivacurium release only small amounts of histamine, and doxacurium and pipecuronium cause virtually no release.(56, 75, 101, 104) Anaphylactic reactions have been reported in human patients given gallamine (113), alcuronium(114), and succinylcholine.(115, 116)

d-Tubocurarine can cause marked histamine release in dogs resulting in hypotension.(65) Atracurium releases small quantities of histamine in dogs, but it is of little significance at doses required to cause neuromuscular block.(65) Bronchoconstriction(117) and hypotension(65) associated with the use of atracurium have been attributed to histamine release in the dog.

CHOLINESTERASE INHIBITION BY RELAXANTS

Neuromuscular blockers by virtue of their structural similarity to acetylcholine interact with cholinesterases, and it seems that all may have some inhibitory activity. Studies have been made on the inhibitory actions of relaxants on cholinesterase enzymes of human origin; however, care is required when extrapolating results from one species to another because enzymes from different species may vary in their substrate and inhibitor specificity.(81)

PLACENTAL TRANSFER OF NEUROMUSCULAR BLOCKERS

Because neuromuscular blocking drugs are highly ionized and have weak lipophilic properties, they cross the placenta from the maternal to fetal circulation very slowly. At clinical doses the quantity of relaxant that enters the fetal circulation is usually minute. Drugs diffuse across the placenta according to the concentration gradient, and time is a major determinant of the concentration that eventually develops in the fetal circulation.

Provided fetal exposure to neuromuscular blockers is not prolonged, that is, the time from anesthetic induction of the mother to removal of the fetus from the uterus is rapid, adverse effects of relaxants in the newborn are unlikely. There is widespread use of muscle relaxants as part of the anesthetic regimen for cesarian section in human patients.

In human patients undergoing cesarian sections there is no evidence of adverse effects in neonates attributable to the use of atracurium(118, 119), vecuronium(120, 121), or pancuronium(122) during anesthesia. With the use of recommended doses of atracurium, its metabolites, including laudanosine, do not show adverse effects in the newborn.(119) Apgar scores and time to sustained respiration are unchanged. Pancuronium is detectable in umbilical venous blood 2 to 3 minutes after injection into the maternal circulation, and peak concentrations occur about 10 to 12 minutes later.(122) The use of succinylcholine, gallamine, pancuronium, and d-tubocurarine in pregnant cats and ferrets does not impair twitch strength in the newborn.(123) Placental transfer of pipecuronium in rats is reported to be less than 0.1% of the dose administered to the pregnant dam.(75)

NEUROMUSCULAR BLOCKERS AND THE CENTRAL NERVOUS SYSTEM

Despite being ionized and weakly lipophilic nondepolarizing muscle relaxants enter the cerebrospinal fluid but at low concentrations. d-Tubocurarine is found in the cerebrospinal fluid within 5 minutes of injection in human patients with central nervous system pathology. The concentrations, although low, increase gradually over time.(124) Large steroidal molecules like pancuronium and vecuronium are unlikely to pass the blood-brain barrier easily.(125)

As previously mentioned, neuromuscular blockers interact with cholinoceptors other than those at the neuromuscular junction. There are many cholinergic pathways within the brain and probably different cholinergic receptor types. The effects of low concentrations of muscarinic inhibitors (gallamine and pancuronium), nicotinic inhibitors (d-tubocurarine and metocurine), and muscarinic and nicotinic stimulators (succinylcholine) on these pathways in the brain is unknown.(126)

Cerebrocortical activity may be altered through the actions of the neuromuscular blockers on muscle spindle afferent input to the reticular activating system. Evidence of arousal shown on the electroencephalogram has been reported in humans(127) and dogs(128) given succinylcholine, an effect that was prevented in patients pretreated with gallamine, alcuronium, or pancuronium. In halothane-anesthetized dogs given succinylcholine, muscle fasciculations occurred simul-

taneously with an increase in cerebral blood flow, raised intracranial pressure, and evidence of some increased cerebral activity on the electroencephalogram.(128) These actions have been explained by the fasciculations stimulating the muscle spindle and impulses being carried to the cerebral cortex. Furthermore, arterial carbon dioxide tensions and cerebral blood flow both increase with the onset of succinylcholine-induced muscle fasciculations, an effect that was reduced by pancuronium or metocurine pretreatment.(129) Because of these actions of succinylcholine, this relaxant should not be given to animals for recordings of an electroencephalogram or animals with an already elevated intracranial pressure.

Minimum alveolar concentration of halothane is reportedly reduced by 25% in patients given pancuronium(130); however, the method of determination and mechanism of action for this effect were unclear.

The atracurium metabolite, laudanosine, crosses the blood-brain barrier easily to induce central nervous system stimulation. In humans and cats the elimination half-life of laudanosine is five to six times that of atracurium. High doses of atracurium (14 to 22 mg/kg IV) induce seizure activity in dogs. This dose is much higher than that required for clinical action.(71)

PROTEIN BINDING

Nondepolarizing neuromuscular blockers bind to plasma proteins to a variable extent.(131-133) Variation in protein binding differs according to experimental design; atracurium, vecuronium, pancuronium, and d-tubocurarine were shown to be strongly bound (77 to 91%) to plasma proteins in one study, although in another a lower proportion of vecuronium, pancuronium, and d-tubocurarine (29 to 56%) were bound to proteins.(131, 133)

In theory, it is only the unbound fraction that is available for action at the receptor, and it is this portion that is filtered at the glomerulus. Relaxants bound to plasma protein cannot be removed by the kidney. Although it is possible that relaxants may bind to other sites such as cartilage and chondroitin, it is difficult to predict the effect of plasma protein binding on muscle relaxant pharmacokinetics.(132) In human patients with cirrhosis of the liver the proportion of d-tubocurarine, pancuronium, and vecuronium bound to plasma protein were similar to that which occurs in patients with normal liver function.(131) Thus, it appears that chronic liver disease does not have a major effect on the plasma protein binding of muscle relaxants. Changes in the proportion of relaxants bound to protein are unlikely to have any significant effect on renal excretion.(134)

NONNEUROMUSCULAR BLOCKING ACTIONS OF SUCCINYLCHOLINE

Succinylcholine administration is frequently accompanied by hyperkalemia, increased intraocular, intragastric, and intracranial pressure, and complications associated with muscle disorders. On occasions this relaxant is contraindicated because of these actions.

Hyperkalemia. Succinylcholine stimulates the muscle end plate region, which sets up local action currents or waves of depolarization that spread to the adjacent excitable membrane. This in turn leads to contraction of the muscle fibers. Prejunctional receptors are also stimulated to cause depolarization of the motor nerve terminal, evoking repetitive discharges of transmitter. Both processes cause muscle fiber contractions, which are seen as fasciculations. During the depolarization process, when receptor ion channels are open, potassium ions efflux from the muscle fiber; at the same time there is an influx of sodium and calcium ions. Serum potassium concentrations rise transiently and are highest after the initial dose of relaxant, but the effect diminishes after each subsequent dose.(135) In healthy human patients, serum potassium concentration increases following succinylcholine. This increase is without serious consequences if the preinjection potassium concentrations are within the normal range and no cardiovascular disease is present.

In patients with burns, direct muscle trauma, tetanus, muscle denervation, spinal cord section, brain damage, and stroke, additional acetylcholine receptor sites develop in the extrajunctional area of the muscle fiber, that is, along the muscle fiber, such that the whole muscle fiber membrane becomes sensitive to acetylcholine or succinylcholine. With these additional receptor sites, sensitivity of the muscle to succinylcholine increases. More important, an increased number of ion channels are now available to release potassium during depolarization from succinylcholine and the increase in serum potassium level is likely to precipitate life–threatening cardiac dysrhythmias. Patients with preexisting increased serum potassium concentrations and renal disease are at greatest risk. Receptor proliferation along the muscle fiber starts about 3 to 15 days after injury and persists for 2 to 3 months following burns or trauma and for 3 to 6 months in patients with tetanus.(136) The dangers of hyperkalemia do not occur in the first 2 days after injury.(137)

Decreased muscle activity or immobilization of a limb increases the sensitivity of the patient to succinylcholine and raises the potential for complications due to hyperkalemia.(138) These changes appear to be due to the development of perijunctional or extrajunctional receptors. In contrast, muscle immobilization or inactivity increases resistance to the paralyzing effects of nondepolarizing relaxants.(139, 140)

Salbutamol, a beta$_2$–adrenoceptor stimulant, can be used to decrease serum potassium following succinylcholine administration.(141) A recent review discusses in greater detail the complications of up–and–down regulation of acetylcholine receptors and hyperkalemia in patients given succinylcholine.(142)

Intraocular Pressure. Extraocular muscles have multiple innervation sites along the muscle fiber surface, and all sites are chemically excitable; consequently, when succinylcholine is given a prolonged state of contracture ensues. This muscle contraction is the likely cause of increased intraocular pressure following succinylcholine administration, which has the danger of causing expulsion of the vitreous humor in patients with penetrating eye injuries (Chapter 24). A single bolus of succinylcholine in human patients increases intraocular pressure significantly for 10 minutes postinjection.(143) By contrast, nondepolarizing relaxants do not raise intraocular pressure.(82) In halothane–anesthetized horses succinylcholine either as a bolus or an infusion does not significantly increase intraocular pressure.(144)

Intragastric Pressure. The muscle fasciculations associated with succinylcholine administration raise the intragastric pressure to a variable extent in human patients. Although it is possible that regurgitation may be increased, a counteracting force of the contracting diaphragm may cause resistance to opening of the lower esophageal sphincter.

Intracranial Pressure. Succinylcholine has been shown to raise intracranial pressure in anesthetized cats and dogs.(145-147) Pressures increase despite thiopental or pentobarbital anesthesia, and it is suggested that the cause of the change is the accompanying increase in cerebral blood flow following muscle fasciculations.(147) Vecuronium injection before succinylcholine decreases the hypertensive response. Succinylcholine should not be given to animals with increased intracranial pressure.

Muscle Responses in Animals Given Succinylcholine. The administration of a bolus dose of succinylcholine is followed by muscle fasciculations; the intensity is determined by the dose and speed of injection. Fasciculations, which precede relaxation, occur following the initial dose only. In human patients these fasciculations can cause postanesthesia muscle pains. There appears to be a good correlation between the intensity of fasciculation and the extent of muscle pain.(148) It is unknown if muscle pain similar to that in human patients is experienced in animals. Pretreatment of dogs with diazepam fails to prevent or reduce succinylcholine–induced fasciculations.(149)

Horses given succinylcholine during anesthesia have increased serum enzyme concentration, and some animals have shown unusual muscle responses. Halothane–anesthetized laterally recumbent horses given a bolus dose of succinylcholine, then an infusion, have slightly raised, but statistically insignificant, concentrations of creatine phosphokinase, lactic dehydrogenase, and aspartate aminotransferase. It was not clear if these enzyme changes were a consequence of muscle fasciculations following succinylcholine or general anesthesia.(150) There have been reports of prolonged muscle fasciculations, increased muscle rigidity, hyperthermia, hypercapnia, tachycardia, increased arterial blood pressure, hyperkalemia, and metabolic acidosis in halothane–anesthetized horses(151, 152) and ponies (153) given succinylcholine. One animal showed signs consistent with those for myositis that improved over the next few days(152), but others showed complications described as being malignant hyperthermia-like reactions. If signs of unusual muscle responses appear the administration of all possible triggering agents, including succinylcholine, should cease immediately, the patient should be cooled, and dantrolene, if available, should be administered.(152) Cardiac dysrhythmias and myoglobinuria are other complications that may occur in horses given succinylcholine.(55)

Malignant hyperthermia is a heritable metabolic disorder of muscles in which there is a defect in the intracellular calcium metabolism (Chapters 11 and 20). It has been reported in humans, pigs, horses, dogs, cats, and captured wild animals. One of the known triggering drugs of malignant hyperthermia is succinylcholine; therefore, this relaxant should not be given to animals known to be susceptible to the condition.

USE OF MUSCLE RELAXANTS IN ANESTHETIZED ANIMALS

Neuromuscular blockers are not used during animal anesthesia as extensively as they are during human anesthesia. Endotracheal intubation is performed in the anesthetized human patient following muscle relaxation, whereas most animals can be intubated easily under general anesthesia without the use of relaxants. Some veterinarians prefer to intubate pigs and cats, which are prone to laryngeal spasm, following a neuromuscular blocker, but the animal must then be ventilated until it can breathe spontaneously.

Veterinary use of muscle relaxants is more common in large practices and teaching hospitals, where staff familiar with the use of these drugs and mechanical ventilators are available. Those practices without the equipment or the expertise to use and monitor the actions of neuromuscular blockers may refer their patients to a well-equipped hospital. Muscle relaxation facilitates surgical exposure, and indeed, many surgical procedures in human patients are performed after neuromuscular blockade. Veterinarians are frequently satisfied with the muscle relaxation provided by general anesthesia. However, deep anesthesia can cause excessive depression of the cardiopulmonary system. Some surgeries, such as laparotomies in horses, and some orthopedic procedures are easier with the addition of muscle relaxation to the anesthetic regimen. If surgical exposure is optimized, the anesthetic time is usually decreased.

Indications for Muscle Relaxants. There are a number of indications for the use of muscle relaxants during animal anesthesia. First, those animals unable to breathe adequately may require ventilation. Surgeries requiring mechanical ventilation include thoracotomies, repair of a ruptured diaphragm, or surgery for severe trauma to the thoracic wall. When anesthetized, excessively obese animals do not breathe properly; the tidal volume and lung compliance, which are compromised initially, progressively decrease with duration of anesthesia, producing hypoxemia, hypercapnia, and further central depression. These animals often require positive pressure ventilation. Animals with pneumothorax, hydrothorax, chylothorax, or hemothorax may require positive pressure ventilation. Extreme care is required in patients with tension pneumothorax because ventilation may exacerbate the problem.

Second, the use of muscle relaxants as an adjunct to anesthesia allows good muscle relaxation without the dangers of deep anesthesia and prolonged recovery. Third, neuromuscular blockers abolish muscle tone, which improves surgical access. Surgeries where the most benefit is achieved are laparotomies, fractures, and dislocations, particularly in horses and well-muscled animals. Intraocular and spinal surgery are delicate procedures, and relaxants eliminate the risk of patient movement. Nondepolarizing relaxants maintain the eye in a central position without raising intraocular pressure. Fourth, endoscopy and endotracheal intubation are occasionally performed in the paralyzed patient. Relaxants that have a rapid onset of action (e.g., succinylcholine) are used frequently for intubation. Some animals in critical care units with severe chest or head injuries can benefit from the use of nondepolarizing muscle relaxants and positive pressure ventilation.

Essential Precautions. Neuromuscular blockers have two important properties that should not be forgotten: First, these agents block neuromuscular function to skeletal muscles, preventing the animal from breathing, and second, they have no sedative or analgesic effects. Some method of adequately ventilating the animal must be available; ventilatory efficiency is maximum in the patient with an endotracheal tube inserted and the cuff inflated, though inflation of the lungs can be provided for short periods with a face mask alone. Mask ventilation has its dangers: Ventilation is inefficient due to a poor seal between the mask and the animal's face, and oxygen may be forced down the esophagus to distend the stomach (meteorism). The most common method of artificial ventilation is intermittent positive pressure ventilation by the use of a mechanical ventilator and anesthetic machine (Chapter 17).

Neuromuscular blockers have no central depressant or analgesic effects, a property highlighted in 1947 when a human volunteer chose to be given d-tubocurarine alone. Despite being ventilated by colleagues, the volunteer anesthesiologist showed no evidence of lack of consciousness, impairment of memory, or presence of analgesia.(154) It is absolutely essential, therefore, that patients given muscle relaxants be unconscious and receive appropriate analgesia for the surgical procedure intended.

In the past muscle relaxants were occasionally used alone for capture of wild animals and restraint for experimental or surgical procedures (e.g., castration). In the present era the use of such inhumane practices cannot be justified on any grounds. Many potent anesthetics, sedatives, and local analgesics are available. The patient should either be given adequate analgesia or be anesthetized so that it is unconscious and unaware.

Choice of Relaxant. The choice of muscle relaxant depends on the species of animal to be paralyzed, the surgical procedure, the duration of muscle relaxation, and any ongoing pathologic processes. For example, in dogs and cats the major disadvantage of d-tubocurarine is marked hypotension. Succinylcholine has a variable duration of action in different species, and it is contraindicated if hyperkalemia is present; if intracranial, intraocular, or intragastric pressures are increased; or if the animal is susceptible to certain muscle disorders. Succinylcholine has many adverse effects in horses; consequently, its use has declined since the introduction of newer nondepolarizing relaxants such as atracurium. Animals in renal failure should not be given gallamine.

Because many factors influence the intensity and duration of neuromuscular block, the monitoring of neuromuscular function during relaxant administration allows the dose to be titrated to effect, thus avoiding overdosing. As was previously mentioned, small, handheld nerve stimulators that deliver different stimulation patterns are readily available (Fig. 13–1), and the evoked muscle responses, usually twitches, are easily measured or observed. To avoid relaxant overdose, up to two thirds or three quarters of the dose is given initially, and more is given as required. It should be emphasized that there is no fixed dose for relaxants but the quantity given is in accordance with the depression of evoked twitches. Monitoring also indicates when neuromuscular function is returning and an additional dose is needed.

Tables 13–2 through 13–6 present summaries of the approximate dose and duration of action of that dose for different muscle relaxants given intravenously to horses, dogs, cats, ruminants, and pigs. In those studies where it was measured, twitch height indicative of the end point for recovery is listed in the tables. Time for

onset of maximum relaxation from a bolus dose of nondepolarizing relaxant producing 90 to 99% decrease in twitch height takes from 5 to 7 minutes. Faster onset times and a longer period of paralysis are produced by higher doses. The onset time for succinylcholine block is more rapid than that for the nondepolarizing relaxants.

Individual muscles respond slightly differently to neuromuscular blockers: The diaphragm is usually the last skeletal muscle to be paralyzed, requiring a slightly higher dose of relaxant than that required to paralyze the limb muscles. With onset of muscle paralysis, muscle twitches to facial nerve stimulation are initially depressed along with limb muscle twitches, but complete elimination of the facial twitch requires a higher dose of relaxant.

Recent clinical reports give details of the use of multiple doses or the infusion of short acting relaxants. In the dog, vecuronium at an initial dose of 0.1 mg/kg and incremental doses at 0.04 mg/kg (172, 173) and atracurium at 0.5 mg/kg and incremental doses of 0.2 mg/kg(174) have been reported. In horses given an initial dose of 0.12 to 0.2 mg/kg followed by additional doses, the advantages of atracurium or pancuronium relaxation have been described.(175) Atracurium and vecuronium administration in dogs and cats has been reviewed.(92, 176)

Atracurium mixed with 0.9% sodium chloride has been infused successfully in horses at a dose of 0.17 $mg \cdot kg^{-1} \cdot h^{-1}$ (177) and in dogs at 0.5 mg/kg initially followed by a flow rate of 0.5 $mg \cdot kg^{-1} \cdot h^{-1}$.(178) Atracurium infusion should be prepared in 0.9% saline to minimize degradation by Hofmann elimination.(179) Monitoring of neuromuscular function allows infusion flow rates to be regulated according to the degree of relaxation required.

The newer neuromuscular blockers, pipecuronium, doxacurium, mivacurium, and rocuronium, are under-

Table 13–2. Use of Muscle Relaxants in Horses. Approximate doses and duration of action of muscle relaxants given intravenously to horses. Twitch recovery applies to those experimental studies where evoked muscle contractions following nerve stimulation were recorded. Values for ponies below dotted line.

Muscle Relaxant	Approximate Dose ($\mu g/kg$)	Approximate Duration (min)	Twitch Recovery Signifying End Point Duration	References
Atracurium	70–85	8–12.2	to 100%	29, 30, 155
Gallamine	793	14–40	to 50%	94
Metocurine	100–150	—	—	156
Pancuronium	82–140	20–35	to 50%	93, 94, 157
Succinylcholine	330	then 2.2 $mg \cdot kg^{-1} \cdot h^{-1}$ infusion	—	108, 150
Vecuronium	108	20–40	to 50%	93
Atracurium	110	24	to 10%	96
Pancuronium	125	16	to 50%	27
Succinylcholine	100	then 2.2 $mg \cdot kg^{-1} \cdot h^{-1}$ infusion	—	153

Table 13–3. Use of Muscle Relaxants in Dogs. Approximate doses and duration of action of muscle relaxants given intravenously to dogs. Twitch recovery applies to those experimental studies where evoked muscle contractions following nerve stimulation were measured

Muscle Relaxant	Approximate Dose (μg/kg)	Approximate Duration (min)	Twitch Recovery Signifying End Point of Duration	References
Alcuronium	100	70	to 100%	158
Atracurium	200–400	17–28.9	to 50%	97
Doxacurium	8			100
Gallamine	400–1,000	29	to 50%	159, 160
Metocurine	63	109	to 50%	89
Pancuronium	22–60	31–108	to 50–100%	89, 159
Pipecuronium	3.7–50	16–80.7	to 50%	75, 99
Succinylcholine	300–400	22–29	to 10–50%	22, 160, 161
Succinylcholine (Greyhound)	300	38	to 50%	22
d-Tubocurarine	130	100	to 50%	89
Vecuronium	14–200	15–42	to 50%	89, 162

going clinical trials in human patients; use in animals has been restricted to experimental investigations.

Some of the older muscle relaxants have a cumulative effect when multiple doses are given, although this is not a problem with drugs like atracurium and vecuronium.(29, 30, 96, 180) Pancuronium has a cumulative effect in humans(181) but not in the horse.(182) Neither mivacurium(79) nor doxacurium(183) have cumulative actions.

The practice of combining relaxants has been common in human anesthesia, where patients are frequently intubated following succinylcholine paralysis and then given a longer-acting nondepolarizing relaxant during the surgical procedure. In animal anesthesia there is little need for mixing relaxants, since they are usually given following induction of anesthesia. Investigations have been made into the interaction between

succinylcholine and vecuronium(184), atracurium(185), pipecuronium(186), alcuronium, gallamine, and pancuronium in dogs.(187, 188)

Factors Affecting Neuromuscular Block

The duration and intensity of neuromuscular block are influenced by a number of factors. When relaxants are administered, close monitoring of neuromuscular function will avoid overdosing.

IMPAIRED METABOLISM AND EXCRETION

Hepatic Disease. The effects of liver cirrhosis and obstructive liver disease on the actions and elimination of muscle relaxants in human patients is unlikely to be of great significance.(82) Impaired liver function may prolong relaxant metabolism and present difficulty in antagonizing residual block. This effect is less significant

Table 13–4. Use of Muscle Relaxants in Cats. Approximate doses and duration of action of muscle relaxants given intravenously to cats. Twitch recovery applies to those experimental studies where evoked muscle contractions following nerve stimulation were measured

Muscle Relaxant	Approximate Dose (μg/kg)	Approximate Duration (min)	Twitch Recovery Signifying End Point of Duration	References
Alcuronium	80	31	to 100%	84
Atracurium	250	29	to 100%	65
Gallamine	1200	24	to 100%	84
Metocurine	40	42	to 100%	84
Pancuronium	20–22	14–15	to 50–100%	72, 84
Pipecuronium	2–2.7	16.5–24	to 50%	75
Succinylcholine	3000–5000 (total)	4–6	—	163
d-Tubocurarine	200	20	to 100%	84
Vecuronium	24–40	5–9	to 75–90%	72, 164

Table 13–5.   Use of Muscle Relaxants in Ruminants. Approximate doses and duration of action of muscle relaxants given intravenously to sheep, calf, cattle and llamas. Twitch recovery applies to those experimental studies where evoked muscle contractions following nerve stimulation were measured

Animal	Muscle Relaxant	Approximate Dose (μg/kg)	Approximate Duration (min)	Twitch Recovery Signifying End Point of Duration	References
Sheep	Alcuronium	0.2 μg $\cdot$ kg^{-1} $\cdot$ h^{-1} infusion	—		165
	Atracurium	5.8 μg $\cdot$ kg^{-1} $\cdot$ h^{-1} infusion	—		166
	Gallamine	6 μg $\cdot$ kg^{-1} $\cdot$ h^{-1} infusion	—		165
	Pancuronium	0.15 μg $\cdot$ kg^{-1} $\cdot$ h^{-1} infusion	—		165
	Pancuronium	5.0	21	to 50%	98
	d-Tubocurarine	0.5 μg $\cdot$ kg^{-1} $\cdot$ h^{-1} infusion	—		165
	d-Tubocurarine	44.5	25.2	to 50%	98
	Vecuronium	4.61	13.8	to 50%	98
Calf	Pancuronium	43	26	to 50%	28
Cattle	Pancuronium	100	30–40	—	163
Llama	Atracurium	150	6	to 10%	26

after a single dose but is more likely if multiple doses are given.

Patients with generalized edema as a result of hepatic disease may show initial resistance to nondepolarizing blockers owing to a larger volume of distribution. Indeed, this effect has been recognized with pancuronium along with prolonged elimination.(189) Similarly, vecuronium elimination is delayed in patients with cirrhosis, causing longer duration of paralysis.(190) Patients with obstructive liver disease have an increased volume of distribution, decreasing relaxant efficacy. Nevertheless, the duration of action of pancuronium is prolonged.(191)

Atracurium is the muscle relaxant of choice in patients with hepatic failure because it relies on other routes of metabolism.(66, 192) In pigs, plasma concentrations and neuromuscular actions of atracurium are not affected by the absence of liver function though laudanosine concentrations increase.(168)

Renal Disease. In patients with renal failure, neuromuscular blockers that rely predominantly on urinary elimination are expected to have a prolonged period of muscle relaxation. Gallamine is not recommended for use in patients with renal failure, and, indeed, prolonged duration of action has been reported in human patients.(82) Because a large proportion of pancuronium is excreted by the kidney, its duration of action also increases with renal failure.(193) Pipecuronium is eliminated predominantly unchanged in the urine, and its duration of action in patients with renal failure is variable.(194)

The muscle relaxants that are most suitable for patients with renal failure are those that are eliminated by other routes. Atracurium has been shown to be free of cumulative actions and adverse cardiovascular actions in human patients with no renal function; consequently, it appears to be the drug of choice in these patients.(195)

ANESTHETIC DRUGS

Volatile anesthetics cause a dose–related potentiation of the duration and intensity of neuromuscular block produced by muscle relaxants. The effects of the volatile drugs are complex, and both central and peripheral

Table 13–6.   Use of Muscle Relaxants in Pigs. Approximate doses and duration of action of muscle relaxants given intravenously to pigs

Muscle Relaxant	Approximate Dose (mg/kg)	Approximate Duration (min)	References
Alcuronium	0.1	30–40	163
Atracurium	0.5–2.5	10–60	163, 167, 168
Gallamine	4	15–20	163
Pancuronium	0.073–0.12	7.3–30	95, 163
Succinylcholine	0.75–2	1.2–3	95, 163
d-Tubocurarine	0.3	25–35	163
Vecuronium	0.1–0.2	5–20	95, 163, 169, 170, 171

mechanisms have been proposed to explain the potentiating action. Although the pharmacokinetics of the muscle relaxants are not altered by the anesthetics, variation in regional muscle blood flow allowing a greater fraction of the injected relaxant to reach a particular site of action may be significant.

The order of potency of the volatile anesthetics to potentiate neuromuscular blockers varies with individual relaxants. Enflurane and isoflurane have a greater effect than halothane on reducing the dose of d-tubocurarine, pancuronium, gallamine, succinylcholine, and vecuronium required to lower twitch height in human patients.(196) The potentiating action of enflurane on d-tubocurarine–induced block is time dependent, even when alveolar concentrations are kept constant.(197) It is possible that different mechanisms at more than one site may be involved. Enflurane potentiates atracurium block in humans.(198) Succinylcholine block is also affected by inhalants; the phase II block develops at a lower cumulative dose in the presence of halothane, isoflurane, or enflurane compared with fentanyl in human patients.(199, 200) When relaxants are given to patients anesthetized with an inhalant, decreased doses of the blocker are required. Monitoring of neuromuscular function allows the appropriate dose of relaxant to be administered.

Most injectable anesthetic agents have little effect on the relaxant properties of neuromuscular blockers. For example, atracurium neuromuscular block is not altered significantly by diazepam, ketamine, alphaxalone/alphadolone, or methohexital in cats.(201)

ACID-BASE DISTURBANCES

The neuromuscular block induced by d-tubocurarine, pancuronium, and vecuronium is potentiated by *respiratory* acidosis and antagonized by *respiratory* alkalosis.(202-204) In contrast, evidence has shown that *metabolic* alkalosis potentiates the relaxant actions of gallamine(205), d-tubocurarine, and pancuronium.(206) The pH changes due to respiratory and metabolic origins have only minor effects on the actions of atracurium(82), though hypocapnia reduces the duration of action of this relaxant.(207)

ELECTROLYTE DISTURBANCES

Differences in the serum concentration of potassium, magnesium, and calcium influence the duration of action of muscle relaxants. The concentration of potassium ions in the intracellular compartment relative to that of the extracellular compartment is the major factor determining the resting membrane potential of the cell wall. Changes in the ratio of potassium concentration inside to that outside the cell alters the resting membrane potential; a decrease in plasma potassium concentration decreases the resting membrane potential of the muscle membrane. Nondepolarizing relaxants may have a prolonged action in hypokalemic patients. This action has been reported in patients with low serum

potassium due to diuresis that were given pancuronium.(206)

Increased magnesium concentrations potentiate neuromuscular block by nondepolarizing relaxants by inhibiting the presynaptic release of the transmitter. Magnesium sulfate is occasionally given to horses for colic, and if the animals are anesthetized soon after, an increased duration of action of muscle relaxants may occur. Magnesium therapy in human patients increases the duration of vecuronium activity.(208) Hypokalemia and hypocalcemia may have effects similar to hypermagnesemia, because these electrolyte derangements depress acetylcholine release from the nerve endings. Hypercalcemia weakly antagonizes the actions of muscle relaxants. Hypercalcemia and hyperkalemia were shown to increase relaxant requirements for d-tubocurarine and pancuronium.(209) The dangers of giving succinylcholine to hyperkalemic patients has been discussed.

HYPOTHERMIA

The effects of hypothermia on neuromuscular block is variable. At a low body temperature, less than 32° C, there is diminished mobilization and release of acetylcholine from the nerve ending and relaxant potentiation is expected. Human patients cooled to approximately 26° C for cardiopulmonary bypass surgery have prolonged periods of paralysis following atracurium (210), pancuronium, and vecuronium administration.(211)

Hypothermia prolongs d-tubocurarine and pancuronium neuromuscular block.(132) However, in vitro studies with pancuronium indicate that it is not affected by hypothermia, to temperatures of 25° C, while the potency of d-tubocurarine, metocurine, and gallamine is decreased.(212) Because the onset of neuromuscular block is delayed during hypothermia, care is required during administration of relaxants to avoid overdose. Hypothermia alters other factors that influence neuromuscular block, such as renal and hepatic clearance and muscle blood flow.(132)

AGE

Age influences the dose requirement of muscle relaxants. During the first two years of life the neuromuscular junction matures physically and chemically, and skeletal muscle contractile properties change causing variation in sensitivity to muscle relaxants. Other factors that influence the dose–response and duration of action of relaxants are changes in the volume of distribution, rate of metabolism, and clearance.(213-216)

Human infants are relatively resistant to succinylcholine while being sensitive to nondepolarizing relaxants. A small single dose of d-tubocurarine has a duration of action in neonates similar to that in adults, but with multiple doses prolonged responses may occur owing to decreased plasma clearance and slower elimination.(217) Neonates are slightly more sensitive to atracurium(218) and pancuronium.(219) Both atracurium and vecuronium have been used successfully in the newborn.(216)

The duration of action of nondepolarizing relaxants is prolonged in older patients. This is attributable to lower volumes of distribution and reduced rates of clearance as a result of slower metabolism and excretion. The age of the patient does not affect the duration of action of vecuronium or atracurium because of its unique method of metabolism.(220, 221)

NEUROPATHY, NEUROMUSCULAR, AND MUSCULAR DISORDERS

Occasionally animals with neuropathy, neuromuscular, or muscular disorders require anesthesia. Because neuromuscular blockers act at the pre– and postsynaptic myoneural junction, patients with these diseases may show unpredictable responses to depolarizing or nondepolarizing relaxants. An indication of the presence of some pathologic process may be suspected from a history of muscle weakness or wasting.(142, 222-224)

Neuropathy. Peripheral neuropathies in small animals have been classified as idiopathic, familial, metabolic, and immune–mediated polyneuropathy.(224) Human patients with peripheral neuropathy frequently show resistance to succinylcholine and increased sensitivity to nondepolarizing relaxants.

Neuromuscular disorders. Presynaptic disorders in which acetylcholine release from the nerve endings is impaired include tick paralysis, botulism, and myasthenic syndrome (in human patients). Postsynaptic disorders include myasthenia gravis and denervation sensitivity. Myasthenia gravis is an autoimmune disease causing a decrease in the number of functional cholinoceptors, thus producing generalized muscle weakness. Patients with neuromuscular disorders, including myasthenia gravis, usually show marked sensitivity to nondepolarizing relaxants though unpredictable responses have been known to occur. Myasthenia gravis patients often show resistance to succinylcholine. Close monitoring of neuromuscular function when using relaxants in myasthenic patients will allow accurate dose titration.

Myasthenic dogs have been given atracurium, at an initial dose of 0.1 mg/kg then increments of 0.02 mg/kg (225), and vecuronium, at 0.02 mg/kg and increments of 0.01 mg/kg(226), without adverse effects. Residual muscle relaxation can be antagonized with neostigmine and atropine. The dangers of life–threatening hyperkalemia in patients with denervation or immobilization-induced up-regulation following succinylcholine should be appreciated.

Muscular Disorders. These disorders include myopathies and myotonias. Animals with myotonia and malignant hyperthermia should not be given succinylcholine. Prolonged muscular contractions are likely. Responses to nondepolarizing relaxants are variable, requiring cautious use. In advanced stages of some disorders, patients become more sensitive to nondepolarizing relaxants, and prolonged relaxation may occur.

Anticholinesterase drugs used to antagonize a nondepolarizing block can trigger muscle contracture in myotonic patients.

If a neuromuscular blocker is required for any of these muscular conditions, atracurium or vecuronium should be considered because of their short half-lives. In anesthetized pigs susceptible to malignant hyperthermia, vecuronium(170, 171), atracurium(167), doxacurium(227), and mivacurium(227) have been given without complications. Pancuronium has been used successfully in patients susceptible to malignant hyperthermia, but neostigmine reversal is not recommended because muscle contracture may be triggered.

Conditioning Exercise. During exercise muscles undergo biochemical changes resulting in down-regulation or decreased cholinergic receptors. These changes are opposite to those that occur with prolonged immobilization. Exercise increases the sensitivity of muscle to the blocking actions of metocurine in dogs (140) but not in horses.(156)

INTERACTION WITH OTHER DRUGS

Antibiotics. A number of antibiotics are known to prolong the duration of action of neuromuscular blockers. Antibiotics potentiate nondepolarizing relaxants by different mechanisms of action.(228-231) Certain antibiotics cause channel block, whereas the aminoglycosides, streptomycin, neomycin, gentamicin, kanamycin, and amikacin, potentiate relaxants by a postsynaptic action and presynaptically by reducing acetylcholine release. Neostigmine and calcium have been beneficial in reversing block due to aminoglycosides. Tobramycin and gentamicin have less neuromuscular blocking action in humans than the other aminoglycosides.(232) However, in the cat gentamicin has demonstrated a strong potentiating action.(233)

The polymixins have both pre– and postjunctional actions, including depression of muscle action potentials. Block is not responsive to calcium or neostigmine. Tetracyclines, lincomycin, and clindamycin (the lincosamides) have a prejunctional action and may directly depress muscle contractility. Calcium and neostigmine may antagonize neuromuscular block enhanced by oxytetracycline and the lincosamides but not tetracycline. Chloramphenicol, sulfadiazine, and penicillin–G have no significant blocking actions in pigs and lambs.(234)

If some residual neuromuscular block is present, neostigmine antagonism is beneficial if continued block is caused by aminoglycoside coadministration. Calcium administration is beneficial in antagonizing block caused by some antibiotics but not the polymixins. Disadvantages of calcium therapy are short duration of action and a possible interference with antibacterial effect. Neuromuscular activity following antibiotic therapy should be carefully monitored if there is a preexisting muscle weakness.

Actions of Other Drugs on Neuromuscular Block. Lithium compounds reduce presynaptic release of acetylcholine, potentiating pancuronium's action. A number of other drugs decrease acetylcholine release and stabilize postsynaptic membranes, thus inhibiting the propagation of muscle action potentials. Those drugs that potentiate neuromuscular block by these actions include local anesthetics, barbiturates, quinidine, procainamide, propranolol, phenytoin, and magnesium compounds. Patients given long-term phenytoin therapy have shown resistance to metocurine, d-tubocurarine, pancuronium, and vecuronium(235), but not to atracurium.(236)

Calcium antagonists used to treat cardiac dysrhythmias prolong nondepolarizing neuromuscular block through a presynaptic action. Dantrolene has a potentiating action of muscle relaxants by blocking muscle excitation–contraction coupling. Diuretics, including furosemide, cause possible presynaptic inhibition of acetylcholine release and hypokalemia, thus potentiating d-tubocurarine block. Ganglionic blockers also enhance d-tubocurarine block. Immunosuppressants, including corticosteroids, decrease the potency of nondepolarizing blockers. Some drugs inhibit cholinesterase enzyme, which prolongs the action of succinylcholine. These compounds include metoclopramide(58), immunosuppressants (cyclophosphamide, meturedepa, and chlorambucil), ganglion blockers (trimetaphan), lithium compounds, and organophosphates.(238)

Interaction between neuromuscular blockers has been reported. The effects of gallamine plus d-tubocurarine and gallamine plus pancuronium are additive without showing signs of potentiation. Some evidence of potentiation has been shown with pancuronium plus d-tubocurarine, metocurine plus pancuronium, metocurine plus d-tubocurarine, and gallamine plus metocurine.(237) In view of these interactions the use of single nondepolarizing neuromuscular blocker is recommended.(56, 82, 238)

Antagonism of Neuromuscular Block

ANTICHOLINESTERASES AND NONDEPOLARIZING BLOCK

Antagonism of a nondepolarizing neuromuscular block is achieved by increasing the concentration of acetylcholine molecules in the junctional cleft between the nerve terminal and muscle end plate. By giving anticholinesterase drugs, the hydrolysis of acetylcholine is slowed, the number of acetylcholine molecules accumulates to compete for position at the receptor site, and as muscle relaxant molecules are forced away from the neuromuscular junction normal neuromuscular transmission returns.

Mechanism of Action. Acetylcholinesterase is found in erythrocytes, nerve, muscle, and in high concentrations at the neuromuscular junction. It is a large protein with two subsites, an anionic and an esteratic site, which bind to the acetylcholine molecule. The acetylcholine molecule has a positively charged quaternary nitrogen atom that binds to the anionic site of the enzyme; the carbon atom of the ester binds to the enzyme esteratic site. Choline is split off, leaving an acetylated enzyme

complex that is acetate-attached to the esteratic site of the enzyme. Acetate is split off to leave free enzyme. In summary, the acetylcholine substrate is hydrolyzed by the enzyme to form choline and acetic acid. Free enzyme and acetylcholine are in dynamic equilibrium in the junctional cleft.

Three anticholinesterase compounds, edrophonium, neostigmine, and pyridostigmine, have been synthesized and are used to inhibit the action of the enzyme. These drugs have different mechanisms of action. Edrophonium forms a complex with the enzyme; the quaternary nitrogen of the inhibitor binds electrostatically with the enzyme anionic site, and the inhibitor imidazole nitrogen binds to the enzyme esteratic site. There is a dynamic equilibrium between the free enzyme, edrophonium, and enzyme–edrophonium complex. The complex will dissociate as edrophonium concentration falls, thus allowing it to bind to more enzyme. Edrophonium inhibition is short–acting and easily reversible.

Neostigmine and pyridostigmine differ from edrophonium in that they combine with the enzyme anionic and esteratic sites to form an intermediate compound. The binding between neostigmine and pyridostigmine and the enzyme is similar to the binding that occurs between acetylcholinesterase and acetylcholine when the substrate is hydrolyzed. A complex is formed between inhibitor (neostigmine or pyridostigmine) and enzyme. The small part of the antagonist molecule (a carbonate) is split off and attaches itself to the esteratic site of the enzyme. Although the carbonate residue is attached to the enzyme, it cannot bind to any acetylcholine molecules to hydrolyze them. A carbamyl enzyme is formed that splits off the carbamyl molecule to leave free enzyme. The free enzyme is then available to hydrolyze acetylcholine. The carbamyl enzyme complex has a half–life of about 30 minutes, which is vastly greater than 40 microseconds, the half–life of the acetylated enzyme formed during physiologic hydrolysis of acetylcholine.

In addition to the inhibition of postjunctional acetylcholinesterase by the mechanisms described, these three drugs also have presynaptic actions contributing to the antagonism of neuromuscular block. Anticholinesterases improve the mobilization of transmitter and induce repetitive firing of the motor nerve terminal to generate a brief train of transmitter release, thus increasing strength of muscle contraction. Anticholinesterases can directly depolarize motor nerve terminals, thereby competing directly with the relaxant.

Metabolism and Elimination. The liver is considered to be the predominant site for metabolism of the anticholinesterases: approximately 50% of neostigmine, 30% of edrophonium, and 25% of pyridostigmine is metabolized. Excretion via the kidneys following glomerular filtration accounts for clearance of about 75% of pyridostigmine, 70% of edrophonium, and 50% of neostigmine. Elimination of anticholinesterase is prolonged in patients with renal failure, as is the case for nondepolarizing relaxants. It is unlikely that in a patient with renal failure, the muscle relaxant will outlast the anticholinesterase; if recurarization takes place, other factors that prolong the action of the relaxant should be investigated.(238)

Comparison of Anticholinesterases. The antagonist effects of edrophonium, neostigmine, and pyridostigmine have been compared in human patients given d-tubocurarine. The time for onset of action is 1 to 2 minutes for edrophonium, 7 to 10 minutes for neostigmine, and 12 to 16 minutes for pyridostigmine. Neostigmine is 4.4 times more potent than pyridostigmine and 5.7 times more potent than edrophonium in human patients for antagonizing nondepolarizing block (239), whereas in cats neostigmine is 12 times more potent than edrophonium.(240) The duration of cholinesterase antagonism is similar for neostigmine and edrophonium, whereas for pyridostigmine it is about 40% longer.(239, 241) Edrophonium reverses neuromuscular block induced by d-tubocurarine (239, 241), pancuronium (242), and vecuronium adequately.(240)

Other Actions of Anticholinesterases. Anticholinesterases allow the buildup of acetylcholine at nicotinic (neuromuscular junction) and muscarinic cholinoceptors. Muscarinic receptor stimulation induces bradycardia; increased gastrointestinal motility; increased secretions from salivary glands, the oropharynx, and airways; and bronchiole constriction. Simultaneous administration of an anticholinergic will prevent these adverse effects. Edrophonium has weaker actions on the cardiac vagus than neostigmine, and it is possible that neostigmine has a greater anticholinesterase action.(240) Pyridostigmine induces fewer autonomic effects than neostigmine, as evidenced by less oropharyngeal secretions and bradycardia.(243)

Because edrophonium induces less muscarinic stimulation than neostigmine or pyridostigmine, a lower dose of atropine, about half, is necessary to prevent these undesirable actions. Glycopyrrolate has a slower onset of action than atropine; consequently, it should be given about 3 or 4 minutes before edrophonium. Atropine should be given before edrophonium, whereas with neostigmine and pyridostigmine it can be given simultaneously.(240, 244)

Several factors influence blockade reversal with anticholinesterases. With deep muscle relaxation shown by a markedly depressed twitch height, reversal of block will be slower. The speed of reversal is directly proportional to the dose of antagonist given and the anticholinesterase chosen. Antagonism of neuromuscular block can be expected to be slower in the elderly patient.

Best responses to anticholinesterases are achieved when there is some spontaneous recovery and twitch heights are rising; with the train–of–four stimulation all four twitches are evident. In human patients a train–of–four ratio of 0.7 is frequently used as a guide for anticholinesterase administration, but in horses this level of spontaneous recovery is insufficient for reversal

of muscle relaxation. In horses, spontaneous recovery needs to progress further before attempting reversal of residual muscle relaxation so that the strength of the limb muscles is sufficient for the animal to stand.(245) In monitored patients at least two twitches of a train of four should be evident before anticholinesterases are administered (Fig. 13–2). When patients are not monitored, obvious diaphragmatic contractions should be present.

If neuromuscular block is too intense, attempts at reversal will be slow and the possibility of recurarization very likely. If the response to one dose of anticholinesterase is inadequate, positive pressure ventilation should continue and the antagonist repeated when there is some evidence of spontaneous recovery.

Use of Anticholinesterases. Anticholinesterases should be given to reverse the neuromuscular effects of all nondepolarizing blockers. Exceptions can be made if all four twitch heights of a train of four have returned to prerelaxant heights or there is minimal fade following tetanic stimulation (Fig. 13–2). Responses to train–of–four or tetanic stimulation provide a more accurate assessment of neuromuscular function. If anticholinesterase therapy is to be avoided, vecuronium or atracurium are recommended because spontaneous recovery is fairly rapid. Edrophonium and neostigmine have been used clinically in many animal species. Pyridostigmine has few advantages over these anticholinesterases.

Simultaneous administration of an anticholinergic is nearly always necessary with neostigmine and pyridostigmine but is less important with edrophonium. In small animals the dose of glycopyrrolate is 20 µg/kg and that of atropine is 40 µg/kg. In horses atropine can be given at a dose of 10 µg/kg.

Neostigmine and edrophonium have been used successfully to reverse nondepolarizing neuromuscular block in anesthetized horses. Edrophonium at a dose of 0.5 mg/kg intravenously reverses block in horses and ponies following atracurium (29, 30, 96, 175, 246) and pancuronium.(175, 247) Neostigmine at a dose between 22 to 44 µg/kg intravenously reverses neuromuscular block in horses and ponies produced by gallamine (93, 94), pancuronium(93, 247), and vecuronium.(93) Edrophonium has advantages over neostigmine: Onset of action is more rapid, and the adverse effects of acetylcholine accumulation at muscarinic receptors, including gastrointestinal effects, cardiac changes, and the increase in salivary and airway secretions, are less than those for neostigmine. In horses, edrophonium administration usually does not require atropine coadministration. A disadvantage with neostigmine reversal is the subsequent increase in airway secretions, often requiring atropine administration. Atropine, in turn, may cause tachycardia and gastrointestinal complications.(248) Anticholinesterases should be given slowly, that is, over a period of at least one minute.

Edrophonium administration increases arterial blood pressure in horses (29, 30, 175) and in ponies by about

20%.(247) Heart rate changes are variable, and a slight bradycardia is the more frequent change. Neostigmine also raises blood pressure, but bradycardia is not usually observed in horses.

In dogs neostigmine (2.5 mg) plus atropine can be used to reverse neuromuscular block following atracurium(97, 174, 225, 249), alcuronium(158), gallamine(159), pancuronium(159), pipecuronium(99), and vecuronium.(162, 172, 226) In the cat edrophonium (0.5 mg/kg) has been used to antagonize vecuronium block.(240) Neostigmine reversal of atracurium neuromuscular block in pigs(167) and d-tubocurarine, pancuronium, and vecuronium block in sheep has been reported.(98, 250)

A second dose of anticholinesterase can be given 5 to 7 minutes after the initial dose if the response is poor. Intravenous calcium can also be tried if response to anticholinesterase injection is poor.

After antagonism of neuromuscular block the patient should be observed closely during the recovery period with particular attention being given to respiratory function. A smooth sustained respiratory effort with a good tidal volume usually indicates adequate muscular function. However, short jerky respirations suggesting the presence of residual block or apnea as a result of recurarization may occur. Even in the presence of strong evoked muscle responses to peripheral nerve stimulation, the ability to breathe may be inadequate. Anesthetized dogs given neostigmine and atropine after atracurium relaxation have become apneic up to 25 minutes after neostigmine injection, requiring reintubation and ventilation.(174, 251)

An indicator of adequate reversal of relaxant in a horse can be obtained from respiratory effort. If the endotracheal tube or inspiratory limb of the anesthetic machine is occluded and the inspiratory effort, measured with an aneroid gauge, generates a pressure of –10 to –25 cm water, then sufficient muscle strength is usually present.(245) Further monitoring of respiratory effort should continue.

If recovery from muscle relaxation is unduly prolonged, likely causes need to be investigated. These include hypothermia, electrolyte disturbances, excessively deep anesthesia, simultaneous administration of antibiotics, and other compounds known to prolong neuromuscular block and decreased renal or hepatic function.

ANTICHOLINESTERASES AND SUCCINYLCHOLINE BLOCK

Anticholinesterases prolong the depolarizing block produced by succinylcholine.(59) When multiple or high doses of succinylcholine are given or the relaxant has a prolonged action, phase II block develops. When this occurs, edrophonium can effectively antagonize phase II block when the muscle responses to train–of–four stimulation are at a ratio of 0.4 or less.(252) Likewise, neostigmine consistently antagonizes succinylcholine phase II block in anesthetized dogs when the train–of–four ratio is 0.38 or less.(253)

Neostigmine reversal of the phase II block in the dog should be attempted only when train–of–four twitch heights are measured and a ratio calculated. Without accurate measurement of the train–of–four ratio, recovery from succinylcholine block should be spontaneous. The patient should be ventilated until it can breathe adequately.

AMINOPYRIDINES

The aminopyridines, of which 4–aminopyridine is a well-known example, can antagonize nondepolarizing neuromuscular block, but the effects are less than those for the anticholinesterases. 4–Aminopyridine facilitates release of transmitter from the nerve ending, but as this is not restricted to cholinergic synapses, some adverse effects of the facilitatory actions at other synapses have occurred. When given along with neostigmine or pyridostigmine, 4–aminopyridine has shown a synergistic action to antagonize vecuronium block.(254)

Central Relaxants

GUAIFENESIN

Guaifenesin (glyceryl guaiacolate), a common decongestant and antitussive, has been used extensively in large animal species as a central muscle relaxant. According to Roberts, its unique advantage is that it produces muscle relaxation with little effect on respiration.(255)

Guaifenesin, which chemically is similar to mephenesin, disrupts impulse transmission at connecting neurons in the spinal cord and brain stem. Although relaxation of the skeletal muscles occurs, the diaphragm continues to function and there is no respiratory paralysis. The respiratory rate may be increased while the tidal volume decreases. The minute volume is unchanged. The pharyngeal and laryngeal muscles are relaxed, facilitating intubation. A state of drowsiness is also induced. Preanesthetic and anesthetic agents are potentiated.

Guaifenesin is most commonly prepared as a 5% solution in 5% dextrose in water. The powder is prepared for injection by dissolving it under aseptic conditions in warm (not to exceed 100° F) sterile water. The pH, osmolality, stability, and bacteriostatic characteristics of 5, 10, and 15% solutions of guaifenesin have been studied.(256) A 10% solution of guaifenesin in sterile distilled water is suitable for use in the adult horse. Recumbency can be induced in the horse by intravenous administration of 160 mg/kg of guaifenesin.(257) The lethal dose in horses is approximately three times that required to induce immobilization.(258)

Guaifenesin (5% in 5% dextrose) given alone intravenously produces gentle, excitement–free relaxation and recumbency in horses. This technique can be used for intubation and induction of gas anesthesia. The duration of recumbency when given at the rate of 1 mL/lb is approximately 9 minutes. The blood pressure during this period is stable, in contrast to the use of succinylcholine, which causes a drastic increase (425/320 mm Hg), and barbiturates, which produce a marked decrease (45/20 mm Hg).(259) The cardiovascular and respiratory effects of guaifenesin, either alone or in combination with pentothal sodium, are relatively benign when compared with the effects of succinylcholine on these systems.(257)

The cardiopulmonary effects of guaifenesin and xylazine–guaifenesin have been examined in horses.(260) Heart rate, respiratory rate, right atrial pressure, pulmonary artery pressure, and cardiac output are unchanged when guaifenesin alone is given. Systolic, diastolic, and mean arterial pressures are decreased, whereas PaO_2 is transiently decreased.

Intravenous xylazine (1.1 mg/kg) prior to guaifenesin administration reduced the dose necessary for lateral recumbency (88 ± 10 mg/kg). Transient decreases in heart and respiratory rates, cardiac output, PaO_2, and arterial blood pressures, and increases in central venous pressure occur.

Like other drugs in the mephenesin group, guaifenesin in high concentration produces hemolysis and hemoglobinuria if given intravenously. This has resulted in the reluctance of many veterinarians to employ a 10% solution of guaifenesin. The drug is conjugated to glucuronide in the liver and largely excreted in the urine. The exact mechanism of inactivation in the body is poorly understood. Significant amounts of guaifenesin pass the placental barrier in the mare.(260)

Davis and Wolff found a pronounced sex difference in duration of action, stallions requiring longer to recover than mares. This was attributed to slower disappearance of the drug from the plasma.(26) There is no antagonist for guaifenesin. Concurrent administration of physostigmine is contraindicated.

Although it is used in the horse, guaifenesin alone is not of value in the dog because of the large volume of solution necessary and the brief, shallow muscular relaxation produced.(262) Guaifenesin in combination with ketamine and xylazine, however, has proven to be an effective immobilizing regimen in dogs.(263)

Today, 5% guaifenesin solutions containing thiopental or ketamine and xylazine are commonly employed as anesthetic mixtures in a variety of species including ruminants, swine, and horses. These anesthetic regimens and techniques are reviewed in more detail in other Chapters 10, 20, and 23.

REFERENCES

1. Dale HH, Feldberg W, Vogt M. Release of acetylcholine at voluntary motor nerve endings. J Physiol (Lond) 86:353, 1936.
2. Goerig M. Pioneering curare in anesthesia. Anesthesiology 73:189, 1990.
3. Hall LW. A report on the clinical use of bis (beta-dimethylaminoethyl)-succinate bisethiodide ("Brevedil E", M and B 2210) during anaesthesia in the dog. Vet Rec 64:491, 1952.
4. Dreyer F. Acetylcholine receptor. Br J Anaesth 54:115, 1982.
5. Standaert FG. Release of transmitter at the neuromuscular junction. Br J Anaesth 54:131, 1982.
6. Bowman WC. The neuromuscular junction: Recent developments. Eur J Anaesthesiol 2:59, 1985.
7. Bowman WC. Neuromuscular block and its antagonism: Basic concepts. In: General Anaesthesia, 5th ed. Edited by JF Nunn, JE Utting, and BR Brown. London: Butterworth, 1989.
8. Peper K, Sterz R. Some aspects of the physiology, pharmacology and immunobiology of the acetylcholine receptor at the neuromuscular junction. In: Monographs in Anaesthesiology: Muscle Relaxants. Edited by S Agoston and WC Bowman. Amsterdam: Elsevier, 1990.
9. Paton WDM, Waud DR. The margin of safety of neuromuscular transmission. J Physiol (Lond) 191:59 1967.
10. Waud BE, Waud DR. The margin of safety of neuromuscular transmission in the muscle of the diaphragm. Anesthesiology 37:417, 1972.
11. Bowman WC, Marshall I G, Gibb AJ, Harborne, AJ. Feedback control of transmitter release at the neuromuscular junction. Trends Pharmacol Sci 9:16, 1988.
12. Standaert FG. Neuromuscular Physiology. In: Anesthesia, 3rd ed. Edited by RD Miller. New York: Churchill Livingstone, 1990.
13. Katz B, Thesleff S. A study of the desensitisation produced by acetylcholine at the motor endplate. J Physiol (Lond) 138:63, 1957.
14. Lee C, Barnes A, Katz, RL. Magnitude, dose-requirement and mode of development of tachyphylaxis to suxamethonium in man. Br J Anaesth 50:189, 1978.
15. Williams NE, Webb SN, Calvey TN. Differential effects of myoneural blocking drugs on neuromuscular transmission. Br J Anaesth 52:1111, 1980.
16. Harvey AM, Masland RL. Method for the study of neuromuscular transmission in human subjects. Bull Johns Hopkins Hosp 68:81, 1941.
17. Berger JJ, Gravenstein JS, Munson ES. Electrode polarity and peripheral nerve stimulation. Anesthesiology 56:402, 1982.
18. Donlon JV, Savarese J J, Ali HH. Cumulative dose response curves for gallamine: Effect of altered resting thumb tension and mode of stimulation. Anesth Analg 58:377, 1979.
19. Heckmann R, Jones RS, Wuersch W. A method for recording evoked electrical and mechanical activity of muscle in the intact dog. Res Vet Sci 23:1, 1977.
20. Cullen LK, Jones RS, Snowdon SL. Neuromuscular activity in the intact dog: Techniques for recording evoked mechanical responses. Br Vet J 136:154, 1980.
21. Bowen, JM. Monitoring neuromuscular function in intact animals. Am J Vet Res 30:857, 1969.
22. Curtis MB, Eicker SE. Pharmacodynamic properties of succinylcholine in greyhounds. Am J Vet Res 52:898, 1991.
23. Cullen LK, Jones RS. Recording of train-of-four evoked muscle responses from the nose and foreleg in the intact dog. Res Vet Sci 29:277, 1980.
24. Klein L, Hopkins AS, Beck E, Burton B. Mechanical responses to peroneal nerve stimulation in halothane anesthetized horses in the absence of neuromuscular blockade and during partial nondepolarizing blockade. Am J Vet Res 44:781, 1983.
25. Jones RS, Prentice DE. A technique for the investigation of the action of drugs on the neuromuscular junction in the intact horse. Br Vet J 132:226, 1976.
26. Hildebrand SV, Hill T. Neuromuscular blockade by atracurium in llamas. Vet Surg 20:153, 1991.
27. Manley SV, Steffey EP, Howitt GA, Woliner, M. Cardiovascular and neuromuscular effects of pancuronium bromide in the pony. Am J Vet Res 44:1349, 1983.
28. Hildebrand SV, Howitt GA. Neuromuscular and cardiovascular effects of pancuronium bromide in calves anesthetized with halothane. Am J Vet Res 45:1549, 1984.
29. Hildebrand SV, Arpin D. Neuromuscular and cardiovascular effects of atracurium administered to healthy horses anesthetized with halothane. Am J Vet Res 49:1066, 1988.
30. Hildebrand SV, Hill T, Holland M. The effect of the neuromuscular blocking activity of atracurium in halothane anaesthetized horses. J Vet Pharmacol Ther 12:277, 1989.
31. Miller RD. Are studies of neuromuscular blocking drugs and their antagonists unnecessarily confusing? Anesthesiology, 65: 569, 1986.

32. Ali HH, Utting JE, Gray TC. Stimulus frequency in the detection of neuromuscular block in humans. Br J Anaesth 42:967, 1970.

33. Ali HH, Utting JE, Gray TC. Quantitative assessment of residual anti-depolarising block (Part I). Br J Anaesth 43:473, 1971.

34. Cullen LK, Jones RS. Residual non-depolarising neuromuscular block assessed by train-of-four stimulation in the dog. Res Vet Sci 32:121, 1982.

35. Waud BE, Waud DR. The relation between the response to "train-of-four" stimulation and receptor occlusion during competitive neuromuscular block. Anesthesiology 37:413, 1972.

36. Torda TA, Graham GG, Tsui D. Neuromuscular sensitivity to atracurium in humans. Anaesth Intensive Care 18:62, 1990.

37. Lee C, Barnes A, Katz RL. Neuromuscular sensitivity to tubocurarine. Br J Anaesth 48:1045, 1976.

38. Ali HH, Savarese JJ, Lebowitz PW, Ramsey FM. Twitch, tetanus and train of four as indices of recovery from non depolarizing neuromuscular blockade. Anesthesiology 54:294, 1981.

39. Bowman WC. Prejunctional and postjunctional cholinoceptors at the neuromuscular junction. Anesth Analg 59:935, 1980.

40. Pearce AC, Casson WR, Jones RM. Factors affecting train-of-four fade. Br J Anaesth 57:602, 1985.

41. Graham GG. et al. Relationship of train of four ratio to twitch depression during pancuronium-induced neuromuscular blockade. Anesthesiology 65:579, 1986.

42. Lee C. Dose relationships of phase II, tachyphylaxis and train-of-four in suxamethonium-induced dual neuromuscular block in man. Br J Anaesth 47:841, 1975.

43. Cullen LK, and Jones RS. The nature of suxamethonium neuromuscular block in the dog assessed by train-of-four stimulation. Res Vet Sci 29:281, 1980.

44. Merton PA. Voluntary strength and fatigue. J Physiol (Lond) 123:553, 1954.

45. Epstein RA, Epstein RM. The electromyogram and the mechanical response of indirectly stimulated muscle in anesthetized man following curarization. Anesthesiology 38:212, 1973.

46. Viby-Morgensen J, et al. Posttetanic count (PTC). A new method of evaluating an intense nondepolarizing neuromuscular blockade. Anesthesiology 55:458, 1981.

47. Bonsu AK, et al. Relationship of posttetanic count and train-of-four response during intense neuromuscular blockade caused by atracurium. Br J Anaesth 59:1089, 1987.

48. Muchhal KK, et al. Evaluation of intense neuromuscular blockade caused by vecuronium using posttetanic count (PTC). Anesthesiology 66:846, 1987.

49. Drench NE, et al. Manual evaluation of residual curarization using double burst stimulation: A comparison with train-of-four. Anesthesiology 70:578, 1989.

50. Nordgren I, Baldwin K, Forney R. Succinylcholine–Tissue distribution and elimination from plasma in the dog. Biochem Pharmacol 33:2519, 1984.

51. Hall LW, Lehmann H, Silk E. Responses in dogs to relaxants derived from succinic acid and choline. Br Med J i:134, 1953.

52. Trucchi G, et al. Correlation between the duration of action of suxamethonium serum levels of pseudocholinesterases and dibucaine number in the dog. J Assoc Vet Anaesth 15:96, 1988.

53. Foldes FF, Rendell-Baker L, Birch JH. Causes and prevention of prolonged apnea with succinylcholine. Anesth Analg 35:609, 1956.

54. Pantuck EJ, Pantuck CB. Cholinesterases and anticholinesterases. In: Muscle Relaxants. Edited by RL Katz. Amsterdam: Excerpta Medica, 1975.

55. Benson GJ, Thurmon JC. Clinical pharmacology of succinylcholine. J Am Vet Med Assoc 176:646, 1980.

56. Miller RD, Savarese JJ. Pharmacology of muscle relaxants and their antagonists. In: Anesthesia, 3rd ed. Edited by RD Miller. New York: Churchill Livingstone, 1990.

57. Hill GE, Wong KC, Hodges MR. Potentiation of succinylcholine neuromuscular blockade by lithium carbonate. Anesthesiology 44:439, 1976.

58. Kao YJ, Turner DR. Prolongation of succinylcholine block by metoclopramide. Anesthesiology 70:905, 1989.

59. Jones RS, Heckmann R, Wuersch W. The effect of neostigmine on the duration of action of suxamethonium in the dog. Br Vet J 136:71, 1980.

60. Reynolds WT. Use of suxamethonium in cats fitted with dichlorvos flea collars. Aust Vet J 62:106, 1985.

61. Short CE, Cuneio J, Cupp D. Organophosphate-induced complications during anesthetic management in the horse. J Am Vet Med Assoc 157:1319, 1971.

62. Meijer DKG, Weitering JG, Vermeer GA, Scaf AHJ. Comparative pharmacokinetics of d-tubocurarine and metocurine in man. Anesthesiology 51:402, 1979.

63. Miller RD, et al. The comparative potency and pharmacokinetics of pancuronium and its metabolites in anesthetized man. J Pharmacol Exp Ther 207:539, 1978.

64. McLeod K, Watson MJ, Rawlins MD. Pharmacokinetics of pancuronium in patients with normal and impaired renal function. Br J Anaesth 48:341, 1976.

65. Hughes R, Chapple DJ. The pharmacology of atracurium: A new competitive neuromuscular blocking agent. Br J Anaesth 53:31, 1981.

66. Fisher DM, et al. Elimination of atracurium in humans: Contribution of Hofmann elimination and ester hydrolysis versus organ based elimination. Anesthesiology 65:6, 1986.

67. Chapple DJ, Miller AA, Wheatley PL. Neurological and cardiovascular effects of laudanosine in conscious and anesthetized dogs. Anesthesiology 63:A311, 1985.

68. Ward S, Neill EAM. Pharmacokinetics of atracurium in acute hepatic failure (with acute renal failure). Br J Anaesth 55:1169, 1983.

69. Fahey MR, et al. Effect of renal failure on laudanosine excretion in man. Br J Anaesth 57:1049, 1985.

70. Ward S, Weatherley BC. Pharmacokinetics of atracurium and its metabolites. Br J Anaesth 58:6S, 1986.

71. Hennis PJ, et al. Pharmacology of laudanosine in dogs. Anesthesiology 65:56, 1986.

72. Durant NN, Houwertjes MC, Crul JF. Comparison of the neuromuscular blocking properties of Org NC 45 and pancuronium in the rat, cat and rhesus monkey. Br J Anaesth 52:723, 1980.

73. Marshall IG, et al. Pharmacology of Org NC 45 compared with other non-depolarizing neuromuscular blocking drugs. Br J Anaesth 52:11S, 1980.

74. Upton RA, Nguyen TL, Miller RD, Castagnoli N. Renal and bilary elimination of vecuronium (Org NC 45) and pancuronium in rats. Anesth Analg 61:313, 1982.

75. Karpati E, Biro K. Pharmacological study of a new competitive neuromuscular blocking steroid, pipecuronium bromide. Arzneimittelforschung 30:346, 1980.

76. Khuenl-Brady KS, et al. Pharmacokinetics and disposition of pipecuronium bromide in dogs with and without ligated renal pedicles. Anesthesiology 71:919, 1989.

77. Cook DR, et al. Pharmacokinetics and pharmacodynamics of doxacurium in normal patients and in those with hepatic or renal failure. Anesth Analg 72:145, 1991.

78. Cook DR. et al. In vitro metabolism of BW B1090U Anesthesiology 67:A610, 1987.

79. Savarese JJ, et al. The clinical neuromuscular pharmacology of mivacurium chloride (BW B1090U). Anesthesiology 68:723, 1988.

80. Cason B, et al. Cardiovascular and neuromuscular effects of three steroidal neuromuscular blocking drugs in dogs (Org 9616, Org 9426, Org 9991). Anesth Analg 70:382, 1990.

81. Bowman WC. Non-relaxant properties of neuromuscular blocking drugs. Br J Anaesth 54:147, 1982.

82. Hunter JM. Adverse effects of neuromuscular blocking drugs. Br J Anaesth 59:46, 1987.

83. Richardson FJ, Agoston S. Side-effects of neuromuscular blocking drugs. In: Monographs in Anaesthesiology: Muscle Relaxants. Edited by S Agoston and WC Bowman. Amsterdam: Elsevier, 1990.

84. Hughes R, Chapple DJ. Effects of non-depolarising neuromuscular blocking agents on peripheral autonomic mechanisms in cats. Br J Anaesth 48:59, 1976.

85. Durant NH, et al. The neuromuscular and autonomic blocking activities of pancuronium, Org NC 45, and other pancuronium analogues in the cat. J Pharm Pharmacol 31:831, 1979.

86. Hughes R. The pharmacological development of neuromuscular blocking agents. Proc Assoc Vet Anaesth Gr Br Ir 10:136, 1982.

87. Vercruysse P, et al. Gallamine and pancuronium inhibit pre-and postjunctional muscarinic receptors in canine saphenous veins. J Pharmacol Exp Ther 209:225, 1979.

88. Reitan JA, Warpinske MA. Cardiovascular effects of pancuronium bromide in mongrel dogs. Am J Vet Res 36:1309, 1975.

89. Booij LH, Edwards RR, Sohn YJ, Miller RD. Cardiovascular and neuromuscular effects of Org NC 45, pancuronium, metocurine and d-tubocurarine in dogs. Anesth Analg 59:26, 1980.

90. Hughes R. Haemodynamic effects of tubocurarine, gallamine and suxamethonium in dogs. Br J Anaesth 42:928, 1970.

91. Marshall RJ, et al. Comparison of the cardiovascular actions of Org NC 45 with those produced by other non-depolarizing neuromuscular blocking agents in experimental animals. Br J Anaesth 52:21S, 1980.

92. Jones RS. New skeletal muscle relaxants in dogs and cats. J Am Vet Med Assoc 187:281, 1985.

93. Klein L, Beck E, Hopkins J, Burton B. Characteristics of neuromuscular blockade by gallamine, pancuronium and vecuronium (Org NC 45) and antagonism with neostigmine in anaesthetized horses. Proc Assoc Vet Anaesth Gr Br Ir 10:173, 1982.

94. Klein L, Hopkins J, Beck E, Burton B. Cumulative dose responses to gallamine, pancuronium, and neostigmine in halothane-anesthetized horses: Neuromuscular and cardiovascular effects. Am J Vet Res 44:786, 1983.

95. Muir AW, Marshall RJ. Comparative neuromuscular blocking effects of vecuronium, pancuronium, Org 6368 and suxamethonium in the anaesthetized domestic pig. Br J Anaesth 59:622, 1987.

96. Hildebrand SV, Howitt GA, Arpin D. Neuromuscular and cardiovascular effects of atracurium in ponies anesthetized with halothane. Am J Vet Res 47:1096, 1986.

97. Jones RS, Hunter JM, Utting JE. Neuromuscular blocking action of atracurium in the dog and its reversal by neostigmine. Res Vet Sci 34:173, 1983.

98. Klein L, Sylvina T, and Beck E. Neuromuscular blockade with d-tubocurarine, pancuronium and vecuronium in halothane anesthetized sheep. Proc 2nd Int Cong Vet Anesth, Sacramento, Calif. 1985:174.

99. Jones RS. Observations on the neuromuscular blocking action of pipecuronium in the dog. Res Vet Sci 43:101, 1987.

100. Savarese JJ, et al. Pharmacology of BW A938U. Anesthesiology 59:A274, 1983.

101. Savarese JJ, et al. Comparative pharmacology of BW B1090U in rhesus monkey. Anesthesiology 61:A306, 1984.

102. Savarese JJ, et al. Neuromuscular and cardiovascular effects of BW B1090U in anesthetized volunteers. Anesth Analg 64:278, 1985.

103. Mehta MP, et al. The neuromuscular pharmacology of BW A938U in anesthetized patients. Anesthesiology 65:A280, 1986.

104. Murray DJ, et al. The neuromuscular blocking and cardiovascular effects of doxacurium chloride in patients receiving nitrous oxide narcotic anesthesia. Anesthesiology 69:472, 1988.

105. Ali HH, et al. Clinical pharmacology of mivacurium chloride (BW B1090U) infusion: Comparison with vecuronium and atracurium. Br J Anaesth 61:541, 1988.

106. Lennon RL, et al. Doxacurium chloride for neuromuscular blockade before tracheal intubation and surgery during nitrous oxide-oxygen-narcotic-enflurane anesthesia. Anesth Analg 68:255, 1989.

107. Magorian T, et al. Pharmacokinetics, onset, and duration of action of rocuronium in humans: Normal vs hepatic dysfunction. Anesthesiology 75:A1069, 1991.

108. Benson GJ, Hartsfield SM, Smetzer DL, Thurmon JC. Physiologic effects of succinylcholine chloride in mechanically ventilated horses anesthetized with halothane in oxygen. Am J Vet Res 40:1411, 1979.

109. Zinn RS, Gabel AA, Heath RB. Effects of succinylcholine and promazine on the cardiovascular and respiratory systems in the horse. J Am Vet Med Assoc 157:1495, 1970.

110. Heath RB, Gabel AA. Evaluation of thiamylal sodium, succinylcholine, and glycerol guaiacolate prior to inhalation anesthesia in horses. J Am Vet Med Assoc 157:1486, 1970.

111. Ertama PM. Histamine release in rats after administration of five neuromuscular blocking agents. Arch Int Pharmacodyn Ther 233:82, 1978.

112. Galletly DC. Comparative cutaneous histamine release by neuromuscular blocking agents. Anaesth Intensive Care 14:365, 1986.

113. Fisher MM. Anaphylactic reactions to gallamine triethiodide. Anaesth Intensive Care 6:125, 1978.

114. Fisher MM, Hallowes RC, and Wilson RM. Anaphylaxis to alcuronium. Anaesth Intensive Care 6:125, 1978.

115. Royston D, and Wilkes RG. True anaphylaxis to suxamethonium chloride. Br J Anaesth 50:611, 1978.

116. Assem ESK, Frost PG, Levis RD. Anaphylaxtic like reaction to suxamethonium. Anaesthesia 36:405, 1981.

117. Mehr EH, Hirshman CA, Lindeman KS. Mechanism of action of atracurium on airways. Anesthesiology 76:448, 1992.

118. Flynn PJ, Frank M, Hughes R. Use of atracurium in Caesarian section. Br J Anaesth 56:599, 1984.

119. Shearer ES, Fahy LT, O'Sullivan EP, Hunter JM. Transplacental distribution of atracurium, laudanosine and monoquaternary alcohol during elective Caesarian section. Br J Anaesth 66:551, 1991.

120. Demetriou M, et al. Placental transfer of Org NC 45 in women undergoing caesarian section. Br J Anaesth 54:653, 1982.

121. Baraka A, et al. Succinylcholine-vecuronium (Org NC 45) sequence for Cesarian section. Anesth Analg 62:909, 1983.

122. Abouleish E, Wingard LB, de la Vega S, Uy N. Pancuronium in Caesarian section and its placental transfer. Br J Anaesth 52:531, 1980.

123. Evans CA, Waud DR. Do maternally administered neuromuscular blocking agents interfere with fetal neuromuscular transmission? Anesth Analg 52:548, 1973.

124. Matteo RS, Pua EK, Khambatta HJ, Spector S. Cerebrospinal fluid levels of d-tubocurarine in man. Anesthesiology 46:396, 1977.

125. Fahey MR, et al. Atracurium, vecuronium and pancuronium do not alter the minimum alveolar concentration of halothane in humans. Anesthesiology 71:53, 1989.

126. Savarese JJ. How may neuromuscular blocking drugs affect the state of general anesthesia? Anesth Analg 58:449, 1979.

127. Mori K, Iwabuchi K, Fujita M. The effects of depolarizing muscle relaxants on the electroencephalogram and the circulation during halothane anaesthesia. Br J Anaesth 45:604, 1973.

128. Lanier WL, Milde JH, Michenfelder JD. Cerebral stimulation following succinylcholine in dogs. Anesthesiology 64:551, 1986.

129. Lanier WL, Iaizzo PA, Milde JH. Cerebral afferent muscle responses to succinylcholine in dogs pretreated with pancuronium. Anesth Analg 67:S266, 1988.

130. Forbes AR, Cohen NH, Eger EI. Pancuronium reduces halothane requirement in man. Anesth Analg 58:497, 1979.

131. Duvaldestin P, Henzel D. Binding of tubocurarine, fazadinium, pancuronium and Org NC 45 to serum proteins in normal man and in patients with cirrhosis. Br J Anaesth 54:513, 1982.

132. Miller RD. Pharmacokinetics of competitive muscle relaxants. Br J Anaesth 54:161, 1982.

133. Foldes FF, Deery A. Protein binding of atracurium and other short-acting neuromuscular blocking agents and their interaction with human cholinesterases. Br J Anaesth 55:31S, 1983.

134. Pollard BJ. Neuromuscular blocking drugs and renal failure. Br J Anaesth 68:545, 1992.

135. Stevenson DE. A review of some side effects of muscle relaxants in small animals. J Small Anim Pract 1:77, 1961.

136. Gronert GA, Theye RA. Pathophysiology of hyperkalemia induced by succinylcholine. Anesthesiology 43:89, 1975.

137. Carter JG, Sokoll MD, Gergis SD. Effect of spinal cord transection on neuromuscular function in the rat. Anesthesiology 55:542, 1981.

138. Gronert GA, Theye RA. Effect of succinylcholine on skeletal muscle with immobilization atrophy. Anesthesiology 40:268, 1974.
139. Gronert GA. Disuse atrophy with resistance to pancuronium. Anesthesiology 55:547, 1981.
140. Gronert GA, White DA, Shafer SL, Matteo RS. Exercise produces sensitivity to metocurine. Anesthesiology 70:973, 1989.
141. Slater RM, McLaren ID. Effect of salbutamol and suxamethonium on the plasma potassium concentration. Br J Anaesth 59:602, 1987.
142. Martyn JAJ, et al. Up-and-down regulation of skeletal muscle acetylcholine receptors. Anesthesiology 76:822, 1992.
143. Cook JH. The effect of suxamethonium on intraocular pressure. Anaesthesia 36:359, 1981.
144. Benson GJ, Manning JP, Hartsfield SM, Thurmon JC. Intraocular tension of the horse: Effects of succinylcholine and halothane anesthesia. Am J Vet Res 42:1831, 1981.
145. Cottrell JE, Hartung J, Giffin JP, Shwiry B. Intracranial and hemodynamic changes after succinylcholine administration in cats. Anesth. Analg 62:1006, 1983.
146. Minton MD, Grosslight K, Stirt JA, Bedford RD. Increases in intracranial pressure from succinylcholine: Prevention by prior nondepolarizing blockade. Anesthesiology 65:165, 1986.
147. Thiagarajah S, et al. Effect of suxamethonium on the ICP of cats with and without thiopentone pretreatment. Br J Anaesth 60:157, 1988.
148. Magee DA, Robinson RJS. Effect of stretch exercises on suxamethonium induced fasciculations and myalgia. Br J Anaesth 59:596, 1987.
149. Raffe MR, Crimi AJ, Ruff J. Effect of diazepam pretreatment on succinylcholine induced muscle fasciculation in the dog. Am J Vet Res 43:510, 1982.
150. Benson GJ, Hartsfield SM, Manning JP, Thurmon J. C. Biochemical effects of succinylcholine chloride in mechanically ventilated horses anesthetized with halothane and oxygen. Am J Vet Res 41:754, 1980.
151. Manley SV, Kelly AB, Hodgson D. Malignant hyperthermia-like reactions in three anesthetized horses. J Am Vet Med Assoc 183:85, 1983.
152. Riedesel DH, Hildebrand SV. Unusual response following use of succinylcholine in a horse anesthetized with halothane. J Am Vet Med Assoc 187:507, 1985.
153. Hildebrand SV, Howitt GA. Succinylcholine infusion associated with hyperthermia in ponies anesthetized with halothane. Am J Vet Res 44:2280, 1983.
154. Smith SM, Brown HO, Toman JEP, Goodman LS. The lack of cerebral effects of d-tubocurarine. Anesthesiology 8:1, 1947.
155. Hildebrand SV, Arpin D. Neuromuscular and cardiovascular effects of atracurium in healthy adult horses anesthetized with halothane. Proc 2nd Int Cong Vet Anesth, Sacramento, Calif. 1985:175.
156. White DA, et al. Determination of sensitivity to metocurine in exercised horses. Am J Vet Res 53:757, 1992.
157. Kalhoro AB, Rex MAE. The dose rate of pancuronium bromide for horses. Aust Vet J 60:348, 1983.
158. Jones RS, Heckmann R, Wuersch W. Observations on the neuromuscular blocking action of alcuronium in the dog and its reversal by neostigmine. Res Vet Sci 25:101, 1978.
159. Gleed RD, Jones RS. Observations on the neuromuscular blocking action of gallamine and pancuronium and their reversal by neostigmine. Res Vet Sci 32:324, 1982.
160. Evans AT, Anderson LK, Eyster GE, Sawyer DC. Cardiovascular effects of gallamine triethiodide and succinylcholine chloride during halothane anesthesia in the dog. Am J Vet Res 38:329, 1977.
161. Jones RS, Heckmann R, Wuersch W. Observations on the duration of action of suxamethonium in the dog. Br Vet J 134:521, 1978.
162. Jones RS. Neuromuscular blocking action of vecuronium in the dog and its reversal by neostigmine. Res Vet Sci 38:193, 1985.
163. Hall LW, Clarke KW. Veterinary Anaesthesia, 9th ed. London: Balliere Tindall, 1991.
164. Lee C, Tran BK, Durant N, Nguyen B. Vecuronium, isoflurane and hypotensive anesthesia in the cat. Anesthesiology 59:A271, 1983.
165. Cass N, Brown WA, Ng KC, Lampard DG. Dosage patterns of non-depolarizing neuromuscular blockers in the sheep. Anaesth Intensive Care 8:13, 1980.
166. Lampard DG, Brown WA, Cass NM, Ng KC. Computer controlled muscle paralysis with atracurium in the sheep. Anaesth Intensive Care 14:7, 1986.
167. Lucke JN. A study of atracurium in malignant hyperthermia susceptible pigs. Proc Assoc Vet Anaesth Gr Br Ir 11:90, 1983.
168. Pittet JF, et al. Plasma concentrations of laudanosine but not atracurium are increased during the anhepatic phase of orthotopic liver transplantation in pigs. Anesthesiology 72:145, 1990.
169. Clutton RE, et al. Conditions for tracheal intubation in pigs using vecuronium compared with succinylcholine. Vet Surg 16:318, 1987.
170. Clutton RE, McGrath CJ, Richards DLS, Lee JC. The effects of vecuronium bromide on single twitch studies in malignant hyperthermia susceptible pigs. Vet Surg 15:458, 1986.
171. Richards DLS, McGrath CJ, Clutton RE, Lee JC. The response of malignant hyperthermia sensitive pigs to vecuronium. J Assoc Vet Anaesth 16:18, 1989.
172. Jones RS, Seymour CJ. Clinical observations on the use of vecuronium as a muscle relaxant in the dog. J Small Anim Pract 26:213, 1985.
173. Young SS, Barnett KC, Taylor PM. Anaesthetic regimes for cataract removal in the dog. J Small Anim Pract 32:236, 1991.
174. Jones RS, Clutton RE. Clinical observations on the use of the muscle relaxant atracurium in the dog. J Small Anim Pract 25:473, 1984.
175. Hildebrand SV, et al. Clinical use of the neuromuscular blocking agents atracurium and pancuronium for equine anesthesia. J Am Vet Med Assoc 195:212, 1989.
176. Jones RS, New muscle relaxants. Vet Annu 24:215, 1984.
177. Hildebrand SV, Hill T. Effects of atracurium administered by continuous intravenous infusion in halothane-anesthetized horses. Am J Vet Res 50:2124, 1989.
178. Jones RS, Brearley JC. Atracurium infusion in the dog. J Small Anim Pract 28:197, 1987.
179. Fisher DM, Canfell C, Miller RD. Stability of atracurium administered by infusion. Anesthesiology 61:347, 1984.
180. Ali HH, et al. Evaluation of cumulative properties of three new non-depolarizing neuromuscular blocking drugs BW A444U, atracurium and vecuronium. Br J Anaesth 55:107S, 1983.
181. Katz RL. Clinical neuromuscular pharmacology of pancuronium. Anesthesiology 34:550, 1971.
182. Hildebrand SV, Howitt GA. Dosage requirement of pancuronium in halothane-anesthetized ponies: A comparison of cumulative and single dose administration. Am J Vet Res 45:2441, 1984.
183. Basta SJ, et al. Clinical pharmacology of doxacurium chloride. Anesthesiology 69:478, 1988.
184. Jones RS. Interactions between vecuronium and suxamethonium in the dog. Res Vet Sci 41:93, 1986.
185. Jones RS. Interaction beween atracurium and suxamethonium in the dog. Res Vet Sci 40:299, 1986.
186. Jones RS. Interactions between pipecuronium and suxamethonium in the dog. Res Vet Sci 43:308, 1987.
187. Jones RS, Gleed RD. Effect of prior administration of a non-depolarising muscle relaxant on the action of suxamethonium in the dog. Res Vet Sci 36:348, 1984.
188. Jones RS, Gleed RD. Effect of prior administration of suxamethonium on non-depolarising muscle relaxants in the dog. Res Vet Sci 36:43, 1984.
189. Duvaldestin P, et al. Pancuronium pharmacokinetics in patients with liver cirrhosis. Br J Anaesth 50:1131, 1978.
190. Lebrault C, et al. Pharmacokinetics and pharmacodynamics of vecuronium (Org NC 45) in patients with cirrhosis. Anesthesiology 62:601, 1985.
191. Westra P, et al. Hepatic and renal disposition of pancuronium and gallamine in patients with extra hepatic cholestasis. Br J Anaesth 53:331, 1981.

192. Miller RD. Pharmacokinetics of atracurium and the nondepolarizing neuromuscular blocking agents in normal patients and those with renal or hepatic dysfunction. Br J Anaesth 58:11S, 1986.

193. Somogyi AA, Shanks CA, Triggs EJ. The effects of renal failure on the disposition and neuromuscular blocking action of pancuronium bromide. Eur J Clin Pharmacol 12:23, 1977.

194. Caldwell JE, et al. The influence of renal failure on the pharmacokinetics and duration of pipecuronium bromide in patients anesthetized with halothane and nitrous oxide. Anesthesiology 70:7, 1989.

195. Hunter JM, Jones RS, Utting JE. Use of atracurium in patients with no renal function. Br J Anaesth 54:1251, 1982.

196. Halsey MJ. Drug interactions in anaesthesia. Br J Anaesth 59:112, 1987.

197. Stanski DR, Ham J, Miller RD. Time dependent increase in sensitivity to d-tubocurarine during enflurane anesthesia. Anesthesiology 51:S269, 1979.

198. Ramsey FM, et al. Clinical use of atracurium during N_2O/O_2, fentanyl, and N_2O/O_2, enflurane anesthesia regimens. Anesthesiology 61:328, 1984.

199. Hilgenberg JC, Stoelting RK. Characteristics of succinylcholine produced phase II neuromuscular block during enflurane, halothane, and fentanyl anesthesia. Anesth Analg 60:192, 1981.

200. Donati F, Bevan DR. Potentiation of succinylcholine phase II block with isoflurane anesthesia. Anesthesiology 58:552, 1983.

201. Chapple DJ, Clark TS, Hughes R. Interaction between atracurium and drugs used in anaesthesia. Br J Anaesth 55:17S, 1983.

202. Gencarelli PJ, Swen J, Koot HWJ, Miller RD. The effects of hypercarbia and hypocarbia on pancuronium and vecuronium neuromuscular blockade in anesthetized humans. Anesthesiology 59:376, 1983.

203. Baraka A. The influence of carbon dioxide on the neuromuscular block caused by tubocurarine chloride in the human subject. Br J Anaesth 36:372, 1964.

204. Payne JP. The influence of carbon dioxide on the neuromuscular blocking activity of relaxant drugs in the cat. Br J Anaesth 30:206, 1958.

205. Hughes R. The influence of changes in acid-base balance on neuromuscular blockade in cats. Br J Anaesth 42:658, 1970.

206. Miller RD, Roderick LL. Diuretic induced hypokalaemia, pancuronium neuromuscular blockade and its antagonism by neostigmine. Br J Anaesth 50:541, 1978.

207. Platt M, Hayward A, Cooper A, Hirsch N. Effect of arterial carbon dioxide tension on the duration of action of atracurium. Br J Anaesth 66:45, 1991.

208. Sinatra RS, Philip BK, Naulty JS, Ostheimer GW. Prolonged neuromuscular blockade with vecuronium in a patient treated with magnesium sulfate. Anesth Analg 64:1220, 1985.

209. Waud BE, Waud DR. Interaction of calcium and potassium with neuromuscular blocking agents. Br J Anaesth 52:863, 1980.

210. Flynn PJ, Hughes R, Walton B. Use of atracurium in cardiac surgery involving cardiopulmonary bypass with induced hypothermia. Br J Anaesth 56:967, 1984.

211. Buzello W, Schluermann D, Schindler M, Spillner G. Hypothermic cardiopulmonary bypass and neuromuscular blockade by pancuronium and vecuronium. Anesthesiology 62:201, 1985.

212. Horrow JC, Bartkowski RR. Pancuronium, unlike other nondepolarizing relaxants, retains potency at hypothermia. Anesthesiology 58:357, 1983.

213. Goudsouzian NG. Maturation of neuromuscular transmission in the infant. Br J Anaesth 52:205, 1980.

214. Goudsouzian NG, Standaert FG. The infant and the myoneural junction. Anesth Analg 65:1208, 1986.

215. Cook DR. Muscle relaxants in infants and children. Anesth Analg 60:335, 1981.

216. Bush GH, Vivori E. Neonates. In: General Anaesthesia, 5th ed. Edited by JF Nunn, JE Utting, and BR Brown. London: Butterworth, 1989.

217. Matteo RS, et al. Distribution, elimination, and action of d-tubocurarine in neonates, infants, children, and adults. Anesthesiology 63:799, 1984.

218. Brandom BW, et al. Clinical pharmacology of atracurium in infants. Anesthesiology 59:A440, 1983.

219. Bennett EJ, Ramamurthy S, Dalal FY, Salem MR. Pancuronium and the neonate. Br J Anaesth 47:75, 1975.

220. D'Hollander AA, Luyckx C, Barvis L, De Ville A. Clinical evaluation of atracurium besylate requirement for a stable muscle relaxation during surgery: Lack of age-related effects. Anesthesiology 59:237, 1983.

221. O'Hara DA, Fragen RJ, Shank CA. The effect of age on the dose-response curves for vecuronium in adults. Anesthesiology 63:542, 1985.

222. Azar I. The response of patients with neuromuscular disorders to muscle relaxants: A review. Anesthesiology 61:173, 1984.

223. Hunter JM. Anaesthesia for patients with neuromuscular disorders. In: General Anaesthesia, 5th ed. Edited by JF Nunn, JE Utting, and BR Brown. London: Butterworth, 1989.

224. Fikes LL, Dodman NH, Court MH. Anaesthesia for small animal patients with neuromuscular disease. Br Vet J 146:487, 1990.

225. Jones RS, Sharp NJH. Use of the muscle relaxant atracurium in a myasthenic dog. Vet Rec 117:500, 1985.

226. Jones RS, Brown A, Watkins PE. Use of the muscle relaxant vecuronium in a myasthenic dog. Vet Rec 122:611, 1988.

227. Sufit RL, et al. Doxacurium and mivacurium do not trigger malignant hyperthermia in susceptible swine. Anesth Analg 71:285, 1990.

228. Singh YN, Marshall IG, Harvey AL. Some effects of the aminoglycoside antibiotic amikacin on neuromuscular and autonomic transmission. Br J Anaesth 50:109, 1978.

229. Singh YN, Marshall IG, Harvey AL. Depression of transmitter release and postjunctional sensitivety during neuromuscular block produced by antibiotics. Br J Anaesth 51:1027, 1979.

230. Singh YN, Marshall IG, Harvey AL. Pre- and postjunctional blocking effects of aminoglycoside, polymyxin, tetracycline and lincosamide antibiotics. Br J Anaesth 54:1295, 1982.

231. Sokoll MD, Gergis SD. Antibiotics and neuromuscular function. Anesthesiology 55:148, 1981.

232. Lippmann M, Yang E, Au E, Lee C. Neuromuscular blocking effects of tobramycin, gentamycin, and cefazolin. Anesth Analg 61:767, 1982.

233. Potter JM, Edeson RO, Campbell RJ, Forbes AM. Potentiation by gentamycin of non-depolarizing neuromuscular block in the cat. Anaesth Intensive Care, 8:20, 1980.

234. Mathew BP, Teske RH, Robinson JA, Adams HR. Neuromuscular blocking effects of certain antibacterial agents in pigs and lambs. J Vet Pharmacol Ther 1:171, 1978.

235. Ornstein E, Matteo RS, Young WL, Diaz J. Resistance to metocurine-induced neuromuscular blockade in patients receiving phenytoin. Anesthesiology 63:294, 1985.

236. Ornstein E, et al. The effect of phenytoin on the magnitude and duration of neuromuscular block following atracurium or vecuronium. Anesthesiology 67:191, 1987.

237. Waud BE, Waud DR. Interaction among agents that block endplate depolarization competitively. Anesthesiology 63:4, 1985.

238. Ali HH. Neuromuscular block and its antagonism: Clinical aspects. In: General Anaesthesia, 5th ed. Edited by JF Nunn, JE Utting, and BR Brown. London: Butterworth, 1989.

239. Cronnelly R, Morris RB, Miller RD. Edrophonium: Duration of action and atropine requirement in humans during halothane anesthesia. Anesthesiology 57:261, 1982.

240. Baird WLM, Bowman WC, Kerr WJ. Some actions of Org NC 45 and of edrophonium in the anaesthetized cat and in man. Br J Anaesth 54:375, 1982.

241. Morris RB, et al. Pharmacokinetics of edrophonium and neostigmine when antagonising d-tubocurarine neuromuscular blockade in man. Anesthesiology 54:399, 1981.

242. Ferguson A, Egerszegi P, Bevan DR. Neostigmine, pyridostigmine and edrophonium as antagonists of pancuronium. Anesthesiology 53:390, 1980.

243. Katz RL. Pyridostigmin (Mestinon) as and antagonism of d-tubocurarine. Anesthesiology 28:528, 1967.

244. Bevan DR. Reversal of pancuronium with edrophonium. Anaesthesia 34:614, 1979.

245. Klein LV. Neuromuscular blocking agents. In: Principles and Practice of Veterinary Anesthesia. Edited by CE Short. Baltimore: Williams & Wilkins, 1987.
246. Klein L, Nann L, Brophy MA. Potency and duration of atracurium in anesthetized horses. In: Advances in Veterinary Anaesthesia. Edited by LK Cullen. St. Lucia, Australia: University of Queensland Press, 1988.
247. Hildebrand SV, Howitt GA. Antagonism of pancuronium neuromuscular blockade in halothane-anesthetized ponies using neostigmine and edrophonium. Am J Vet Res 45:2276, 1984.
248. Ducharme NA, Fubini SL. Gastrointestinal complications associated with use of atropine in horses. J Am Vet Med Assoc 182:229, 1983.
249. Jones RS. Reversal of atracurium neuromuscular block with neostigmine in the dog. Res Vet Sci 48:96, 1990.
250. Cass N, Brown WA, Ng KC, Lampard DG. Reversal of nondepolarizing block by neostigmine. Anaesth Intensive Care 8:16, 1980.
251. Hall LW, Kellagher REB, Watkins SB. Respiratory problems after atropine and neostigmine in dogs. Br J Anaesth 57:1046, 1985.
252. Lee C. Train-of-four fade and edrophonium antagonism of neuromuscular block by succinylcholine in man. Anesth Analg 55:663, 1976.
253. Cullen LK, Jones RS. The effect of neostigmine on suxamethonium induced neuromuscular block in the dog. Res Vet Sci 29:266, 1980.
254. Booij LH, van der Pol F, Crul JF, Miller RD. Antagonism of Org NC 45 neuromuscular blockade by neostigmine, pyridostigmine and 4-aminopyridine. Anesth Analg 59:31, 1980.
255. Roberts D. The role of glyceryl guaiacolate in a balanced equine anesthetic. Vet Med Small Anim Clin 63:157, 1968.
256. Grandy JL, McDonell WN. Evaluation of concentrated solutions of guaifenesin for equine anesthesia. J Am Vet Med Assoc 176:619, 1980.
257. Tavernor WD. The influence of guaiacol glycerol ether on cardiovascular and respiratory function in the horse. Res Vet Sci 11:91, 1970.
258. Gertsen KE, Tillotson PJ. Clinical use of glyceryl guaiacolate in the horse. Vet Med Small Anim Clin 63:1062, 1968.
259. Heath RB. Personal communication. Colorado State University, Fort Collins, Colorado, 1970.
260. Hubbell JAE, Muir WW, Sams RA. Guaifenesin: Cardiopulmonary effects and plasma concentrations in horses. Am J Vet Res 41:1751, 1980.
261. Davis LE, Wolff WA. Pharmacokinetics and Metabolism of Glyceryl Guaiacolate in Ponies. Am J Vet Res 31:469, 1970.
262. Tavernor WD, Jones EW. Observations on the cardiovascular and respiratory effects of guaiacol glycerol ether in conscious and anaesthetized dogs. J Small Anim Pract 11:177, 1970.
263. Benson GJ, Thurmon JC, Tranquilli WJ, Smith CW. Cardiopulmonary effects of an intravenous infusion of guaifenesin, ketamine, and xylazine in dogs. Am J Vet Res 46:1896, 1985.

ANESTHETIC EQUIPMENT AND MONITORING

chapter 14

ANESTHETIC MACHINES AND BREATHING SYSTEMS

Sandee M. Hartsfield

Introduction

The halogenated hydrocarbon anesthetics are liquids that must be vaporized for administration (Chapter 11). These volatile drugs are potent and should be delivered with accuracy. Nitrous oxide is a gas anesthetic, normally used in high concentrations. It should be administered with enough oxygen to assure an adequate inspired concentration of O_2 (F_IO_2). Using contemporary methods, anesthesia machines and breathing systems are required for administration of inhalant anesthetics. Standards for performance and safety of anesthesia machines designed for human use have been published.(1-4) New veterinary anesthesia machines meet some of these standards, but are not required to fully comply with the American Society for Testing and Materials (ASTM) guidelines.

Anesthesia Machines

Anesthesia machines have certain basic components, and are compatible with various breathing systems. An anesthesia machine prepares a precise but variable gas mixture (O_2 and anesthetic) for delivery to a breathing system.(2) The breathing system supplies oxygen and anesthetic to the patient, eliminates CO_2 from exhaled gases, and provides a means for controlled ventilation. Sources for medical gases (e.g., cylinders for O_2 and N_2O), a regulator and a flowmeter for each gas, and a vaporizer for each volatile anesthetic are fundamental to the operation of an anesthesia machine.(5)

Pressures of gases vary at different locations in an anesthesia machine (2, 3), and knowledge of these pressures facilitates the evaluation and safe operation of an anesthesia machine. There are low-, intermediate-, and high-pressure areas. The high-pressure area accepts gases at cylinder pressure and reduces and regulates the pressure; this area includes gas cylinders, hanger yokes, yoke blocks, high-pressure hoses, pres-

sure gauges, and regulators, and the pressure may be as high as 2200 pounds per square inch (psi). The intermediate pressure area accepts gases from the central pipeline or from the regulators on the anesthesia machine and conducts them to the flush valve and flowmeters; this area includes pipeline inlets, power outlets for ventilators, conduits from pipeline inlets to flowmeters, and conduits from regulators to flowmeters, the flowmeter assembly, and the O_2 flush appara-

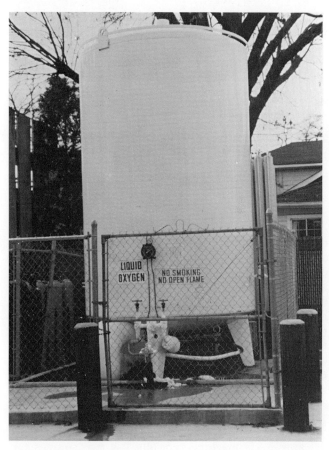

Fig. 14–2. An outside bulk container for liquid oxygen supplying the central medical gas pipeline system of a large human hospital.

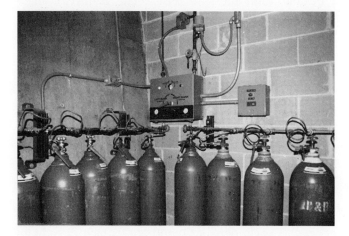

Fig. 14–1. Primary and reserve banks of large oxygen cylinders supplying the central medical gas pipeline system at a veterinary teaching hospital. The primary bank supplies oxygen to the pipeline system until the cylinders are depleted, at which time the system is automatically switched to the reserve bank.

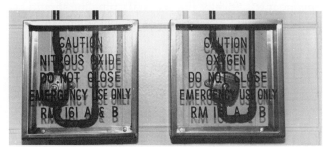

Fig. 14–3. A set of emergency shutoff valves for oxygen and nitrous oxide in a central pipeline system for medical gases in a veterinary teaching hospital. These valves should be placed strategically throughout the gas distribution system to control the flow of gases during emergencies or maintenance.

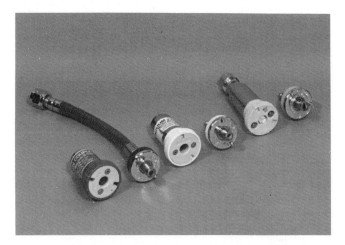

Fig. 14–4. A set of proprietary (Ohio or Ohmeda, Madison, Wisconsin) quick connects (quick couplers) for oxygen (male and female on the left), vacuum (male and female in the center), and air (male and female on the right). The female connectors are usually present at the site of use (station outlet) for attachment to the male counterparts from the anesthesia machine or other equipment via high-pressure flexible hose. Inadvertent interchange of the gases is prevented by variations in the spacing of corresponding components of the couplers.

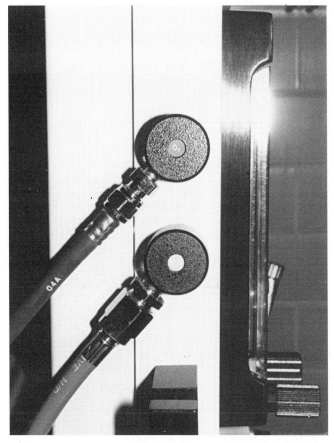

Fig. 14–5. Pipeline inlets for oxygen (upper connector labeled as O_2) and nitrous oxide (lower, larger connector) on a Drager anesthesia machine (North American Drager, Telford, Pennsylvania). The female DISS connectors from the high-pressure hoses couple to the male DISS pipeline inlets on the anesthesia machine.

tus. The pressure usually ranges from 37 to 50 psi, although it may be lower on newer anesthesia machines. The low-pressure area consists of the conduits and components between the flowmeter and the common gas outlet; this area includes vaporizers located outside the breathing system, piping from the flowmeters to the vaporizer, conduit from the vaporizer to the common gas outlet, and conduit from the common gas outlet to the breathing system, and the pressure is only slightly above ambient. Pressures in the breathing system itself vary, but usually range from 0 to 30 cm of H_2O when used with normal, healthy patients.

Medical Gases

An anesthesia machine typically has two sources for each medical gas. First, small compressed-gas cylinders attach to the machine at the hanger yokes, and second, the hospital's central gas supply enters the machine at pipeline inlets. Ideally, the hospital's pipeline should be the primary source of medical gases, and small cylinders should be reserved for emergencies or transport.(6) Generally, bulk sources of medical gases are more economic than small cylinders.

The pipeline source for N_2O originates from a bank of large (G or H) compressed gas cylinders, and O_2 may be supplied similarly (Fig. 14–1). Alternately, the central source of O_2 may emanate from a bulk tank of liquid O_2 (Fig. 14–2) or possibly from an O_2-concentrating system. The latter will not reliably deliver 100% O_2. Pipeline systems (Fig. 14–3) convey gases from the central source to terminal units (station outlets) throughout the hospital. A noninterchangeable gas-specific connector at the station outlet accepts only its corresponding connector, which attaches to

the pipeline inlet of an anesthetic machine through a flexible, high pressure hose. "The connector may be a threaded Diameter Index Safety System (DISS) or a proprietary (manufacturer-specific) non-threaded, noninterchangeable quick connector" (Fig. 14–4).(3) The high-pressure hose connects to the anesthesia machine at a pipeline inlet, which is usually a DISS male connector (Fig. 14–5).

Gases move to and from a cylinder through a brass valve (Fig. 14–6). The valve stem controls flow, and a safety relief device (e.g., a fusible plug with a low melting point) allows emergency escape of gas to prevent bursting of a cylinder during exposure to high temperatures.(2) The threaded outlets of the valve bodies on large cylinders (G and H) are designed to prevent the accidental interchange of O_2, N_2O, and other gases at regulators or manifolds. The valve bodies of small (E) cylinders of O_2 and N_2O attach directly to anesthesia machines at the hanger yokes, and they utilize the Pin Index Safety System (Fig. 14–7) to prevent interchange of O_2 and N_2O. Two pin holes and a port in the valve body correspond to two pins and a nipple on the hanger yoke. Specific spacing of the pins for each medical gas precludes the interchange of gases under ordinary conditions (Fig. 14–8).

Although the pin-index system is effective, the system can be defeated.(2) The pins can be removed (Fig. 14–9), bent, broken, or forced deeper into the yoke. The nipple can be stacked with enough washers to allow attachment of the wrong cylinder. Yoke blocks coupled to high pressure hoses will accommodate alternate gas sources. Some of the older yoke blocks do not have pin holes, and some short blocks can be attached upside down (Fig. 14–9), allowing connection of the wrong gas. Older anesthesia machines should be inspected to assure the integrity of the pin-index system for oxygen

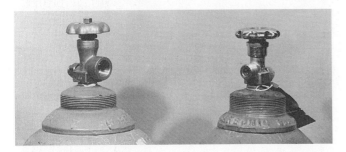

Fig. 14–6. Brass valves on large gas cylinders. The valve outlets on these two cylinders are designed to prevent the inadvertent interchange of gases. The valve on the right has external threads, while the one on the left has internal threads. The valve outlet for a large cylinder is distinguished by diameter, number of threads per inch, and type of threads (right-hand or left-hand and internal or external).

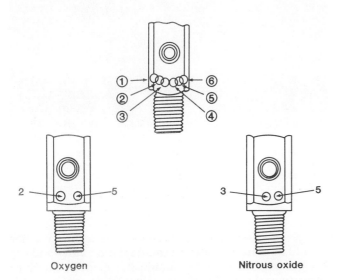

Fig. 14–7. Diagram of the Pin Index Safety System. The spacing between the valve outlet and the pin holes in the valve bodies for oxygen and nitrous oxide cylinders are illustrated. The pin holes and outlets correspond to the nipple and pins of hanger yokes on anesthesia machines and function to prevent inadvertent interchange of medical gases. Pin holes 2 and 5 are used for oxygen, and pin holes 3 and 5 are used for nitrous oxide.(2) (From Hartsfield, S.M. Machines and Breathing Systems for Administration of Inhalation Anesthetics. In: Principles and Practice of Veterinary Anesthesia. Edited by C.E. Short. Baltimore: Williams & Wilkins, 1987)

and nitrous oxide. Small cylinders should be aligned correctly to the hanger yoke to prevent the creation of a potential hazard. Directing the retaining screw into the safety relief device instead of the conical depression has caused rapid decompression of a cylinder (Fig. 14–10).(7, 8) If an anesthesia machine has multiple hanger yokes, each yoke should be fitted with a cylinder or a yoke plug (Fig. 14–11) when the machine is in operation.

An O_2 cylinder's service pressure is about 2200 psi. An E cylinder contains about 700 L of gaseous O_2 and an H cylinder about 7000 L (Table 14–1). The pressure is proportional to the contents, and an E cylinder with a pressure of 1100 psi contains about 350 L of O_2. The pressure in a full N_2O cylinder is about 750 psi at normal room temperature, with N_2O in both liquid and gaseous phases (Chapter 11). The vapor pressure of N_2O varies with temperature and determines the pressure in the cylinder. In a full cylinder, 95% of the volume is liquid (9), an E cylinder containing about 1600 L of gaseous N_2O and an H cylinder about 16,000 L (Table 14–1). As liquid N_2O vaporizes, the cylinder cools, and frosting may occur. The content of a N_2O cylinder is not directly proportional to the pressure. As pressure starts to decrease after all liquid N_2O has vaporized, about 25% of the original contents remains. The remaining gas will then be depleted based on rate of flow.(10) Although the amount of N_2O is not directly related to pressure, the content of any cylinder can be determined by weight regardless of the state of the material in the cylinder.(3)

In the United States, the Department of Transportation (DOT) controls the construction and testing of gas cylinders. The service pressure, defined as the maximum filling pressure at 70° F (2), is typically 1900 to 2200

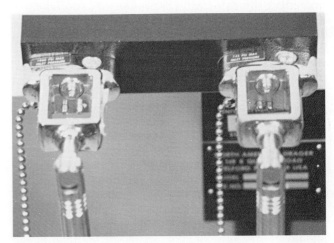

Fig. 14–8. Comparison of the yokes for small cylinders of oxygen (left) and nitrous oxide (right). The relationship of the pins and the nipple on each yoke show how the inadvertent interchange of oxygen and nitrous oxide is prevented. (From Hartsfield, S.M. Machines and Breathing Systems for Administration of Inhalation Anesthetics. In: Principles and Practice of Veterinary Anesthesia. Edited by C.E. Short. Baltimore: Williams and Wilkins, 1987) .

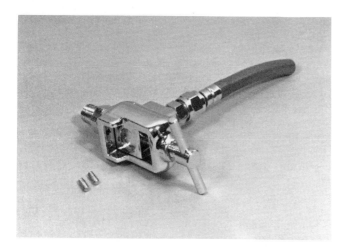

Fig. 14–9. An oxygen yoke illustrating ways in which the pin-index system for small gas cylinders can be defeated. The pins have been removed, and a short yoke block has been inserted upside down. Both will defeat the effectiveness of the pin-index system and allow connection to an inappropriate cylinder.

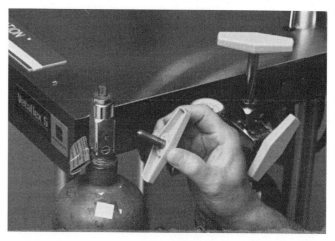

Fig. 14–10. The retaining screw of the yoke and a small (E) cylinder of oxygen next to a Vetaflex 5 Veterinary Anesthesia Machine (Pitman-Moore, Washington Crossing, New Jersey). The retaining screw has been removed from the yoke to illustrate the pointed shape, which is intended to correspond to the conical depression of the cylinder valve and to secure the cylinder in the yoke. If the cylinder is positioned incorrectly in the yoke and the retaining screw is tightened into the fusible plug (round, slotted device below the conical depression), rapid decompression of the cylinder may occur.

psi for O_2. Cylinders are designated alphabetically, size A being the smallest. Sizes E, G, and H are common for medical O_2 and N_2O (Table 14–1). Permanent markings near the top of the cylinder indicate the DOT specification number, the type of material used in construction (e.g., steel or aluminum), service pressure in pounds per square inch, serial number, identification of the manufacturer, and testing dates. A five-point star after the last testing date qualifies the cylinder to be retested after 10 years.(3)

A color-coded (green for O_2 and blue for N_2O) label on the wall of the cylinder indicates the gas contents, warns of potential hazards (e.g., oxidizing agent), and names the manufacturer or distributor (Fig. 14–12). A signal word appears on the label; *danger* means an immediate threat to health or property if gas is released, *warning* indicates a less than immediate threat, and *caution* means no immediate hazard to health or property. A diamond-shaped area on the label indicates the hazard class of the gas by words (oxidizer, nonflammable, or flammable) and color code (yellow, green, and red, respectively).(3) Distributors often attach a color-coded tag to the valve body, identifying a cylinder's contents. Tags incorporate sequential perforated tabs imprinted with the terms *full*, *in use*, and *empty* to track the use of the cylinder.

Extensive descriptions of the appropriate handling, storage, and use of compressed gas cylinders have been published.(2, 3, 4, 8, 11) Briefly, cylinders should not be stored near flammable materials and should be properly secured at all times, even during transport. Cylinders should be stored in "a cool, dry, clean, well-ventilated room that is constructed of fire-resistant materials." (3) Before using a cylinder, the contents should be clearly identified from the label. The valve port should be pointed away from the operator, opened briefly to clear possible debris, and then closed before connection to a

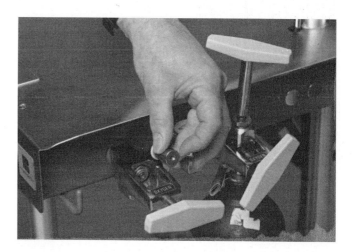

Fig. 14–11. Preparation for inserting a yoke plug into a yoke intended for a small (E) cylinder prior to use of the anesthesia machine. Since only one cylinder is present, the open yoke should be blocked with a yoke plug to prevent gas leaks, even if a check valve is present immediately upstream from the cylinder.

hanger yoke, regulator, or manifold. A sealing washer should be placed between a small cylinder valve and the hanger yoke. The valve should be opened slowly to pressurize the regulator and then fully opened.(2, 3) Defective cylinders should not be used.

Pressure Gauges

Each compressed gas supplied to an anesthesia machine should have a corresponding pressure gauge (Fig. 14–13) (1-3) that is attached to the regulators for large cylinders and to manifolds for banks of cylinders. The

Table 14–1. Characteristics of Medical Gas Cylinders (3)

Size	Gas	Gas Symbol	Color Code (U.S.)	Capacity and Pressure (at 70° F)	Empty Cylinder Weight
E	Oxygen	O_2	Green	660 L 1900 psi	14 lb
E	Nitrous Oxide	N_2O	Blue	1590 L 745 psi	14 lb
G	Nitrous Oxide	N_2O	Blue	13,800 L 745 psi	97 lb
H	Oxygen	O_2	Green	6900 L 2200 psi	119 lb
H	Nitrous Oxide	N_2O	Blue	15,800 L 745 psi	119 lb

psi, pounds per square inch

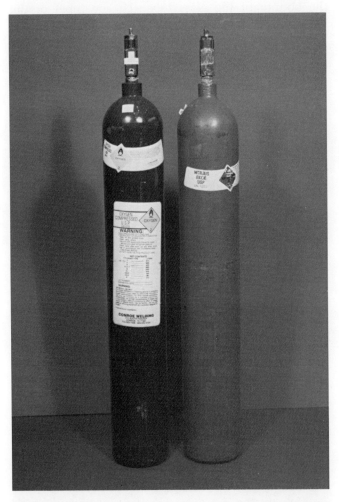

Fig. 14–12. Small (E) cylinders of oxygen and nitrous oxide, with labels and warnings. The diamond-shaped figure on each cylinder's label is indicative of the hazard class of the contents (yellow for oxygen, an oxidizer; green for nitrous oxide, a nonflammable gas).

gauge indicates pressure on the cylinder side of the regulator. Gauges are identified by the gas's chemical symbol or name, and are usually color-coded. The scale is graduated to indicate the units of measure in kilopascals (kPa) and pounds per square inch (1); Bourdon tube–type gauges are typical for anesthesia machines.(12) Earlier standards for anesthesia machines required that the gauge's full-scale reading should be at least one third greater than the maximum cylinder pressure, and that on a given anesthesia machine, all gauges should displace a similar arc from the lowest to highest readings.(2) Pressure gauges are also incorporated into pipeline distribution systems at various locations. In addition, pressure gauges may be used on anesthesia machines to report pipeline pressure.(1, 3) Pressure gauges do not accurately report the quantitative contents of a cylinder containing liquified gas.(1)

Regulators

An anesthesia machine should have a regulator for each medical gas supplied to the machine (Fig. 14–14).(1) The pressure in a gas cylinder varies with its content and temperature, and the pressure in a full cylinder is relatively high (e.g., 2000 psi in an O_2 cylinder). A regulator reduces the high and variable storage pressure to a lower and more constant pressure that is appropriate for the anesthesia machine.(6) By reducing and controlling pressure as gas exits a cylinder, a regulator maintains constant flow to the flowmeter, even though the pressure in the cylinder decreases as the contents are depleted.

Although regulators on newer anesthesia machines designed for human beings may be quite sophisticated, a simple regulator has a high-pressure chamber separated by a valve port from a low-pressure chamber (Fig. 14–15).(12) Movement of a flexible diaphragm opens or closes the valve, regulating a variable opening, and consequently, the pressure in the low-pressure chamber. Increasing pressure on the low pressure side tends to close the valve. The amount of pressure required to close the valve depends on a spring opposite the diaphragm. The exact construction varies in regulators, but function is consistent. Regulators are designed for safety relief, at two to four times the pressure in the low-pressure chamber, protecting equipment and personnel.(3, 12)

Regulators produce a safe operating pressure, prevent flowmeter fluctuations as cylinders empty, and decrease the sensitivity of the flowmeter's indicator to slight movements of the control knob. The ASTM standard requires that regulators on anesthesia machines be set so that the pipeline gases are used preferentially.(1) Therefore, regulators may be set at about 45 psi (if a power outlet is present for a ventilator) or at 37 to 42 psi (without a power outlet), since pipeline pressure is usually 50 psi. Older anesthesia machines may have regulators set at 50 psi, and open E cylinders on the machine may flow instead of pipeline gases if no check valve is present, possibly depleting gases from the cylinder that should be saved for emergency situations (e.g., pipeline failure). Contemporary anesthesia machines designed for human beings have additional regulators (second-stage) that deliver gases to the flowmeters at much lower pressures (e.g., 12–16 psi) to increase the constancy of the flowmeter.(3, 6)

Flowmeters

Flowmeters for medical gases are positioned downstream from the regulators for their corresponding gases and the portion of the flowmeter that is downstream from the flow control valve is part of the low-pressure system of an anesthesia machine. A flowmeter measures and indicates the rate of flow of gas (3), and allows precise control of O_2 or N_2O delivery to an out-of-system vaporizer and to the common gas outlet.

Gas moves through the flow-control valve to enter the bottom of the glass tube (Thorpe tube) of the flowmeter assembly. The gas then courses around a moveable indicator (float) in the annular space between the float and the wall of the tube, and exits at the top of the tube (Fig. 14–16). The tube is larger at the top than at the bottom, and a greater volume of gas moves around the indicator as it rises.(2) The scale associated with the tube indicates rate of gas flow in mL/min or in L/min. Some flowmeters, especially those on older anesthesia machines, have double tapers (Fig. 14–16). A slight taper in the lower part of the tube promotes accuracy at low flows (mL/min), and a greater taper at the top allows higher flow rates (L/min). The current machine standard requires that the scale be on the glass tube itself or be located to the right of the tube (viewed from the front of the anesthesia machine).(1) The scale may be on the left in older anesthesia machines, and the operator should assure the proper adjustment of flowmeter control knobs when older equipment is used.(3)

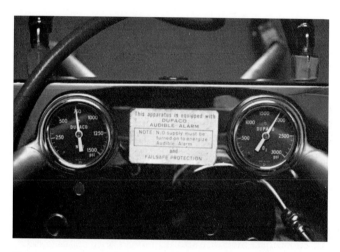

Fig. 14–13. Pressure gauges for oxygen (1900 psi) and nitrous oxide (750 psi) on a veterinary anesthesia machine.

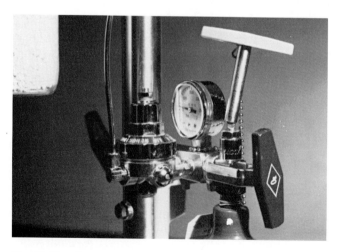

Fig. 14–14. Pressure regulator on a Pitman-Moore 970 Veterinary Anesthesia Machine (Pitman-Moore, Washington Crossing, New Jersey). The triangular-shaped regulator for oxygen is shown in-line between the yoke for the oxygen cylinder and the small-diameter oxygen line to the flowmeter. The pressure gauge indicates the pressure in the cylinder, and the pressure downstream from the regulator is reduced to 50 psi by the regulator.

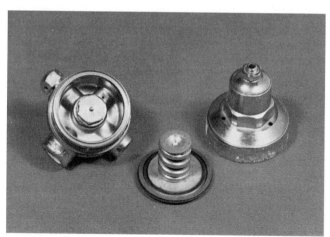

Fig. 14–15. A simple pressure regulator for oxygen that has been separated into its component parts. The body of the regulator with the entry port for high-pressure gas at 7 o'clock (left), the diaphragm and spring (center), and the cover (right) with holes for pressure relief through the diaphragm and the adjusting screw are shown.

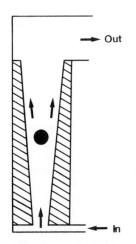
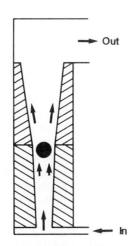

Single taper flowmeter   Double taper flowmeter

Fig. 14–16. Flowmeter diagram illustrating gas flow from bottom to top through flowmeters with single and double tapers. As the indicator (black dot) rises, flow increases because orifice size increases. The double taper tube allows increased accuracy at the lower end of the tube while metering high flows at the top. (From Hartsfield, S.M. Machines and Breathing Systems for Administration of Inhalation Anesthetics. In: Principles and Practice of Veterinary Anesthesia. Edited by C.E. Short. Baltimore: Williams and Wilkins, 1987.)

Flowmeters are calibrated at 760 mm Hg and 20° C, and accuracy may change under other conditions.(3) Generally, the effects of temperature on flowmeter function are minimal, but changes in barometric pressure may be significant, producing a higher flow than indicated at lower barometric pressure (altitude) and a lower flow at higher pressure (i.e., in a hyperbaric chamber).(3) Since a flowmeter (tube, indicator, scale) is calibrated as a unit, parts from different flowmeters should not be interchanged. If a flowmeter fails, the glass tube, indicator, and scale should be replaced as a unit. The lowest mark on the scale is the first accurate setting, and extrapolation to lower flow rates is not reliable.(2) A flowmeter's indicator should be read at the top (Fig. 14–17), except for a ball-type float, which is read at the center (Fig. 14–18). Recent standards require the point of reference for reading the indicator be shown on the flowmeter assembly.(1) Flowmeters should be used in the position for which originally designed (e.g., vertical on most newer machines or slanted in some older machines).

The flow-control knob for oxygen on contemporary anesthesia machines should be as large or larger than other flow control knobs, it should have a fluted profile (Figs. 14–17 and 14–18) as dictated by the ASTM standard, and it should project beyond the control knobs for other gases.(1) This allows the operator to "feel" which gas is being adjusted ("touch-coded").(2) A control knob is labeled with the gas symbol and is color-coded (Figs. 14–17 and 14–18). Good flow controls have fine threads for accuracy and stops to prevent overtightening and damage to flow control valves.

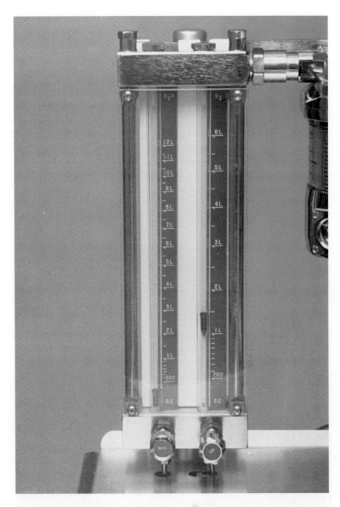

Fig. 14–17. Oxygen and nitrous oxide flowmeters on a Vetaflex 5 Veterinary Anesthesia Machine. The oxygen flowmeter is located to the right in the cluster, and the indicator should be read at the top (1.5 L/min). The indicator is relatively long compared to the calibrations on the scale. Erroneously reading the bottom of the indicator would result in a flow of oxygen that was 600 mL/min lower than intended. The O_2 flow-control knob is fluted and color coded.

The size of the flowmeter's indicator in relation to the scale influences accuracy. Floats may be more than one centimeter long, and reading the scale at the wrong location may affect the flow rate significantly (Fig. 14–17). Errors in reading the flowmeters for flowmeter-controlled vaporizers such as Copper Kettles and Verni-Trols may dangerously alter the inspired concentration of anesthetic. Dirt, static electricity, or a damaged float may impair movement and cause erroneous readings. The indicator should move freely in the glass tube, and a sluggish or sticking float indicates a need for cleaning or replacement. A sticking float, indicating O_2 flow when the O_2 cylinder was empty, has been reported as a cause of hypoxia.(2, 13) Flowmeters should be "off" when not in use to prevent the sudden application of pressure to the glass tube and indicator when a cylinder valve is opened. Sudden high pressure may force the indicator upward, damaging the indicator or the stop. The indicator may jam at the top of the tube, where it may go unnoticed.(2)

The standard for modern anesthesia machines requires the presence of only one flow adjustment control for each gas delivered to the common gas outlet.(1) Ideally, when there are two flowmeters for one gas, they should be connected in series and controlled by a single flow-control knob.(3) Some newer veterinary anesthesia machines (Fig. 14–19) and older human and veterinary machines may have multiple flow controls for multiple flowmeters with different scales in a parallel arrangement, and the operator should assure proper settings with both control knobs. Similarly, the sequence of flowmeters is important with multiple gases on a single anesthesia machine. The machine standard requires that O_2 be delivered downstream of other gases when all gases utilize a common manifold.(1) If O_2 enters the manifold upstream from the other gases, the possibility exists for delivering hypoxic mixtures, and

this complication has been reported several times.(2) The U.S. and Canadian standard locates the O_2 flowmeter to the right in a cluster of flowmeters as viewed from the front of the anesthesia machine. If a flowmeter for a vaporizer is required, it should be to the right of the cluster, at least 10 cm from the O_2 flowmeter (2), although flowmeter-controlled vaporizers are no longer covered in the ASTM standard.(1) For flowmeter-controlled vaporizers, this arrangement standardizes the location of control knobs and decreases the likelihood of adjusting the incorrect flowmeter. Standardization of location of the flowmeters for O_2 and for vaporizers and requiring "touch-coded" flow-control knobs for O_2 flowmeters were intended to reduce errors in adjusting O_2 flow rates. Locating the O_2 flowmeter to the right in a cluster of flowmeters is a fairly recent North American standard, and the location may vary on older machines and in machines manufactured in other countries.(3) Other arrangements of flowmeters may exist in older anesthesia machines (e.g., O_2 flowmeter located to the left, to the right, or in the center in a cluster), and the danger of delivering hypoxic mixtures by adjusting the wrong control knob should be considered when using both N_2O and O_2.

The arrangement of flowmeters on older models of Drager anesthesia machines allowed delivery of hypoxic mixtures if both O_2 and N_2O were used and a leak developed at the base of the O_2 flowmeter (Fig. 14–20). This malfunction resulted in the death of a horse.(14)

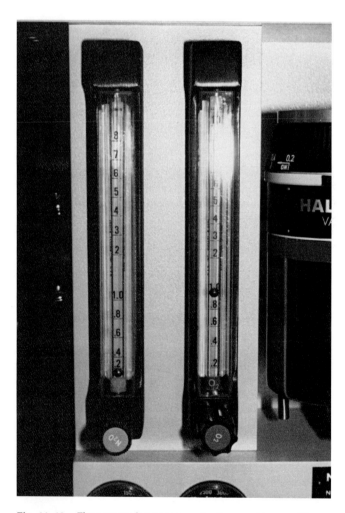

Fig. 14–18. Flowmeters for oxygen and nitrous oxide on a Drager anesthesia machine (North American Drager, Telford, Pennsylvania). The oxygen flowmeter is located to the right of the nitrous oxide flowmeter, and the ball-type indicator should be read in the center (1 L/min). The flow-control knob for oxygen is fluted in design, is color coded, and is larger than the flowmeter for nitrous oxide.

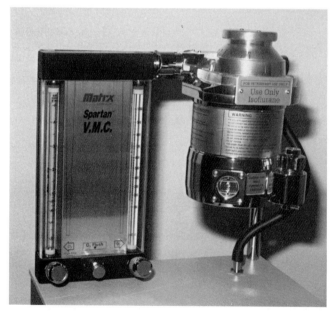

Fig. 14–19. Double oxygen flowmeters on a Matrx Spartan V.M.C. Veterinary Anesthesia Machine (Matrx, Orchard Park, New York). One flowmeter (left) is graduated from 0 to 1000 mL/min, and the other is graduated from 0.2 to 4 L/min. The intent is to increase accuracy at low flows, but two flow-control knobs in parallel offer an opportunity for setting an incorrect flow of oxygen. With two flowmeters in parallel, the total flow is the sum of the flows from each flowmeter.

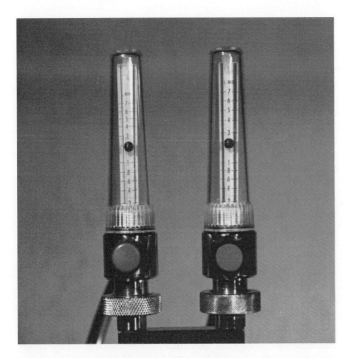

Fig. 14–20. Flowmeters for oxygen and nitrous oxide on a Drager Narkovet Stand Model Anesthesia Machine (North American Drager, Telford, Pennsylvania) for small animals. A leak at the seal created by the nut below the flowmeter could result in delivery of an inadequate amount or a hypoxic concentration of oxygen to the breathing system.

Similarly, cyanosis and light anesthesia occurred shortly after intubation and attachment of a dog to an anesthesia machine; (15) evaluation of the oxygen flowmeter revealed a leak at its base caused by a faulty seal with a folded washer. Because of this flowmeter's design, the indicator showed a correctly adjusted flow rate for O_2, although total gas flow to the vaporizer and breathing system was very low. Leaks associated with the flowmeter can occur at several locations, including cracks in the glass tube as well as problems with O-rings and gaskets.(6) Leaks in the flowmeter should be detected by leak tests performed on the low-pressure area of an anesthesia machine.(16)

Flowmeters should be adjusted to assure an adequate total volume and an appropriate concentration of each medical gas. Flow rates should meet or exceed the patient's oxygen consumption and deliver an adequate inspired oxygen concentration (usually an $F_IO_2 \geq 0.3$). Delivery of an appropriate concentration of O_2 as well as an adequate quantity of O_2 is essential for saturating hemoglobin and for supplying the patient's metabolic needs (Chapters 5 and 6). Accuracy becomes especially important with the administration of nitrous oxide and with closed and low-flow breathing systems. The accuracy of flowmeters significantly decreases with flows lower than 1 L/min.(2) With low-flow systems, scrutiny of F_IO_2 becomes important; continuous monitoring of O_2 concentration on the inspiratory limb of the breathing system has been recommended. Indeed, to meet the ASTM standard, an oxygen analyzer is a required component of the anesthesia machine.(1, 6)

Safety Devices for Pressure and Flow of Oxygen

Anesthesia machines may be designed to alert the operator to a dangerously low pressure or flow of oxygen.(3, 4) When the pressure of oxygen reaches a certain value, the machine may alert the user with an alarm, or the machine may be engineered to cut off the supply of all other gases (e.g., nitrous oxide) to prevent the delivery of hypoxic mixtures. In addition, some anesthesia machines incorporate proportioning devices to assure that oxygen is flowing at some preset minimum portion of the total fresh gas flow. Dupaco anesthesia machines with oxygen and nitrous oxide were popular in veterinary anesthesia and incorporated an audible alarm if the pressure of oxygen was dangerously low, and the Metomatic Veterinary Anesthesia Machine reduced the flow of other gases (e.g., flow through the Verni-Trol) if oxygen flow was reduced. These safety mechanisms may malfunction, and continuously monitoring gases on the inspiratory limb of the breathing system is probably a more reliable way to assure the delivery of an adequate concentration of oxygen.

Flush Valves

Oxygen is supplied to the flush valve of an anesthesia machine at approximately 50 psi. The flush valve delivers a high but unmetered flow (35 to 75 L/min is the ASTM standard) (1) of O_2 to the common gas outlet or directly to the breathing system in some simple veterinary machines (e.g., Matrx VMS Small Animal Anesthesia Machine). The contemporary machine standard does not allow piping of O_2 from the flush valve through the vaporizer. However, older anesthesia machines, especially those with precision vaporizers added after the machine was manufactured, may direct O_2 through the vaporizer with the potential for increased output of anesthetic.(6)

At a flow rate of 50 L/min, O_2 from the flush valve can quickly fill the breathing system. In general, pediatric breathing systems (i.e., pediatric circles, Mapleson systems, or valved nonrebreathing systems) should not be filled via the flush valve due to the danger of overpressurizing the patient's respiratory system. Current machine standards require that the actuating device for the flush valve be recessed to prevent inadvertent activation and delivery of a high volume of gas to the breathing system (Fig. 14–21).(1) Other problems involving the flush valve include leaks in the flush valve assembly and sticking of the flush valve in the on position.(3) A leak at the flush valve in a human anesthesia machine used for small veterinary patients resulted in loss of anesthetic and O_2 at flow rates less than 1 L/min, making it impossible to maintain surgical anesthesia at normal fresh gas flow rates for a semiclosed circle breathing system.(17)

Vaporizers

Except for N_2O, modern inhalant anesthetics are delivered with vaporizers. Currently, concentration-calibrated, variable-bypass vaporizers, which are tem-

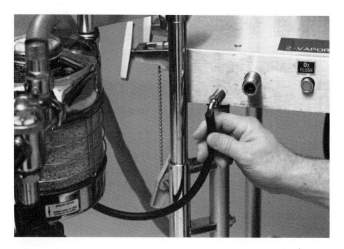

Fig. 14–21. Flush valve and common gas outlet on a Vetaflex 5 Veterinary Anesthesia Machine. The flush valve (labeled on the machine) is protected from inadvertent activation by a circular stainless steel guard. The common gas outlet (open hole) receives a connector to link the anesthesia machine through rubber hose to the fresh gas inlet of the breathing system.

perature, flow, and back-pressure compensated are standard in human anesthesia, and are recommended for delivery of volatile inhalant anesthetics to veterinary patients. However, a nonprecision, uncompensated vaporizer (Stephens vaporizer) is currently marketed to veterinarians as a part of a complete anesthesia machine. In addition, an obsolete vaporizer (Ohio #8 glass bottle) modified by removal of the wick has been recommended for the delivery of halothane and isoflurane to veterinary patients.(18, 19) Administering highly volatile, highly potent inhalant anesthetics with nonprecision, uncompensated vaporizers is associated with a high degree of risk unless instrumental monitoring (e.g., inspired or expired anesthetic concentration) is available.

A vaporizer is designed to change a liquid anesthetic into its vapor and to add a specific amount of vapor to the gases being delivered to the patient.(2) Carrier gas, O_2 alone or with N_2O, passes through the vaporizer to acquire anesthetic vapor. Because the saturated vapor pressures of most inhalant anesthetics are significantly greater than the partial pressures required for clinical anesthesia (i.e., significantly greater than the minimum alveolar concentration [MAC]) (Chapter 11), a vaporizer should deliver a concentration that is close to the setting on the vaporizer control dial. Otherwise, the inspired concentration of anesthetic should be monitored. In general, the design of precision vaporizers allows dilution of a high concentration of anesthetic vapor from the vaporization chamber to a clinically useable, relatively safe concentration.

PHYSICS OF VAPORIZER DESIGN AND FUNCTION

Several principles of physics are involved in the function of a vaporizer for inhalant anesthetics.(2-4) Heat is required for vaporization of liquid anesthetics;

the latent heat of vaporization is defined as the number of calories required to change 1 g of liquid into its vapor. This heat requirement causes liquid anesthetic to cool during vaporization. The vapor pressure of an anesthetic is the partial pressure of the anesthetic gas above the liquid at equilibrium, and vapor pressure varies directly with temperature. Thus, uncontrolled cooling limits a vaporizer's maximum output. A vaporizer made of a substance (e.g., copper) with a high specific heat (the quantity of heat required to raise the temperature of 1 g of the substance 1° C) supplies heat to the liquid anesthetic during vaporization, retarding the cooling process. If a vaporizer is constructed of a material with a high thermal conductivity (rate at which heat flows through a substance) such as copper, heat flows from warmer ambient air into the vaporizer to impede cooling. Materials including copper and bronze are used in the construction of vaporizers because of their favorable values for specific heat and thermal conductivity. More recently, stainless steel has been used in the construction of vaporizers.(4) The output of concentration-calibrated vaporizers is generally expressed as volumes percent of anesthetic vapor in the gases exiting the vaporizer. This relative value changes with variations in barometric pressure (BP) (Chapter 11).

COMPENSATORY MECHANISMS FOR VAPORIZERS

The conditions of use affect the performance of vaporizers and must be stated in the operation manual for a concentration-calibrated vaporizer to meet the ASTM standard.(1) The effects of changes in carrier gas flow, temperature, ambient pressure, and back-pressure should be delineated. Vaporizers compensate for changes in flow, temperature, and pressure in various ways.(2-4)

Compensation for variations in temperature of the liquid anesthetic during vaporization can be accomplished by several mechanisms. As previously mentioned, copper and bronze materials with high specific heat and thermal conductivity values, supply and conduct heat efficiently to the liquid anesthetic to promote a relatively constant temperature; this "heat sink" mechanism attenuates changes in temperature, producing a degree of thermostability. Bimetallic strip valves in Tec vaporizers, a gas-filled bellows linked to a valve in the bypass gas flow in Ohio calibrated vaporizers, and an expansion member (silicone cone) in Vapor vaporizers expand and contract with temperature changes, altering carrier gas flow through the vaporization chamber and controlling anesthetic output.(4) Manual adjustments in carrier gas flow are required to compensate for temperature variations in measured-flow vaporizers (e.g., Verni-Trol vaporizer) and older Vapor vaporizers. Other vaporizers are electrically heated, and the mechanism for control of the temperature of the anesthetic is supplied heat (e.g., Verni-Trol vaporizer on the Ohio DM 5000 anesthesia machine). The ultramodern Tec 6 vaporizer for desflurane is electrically heated and thermostatically controlled to 39° C.(16)

Differences in carrier gas flow rates alter the output of uncompensated vaporizers. Modern flow-compensated vaporizers produce relatively accurate anesthetic concentrations over an approximate range of 250 mL/min to 15 L/min.(6) The splitting ratio (ratio of the bypass gas to the gas passing through the vaporization chamber) determines the output of vapor (4), and the resistance to flow through each of the two channels in the vaporizer allows the splitting ratio to be maintained at various rates of flow.(3) Below 250 mL/min and above 15 L/min, the output from most concentration-calibrated vaporizers is variable, and performance data outside that range may not be available. Output from older variable-bypass vaporizers (e.g., Fluotec 2) may vary significantly from the setting on the control dial at flow rates less than 4 L/min. Measured-flow (flowmeter controlled) vaporizers (e.g., Copper Kettle) require adjustments in flow of oxygen to the vaporization chamber when the total flow of gas is changed.

Vaporizer output may vary with the composition of the carrier gas; the output of anesthetic with O_2 as the carrier gas may differ from the output with a combination of O_2 and N_2O as the carrier gas.(2, 4) The magnitude of effect is variable, depending on the specific vaporizer. With N_2O, newer vaporizers initially deliver concentrations that are less than the control dial setting. With the Fluotec Mark 3, N_2O had little effect on output. However, N_2O as the carrier gas in the Fluotec Mark 2 increases the output of halothane.(2)

Back-pressure compensation is a design feature of modern vaporizers. Intermittent pressure transmitted to a vaporizer during activation of the flush valve and during application of positive pressure ventilation may increase vaporizer output compared to output of anesthetic during free flow of gases through the vaporizer.(6) Newer vaporizers prevent or minimize this "pumping effect" by use of small vaporization chambers (e.g., Tecs), long spiral tubes at the inlet to the vaporization chamber (e.g., Vapor), pressure check valves just downstream from the vaporizer, and relief valves at the vaporizer outlet.(2, 3, 6)

EFFECTS OF BAROMETRIC PRESSURE ON VAPORIZER FUNCTION

Variations in barometric pressure (e.g., high altitude or hyperbaric chambers) alter vaporizer output expressed in volume percent. A specific partial pressure of inhalant anesthetic (e.g., 1 MAC) represents the same anesthetic potency (partial pressure) at various barometric pressures.(20) However, anesthetic concentration is expressed as volume percent on most vaporizers, and MAC expressed as volume percent increases as barometric pressure decreases. Changing the barometric pressure also alters the viscosity and density of gases flowing through vaporizers and flowmeters and affects the output concentration.(20) The current ASTM standard states that the effects of barometric pressure on the performance of a vaporizer must be described in catalogs and operation manuals.(1, 3)

With decreasing barometric pressure, most concentration-calibrated vaporizers (e.g., Fluotec III) are considered "self-compensating" and deliver about the same partial pressure, but an increasing volume percent of anesthetic.(3, 20) Basically, the vaporizer can be set normally in volume percent despite the fact that the volume percent setting on the control dial is inaccurate.(20) In theory, a halothane vaporizer at an ambient pressure of 500 mm of Hg should deliver twice the concentration on the control dial in volume percent and approximately 1.3 times the dialed concentration in terms of MAC or potency.(4) Since small changes occur in concentration output caused by variations in resistance of flow through the vaporizer at differing ambient pressures (3), the best approach is to measure partial pressure of anesthetic in inspired or expired gases when working at atypical barometric pressures.

With measured-flow vaporizers (e.g., Copper Kettle), changes in barometric pressure affect both partial pressure and volume percent of the delivered anesthetic.(20) If barometric pressure is low, the output expressed as volume percent and as partial pressure increases. When the barometric pressure is high, measured-flow vaporizers deliver a lower anesthetic concentration, expressed as either volume percent or partial pressure. Temperature, barometric pressure, and vapor pressure of the anesthetic affect the final anesthetic concentrations, but the greatest effects are on anesthetics with low boiling points and with vapor pressures that are near the barometric pressure.(3, 20)

Changes in BP also affect the function of flowmeters. Actual flow increases, becoming higher than the indicator and scale of the flowmeter show, as barometric pressure decreases.(20) In contrast, a flowmeter will deliver less flow than indicated when ambient pressure is higher than the barometric pressure at which the flowmeter was calibrated.(3)

POTENTIAL PROBLEMS WITH VAPORIZERS

The arrangement of vaporizers on anesthesia machines and how vaporizers are maintained affect their safety under clinical conditions. Filling errors, improper transport, using vaporizers in series, and improperly connecting a vaporizer to a machine may cause significant variations in output.

Veterinary practices often stock more than one inhalant anesthetic, and a vaporizer may be inadvertently filled with the wrong drug, especially if the vaporizer has a screw-cap filler port in contrast to a keyed filler port. Keyed filler systems are designed to prevent the introduction of the wrong anesthetic into a vaporizer (Fig. 14–22). However, they are more inconvenient, and screw-cap filler ports and a simple bottle adapter will decrease spillage (Fig. 14–23). Admittedly, there is an increased chance for incorrect filling of vaporizers (Fig. 14–24). If an agent-specific vaporizer for a drug with a low vapor pressure (e.g., methoxyflurane)

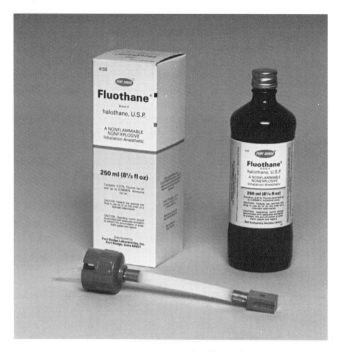

Fig. 14–22. Bottle adapter for halothane vaporizers with keyed filler systems. Such systems reduce the likelihood of introducing an inappropriate anesthetic into an agent-specific vaporizer. The larger end (left) of the device attaches to a bottle of halothane and the opposite end corresponds to the vaporizer filler receptacle. A screw in the receptacle allows a tight seal to be created during the filling process. Newer bottles have a color-coded collar to accept only the correct bottle adapter (Fig. 14–23).

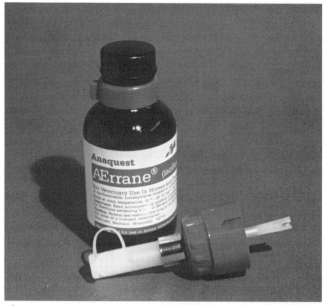

Fig. 14–23. Bottle adapter (Southmedic, Inc., Beaumont, Texas) for filling isoflurane vaporizers with screw-cap filler ports. The isoflurane bottle has a color-coded collar corresponding to the color on the bottle's label and the color of the bottle adapter. This type of bottle adapter is intended to reduce spillage during the filling of vaporizers with screw-cap filler ports.

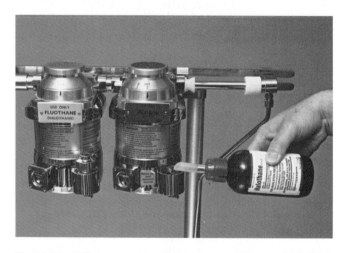

Fig. 14–24. Filling a vaporizer with a screw-cap filler port. Halothane is about to be poured into an isoflurane vaporizer illustrating the possibility of filling a vaporizer with a screw-cap filler port with the wrong anesthetic. Tec 3 vaporizers for halothane (Fluotec 3) and isoflurane (Isotec 3) are shown in series. The ideal order would be to reverse these vaporizers with the isoflurane immediately downstream from the flowmeters followed by the halothane vaporizer.

is filled with a potent, highly volatile anesthetic, dangerously high concentrations may be produced. If this occurs, the vaporizer should be decontaminated before it is used for a patient. The best approach is to have the vaporizer serviced by a qualified vaporizer technician. For Ohio calibrated vaporizers, service is required because the paper wicks must be replaced. For a contaminated Tec vaporizer, an option is to drain the vaporizer, flush it with an O_2 flow of 5 L/min for 45 minutes or until no trace of a contaminant is present, allow it to stabilize thermally for about 2 hours, and refill it with the appropriate anesthetic. Vaporizers contaminated with a nonvolatile contaminant (e.g., water or thymol) should be drained and serviced.(4)

Filler ports and sight glasses are designed to preclude overfilling of modern vaporizers, primarily to prevent liquid anesthetic from entering the fresh gas line of the vaporizer (Fig. 14–25). Recent designs for some vaporizers prevent liquid from entering the fresh gas line even during tipping or inversion. However, tipping of certain vaporizers may introduce liquid anesthetic into the bypass channel.(3) If this occurs, a high concentration of anesthetic vapor may be delivered; tipping a vaporizer that was not securely attached to an anesthetic machine resulted in a cardiac arrest in a human patient.(21) Also, moving a vaporizer on a mobile anesthesia machine may alter vaporizer output if the

machine is tipped or liquid anesthetic is sloshed as the machine is moved over doorway thresholds. Generally, vaporizers should be emptied before transport. Even portable anesthesia machines should be moved with care. If tipping occurs, a high flow of oxygen through the vaporizer for 20 minutes with the control dial at a low setting has been recommended, but servicing may be required.(2)

One anesthesia machine may be fitted with multiple vaporizers (Fig. 14–24). Modern anesthesia machines designed for human use are equipped with interlocking mechanisms that do not allow two vaporizers to be "on" simultaneously.(6) Few veterinary practices have the luxury of owning anesthesia machines with interlocking vaporizers. In-line, noninterlocked vaporizers offer the possibility of operating two vaporizers concurrently, conceivably resulting in excessive depth of anesthesia.(2) The simultaneous use of more than one vaporizer in series also increases the probability of contamination of a vaporizer with an inappropriate agent. If vaporizers are placed in series, the best order is methoxyflurane, enflurane, isoflurane, and halothane from upstream to downstream; this reduces the chance of contamination by taking into account both vapor pressure and po-

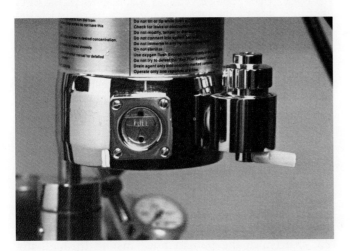

Fig. 14–25. Screw-cap filler system and sight glass for a Fluotec Mark III vaporizer. The location of the filler port prevents the operator from filling the vaporizer excessively because liquid will overflow if the maximum level on the sight glass is exceeded significantly. The plastic tubing on the bottom of the filler system facilitates drainage of the vaporizer.

tency.(3, 4) Anesthesia machines with vaporizers in series should be used carefully if an interlocking mechanism is not in place.

Occasionally, veterinarians will use a freestanding, concentration-calibrated vaporizer that is periodically connected between the common gas outlet and the breathing system or between the outlet of another vaporizer and the breathing system. Also, freestanding vaporizers are commonly used with pump oxygenators for cardiopulmonary bypass procedures.(4) A freestanding vaporizer offers a greater opportunity for tipping. Inadvertently reversing the flow through the vaporizer is possible when vaporizer connections are changed periodically, and forcing O_2 through the vaporizer with the flush valve may occur if the vaporizer is located downstream from the flush valve. All of these situations lead to a significant increase in the output concentration.(6) Use of a freestanding vaporizer is not the safest approach for access to a second inhalant anesthetic.

In anesthesia machines designed for veterinary use, it is possible to connect a concentration-calibrated vaporizer in reverse, even though the connections are labeled and are of different sizes. In this configuration, the vaporizer output can potentially be twice that indicated on the control dial.(6)

CLASSIFICATION OF VAPORIZERS

Vaporizers have been classified according to several major characteristics:
1. Method of output regulation
2. Method of vaporization
3. Location
4. Mechanism of temperature compensation
5. Agent specificity
6. Resistance

Even though some authors have classified vaporizers using only one feature, such schemes are incomplete because of the variations among vaporizers.(3) The

Table 14–2. Classification Characteristics of Some Vaporizers Used in Veterinary Anesthesia (2, 3, 4)

Vaporizer	Method of Output Regulation	Method of Vaporization	Location	Temperature Compensated	Resistance	Specificity
Ohio #8	VBP CC −	FO/wick	VIC	No	Low	No
Stephens	VBP CC −	FO/wick	VIC	No	Low	No
Tec 2	VBP CC + *	FO/wick	VOC	Yes	High	Yes
Tec 3	VBP CC +	FO/wick	VOC	Yes	High	Yes
Vapor	VBP CC +	FO/wick	VOC	Yes	High	Yes
Vapor 19.1	VBP CC +	FO/wick	VOC	Yes	High	Yes
Ohio Calibrated	VBP CC +	FO/wick	VOC	Yes	High	Yes
Siemens	NA CC +	Inject	VOC	No	High	Yes
Copper Kettle	MF CC −	Bubble-through	VOC	Yes	High	No
Verni-Trol	MF CC −	Bubble-through	VOC	Yes	High	No

VBP, variable bypass; CC +, concentration calibrated; CC −, not concentration calibrated; FO, flow-over; VIC, vaporizer-in-the-system; VOC, vaporizer-out-of-the-system; NA, not applicable; MF, measured flowthrough vaporizer.

*A Tec 2 vaporizer is concentration-calibrated at higher flows of carrier gas, but output varies with low flows.

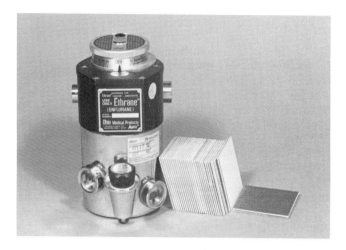

Fig. 14–26. Ohio Calibrated Vaporizer with paper wicks and copper spacers. The wicks function to increase the surface area for vaporization of inhalant anesthetic.

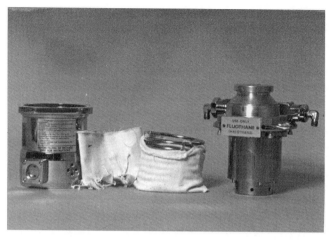

Fig. 14–27. Fluotec Mark 3 Vaporizer with cloth wicks. The wicks function to increase the surface area for vaporization of inhalant anesthetic. (From Hartsfield, S.M. Machines and Breathing Systems for Administration of Inhalation Anesthetics. In: Principles and Practice of Veterinary Anesthesia. Edited by C.E. Short. Baltimore: Williams & Wilkins, 1987.)

characteristics of the vaporizers to be discussed are summarized in Table 14–2.

Regulation of Output. Regulation of anesthetic output in volume percent is accomplished by variable-bypass or measured-flow mechanisms.(3, 4) With variable-bypass vaporizers, all fresh gas flows into the vaporizer, part being directed through and part bypassing the vaporization chamber. The gases rejoin before exiting the vaporizer, establishing the anesthetic concentration dialed with the control knob. The standard for these vaporizers is for the control dial to be turned on in a counterclockwise direction.(1) Concentration-calibrated variable-bypass vaporizers are quite accurate (e.g., Tecs), but uncalibrated variable-bypass vaporizers (e.g., Ohio #8) are inaccurate.

Measured-flow (flowmeter-controlled) vaporizers are considered non-concentration-calibrated.(4) They route a small flow of carrier gas (oxygen) through the vaporizer, and this gas becomes fully saturated with anesthetic. A second source of gas (O_2 and possibly N_2O) that never enters the vaporizer dilutes the saturated gas to the desired concentration. Calculations are necessary to determine the concentration of anesthetic that is delivered to the common gas outlet and breathing system.

Method of vaporization. The method of vaporization can be flow-over, bubble-through, or injection.(2-4) Flow-over vaporizers direct carrier gas over the surface of the liquid anesthetic. The surface area may be increased with wicks to improve the efficiency of vaporization (Figs. 14–26 and 14–27). The Stephens vaporizer can be used with or without a wick, depending on the anesthetic and the decision of the anesthetist.(22) The bubble-through method of vaporization delivers carrier gas below the surface of the liquid through a diffuser (a sintered bronze disc in the Copper Kettle) that disperses bubbles of carrier gas through the liquid anesthetic to increase the liquid gas interface.(4) Efficiency of vaporization increases with

smaller bubbles, deeper bubble dispersion, and slower carrier gas flow.(2) Injection vaporizers deliver a known amount of liquid anesthetic or pure vapor into a known volume of gas to deliver an accurate concentration.(3)

Vaporizer Location. In relation to the breathing system, a vaporizer may be located either out of the system (VOC) (Fig. 14–28) or in the system (VIC) (Fig. 14–29).(2) High-resistance vaporizers are used as VOC units, and low-resistance vaporizers are necessary for VIC use (since the patient must inspire through the vaporizer). Traditionally, highly potent, highly volatile anesthetics have been administered with VOC vaporizers. However, use of VIC vaporizers for delivery of isoflurane and halothane to veterinary patients has been and continues to be advocated. No VIC-type vaporizers are being manufactured in the United States at present; "unpredictable output" is cited as an unsolved problem with these vaporizers.(3, 23)

Temperature Compensation. As discussed previously, heat is required to vaporize liquid anesthetics. To prevent or compensate for cooling, which alters the rate of vaporization of the liquid anesthetic, heat must be supplied to maintain the temperature of the liquid anesthetic, or the flow of carrier gas through the vaporizer must be adjusted to account for changing rate of vaporization. Heat may be supplied from the vaporizer itself if it is made of a material with high specific heat and high thermal conductivity (thermostability).(4) Electric heaters and warm water jackets were used to supply heat for older vaporizers, and an electric heating device has been incorporated into a new vaporizer (Tec 6) designed for desflurane.(16) In other vaporizers, thermostatic mechanisms (e.g., a bimetallic strip valve) automatically vary the flow of carrier gas through the vaporization chamber to counterbalance changes in temperature and vaporization.

Manual adjustments of flow through the vaporization chamber are made to offset variations in temperature that occur with measured-flow vaporizers.

Agent Specificity. Vaporizers can be either agent-specific (designed for a particular inhalant anesthetic) or multipurpose (used with any volatile liquid anesthetic).(2) If a vaporizer is designed and used for multiple agents, it should be clearly labeled with the name of the agent currently in the vaporizer. If the anesthetic is changed, the vaporizer should be cleared of the original anesthetic before another anesthetic is introduced into the vaporizer, and draining alone may not eliminate all of the original anesthetic.(3) The trend in vaporizers for anesthesia in human and animal patients has been toward agent-specific, concentration-calibrated vaporizers.

Resistance. Vaporizers have been classified according to resistance to flow.(3) Plenum-type vaporizers are high resistance vaporizers designed for location outside of the breathing system, and high resistance is characteristic of contemporary concentration-calibrated, variable bypass vaporizers. Low-resistance vaporizers are those designed for incorporation into the breathing system (3) and include the Ohio #8 and the Stephens vaporizers.

VIC VAPORIZERS FOR VETERINARY ANESTHESIA

Nonprecision, draw-over, VIC vaporizers have been common in veterinary anesthesia for many years. Until the introduction of isoflurane into veterinary anesthesia, perhaps the most widely used vaporizer for veterinary patients in the United States was the Ohio #8 glass bottle. Although it is no longer manufactured, it was the basic vaporizer on many veterinary anesthesia machines (Pitman-Moore Models 960 and 970) sold in the 1970s for administration of methoxyflurane, many of which remain in use. More recently, the Stephens vaporizer has been advocated for veterinary patients. In the past for maximum safety, VIC vaporizers have been recommended for anesthetics low in potency (e.g., ether) or low in vapor pressure (e.g., methoxyflurane), and in human anesthesia, the Ohio #8 glass bottle was used most for diethyl ether and to a lesser extent for methoxyflurane. However, the use of halothane and isoflurane in VIC vaporizers has been described, specifically for low-flow and closed breathing systems.(24)

With VIC vaporizers, the inspired anesthetic concentration varies with the patient's respiratory minute volume, use of positive pressure ventilation, changes in carrier gas flow rate, and variations in temperature. At a given vaporizer setting, increased spontaneous ventilation, positive pressure ventilation, and lower fresh gas flows increase the inspired anesthetic concentration. As stated specifically for the Ohio #8 vaporizer, "The delivered concentration is unknown and changes unpredictably with use." (23) Without instrumental monitoring of the inspired or expired anesthetic concentration, the anesthetist is completely dependent on the response of the patient to determine appropriate settings for the vaporizer. This is often referred to as *qualitative anesthesia* in contrast to *quantitative anesthesia*, where a known concentration of inhalant is continually delivered to the patient.

Ohio #8 Glass Bottle Vaporizer. The Ohio #8 vaporizer is classified as variable-bypass, flow-over with wick, non-temperature-compensated, VIC, low-resistance, and multipurpose.(2) It is designed very simply; the vaporization chamber is made of glass, and a cloth wick creates a large surface area for vaporization (Fig. 14–30). The vaporizer is not calibrated; it is considered nonprecision. The vaporizer has no method for controlling the temperature of the liquid. Its low resistance allows it to be situated in the breathing system (VIC), usually on the inspiratory side of the circle. If positioned on the expiratory limb, the vaporization chamber may become contaminated with water condensing from expired gases. The control arm or lever is adjustable from 0,

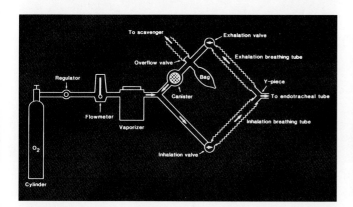

Fig. 14–28. Diagram of a vaporizer located outside the breathing system (VOC) and its relationship to other basic components of the anesthesia machine and circle system. (From Hartsfield, S.M. Machines and Breathing Systems for Administration of Inhalation Anesthetics. In: Principles and Practice of Veterinary Anesthesia. Edited by C.E. Short. Baltimore: Williams & Wilkins, 1987.)

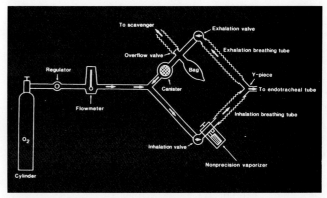

Fig. 14–29. Diagram of a vaporizer located inside the breathing system (VIC) and its relationship to other basic components of the anesthesia machine and circle system. (From Hartsfield, S.M. Machines and Breathing Systems for Administration of Inhalation Anesthetics. In: Principles and Practice of Veterinary Anesthesia. Edited by C.E. Short. Baltimore: Williams & Wilkins, 1987.)

corresponding to no gas flow through the vaporization chamber, to 10, corresponding to total inspiratory flow through the vaporization chamber (Fig. 14–31). The possibility of diverting all gas flow through the vaporization chamber makes the use of highly volatile anesthetics particularly dangerous, especially if the wick is in place. The delivered concentration is un-

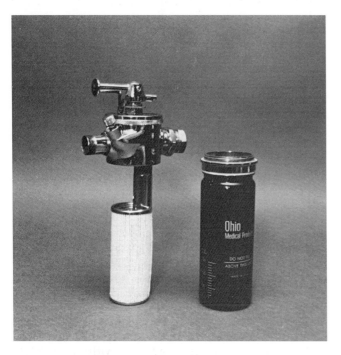

Fig. 14–30. Partially disassembled Ohio #8 glass bottle vaporizer. The cloth wick on left functions to increase the surface area for vaporization of the anesthetic.

known and may change unpredictably. The function of this vaporizer is probably best summarized by the following: "Because of the variability associated with an in-system vaporizer, it is not possible to give performance data." (2) The Ohio #8 vaporizer is no longer being manufactured, and finding expertise and parts for repairing the vaporizer may be difficult.

In veterinary medicine, the Ohio #8 vaporizer continues to be used for the administration of methoxyflurane. Modified by the removal of the wick, the vaporizer has been proposed as an inexpensive alternative for administration of isoflurane (18) and halothane.(19) Use of an Ohio #8 vaporizer for halothane or isoflurane with the wick in place is dangerous owing to the high concentration of anesthetic that may be delivered in the inspired gases, especially if all carrier gases are diverted through the vaporization chamber. Even with the wick removed, recommendations for using the Ohio #8 vaporizer for isoflurane include "familiarity with guidelines for its use and understanding of its limitations." (18) The Ohio #8 vaporizer also has potential for leaking anesthetic into the breathing system when the control lever is off.(2) With age, the vaporizer's valves may not seat properly (Fig. 14–32), allowing continuous passage of fresh gases through the vaporization chamber and production of anesthetic-rich gases.

Stephens Vaporizer. The Stephens vaporizer is classified as variable-bypass, flow-over, non-temperature-compensated, VIC, low-resistance, and multipurpose. It is not a precision vaporizer. The vaporizer's low resistance allows it to be located within the breathing system on the inspiratory side. The vaporization cham-

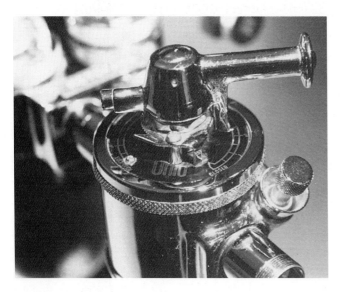

Fig. 14–31. Control lever for the Ohio #8 vaporizer set at position #2. The numbered positions (0 to 10) on the vaporizer correspond to increasing flow of carrier gas through the vaporization chamber. At the closed position (0), all gas entering the vaporizer should bypass the vaporization chamber, and at full open (10), all gas entering the vaporizer should move through the vaporization chamber.

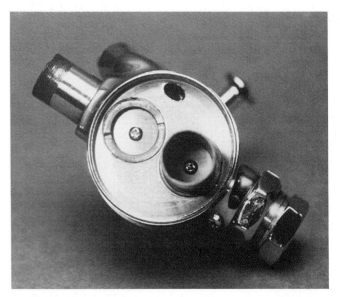

Fig. 14–32. Underside of the head of an Ohio #8 vaporizer showing valves and seats through which gases enter and leave the vaporization chamber. The integrity of these valves in the off position may be lost because of wear or corrosion leading to flow of carrier gas through the vaporization chamber, even when the control lever is in the off position.

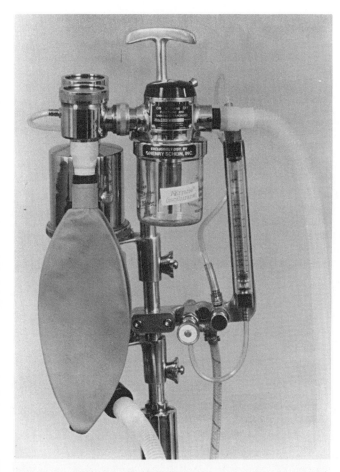

Fig. 14–33. Stephens Anesthesia Machine and Vaporizer (Henry Schein, Inc., Port Washington, New York). The glass vaporizer can be set at the off and full-on positions with incremental settings marked in eighths. The vaporizer has been recommended for methoxyflurane with a wick in place and for halothane or isoflurane with the wick removed.

ber is made of glass (Fig. 14–33), and a wick is provided for administration of methoxyflurane. The wick should not be used for halothane or isoflurane.(22) The vaporizer is not calibrated and has no method for controlling the temperature of the liquid. The control knob is adjustable from the off to the full-on position in increments of eighths. The off position indicates no flow through the vaporization chamber, and the on position corresponds to complete flow through the vaporization chamber. The Stephens vaporizer is intended for use in a low-flow or closed circle breathing system.(22)

VOC VAPORIZERS IN VETERINARY ANESTHESIA

Modern concentration-calibrated vaporizers located outside of the breathing circuit are considered precision vaporizers; any of the volatile liquid anesthetics can be administered safely with a concentration-calibrated, agent-specific, VOC vaporizer. Several brands of VOC-type vaporizers are common in veterinary anesthesia. Many older models of vaporizers, although no longer being manufactured, remain serviceable and may be

purchased as "used" equipment. Newer VOC-type vaporizers are temperature, flow, and back-pressure compensated. The performance of older VOC-type vaporizers varies with changes in temperature, flow, and back-pressure, and performance data should be reviewed before using them. The concentration control dial and the vaporizer output generally are linear over a wide range of flow rates and temperatures in newer VOC-type vaporizers. The following discussion, though not exhaustive, includes information about several of the VOC-type vaporizers that are commonly used in veterinary anesthesia.

Tec Vaporizers. "Tec" vaporizers for halothane and isoflurane, particularly the Fluotec Mark 3 and Isotec 3, are common in veterinary anesthesia and are presently available through veterinary anesthesia equipment companies. They are considered reliable because they are temperature, flow, and back-pressure compensated under normal operating conditions. The Fluotec Mark 3's predecessor, the Fluotec Mark 2, is no longer being manufactured, but may still be available as used equipment. In some veterinary practices, Fluotec Mark 2 vaporizers remain in use. Tec 4, 5, and 6 vaporizers have superseded the Tec 3 vaporizers for contemporary human anesthesia machines.(6, 16) Tec 4, 5, and 6 vaporizers are not common in veterinary anesthesia at the present time; various publications and the specific operation manuals offer information about the use and performance of each of these vaporizers.(3, 4, 6, 16)

Fluotec Mark 2. This vaporizer (Fig. 14–34) is classified as variable bypass, flow-over with wick, VOC,

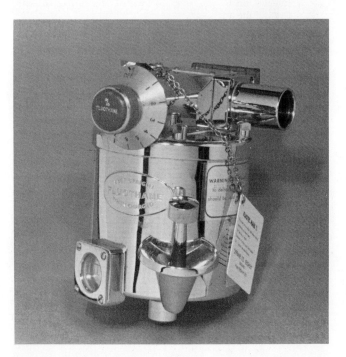

Fig. 14–34. Fluotec 2 Vaporizer. The performance characteristics for variations in carrier gas flow are included on the plastic card attached to the vaporizer (Figure 14-35).

Table 14–3.   Approximate Output (vol %) from a Fluotec Mark 2 at Various Flow Rates and Dial Settings (15)

Dial Setting	1 L/min	2 L/min	3 L/min	4 L/min	6 L/min	8 L/min
0.5%	0	0	0	0.5	0.5	0.5
1.0%	0	0.5	1.0	1.0	1.0	1.0
1.5%	0.5	1.5	1.5	1.5	1.5	1.5
2.0%	1.8	2.0	2.0	2.0	2.0	2.0
2.5%	3.0	2.5	2.5	2.5	2.5	2.5
3.0%	4.0	3.1	3.0	3.0	3.0	3.0
3.5%	5.0	4.0	3.5	3.5	3.5	3.5
4.0%	6.5	5.0	4.1	4.0	4.0	4.0

temperature-compensated, high-resistance, and agent-specific.(2) Temperature compensation is with a bimetallic strip valve at the outlet to the vaporization chamber.(3) Performance data show that the Mark 2 becomes imprecise at flow rates below 4 L/min, and inaccuracy increases distinctly below 2 L/min.(2) At flow rates and dial settings likely to be selected for small veterinary patients, the Mark 2's output tends to be lower than control dial settings of less than 2% and higher than dial settings of 2% or greater (Table 14–3).

At the very low flow rates required for closed and low-flow maintenance techniques, the Mark 2's output may decrease to zero or increase to concentrations much higher than dial settings. Because of its unpredictable output characteristics, the Mark 2 has been categorized as unsuitable and unreliable for use with low fresh gas flow rates.(2, 22, 25) Back pressure (e.g., positive pressure ventilation) increases the output of the Mark 2 dramatically at flow rates less than 2 L/min.(2, 26) A pressurizing valve was developed for the Mark 2 to minimize the effects of back pressure (2), but it may not be present on all anesthesia machines with the Mark 2 vaporizer. The operator should fully understand the Mark 2's performance characteristics before using the vaporizer clinically, and the output diagram for the Mark 2 should be available for consultation during clinical use (Fig. 14–35).

Tec Mark 3 Vaporizers. These vaporizers are classified as variable-bypass, flow-over, temperature-compensated, agent-specific, high-resistance, and VOC.(2, 3) This model includes the Fluotec Mark 3, the Pentec Mark 2, and the Isotec 3 (Fig. 14–24). The Tec 3 vaporizer is temperature-compensated with a bimetallic, temperature-sensitive element associated with the vaporization chamber. Output from the Tec 3 vaporizer is nearly linear over the range of concentrations and flow rates that would typically be selected for veterinary patients (250 mL/min to 6 L/min). Back-pressure compensation is accomplished in the internal design of the vaporizer with a long tube leading to the vaporization chamber, an expansion area in the tube, and exclusion of wicks from the area of the vaporization chamber near the inlet.(2)

Vapor Vaporizers. **Vapor 19.1.** The Vapor 19.1 vaporizer (Fig. 14–36) is classified as variable-bypass, flow-over with wick, temperature-compensated, high-

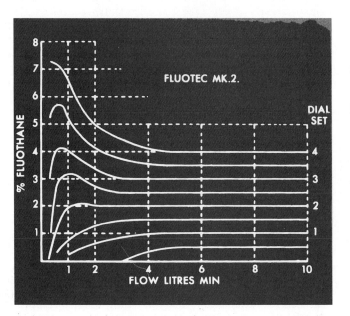

Fig. 14–35. Performance diagram for a Fluotec 2 Vaporizer. The diagram indicates expected output of halothane in volume percent for specific control dial settings and specific carrier gas flow rates.

resistance, agent-specific, and VOC.(2, 3) Specific vaporizers are available for isoflurane, halothane, and enflurane. Temperature compensation is automatic with an "expansion member" that varies the flow of gas through the vaporization chamber with changes in temperature. Pressure compensation is accomplished by the presence of a long spiral inlet tube to the vaporization chamber.(4) This vaporizer is accurate from 0.3 to 15 L/min of fresh gas flow at the lower settings on the control dial, but complete saturation may not occur at higher settings with higher flows. The vaporizer is designed for operation (temperature compensation) in the range of 10 to 40° C.(2)

Vapor. The Vapor vaporizer (Fig. 14–37) preceded the Vapor 19 and 19.1, and has been called "semiautomatic," since manual adjustments are required for complete temperature compensation (Fig. 14–38).(5) The unit is no longer being manufactured, but some vaporizers may still be in operation in veterinary practices. The vaporizer was available for both methoxyflurane and halothane. It is classified as variable-bypass, flow-over with wick, VOC, temperature-compensated by manual flow alteration, high-resistance, and agent-specific, and is considered to be very accurate.(2) It was designed for thermostability and is constructed of a large mass of copper as a heat sink to prevent excessive cooling during vaporization (2, 27) The concentration dial must be manually adjusted to the temperature of the vaporizer and the liquid between 16 and 28° C (Fig. 14–38).(28) The unit is flow-compensated over a wide range (approximately 250 mL/min to 10 L/min) with some deviation at high concentrations at high flows. The mechanism for back-pressure compensation involves a long coiled tube at the inlet to the vaporization chamber.(2)

Other Vaporizers. **Ohio Calibrated Vaporizer.** This vaporizer (Fig. 14–26) has been available for veterinary use and is common on used human anesthesia machines. This vaporizer is classified as variable-bypass, flow-over with wick, automatically temperature compensated, agent-specific, VOC, and high-resistance.(2, 3) Specific units were manufactured for isoflurane, halothane, and enflurane. These vaporizers were designed for accuracy at fresh gas flows between 0.3 to 10 L/min, and temperature compensation occurs between 16° and 32° C. Tilting these vaporizes up to 20° while in use or up to 45° when not in use does not cause problems. Greater tipping of the vaporizer may result in delivery of high concentrations. The vaporizer has plastic spacers between paper wicks that may react with enflurane or isoflurane to cause discoloration of the liquid anesthetic, apparently without significant consequences.(3)

Siemens Vaporizer. This vaporizer is a concentration-calibrated, injection-type, nonthermocompensated, agent-specific, plenum (high-resistance) vaporizer.(3) It has not had extensive use in clinical veterinary anesthesia, except in laboratory animal facilities associated with human hospitals. The vaporizer was designed to couple with a specific Siemens ventilator. The function and evaluation of this vaporizer have been reviewed.(3)

Measured-Flow Vaporizers. Verni-Trols and Copper Kettles (Fig. 14–39), are flowmeter-controlled vaporizers that formerly were popular in human anesthesia.(2-4)

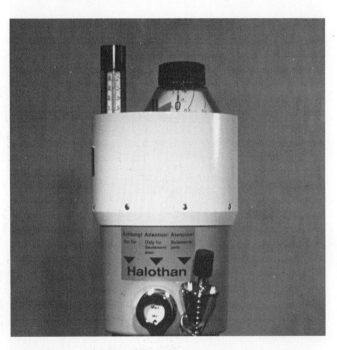

Fig. 14–37. Vapor Vaporizer for halothane (North American Drager, Telford, Pennsylvania).

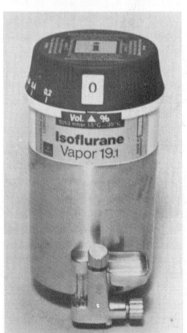

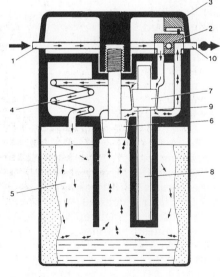

1 Fresh Gas Inlet
2 Turn On and Turn Off Control
   (Actuated by Concentration Knob)
3 Concentration Knob
4 Pressure Compensation (Patented)
5 Vaporizing Chamber
6 Control Cone
7 Vaporizing Chamber By-pass Cone
8 Expansion Member for Temperature
   Compensation
9 Mixing Chamber
10 Fresh Gas Outlet

Fig. 14–36. Vapor 19.1 Vaporizer (North American Drager, Telford, Pennsylvania) for isoflurane and a cross-sectional diagram of the vaporizer: 1, Fresh gas inlet; 2, On and off control (activated by concentration knob); 3, Concentration knob; 4, Pressure compensation; 5, Vaporizing chamber; 6, Control cone; 7, Vaporizing chamber bypass cone; 8, Expansion member for temperature compensation; 9, Mixing chamber; 10, Fresh gas inlet. (From Lumb, W.V., and Jones, E.W. Veterinary Anesthesia, 2nd ed. Philadelphia: Lea & Febiger, 1984.)

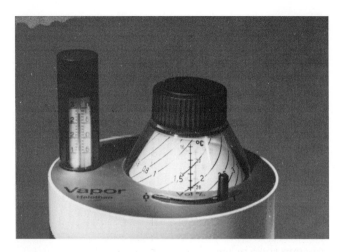

Fig. 14–38. Vapor Vaporizer with a control dial setting of 2% at 28° C. The thermometer (left) indicates the temperature of the vaporizer (liquid anesthetic), and the control dial is used to manually align the curved line corresponding to the desired anesthetic concentration with the temperature of the vaporizer (vertical line with hash marks). (From Hartsfield, S.M. Machines and Breathing Systems for Administration of Inhalation Anesthetics. In: Principles and Practice of Veterinary Anesthesia. Edited by C.E. Short. Baltimore: Williams & Wilkins, 1987.)

Copper Kettles were the first devices to allow precise vaporization of liquid anesthetics.(2) These flowmeter-controlled vaporizers are classified as measured-flow, bubble-through, high-resistance, VOC, temperature-compensated (thermally stable with manual flow adjustments based on temperature of the liquid anesthetic), and multipurpose. They have been classified as saturation vaporizers. These vaporizers are constructed of copper (Copper Kettle) or silicon bronze (Verni-Trol) for thermostability; back-pressure compensation mechanisms are present on more recent models and can be fitted on older models (e.g., check valves). These vaporizers are not being manufactured in the United States and are not covered by the ASTM standard of 1989.(6) However, they are available on used anesthesia machines and can be purchased economically for veterinary practices. Since the vaporizers are multipurpose, they will accurately vaporize halothane, isoflurane, enflurane, or methoxyflurane, but they should be clearly labeled for the agent in use.

With measured-flow vaporizers, manual adjustments in flow rates are required to account for variations in total gas flow, day-to-day changes in temperature, and changes in liquid temperature during use, especially with high fresh gas flow rates. In most cases, a calculator or slide rule (Fig. 14–40) is supplied with each vaporizer for determining proper flow rates. Anesthesia machines with measured-flow vaporizers have oxygen flowmeters for two purposes. One flowmeter routes all of its oxygen through the vaporization chamber, where it is fully saturated with anesthetic; the other flowmeter supplies oxygen that bypasses the vaporizer and supplies oxygen to meet the patient's requirements. Both sources of gas combine at a mixing valve to achieve the

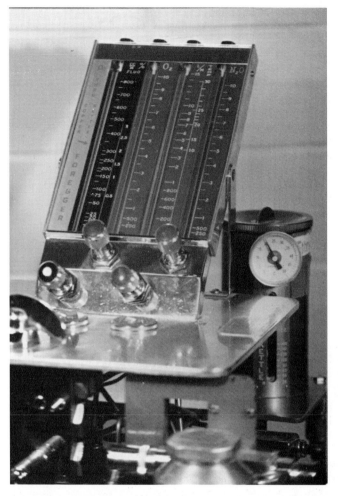

Fig. 14-39. Copper Kettle Vaporizer (Foregger, Allentown, Pennsylvania). The vaporization chamber (copper kettle) with its thermometer is behind the table top (right rear), and the vaporizer circuit control valve is attached to the left front corner of the table top. The flowmeter cluster from left to right includes the oxygen flowmeter to the vaporization chamber (black scale), two bypass oxygen flowmeters (green), and one nitrous oxide flowmeter (blue). This cluster does not meet recent standards for the arrangement of flowmeters. (From Hartsfield, S.M. Machines and Breathing Systems for Administration of Inhalation Anesthetics. In: Principles and Practice of Veterinary Anesthesia. Edited by C.E. Short. Baltimore: Williams & Wilkins, 1987.)

proper anesthetic concentration before gases enter the breathing system.

Since the output of a measured-flow vaporizer is oxygen fully saturated with anesthetic, the concentration of halothane or isoflurane approaches 32%. Dangerously high concentrations of anesthetic can be delivered to the breathing system if flowmeters are set carelessly or if the diluent flow is not turned on. It is also possible to misread the slide rule and set incorrect flows.(2) Because such high concentrations can be achieved and because errors in adjustment of flowmeters are possible, the use of continuous monitoring of the inspired anesthetic agent concentration with an infrared analyzer has been recommended.(4) For standard Copper Kettles and Verni-Trols, Table 14–4 provides flow rates for the vaporizer flowmeter to produce various delivered concentrations at several total fresh gas flow rates at 21° C.

In addition to using a slide rule, the output from measured-flow vaporizers can be calculated or estimated. Methods, including formulas, for calculating flow requirements for measured-flow vaporizers have been reviewed.(22) The vaporization chamber produces an anesthetic concentration equal to the anesthetic's saturated vapor pressure. Thus, if halothane's vapor pressure is 243 mm Hg at 20° C, approximately 32% halothane is delivered to the mixing valve. This concentration is diluted by bypass gases to an appropriate concentration for the patient.

If a patient is to be maintained with a total gas flow of 2 L/min and a halothane concentration of 1.5%, then 30 mL/min of halothane vapor (1.5% times 2000

mL = 30 mL) must be delivered to the breathing system along with 1970 mL/min of O_2. About 64 mL of O_2 must enter the vaporization chamber each minute to produce an output of 30 mL/min of halothane (30 mL = 32% · X, where X is the total gas flow exiting the vaporization chamber; thus, X = 94 mL, and 94 mL – 30 mL = 64 mL). The bypass oxygen flow must equal (2000 mL/min – 94 mL/min) or 1906 mL/min. In all calculations, the total gas flow to the patient must be considered, including oxygen, nitrous oxide, and vaporizer flows, for determination of anesthetic requirements.

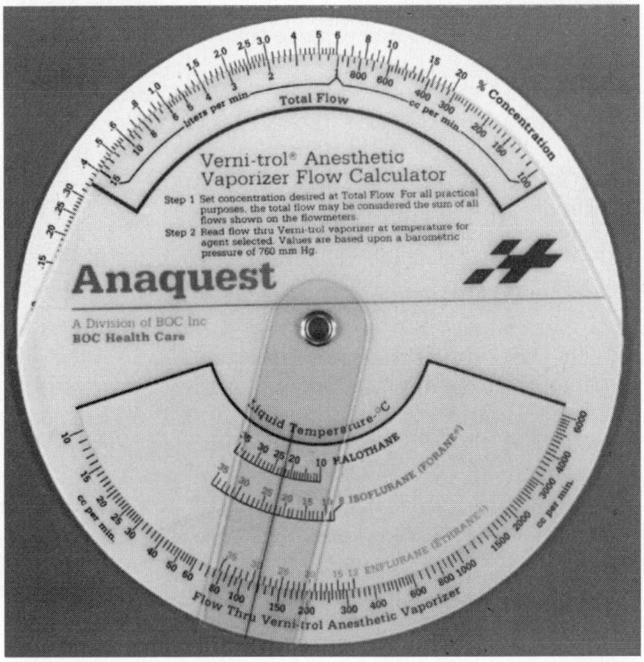

Using similar computations for methoxyflurane at 20° C (VP = 23 mm Hg), a maximum vaporizer output of 3% can be predicted. Thus, with 2 L/min of total fresh gas flow to the breathing system and a desired concentration of 1%, 20 mL/min of methoxyflurane (1% times 2000 mL = 20 mL) must be delivered to the breathing system. About 647 mL of oxygen must enter the vaporization chamber to deliver 20 mL/min of methoxyflurane (20 mL = 3% · X, where X is the total gas flow exiting the vaporization chamber; thus, X = 667 mL, and 667 mL – 20 mL = 647 mL). Therefore, 647 mL/min of oxygen must be delivered to the vaporization chamber to produce a total output of 667 mL/min, including 20 mL of methoxyflurane. The bypass flow must then be equal to 1333 mL/min, for a total flow of 2 L/min to the breathing system.

Most of the hazards associated with measured-flow vaporizers relate to incorrect use, including errors in calculation of the output of vapor, failure to turn on the vaporizer flowmeter or the vaporizer circuit control valve, and careless handling of the vaporizer during filling and transport. With tipping, liquid anesthetic may enter the discharge tube of the vaporizer, ultimately delivering very high concentrations of anesthetic to the breathing system. Overfilling is also possible in older models.(2) Older vaporizers may not be equipped for back-pressure compensation, and application of positive pressure ventilation may significantly increase the delivered concentration.(2) Reduced O_2 concentration and hypoxia were reported in human patients caused by an inflowing gas leak at a faulty O-ring on the base of a sidearm Verni-Trol.(29) Later models of the same machine incorporated a check valve to prevent loss of fresh gas flow. Finally, flow rates below the lowest mark on the scale for the vaporizer's flowmeter should not be extrapolated.

Fig. 14–40. A circular slide rule for calculation of oxygen flows for an anesthetic machine with a measured-flow vaporizer. The rule can be used for several different anesthetics at various total flow rates over a range of temperatures. This circular slide rule shows that 120 mL of oxygen must be supplied to the vaporizer to produce 3% halothane at a total gas flow rate of 2 L/min at a vaporizer temperature of 23° C.

Table 14–4. Flow Rates of O_2 (mL/min) from the vaporizer flowmeter of a measured-flow (saturation) vaporizer required to deliver 1%, 2%, 3%, 4%, and 5% halothane to the breathing system when the total maintenance flow rates (O_2, N_2O, and halothane) are 1, 2, 3, 4, and 5 L/min and the temperature of the liquid halothane is 21° C (15)

Total Flow →	1 L/min	2 L/min	3 L/min	4 L/min	5 L/min
1% Halothane	20	40	60	80	100
2% Halothane	40	80	120	160	200
3% Halothane	60	120	180	240	300
4% Halothane	80	160	240	320	400
5% Halothane	100	200	300	400	500

Some measured-flow vaporizers, including the Verni-Trol on the Ohio DM 5000 anesthesia machine (2) and the vaporizer on the Pitman-Moore 980 veterinary anesthesia machine (Fig. 14–41), which was designed specifically for methoxyflurane (22, 30), were calibrated for the flowmeter to the vaporizer to measure in cubic centimeters (milliliters) per minute of anesthetic vapor, rather than in mL/min of oxygen flow to the vaporizer. Applying the common calculations (22, 31) or slide rule calculators for Copper Kettles or Verni-Trols to determine output for these vaporizers will result in a delivered concentration that is greater than expected. Volatile anesthetics other than methoxyflurane should not be used in the Pitman-Moore 980 machine's vaporizer.(22, 30)

MAINTENANCE OF VAPORIZERS

Vaporizers should be conscientiously maintained. In general, the best policy is to follow the manufacturer's guidelines for care and servicing of vaporizers. Recom-

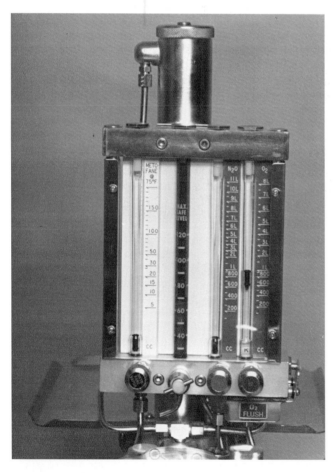

Fig. 14–41. Pitman-Moore 980 Veterinary Anesthesia Machine (Washington Crossing, New Jersey). This machine includes a Verni-Trol vaporizer with the oxygen flowmeter (left, white background) to the vaporization chamber calibrated in milliliters per minute of methoxyflurane vapor. (From Hartsfield, S.M. Machines and Breathing Systems for Administration of Inhalation Anesthetics. In: Principles and Practice of Veterinary Anesthesia. Edited by C.E. Short. Baltimore: Williams & Wilkins, 1987.)

mendations for maintenance vary. Returning a vaporizer to the manufacturer yearly for cleaning and calibration has been suggested.(32) One source recommends calibration and testing for leaks every 3 to 6 months.(3) Maintenance should be performed on a vaporizer if, based on the responses of patients, the dialed anesthetic concentration is suspected to be erroneous or if any of the components of the vaporizer function improperly (e.g., control dial is difficult to adjust). Servicing, as recommended by the manufacturer, includes an evaluation of operation, cleaning, changing of filters, replacement of worn parts, and recalibration.(2) Halothane and methoxyflurane contain preservatives (thymol and butylated hydroxytoluene, respectively) that do not vaporize and collect in the vaporization chambers and on the wicks, potentially affecting anesthetic output. Vaporizers should be periodically drained to eliminate these preservatives. Vaporizers should not be overfilled or tipped when filled. Vaporizers should be emptied before removal from the anesthesia machine for service. In the past, flushing a vaporizer with ether to dissolve preservatives that collect in the vaporizer has been recommended. Owing to the flammability and explosiveness of ether, extreme caution should be exercised. Flushing the vaporizer does not eliminate the need for regular service by a certified vaporizer technician.

USE OF THE WRONG ANESTHETIC IN AN AGENT-SPECIFIC VAPORIZER

Using an agent-specific vaporizer for an anesthetic for which the vaporizer is not calibrated is problematic, especially if the introduction of the wrong anesthetic is unintentional (i.e., the operator does not realize the mistake). A low output of anesthetic is the expected result if an anesthetic with a low vapor pressure is placed into a vaporizer designed for a drug with a higher vapor pressure. Conversely, a highly volatile anesthetic in an agent-specific vaporizer designed for a drug with a lower vapor pressure is likely to produce a high, potentially lethal concentration. The differential potencies of the drugs in question would be expected to affect the depth of anesthesia in either situation.

During the introduction of isoflurane into veterinary anesthesia, it was commonly administered with agent-specific, halothane vaporizers that were not recalibrated for isoflurane. Because the vapor pressures of halothane and isoflurane are similar, the output was not expected to differ greatly from the control dial setting. Indeed, halothane vaporizers produce concentrations of isoflurane that are reasonably close to the dial setting for halothane.(33) Nevertheless, current manufacturer recommendations are against the use of isoflurane in halothane-specific vaporizers, and vice versa.(3) Depending on the vaporizer and conditions of operation, isoflurane in a halothane vaporizer may produce 25 to 50% more vapor than expected, and halothane in an isoflurane-specific vaporizer usually yields a delivered concentration that is lower than

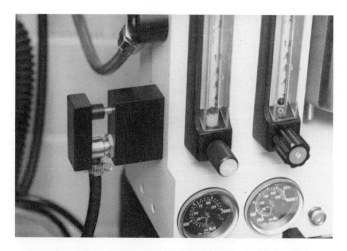

Fig. 14–42. Common gas outlet on a Drager Anesthesia Machine. The retaining device designed to prevent an accidental disconnection at the common gas outlet is in the closed position.

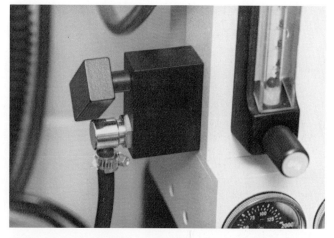

Fig. 14–43. Common gas outlet on a Drager Anesthesia Machine. The retaining device designed to prevent an accidental disconnection at the common gas outlet is in the open position.

expected.(3) If isoflurane is to be used in an agent-specific halothane vaporizer, the vaporizer should be serviced and completely recalibrated for isoflurane. Complete calibration implies that the vaporizer has been tested for accuracy with an anesthetic gas analyzer (e.g., Beckman LB2 Medical Gas Analyzer) at various carrier gas flows and various temperatures to assure reliable function.

Common Gas Outlet

The common gas outlet is the site from which gases that have passed through the flowmeters, vaporizer (VOC), and flush valve exit the anesthesia machine on the way to the breathing system. Typically, there is a 15-mm i.d. opening to which a fitting with rubber tubing attaches (Fig. 14–21). The other end of the tubing connects to the fresh gas inlet of the breathing circuit. In some simple veterinary anesthesia machines with VOC vaporizers, all gases flow directly from the vaporizer outlet to the fresh gas inlet of the breathing system.

Disconnections at the common gas outlet, the vaporizer outlet, or the fresh gas inlet can cause loss of gas flow to the breathing system. The ASTM standard requires that the common gas outlet incorporate a retaining device to prevent accidental disconnection (Figs. 14–42 and 14–43).(1) Disconnects should be detected during the checkout of the machine and breathing system before each case, but disconnects can occur during use of the machine if a retaining mechanism is not present.

A disconnection from the common gas outlet or from the outlet of the vaporizer (Fig. 14–44) during an anesthetic procedure may not be recognized immediately in a spontaneously breathing patient. With a circle system and a VOC, low F_IO_2, increased respiratory efforts, and light anesthesia are likely. Some circle systems (Matrx VMS Small Animal Circle) incorporate an air intake valve (negative pressure relief valve; Fig. 14–45) to entrain room air when the fresh gas flow is inadequate. With a nonrebreathing system and an

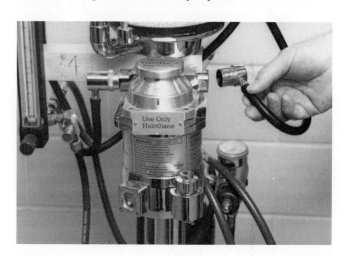

Fig. 14–44. Outlet on a Fluotec 3 vaporizer on a Fraser Harlake Small Animal Anesthesia Machine (Orchard Park, New York). The outlet connector is attached to a rubber hose that directs anesthetic and carrier gas to the circle system. Alternately, the rubber hose could be attached to one of the Mapleson systems. A faulty connection to the vaporizer or disconnection of the rubber hose could be responsible for interfering with the delivery of oxygen and anesthetic to the breathing system.

outlet disconnect, exhaled CO_2 will be rebreathed, low F_IO_2 is probable, and the patient will appear lightly anesthetized with increased respiratory efforts. The use of an O_2 analyzer for continuous evaluation of inspired gases allows early detection of this problem.

Breathing Systems

Anesthetic breathing systems deliver anesthetic gases and oxygen to the patient, remove carbon dioxide from exhaled gases, and usually provide a means to manually support ventilation. Spontaneously breathing patients inhale and exhale through the breathing system, and the breathing system should be able to supply enough gases to meet the peak inspiratory demands of the patient.

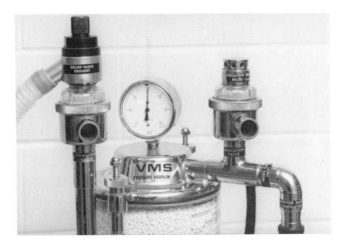

Fig. 14–45. Air-intake valve (negative pressure relief valve) on the dome of the inspiratory one-way valve of a circle system on a Fraser Harlake Small Animal Anesthesia Machine. The valve is designed to entrain room air if the supply of fresh gas to the circle breathing system is interrupted. In addition, the pop-off valve is attached to the expiratory one-way.

The breathing system adds resistant to the flow of gases, and the diameter of the breathing tubes and other conduits is a major factor in determining the amount of resistance. Doubling the radius decreases the resistance 16 times. Halving the length of the circuit halves the resistance. Changing the direction of gas flow or routing gases through restrictive orifices creates turbulent flow and increases resistance. Therefore, breathing systems should be as short as practical, with maximum diameters in the conduits and the fewest bends and restrictions in the path of gas flow.(2) Generally, the endotracheal tube has the smallest luminal diameter of the breathing apparatus, and the largest tube that is practical should be selected.

Classification of breathing systems has been called "a favorite pastime among anesthesiology personnel." (3) Most systems of classification are confusing, not exclusive, and not helpful to veterinary students or personnel. When referring to a breathing system in the veterinary or medical literature, the system should be named and physically described, the fresh gas flow rates should be stated, and the patient's body weight and/or oxygen consumption should be listed.(5, 34) This eliminates the need for cumbersome, obscure classification systems.

SYSTEMS USING CHEMICAL ABSORPTION OF CARBON DIOXIDE

Circle and to-and-fro breathing systems utilize a chemical absorbent for exhaled carbon dioxide. They are termed *rebreathing* systems because part or all of the exhaled gases, after extraction of carbon dioxide, flow back to the patient. In contrast to *nonrebreathing* systems, rebreathing systems conserve anesthetic, oxygen, heat, and moisture, but impart more resistance to ventilation. Rebreathing systems are relatively expen-

sive to purchase, but comparatively economic to operate.

Circle Systems. Pediatric, standard adult (small animal), and large animal circles differ primarily in their internal diameters and volumes. Arbitrarily, pediatric circles have been recommended for veterinary patients weighing less than 6.8 kg (15 lb), standard adult circles for patients between 6.8 kg and 135 kg (300 lb), and large animal circles for larger patients.(5) However, choosing the size of circle system for a veterinary patient may be influenced by the species, the practical availability of equipment, the type of ventilation used, and the anesthesiologist's preferences. Special pediatric circles with small absorbers are no longer commercially available.(3) Currently in human anesthesia, a pediatric circle usually refers to a standard (adult) absorber assembly, short breathing tubes of small diameter (15 mm i.d.), and a small bag.(3)

All circle systems have the same basic components, arranged so that gases move in only one direction (Figs. 14–28 and 14–29). Exhaled gases enter the Y-piece and flow through the expiratory breathing tube and the expiratory one-way valve. Gases may enter the reservoir bag before or after coursing through the CO_2 absorbent canister. On inspiration, gases exit the reservoir bag and travel through the inspiratory one-way valve, the inspiratory breathing tube, and the Y-piece to the patient.

Components of the Circle System

Y-Piece. The Y-piece is usually constructed of plastic and unites the endotracheal tube connector and the inspiratory and expiratory breathing tubes. The Y-piece contributes to the system's mechanical dead space, but a septum may be present in the Y-piece to decrease dead space. It has been argued that the amount of dead space in a standard, adult (small animal) Y-piece is not significantly greater than that in a nonrebreathing system.(35) A standard adult Y-piece has a 15-mm female port for the endotracheal tube connector, and this port may have a 22-mm o.d. to accept a mask. The two 22-mm male ports connect to the breathing tubes. Disposable systems may have the Y-piece and the breathing tubes permanently attached to each other. The dimensions of the Y-piece in large animal circles vary between manufacturers, but approximate 50 mm (2 inches).

Breathing Tubes. Breathing tubes are usually made of rubber or plastic, and serve as flexible, low-resistance conduits between the Y-piece and the one-way valves. Corrugations reduce the likelihood of obstructions if the tubes are bent. Breathing tubes add length and volume to the system, and increase resistance to ventilation; the tubes should have an internal diameter larger than the internal diameter of the patient's endotracheal tube. Standard adult breathing tubes have an internal diameter of 22 mm, and have been recommended for small animals weighing more than 7 kg.(36) Fifteen-mm i.d. tubes are available for smaller patients, and 50-mm i.d. (2-inch) breathing tubes are used with large animal circle systems. Breathing tubes do not contribute to mechanical dead space if the one-way valves are functional.

One-Way (unidirectional) Valves. These paired valves direct gas flow away from the patient on expiration and toward the patient on inspiration, preventing the rebreathing of exhaled gases before they pass through the absorbent canister. Gases enter a unidirectional valve from below, raise the disc, and pass under the dome (Fig. 14–46) to the reservoir bag, the absorbent canister, or the inspiratory breathing tube, depending on the location of the valve and the design of the circle. The one-way valves are usually attached to the canister on modern circle systems, but some older systems located the one-way valves within the Y-piece where they were more likely to become incompetent. Valves contribute to the resistance of breathing and should be inspected regularly to assure proper function.

Fresh Gas Inlet. The fresh gas inlet is the location at which gases from the common gas outlet of the anesthesia machine or from the outlet of the vaporizer enter the circle system. The fresh gas inlet is located on the absorbent canister near the inspiratory one-way valve or on the inspiratory one-way valve. Entry of fresh gases on the inspiratory side of the circle minimizes dilution of fresh gases with exhaled gases with a VOC, prevents absorbent dust from being forced toward the patient, and reduces loss of fresh gases through the pop-off valve.

Pop-Off Valve. The pop-off valve (adjustable pressure-limiting valve, relief valve, or overflow valve; Fig. 14–47) vents gases to the scavenger system to prevent the buildup of excessive pressure within the circle, and it allows rapid elimination of anesthetic gases from the circle when 100% oxygen is indicated. The

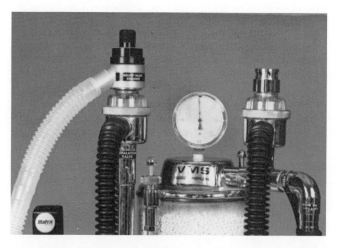

Fig. 14–47. Pop-off valve and manometer on a circle breathing system of a Fraser Harlake VMS Anesthesia Machine. The exhaust port (19 mm o.d.) of the pop-off valve is attached to clear corrugated tubing, which directs waste gases to the scavenging system. The air intake valve is mounted on the top of the dome for the inspiratory (right) one-way valve, and functions to entrain room air if the fresh gas supply to the circle system fails.

exhaust port of the pop-off valve through which overflow gases enter the scavenger system is designated to have a 19- or 30-mm male connector according to ASTM standards (1, 3), although older overflow valve ports were sized at 22 mm o.d. A pop-off valve should vent gases at pressures of 1 to 2 cm H_2O when it is fully opened. Several types of pop-off valves are available, but those with a spring-loaded disc are common. The pop-off valve is most convenient and relatively conservative with absorbent if it is located between the expiratory one-way valve and the absorbent canister. This location limits waste of fresh gases during exhalation. The pop-off valve is a major safety feature of a circle breathing system regardless of the mode of operation of the circle (e.g., closed, low-flow, or semi-closed fresh gas flow rates). The pop-off valve is designed to prevent the inadvertent buildup of pressure, and it should remain open except during the administration of positive pressure ventilation.

Reservoir Bag. The reservoir bag is located on the absorber side of the circle, either upstream or downstream from the canister depending on the manufacturer. The reservoir bag attaches to the bag port, the outside diameter being 22 mm for small animal circles and 50 mm (2 inches) for large animal circle systems. Gas from an appropriately sized reservoir meets the patient's peak inspiratory flow demands and provides compliance in the system during exhalation.(3) The bag also provides a mechanism for assisted or controlled ventilation. Excursions of the bag during spontaneous ventilation allow the anesthetist to assess respiratory rate and to roughly estimate the tidal volume. In addition, if the pop-off valve is inadvertently left closed, the bag provides a compliant area of the system to prevent the immediate buildup of excessive pressure.

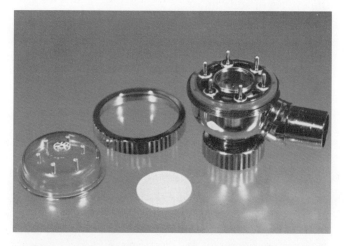

Fig. 14–46. Components of a unidirectional valve (North American Drager, Telford, Pennsylvania) of a circle breathing system. From the left, the plastic dome, the retaining ring for the dome, the valve itself, and the valve housing are depicted. (From Hartsfield, S.M. Machines and Breathing Systems for Administration of Inhalation Anesthetics. In: Principles and Practice of Veterinary Anesthesia. Edited by C.E. Short. Baltimore: Williams & Wilkins, 1987.)

Ideally, the bag should not allow pressures to exceed about 60 cm of H$_2$O.(3) The minimum size of the reservoir should be six times the patient's tidal volume, but as a matter of practicality, the bag's volume should exceed the patient's inspiratory capacity. Therefore, "a spontaneous deep breath should not empty the bag." (4) One-, 2-, 3-, and 5-liter bags are common for small animal circle systems, and 15-, 20-, or 30-liter bags are used for large animals. An optimally sized bag allows the anesthetist to manually support ventilation comfortably and to observe ventilatory excursions. An unnecessarily large bag is cumbersome, impairs monitoring, and slows changes in the inspired anesthetic concentration when settings on a VOC vaporizer are altered.

Manometer. A manometer (Fig. 14–47) is a pressure gauge that is usually attached to the top of the absorber assembly. It is calibrated in cm of H$_2$O, although it may have a scale in kPa or in mm of Hg. Primarily, the manometer is used to assess pressures during assisted or controlled ventilation.

Air Intake Valve. The air intake valve (negative pressure relief valve) is present on some veterinary anesthesia machines (Matrx VMS Small Animal) (Fig. 14–47). Located on the dome of the inspiratory one-way valve in these small animal circle systems, the valve will entrain room air in emergencies (i.e., absence of fresh gas inflow). If fresh gas flow is interrupted, the valve allows ambient air (21% oxygen) to enter the circle and prevents the patient from inspiring against a negative pressure and becoming hypoxic.

Vaporizers (VIC). Vaporizers can be located within the breathing system (Fig. 14–29), the Ohio #8 glass bottle and the Stephens vaporizer being the most likely ones located in this position. The primary requirement is that the VIC vaporizer be of a low-resistance type, since the patient must inspire through the vaporizer.

Absorber. The absorber assembly contains the canister for the chemical absorbent for carbon dioxide and is located between the one-way valves, on the side of the circle opposite the patient (Fig. 14–48). The canister is usually one plastic container or two stacked containers. For a specific patient, the canister should be large enough to contain an airspace between chemical granules that is equal to or greater than the patient's maximum tidal volume. The intergranular space is approximately 50% when a canister is filled with standard absorbent (4 to 8 mesh size).(4) Exhaled gases may enter the top or bottom of a canister, and baffles or annular rings (Fig. 14–49) in many absorbers move gases toward the center of the canister to compensate for lower resistance to gas flow near the canister wall. Without baffles or annular rings, channeling of gases and inefficient absorption of the CO$_2$ may occur. Internal tubes for gas return from an absorber may enhance the wall effect and gas channeling.(2) Some absorber units, especially those for large animals, have a drain in the bottom to discharge water that condenses from exhaled gases.

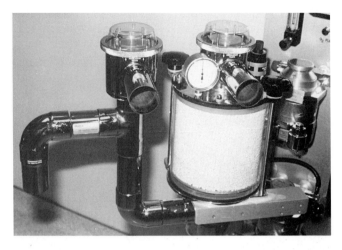

Fig. 14–48. Absorber assembly for a Matrx (Orchard Park, New York) large animal circle breathing system. Attached to the absorber are the unidirectional valves, the manometer, the ports for the breathing hoses and reservoir bag, and the pop-off valve.

The canister filled with absorbent, besides being a source of resistance during ventilation, is an important area for malfunctions in circle systems. The canister is removed regularly for changing the absorbent, and failure to adequately create a seal when replacing the canister causes leaks. Normal wear and tear may damage the canister, the caustic effects of soda lime may corrode metal parts, and aging results in deterioration of gaskets. Simply leaving soda lime granules on the gaskets can make a tight seal impossible. One report described the bypass of soda lime with resultant hypercarbia because of the disconnection of the diffuser foot from the conduction tube in the canister on a veterinary anesthesia machine.(37) Newer circle systems are constructed with materials less vulnerable to the effects of soda lime.

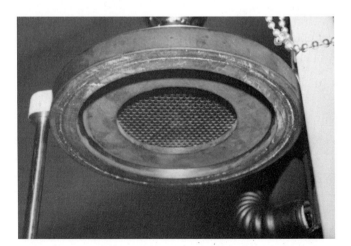

Fig. 14–49. An absorber assembly with an annular ring. The diameter of the ring, being smaller than the diameter of the canister, promotes dispersion of gases throughout the canister and helps to prevent preferential flow of gases next to the wall of the canister leading to the development of dead space.

Some circle systems were designed with a mechanism for purposely bypassing the absorbent canister (Fig. 14–50). The bypass was intended for use during the changing of soda lime and for intentionally elevating the inspired concentration of carbon dioxide.(2) If these obsolete systems are used in veterinary practices, the operator should understand the function of the bypass and its control apparatus and should not operate the circle in the bypass mode.

Chemical absorption of carbon dioxide is a fundamental function of circle and to-and-fro breathing systems. Depending on the fresh gas inflow, all or part of the exhaled CO_2 may be absorbed chemically. If the fresh gas flow approximates the patient's O_2 consumption, almost all exhaled CO_2 will be chemically neutralized. Chemical absorption of CO_2 allows lower fresh gas flows, reduces wastage of anesthetics and oxygen, and lowers the cost for anesthesia. With high fresh gas flows, much of the exhaled CO_2 escapes through the pop-off valve and into the scavenger system, and the dependence on chemical absorption of CO_2 is decreased.

Chemical Absorption of Carbon Dioxide

Calcium hydroxide is the primary component of soda lime and barium hydroxide lime, the two most common absorbents for carbon dioxide. Small amounts of sodium and potassium hydroxide in soda lime activate the reaction, and silica and kieselguhr are included to give hardness to the granules.(2, 3) Barium hydroxide lime is inherently hard owing to bound water molecules and does not require silica.(2) Fourteen to nineteen percent water is required in soda lime for optimal absorption of CO_2. Water formed during granule reactions with CO_2 can be useful in humidifying dry gases from the fresh

gas inlet but does not participate in the reactions of chemical absorption of CO_2. The overall chemical reaction of CO_2 with soda lime includes multiple steps (e.g., CO_2 first reacts with water to form carbonic acid), but can be summarized as follows:

$$2\,NaOH + 2\,H_2CO_3 + Ca(OH)_2 \rightarrow$$
$$CaCO_3 + Na_2CO_3 + 4H_2O + Heat$$

The granule size for chemical absorbents is typically 4 to 8 mesh and represents a compromise between absorptive activity and air flow resistance.(2) Small granules offer the most surface area for chemical reactions, but large granules impose less resistance to gas flow through the canister. Proper packing of a canister is necessary to prevent flow of gases over a single pathway in the canister, creating excessive dead space. Gentle shaking of the canister upon filling it with an absorbent will avoid loose packing and reduce channeling. Packing too tightly should be avoided to prevent formation of dust and increased resistance to ventilation.(4)

During evaluation of a rebreathing system, the anesthetist should confirm that the absorbent is functional. Fresh granules of $Ca(OH)_2$ are soft enough to be easily crushed, while expended granules have chemically changed to $CaCO_3$ and are hard (Fig. 14–51). Indicators of pH are added to absorbents to show color changes as chemical reactions proceed. Soda lime changes from white to violet as the granules are exhausted. The violet color may revert to white during storage but will reappear when the granules are exposed to CO_2 again. The absorption of CO_2 is an exothermic reaction, and a "heat line" should be detectable on the wall of the canister if CO_2 absorption is effective. Heat is particularly notable in canisters for large animals. The amount of CO_2 absorption is about 26 L/100 g (4), but efficiency may vary depending on the

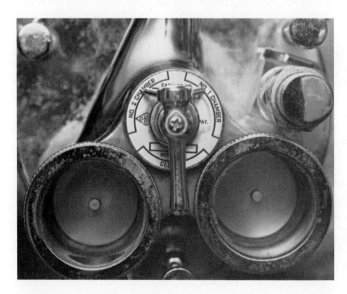

Fig. 14–50. The top of an absorber from an obsolete circle breathing system. The control on the absorber functions to direct exhaled gases through one or both chambers of the canister. With both indicators in the closed position, exhaled gases bypass the carbon dioxide absorbent completely.

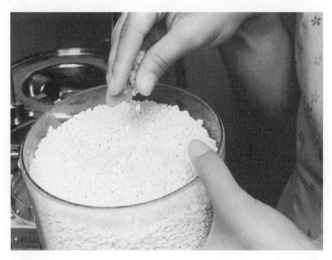

Fig. 14–51. Evaluation of the consistency of soda lime granules. Functional granules are relatively soft and easily crushed, while expended granules are hard.

Table 14–5. Values Reported for the Consumption of O_2 in Dogs

O_2 Consumption ($mL \cdot kg^{-1} \cdot min^{-1}$)	Conditions	Author
6 to 8 mL $\cdot$ kg^{-1} $\cdot$ min^{-1}	Anesthetized	Soma (46)
10 to 11 mL $\cdot$ kg^{-1} $\cdot$ min^{-1}	Anesthetized	Soma (46)
4 to 8 mL $\cdot$ kg^{-1} $\cdot$ min^{-1}	Awake, resting	Haskins (63)
9 to 14 mL $\cdot$ kg^{-1} $\cdot$ min^{-1}	Ketamine anesthesia	Haskins (63)
3 to 7 mL $\cdot$ kg^{-1} $\cdot$ min^{-1}	Barbiturate and inhalant anesthesia	Haskins (63)
4 to 7 mL $\cdot$ kg^{-1} $\cdot$ min^{-1}	Basal metabolic rate	Wagner and Bednarski (24)

design of the canister and the method of packing. When using a circle system with a chemical absorbent, the inspired carbon dioxide should be near zero.(2) Measuring the concentration of CO_2 in inspired gases, with 0.1 to 1.0% being acceptable (38, 39), is the most accurate way to determine if the absorbent is functional.(2, 3) Without such measurements, the absorbent should be exchanged when the color reaction is apparent in approximately two thirds of the absorbent.(2, 36)

Fresh Gas Flows for Circle Breathing Systems

The most appropriate fresh gas flow rates for circle systems are controversial. Semiclosed, low-flow, and closed circles are the options, and when all factors are considered, the anesthetist's personal preference usually determines the flow of fresh gas. Nevertheless, there are advantages to each mode of fresh gas flow. The terms *closed, low-flow* and *semiclosed,* in reference to circle breathing systems, refer to the fresh gas inflow compared to the metabolic needs of the patient. The terms do not denote any structural differences among the breathing systems, and they do not relate any information about the state of the pop-off valve (open or closed).

Closed Circle System. "Closed system anesthesia is a form of low-flow anesthesia in which the fresh gas flow equals uptake of anesthetic gases and oxygen by the patient and system." (3) Thus, the flow of O_2 into a closed circle approximates the patient's O_2 consumption, which varies with the patient's metabolic rate. Metabolic rate and O_2 consumption are influenced by the patient's body weight and body surface area, its temperature, its state of consciousness, and the type of anesthetic. Table 14–5 lists values for O_2 consumption in dogs as summarized in several publications on the use of breathing systems. Table 14–6 includes published recommendations for fresh gas flows for closed circle systems in dogs, and all fall within the minimum and maximum rates of O_2 consumption for dogs as listed in Table 14–5. In practice, observation of the reservoir bag allows the anesthetist to adjust the fresh gas flow to approximate the patient's uptake of gases when using a closed system.

Although a patient's O_2 consumption is used to guide the rate of fresh gas flow into a closed system, the minimum flow of carrier gas for accurate function of the vaporizer should be considered. Concentration-calibrated, variable-bypass vaporizers (VOC) require a certain minimum flow to assure proper performance, and flow below the minimum may cause erratic output of anesthetic. With a vaporizer, the lowest flow known to produce a reliable output should be the minimum acceptable flow for the breathing system. Strategies for using closed system anesthesia with both VIC and VOC vaporizers have been reviewed.(24)

Generally, N_2O is not used in a closed breathing system because of the potential for developing hypoxic gas mixtures with low inflow of O_2. If N_2O is administered in a closed system, continuous monitoring of F_IO_2 is imperative. With closed systems, denitrogenation of the system by emptying the reservoir bag through the pop-off valve and refilling the system with fresh gas should be done two to four times during the first 15 minutes of anesthesia and each 30 minutes thereafter to prevent exhaled nitrogen from diluting O_2 in the system.(31, 40) A closed system is completely dependent on chemical CO_2 absorption, and the quality of the absorbent should be assured before each use. Ideally, the inspired concentration of CO_2 should be monitored to assure proper function of the absorbent. Closed systems are more economic, retain more heat and humidity, and are less likely to produce operating room pollution than other systems.

Low-Flow Circle Systems. Low-flow anesthesia for small animals has been defined as an O_2 flow rate greater than the patient's O_2 consumption (4 to 7 mL $\cdot$ kg^{-1} $\cdot$ min^{-1}) but less than 22 mL $\cdot$ kg^{-1} $\cdot$ min^{-1}.(24) In the definition, 22 mL $\cdot$ kg^{-1} $\cdot$ min^{-1} was used because it is the lower limit of the traditional range of flow for a semiclosed circle system.(41) The advantages of a low-flow system are similar to those for a closed system, including economy, reduced waste gas, and some retention of heat and moisture.(42) The primary disadvantage of both closed and low-flow techniques relates to inadequate delivery of anesthetic from a con-

Table 14–6. Recommendatinos for O_2 Flow for Closed Circle Systems in Veterinary Anesthesia

Flow rate of O_2	Author(s)
11 mL $\cdot$ kg^{-1} $\cdot$ min^{-1}	Hartsfield (5)
4.4 to 11 mL $\cdot$ kg^{-1} $\cdot$ min^{-1}	Muir and Hubbell (41)
4 to 7 mL $\cdot$ kg^{-1} $\cdot$ min^{-1}	Wagner and Bednarski (24)
4.4 to 6.6 mL $\cdot$ kg^{-1} $\cdot$ min^{-1}	Muir and Hubbell (32)

centration-calibrated, variable bypass (VOC) vaporizer during mask induction or during the transition from injectable induction to inhalant maintenance. The suggested solution for this problem is the use of higher flows for the first 15 to 30 minutes of anesthesia followed by a change to low-flow technique after the uptake of inhalant anesthetic by the patient has decreased.(24) Similarly, changing depth of anesthesia is slower with low fresh gas flow rates. To increase anesthetic concentration in the system with a concentration-calibrated (VOC) vaporizer, the fresh gas flow should be increased temporarily to speed the process. To lower the anesthetic concentration in the system, anesthetic concentration should be decreased and fresh gas inflow should be increased with either a VOC- or a VIC-type vaporizer. For small animals, 10 to 15 mL · kg^{-1} · min^{-1} has been suggested as an appropriate flow rate for a low-flow system.(24)

Semiclosed Circle Systems. A semiclosed circle system is one in which the fresh gas inflow exceeds the uptake of oxygen and anesthetic by the patient, and traditional flows for semiclosed circle systems range from 22 to 44 mL · kg^{-1} · min^{-1}.(24, 41) A significant quantity of excess gas must be eliminated through the pop-off valve. The choice of flow rate for a semiclosed circle is based primarily on personal preference, but the patient's O$_2$ consumption times three has been a common guideline. For example, if a dog's O$_2$ consumption is 7 mL · kg^{-1} · min^{-1}, the fresh gas flow would be 21 mL · kg^{-1} · min^{-1}. Use of N$_2$O will increase total gas flow requirement. For 50% N$_2$O, O$_2$ flow would equal 21 mL · kg^{-1} · min^{-1} and N$_2$O flow, 21 mL · kg^{-1} · min^{-1}, with a total fresh gas flow of 42 mL · kg^{-1} · min^{-1}. With a semiclosed circle, nitrogen accumulation within the system is not significant because gases are rapidly eliminated through the pop-off valve. Nitrous oxide can be used safely, the inspired anesthetic concentration can be changed rapidly, and dependency on the CO$_2$ absorbent is less since CO$_2$ is partly eliminated through the pop-off valve into the scavenging system. However, retention of heat and humidity is reduced, and economy is less, compared to closed and low-flow systems.

Breathing systems inducing the least resistance to gas flow should be chosen for spontaneously breathing patients. Resistance to gas flow through a circle breathing system is influenced primarily by the pop-off valve, unidirectional valves, and CO$_2$ absorbent canister.(2) The total resistance in a circle system varies with fresh gas flow rate and the type of ventilation. High fresh gas flow rates can increase flow through the pop-off valve and therefore may increase resistance to ventilation. The pattern of ventilation affects the flow rate and therefore the resistance through the soda lime canister and the unidirectional valves.(2)

Resistance to breathing has been cited as a reason for not using adult circle systems for pediatric patients. However, Dorsch and Dorsch suggest that the use of circle systems in spontaneously breathing pediatric

patients may not be contraindicated solely on the basis of resistance.(2) For veterinary patients, it has been recommended that circle breathing systems are appropriate for healthy animals as small as 2.5 to 3.0 kg in body weight.(24, 43, 44)

In breathing circuits designed for large animals total resistance to constant flow in nine breathing circuits and measured resistance in certain component parts have been assessed.(45) Greater resistance occured with higher flows through all of the breathing circuits. The Drager and Fraser Sweatman circuits were intermediate in total resistance when all nine circuits were compared, and each circuit had individual parts that contributed significantly to resistance. The inspiratory and expiratory breathing tubes, absorbent canister, and inspiratory and expiratory valves each contributed significantly to resistance in at least one of the circuits. Low resistance was considered an advantage, and some components of large animal breathing circuits should be redesigned to decrease resistance.

To-and-Fro System. A to-and-fro system (Fig. 14–52) is a rebreathing system that is much less popular than circle and Mapleson systems. The to-and-fro system has a CO$_2$ absorbent canister located between the endotracheal tube connector and a reservoir bag. A pop-off valve and the fresh gas inlet are positioned between the canister and the endotracheal tube connector. A to-and-fro system is suitable for both large and small animals if proper canisters are available.(28, 46) In a to-and-fro system, gases pass back and forth through the absorbent during ventilation. Fresh gas flow rates in a to-and-fro system should be selected on the same basis as for circle systems. With low flows approximating the patient's O$_2$ consumption, CO$_2$ removal depends on chemical absorption. With higher flows, part of the expired CO$_2$ is vented through the pop-off valve.

Portability, simplicity, and ease of disassembly for cleaning are advantages of the to-and-fro system. Disadvantages are related to the position of the system, including the canister, next to the patient. Heat produced during CO$_2$ absorption may be transferred to the patient during inspiration, there is greater potential for inhalation of alkaline dust from the absorbent than with a circle system, and the system is quite cumbersome. Over time, channeling of gases through the canister may create dead space in the absorbent, causing inefficient absorption of CO$_2$. The horizontal position of the canister is probably less desirable than the vertical position used in most circle systems.(4) As with circle systems, denitrogenation during the early phases of anesthesia is important with low fresh gas flows.

MAPLESON SYSTEMS

Breathing systems that use no chemical absorbent for CO$_2$, but depend primarily on high fresh gas flow rates to flush exhaled CO$_2$ from the system, have been classified as Mapleson systems. They have been called *nonrebreathing systems* as a group; this terminology is technically incorrect because some rebreathing of exhaled gases occurs in most of these systems, especially with lower recommended flow rates.(5)

The Mapleson systems are simple and easy to use, are easily cleaned and sterilized, are lightweight and compact, can be positioned conveniently, have few moving parts, are relatively inexpensive, impart little resistance to respiration, do not require carbon dioxide absorbents, add minimal mechanical dead space, and allow the inspired concentration of anesthetic to be changed rapidly. The main disadvantage of the Mapleson systems is the requirement for higher flow rates of fresh gas, which decreases economy. High flow rates also promote hypothermia and drying of the respiratory tract. The Mapleson systems are diagrammed in Figure 14–53, and characteristics of the Mapleson systems are listed in Table 14–7.

Magill System. A Magill system (Fig. 14–54) is classified as a Mapleson A system and is characterized by a fresh gas inlet, an overflow valve near the patient, and a corrugated tube connecting the patient end of the system to a reservoir bag.(46) Fresh gas flows continuously into the reservoir bag and into the corrugated tubing, moving CO_2-rich gases through the overflow valve. The system is efficient during spontaneous ventilation, but during controlled ventilation, some rebreathing of expired gases occurs. Fresh gas inflow should approximate the patient's minute volume, (9), with flows less than 0.7 of minute volume leading to some rebreathing.(2) The flow of nitrous oxide should be calculated as a part of the total fresh gas inflow. The volume of the corrugated tubing and the reservoir bag should be equal to or greater than the patient's tidal volume. Because of the location of the overflow valve, the system is relatively cumbersome during controlled ventilation.

Bain Coaxial System. The Bain coaxial system (Fig. 14–55) is a modified Mapleson D system. It is designed as a tube within a tube.(9) The internal tube (0.7 mm i.d.) supplies fresh gases to the patient end of the system (Fig. 14–56), minimizing mechanical dead space. The Bain system accepts an endotracheal connector (15 mm) or a mask (22 mm). The external corrugated tube conducts exhaled gases from the patient to a reservoir bag. The reservoir bag may attach directly to the

corrugated tubing, in which case the pop-off valve is built into the bag, or the corrugated tubing may attach to a metal head with drilled channels and accommodations for the reservoir bag, the overflow valve, and optionally a manometer.(2, 3)

Recommendations for total fresh gas flow into a Bain system are variable for both human beings and animals. Recommendations have been based on minute volume, body weight, and body surface area.(2) During spontaneous ventilation, 200 to 300 $mL \cdot kg^{-1} \cdot min^{-1}$ has been recommended for human anesthesia (9), and 100 to 150 $mL \cdot kg^{-1} \cdot min^{-1}$ (36) and 100 to 130 $mL \cdot kg^{-1} \cdot min^{-1}$

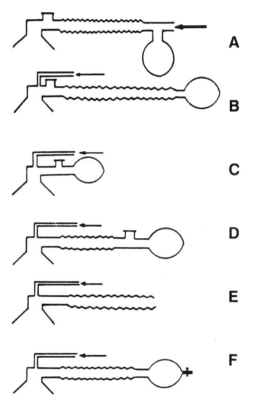

Fig. 14–53. Diagrams of each of the Mapleson breathing systems (A through F Mapleson systems). (From Rayburn, R.L. Pediatric anesthesia circuits. Annual Refresher Course Lectures, Lecture No. 117, Am Soc Anesth, 1981)

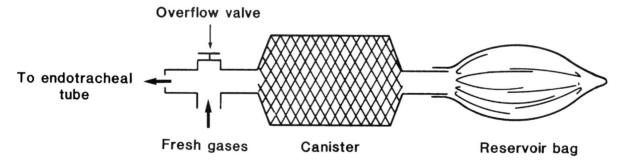

Fig. 14–52. Diagram of a to-and-fro system showing the basic component parts: patient connector, pop-off valve, fresh gas inlet, canister, and reservoir bag. (From Hartsfield, S.M. Machines and Breathing Systems for Administration of Inhalation Anesthetics. In: Principles and Practice of Veterinary Anesthesia. Edited by C.E. Short. Baltimore: Williams & Wilkins, 1987.)

Table 14–7. Characteristics of the Mapleson Breathing Systems

Class	Fresh Gas Inlet	Overflow Location	Presence of a Reservoir	Corrugated Tubing	Example System
A	Near the reservoir	Near the patient	Yes	Yes	Magill
B	Near the patient	Near the patient	Yes	Yes	*
C	Near the patient	Near the patient	Yes	No	*
D	Near the patient	Away from the patient†	Yes	Yes	*
MD‡	Near the patient	Away from the patient	Yes	Yes	Bain
E	Near the patient	Away from the patient	No	Yes	T-piece
F	Near the patient	Away from the patient†	Yes	Yes	Jackson-Rees

*No system in this classification is commonly used in veterinary anesthesia.
†The overflow may be located between the reservoir and the corrugated tubing of the system.
‡MD, modified Mapleson D system

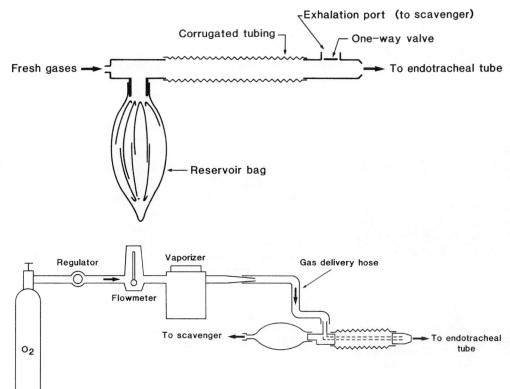

Fig. 14–54. Diagram of a Magill system illustrating the basic components and the entry of fresh gases. (From Hartsfield, S.M. Machines and Breathing Systems for Administration of Inhalation Anesthetics. In: Principles and Practice of Veterinary Anesthesia. Edited by C.E. Short. Baltimore: Williams & Wilkins, 1987.)

Fig. 14–55. Diagram of a Bain coaxial system attached to an anesthesia machine. Fresh gas flows from the outlet of the vaporizer or the common gas outlet of the anesthesia machine to enter the Bain system near the reservoir. Moving through the Bain's inner tube, fresh gas is delivered near the patient end of the system. Exhaled gases flow through the corrugated tubing to the reservoir and the overflow to the scavenging system.

(47) have been recommended for veterinary patients. Others have suggested 200 mL · kg⁻¹ · min⁻¹ (48) for patients weighing less than 7 kg, and a range of flow of 220 to 330 mL · kg⁻¹ · min⁻¹.(32) The fresh gas flow that will eliminate rebreathing during spontaneous ventilation with a Bain system differs significantly from patient to patient. After reviewing numerous references, Dorsch and Dorsch concluded that most studies recommended fresh gas flows of 1.5 to 3 times minute volume.(3) Less than 2 to 3 times the minute volume will result in some rebreathing of CO_2, but end-tidal CO_2 concentration may remain normal even with some

rebreathing of CO_2.(3) For spontaneously breathing patients, 440 to 660 mL · kg⁻¹ · min⁻¹ may be used for maintenance of anesthesia with the Bain system to assure that rebreathing of exhaled gases does not contribute to increases in $PaCO_2$. Without regular monitoring of carbon dioxide tensions or expired CO_2 values, the exact flow requirements are difficult to define for an individual patient. Minute volumes for dogs and cats range from 170 to 350 mL · kg⁻¹ · min⁻¹ and 200 to 350 mL · kg⁻¹ · min⁻¹, respectively.(49) Using these values for minute volume, an argument can be made for even higher flows than 660 mL · kg⁻¹ · min⁻¹.

In general, a total fresh gas flow of less than 500 mL/min or more than 3 L/min with a Bain system for animals that weigh less than 6.8 kg is not recommended. With controlled ventilation, $100 \text{ mL} \cdot \text{kg}^{-1} \cdot \text{min}^{-1}$ is apparently an adequate flow for fresh gases.(50) For larger patients maintained with an adult Bain system, lower total fresh gas flow (e.g., $100 \text{ mL} \cdot \text{kg}^{-1} \cdot \text{min}^{-1}$) may be appropriate. Use of Bain systems has been effective in dogs weighing up to 35.5 kg.(47) Fresh gas flows higher than usually recommended are indicated in situations of increased CO_2 production, increased dead space, and decreased minute ventilation.(3) Flow rates of two to three times minute volume have been recommended for hypoventilating animals in which controlled ventilation was not corrective.(47)

During spontaneous ventilation, a Mapleson D system has been shown to function identically to a Mapleson F system.(2) The Bain's coaxial design has been shown to be effective in reducing loss of heat and humidity (2), although the overall benefit in small veterinary patients maintained with relatively high fresh gas flow rates is questionable.

Ayre's T-Piece and Norman Mask Elbow Systems. Ayre's T-piece and Norman mask elbow systems (Fig. 14–57) equipped with an expiratory limb (corrugated tubing) and reservoir bag are classed as Mapleson F systems.(2) Without a reservoir bag, they are Mapleson

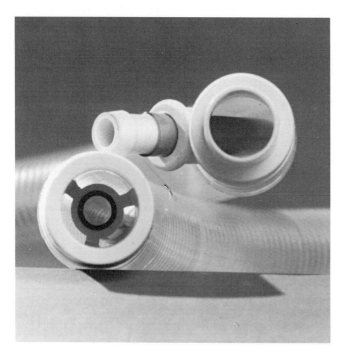

Fig. 14–56. The two ends of a Bain coaxial system showing the location for attachment of the reservoir bag (top right) and the endotracheal tube (lower left). Fresh gases enter at the reservoir end (Y-connection at the upper left) and move through the small inner tube to the patient end of the system (triangular supports). (From Hartsfield, S.M. Machines and Breathing Systems for Administration of Inhalation Anesthetics. In: Principles and Practice of Veterinary Anesthesia. Edited by C.E. Short. Baltimore: Williams & Wilkins, 1987.)

E systems. The T-piece itself is a T-shaped tube with an internal diameter of 1 cm. Fresh gas enters the tube from the side, perpendicular to the direction of gas flow during ventilation (Fig. 14–57). One end of the tube attaches to the endotracheal tube connector, and the other end attaches to an expiratory arm (corrugated tubing equivalent to one third of the patient's tidal volume) to which a reservoir bag may or may not be attached. The reservoir bag has an overflow valve. An Ayre's T-piece with an expiratory tube and reservoir is a Rees modification of an Ayre's T-piece or a Jackson-Rees system.(2)

During spontaneous ventilation, fresh gas flows to the patient during inspiration; during expiration and prior to the next inspiration, gas flows toward the reservoir. Gas flow follows the path of least resistance. Inspiratory flow requirements in excess of the fresh gas flow are obtained from the expiratory arm and reservoir. During expiration and before inspiration, high gas flow clears exhaled gases from the expiratory tube and washes out carbon dioxide. Such a system should have an internal diameter of at least 1 cm to minimize resistance.

Generally, two to three times the patient's minute volume is recommended to prevent dilution of the inspired anesthetic concentration and rebreathing of carbon dioxide with Mapleson F systems. If N_2O is used, the desired concentration is calculated using N_2O as a portion of the total fresh gas flow. Variable recommendations for the most appropriate flow rates to use with these systems exist in the veterinary literature.

In a Norman mask elbow system, the direction of gas flow into the system is parallel to the flow of gases into the endotracheal tube during inspiration and expiration (Fig. 14–57). The fresh gas inlet is located in the center of the patient end of the system. This location probably reduces dead space slightly more than the Ayre's T-piece system. Also, the patient end of the elbow accepts a standard mask (22 mm). Recommendations for flow rates, tube sizes and volumes, and reservoir sizes and volumes are similar to the Ayre's T-piece system. Controlled ventilation can be used with either system by closing the overflow valve and compressing the reservoir bag. To prevent rebreathing during controlled ventilation, the expiratory tube's volume should be greater than the patient's tidal volume.

Resistance to ventilation in the Mapleson systems is minimal (2), and this may be advantageous for small patients. The advantages of modern "nonrebreathing" systems for very small patients include decreased resistance to ventilation, better gas exchange, greater control of the depth of anesthesia, and fewer mechanical problems.(48) Hazards of nonrebreathing systems relate primarily to outflow occlusion, development of excessive airway pressure, and barotrauma to the lungs, including development of pneumothorax.

Care in positioning the Mapleson systems and judicious use of overflow valves during positive pressure ventilation are important considerations. Activation of

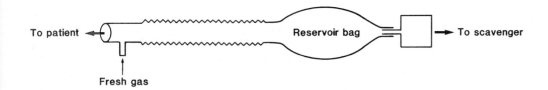

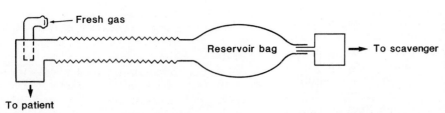

Fig. 14–57. Diagrams of Norman Mask Elbow (bottom) and Ayre's T-piece systems (top). (From Hartsfield, S.M. Machines and Breathing Systems for Administration of Inhalation Anesthetics. In: Principles and Practice of Veterinary Anesthesia. Edited by C.E. Short. Baltimore: Williams & Wilkins, 1987.)

the flush valve when a nonrebreathing system is being used can result in overpressurizing the respiratory system, volotrauma and subsequent pneumothorax. Therefore, the machine's flush valve should not be used when one of the Mapleson systems is connected to a patient.

SYSTEMS WITH NONREBREATHING VALVES

Numerous nonrebreathing valves (e.g., Stephens-Slater, Fink, Digby-Leigh) were designed for anesthesia breathing systems, but they are not commonly used today.(3) These breathing systems with one-way valves were cumbersome, and essentially have been replaced by the Mapleson and circle systems. Presently, nonrebreathing valves are used most in self-inflating bags for resuscitation or transport of patients requiring manual ventilation.

Stephens-Slater System. The Stephens-Slater system (Fig. 14–58) was common in veterinary anesthesia in the 1970s, but today is mainly of historical interest. The system was designed with two one-way valves, one directing gas from the reservoir to the patient and blocking exhaled gases from the reservoir and a second valve directing exhaled gases away from the system and preventing entry of ambient gases during inspiration. Fresh gases enter the system through the reservoir bag and move through the inspiratory valve to the patient. The recommended total fresh gas flow is equal to the patient's minute volume.(2, 46) The flow of N_2O, if used, is calculated as a part of the total fresh gas flow. Since the valves are located near the patient, the system is cumbersome, especially with manual ventilation during which the exhalation valve is held closed while the reservoir bag is compressed. The reservoir must be monitored closely to assure sufficient gas to meet inspiratory demands. This valved system added minimal dead space and resistance to respiration. However,

the valve flaps could stick and obstruct ventilation. The system was popular prior to the advent of scavenging, which presents some difficulty with the Stephens-Slater system.

Resuscitation Bags. Self-inflating resuscitation bags incorporate nonrebreathing valves (Chapter 17). As an example, an Ambu bag facilitates resuscitation and transport of apneic or anesthetized patients. Oxygen can be flowed into the reservoir bag to increase F_1O_2. When the bag is compressed, the increase in pressure closes the exhalation port and gases enter the patient's respiratory system. When pressure on the bag is released, gas flows from the patient's respiratory system through the exhalation port. With spontaneous breathing, the Ambu valve allows the patient to inhale room air only. The Ambu E2 is a modification that allows the patient to inhale both from the reservoir and from the exhalation port, creating a mixture of fresh gas and air. During controlled ventilation, all gases originate from the reservoir.(2) Other similar valves are also available.(2, 3)

CLOSED CONTAINERS AND MASKS

Closed Containers. Closed containers are used for oxygenation and inhalant inductions in small veterinary patients. Inhalant inductions have decreased in popularity because of the difficulty associated with scavenging of waste gases, especially as the anesthetized patient is removed from the chamber. Perhaps, the only completely effective way to assure elimination of waste anesthetic gases with this system is the concurrent use of a fume hood. The primary advantage of induction in a closed container is the reduced requirement for physical restraint of the patient. Induction in a closed container is very effective for aggressive cats and for some laboratory and small wild or exotic species. Often, the container can be placed

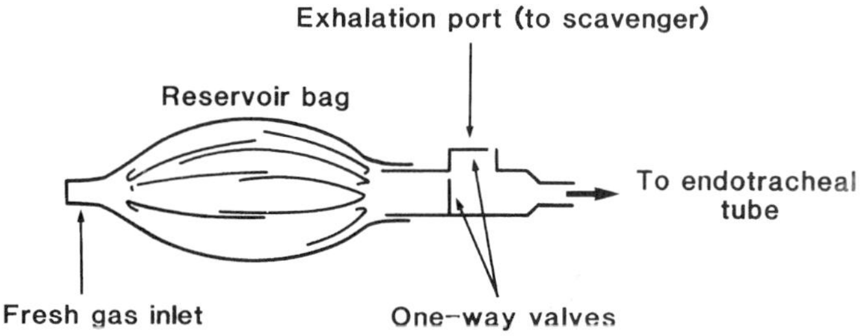

Fig. 14–58. Diagram of a Stephens-Slater system. (From Hartsfield, S.M. Machines and Breathing Systems for Administration of Inhalation Anesthetics. In: Principles and Practice of Veterinary Anesthesia. Edited by C.E. Short. Baltimore: Williams & Wilkins, 1987.)

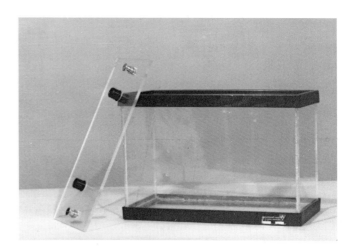

over the animal, eliminating the need for any physical restraint.

Most containers for inhalant inductions are constructed of glass, plexiglass, or other clear plastic materials (Fig. 14–59), allowing the patient to be observed during induction. Since obstruction of the airway is possible during a closed container induction, ventilatory efforts should be monitored throughout the process. The chamber should be no larger than necessary, but the animal should be able to lie in lateral recumbency without having to flex its neck. A chamber that is too small for the patient promotes airway obstruction. Excessive chamber volume slows the rate of rise of anesthetic concentration and the onset of induction. When the patient is induced and is manageable, it should be removed from the chamber, and the induction should be completed by mask.

Relatively high flows of fresh gas facilitate inductions in closed containers. The outlet of the chamber should be attached to a scavenger system when anesthetic is being administered. Chamber inductions should be done in a well-ventilated area, ideally, under a fume hood that vents all waste gases from the working environment. Depending on the size of the chamber and the body weight of the patient, total flow of fresh gas into the chamber should be approximately 2 to 5 L/min.(51) Low flow rates of fresh gases slow induction and contribute to the development of excitement. Oxygen should be administered for about 5 minutes before the introduction of inhalant anesthetic. Then, the concentration of the inhalant should be increased at 0.5% increments every 10 seconds until 4% to 4.5% halothane or isoflurane is being administered. Unless N_2O is contraindicated because of patient pathology, it can be used in concentrations of 60 to 70%.

Masks. Mask inductions (Fig. 14–60) are facilitated by anesthetic concentrations and fresh gas flows that are similar to those for closed containers. Mask inductions are smoothest in depressed, tranquilized, or sedated patients. Masks should fit snugly over the muzzle to minimize dead space, and the appropriate size for the patient should be used. A tight-fitting mask promotes a rapid induction and minimal contamination of the workplace with waste gases. A clear mask with a rubber diaphragm (Fig. 14–61) allows visualization of the nares and mouth during induction and creates a good seal around the animal's muzzle. The mask should be attached to a breathing system to provide a reservoir of

Fig. 14–59. Closed container for oxygenation and inhalant inductions in small patients. The container is clear so that the animal can be monitored during the induction process. The ports for the entrance of fresh gases and for attachment of a scavenging system are present on the lid.

gases to meet the patient's peak inspiratory flow demands, which may exceed the inflow of fresh gases. Most excess gases can be scavenged through the pop-off valve of the breathing system, but masking procedures should be done in a well-ventilated environment. High fresh gas flows (e.g., 3 to 5 L/min for most dogs and cats) during masking supply the oxygen demands of the patient, dilute and eliminate exhaled carbon dioxide, and provide inhalant anesthetic concentrations equivalent to the vaporizer setting (3–5%) for a relatively rapid induction.

Scavenging Waste Anesthetic Gases

Over the last two decades, the exposure of medical and veterinary personnel to waste anesthetic gases has become a significant concern. A bulletin from the American Veterinary Medical Association's Liability Insurance Trust recently stated the following: "Numerous studies in the United States and abroad have found no conclusive evidence that waste gases or trace amounts of waste gas cause specific health problems. There is enough evidence, however, to suggest that removal of gases from veterinary facilities will improve the occupational health of the veterinary staff." (52)

At present, the Occupational Safety and Health Administration (OSHA) has no set limits for exposure to anesthetics, but OSHA can enforce NIOSH (National Institute for Occupational Safety and Health) recommendations under the "general duty clause." The general duty of an employer is provision of a work environment that is "free from recognized hazards that are likely to cause death or serious physical harm." (53, 54) The recommended exposure limits from NIOSH vary from a maximum of 2 parts per million (ppm) for halogenated hydrocarbon anesthetics like halothane and isoflurane to an 8-hour time-weighted average exposure to N_2O of 25 ppm. Used together, 0.5 ppm is the limit for the halogenated agent with 25 ppm the limit for N_2O.(55) The American Conference of Governmental Industrial Hygienists (ACGIH) has recommended threshold limit values of 50 ppm for halothane and N_2O as 8-hour time-weighted averages.(56)

RECOMMENDATIONS FOR CONTROLLING WASTE GASES

Veterinary workers should be aware of potential risks so that they can take steps to minimize their exposure to the inhalant anesthetics. Women in the first trimester of pregnancy, individuals with hepatic or renal disease, and persons with compromise of the immune system appear to be at greatest risk.(57) The following considerations are important in regard to managing waste anesthetic gases:

1. All personnel should be educated about the potential health hazards associated with exposure to waste anesthetic gases.
2. Scavenger systems should be used with all anesthesia machines and breathing systems.
3. All rooms in which anesthetic gases are used should be well ventilated with an appropriate number of air exchanges (e.g., 15 air changes per hour).
4. Anesthetic machines and breathing systems should be maintained as leak-free as possible, and

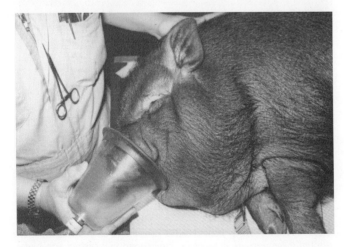

Fig. 14–60. Masking a tranquilized potbellied pig with isoflurane in oxygen administered with a transparent veterinary mask. The rubber diaphragm allows a good seal between the patient's snout and the mask, minimizing leakage.

the leakage tolerances should comply with established criteria (e.g., <300 mL/min at 30 cm of H_2O for a circle breathing system with the pop-off valve closed).(3)
5. A log documenting the performance and maintenance procedures for anesthesia machines, vaporizers, and breathing systems should be maintained.
6. Personnel should minimize spillage when filling vaporizers, and keyed filling mechanisms should be considered.
7. Periodic monitoring of anesthetic concentrations in induction, operating, and recovery rooms should be done to assure the efficacy of scavenging and other efforts to reduce contamination in the workplace.

Several ways of decreasing contamination of the occupational environment with anesthetic gases have been suggested:

1. Avoid spills when filling vaporizers.
2. Start gas flows only after intubation of the patient.
3. Use endotracheal tubes with inflated cuffs.
4. Occlude the Y-piece of the circle or the patient end of a Mapleson system if the system is disconnected from the patient.
5. Use a scavenging pop-off (APL) valve.
6. Discharge all gases through an effective scavenger system.
7. Flush breathing systems with O_2 before disconnecting the patient.
8. Use the minimum gas flow that promotes safe anesthesia.
9. Minimize the use of masks and closed containers. When using masks, be sure that they fit well, and use closed containers only in well-ventilated areas. Ideally, they should be used under a fume hood.
10. Maintain proper ventilation in work areas and minimize exposure to exhaled gases during the initial phases of the recovery period whenever possible.

Having anesthetic machines and breathing systems properly outfitted and functional for administration of anesthetic gases is essential for assuring the minimum amount of environmental pollution. Each machine should be leak-free, and each machine-breathing system combination should connect with a functional scavenger system. An efficient scavenging system is the most important factor in reducing trace gases, lowering ambient concentrations as much as 90%.(3)

Scavenging Systems

A scavenging system collects waste gases from the anesthetic breathing system and eliminates them from the workplace.(3, 57) The scavenger system is composed of a gas-collecting assembly, an interface, and a disposal system (Figs. 14–62 and 14–63). Depending on the system, various types of tubing connects these parts.

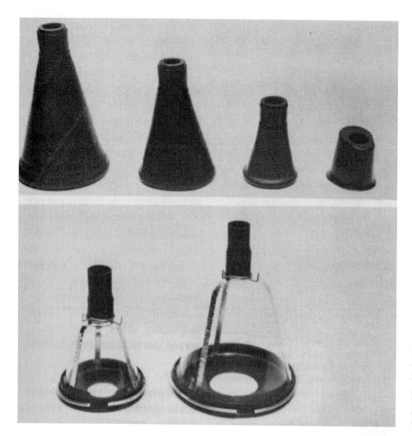

Fig. 14–61. Small animal masks of varying sizes. The clear masks with rubber diaphragms facilitate monitoring during the masking procedure, and they allow a good seal around the muzzle. A conical rubber mask of the correct size minimizes dead space under the mask. (From Lumb, W.V., and Jones, E.W. Veterinary Anesthesia, 2nd ed. Philadelphia: Lea & Febiger, 1984.)

THE GAS-COLLECTING ASSEMBLY

The gas-collecting assembly gathers waste gases from the breathing system. At present, the exhaust outlet from the pop-off valve (Fig. 14–47) on a circle system must be either 19 mm or 30 mm in diameter. The latter has been proposed as an international standard and "may be the only size available on future U.S. machines." (3) Twenty-two-millimeter connectors were used on older anesthesia machines, which permitted inadvertent interchange of scavenging hoses and breathing tubes. Depending on the location of the overflow in Mapleson systems (e.g., Bain system), devices connecting to the tail or the side of the reservoir bag serve as the gas-collecting assembly and attach to transfer tubing leading to the interface.

THE INTERFACE

The interface is intended to prevent the transfer of pressure changes in the scavenging system to the breathing system. The inlet to the interface should be 19 mm or 30 mm o.d., and the outlet can be of variable diameter (not 15 mm or 22 mm). Various interfaces are available (Fig. 14–62). An interface should provide positive pressure relief to protect the patient from occlusions of the scavenging system, negative pressure relief to limit the pressure effects of an active disposal system, and a reservoir for excess waste gas for use with active disposal systems. Interfaces may be opened or closed.(3)

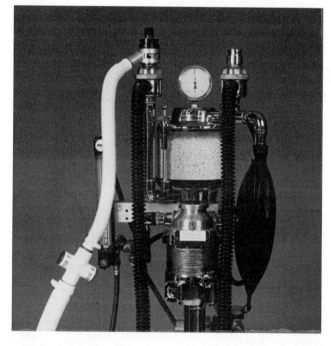

Fig. 14–62. A scavenging system (Vetroson, Summitt Hill Laboratories, Navesink, New Jersey) on a veterinary anesthesia machine showing the pop-off valve of the circle breathing system attached to the corrugated tubing of the scavenging system that directs waste gases to the disposal system. The T-shaped component includes air intake valves and is part of the interface that assists in the regulation of pressure in the scavenging system.

THE DISPOSAL SYSTEM

The disposal system can be passive or active. Passive systems include nonrecirculating ventilation systems, piping directly to the atmosphere, and absorption devices. Active systems include piped vacuum and active duct systems. A nonrecirculating ventilation system for the room allows the discharge of waste gases through an exhaust vent or grille. Discharging waste gases directly to the atmosphere is suitable for many veterinary hospitals because the distance from the gas-collecting assembly on the breathing system to the outside can be relatively short. Such systems can be affected by wind currents, and should be designed so that water, wind, dust, and insects and other pests cannot enter the system from the outside.

Canisters containing activated charcoal (Fig. 14–63) will adsorb halogenated hydrocarbon anesthetics with a varying degree of efficiency. They are simple to use and portable. The effectiveness of absorption varies with different brands, styles of canisters, and rates of flow through the canisters. These devices must be changed regularly, making them rather expensive to use, and they do not absorb N_2O.(3) In general, other methods for scavenging waste gases are preferable, with absorption systems reserved for situations where more reliable methods are not accessible.

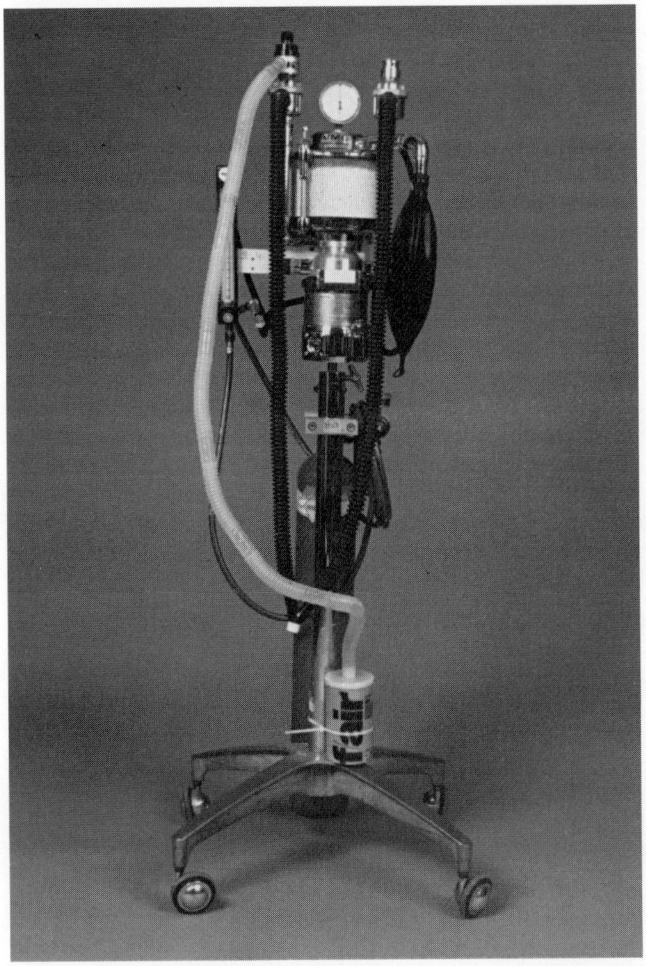

Central vacuum systems provide convenient disposal systems for hospitals with such systems already in place. The system should be able to create a flow of at least 30 L/min, and the system functions best when the operator can manually adjust the flow.(3) The location for discharge of waste gases must be in an appropriate location, and not situated where waste gases can reenter the ventilation system of the hospital. Ideally, a central vacuum system dedicated to scavenging, with another system to provide suction for other hospital needs (e.g., surgical suction), is most desirable.

An active duct system with a high volume of flow and a low negative pressure provides an excellent means of gas-disposal (Fig. 14–64). Negative pressure is generated by a fan, pump, or other device in a large duct that is connected to smaller ducts that open into the room at the site of use. Such systems are effective, but regular maintenance is required to assure that the fan or pump is operational. This system is not affected by wind currents.

With any disposal system, the ultimate elimination of gas must be at a point that prevents reentry

Fig. 14–63. A scavenging system including the pop-off valve, which is connected to a canister containing activated charcoal (F/air, Omnicon, Critical Care Products, Houston, Texas). This system can be used for halogenated hydrocarbon anesthetics, but not for nitrous oxide.

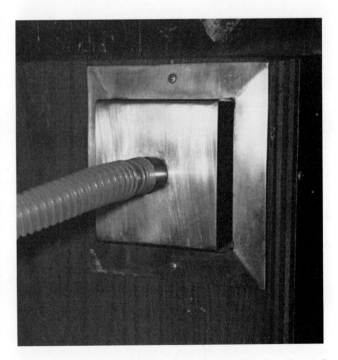

Fig. 14–64. Corrugated tubing from the pop-off valve of a circle breathing system attached to a high-volume, low-pressure scavenging system (an active duct system). Air is constantly entrained on each side of the stainless steel plate, while waste gas from the breathing system enters the scavenging system through the corrugated tubing.

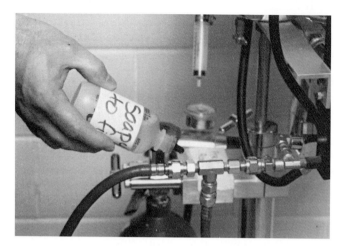

Fig. 14–65. Searching for leaks in the gas piping system of an anesthesia machine. With the cylinder valve on and pressure on the system, soapy water is applied to areas with potential for leaks. Bubbles will form if gas leaks are present.

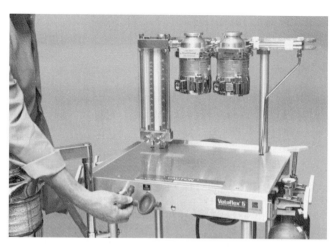

Fig. 14–66. Universal Negative-Pressure Leak Test. With all gases off and the vaporizer off, a compressed rubber bulb is attached to the common gas outlet of the anesthesia machine. The bulb should not reinflate in less than 10 seconds. The test should be repeated with the vaporizer control on.(16)

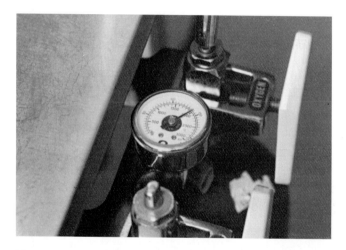

Fig. 14–67. Oxygen cylinder with the pressure gauge reading 2000 psi. An oxygen cylinder should have at least 500 psi before using the cylinder and anesthesia machine for a patient. With oxygen flowmeters off, the cylinder valve should remain on to allow evaluation of the machine for slow leaks.

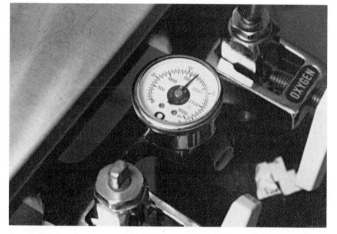

Fig. 14–68. Oxygen cylinder with the pressure gauge reading at 1700 psi after 15 minutes with the cylinder valve open. If the cylinder pressure was 2000 psi at the start of the test and the flowmeters were off, a significant leak is present and should be corrected before using the anesthesia machine for a patient.

of gases to any area of the hospital. The discharge site should be located away from any air intake vents for the building, and the prevailing winds should not direct exhausted gases toward the air intake vents for the building.

Anesthesia Apparatus: Checkout Recommendations

Evaluation of anesthesia machines and breathing systems is important to ensure safety for personnel and patients. For the patient, delivery of appropriate concentrations and amounts of oxygen and anesthetics is essential. For personnel, the machine and breathing system should be maintained to prevent contamination of the workplace with anesthetics. The Food and Drug Administration published "Anesthesia Apparatus

Checkout Recommendations" for the anesthesia gas delivery system in 1986 and recommended that this checkout or a reasonable equivalent be conducted before administering anesthesia. The intent was improvement of patient safety.(58, 59) Recommendations for checkout of veterinary machines have been published.(60)

The high-, intermediate-, and low-pressure areas of the anesthesia apparatus should be evaluated.(1-3) The high-pressure area includes gas cylinders, hanger yokes, yoke blocks, high-pressure hoses, pressure gauges, and regulators. These components are exposed to pressures up to 2200 psi for O_2 and up to 745 psi for N_2O. Testing should include inspection for loose connections and audible leakage, pressure checks (loss of pressure when cylinder valves are open and flow-meters are off), and use of soapy water solutions to "snoop" for leaks (creation of bubbles) especially at joints (Fig. 14–65). The intermediate pressure area (approximately 40 to 50 psi) includes pipeline inlets, conduits from pipeline inlets to flowmeters, and con-duits from regulators to flowmeters, the flowmeter assembly, and the O_2 flush apparatus. Tests include visual inspection, listening for leaks, and use of soapy water solutions. The low-pressure area includes the VOC vaporizer(s), conduits from the flowmeters to the vaporizer, a conduit from the VOC to the common gas outlet, and a conduit from the common gas outlet to the breathing system. Pressures are slightly above atmospheric. Routine tests include visual inspection and pressure checks with the breathing system. In many anesthesia machines, pressure applied to the breathing system affects the low-pressure area of the machine. Some newer anesthesia machines have check valves near the common gas outlet.

A universal negative-pressure leak test has been proposed for contemporary anesthesia machines to evaluate the low-pressure area. The test requires a simple suction bulb.(16) The flowmeters and vaporizers are off during the test. The suction bulb is attached at the common gas outlet and squeezed until it fully collapses, creating a vacuum in the low-pressure area (Fig. 14–66). If the bulb reinflates in less than 10 seconds, a significant leak is present. The test is repeated with the control dial of the vaporizer on to detect any internal leaks that might not be found with the vaporizer off. This test differentiates between leaks in the low-pressure area of the machine (vaporizer) and the breathing system. The test is capable of detecting leaks as small as 30 mL/min and has been described as extremely reliable.

Anesthetic machines should be checked out each day before anesthetizing the first patient, and the breathing system should be evaluated before each patient. The operation manual for individual anesthesia machines

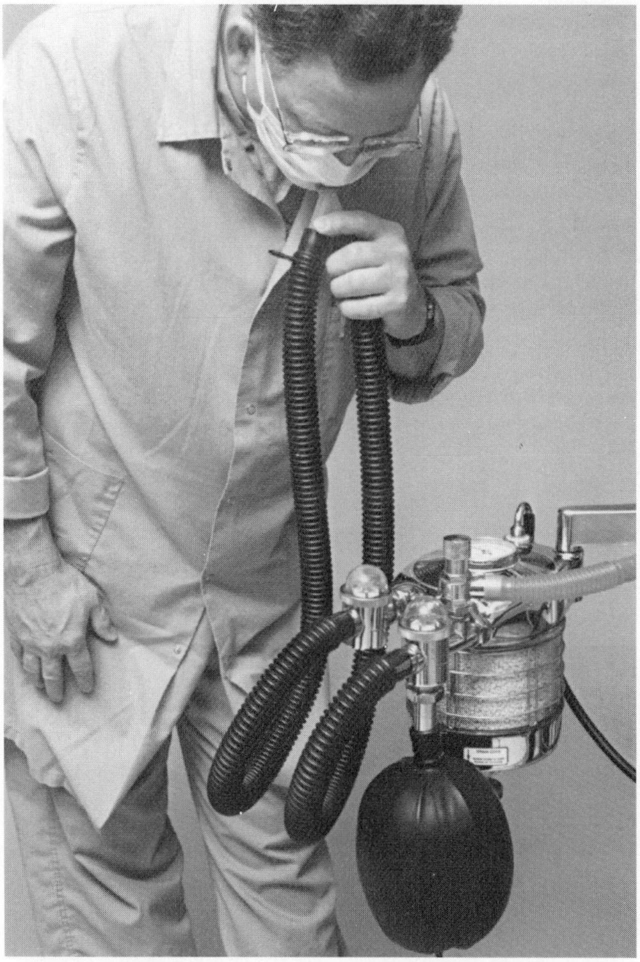

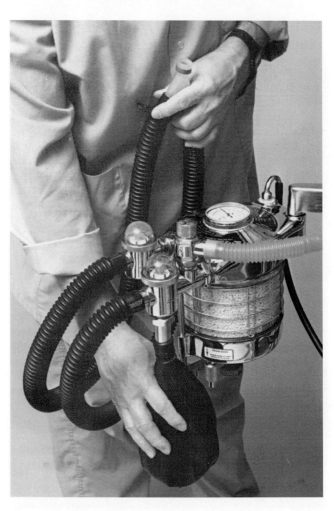

Fig. 14–69. Checking the function of the expiratory one-way valve of a circle system. Wearing a surgical mask, the evaluator exhales through the Y-piece and observes the expiratory one-way valve to be sure that the valve disc moves appropriately. The reservoir bag should expand as air moves through the valve.

Fig. 14-70. Checking the function of the inspiratory one-way valve of circle system. With the pop-off valve closed, the reservoir bag is compressed, and the valve disc of the inspiratory one-way valve should move appropriately.

gives specific guidelines for evaluation and checkout, and machines with special features require individualized attention. Ventilators on anesthesia machines and monitoring equipment should also be evaluated before beginning anesthesia, but will not be included in this discussion. The following procedures are modified from the "Anesthesia Apparatus Checkout Recommendations" from the FDA's Center for Devices and Radiological Health (1) and are appropriate for evaluation of anesthesia machines and breathing systems before the first case of the day.

1. Check central O_2 and N_2O supplies for adequate quantities of gases and pipeline pressures.
2. Inspect the flowmeters, vaporizers, gauges, and supply hoses. Assure correct mounting of cylinders in the hanger yokes; the presence of a wrench for the cylinder valve; and a complete, undamaged breathing system with adequate absorbent for CO_2.
3. Assure that the waste scavenging system is connected to the pop-off valve and is working properly. Leak tests for the scavenger system have been recommended.(3) If a charcoal canister is being used, confirm that it is not exhausted.
4. Turn off the flow-control valves for the flowmeters.
5. Assure that the vaporizer is properly filled with the filler cap sealed and the control dial off.
6. Check O_2 cylinders on the machine. With the pipeline supply disconnected, O_2 cylinder valve

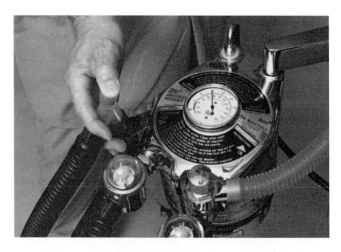

Fig. 14–71. Evaluation of the integrity of a circle breathing system. The pop-off valve is closed, the patient port is occluded, and the system is filled to a pressure of 30 cm of H_2O. The pressure should remain at 30 cm of H_2O for at least 10 seconds, or the leak as determined by use of the oxygen flowmeter should be less than 250 mL/min.

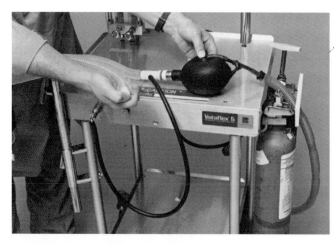

Fig. 14–72. Evaluation of a Bain breathing system (Kendall Co., Boston, Massachusetts) with a complete system check. With all gas flows off, the overflow valve is closed, and the patient port is occluded. The bag is filled with the flush valve to a pressure of 30 cm of H_2O, and a leak-free system should maintain this pressure for at least 10 seconds. If a leak is present, it can be quantified with the oxygen flowmeter and should not exceed 300 mL/min.(3)

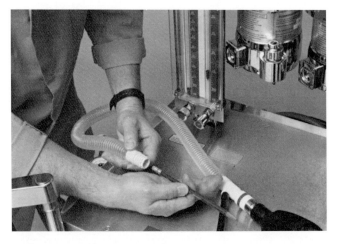

Fig. 14–73. Evaluation of the inner tube of a Bain breathing system. The first step is to turn on the oxygen flowmeter. In this example, the flow of oxygen was set at 1 L/min.

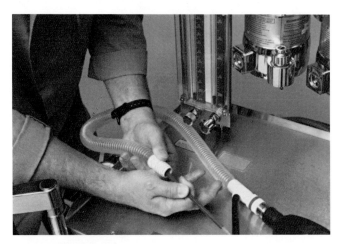

Fig. 14–74. Evaluation of the inner tube of a Bain breathing system. The second step is to occlude the patient end of the inner tube. If the inner tube is intact, the oxygen flowmeter's indicator (e.g., ball or bobbin) should fall.(3)

off, and pressure gauge at zero, slowly open the valve to check the pressure (500 psi) and determine the presence of leaks (a slow drop in pressure on the gauge) (Figs. 14–67 and 14–68). With multiple O_2 cylinders, each cylinder should be checked.

7. Check the N_2O supply (if present) as in step 6. If they are present, fail-safe devices to assure that N_2O cannot be delivered without an adequate amount of O_2 should be tested.
8. Test the flowmeters for each gas. With the flow-control valve off, the float should rest at the bottom of the glass tube. Adjust flow through the full range to assure proper function (no sticking or erratic movements).
9. Test the central pipeline supplies of O_2 and N_2O. With small (E) cylinders off and pipeline inlets connected to the central gas supply, adjust flows to a mid-range and assure that supply pressures remain near 50 psi.
10. With the vaporizer off, no odor of anesthetic should be present when the O_2 flowmeter is on.
11. For a circle system, test the function of the unidirectional valves. Wearing a surgical mask (Fig. 14–69), exhale through the exhalation limb to check the exhalation valve, and compress the reservoir bag (pop-off valve closed and Y-piece open) to check the inhalation valve (Fig. 14–70). Valve discs should be present and should rise and fall appropriately.
12. Test for leaks in the circle breathing system and the anesthesia machine. Close the pop-off valve, occlude the Y-piece, fill the system with O_2, and turn the O_2 flow to 5 L/min. As the pressure in the system reaches 20 cm of H_2O, reduce the flow until the pressure in the system (manometer) no longer rises. The O_2 flow should be negligible; a high leakage rate is unacceptable. Squeeze the reservoir bag to create a relatively high pressure (40 to 50 cm of H_2O), and assure a tight system. In checking the circle system for leaks, one recommendation is to fill the circle (pop-off valve closed and Y-piece occluded) to a pressure of 30 cm of H_2O and assure that the leak rate is less than 250 mL/min (39) or that the pressure drop is less than 5 cm of H_2O in 30 seconds or that the pressure remains at 30 cm of H_2O for at least 10 seconds (Fig. 14–71).(3) Others have recommended similar testing procedures with slightly different values for testing pressures and acceptable leak rates.(61, 62)
13. Open the pop-off valve slowly, and observe the release of pressure. Occlude the Y-piece, and verify that only a negligible positive or negative pressure develops with an O_2 flow rate of zero or 5 L/min.
14. Assure that the pop-off valve provides relief of pressure when the flush valve is activated.

Similar to the circle system, nonrebreathing systems should be tested before use. For a complete system check of a Bain system, the patient port should be occluded, the relief valve closed, and the reservoir bag distended. The bag should remain fully distended, and pressure within the system should not decrease (Fig. 14–72). The complete system check does not assure a leak-free inner tube of the coaxial system. Therefore, the inner tube is evaluated by temporarily occluding the inner tube at the patient end with oxygen flowing at approximately 1 to 2 L/min (Fig. 14–73). During a short period of occlusion with an instrument such as the plunger of a syringe, the float in the O_2 flowmeter should fall (Fig. 14–74).(2, 3) The complete system check will usually suffice for other nonrebreathing systems (e.g., Norman mask elbow and Ayre's T-piece systems).

The tests mentioned here should be considered the minimum. The operation manual for a specific anesthesia machine usually provides appropriate preuse checkout procedures, and numerous other tests have been described to evaluate anesthesia apparatus.(3) Depending on the type of anesthesia machine, breathing system, ventilator (manual or mechanical), and monitoring equipment, other tests may be indicated. Veterinarians should familiarize themselves with the evaluation procedures that are most appropriate for their specific anesthesia apparatus.

References

1. American Society for Testing and Materials. Minimum performance and safety requirements for components and systems of anesthesia gas machines (ASTM F1161–88). Philadelphia: American Society for Testing and Materials, 1989.
2. Dorsch JA, Dorsch SE. Understanding anesthesia equipment, 2nd. ed. Baltimore: Williams & Wilkins, 1984.
3. Dorsch JA, Dorsch SE. Understanding anesthesia equipment, 3rd. ed. Baltimore: Williams & Wilkins, 1994.
4. Ehrenwerth J, Eisenkraft JB. Anesthesia equipment, principles and application. St. Louis: CV Mosby, 1993.
5. Hartsfield SM. Machines and breathing systems for administration of inhalation anesthetics. In: Short CE, ed. Principles and practice of veterinary anesthesia. Baltimore: Williams & Wilkins, 395:1987.
6. Andrews JJ. Inhaled anesthetic delivery systems. In: Miller RD, ed. Anesthesia, 3rd ed. New York: Churchill Livingstone, 171:1990.
7. Fox JWC, Fox EJ. An unusual occurrence with a cycloproprane cylinder. Anesth Analg 47:624, 1968.
8. Webb AI, Warren RG. Hazards and precautions associated with the use of compressed gases. J Am Vet Med Assoc 181:1491, 1982.
9. Stoelting RK, Miller RD. Basics of anesthesia. New York: Churchill Livingstone, 1984.
10. Haskins SC, Sansome AL. A timetable for exhaustion of nitrous oxide cylinders using cylinder pressure. Vet Anesth 6:6, 1979.
11. Grant WJ. Medical gases, their properties and uses. Chicago: Year Book, 1978.
12. Schreiber P. Anesthesia equipment. New York: Springer-Verlag, 1972.
13. Mazzia VDB et al. Oxygen and the anesthesia machine. N Y State J Med 62:2845, 1962.
14. Gray PR et al. Anesthetic machine leak . J Am Vet Med Assoc 179:1348, 1981.
15. Hartsfield SM. Practical problems with veterinary anesthesia machines. Proc 5th Intl Cong Vet Anesth, Guelph, Ontario, 1994:21.
16. Andrews JJ. Understanding your anesthesia machine. In: Annual refresher course lectures 163:1. Washington, DC: American Society of Anesthesiologists, 1993.

17. Hartsfield SM, Thurmon JC. Reduced anesthetic vapor concentration in a breathing circuit related to a leak in the oxygen flush apparatus. Vet Anesth 5:35, 1978.
18. Bednarski RM, Gaynor JS, Muir WW III. Vaporizer in circle for delivery of isoflurane to dogs. J Am Vet Med Assoc 202:943, 1993.
19. Gallagher LV, Klavano PA. Scavenging waste anesthetic gases from obsolescent anesthetic machines. J Am Vet Med Assoc 179:1393, 1981.
20. Schreiber PJ. Effects of barometric pressure on anesthetic equipment. Audio Digest (Anesthesiology) 17:14, 1975.
21. Munson WM. Cardiac arrest: hazard of tipping a vaporizer. Anesthesiology 26:235, 1965.
22. Ludders JW. Vaporizers used in veterinary anesthesia. Semin Vet Med Surg Small Anim 8:72–81, 1993.
23. Orkin FK. Anesthetic systems. In: Miller RD, ed. Anesthesia, 2nd ed. New York: Churchill Livingstone, 1986:117.
24. Wagner AE, Bednarski RM. Use of low-flow and closed-system anesthesia. J Am Vet Med Assoc 200:1005, 1992.
25. Lin C. Assessment of vaporizer performance in low-flow and closed-circuit anesthesia. Anesth Analg 59:359, 1980.
26. Hill DW, Lowe HJ. Comparison of concentration of halothane in closed and semiclosed circuits during controlled ventilation. Anesthesiology 23:291, 1962.
27. Hill DW. The design and calibration of vaporizers for volatile anesthetic agents. In: Scurr C, Feldman S, eds. Scientific foundations of anaesthesia. Chicago: Year Book, 1974.
28. Thurmon JC, Benson GJ. Inhalation anesthetic delivery equipment and its maintenance. Vet Clin North Am Large Anim Pract 3:73, 1981.
29. Mulroy M, Ham J, Eger EI II. Inflowing gas leak, a potential source of hypoxia. Anesthesiology 45:102, 1976.
30. Operation and Maintenance Manual for the Metomatic Model 980 Veterinary Anesthesia Machine. Madison, WI: Ohio Medical Products.
31. Lumb WV, Jones EW. Veterinary anesthesia, 2nd ed. Philadelphia: Lea & Febiger, 1984.
32. Muir WW III et al. Handbook of veterinary anesthesia, 2nd. ed. St. Louis: Mosby, 1995.
33. Steffey EP, Woliner MJ, Howland D. Accuracy of isoflurane delivery by halothane-specific vaporizers. Am J Vet Res 44:1072, 1983.
34. Hamilton WK. Nomenclature of inhalation anesthetic systems. Anesthesiology 25:3, 1964.
35. Dunlop CI. The case for rebreathing circuits for very small animals. Vet Clin North Am Small Anim Pract 22:400, 1992.
36. Bednarski RM. Anesthetic breathing systems. Sem Vet Med Surg Small Anim 8:82, 1993.
37. Menhusen MJ. Anesthetic machine malfunction resulting in soda lime bypass and hypercarbia. J Am Anim Hosp Assoc 15:507, 1979.
38. Jorgensen B, Jorgensen S. Carbon dioxide elimination from circle systems. Acta Anaesth Scand Suppl 53:86, 1973.
39. Bednarski RM. Anesthetic equipment. In: Muir WW III, Hubbell JAE, eds. Equine anesthesia, monitoring and emergency therapy. St. Louis: Mosby Year Book, 1991:325.
40. Tevik A et al. Effect of nitrogen in a closed circle system with low oxygen flows for equine anesthesia. J Am Vet Med Assoc 154:166, 1969.
41. Muir WW III, Hubbell JAE. Handbook of veterinary anesthesia. St. Louis: CV Mosby, 1989.
42. Klide AM. The case for low gas flows. Vet Clin North Am Small Anim Pract 22:384, 1992.
43. Hartsfield SM, Sawyer DC. Cardiopulmonary effects of rebreathing and nonrebreathing systems during halothane anesthesia in the cat. Am J Vet Res 37:1461, 1976.
44. Suter CM et al. Resistance and work of breathing in the anesthetized cat: comparison of a circle breathing circuit and a coaxial breathing system. Proc Annu Mtg Am Coll Vet Anesthesiol, 1989.
45. Hodgson DS, McMurphy RM. Resistance to flow in large animal anesthetic machine breathing circuits. Proc Annu Mtg Am Coll Vet Anesthesiol, Washington, DC, 1993.
46. Soma LR. Textbook of veterinary anesthesiology. Baltimore: Williams & Wilkins, 1971.
47. Manley SV, McDonell WN. Clinical evaluation of the Bain breathing circuit in small animal anesthesia. J Am Anim Hosp Assoc 15:67, 1979.
48. Hodgson DS. The case for nonrebreathing circuits for very small animals. Vet Clin North Am Small Anim Pract 22:397, 1992.
49. Haskins SC. Monitoring the anesthetized patient. In: Chort CE, ed. Principles and practice of veterinary anesthesia. Baltimore: Williams & Wilkins, 1987.
50. Manley SV, McDonell WN. A new circuit for small animal anesthesia: the Bain coaxial circuit. J Am Anim Hosp Assoc 15:61, 1979.
51. Sawyer DC. The practice of small animal anesthesia. Philadelphia: WB Saunders, 1982.
52. Anesthetic gases. AVMA Professional Liability Insurance Trust Safety Bulletin 1(1):1, 1992.
53. OSHA-Occupational Safety and Health Administration. DVM issues. Austin, TX: Texas Veterinary Medical Association, May 1991.
54. Quick BA, Fountain BL. OSHA and the veterinary practice establishment. J Am Vet Med Assoc 195:302, 1989.
55. Criteria for a recommended standard occupational exposure to waste anesthetic gases and vapors. HEW Publication Number N105H US Department of Health, Education, and Welfare, Public Health Service, Centers for Disease Control, National Institute for Occupational Safety and Health. Washington, DC: US Government Printing Office, 1977.
56. Milligan JE. Anesthetic Gas Hazards. In: Heidelbaugh ND, Murnane TG, Rosser WW, eds. Health hazards in veterinary practice, 2nd ed. Austin, TX: Texas Department of Health, 1989:101.
57. Smith JA. Anesthetic pollution and waste anesthetic gas scavenging. Sem Vet Med Surg Small Anim 8:90, 1993.
58. Anesthesia apparatus checkout recommendations; availability. Washington, DC: Federal Register 52:5583, 1987.
59. March MG, Crowley JJ. An evaluation of anesthesiologists' present checkout methods and the validity of the FDA checklist. Anesthesiology 75:724, 1991.
60. Mason DE. Anesthesia machine checkout and troubleshooting. Sem Vet Med Surg Small Anim 8:104, 1993.
61. Paddleford RR. Exposure of veterinary personnel to waste anesthetic gases. Sem Vet Med Surg 1:249, 1986.
62. Manley SV, McDonell WN. Recommendations for reduction of anesthetic gas pollution. J Am Vet Med Assoc 176:519, 1980.
63. Haskins SC. Opinions in small animal anesthesia. Vet Clin North Am Small Anim Pract 22(2):245–260, 1992.

chapter 15

MONITORING THE ANESTHETIZED PATIENT

Steve C. Haskins

Introduction

The purpose of anesthesia is to provide reversible unconsciousness, amnesia, analgesia, and immobility, with minimal risk to the patient. Anesthetic drugs and adjuvants may, however, compromise patient homeostasis at unpredictable times and in unpredictable ways. Anesthetic crises, unfortunately, tend to be rapid in onset and devastating in nature. The purpose of monitoring is to provide information that can be used to maximize the safety of anesthesia and minimize the decrement of organ function, thereby improving the likelihood of an uneventful recovery.

Monitoring begins in the preoperative period, when the patient is assessed to determine the existence of any abnormal processes. The magnitude of pathology and the extent to which it may compromise the patient's response to anesthesia and the operative procedure are estimated (ASA classification; Chapter 2). This preoperative evaluation provides the basis for tailoring drug selection, monitoring, and support to the specific needs of the patient.

Questions to Ask When Monitoring

There are several questions that can be answered by utilizing intraoperative monitoring: (a) Is the animal adequately anesthetized/amnesic? (b) Is the animal adequately analgesic, and is the autonomic response adequately subdued? (c) Is the animal adequately immobilized? (d) What are the physiologic consequences of the anesthetic state? (e) Are any of the identified intraoperative abnormalities serious enough to warrant treatment? The pharmacologic characteristics of various anesthetic drugs differ in their ability to accomplish all of these effects; some drugs are good

ANESTHETIC EQUIPMENT AND MONITORING

410

CNS depressants (anesthesia) but are not particularly good analgesics (barbiturates and halothane); some agents are good analgesics but are not particularly good CNS depressants (opioids and nitrous oxide).

IS THE ANIMAL ADEQUATELY ANESTHETIZED/AMNESIC?

Anesthesia must provide unconsciousness and amnesia. With the traditional anesthetics (barbiturates, etomidate, propofol, and the inhalationals), unconsciousness is generally achieved at the top of the excitement stage. Because procedures cannot be implemented until spontaneous movement ceases, immobilized patients should be unconscious and amnesic. Deeper levels of anesthesia may be required to provide better muscle relaxation, diminished muscular response to surgical stimulation, and diminished autonomic response to surgical stimulation. The same can probably be said of ketamine, even though its pattern of inducing unconsciousness is somewhat different from that of the traditional anesthetics. Opioid-based anesthetic protocols are an exception in that they are not unconsciousness-producing, muscle-relaxing agents as compared to traditional anesthetics.

The signs of anesthetic depth depend, for the most part, upon the evaluation of muscular tone and muscular reflexes. The signs of anesthetic depth will vary among species and anesthetic drugs.(1–8) These signs also vary from individual to individual and from moment to moment during a single anesthetic episode because of adjunctive events such as surgical stimulation, hypotension, or hypothermia. All evaluations of anesthetic depth should be interpreted as single-point-in-time measurements. When the signs of anesthetic depth are unclear and contradictory, the anesthetic depth should be lightened a little until the signs change sufficiently that it is clear that the animal is lightly anesthetized.

Prior anesthetic dosing (e.g., the vaporizer setting) is important when evaluating anesthetic depth. Large doses, compared to those normally recommended/used, would be expected to induce a deeper level of anesthesia and vice versa. The anesthetic dose must also be evaluated in the light of adjunctive diseases: Critically ill or hypothermic animals require smaller-than-normal dosages, and they would be overanesthetized with "normal" dosages.

Minimum alveolar anesthetic concentrations of an inhalational anesthetic to prevent muscular movement in response to a strong surgical stimulus define the average anesthetic concentration needed to conduct a surgical procedure in 50% (MAC_{50}) or 95% (MAC_{95}) of an average patient population (Chapters 2 and 11).(8) MAC_{awake} is the average anesthetic concentration at which a human will open his or her eyes in response to verbal command; it is lower than $MAC_{incision}$ (the standard stimulus in humans). Both $MAC_{intubation}$ (coughing in response to endotracheal intubation) and MAC_{BAR} (blockade of autonomic response to skin incision) are higher than $MAC_{incision}$.(8) MAC designations presume equilibration of the anesthetic agent

between the alveoli and the brain, and have little relevance to anesthetic depth during states of transition (induction or recovery). MAC is a means of comparing anesthetic potency so that different studies (e.g., cardiovascular effects of) can be compared. MAC is not, however, the *definition* of anesthetic depth in an individual patient, owing to individual variations and adjunctive diseases that may raise or lower anesthetic requirements.

Awareness under general anesthesia and recall of intraoperative events has been reported in humans.(8) However, recall has been reported to be associated with virtually all anesthetics, including thiopental and inhalational anesthetics.(8) Patient-to-patient anesthetic requirements probably vary greatly, and these variations are not always imminently apparent to the anesthetist or veterinarian. Thus, there is a common tendency to err on the side of overanesthetizing the patient somewhat just to make sure that it is fully unconscious, amnesic, and analgesic. In normal animals, there is a fairly wide range between cessation of spontaneous movement and serious, drug-induced decompensation, so some "overanesthetization" can be done with relative impunity. This range narrows as the patient becomes progressively compromised by disease. It is in these marginal patients that "standard" anesthetic techniques may cause problems. And it is for this reason that the preanesthetic exam, to quantitate the degree of the compromise, is so important.

The opioids are not particularly good CNS depressants in dogs and humans, and there is a ceiling effect with regard to their ability to decrease MAC in dogs anesthetized with inhalational anesthetics.(8) There is a higher incidence of intraoperative recall associated with opioid/nitrous oxide/neuromuscular blocking agent cocktails compared to other anesthetics. There is also a high incidence of spontaneous muscular movements reported with oxymorphone-alone "anesthesia" in dogs.(9) Both recall and spontaneous movement are minimized by the adjunctive administration of a small dose of a benzodiazepine or inhalational agent.(8, 9)

The unconsciousness/amnesia issue has been perceived as more problematic with ketamine, which induces an anesthetic state that is clearly different from that of the "traditional anesthetics" (Chapters 2 and 10). Dreams and hallucinations are commonly induced by ketamine, and these must be differentiated from awareness or pain during or following surgery.

Unconsciousness is associated with the appearance of high-amplitude, slow-wave EEG activity in humans (Chapter 7).(10) In Winter's EEG classification of the cataleptic-anesthetic state, unresponsiveness occurred at anesthetic state IIC.(11) States IIA and IIB were considered hallucinatory states associated with excitation of the reticular formation. Cats given ketamine were responsive to external stimuli, but whether or not conscious perception of the stimulus was achieved could not be evaluated. Because ketamine has the potential to induce EEG states IIC and beyond, it can only be concluded that ketamine, when used in an adequate dose, has the potential of inducing a true anesthetic state. Ketamine provides profound analgesia in subanesthetic doses in humans, and recall is considered to be a minimal problem.(12) Ketamine has been associated with a lower incidence of recall when compared with thiopental.(13) Emergence reactions and intraoperative awareness are diminished by the adjunctive administration of benzodiazepines or low concentrations of inhalational anesthetics in humans.(5, 12) In animals, the adjunctive use of a benzodiazepine, a phenothiazine, or an alpha$_2$-agonist diminishes muscle hypertonus, achieving better muscle relaxation and anesthesia. Regardless of technique, the problem of awareness or recall during general anesthesia in animals is unresolvable per se, so we are left to extrapolate anesthetic protocols that have been reported to be efficacious in humans.

IS THE ANIMAL ANALGESIC?

If the animal is truly anesthetized (unaware/detached from environmental stimuli), it can be concluded that it is analgesic as well (not consciously perceiving pain). If the animal is lightly anesthetized with a traditional anesthetic, reflex or spontaneous movement may occur; however, it is extremely unlikely that pain is being consciously perceived. It is a common practice to deepen anesthesia or add an adjuvant drug if there is spontaneous movement, movement in response to surgical stimulation, or a sympathetic response to surgical stimulation. Although probably unnecessary for pain relief, this is an acceptable procedure, as long as the patient can tolerate the deeper anesthesia. An increased depth of anesthesia may be necessary if the movement interferes with the surgical procedure. If neuromuscular blocking drugs are used, movement, of course, is not a reliable indicator of a light level of anesthesia, and then the sympathetic response to surgical stimulation is the only sign that can be used.

Opioid-based anesthetic protocols are considered to provide excellent analgesia even though muscular relaxation and CNS depression require reinforcement with adjunctive drugs. Ketamine is considered to be a good analgesic in human beings.(10, 12, 14, 15) Analgesia is associated with a plasma ketamine concentration of 0.1 μg/mL (15) and with theta-wave EEG activity.(10) Ketamine has been reported to be less efficacious for visceral pain than somatic pain.(10) This does not mean that it is ineffective, only less effective. And it certainly doesn't mean that it is inappropriate to use ketamine anesthesia for abdominal procedures; only that higher doses or additional drugs to assure analgesia may be required. There is electroencephalographic evidence that ketamine has antinociceptive qualities in animals (10, 16, 17) and that it is a good analgesic for many surgical procedures when given in adequate doses.

IS THERE ADEQUATE MUSCLE RELAXATION?

The required degree of muscle relaxation is that amount which is compatible with the completion of the surgical procedure. A little movement, as long as it does not interfere with the surgical procedure, should be acceptable, since it is not generally associated with the conscious perception of pain. It is generally considered that consciousness is lost at the top of the excitement stage (a long time prior to the cessation of spontaneous muscular activity). The incidence of movement during anesthesia is much higher than the incidence of recall.(8)

Intraocular surgeries clearly constitute an exception to the rule that a little bit of movement is OK (Chapter 24). It may also be desirable to minimize muscle tone during extensive laparotomies or thoracotomies, or during long bone fracture repair. In these situations, neuromuscular blocking drugs, rather than very deep anesthesia, should be used.

WHAT ARE THE PHYSIOLOGIC CONSEQUENCES OF THE ANESTHETIZED STATE?

Animals can experience adverse physiologic responses to anesthetic drugs at any anesthetic depth. Although the pharmacodynamic effects of anesthetics vary, the mechanisms by which they cause anesthetic emergencies are usually the same: excessive hypotension, bradycardia, arrhythmias, myocardial depression, vasodilation or vasoconstriction, hypoventilation, hypoxemia, and so on. It is the purpose of the preanesthetic examination to determine to what extent the existing underlying disease processes predispose to these problems. Selection of anesthetic drugs should be made to minimize the effects of anesthesia on the development of these problems, and it is the purpose of the monitoring procedures to determine to what extent these problems develop in the perioperative period. Ongoing, automatic, audible monitors of organ function are the mainstays of intraoperative monitoring and crisis prevention.

It is important to understand the physiologic significance of each monitored parameter so that it is not over- or underinterpreted. Unless the measurement is extremely low or high, its proper interpretation, its clinical importance, and its indication of the overall adequacy of the function of the organ system, can only be assessed by correlating its current value with those previously taken (trends), with other organ system measurements, and with consideration of the patient's recent history.

Pulmonary Monitoring

BREATHING RATE, RHYTHM, NATURE, AND EFFORT

The breathing rate per se is of limited value without some reference to tidal volume and previous trends because normal rates can vary so widely. A change in breathing rate is, however, often a sensitive indicator to an underlying physiologic change (Table 15–1).

The rhythm, nature, and effort of breathing should be characterized. Arrhythmic breathing patterns are indicative of a medullary respiratory control problem. However, a Cheyne-Stokes breathing pattern (cycling between hypoventilation and hyperventilation) may be seen in otherwise healthy anesthetized horses, and

Table 15–1. Causes of Perioperative Tachypnea

1. Too lightly anesthetized
2. Too deeply anesthetized
3. Hypoxemia (Table 15-6)
4. Hypercapnia (Table 15-3)
5. Hyperthermia
6. Hypotension
7. Atelectasis
8. Postoperative recovery phase
9. Postoperative pain
10. Drug-induced (opioids)
11. Individual variation

apneustic breathing (inspiratory hold) may be seen in otherwise healthy dogs, cats, and most other species anesthetized with ketamine.

VENTILOMETRY

Ventilation volume can be estimated by visual observation of chest or rebreathing bag excursions, or measured by ventilometry (Fig. 15–1). Normal tidal volume ranges between 10 and 20 mL/kg. A small tidal volume may be acceptable if the breathing rate is fast enough to accomplish normal alveolar minute ventilation. Normal total minute ventilation ranges between 150 and 250 $mL \cdot kg^{-1} \cdot min^{-1}$. Alveolar minute ventilation is more important than total minute ventilation (Chapter 6). Alveolar minute ventilation may be as low as 20% of the total minute ventilation in animals breathing rapidly and shallowly or that have added upper airway dead space, and may be as high as 70% of the total if an animal is breathing slowly and deeply, and is endotracheally intubated.

BLOOD GAS ANALYSIS

The analysis of carbon dioxide and oxygen in an arterial blood sample defines pulmonary function.(18, 19) Venous samples interpose a tissue bed between the lungs and the sample site, and provide little information about pulmonary function. A blood sample should be analyzed as soon as possible to minimize in vitro metabolism changes, but can be maintained in ice water for several hours before significant changes occur. The arterial partial pressure of carbon dioxide ($PaCO_2$) and oxygen (PaO_2) are normally measured with a blood gas analyzer. Economic, portable, reliable, battery-operated blood gas analyzers are available.[1]

THE PARTIAL PRESSURE OF CARBON DIOXIDE (PCO_2)

The arterial PCO_2 ($PaCO_2$) is a measure of the ventilatory status of the patient and normally ranges between 35 and 45 mm Hg. A $PaCO_2$ below 35 mm Hg indicates hyperventilation; a $PaCO_2$ above 45 mm Hg indicates hypoventilation. A $PaCO_2$ in excess of 60 mm Hg may be associated with excessive respiratory acidosis and hypoxemia (when breathing room air) and usually

represents sufficient hypoventilation to warrant mechanical ventilatory support. $PaCO_2$ values below 20 mm Hg are associated with severe respiratory alkalosis and a decreased cerebral blood flow, which may impair cerebral oxygenation. Venous PCO_2 is usually 3 to 6 mm Hg higher than arterial in stable states. It is variably higher in transition states, during anemia, and carbonic anhydrase inhibitor therapy. It is a reflection of tissue PCO_2, which represents some combination of arterial PCO_2 and tissue metabolism.

$PaCO_2$ may also be estimated by measuring the carbon dioxide in a sample of gas taken at the end of an exhalation. The analyzer should be calibrated and periodically correlated to an actual $PaCO_2$ measurement. The accuracy of these instruments can be impaired by many factors.(20, 21) The presumption in correlating end-tidal PCO_2 with $PaCO_2$ is that alveolar and capillary PCO_2 are equilibrated. End-tidal PCO_2 is usually somewhat lower than $PaCO_2$, but the difference is usually inconsequential for clinical purposes. Capnography allows the anesthetist to continually evaluate adequacy of ventilation as well as many other problems (Table 15–2).(20-23) Whenever possible, the capnographic waveform should be displayed, as it will reveal more information than just the end-tidal CO_2

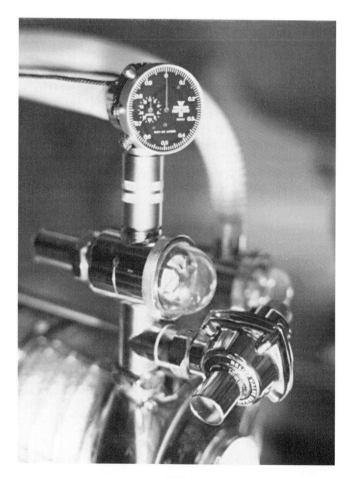

Fig. 15–1. A ventilometer can be attached to an anesthetic machine for the measurement of expired tidal volume.

Table 15–2. Potential Causes of Changes in the Capnogram (18, 19, 21)

End-Tidal CO$_2$ Change	Potential Causes
Sudden decrease to zero	Airway obstruction
	Airway disconnect
	Ventilator failure
	Capnograph malfunction
	Obstructed aspirating tube
Sudden decrease to low plateau values	Airway leaks
Exponential decrease in plateau values	Severe cardiovascular disturbance
	Inadvertent sudden hyperventilation
Slow decrease in plateau values	Hyperventilation
	Hypothermia
	Vasoconstriction
Low measurement without a good plateau—slow rate of rise	Exhalation not complete before next inhalation (partial obstruction; bronchospasm; rapid breathing rates)
	Low aspirating flow rate
	Fresh gas contamination
Low measurement with a good plateau	Uncalibrated capnograph
	Large physiologic dead space
Increased plateau	Hypoventilation
	Increased rate of metabolism
Increased baseline	Contaminated sample cell
Increased baseline and plateau	Rebreathing
Increased P(a-A)co$_2$	Dead space ventilation

measurement. Hypercapnia may be caused by hypoventilation or dead space rebreathing (Table 15–3).

THE PARTIAL PRESSURE OF OXYGEN (PO$_2$)

The PaO$_2$ is a measure of the oxygenating efficiency of the lungs. The PaO$_2$ measures the tension of oxygen dissolved in physical solution in the plasma, irrespective of the hemoglobin concentration. Hemoglobin saturation measures the percent saturation of hemoglobin and is related to the PaO$_2$ by a sigmoid curve. The clinical information derived from the measurement of hemoglobin saturation (SaO$_2$) is similar to that obtained from a PaO$_2$ measurement in that they are both a mea-

Table 15–3. Causes of Hypercapnia

I. Hypoventilation
   A. Neuromuscular disorder
     1. Excessive depths of anesthesia
     2. Intracranial disease
     3. Cervical disease
     4. Neuromuscular junction disorder
   B. Airway obstruction
     1. Big airway
     2. Bronchoconstriction
   C. Thoracic or abdominal restrictive disease
   D. Pleural space filling disorder
     1. Air
     2. Fluid
   E. Pulmonary parenchymal disease (terminal)
   F. Inappropriate ventilator settings
II. Dead space rebreathing
III. Hyperthermia, increased CO$_2$ production
IV. Recent bicarbonate therapy

sure of the ability of the lung to deliver oxygen to the blood stream. However, "the values of importance" for evaluating hypoxemia differ as shown in Table 15–4.

Oxygen content is dependent upon both hemoglobin concentration and PO$_2$: O$_2$ content = ([Hb · 1.34] · % saturation) + (0.003 – PO$_2$). Oxygen content is difficult to measure, whereas oxygen saturation and PO$_2$ are easy. Oxygen partial pressure, saturation, and content (CaO$_2$) are related, but depending upon the underlying condition, any one measurement may be misleading (Table 15–5).

In vitro oxygen-hemoglobin saturation analyzers are commercially available, economical, and easy to operate. They could be used to evaluate blood oxygenation if the cost of a blood gas analyzer is prohibitive.

PULSE OXIMETRY

Pulse oximeters attach to a patient externally (tongue, lips, tail, toenail) (Fig. 15–2). These devices are very popular in human anesthesia, and there are many from which to choose. Performance in horses, dogs, and cats has been sporadic in that it has been difficult to obtain a signal with some instruments. Purchasers should assure that instruments perform satisfactorily.[2] A pulse oximeter is an ideal perioperative monitor in that it is an automatic, continuous, audible monitor of mechanical cardiopulmonary function. It specifically measures pulse rate and hemoglobin saturation and requires

---

2. Sensor Devices, Inc., 21850 Watertown Road, Building D, Waukesha, WI 53186r, (414) 524-1000. Nelcor, Inc., 4280 Hacienda Drive, Pleasanton, CA 94588, (510) 463-4022.

reasonable pulmonary and cardiovascular function in order to achieve a measurement. One of the common reasons for poor instrument performance has been peripheral vasoconstriction; the instrument will not be able to pick up a pulse. Its value as an ongoing monitor in detecting hypoxemia has been established.(22, 24) Accuracy should be verified from time to time with an arterial blood gas measurement.(25)

Oximetry is based on the absorption of infrared light transmitted through a blood sample. Oxyhemoglobin, reduced hemoglobin, methemoglobin, and carboxyhemoglobin absorb red to infrared light differently.(24) One wavelength of light is required to identify each species of hemoglobin, preferably one that maximizes the difference between the different hemoglobin species. If methemoglobin or carboxyhemoglobin were present in high concentrations, they would absorb light and would impact the measurement made by a two-wavelength oximeter designed to measure only oxyhemoglobin and reduced hemoglobin. Because of the biphasic absorption of methemoglobin at both the 660- and 940-nm wavelengths, abnormal accumulation of this hemoglobin species tends to push the oximeter reading toward 85% (underestimating measurements when SaO_2 is above 85% and overestimating it when below 85%).(26) Carboxyhemoglobin absorbs light similarly to oxyhemoglobin at 660 nm but hardly at all at 940 nm, and this would increase the apparent oxyhemoglobin measurement.(27) Fetal hemoglobin produces very little effect on measured hemoglobin saturation.(24) Indocyanine green dye and methylene blue dye absorb light and will generate falsely low saturation measurements.(24)

Tissue, venous and capillary blood, nonpulsatile arterial blood, and skin pigment also absorb infrared light. Pulse oximeters have different ways of separating this background absorption from the change in light absorbance associated with pulsatile arterial blood. There is a fairly narrow spectrum of wavelengths that both pass through skin and yet are absorbed by hemoglobin. It has been an observation that many pulse oximeters that work well in humans do not work well in animals. Differences in tissue absorption or scatter of light, different thicknesses of tissue, smaller pulsatile flow patterns and small signal-to-noise ratios, and incompletely compensated light emitting diodes may account for species differences in efficacy. Inaccuracies may also generate from baseline read errors (motion), differences in sensor location, and electric or optical interference. The accuracy of a pulse oximeter is

Table 15–4. Relationship Between Pao_2 and Sao_2 with Respect to Hypoxemia

Pao_2	Sao_2	Importance
>80	>95	Normal
<60	<90	Serious Hypoxemia
<40	<75	Very serious hypoxemia

Table 15–5. Changes Observed in Arterial Blood Oxygen Partial Pressure, Saturation and Content with Various Diseases and During Anesthesia

Condition	Pao_2	Sao_2	Cao_2
Anemia	Normal	Normal	Reduced
Polycythemia	Normal/reduced	Normal/reduced	Increased
Methemoglobinemia	Normal	Reduced	Reduced
Severe pulmonary disease	Reduced	Reduced	Reduced
Hyperoxemia (Anesthesia)	Increased	Normal	Slightly increased

greatest within the range of 80 to 95% hemoglobin saturation, and is determined by the accuracy of the empiric formula that is programmed into the instrument.(24) For most clinical purposes, most pulse oximeters are sufficiently accurate *approximations* of hemoglobin saturation, but their accuracy should be verified by an in vitro standard. There are substantial bias and precision variations and response times between products at different levels of saturation.(22)

For the most part, SaO_2 is as informative as PaO_2; each is a measure of the ability of the lungs to deliver oxygen to the blood. The two measurements are related via the sigmoid oxygen-hemoglobin saturation curve, and to the extent that the curve is normal, one can be derived from the other. This extrapolation will be in error to the extent that the curve is shifted to the left or right. SaO_2 may not be too discriminating when an animal is breathing an enriched oxygen mixture, since such measurements would most likely be positioned on the upper plateau of the dissociation curve. The difference between a PaO_2 of 500 and 100 mm Hg in an animal breathing 100% oxygen is very important; the corresponding decrease in SaO_2, from 99 to 98%, would hardly be noticed.

The normal PaO_2 is considered to range between 80 and 110 mm Hg. A PaO_2 of 50 to 60 mm Hg is a commonly selected minimum value at which support procedures such as enriching the inspired oxygen concentration and/or ventilation therapy should be instituted. Hypoxemia, herein defined as a PaO_2 below 80 mm Hg, could be caused by a low inspired oxygen concentration, hypoventilation while breathing 21% oxygen, and lung disease (venous admixture) (Table 15–6).

Venous PO_2 reflects tissue PO_2 and bears no correlation to arterial PO_2. Mixed or central venous PO_2 ranges between 40 and 50 mm Hg. Values below 30 mm Hg may be caused by anything that decreases the delivery of oxygen to the tissues (hypoxemia, low cardiac output, vasoconstriction); values above 60 mm Hg (while breathing room air) suggest reduced tissue uptake of oxygen (shunting, septic shock, metabolic

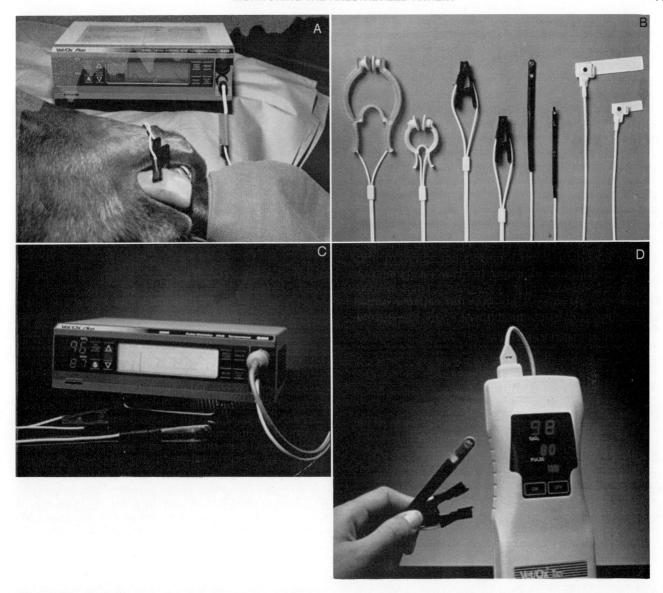

Fig. 15–2. Pulse oximeters can be attached to the tongue (A), lip, toenail, ear, or tail–anyplace where the underlying pulse can be detected. A variety of probes (B) and display units (C and D) are available.

poisons). Venous blood for such evaluations must be from a central vein such as the jugular, anterior vena cava, or pulmonary artery. Continuous mixed–venous oxygen–hemoglobin saturation can be measured via a pulmonary artery catheter containing a fiber-optic infrared light source.(28) The reflected light beam is proportional to the degree of hemoglobin oxygenation.

Tissue oxygen can be measured by transcutaneous oximetry and, experimentally, by near–infrared spectro-photometry, magnetic resonance spectroscopy, magnetic resonance imaging, and time–of– flight absorbance (TOFA) spectrophotometry.(29)

Blood gases are measured at the temperature of the blood gas analyzer water bath. Ideally the animal's body temperature would be identical to the water bath temperature, but this seldom occurs. When the animal's body temperature is different from that of the water

Table 15–6. **Causes of Hypoxemia**

I. Decreased inspired oxygen concentration
    A. Improper functioning equipment
II. Hypoventilation (while inspiring 21% oxygen)
III. Venous admixture
    A. Low ventilation/perfusion regions (bronchoconstriction)
    B. No ventilation/perfusion regions (atelectasis)
    C. Diffusion impairment (inhalation toxicity)
    D. Anatomic right-to-left shunt

bath, there will be in vitro temperature changes in the measured pH and blood gases. It has been conventional for several years to correct for these changes so that the clinician would know what the values would be at the patient's existing body temperature at the time of sampling. There is some debate about whether or not to correct for these temperature changes. If one wants to know what is actually happening in the patient and wants to compare the current measurement with previous measurements, even though there has been a substantial change in body temperature, the temperature-corrected values should be used. If the clinician is contemplating therapy to "fix" an abnormality, using normothermic reference points, then the uncorrected values should be used. "Normal values" for a hypothermic/hyperthermic patient are probably different than those for the normothermic patient, but these reference values have not been established for each level of hypothermia/hyperthermia. Under most clinical circumstances, it is recommended to use the uncorrected values.(18)

VENOUS ADMIXTURE

Venous admixture is the collective term for all of the ways in which blood can pass from the right side of the circulation to the left side of the circulation without being properly oxygenated (Table 15–6). Venous admixture can be estimated via the alveolar air equation: Alveolar PO_2 = Inspired PO_2 – $PaCO_2$(1.1), where inspired PO_2 = $(P_B - P_{H_2O}) \times 21\%$ and 1.1 = 1/RQ, assuming RQ = 0.9. The difference between the alveolar PO_2 and the measured arterial PO_2 is the A – a PO_2 difference. The normal A – a PO_2 = 10 mm Hg when the animal is breathing 21% oxygen and 100 mm Hg when the animal is breathing 100% oxygen. Larger A – a PO_2 differences when breathing room air or 100% oxygen are indicative of a decreased ability of the lung to oxygenate blood or venous admixture. If a dog or cat is breathing 21% oxygen at sea level and has an approximately normal body temperature, a simplified version of the alveolar air equation is to add the measured PaO_2 and $PaCO_2$ values. If the added value is less than 120 mm Hg, there is venous admixture; the lower the added value, the greater the magnitude of the venous admixture.

Patients breathing an enriched oxygen mixture should have an elevated PaO_2. A rough estimate of the expected PaO_2 can be obtained by multiplying the inspired oxygen concentration by 5. A PaO_2 measurement below this value indicates venous admixture. A more accurate estimate can also be obtained via the alveolar air equation given earlier.

A simplified formula that is relatively independent of inspired oxygen concentration is the a/A value (PaO_2/P_AO_2).(30) An a/A value of less than 0.85 is indicative of venous admixture.

The "shunt formula" is the most accurate way to quantitate venous admixture, since it is less susceptible to errors in assumptions, transitional disequilibrium, and variations in venous oxygen content. Venous admixture = $(CcO_2 - CaO_2)/(CcO_2 - CvO_2)$; where C = content of oxygen in capillary (c), arterial (a), and pulmonary artery (mixed venous) (v) blood. Capillary PO_2 is assumed to equal alveolar PO_2 for the

purposes of this calculation. This is a calculation of the percentage of cardiac output that would have to bypass the lung (and be totally unoxygenated, assuming that the remainder was perfectly arterialized) in order to account for the observed blood gas measurements. This is a contrived number, since much of the blood is, in reality, partially arterialized (Chapter 6, Figure 13). Venous admixture assessed by this calculation is less than 5 percent in the normal, awake human or dog. Anesthesia impairs the ability of the otherwise normal lung to oxygenate the blood, and this change would be reflected by all of the preceding measurements. Venous admixture, for instance, in the anesthetized human being with normal lung function is 5 to 10%.

When mixed-venous blood is not available, the *estimated shunt equation* will provide a close approximation of the venous admixture as calculated by the real shunt equation: $Qs/Qt = (CcO_2 - CaO_2)/3.5 + (CcO_2 - CaO_2)$.(31)

Cardiovascular Monitoring

Oxygen delivery to the tissues is dependent upon the coordinated interaction of several physiologic events: The lungs must effectively move oxygen from the environment to the plasma; hemoglobin must be present in adequate amounts; cardiac output must provide sufficient flow of the oxygenated hemoglobin toward the tissues; arterial blood pressure must be adequate to maintain cerebral and coronary perfusion pressure; and vasomotor tone must not be excessive to maintain visceral organ perfusion (Chapters 5 and 6). This overall perspective of cardiopulmonary function is illustrated in Figure 15–3, and the integrated function of these events is the overall focus of perioperative cardiopulmonary monitoring and support (Tables 15–7 and 15–8). Monitoring individual components provides but one window to the big picture but does not define overall function. The importance of any one measured parameter to overall function can only be determined by reference to previous measurements of that parameter, to recent therapeutic (or disease-induced) events, and to as many other measured parameters as are available.

ELECTRICAL ACTIVITY

Abnormal electric activity includes bradycardia (Table 15–9), tachycardia, and arrhythmias (Table 15–10). The electrocardiogram does not measure mechanical performance and can appear quite normal in the face of poor myocardial performance and tissue perfusion. Precise ECG electrode placement of the ECG leads is not necessary for monitoring purposes. The major concern is whether the PQRST wave forms appear to be approximately normal and whether they change with time.

Ectopic pacemaker activity (Fig. 15–4) does not necessarily require treatment. It indicates the presence of an underlying abnormality that should be identified (Table 15–10), if possible, and treated. Specific treatment is indicated when there is evidence of impaired myocardial performance, cardiac output, or tissue perfusion. Specific treatment is also indicated if there is concern regarding the progression of the arrhythmia to ventricular fibrillation (when the rate exceeds the upper limit of normal for the species, when it is multifocal, and when the ectopic beat occurs over the preceding T wave). Total elimination of the arrhythmia is not necessarily the objective of therapy, since large doses of antiarrhythmic drugs may have deleterious effects. A simple decrease in the rate or severity of the arrhythmia may be a suitable end point to the titration of the antiarrhythmic drugs.

PERIPHERAL PERFUSION

Perfusion of visceral and other peripheral organs is primarily regulated by vasomotor tone. Vasodilation improves peripheral perfusion but, if excessive, causes hypotension. Vasoconstriction may increase blood pressure but decreases peripheral perfusion. Vasomotor tone is assessed by mucous membrane color, capillary refill time, urine output, and toe-web/core temperature gradient.

CENTRAL VENOUS PRESSURE

Central venous pressure (CVP) is the luminal pressure of the intrathoracic vena cava (Fig. 15–5). Peripheral venous pressure is variably higher than CVP, is subject to unpredictable extraneous influences, and is not a reliable indicator of CVP. Catheters are usually positioned via the jugular vein into the anterior vena cava. Contact with the endocardium of the right atrium or ventricle should be avoided, since this may stimulate ectopic pacemaker activity. Verification of a well-placed, unobstructed catheter can be ascertained by observing small fluctuations in the fluid meniscus

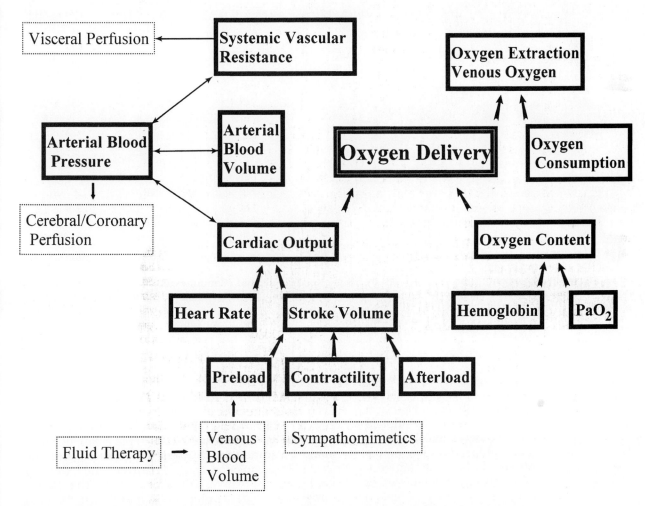

Fig. 15–3. Proper interpretation of individual cardiopulmonary measurements depends upon the integration of the measurement with all of the other measured parameters. Oxygen delivery is determined by cardiac output (heart rate and stroke volume) and oxygen content (hemoglobin and PO_2). Stroke volume is determined by preload, contractility, and afterload. The purpose of preload is to optimize stroke volume whereas sympathomimetic therapy is used to optimize contractility (and systemic resistance). Arterial blood pressure is determined by arterial blood volume, cardiac output, and peripheral vasomotor tone. Arterial blood pressure is a primary determinant of coronary and cerebral perfusion, and vasomotor tone is a primary determinant of peripheral and visceral perfusion. Venous oxygen is a reflection of the relationship between oxygen delivery and oxygen consumption.

Table 15–7. Cardiopulmonary and Oxygenation Parameters in Awake and Anesthetized Dogs

Parameter	Awake[a] (n = 60)	Ketamine[b] (n = 18)	Oxymorphone[c] (n = 10)	Halothane[d] (n = 11)	Pentobarbital[e] (n = 7)
Weight (kg)	22 ± 5	24 ± 6	23 ± 3	23 ± 3	21 ± 5
Temperature (°C)	38.6 ± 0.5	38.9 ± 0.6	38.2 ± 0.6	38.7 ± 0.1	38.5 ± 0.7
Heart rate (beats/min)	90 ± 21	166 ± 44	72 ± 14	97 ± 13	107 ± 20
Arterial pressure (mm Hg)	104 ± 12	139 ± 13	112 ± 10	64 ± 9	118 ± 18
Pulmonary arterial pressure (mm Hg)	15 ± 4	17 ± 6	21 ± 4	10 ± 2	17 ± 3
CVP (cm H_2O)	3 ± 4	2 ± 4	12 ± 4	2 ± 1	NR
Wedge pressure (mm Hg)	5 ± 2	NR	15 ± 2	5 ± 2	NR
Cardiac Output					
($mL \cdot kg^{-1} \cdot min^{-1}$)	167 ± 39	250 ± 85	154 ± 42	120 ± 23	149 ± 18
($L \cdot m^{-2} \cdot min^{-1}$)	4.67 ± 1.37	NR	NR	NR	NR
Stroke volume					
($mL \cdot beat^{-1} \cdot kg^{-1}$)	1.86 ± 0.4	1.5 ± 0.4	2.1 ± 0.3	(1.2)	(1.4)
($mL \cdot beat^{-1} \cdot m^{-2}$)	52.4 ± 12.1	NR	NR	NR	NR
Systemic resistance					
($mm Hg \cdot mL^{-1} \cdot kg^{-1} \cdot min^{-1}$)	0.64 ± 0.16	0.61 ± 0.21	0.65 ± 0.14	0.55 ± 0.11	0.79 ± 0.13
($dynes \cdot s^{-1} \cdot cm^{-5}$)	1912 ± 526	NR	NR	NR	NR
Pulmonary resistance					
($mm Hg \cdot mL^{-1} \cdot kg^{-1} \cdot min^{-1}$)	0.05 ± 0.01	NR	0.054 ± 0.031	NR	NR
($dynes \cdot s^{-1} \cdot cm^{-5}$)	186 ± 69	NR	NR	NR	NR
Pao_2 (mm Hg)	100 ± 6	96 ± 7	81 ± 6	540 ± 46	90 ± 7
Pvo_2 (mm Hg)	50 ± 5	50 ± 5	NR	81 ± 8	51 ± 3
$Paco_2$ (mm Hg)	40 ± 3	41 ± 6	50 ± 2	45 ± 8	43 ± 5
(A-a) Po_2 (mm Hg)	10 ± 5	6 ± 3	(14)	NR	12 ± 5
Qs/Qt (%)	4 ± 3	3 ± 3	13 ± 6	6 ± 1	7 ± 3
Hemoglobin (g/dL)	13.1 ± 1.7	14.9 ± 1.9	16.3 ± 1.8	14.0 ± 2.2	14 ± 1
Do_2 ($mL \cdot kg^{-1} \cdot min^{-1}$)	29 ± 9	47 ± 16	(30)	23.7 ± 5.9	(28)
($mL \cdot m^{-2} \cdot min^{-1}$)	811 ± 252	NR	NR	NR	NR
Vo_2 ($mL \cdot kg^{-1} \cdot min^{-1}$)	8 ± 2	11.9 ± 4.6	NR	4.5 ± 0.7	5.3 ± 1.5
($mL \cdot m^{-2} \cdot min^{-1}$)	217 ± 71	NR	NR	NR	NR
O_2 extraction (%)	25 ± 3	(25)	NR	20 ± 4	(19)

[a]Unmedicated, untrained, left lateral recumbency, breathing room air. Data expressed as mean ± 1 standard deviation.(25–30)
[b]15 minutes after ketamine (10 mg/kg) administered IV.(26)
[c]75 minutes after 0.4 mg/kg oxymorphone IV, followed by 0.2 mg/kg at 20, 40, and 60 minutes.(25)
[d]40 minutes after first exposure to halothane via mask; approximately 30 minutes after intubation.(30)
[e]40 ± 18 minutes after pentobarbital induction.(31)
Numbers in parentheses were not reported but were calculated from the relevant mean values.
NR, not reported.

within the manometer synchronous with the heartbeat, and larger excursions synchronous with ventilation. Large fluctuations synchronous with each heartbeat may indicate that the end of the catheter is positioned within the right ventricle. Direct observation of the CVP waveform may help identify proper location of the catheter tip. Measurements should be made between ventilatory excursions (either during spontaneous or positive pressure ventilation), since changes in pleural pressure affect the luminal pressure within the anterior vena cava. A horizontal line drawn between the estimated level of the end of the catheter (the manubrium or thoracic inlet) and the manometer establishes the "zero" reference level. The vertical difference between the zero level and the meniscus of fluid in the column manometer, after equilibration, represents the CVP.

The normal CVP in small animals is 0 to 10 cm H_2O. In laterally recumbent horses, it is 15 to 25 cm H_2O, and it is 5 to 10 cm H_2O in dorsally recumbent horses.(7) Low-range or below-range values indicate relative hypovolemia and suggest that a rapid bolus of fluids should be administered. Above-range values indicate relative hypervolemia and that further fluid therapy should be conservative. CVP is a measure of the relative ability of the heart to pump the venous return; it should be measured when a component of heart failure is suspected. CVP is also an estimate of the relationship between blood volume and blood volume capacity; it should be measured as an end-point to very large fluid infusions.

Preload is defined as end-diastolic muscle stretch, which, in vivo, is most closely related to end-diastolic volume (Chapter 5). CVP is a measure of pressure, not volume, and therefore may not truly be representative of preload in diseases associated with reduced ventricular compliance (hypertrophy, tamponade, fibrosis). Diastolic performance (relaxation) is adversely affected by some anesthetics (40).

Central venous pressure measurements are used to determine whether there is "room" for additional fluid therapy. Subcutaneous edema is not an indication that fluid therapy has been excessive (only that crystalloid therapy has been excessive) and is not an indication of an effective circulating blood volume. Edema may occur in the face of hypovolemia if the patient is hypoproteinemic or if there is increased vascular permeability.

ARTERIAL BLOOD PRESSURE

Arterial blood pressure is the product of cardiac output, vascular capacity, and blood volume. Adequate arterial blood pressure establishes a perfusion pressure for the brain and the heart. Since anesthetic drugs and operative procedures can greatly compromise cardiovascular homeostases (Tables 15–7 and 15–8) and since excessive hypotension is not an uncommon cause of perioperative morbidity, the measurement and support of arterial blood pressure in patients at risk is extremely important.

Digital palpation of the quality of the pulse amplitude in a peripheral artery reflects stroke volume and may bear little correlation to the arterial blood pressure. The weak, thready pulse that occurs with hypovolemia is caused by a small stroke volume; such patients may

Table 15–8. Cardiopulmonary Values in Awake and Anesthetized Horses (39)

Parameter	Awake	1.2 MAC Isoflurane
Temperature	37.9 ± 0.2	37.5 ± 0.3
Heart rate (beats/min)	37 ± 2	43 ± 5
Arterial pressure (mm Hg)	133 ± 4	92 ± 5
Pulmonary arterial pressure (mm Hg)	29 ± 2	25 ± 2
Cardiac output ($mL \cdot min^{-1} \cdot kg^{-1}$)	69 ± 3	59 ± 7.8
Stroke volume (mL)	889 ± 55	649 ± 45
Systemic resistance ($dynes \cdot s \cdot cm^{5^{-1}}$)	333 ± 18	285 ± 28
Pao_2 (mm Hg)	507 ± 14	318 ± 46
Pvo_2 (mm Hg)	52 ± 6	57 ± 4
$Paco_2$ (mm Hg)	45 ± 1	73 ± 4
Q_s/Q_t (%)	(9.3)	(28.0)
Packed cell volume (%)	32 ± 2	35 ± 2
Do_2 ($mL \cdot min^{-1} \cdot kg^{-1}$)	(10.7)	(9.8)
Vo_2 ($mL \cdot min^{-1} \cdot kg^{-1}$)	(2.2)	(1.4)
O_2 extraction (%)	(20.7)	(14.2)

Data expressed as mean $\pm$ 1 standard error of the mean. Numbers in parentheses were not reported but were calculated from the relevant mean values.

Table 15–9. Causes of Bradycardia

1. Anesthetic drugs: opioids, alpha$_2$-agonists, or excessive doses of any general anesthetic
2. Excessive vagal tone, which may be caused by pharyngeal, laryngeal, or tracheal stimulation by foreign bodies; by pressure on the eyeball or rectus muscles; and by visceral inflammation or distention
3. Hypoxia—as a terminal event
4. Exogenous toxemia (digitalis, organophosphates)
5. Endogenous toxemia (hypothermia, hypothyroidism, hyperkalemia, or visceral organ failure)
6. Sick sinus syndrome

actually be normotensive depending upon other cardiovascular changes.

Arterial blood pressure can be measured in animals by indirect and direct techniques.(4, 7, 42, 43) Indirect sphygmomanometry involves the application of an occlusion cuff over an artery in a cylindrical appendage (Fig. 15–6). The width of the occlusion cuff should be about 40% of the circumference of the leg to which it is applied. The occlusion cuff should be placed snugly around the leg. If it is applied too tightly, the pressure measurements will be erroneously low, since the cuff itself will partially occlude the underlying artery. If the cuff is too loose, the pressure measurements will be erroneously high, since excessive cuff pressure will be required to occlude the underlying artery.

Inflation of the cuff applies pressure to the underlying tissues and will totally occlude blood flow when the pressure exceeds the systolic blood pressure. As the cuff pressure is gradually decreased, blood will begin to flow intermittently when the cuff pressure falls below the luminal systolic pressure.

The appearance of needle oscillations on the manometer during cuff deflation is caused by the pulse wave hitting the cuff and corresponds approximately to

Table 15–10. Causes of Paroxysmal or Persistent Atrial or Ventricular Ectopic Pacemaker Activity

1. Endogenous release of catecholamines secondary to any stress, exogenous catecholamine therapy
2. Hypoxia or hypercapnia
3. Hypovolemia or hypotension
4. Digitalis toxicity (potentiated by hypokalemia and hypercalcemia)
5. Hypokalemia (potentiated by respiratory or metabolic alkalosis, glucose, or insulin therapy)
6. Hyperkalemia (potentiated by acidosis, hypocalcemia, or succinylcholine, or may be iatrogenic)
7. Some anesthetics lower the threshold to endogenous or exogenous catecholamines (inhalants, xylazine, thiamylal, thiopental)
8. Myocardial inflammation, disease or stimulation (intracardiac catheters, pleural tubes)
9. Thoracic and nonthoracic trauma
10. Congestive or hypertrophic heart failure
11. Visceral organ disease (gastric volvulus/torsion)
12. Intracranial disorders (increased pressure, hypoxia)

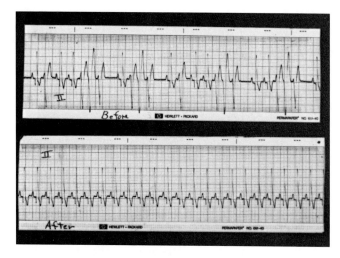

Fig. 15–4. Ventricular arrhythmias should be treated when they interfere with cardiac output or if they are sufficiently severe to threaten ventricular fibrillation. PVCs in top strip were successfully treated with lidocaine (bottom strip).

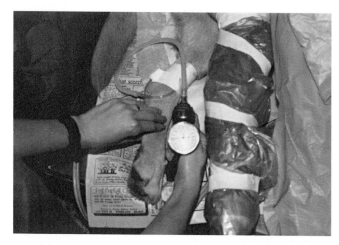

Fig. 15–6. Systolic arterial blood pressure can be estimated with an occlusion cuff placed snugly around a peripheral appendage. Detection of a pulse can be accomplished with a finger, a Doppler blood flow detector, or an oscillometer.

systolic blood pressure; however, the values are slightly higher than those derived by direct arterial measurement. Digital palpation of a pulse distal to the cuff corresponds approximately to the systolic blood pressure, although measurements are usually slightly lower than corresponding direct arterial measurements.

Doppler instrumentation involves the application of a small piezoelectric crystal over an artery. Energy is transmitted into the underlying tissue. The energy frequency reflected from moving tissues is shifted slightly from that which was transmitted, and this frequency difference is converted electronically to an audible signal. Some Doppler instruments measure blood flow and are used for the measurement of systolic blood pressure; other instruments generate signals from the movement of the arterial wall and can be used to measure both systolic and diastolic blood pressures. Doppler instrumentation has been shown to correlate closely with direct arterial measurements in a variety of animal species.

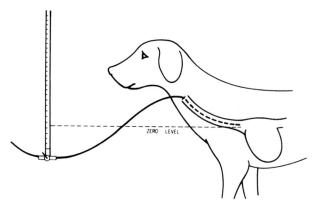

Fig. 15–5. The pressure in a central vein is dependent upon venous blood volume, venous vessel tone, and cardiac output. Filling pressure is utilized as an estimate of preload volume.

Oscillometric technology involves simply the placement of a cuff around an appendage. The changes in intracuff pressure caused by the changes in appendage size associated with each pulse wave as the cuff is slowly deflated are measured and computed, and then systolic, mean, and diastolic blood pressure, and heart rate are digitally displayed. Most of these instruments can be set to recycle (remeasure) at discrete time intervals. There are many of these instruments on the market because of their popularity in human medicine. Not all of these instruments work well in small dogs and cats (measurements are more consistent in medium-sized and large animals). All of these instruments are easily confused by motion artifact. Notwithstanding motion and variation of cuff application, when the instrument can make a measurement, repeat measurements should be within about 20%.

All external techniques are least accurate when vessels are small, when the blood pressure is low, and when the vessels are constricted. Direct measurement of arterial blood pressure is more accurate and continuous than indirect methods, but requires the introduction of a catheter into an artery by percutaneous or cutdown procedure. The dorsal metatarsal artery in dogs and cats, and the facial, auricular, and metatarsal arteries in horses and ruminants, are commonly used for percutaneous catheterization. The subcutaneous tissues around these arteries are relatively tight, so hematoma formation at the time of catheter removal is rarely a problem.

Following a wide depilation and surgical scrub of the area over the artery, the artery to be percutaneously catheterized is palpated with one or two fingers of one hand. A relief incision is made completely through the skin with the beveled edge of a hypodermic needle without entering the artery. A thin-wall catheter-outside-the-needle system (20 to 24 ga) is positioned subcutaneously on top of the artery with the bevel up.

The needle tip and the artery are simultaneously palpated with the opposite hand, and the catheter is inserted into the artery, steeply at first so that the tip of the needle just penetrates the upper wall of the artery and then flat against the skin surface and parallel with the longitudinal axis of the artery so that the bevel of the needle and end of the catheter come to lie entirely within the lumen of the artery without penetrating the deep wall. The presence of the needle tip within the lumen can be verified by the reflux of blood into the hub of the needle. At this point neither vessel nor needle should be moved while the catheter is gently rotated into the artery to its full length. The needle is then rapidly removed, replaced with an infusion plug and gently flushed with heparinized saline.

For cutdown procedures, the artery is surgically isolated and a catheter-outside-the needle system is inserted into the lumen of the artery, the needle is removed and replaced with an infusion plug, and the catheter flushed with heparinized saline. Generally, no circumferential sutures are placed around the artery. The incision is closed, and the catheter hub is sutured or glued to the skin at the entrance site.

Once the catheter is placed, it is connected to a monitoring device. The catheter must be flushed with heparinized saline at frequent intervals (hourly) or continuously. The measuring device could be comprised of a long fluid administration set suspended from the ceiling and operated like a central venous pressure measurement. Fluid is instilled into the tubing via a 3-way stopcock to a very high level and then allowed to gravitate into the artery until the hydrostatic pressure of the column of water is equalized with the mean arterial blood pressure of the patient. Never allow blood to flow into the catheter, because it will clot. Since blood pressure oscillates, leaving the system open between measurements is not advised, because it will allow blood to enter the catheter.

The measuring device could also be an aneroid manometer (Fig. 15–7). Water or blood must not be allowed to enter the manometer. The manometer can be attached to the catheter by a couple of lengths of sterile extension tubing. Sterile saline is injected into the tubing toward the manometer via a 3-way stopcock until the compressed air increases the registered pressure to a level above that of mean blood pressure. The pressurized manometer system is then allowed to equilibrate with the mean blood pressure of the patient.

The arterial catheter can also be attached to a commercial transducer and recording system, which, although more expensive than the homemade systems described earlier, is much easier to use for continuous pressure measurement. The extension tubing between the catheter and the transducer should not be excessively long and should be constructed of nonexpansible plastic to avoid dampened signals. The transducer should be zeroed periodically and calibrated with a mercury manometer to verify accurate blood pressure measurements. With modern patient monitors, the transducer can be placed anywhere with reference to the patient as long as this relative vertical position does not change (in which case the transducer needs to reze-roed) and the stopcock that is opened to room air is at the level of the heart. The patient monitor will compensate internally with an "offset pressure" for any vertical differences between the patient and the transducer, and for transducer variances. With older patient monitors without this offset feature, the transducer and the zeroing stopcock should be placed at the level of the heart.

Normal systolic, diastolic, and mean blood pressures are approximately 100 to 160, 60 to 100, and 80 to 120 mm Hg, respectively. Systolic pressures below 80 and mean pressures below 60 are assumed to result in inadequate cerebral and coronary perfusion and warrant therapy.

Hypotension may be caused by hypovolemia, peripheral vasodilation, or reduced myocardial contractility. Hypovolemia (vasodilation causes a relative hypovolemia as well) is the most common cause and should be treated with crystalloids and colloids. Decreased cardiac output may be due to a variety of disorders. The underlying cause should be identified and corrected prior to anesthesia if possible. The immediate management of heart failure may require sympathomimetic therapy in addition to correction of the underlying systemic disease. A sympathomimetic agent that causes minimal peripheral vasoconstriction should be utilized for prolonged support (dobutamine, dopamine, mephenteramine, or ephedrine). Alpha-receptor agonists may be indicated initially to pharmacologically support blood pressure and to provide time for blood volume restoration (Chapters 5, 23, and 24).

CARDIAC OUTPUT

Arterial blood pressure may, however, be normal in the face of very low cardiac output and very high peripheral vascular resistance, and therefore is not the total

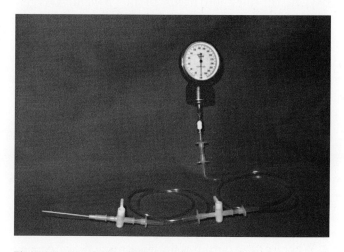

Fig. 15–7. A catheter can be placed percutaneously into an artery and attached to an aneroid manometer or transducer. Aneroid manometer is shown and provides mean blood pressure data.

definition of cardiovascular function. Cardiac output is a flow parameter and is more relevant to systemic perfusion than is a pressure parameter. Cardiac output is most easily determined clinically by thermodilution techniques.(32, 44, 45-47) When these measurements are not available, changes in pulse quality (height and width of the pulse pressure wave) provide a rough clinical index to stroke volume.

Cardiac output may be reduced by insufficient venous return and end-diastolic ventricular filling volume (hypovolemia, positive pressure ventilation, or disease-induced or surgical inflow occlusion); by ventricular restrictive disease (hypertrophic or restrictive cardiomyopathy, pericardial tamponade, or pericardial fibrosis); by decreased contractility; by excessive bradycardia, tachycardia, or arrhythmias; by regurgitation (retrograde flow) of part of the end-diastolic blood volume owing to insufficient atrioventricular valves; or by outflow tract obstruction (stenosis).

Poor cardiac output should be improved by correcting the underlying problem when possible. The dose of anesthetic should be optimized (the least amount that will allow the completion of the surgical procedure). Preload should be optimized. Sympathomimetic therapy is indicated when fluid therapy alone has failed to restore acceptable arterial blood pressure, cardiac output, or tissue perfusion. Adequate blood volume restoration may be functionally defined as a central venous pressure of about 10 cm H_2O.

OXYGEN DELIVERY

Oxygen delivery is the product of cardiac output and blood oxygen content (Fig. 15–3). It is the "bottom line" of cardiopulmonary function. Disease becomes life-threatening when, in spite of compensatory mechanisms, oxygen delivery is reduced below the critical level for the patient. Therapeutic intervention is adequate when oxygen delivery is adequate to meet the oxygen consumption needs of the patient. Oxygen consumption is generally reduced during general anesthesia in association with muscular inactivity and hypothermia.(48, 49) Critical oxygen delivery (oxygen delivery below which oxygen consumption begins to decrease) is therefore lower during general anesthesia compared to unanesthetized states, and varies among patients and anesthetics (Table 15–5). In critically ill human patients, a minimum oxygen delivery of 550 to 600 mL · min^{-1} · m$^{2^{-1}}$ has been recommended (Chapter 24).(50, 51) Mixed or central venous PO_2 and oxygen extraction reflect the relationship between oxygen consumption and oxygen delivery. A low venous PO_2 or a high oxygen extraction calculation, notwithstanding arteriovenous shunts, suggest either that oxygen delivery is impaired or that oxygen consumption exceeds the amount delivered.

When cardiac output is not measured, the adequacy of oxygen delivery must be extrapolated from parameters that are measured, such as pulse quality, capillary refill time, urine output, toe-web/core temperature gradient, base deficit, venous PO_2, or blood lactate concentration.

Renal Function

The presence of urine output is used as an indirect measure of renal blood flow; renal blood flow is used as an indirect measure of visceral blood flow. Urine output can be assessed by serial palpation of the urinary bladder or by actual measurement following the aseptic placement of a urinary catheter. Normal urine output should be 1 to 2 mL · kg^{-1} · h^{-1} in the awake healthy patient.

Laboratory Evaluations

Certain parameters including packed cell volume/hemoglobin, total protein/albumin/colloid oncotic pressure, platelets/coagulation parameters, and core temperature may be impacted sufficiently during and immediately following the operative period, and they should also be monitored at regular intervals in patients at risk.

ARE ANY OF THE IDENTIFIED ABNORMALITIES SERIOUS ENOUGH TO WARRANT TREATMENT?

Most parameters do not merit specific treatment when they are "just a little bit abnormal." All such abnormalities, when carried to an extreme, however, may harm the patient and therefore warrant specific therapy. Drawing the ever-important line between "just a little bit abnormal and not warranting therapy" and "a lot abnormal and warranting therapy" is not always an easy task. There is much patient-to-patient variation, and generic definition of a "critical point" is probably not possible (Chapter 2). For instance, the critical packed cell volume is commonly defined as 20%, but animals with chronic, singular anemic diseases (autoimmune hemolytic anemia) can probably safely go below 20%, whereas animals with acute, systemic diseases (septic shock) associated with impaired myocardial contractility might be better served with a packed cell volume of 30%. A heart rate of 60 beats/min, for instance, is a commonly recommended critical point; however, the actual heart rate at which oxygen delivery becomes insufficient is dependent upon the interplay of all of the other determinants of oxygen delivery (Fig. 15–3). Lower heart rates have been associated with lower cardiovascular parameters, but heart rates of about 50 beats/min are not necessarily associated with unacceptable cardiovascular function.(52, 53) For most parameters, there is not a critical point, but rather a critical range, depending upon the other "goings on" in the patient. When a patient is found to have an abnormal measurement, the impact of the abnormality on the overall performance of that organ system should be evaluated, if possible. Specific therapy is warranted if (a) the abnormal value is indicative of negative overall performance of the organ system, or (b) the performance of the organ system could be improved by specific therapy. A negative impact does not need to be *proven* before therapy can be instituted. If the *potential* for improving overall organ system performance outweighs the *risks and disadvantages* of the therapy, it should be given strong consideration.

References

1. Hall LW, Clarke KW. Veterinary anaesthesia. London: Balliere Tindall, 1983.
2. Thurmon JC. Anesthesia. Veterinary Clinics of North America, Food Animal. Philadelphia: WB Saunders, 1986.
3. Haskins SC. Monitoring. In: Paddleford RR, ed. Manual of small animal anesthesia. New York: Churchill Livingstone, 1988:119–145.
4. Haskins SC. Monitoring the anesthetized patient. In: Short CS, ed. Principles and practice of veterinary anesthesia. Baltimore: Williams & Wilkins, 1987:455–477.
5. Stanski DR. Monitoring depth of anesthesia. In: Miller RD, ed. Anesthesia, 3rd ed. New York: Churchill Livingstone, 1990:1001–1029.
6. Riebold TW. Monitoring equine anesthesia. In: Riebold TW, ed. Principles and techniques of equine anesthesia. Veterinary Clinics of North America, Food Animal. Philadelphia: WB Saunders, 1990:607–624.
7. Hubbell JAE. Monitoring. In: Muir WW, Hubbell JAE, eds. Equine anesthesia monitoring and emergency therapy. St. Louis: Mosby Year Book, 1991:153–178.
8. Haskins SC, Klide AM. Opinions in Small Animal Anesthesia, Veterinary Clinics of North America, Small Animal Practice, 1992:435–438.
9. Copland VS, Haskins SC, Patz JD. Oxymorphone: Cardiovascular, pulmonary, and behavioral effects in dogs. Am J Vet Res 48:1626–1630, 1987.
10. Corssen G, Reves JG, Stanley TH, eds. Intravenous anesthesia and analgesia. Philadelphia: Lea & Febiger, 1988:99–173.
11. Winters WD, Ferrar-Allado T, Guzman-Flores C, et al. The cataleptic state induced by ketamine: a review of the neuropharmacology of anesthesia. Neuropharmacology 11:303–315, 1972.
12. Reves JG, Glass PSA. Nonbarbiturate intravenous anesthetics. In: Miller RD, ed. Anesthesia, 3rd ed. New York: Churchill Livingstone, 1990:254–258.
13. Schultetus RR, Hill CR, Dharmaraj CM, et al. Wakefulness during cesarean section after anesthetic induction with ketamine, thiopental, or ketamine and thiopental combined. Anesth Analg 65:723–728, 1986.
14. Sadove MS, Shulman M, Hatano S, et al. Analgesic effects of ketamine administered in subdissociative doses. Anesth Analg 50:452–457, 1971.
15. Nimmo WS, Clements JA. Ketamine. In: Prys-Roberts C, Hug CC, eds. Pharmacokinetics of anesthesia. Boston: Blackwell,1984:235–245.
16. Miyasaka M, Domino EF. Neuronal mechanisms of ketamine-induced anesthesia. Int J Neuropharmacol 7:557–573, 1968
17. Sparks DL, Corssen G, Sides J, et al. Ketamine-induced anesthesia: neural mechanisms in the Rhesus monkey. Anesth Analg 51:288–297, 1973.
18. Shapiro BA, Peruzzi WT, Templin R. Clinical application of blood gases, 5th ed. Chicago: Mosby-Yearbook, 1994.
19. Haskins SC. Blood gases and acid-base balance: clinical interpretation and therapeutic implications. In: Kirk RW, ed. Current veterinary therapy, vol. 8, 1983. Philadelphia: WB Saunders, 201–215.
20. Swedlow DB. Capnometry and capnography: the anesthesia disaster early warning system. Semin Anesth 5:194–205, 1986.
21. Raemer DB, Calalang I. Accuracy of end-tidal carbon dioxide tension analyzers. J Clin Monit 7:195–208, 1991.
22. Weingarten M. Respiratory monitoring of carbon dioxide and oxygen: a ten-year perspective. J Clin Monit 6:217–225, 1990.
23. Gravenstein JS, Paulu DA, Hayes TJ. Capnography in clinical practice. London: Butterworth, 1989.
24. Tremper KK, Barker SJ. Pulse oximetry. Anesthesiology 70:98–108, 1989.
25. Whitehair KJ, Watney GCG, Leith DE, et al. Pulse oximetry in horses. Vet Surg 19:243–248, 1990.
26. Barker SJ, Tremper KK, Hyatt J, Zaccari J. Effects of methemoglobinemia on pulse oximetry and mixed venous oximetry. Anesthesiology 67:A170, 1987.
27. Barker SJ, Tremper KK. The effect of carbon monoxide inhalation on pulse oximeter signal detection. Anesthesiology 78:599–603, 1987.
28. Moon RE, Camporesi EM. Respiratory monitoring. In: Miller RD, ed. Anesthesia, 3rd ed. New York: Churchill Livingstone, 1990:1165–1184.
29. Benaron DA, Benitz WE, Ariagno RL, et al. Noninvasive methods for estimating in vivo oxygenation. Clin Pediatr 5:258–272, 1992.
30. Gilbert R, Keighley JF. The arterial/alveolar oxygen tension ratio. An index of gas exchange applicable to varying inspired oxygen concentrations. Am Rev Resp Dis 109:142–145, 1974.
31. Cane RD, Shapiro BA, Templin R, et al. The unreliability of oxygen tension based indices in reflecting intrapulmonary shunting in the critically ill. Crit Care Med 12:1243–1245, 1988.
32. Haskins SC, Farver TB, Patz JD. Ketamine in dogs. Am J Vet Res 46:1855–1860, 1985.
33. Copland VS, Haskins SC. Oxymorphone: cardiovascular, pulmonary, and behavioral effects in dogs. Am J Vet Research 48:1626–1630, 1987.
34. Ilkiw J, Haskins SC, Patz JD. Cardiovascular and respiratory effects of thiopental administration in hypovolemic dogs. Am J Vet Res 52:576–580, 1991.
35. Pascoe PJ, Ilkiw JE, Haskins SC, Patz JD. Cardiopulmonary effects of etomidate in hypovolemic dogs. Am J Vet Res 53:2178–2182, 1992.
36. Ilkiw JE, Pascoe PJ, Haskins SC, and Patz JD. Cardiovascular and respiratory effects of propofol administration in hypovolemic dogs. Am J Vet Res 53:2323–2327, 1992.
37. Haskins SC, Ilkiw JE, Guilford WG, Komtebedde J. The cardiopulmonary effects of halothane induction in dogs. Unpublished data.
38. Haskins SC, Patz JD. Long-term cardiopulmonary effects of pentobarbital in dogs. Proc 2nd Intl Cong Vet Anesth, Sacramento, California, 1985:74.
39. Steffey EP, Dunlop CI, Farver TB, et al. Cardiovascular and respiratory measurements in awake and isoflurane-anesthetized horses. Am J Vet Res 48:7–12, 1987.
40. Pagel PS, Kampine JP, Schmeling WT, et al. Alteration of left ventricular diastolic function by desflurane, isoflurane, and halothane in the chronically instrumented dog with autonomic nervous system blockade. Anesthesiology 74:1103–1114, 1991.
41. Pagel PS, Kampine JP, Schmeling WT, et al. Comparison of the systemic and coronary hemodynamic actions of desflurane, isoflurane, halothane, and enflurane in the chronically instrumented dog. Anesthesiology 74:539–551, 1991.
42. Henneman EA, Henneman PL. Intricacies of blood pressure measurement: reexamining the rituals. Heart Lung 18:263–273, 1989.
43. Stanley TE, Reeve JG. Cardiovascular monitoring. In: Miller RD, ed. Anesthesia, 3rd ed. New York: Churchill Livingstone, 1990:1031–1099.
44. Sprung CL. The pulmonary artery catheter. Methodology and clinical applications. Baltimore: University Park Press, 1983.
45. Dyson DH, Allen DG, McDonnell WN. Evaluation of three methods for cardiac output determination in cats. Am J Vet Res 46:2546–2552, 1985.
46. Muir WW, Skarda RT, Milne DW. Estimation of cardiac output in horses by thermodilution techniques. Am J Vet Res 37:697–700, 1976.
47. Dunlop CI, Hodgson DS, Chapman PL, et al. Thermal dilution estimation of cardiac output at high flows. FASEB J 2:A1287, 1988.

48. Mikat M, Peters J, Zindler M, et al. Whole body oxygen consumption in awake, sleeping, and anesthetized dogs. Anesthesiology 60:220–227, 1984.
49. Rock P, Beattie C, Kimball AW, et al. Halothane alters the oxygen consumption-oxygen delivery relationship compared with the conscious state. Anesthesiology 73:1186–1197, 1990.
50. Shoemaker WC, Kram HB, Waxman K, et al. Prospective trial of supranormal values of survivors as therapeutic goals in high-risk surgical patients. Chest 94:1176–1186, 1988.
51. Yu M, Levy MM, Smith P, et al. Effect of maximizing oxygen delivery on morbidity and mortality rates in critically ill patients: a prospective randomized, controlled study. Crit Care Med 21:830–838, 1993.
52. Copland VS, Haskins SC, Patz JD. Atropine reversal of oxymorphone induced bradycardia. Vet Surg 21:414–417, 1992.
53. Ilkiw JE, Pascoe PJ, Haskins SC, et al. The cardiovascular sparing effect of fentanyl, administered to enflurane anesthetized dogs. Can J Vet Res 58(4):248–253, 1994.

SELECTED ANESTHETIC TECHNIQUES

chapter 16A

LOCAL AND REGIONAL ANESTHETIC AND ANALGESIC TECHNIQUES: DOGS

Roman T. Skarda

Introduction

The popularity of local anesthetic-induced neural blockade in dogs has waned with the development of new injectable and inhalant anesthetics. This is especially true for dogs that are considered difficult to sedate and restrain for surgery. General anesthesia may be advantageous where complete immobilization and relaxation of the patient are required; however, topical anesthesia, infiltration anesthesia, field blocks, selected nerve blocks (anesthesia of the maxilla, upper teeth, eye and orbit, mandible, and lower teeth), anesthesia of the foot, (ring block, brachial plexus block, and intravenous regional anesthesia), multiple intercostal nerve blocks, lumbosacral epidural anesthesia, and continuous epidural anesthesia are all logical techniques for providing surgical anesthesia in dogs that are considered at risk for inhalant or intravenous anesthesia. The techniques described in this discussion should be considered and used more often in appropriate surgical and postoper-

ative situations to provide analgesia (Table 16A–1). Continuous interpleural analgesia and epidural opioid analgesia, for example, can be used to provide postoperative pain relief following general anesthesia.

The purpose of this chapter is to discuss the techniques, pharmacology (Chapter 12), advantages, and disadvantages of the most commonly used local and regional anesthetic techniques for surgical and postoperative pain relief in dogs.

Topical Anesthesia

Many local anesthetics are effective when placed topically on mucous membranes and may be used in the mouth, tracheobronchial tree, esophagus, and genitourinary tract. Local anesthetics used topically include lidocaine (2 to 5%), proparacaine (0.5%), tetracaine (0.5 to 2%), butacaine (2%), and cocaine (4 to 10%). Preparations include injectables applied topically, cream, ointment, jelly, powder, and aerosol. Injectable prepa-

426

Table 16A–1. Classification and Degree of Required Dexterity for Producing Local and Regional Anesthetic Techniques in Dogs

Classification	Techniques	Required Manual Dexterity and Experience
Terminal anesthesia	Topical	+
	Intravenous regional anesthesia	+ +
Infiltration anesthesia	Subcutaneous, intramuscular injection	+
	Subpleural injection	+ +
	Ring block	+
Perineural anesthesia	Nerve blocks on the head	+ +
	Nerve blocks on the legs	+ + +
	Brachial plexus block	+ +
	Intercostal nerve block	+
Spinal anesthesia	Lumbosacral epidural anesthesia	+ +
	Continuous epidural anesthesia (catheter technique)	+ + +
	Lumbar subarachnoid anesthesia	+ + +
Postoperative analgesia	Epidural opioid analgesia	+ +
	Continuous epidural opioid analgesia (catheter technique)	+ + +
	Interpleural regional analgesia (catheter technique)	+ + +
Therapeutic analgesia	Anesthesia of the cervicothoracic ganglion	+ + +
	Anesthesia of the lumbar sympathetic ganglia	+ + +

+, little; + +, some; + + +, considerable

rations of lidocaine (0.5 to 5%), available in ampules and vials, with and without epinephrine (1:50,000 to 1:200,000), can be used for infiltration (0.5 to 1%) and nerve block (1 to 2%), and applied topically to mucous membranes (1 to 5%). Topical local anesthetic agents can relieve pain during cleaning or dressing of wounds, although their effect is highly variable. The lowest effective dose of topical anesthetic should always be used in order to prevent toxicity from excessive drug plasma concentrations.(1) The time between application of topical anesthetics and onset of anesthesia is generally longer and pain relief less than for infiltration anesthesia. A 2 to 4% solution of lidocaine used for topical anesthesia on mucous membranes produces effects in approximately 5 minutes and lasts for 30 minutes. Local instillation of proparacaine (0.5%), tetracaine (0.5% to 1%), butacaine (2%), piperocaine (2%), oxybuprocaine (0.4%), or cocaine (1 to 4%) into the conjunctival sac anesthetizes the cornea and conjunctiva for short procedures (e.g., removal of hypertrophied gland of the third eyelid). Proparacaine (0.5%) has been advocated as an excellent topical anesthetic for examination of the painful eye, removal of foreign bodies, sutures, obtaining conjunctival scrapings, and subconjunctival injections.(2) Anesthesia occurs rapidly (1–6 minutes), lasts for 10 to 15 minutes after single instillation, and may last for up to 2 hours after repeated instillation without untoward effects (e.g., irritation, epithelial damage).(3) A series of 3 to 5 instillations of 1 or 2 drops of proparacaine at approximately 1-minute intervals may be necessary to produce satisfactory anesthesia of the cornea and conjunctiva. Topical anesthesia is very safe, is simple to apply, and can be repeated, although dogs may resent the application of cold solutions. Data on vascular uptake and maximum blood concentration are not available, large interpatient variability should be expected, and potential for bacterial contamination exists.(4)

Local anesthetic sprays (10% lidocaine, 14 to 20% benzocaine) produce anesthesia of the mucosa up to a depth of 2 mm within 1 to 2 minutes after application. Anesthesia lasts for approximately 15 to 20 minutes. The movable nozzle (Jetco nozzle) of the spray can enables easy access to the site of application. Pressure on the nozzle with the forefinger delivers a specific quantity of the anesthetic each second (10 mg of lidocaine from a 10% lidocaine spray can). The average expulsion rate from a benzocaine (Cetacaine) spray can is 200 mg/s.

Endotracheal tubes are frequently coated with local anesthetic jells but should not be lubricated with jelly containing 20% benzocaine HCl. Topical sprays and ointments containing 14 to 20% benzocaine reproducibly cause dose-dependent methemoglobinemia. Preparations with over 8% benzocaine include Hurricane Spray (20%), Hurricane Topical Anesthetic Gel (20%) and Liquid (20%), Camphophenique Sting Relief Formula (20%), Dermoplast Anesthetic Pain Relief (20%), and Cetacaine Spray (14%).(5) Exposure of the tracheal mucosa to topical benzocaine oxidizes blood hemoglobin in dogs in proportion to the absorbed dose within 10 minutes. Methemoglobin is not capable of binding oxygen or carbon dioxide.(6) Dogs are usually asymptomatic when concentrations of methemoglobin are less than 20%, but show fatigue, weakness, dyspnea, and tachycardia at concentrations between 20 to 50%.(7) Laryngeal sprays containing benzocaine should be used with caution in cats, and if signs of cyanosis and respiratory distress develop, methemoglobinemia should be considered.(8) In general, benzocaine should be used sparingly and cautiously using continuous

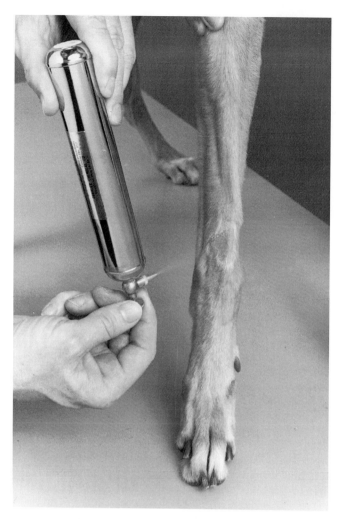

Fig. 16A–1. Ethylchloride is sprayed on the skin to produce surface anesthesia.

monitoring for cyanosis. Patients at risk of hypoxia after using benzocaine topical anesthesia should receive oxygen (5) and methylene blue (1.5 mg/kg) intravenously.(7)

One of the oldest forms of topical anesthesia is superficial cooling. Ethylchloride can be used to freeze a small local area of skin for punctures, skin biopsy, or incision of small abscesses. Ethylchloride is sprayed on the skin for 2 to 5 seconds from a distance of approximately 20 cm (Fig. 16A–1). Surface anesthesia results from cooling (<4° C), which occurs during the evaporation process. Attempts to freeze large skin areas using ethylchloride is contraindicated because of the potential for frost bite. Ethylchloride's short duration of action (<3 minutes), ability to produce a freezing sensation, and flammability when exposed to open flames and electric sparks (electrocauterization), limit its use.

Pontocaine cream and a liposomal tetracaine preparation (0.5% tetracaine encapsulated into phospholipid vehicles) effectively penetrate the skin of humans

within 30 to 60 minutes of application, producing long-lasting (>4 h) analgesia.(9) The most clinically utilizable cream contains a 5% eutectic mixture of lidocaine and prilocaine (EMLA), which overcomes the stratum corneum barrier of man within 1 hour of topical application without adverse effects.(10) The usefulness of EMLA cream in dogs, which have a different type of skin than humans, has not been reported.

Infiltration Anesthesia

Local infiltration of local anesthetics requires their extravascular placement by direct injection and may be the most reliable and safest of all the local anesthetic techniques (Table 16A–1). Lidocaine (0.5 to 2.0%) is the local anesthetic most often used for infiltration. Only sharp and sterile needles should be used. Local anesthesia can be produced by multiple intradermal or subcutaneous injections of 0.3 to 0.5 mL of local anesthetic solution, using a 2.5-cm, 22- to 25-gauge needle, or by using a longer needle (3.75 to 5 cm) and slowly injecting local anesthetic while advancing the needle along the line of proposed incision (linear infiltration). Pain is minimal if the needle is advanced slowly into the first desensitized wheal and successive injections are made at the periphery of the advancing wheal. This technique assures that the dog senses only the initial needle insertion. Intradermal deposition of local anesthetic over a superficial abscess, cyst, or hematoma is a routine procedure. Infection along the filtration site will not occur if the needle has not entered the abscess. The amount of local anesthetic used for infiltration anesthesia depends upon the size of the area to be anesthetized. Approximately 2 to 5 mg/kg of lidocaine or mepivacaine and 4 to 6 mg/kg of procaine without epinephrine may be used for infiltration. Alternatively, approximately 5 to 8 mg/kg of local anesthetic with epinephrine (1:200,000) may be used for infiltration (Table 16A–2). The lowest possible concentration of local anesthetic that will produce the desired effect should be administered. For example, an average dog (20 kg) will tolerate approximately 50 mL of 0.5% lidocaine without demonstrating signs of toxicity, whereas only 20 to 30 mL of 1% lidocaine or 10 to 15 mL of 2% lidocaine can be injected. The local anesthetic may be diluted in 0.9% NaCl solution (not with sterile water) to a 0.25% solution if a large volume of local anesthetic is needed for infiltration of a large operative area. The total dose of drug administered should be reduced by 30 to 40% in old dogs (>8 years) and sick or cachectic dogs in poor condition.(11) Epinephrine (1:200,000) is often added to local anesthetic solutions to produce local vasoconstriction, which reduces absorption rates (30%) and helps to maintain a high drug concentration at the nerve fiber, thus increasing the local anesthetic effect and duration (50%). Local anesthetics containing epinephrine should not be injected into tissues supplied by end arteries (e.g., ears, tail) or in thin and dark-skinned dogs (e.g. poodle) because of the risk of

Table 16A–2. Commonly Used Local Anesthetic Drugs and Doses for Peripheral and Epidural Block Procedures in Conscious Dogs

Local Anesthetic		Concentration (%)	Usual Doses (mg/kg)		Toxic Doses, IV (mg/kg)		Approximate Onset of Motor and Sensory Block (min)	Approximate Duration of Motor and Sensory Block (h)	Motor Block
Generic Name	Trade Name (Manufacturer)		With Epinephrine	Without Epinephrine	Convulsive	Lethal			
Ester-Linked									
Procaine	Novocaine (Withrop Laboratories)	1–2	8	6	36	100	10–15	0.5	±
Chloroprocaine	Nesacaine (Pennwalt, Inc.)	1–1.5	8	6	—	—	7–15	0.5–1	±
Amide-Linked									
Lidocaine	Xylocaine (Astra Pharmaceutical Products)	0.5–2	7	5	11–20	16–28	10–15	1–2	+
Mepivacaine	Carbocaine (Breon Laboratories, Inc.)	1–2	7	5	29	—	5–10	2–2.5	+
Bupivacaine	Marcaine (Breon Laboratories, Inc.)	0.25–0.5	3	2	3.5–4.5	5–11	20–30	2.5–6	±
Ropivacaine	(LEA 103) (Breon Laboratories, Inc.)	0.5	5	3	4.9	—	5–15	2.5–4	+
Etidocaine	Duranest (Astra Pharmaceutical Products)	0.5–0.75	5	3	4.5	20	5–10	2–5	+++

±, inconsistent motor nerve block; +, weak motor nerve block; +++, strong motor nerve block

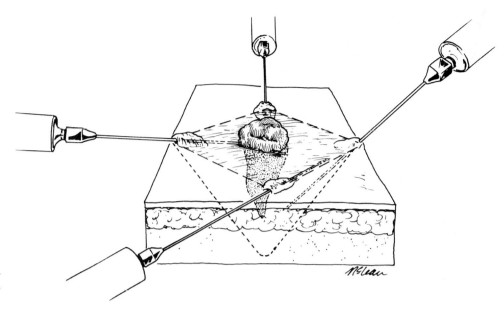

Fig. 16A–2. Field block: the production of walls of anesthesia enclosing the surgical field.

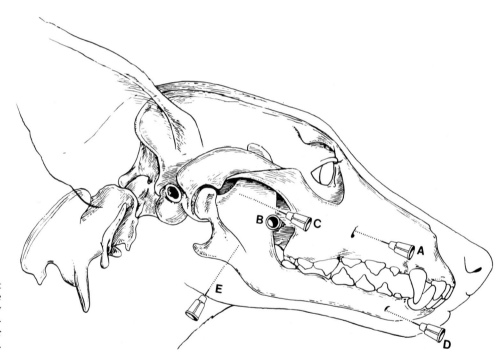

Fig. 16A–3. Needle placement for producing nerve blocks on the head: Infraorbital (A), maxillary (B), zygomatic, lacrimal, and ophthalmic (C), alveolar mandibular (D), and mandibular (E) nerves.

severe vasoconstriction, local ischemia, and necrosis. Epinephrine increases the potential risk of cardiac arrhythmias (e.g., sinus tachycardia, ventricular tachycardia, and ventricular fibrillation in a halothane-sensitized heart), although this has not been a problem when administered in conjunction with lidocaine in dogs. Hearts sensitized to ventricular arrhythmias with halothane do not develop serious ventricular arrhythmias when given lidocaine (1.3 to 7.9 mg/kg) containing epinephrine (0.3 to 1.9 mg/kg) in doses found in lidocaine-epinephrine mixtures used commonly for local anesthesia.(12) Subfascial and intraarterial injections must be avoided.

Field Blocks

Field block is a technique for anesthetizing large areas. First, intradermal or subcutaneous linear infiltration is produced around the lesion as previously described. Local anesthetic is then deposited in the deeper tissues by passing the needle through the desensitized skin far enough to infiltrate the deep nerves supplying the area (Fig. 16A–2).(13)

Nerve Blocks

Injection of local anesthetic solution into the connective tissue surrounding a particular nerve produces loss of sensation (sensory nerve block) and/or paralysis (motor nerve block) in the region supplied by the nerves (regional anesthesia). Smaller volumes (1 to 2 mL) of local anesthetic are needed to produce nerve block compared to field block, therefore reducing the danger of toxicity.

Regional Anesthesia of the Head

Nerves in the head of dogs that do not object to physical restraint or oral examination are occasionally desensitized. Administration of local anesthetic drugs around the infraorbital, maxillary, ophthalmic, mental, and alveolar mandibular nerves can provide extremely valuable and practical advantages over general anesthesia when combined with effective sedation (Fig. 16A–3). Each nerve may be desensitized by injecting 1 to 2 mL of a 2% lidocaine hydrochloride solution using a 2.5- to 5-cm, 20- to 25-gauge needle.

The infraorbital nerve is desensitized at its point of emergence from the infraorbital canal. The needle is inserted either intra- (14) or extraorally approximately 1 cm cranial to the bony lip of the infraorbital foramen.(15) The needle is advanced to the infraorbital foramen, which can be found between the dorsal border of the zygomatic process and the gum of the upper canine tooth (Fig. 16A–3A). Successful injections desensitize the upper lip and nose, the roof of nasal cavity, and the surrounding skin up to the infraorbital foramen.

The maxillary nerve must be desensitized in order to completely desensitize the maxilla, upper teeth, nose, and upper lip. The needle is placed percutaneously along the ventral border of the zygomatic process approximately 0.5 cm caudal to the lateral canthus of the eye and is advanced into close proximity of the pterygopalatine fossa (Fig. 16A–3B). Local anesthetic is administered at the point where the maxillary nerve courses perpendicular to the palatine bone between the maxillary foramen and foramen rotundum.(14, 15)

EYE AND ORBIT

Anesthesia of the eye and orbit is produced by desensitizing the ophthalmic division of the trigeminal nerve. A 2.5-cm, 22-gauge needle is inserted ventral to the zygomatic process at the level of the lateral canthus. The point of the needle should be approximately 0.5 cm cranial to the anterior border of the vertical portion of the ramus of the mandible. The needle is advanced medial to the ramus of the mandible in a mediodorsal and somewhat caudal direction until it reaches the lacrimal, zygomatic, and ophthalmic nerves at the orbital fissure (Figs. 16A–3C and 16A–4). Deposition of 2 mL of local anesthetic at this site produces akinesia of the globe because of the proximity of the abducens, oculomotor, and trochlear nerves to the ophthalmic nerve. Other methods for producing local anesthesia of the eye (retrobulbar anesthesia) run the risk of direct subarachnoid injection, intravascular injection, and systemic absorption (Chapter 24).(4, 16)

The risk of puncturing the globe is minimal if a 7.5-cm, 20-gauge needle is inserted at the lateral canthus through the anesthetized conjunctiva and is advanced past the globe toward the opposite mandibular joint until the base of the orbit is encountered.(14) The potential for puncturing ciliary and scleral blood vessels is minimal if a 5-cm curved needle (0.5 mm i.d.) conformed to the roof of the orbit is inserted through the anesthetized conjunctival sac at the vertical meridian (Fig. 16A–5).(17)

Injection of local anesthetic into the optic sheath can cause respiratory arrest attributable to the infiltration of local anesthetic into the subarachnoid space of the central nervous system.(16) The pressure generated by injection into the optic nerve sheath or intrascleral injection is 3 or 4 times that produced by injection into the retrobulbar adipose tissue (135 vs 35 mm Hg).(16) Increased resistance encountered during retrobulbar block should serve as a warning, mandating redirection of the needle in order to prevent subarachnoid injection.

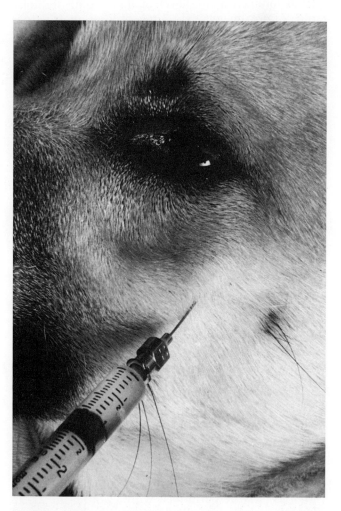

Fig. 16A–4. Anesthesia of ophthalmic nerves. The site and direction of inserted needle.

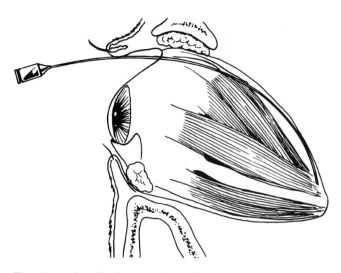

Fig. 16A–5. Needle placement for producing retrobulbar anesthesia

LOWER LIP

The lower lip can be desensitized by percutaneously inserting a 2.5-cm, 22- to 25-gauge needle rostral to the mental foramen at the level of the second premolar tooth. Approximately 1 to 2 mL of local anesthetic is deposited in close proximity to the alveolar mandibular nerve (Fig. 16A–3D).

MANDIBLE AND LOWER TEETH

The mandible, including molars, premolars, canine, incisors, skin, and mucosa of the chin and lower lip, can be desensitized by injecting 1 to 2 mL of the local anesthetic in close proximity to the inferior alveolar branch of the mandibular nerve as it enters the mandibular canal at the mandibular foramen (Fig. 16A–3E). A 2.5-cm, 22-gauge needle is inserted at the lower angle of the jaw approximately 0.5 cm rostral to the angular process and is advanced 1 to 2 cm dorsally along the medial surface of the ramus of the mandible to the palpable lip of the mandibular foramen.(14)

Anesthesia of the Foot

Several techniques may be used to successfully induce anesthesia of the foot: (a) infiltration of tissues around the limb using local anesthetic solution (ring block), (b) infiltration of the branchial plexus with local anesthetic solution (brachial plexus block), (c) injection of local anesthetic into an accessible superficial vein in an extremity that is isolated from the general circulation by placing a tourniquet proximal to the injection site (intravenous regional anesthesia), (d) injection of local anesthetic solution into the lumbosacral epidural space to induce anesthesia of the hindlegs, and (e) perineural infiltration of sensory nerves in the limbs (nerve block).

RING BLOCK

Local infiltration and field blocks around the distal extremity may be performed with a 2- to 5-cm, 22- to 23-gauge standard needle. Intradermal wheals around a superficial lesion and subcutaneous infiltration around the limb are performed using a short (<3 cm) and fine (23- to 25-gauge) needle.

Brachial Plexus Block

Brachial plexus block is suitable for operations on the front limb within or distal to the elbow.(18, 19) The technique should be done in well-sedated standing or laterally recumbent dogs. A 7.5-cm, 20- to 22-gauge needle is inserted medial to the shoulder joint and directed parallel to the vertebral column toward the costochondral junction (Fig. 16A–6). In larger dogs approximately 10 to 15 mL of 2% lidocaine HCl solution with 1:200,000 epinephrine is slowly injected as the needle is withdrawn, if no blood is aspirated into the syringe, thereby placing local anesthetic in close proximity to the radial, median, ulnar, musculocutaneous, and axillary nerves. Gradual loss of sensation and motor function occurs within 10 to 15 minutes. Anesthesia lasts for approximately 2 hours, and total recovery requires approximately 6 hours. Brachial plexus block is relatively simple and safe to perform and produces selective anesthesia and relaxation of the limb distal to the elbow joint (Fig. 16A–7). The relatively long waiting period (15 to 30 minutes) required to attain maximal anesthesia and some occasional failures to obtain complete anesthesia, particularly in fat dogs, are disadvantages of the technique.

Intravenous Regional Anesthesia

Intravenous regional anesthesia (IVRA) is a rapid and reliable method for producing short-term (<2 hours) anesthesia of the extremities. The clinical value of IVRA

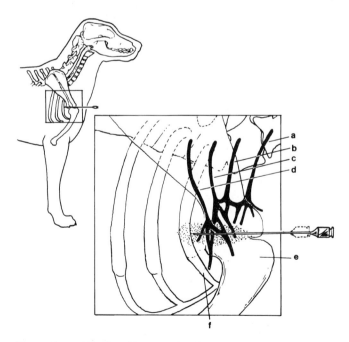

Fig. 16A–6. Needle placement for brachial plexus block. Inset: ventral branches of (a) sixth, (b) seventh, (c) eighth cervical, and (d) first thoracic spinal nerve; (e) tuberosity of humerus; (f) first rib.

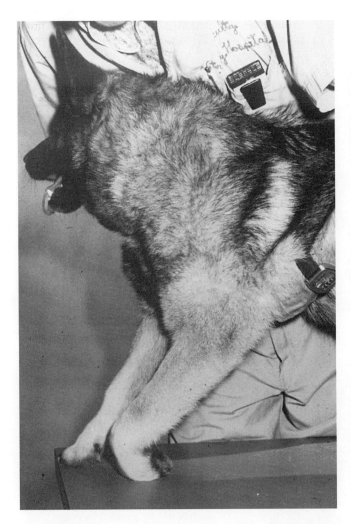

Fig. 16A–7. Anesthesia of brachial plexus of left thoracic limb in the conscious dog.

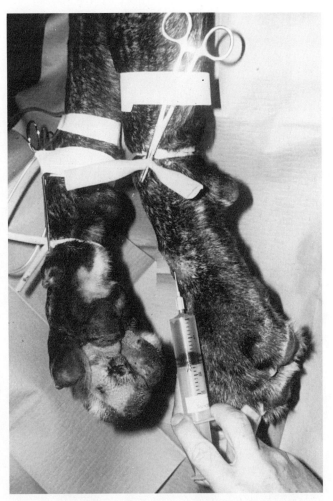

Fig. 16A–8. Intravenous regional anesthesia in a sedated bullmastiff (80 kg) in right lateral recumbency for skin biopsies at the palmar paws of both front legs. A rubber tourniquet is placed distal to the carpus (right foot) and proximal to the carpus (left foot). The tourniquets are secured with hemostatic forceps, which are taped to the skin. Injection of 12 mL of 1% lidocaine hydrochloride solution (1.5 mg/kg per leg) into the cephalic vein is shown.

in humans is well established. The IVRA technique is also known as "BIER block."(20) Little information on clinical experiences with IVRA in dogs exists, even though it appears to be a simple, safe, and practical method for providing 60 to 90 minutes of regional anesthesia in an extremity distal to a tourniquet (Fig. 16A–8).(21) The technique is best accomplished in dogs by placing an intravenous catheter in an appropriate and accessible vein (e.g., the cephalic or lateral saphenous vein) distal to the tourniquet. The limb is first desanguinated by wrapping it with an Esmarch bandage. A rubber tourniquet is placed around the limb proximal to the Esmarch bandage. The tourniquet must be tight enough to overcome arterial blood pressure.(22) Once the tourniquet is secured, the Esmarch bandage is unwrapped, and 2.5 to 5 mg/kg of lidocaine is injected intravenously with light pressure. Five to 10 minutes are required to achieve maximum anesthesia before beginning the surgical procedure. Diluted concentrations (0.25% and 0.5%) of lidocaine produce adequate sensory blockade as long as the tourniquet is applied. By

avoiding leakage and keeping the local anesthetic isolated in the limb, the incidence and severity of toxic symptoms are decreased and the percentage of successful blocks increased.(22) Complications resulting from blood flow deprivation to the limb or the dose of anesthetic used do not occur if the procedure is limited to 90 minutes.

Once the tourniquet is removed, sensation returns within 5 to 15 minutes and residual analgesia remains for up to 30 minutes. Minimal effects on the heart rate, respiratory rate, or electrocardiogram are noted in dogs after removal of the tourniquet.(21) The site and mechanism of local anesthetic action in IVRA is unclear but may involve desensitization of major nerve trunks and/or sensory nerve endings.(23) Unlike the desensitization described by other nerve blocks, the onset of anesthesia and muscle paralysis begins distally and

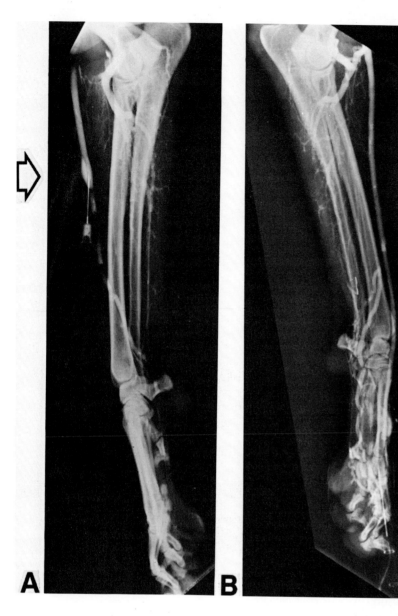

Fig. 16A–9. Radiographs of the left forelimb of a German shepherd dog (35 kg); A, a mixture of 3 mL 2% lidocaine hydrochloride solution and 3 mL of Omnipaque 300 was injected into the cephalic vein at a proximal site. Retrograde dissipation of the anesthetic was prohibited by venous valves; thus, anesthesia of the limb did not develop. B, The injection was repeated at a distal site 1 week later, thereby inducing anesthesia of the limb distal to the tourniquet.

progresses proximally; thus, the local anesthetic should be injected as distally as possible in the limb to be anesthetized (Fig. 16A–9). The blood-free surgery site is ideal for taking biopsies and removing a foreign body from the paws. Prolonged procedures (>90 minutes) may produce tourniquet-induced ischemia, which is associated with pain and increased blood pressure. If pain occurs, it is often difficult to control and requires induction of general anesthesia.(24) Reversible shock occurs if the tourniquet is removed after 4 hours; and sepsis, endotoxemia, and death occur if the tourniquet is removed after 8 to 10 hours. Bupivacaine should not be used for this technique because of cardiovascular collapse and death associated with its use.(25-28)

Lumbosacral Epidural Anesthesia

Lumbosacral epidural anesthesia is noted for its simplicity, safety, and effectiveness, and is one of the most frequently used regional anesthetic techniques de-scribed for surgical procedures caudal to the umbilicus in dogs.(29-51) Epidural anesthesia is frequently recommended for cesarean section because, unlike other anesthetic techniques, it does not depress the puppies (Chapter 24). The bitch remains awake and able to take care of her puppies immediately after surgery.

Dogs are generally sedated or tranquilized to reduce fear and apprehension and then are placed either in sternal recumbency (for bilateral anesthesia) or in lateral recumbency (for ipsilateral anesthesia). The hind limbs can be extended cranially to maximally separate the lumbar vertebrae.

The anesthetic procedure is not technically difficult when performed by an experienced clinician. Local anesthetic solution is injected through a disposable 2.5- to 7.5-cm, 20- to 22-gauge spinal needle as a single dose or is injected through a catheter that is inserted 1.5 to 2 cm beyond the end of an 18- or 17-gauge Huber point (Tuohy) or 18-gauge Crawford needle (continuous technique; Fig. 16A–10). A 2.5-cm, 22-gauge spinal needle is used for small dogs, a 3.8-cm, 20-gauge needle for medium dogs, and a 7.5-cm 18-gauge needle for large dogs. Important landmarks for needle placement are easily identified in most dogs. The iliac prominences on either side of the spine are palpated by using the thumb and middle finger of one hand (Fig. 16A–10). The spinous process of the seventh lumbar (L7) vertebra is located with the index finger. The lumbosacral (L7-S1) interspace should be palpated from both the cranial and caudal directions by moving the finger on the dorsal spinous processes of L6 to L7 and S2 to S1. This will help to avoid inadvertent placement of the needle into the L6 to L7 interspace. The needle must be correctly placed on the midline and caudal to the L7 spinous process, and is inserted until a distinct popping sensation is felt as the needle point penetrates the interarcuate ligament. Movement of the tail may indicate that the needle has engaged nerve tissue. The epidural space is best identified by the "loss of resistance test," using either an air- or a saline-filled syringe. Deliberate injection of 3 to 4 mL of air into the epidural space of dogs weighing 20 to 27 kg results in bubble formation that can persist for 24 hours. The bubbles, however, are not large or numerous enough to impede transfer of local anesthetic across the meninges and into the CSF, spinal roots, and cord, nor do they localize in any particular region (e.g., nerve roots); thus, subsequent injection of local anesthetic does not result in patchy anesthesia or inadequacies attributable to bubbles.(52) Subcutaneous crepitation may be felt at the site of skin penetration if air has been injected outside the epidural space.

The needle or catheter should be carefully inspected for flow of cerebrospinal fluid (CSF) or blood before the local anesthetic is administered. Presence of CSF indicates inadvertent subarachnoid puncture. Presence of blood indicates penetration of the ventral venous plexus. The possibility of obtaining CSF at the L7 to S1 site is minimal because the subarachnoid space of dogs usually ends cranial to the lumbosacral interspace. The spinal cord and meninges in younger and smaller dogs may occasionally extend into the lumbosacral vertebral junction.(53) A subarachnoid injection may be made if CSF is encountered, with the precaution that only 50% of the intended epidural dose is needed: 1 mL of local anesthetic per 10 kg of body weight injected over a 1-minute period.(45, 48) The reduced dose should avoid "total spinal anesthesia" with cardiovascular and respiratory depression or collapse. The needle is withdrawn and cleansed, and another attempt is made to place it into the epidural space if blood is encountered. Intravascular injection of local anesthetic can result in systemic toxicity, which is characterized by convulsions, cardiopulmonary depression, and the absence of regional anesthesia.(26, 27, 54) Inadvertent subarachnoid administration of small amounts (2 mL) of fresh autologous blood aspirated from the venous plexus during attempted lumbar epidural puncture will cause spasm of the pelvic limbs in dogs. The dogs, however, are able to stand unassisted within 20 minutes after blood injection and demonstrate no signs of meningeal irritation, long-term neurologic sequelae, or neuropathologic changes.(55)

The shape and bevel orientation of the spinal needle affects the size of the dural defect. Large dural defects in humans may result in post–lumbar puncture headache attributable to a postulated increased CSF leak. The dural defect produced by a 22-gauge Whitacre

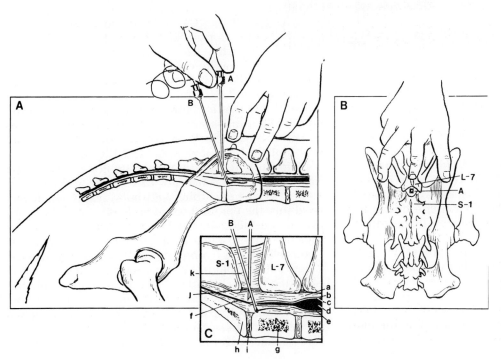

Fig. 16A–10. A, Needle placement into the lumbosacral epidural space of the dog (A) and catheter placement for continuous epidural anesthesia using a local anesthetic and/or analgesia using an opioid (B). B, Dorsal view. Palpation of the dorsal spinous process of L7 vertebra and dorsoiliac wings. C, Inset: (a) epidural space with fat and connective tissue, (b) dura mater, (c) arachnoid membrane, (d) spinal cord, (e) cerebrospinal fluid, (f) cauda equina, (g) seventh lumbar (L7) vertebra, (h) first sacral (S1) vertebra, (i) intervertebral disc, (j) interarcuate ligament (ligamantum flavum), (k) interspinous ligament.

needle is smaller than that produced by a 22-gauge Quincke needle (27,400 vs 39,400 sq. microns). Likewise, a bevel orientation parallel rather perpendicular to the dural fibers results in smaller dural defects (39,400 vs 73,300 sq. microns), because the needle is splitting rather than cutting the longitudinal dural fibers.(56) It is necessary to administer the calculated dose of local anesthetic at the body temperature of the dog and slow enough (over 45 to 60 seconds) to avoid causing pain.

A variety of local anesthetics of different concentrations and doses have been used to produce epidural anesthesia in dogs and have induced a wide spectrum of sensory and motor blockades. The selected local anesthetic and dosage (concentration, volume) depends upon the dog's size, the desired extent of anesthesia, and the desired onset and duration of anesthetic effect. A test dose of 0.5 to 1.0 mL of 2% lidocaine hydrochloride solution produces almost immediate dilation of the external anal sphincter, followed by relaxation of the tail and ataxia of pelvic limbs within 3 to 5 minutes. Approximately 1 mL of 2% lidocaine per 4.5 kg of body weight will completely anesthetize the pelvic limbs and posterior abdomen caudal to the first lumbar (L1) vertebra within 10 to 15 minutes after administration.(36) The flexor pinch reflex of pelvic limbs will be absent in 5 to 10 minutes after injection.(32) Clinical experience indicates that the disappearance of the toe reflexes is associated with surgical anesthesia from midthorax to coccyx sufficient for abdominal surgery.(33) The latent period is prolonged to 20 to 30 minutes if 0.75% bupivacaine hydrochloride is administered and is attributable to the drug's low solubility and slow uptake by nervous tissue.(48) Good anesthesia for abdominal and orthopedic surgeries caudal to the diaphragm is generally achieved by administering 1 mL/5 kg (maximum 20 mL) of 2% lidocaine or 0.5% bupivacaine, both with freshly added 1:200,000 epinephrine.

A reduced volume of 2% lidocaine (1 mL/6 kg) is generally satisfactory for epidural anesthesia in dogs for cesarean section. The reason for the (approximately 25%) decrease in dose requirement during pregnancy is unclear.(57) Several theories have been proposed: (a) distension of epidural veins, which decreases the size of the epidural space and/or increase in the spread of local anesthetic (58), (b) hormonal changes, which influence proteins that affect membrane sensitivity (59), and (c) chronic exposure to progesterone, which alters the permeability of intercellular connective tissue matrix, thereby facilitating diffusion of local anesthetics across the nerve sheath.(60) It is rarely necessary to inject more than 3 mg lidocaine/kg body weight for epidural anesthesia during cesarean section in dogs.

The duration of anesthesia obtained from the deposition of epidural local anesthetic drugs is primarily dependent upon the drug selected, the dermatomal level of anesthesia, and the presence or absence of epinephrine (Table 16A–2). The duration of postoperative analgesia (after general anesthesia) is longer when epidural anesthesia is performed at the end of surgery,

and is attributable to a diminished intensity of the painful stimulus (Chapter 4). Two percent solutions of procaine, lidocaine, and carbocaine have provided satisfactory anesthesia and muscle relaxation for 60 to 120 minutes. Epidural bupivacaine (0.75%) and etidocaine (1%) have induced surgical anesthesia for periods lasting from 4 to 6 hours. Surgical anesthesia caudal to the last rib is produced and is gradually converted into a phase of postoperative analgesia lasting for 24 hours without affecting motor activity or cardiopulmonary function, if a combination of 0.7 to 1.0 mL/10 cm vertex-coccyx distance of 0.5% bupivacaine hydrochloride solution and 0.1 mg/kg morphine hydrochloride is injected epidurally.(61)

The efficacy of bupivacaine and ropivacaine for producing lumbar epidural and subarachnoid anesthesia in dogs has been compared.(62) Various concentrations of ropivacaine (0.25, 0.5, 0.75, 1%) and bupivacaine (0.25, 0.5, 0.75%) using a constant 3-mL epidural volume and 1-mL subarachnoid volume of ropivacaine and bupivacaine were used. Epidural blockade was also performed utilizing solutions of ropivacaine and bupivacaine that contained epinephrine (1:200,000). There were no signs of adverse reactions, irreversible block, or other sequelae in any of the dogs studied. Onset of motor blockade (time from the completion of the injection until the dog's pelvic limbs were unable to support weight), ranged from 1.7 to 4.1 minutes following subarachnoid injection (mean weight 19.1 ± 0.9 kg of 8 dogs). There were no differences in the onset of motor blockade between various anesthetic solutions. Duration of motor blockade (time from onset of motor blockade until the dog was able to support its own weight) ranged from 103 minutes (0.75% ropivacaine) to 163 minutes (0.75% bupivacaine).

Solutions of 0.25% ropivacaine and 0.25% bupivacaine failed to induce complete loss of weight support (mean weight 18.7 ± 1.4 kg) following epidural injection. Onset of motor blockade varied between 5 and 9 minutes with the use of higher concentrations (>0.25%), and was inversely related to dose. Duration of motor blockade ranged from 141 minutes (0.5% ropivacaine) to 258 minutes (0.75% bupivacaine). The similar onset times for both drugs were related to their similar pKa (ropivacaine, 8.0; bupivacaine, 8.1). The decreased motor blocking potency of ropivacaine is consistent with its low lipid solubility. Epinephrine failed to prolong the duration of motor blockade for either drug. Little difference in vascular activity may exist between ropivacaine and bupivacaine when injected into the epidural space of dogs.

Local anesthetics injected epidurally in the dog may enter the cerebrospinal fluid (29, 63) and the epidural venous blood and lymph (35), and become partitioned in epidural fat. Epidurally administered drugs enter the lymphatic system by diffusion into the dural lymphatic vessels located at the level of the nerve roots, leakage of local anesthetic drug out of the vertebral canal through the intervertebral foramina, and vascular absorption and systemic redistribution.(64)

The pharmacokinetics of bupivacaine and ropivacaine after lumbar epidural administrations of either drug, (0.75% solution, 3-mL volume with or without 1:200,000 epinephrine) in dogs have been determined.(25) Both drugs have a similar pharmacokinetic profile. Peak arterial concentrations of bupivacaine and ropivacaine occur within 5 to 10 minutes after injection and were less than 1 μg/mL. The addition of epinephrine did not consistently decrease the C_{max} of either agent.

Selective epidural anesthesia that extends as far cranially as the anterior thoracic dermatomes (T3 to T5) does not adversely change cardiovascular function, respiratory rate, arterial blood pH, and gas tensions (PaO_2, $PaCO_2$) in conscious dogs or dogs that are premedicated with methadone (0.8 mg/kg), acepromazine (0.3 mg/kg), and atropine (0.6 to 1.2 mg).(44) Likewise, awake and unsedated healthy dogs compensate for markedly attenuated spinal sympathetic outflow, which might occur during thoracic epidural anesthesia, by increasing endogenous vasopressin concentrations, thus supporting arterial blood pressure.(65, 66) Severe hypotension (with mean arterial blood pressure < 60 mm Hg) can occur in aged and sick dogs with suppressed neurally mediated renin release or in dogs when endogenous vasopressin is prevented from acting on its (V1)-vasopressin receptors.(34, 66) Hypotension should be treated with intravenous crystalloid solutions (20 to 30 mL/kg) and/or a vasopressor (phenylephrine, methoxamine).(67)

High epidural anesthesia to T1 myotomal level in 5 pentobarbital-anesthetized dogs (8 to 13 kg) in dorsal recumbency, has recently been documented to be associated with increased intrathoracic volume at end-expiration (76 ± 35 mL, mean ± SD) by increasing intrathoracic tissue volume (33 ± 15 mL) and the amount of gas in the lungs at end expiration [functional residual capacity (FRC)].(68) The increases in thoracic tissue volume were probably attributable to increases in intrathoracic blood volume. High epidural anesthesia (coccyx to T1) in these dogs was achieved by injecting 0.5 mL increments of 1.5% etidocaine with epinephrine 1:200,000 into a catheter, which was placed percutaneously through the vertebral arch of the second coccygeal vertebra and advanced until the tip was near the L4 to L5 vertebrae in the epidural space.(68)

Thoracic epidural block in dogs before the production of experimental hemorrhagic shock has been advocated as potentially therapeutic.(50) Endocardial blood flow improves, and determinants of myocardial oxygen consumption decrease.(69)

Rectal temperature usually remains unchanged during epidural anesthesia in dogs. If hypothermia occurs after epidural injections, it may result from redistribution of heat within the body.(70) Fluctuation in skin temperature of the limbs (but not the trunk) and an absence of sweating (dogs have no sweat glands except in the paws(71), may reflect changes of sympathetic activity after epidural nerve blockade.(49, 72) Increased skin temperature in the pelvic limbs (1.2° C) and paw

(2.0° C), decreased skin temperature in the thoracic limbs and thorax (−0.6° C), and no change in rectal temperature were produced when small doses of bupivacaine (3.5 mL, 0.5%) were administered into the lumbar epidural space of conscious dogs.

Epidural anesthesia is likely to suppress the markers of stress as represented by serum levels of ACTH, beta endorphin, epinephrine, and norepinephrine.(65, 73) In addition, epidural anesthesia could play a role in host defense mechanisms against various microorganisms.(74)

Adverse effects associated with epidural and subarachnoid anesthesia in dogs include (a) hypoventilation secondary to respiratory muscle paralysis, which is attributable to the spread of local anesthetic to the cervical spinal segments; (b) hypotension, Horner's syndrome (Fig. 16A–11), and hypoglycemia caused by sympathetic blockade; (c) Shiff-Sherrington-like reflexes; and (d) muscular twitches, coma, convulsion, and

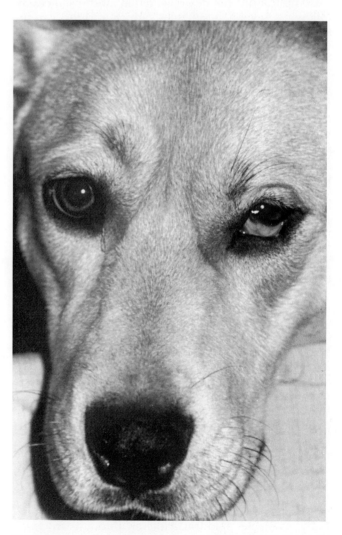

Fig. 16A–11. Unilateral Horner's syndrome (e.g., ptosis, miosis, and enophthalmus in a Golden Retriever (35 kg) with ipsilateral paresis of the left thoracic limb, after overdosage (12 mL) of the lumbosacral epidural anesthetic.

circulatory depression due to toxic plasma concentrations of local anesthetic. Delay in onset of anesthesia, unilateral hind limb paresis, partial anesthesia of tail or perineal region, and sepsis can result from improper injection technique.(75, 76)

Although epidural anesthesia has been referred to as the ideal anesthetic procedure for bitches in dystocia (32, 77, 78), respiratory depression can be a serious complication. Changes from a thoracic to a diaphragmatic (abdominal) pattern of breathing indicate at least partial motor block of the intercostal musculature, which may not be reflected by changes in arterial pH, PaO_2, or $PaCO_2$. The use of preblock oxygenation, proper doses of local anesthetic, and slight elevation of the head, neck, and thorax minimize this problem. The presence of paresis of the nictitating membrane of the eye (Fig. 16A–11), which derives its sympathetic nerve supply from the first three thoracic spinal segments is evidence that most, if not all, of the sympathetic outflow has been blocked by extensive epidural spread.

Complications can be prevented in most instances by following several basic rules, which include careful selection of drugs and dosage, aspiration before injection (to assure that the tip of the needle is not in a blood vessel or subarachnoid space), and injection of test doses.(51)

Absolute contraindications for epidural anesthetic techniques include infection at the lumbosacral puncture site, uncorrected hypovolemia, bleeding disorders, therapeutic or physiologic anticoagulation, degenerative central or peripheral axonal diseases, and anatomic abnormalities that would make epidural anesthesia difficult. Bacteremia, neurologic disorders, and minidose heparin therapy are relative contraindications. The benefits of epidural anesthesia often outweigh the risks.(79)

Continuous Epidural Anesthesia

The indications, advantages, contraindications, and complications associated with continuous epidural anesthesia in dogs are similar to those of the single-injection method. Additional advantages of continuous epidural anesthesia are the ability to tailor the duration of anesthesia to the length of operation and to maintain a route for injecting epidural opioids during surgery and postoperatively.(41, 61, 80)

Despite numerous reports describing continuous epidural anesthesia in dogs, epidural catheters are not used routinely because of technical difficulties; the potential to produce damage of the spinal cord, meninges, and nerves; the risk of infection; and catheter-related problems. Nevertheless, insertion of plastic catheters into the epidural space of dogs is a relatively simple and safe procedure once practiced. Local anesthetics and/or opioids may be administered to produce continuous epidural anesthesia by placing a commercially available epidural catheter through an 18-or 17-gauge Huber-point (Tuohy) needle or 18-gauge Crawford needle into the epidural space (Fig. 16A–10).

Self-prepared sterile 20-gauge catheters (e.g., polyethylene tubing PE 160) may also be used.

A comprehensive selection of epidural products and accessories exists for use in humans and can be adapted for dogs, thus making the technique in dogs easier and safer. Epidural trays contain a 7.5-cm, 17-gauge Tuohy needle and an 18-gauge catheter set with a luer slip glass syringe, a polyamide radiopaque catheter that resists kinking, with either an open tip–rounded or a closed tip–atraumatic catheter with lateral flow side ports, a thread assist guidewire that eliminates the need for a stylet, a catheter connector that attaches quickly and securely without possibility of crushing the catheter, and a variety of syringes, needles, sterile preparation solutions, and sponges (Fig. 16A–12). The theoretical advantages of the multiple side port epidural catheter include even distribution of local anesthetic, less chance of clotting (because fibrins are less likely to collect on the side), and the ability to have a completely

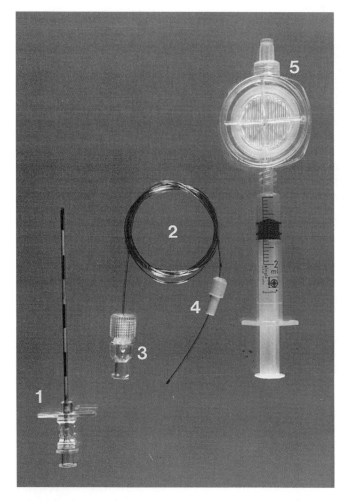

Fig. 16A–12. Epidural trays for continuous epidural anesthesia. The basic Perifix 300 set contains (1) Tuohy needle (1.3 × 80 mm, 18G × 3 1/4″), (2) radiopaque polyamide catheter (0.45 × 0.85 × 1000 mm), (3) screw connector (4), introducing aid, and (5) Luer Lock antibacteria injection filter (0.2 μm).

rounded and therefore atraumatic tip. Although these accessories can increase the convenience of placing an epidural catheter, they add to the cost of an epidural tray.

The Tuohy needle is placed into the epidural space between the L7 and S1 intervertebral space, similar to the single-injection epidural block technique. Catheterization is facilitated by first desensitizing the lumbosacral space with a small amount (2 mL) of 2% lidocaine. The Tuohy needle is inserted at a 15 to 45° angle from the vertical position with the bevel directed cranially (Fig. 16A–10). Catheters with a stylet are preferred. A slight resistance is usually encountered when the catheter passes through the tip of the Tuohy needle. Special markings on the catheter denote the distance the catheter has been advanced. The catheter is advanced at least 2 to 3 markings beyond the hub of the needle, which ensures that at least 2 to 3 cm of catheter has entered the epidural space. Flushing the needle with saline, rotating the needle, and advancing the catheter while slowly withdrawing the needle help to overcome the problem of failure of the catheter to thread into the epidural space. If these maneuvers fail, the needle and catheter should be withdrawn together. No attempt should be made to withdraw the catheter back through the needle, since this may sever the catheter. Most authorities believe that no attempt should be made to retrieve severed catheters.(81) Wire-reinforced catheters can be inserted epidurally to the anterior lumbar (L4) (82) or thoracic (T1) (63) vertebrae with minimal resistance and without coiling, turning on themselves, kinking, or knotting.

Tuohy needles have been epidurally placed at the second coccygeal (Co3 to Co2), third coccygeal (Co4 to Co3), or fourth coccygeal (Co5 to Co4) intervertebral space of dogs. A wire-reinforced catheter can then be threaded epidurally for up to 15 cm in order to reach the thoracic vertebrae.(64) Inserting a catheter for long distances increases the risk that the catheter tip may exit a paravertebral foramen. Fluoroscopy can be used to facilitate catheter guidance.

Nerve Blocks in the Limb

Specific nerve blocks in the front limbs (radial, ulnar, median, musculocutaneous nerve block.) and hind limbs (tibial, peroneal, saphenous) of the dog have been described.(83) These techniques are rarely used in clinical practice because of difficulty in locating the proper site for injection of local anesthetic and the substitution of simpler methods (e.g., intravenous regional anesthesia, epidural anesthesia).

Intercostal Nerve Blocks

Intercostal nerve blocks may be used for relieving pain during and after thoracotomy, pleural drainage, and rib fractures. They are not recommended for dogs with pulmonary diseases, which impair blood gas exchange, or for dogs that cannot be observed for several hours

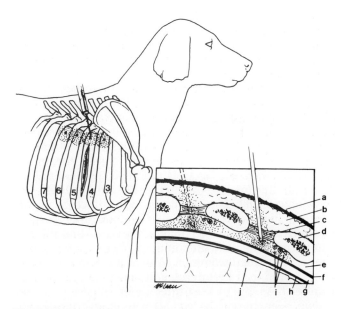

Fig. 16A–13. Needle placement for inducing intercostal nerve blocks. Inset: (a) skin, (b) subcutaneous tissue, (c) intercostal muscles, (d) rib, (e) subcostal space, (f) pleura costalis and fascia, (g) interpleural space, (h) pleura pulmonalis, (i) intercostal artery, vein and nerve, (j) lung.

after injection because of the chance of clinically delayed pneumothorax.

A minimum of two adjacent intercostal spaces both cranial and caudal to the incision or injury site are selectively blocked because of overlap of nerve supply. The site for needle placement is the caudal border of the rib (R3-6) near the intervertebral foramen (Fig. 16A–13). Approximately 0.25 to 1.0 mL of 0.25% or 0.5% bupivacaine hydrochloride/site, with or without epinephrine 1:200,000, is deposited. Small volumes and/or diluted local anesthetic solutions should be used as initial pain therapy so that the total dose does not exceed 3 mg/kg. Small dogs receive 0.25 mL/site, medium dogs 0.5 mL/site, and large dogs 1.0 mL/site. Postthoracotomy pain is generally controlled for 3 to 6 hours following successful block.(84) Heart rate, respiratory rate, hematocrit, plasma protein, blood pH, PaO_2 and $PaCO_2$ in halothane-anesthetized dogs following intercostal nerve block do not change significantly.(84) Prolonged analgesia may be achieved by repeated administrations of local anesthetics, although the patient may not tolerate multiple percutaneous injections. Intercostal nerve block produces high blood concentrations of local anesthetic for a given dose; (85, 86) therefore, the risk for toxic blood concentrations is a possibility.

Selective intercostal nerve block is easily performed because of the proximity of each nerve to its adjacent rib. The intercostal nerves can be visualized beneath the parietal pleura during thoracotomy. The technique provides consistent analgesia and does not produce respiratory depression, with subsequent hypercarbia and hypoxemia being a frequent problem in dogs administered intramuscular or intravenous opioids.(84, 87)

Interpleural Regional Analgesia

Interpleural injection of local anesthetics is a relatively new option for managing certain types of acute and chronic pain originating from thoracic and upper abdominal structures in humans.(88) Pain from lateral and posterior thoracotomies, rib fractures, metastasis to the chest wall, pleura, and mediastinum, mastectomy, chronic pancreatitis, cholecystectomy, renal surgery, abdominal cancer, and posthepatic neuralgesia can be relieved by intermittent or continuous administration of local anesthetic into the pleural space through a catheter, without the systemic effects commonly observed after the use of parenterally administered (IM, IV) opioids.(89) Most clinical studies have been performed in patients recovering from gallbladder surgery. Less frequently, this technique has been used for pain relief in patients with multiple fractured ribs; other indications are uncommon.(90) The mechanisms of pain relief produced by interpleural analgesia are not fully understood, but at least three different sites of actions have been hypothesized: (a) retrograde diffusion of local anesthetic through the parietal pleura causing intercostal nerve block (91, 92), (b) unilateral block of the thoracic sympathetic chain and splanchnic nerves (93), and (c) diffusion of the anesthetic into the ipsilateral brachial plexus resulting in a parietal block.(88)

The technique requires the insertion of a catheter into the pleural space of a sedated or anesthetized dog. The catheter is placed into the pleural space either percutaneously or prior to closure of a thoracotomy (Fig. 16A–14). Percutaneous placement of a catheter into the pleural space is difficult to perform on dogs with pleural fibrosis, since thickening of the pleura makes identifi-

cation of the pleural space guesswork. The dog should be sedated, and the skin, subcutaneous tissues, periosteum, and parietal pleura over the caudal border of the rib should first be desensitized with 1 to 2 mL of 2% lidocaine solution, using a 2.5-to 5-cm, 20- to 22-gauge needle. A 5 cm × 1.4 mm o.d., 17-gauge Huber point (Tuohy) needle is then used for catheter placement. The stylet is removed and the needle filled with sterile saline until a meniscus is seen at the needle's hub. The needle is then advanced until a clicking sensation is perceived as the needle tip perforates the parietal pleura or until the meniscus disappears when the needle tip enters the pleural space (hanging-drop technique).

The hanging-drop technique for the identification of the subatmospheric pleural pressure is not always reliable because the meniscus may also disappear when the needle passes through the intercostal muscles. Alternatively, a freely moving 10 mL glass syringe is attached to the needle. The syringe and needle are then advanced as a unit. On entering the pleural space, the plunger of the syringe is drawn inward by the negative pressure of the interpleural space.(89) Some veterinarians place the catheter in the tissue plane superficial to the parietal pleura, close to or in the paravertebral space in order to produce a more effective block attributable to a decreased loss of local anesthetic through thoracic drainage tubes.(90) A catheter (6- to 10-cm length of fenestrated medical grade silastic tubing, 2-mm inside diameter) can be introduced and advanced 3 to 5 cm beyond the needle tip with minimal resistance after the needle tip is placed subpleurally.

A new technique has recently been developed to insert the catheter without disconnection to minimize

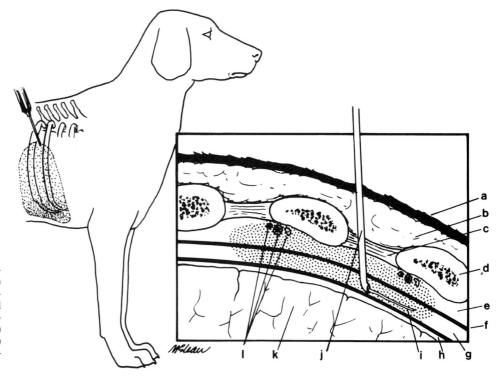

Fig. 16A–14. Interpleural catheter placement. Inset: (a) skin, (b) subcutaneous tissue, (c) intercostal muscles, (d) rib, (e) subcostal space, (f) pleura costalis and fascia, (g) interpleural space, (h) pleura pulmonalis, (i) catheter, (j) Tuohy needle, (k) lung, (l) intercostal artery, vein and nerve.

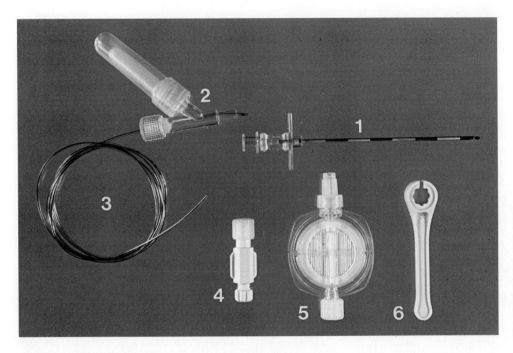

Fig. 16A–15. Interpleural tray for continuous interpleural analgesia. The basic Pleurocert procedure set contains (1) Tuohy needle (1.7 × 80 mm, 16G × 3 1/4", (2) Y-piece with control-balloon, (3) radiopaque polyamide catheter (0.65 × 1.05 × 1000 mm, (4) screw connector, (5) Luer Lock antibacteria injection filter (0.2 μm), and (6) wrench.

the risk of pneumothorax.(94) The technique involves the use of a Tuohy needle to which a Y-piece with a latex balloon and catheter is attached. The needle is inserted until the balloon collapses under the negative pressure of the pleural cavity, the catheter is then advanced as required. The needle is then carefully withdrawn over the catheter and the catheter is left in place.

Approximately 1 to 2 mg bupivacaine/kg (0.5%, with or without 5 μg epinephrine/mL) is injected over 1 to 2 minutes following negative aspiration of air or blood through the catheter. The catheter is then cleared with 2 mL of physiologic saline solution. Bolus interpleural bupivacaine is effective in relieving postthoracotomy pain for 3 to 12 hours.(84) The addition of epinephrine (5 μg/mL) to the local anesthetic solution may or may not increase the duration of analgesia and decrease the plasma concentration of the local anesthetic.

Complications, such as lung trauma, bleeding, and pneumothorax, are occasionally reported with the blind percutaneous insertion technique in humans.(95) The balloon technique is superior to other methods (e.g., loss-of-resistance technique, low-friction syringe-piston movement, infusion technique). Sterile sets for single continuous interpleural analgesia are available. They contain a Tuohy needle, catheter, control-balloon, flat antibacteria injection filter, screw connector, screw-driver, and drape (Fig. 16A–15).

Catheter placement in the open chest is accomplished by inserting the Tuohy needle through the skin over the rib at a site that is at least two intercostal spaces caudal to the incision while taking care to retract the lung. The catheter is then passed through the needle and placed 3 to 5 cm subpleurally under direct vision. Local anesthetic is injected in the usual manner. The ventral tip of the catheter is best anchored using one encircling suture of surgical gut (3-0) in the intercostal space at the site of puncture.

Positioning of the catheter will affect the site of intercostal nerve blockade and is attributable to gravity-induced pooling of the local anesthetic within the interpleural space.(96-98) Dogs that recover from lateral thoracotomy should be placed with the incision side down. Dogs that have had a sternotomy should be placed in sternal recumbency for approximately 10 minutes to allow the local anesthetic to pool near the incision and adjacent intercostal nerves. The external portion of the catheter should be anchored with tape, sutured to the skin, and covered with a nonocclusive type dressing that allows air circulation. Analgesia produced by interpleural infusion in dogs is similar to analgesia produced by morphine (0.5 mg/kg subcutaneously) or selective intercostal nerve block with bupivacaine (0.5 mL of 0.5% bupivacaine per site), but lasts longer (3 to 12 hours).(84) Dogs that are treated with 1.5 mg interpleural bupivacaine/kg through an interpleural catheter do not demonstrate significant changes of heart rate, respiratory rate, hematocrit, plasma protein, blood pH, or $PaCO_2$.(84)

The optimum total dose, concentration, or volume of interpleural bupivacaine in sick dogs has not been reported. Theoretically, it is possible to block one or two of the three branches of the phrenic nerve, leaving the remaining branch(es) intact. Isolated contraction of the costal portion of the diaphragm without contraction of the crural portion may result in paradoxical respiration with negative intraabdominal pressures.(99) The catheter is usually removed 24 hours after thoracotomy when postoperative pain has normally decreased. Long-term use (over several weeks) of an interpleural catheter is possible if the catheter is subcutaneously tunneled.(100)

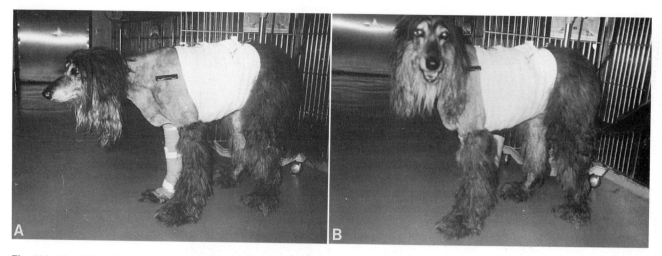

Fig. 16A–16. Afghan hound (35 kg) recovering from bilateral thoracotomy: A, before; B; 15 minutes after interpleural bupivacaine (0.5%, 35 mg = 7 mL) administration into each of the two chest tubes (total dose 70 mg).

The administration of interpleural bupivacaine is greatly facilitated in dogs in which a chest-tube has been placed for evacuation of air (Fig. 16A–16). Interpleural regional analgesia has limitations but also several distinct advantages over the more traditional intercostal nerve blocks and administration of parenteral opioids. The procedure is technically simple to perform. Only one needle stick is needed, in contrast to multiple intercostal nerve blocks. Pain relief lasts longer and is less likely to produce central nervous system and respiratory depression than after the use of parenteral opioids.

Infection, tachyphylaxis to local anesthetic, high anesthetic blood concentration, systemic toxicity from local anesthesia, unilateral sympathetic block (evidenced as a Horner's syndrome) and increased subcutaneous skin temperature of the affected side, pleural effusion, phrenic nerve paralysis or paresis, and catheter-related complications (e.g., intrapulmonary placement of catheter) do not occur if the procedure is performed properly. Pain relief is minimal in dogs with a misplaced catheter, excessive bleeding into the pleural space, or pleural effusion. Care must be taken to avoid the serious potential complication of pneumothorax, particularly when this method is used bilaterally.(101)

Epidural Opioid Analgesia

The presence of a large number of opiate receptors in the substantia gelatinosa of the dorsal horn of the spinal cord suggests that the administration of small doses of opioids into the epidural space should be effective in producing analgesia (Chapters 4 and 7).(102) The administration of epidural opioids offers the advantages of producing more profound and prolonged analgesia with significantly smaller doses and less sedation than the analgesia produced by comparable parenterally administered (intramuscular, intravenous) opioids (Chapter 8). Epidural opioids relieve somatic and visceral pain by selectively blocking nociceptive

impulses without interfering with sensory and motor function or depressing the sympathetic nervous system (selective spinal analgesia).(79, 103-107) Studies using subanalgesic doses of the mu-specific agonist (DAGO) and the delta-specific agonist (DPDPE) in cats demonstrate a supraadditive interaction that results in significant suppression of noxious stimuli.(108)

The major advantages of selective nociceptive blockade are long-term pain relief without producing muscle paralysis or weakness, or significant hemodynamic effects. For example, a single dose of morphine (1 mg, diluted in 3 to 4 mL physiologic saline solution), administered via a catheter introduced into the epidural space between the lumbosacral vertebrae (Fig. 16A–17) and advanced to the fourth and fifth lumbar vertebrae in dogs weighing 10 to 15 kg produced pain relief caudal to the costal arch for up to 22 hours, without affecting heart rate, arterial blood pressure, pulmonary arterial pressure, cardiac output, systemic vascular resistance, PaO_2, PvO_2, $PaCO_2$, and pHa.(82) Similarly, 0.1 mg oxymorphone/kg in 3 mL 0.9% NaCl solution administered epidurally in dogs via a catheter positioned between the lumbar L5-6 or L6-7 intervertebral space, alleviated postthoracotomy pain for 10 hours without affecting heart rate, respiratory rate, systolic and diastolic blood pressure, PaO_2 and $PaCO_2$.(109)

Most recently, the effects of epidural and intravenous morphine on analgesic effectiveness, vital signs, and cortisol and catecholamine concentrations in dogs (18 to 26 kg) after experimental thoracotomy were compared.(110) In this study, the dogs were randomly assigned to two groups: group 1 (6 dogs) received 0.15 mg/kg of preservative-free morphine (Duramorph, Elkins-Sinn) epidurally in 5 to 6 mL 0.9% NaCl administered via catheter 8 to 10 cm cranial to the entrance of the epidural space at L5-6 or L6-7 interspace at 30 to 40 minutes before the end of surgery. Group 2 received 0.15 mg/kg morphine intravenously (IV) 5 to 10 minutes before the end of surgery. The efficacy of the

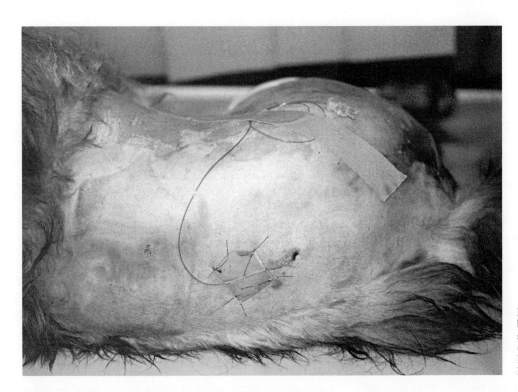

Fig. 16A–17. Epidural catheter is butterfly taped and sutured to the skin of a severely traumatized dog (multiple fractures of pelvis and humerus, and pneumothorax) in left lateral recumbency.

opioid is increased if it is given before onset of pain. In comparison, dogs with epidural morphine demonstrated lower subjective pain scores and lower serum cortisol concentrations, plasma adrenaline and noradrenaline concentrations, noninvasive systolic arterial blood pressure, heart rates, and respiratory rates than dogs with intravenous morphine when observed hourly for the first 10 hours postoperatively.(110) The single epidural injection of morphine was effective in preventing physiologic responses to postthoracotomy pain, one of the most severe causes of stress in the early postoperative period, for up to 24 hours. In contrast, 5 out of 6 dogs in the morphine intravenous group required supplemental morphine for pain relief by the fourth postoperative hour. Similarly, cortisol concentrations and heart rates in 12 dogs were unchanged at 6, 12, 18, and 24 hours after hindlimb orthopedic surgery when 0.1 mg morphine/kg body weight (1.0 mg/mL) was injected epidurally via lumbosacral catheter at wound closure.(111)

Epidural morphine (0.1 mg/kg diluted in 0.26 mL/kg of saline) results in a decrease in the minimum alveolar concentration (MAC) of halothane and improvement of arterial blood pressure, cardiac index, stroke volume, left ventricular work, and pulmonary artery pressure in dogs.(112) Increasing the volume of 0.9% NaCl solution from 0.13 to 0.26 mL/kg and thus injecting a less concentrated morphine solution (0.1 mg/kg) did not affect the degree or spread of analgesia.(113) The explanation for these findings may be related to the low lipid solubility of morphine. Epidural administration of morphine or oxymorphone (0.1 mg/kg) are equivalent to one tenth of systemically administered doses. Anal-

gesia lasts a significantly longer period of time than that provided by the intramuscular route (10 to 22 hours vs 2 hours).

The physiochemical properties of opioids, particularly their lipid solubility, molecular weight, pKa, and receptor-binding affinity, are important in determining their pharmacokinetic and pharmacodynamic properties and the onset and duration of analgesia (Table 16A–3). Oxymorphone, for example, is a relatively lipid soluble opioid that binds more rapidly to opiate receptors in the spinal cord and has a small volume of distribution in the CSF (segmental analgesia). In contrast, the relatively hydrophilic morphine (oil-water partition coefficient, 1:42) remains in the CSF for long periods, allowing rostral spread and analgesia distant from the site of injection (nonsegmental distribution of analgesia). Lumbosacral epidural administration of 0.1 mg morphine/kg has been reported to produce adequate postthoracotomy analgesia in dogs.(113, 114)

Epidurally administered morphine or oxymorphone is distributed by at least four different pathways: (a) transdural passage to the CSF and neural axis; (b) vascular uptake by epidural venous plexi and spinal radicular arteries; (c) lymphatic uptake; and (d) deposition into epidural fat.(64, 115-117) The distribution in CSF, blood, and lymph of lumbar epidurally administered morphine (MW, 285; pKa, 7.9) into the lumbar area in dogs has been determined.(64) The fraction of morphine crossing the dura after epidural injection of 2 mg/30 kg dog has been calculated to be 0.3%.(64) Maximal morphine concentration in lumbar CSF ranged between 5 and 93 ng/mL and was reached 5 to 60 minutes after injection. Morphine clearance from the

Table 16A–3. Physiochemical Properties and Doses of Opioids for Epidural Analgesia in the Dog

Opioid	Molecular Weight of Base	pKa (25° C)	Partition Coefficient*	Dose (mg/kg)	Approximate Time for Pain Relief (min)	Approximate Duration of Analgesia (h)
Morphine sulfate	285	7.9	1.42	0.05–0.15	30–60	10–24
Meperidine hydrochloride	247	8.5	38.8	0.5–1.5	10–30	5–20
Methadone hydrochloride	309	9.3	116	0.05–0.15	15–20	5–15
Oxymorphone hydrochloride	301	–	–	0.05–0.15	20–40	10–22
Fentanyl citrate	336	8.4	813	0.001–0.01	15–20	3–5

*Octanol/pH 7.4 buffer partition coefficient

CSF was 14.7 minutes (mean t-alpha) and 106 minutes (mean t-beta), respectively, independent of the dose.(64) Maximal concentration of morphine in cisternal CSF was 102.3 ± 28.0 ng/mL, (mean ± SEM)) 180 minutes after lumbar epidural administration of 0.1 mg morphine/kg diluted in 0.26 mL saline/kg in 5 anesthetized dogs (25 to 31 kg body weight).(117) The maximal concentration of morphine in serum of these same dogs was 95.7 ± 27.0 ng/mL at 31.0 ± 15.2 minutes.

The variability in CSF and plasma concentrations of morphine in dogs is a striking finding and emphasizes the need to adjust the dose of epidural morphine for each patient. Practically, this can be accomplished by using an epidural catheter, observing the degree of analgesia and the severity of side effects. Pharmacodynamic studies evaluating the degree of analgesia and CSF and plasma drug concentrations of epidurally administered morphine support a spinal mechanism of action. These studies also indicate that rapid but short-lasting serum concentrations and delayed long-lasting CSF concentrations are achieved in dogs with epidurally administered doses of morphine.

The analgesic efficacy, duration of action (107), and adverse side effects of epidurally administered morphine are dose related.(118) The most serious adverse effect is respiratory depression, which is biphasic. Respiratory depression is speculated to be caused by absorption of morphine into epidural veins and subsequent circulatory redistribution to the brain (early depression), and cephalad movement of morphine in CSF to the brain stem (late respiratory depression).(119) Lumbar epidural administration of excessive doses of morphine (20 mg morphine sulfate in 3 mL saline solution) in awake dogs (30 kg) increased $PaCO_2$ by 10 mm Hg 1.5 to 2 hours after administration, with no further ventilatory depression occurring thereafter.(116) Maximal concentration of morphine in the CSF of these dogs was 64 ng/mL at 45 minutes after administration but gradually declined to 50% of maximum concentration at 6 hours. The morphine concentration in arterial plasma was maximal at 30 minutes and declined to 20% of maximal by 6 hours.

Administration of increasing concentrations (0.1 to 100 ng/mL) of morphine into the fourth ventricle or cisterna magna in awake dogs produced a reduction in tidal volume but did not reduce respiratory rate,

suggesting that large doses (20 mg) of epidural morphine produce respiratory depression in dogs. This effect is most likely caused by the delivery of morphine to the brain-stem respiratory centers via the blood rather than the CSF.(120) The time course of ventilatory depression following subarachnoid administration of morphine in dogs corresponded poorly with morphine concentration changes in CSF.(106) Severe respiratory depression should not occur in dogs when therapeutic doses (0.1 mg/kg) of morphine are administered epidurally.

The administration of alpha₂-adrenoceptor agonists (xylazine, medetomidine) alone or in combination with morphine into the epidural space of isoflurane-anesthetized dogs is a new procedure. Morphine (0.11 mg/kg), alone or with medetomidine (5 μg/kg), was epidurally administered at the lumbosacral intervertebral space in six healthy beagle dogs, using a randomized complete block design.(121) The drugs were diluted in sterile 0.9% NaCl solution to make the volume injected 1 mL/4.5 kg. Dogs receiving low-dose medetomidine alone did not show evidence of analgesia, as evidenced by response to a tail clamp. The addition of medetomidine to morphine prolonged the duration of analgesia beyond that achieved with morphine alone (13.1 ± 3.1 vs 6.3 ± 1.2 hours, mean ± SD), indicating the supraadditive effects of both drugs.

Most recently, the cardiovascular effects of lumbosacral-epidurally administered morphine (0.1 mg/kg), xylazine (0.02 mg/kg) (122), or morphine (0.1 mg/kg) and xylazine (0.02 mg/kg) combination (123), and 5 mL 0.9% NaCl solution (controls) were assessed in six healthy dogs during 2 hours of 2.0% end-tidal concentrations of isoflurane anesthesia. The EKG, heart rate, body temperature, cardiac index, central venous pressure, mean pulmonary artery pressure, pulmonary capillary wedge pressure, systemic vascular resistance, arterial HCO_3^-, and base excess were not significantly ($P < 0.05$) different among the treatments and controls. These results indicate that epidural morphine, xylazine, or morphine/xylazine is not associated with cardiovascular side effects during isoflurane anesthesia in dogs.

The therapeutic benefits achieved following the epidural administration of opioids include profound analgesia, modification of the endocrine-metabolic stress response, improvement in pulmonary function, decreased morbidity, and a comparatively short recovery. Contraindications to epidural opioid analgesia are primarily associated with the technique of epidural catheterization. Potential side effects in humans include respiratory depression, urinary retention, delayed gastrointestinal motility, vomiting, itching, and catheter-related problems such as catheter displacement, occlusion, and infection.(124) Side effects are more common when intrathecal injection is performed as opposed to epidural injection, and they can be reversed by a low-dose intravenous infusion of the opioid antagonist naloxone, with minimal effect on the analgesia produced.(125) These side effects, with the exception of pruritus (113), have not been reported in dogs, and for the most part are preventable by careful patient selection, using appropriate dosages, and proper patient management.

Ganglion Blocks

Anesthesia of the cervicothoracic ganglion (CTG) and lumbar sympathetic chain in dogs has been described to treat paralysis of the radial, facial, and trigeminal nerves and muscle and joint diseases.(126, 127) Five to 8 mL of procaine HCl solution (0.5%) has been administered in close proximity to the CTG and lumbar sympathetic chain without ill effects.

Conclusion

Local and regional anesthetic techniques can be used to provide intra- and postoperative pain relief in dogs. Appropriately selected techniques provide safe, effective, and reliable analgesia with minimal physiologic alterations. Similarly, the interpleural administration of local anesthetic drugs or the epidural administration of opioids can provide unparalleled long-term relief of pain in dogs with preservation of consciousness while maintaining normal physiologic function. The selection of the appropriate local anesthetic technique and drug must be tailored to the patient in order to maximize beneficial effects.

References

1. Ritchie JM, Cohen PJ. Local anesthetics. Cocaine, procaine and other synthetic local anesthetics. In: Goodman LS, Gilman AG, Gilman A, eds. The pharmaceutical basis of therapeutics, 5th ed. New York: Macmillan, 1975.
2. Formstom C. Ophthaine (proparacaine hydrochloride)–a local anesthetic for ophthalmic surgery. Vet Rec 76:385, 1964.
3. Magrane WG. Investigational use of ophthaine as a local anesthetic in ophthalmology. North Am Vet 34:568–569, 1953.
4. Überreiter O. Zur Technik der Augenoperationen beim Hunde. Arch Wiss Prakt Tierheilk 74:235–332, 1937.
5. Severinghaus JW, Xu FD, Spellman MJ. Benzocaine and methemoglobin: recommended actions. Anesthesiology 74:385–386, 1991.
6. Harvey JW, Sameck JH, Burgard FJ. Benzocaine induced methemoglobinemia in dogs. J Am Vet Med Assoc 175:1171–1175, 1979.
7. Paddleford RP, Krahwinkel DJ, Fuhr JE, et al. Experimentally induced methemoglobinemia in the dog following exposure to topical benzocaine HCl. Proc 2nd Intl Cong Vet Anesth [Abstract]. Sacramento, California, 1985:98–99.
8. Wilkie DA, Kirby R. Methemoglobinemia associated with dermal application of benzocaine cream in a cat. J Am Vet Med Assoc 192:85–91, 1988.
9. Gesztes A, Mezei M. Topical anesthesia of the skin by liposome-encapsulated tetracaine. Anesth Analg 67:1079–1081, 1988.
10. Ehrenstrom-Reiz GME, Reiz SLA. EMLA–a eutectic mixture of local anesthetics for topical anaesthesia. Acta Anaesthesiol Scand 26:596–598, 1982.
11. Wilcke JR, Davis LE, Neff-Davis CA, et al. Pharmacokinetics of lidocaine and its active metabolites in dogs. J Vet Pharmacol Ther 6:49–58, 1983.
12. Hamlin RL, Bishop MA, Hadlock DJ, et al. Effects of lidocaine, with or without epinephrine on ventricular rhythm. J Am Anim Hosp Assoc 24:701–704, 1988.
13. Ott RL. Local anesthesia in the dog. Fed Proc 28(4):1450–1455, 1969.
14. Barth P. Die Leitungsanästhesie am Kopf des Hundes [Dissertation]. Vet Med Faculty, University of Zürich, Switzerland, 1948.
15. Frank ER. Dental anesthesia in the dog. J Am Vet Med Assoc 73:232–233, 1928.
16. Wang BC, Bogart BB, Hillman DE. Subarachnoid injection–a potential complication of retrobulbar block. Anesthesiology 71:845–847, 1989.
17. Dietz O. Eine retro-bulbäre Anästhesie beim Hund zur Erzeugung einer Mydriasis. Berlin Münch Tierärztl Wochenschr 15:235–237, 1954.
18. Tufvesson G. Anestesi av plexus brachialis. Nord Veterinaermed 3:183–193, 1951.
19. Nutt P. Brachial plexus analgesia in the dog. Vet Rec 74:874–876, 1962.
20. Bier A. Ueber einen neuen Weg Lokalanästhesie an den Gliedmassen zu erzeugen. Arch Klin Chir 86:1007–1016, 1908.
21. Küpper W. Die intravenöse Regionalanästhesie (BIER) beim Hund. Zentralbl Veterinärmed [A] 24:287–297, 1977.
22. Grice SC, Eisenach JC, Prough DS. Intravenous regional anesthesia. Effect of tourniquet site and type on leakage under the tourniquet. Anesth Analg 66:S191, 1987.
23. Cotev S, Robin GC. Experimental studies on intravenous regional anaesthesia using radioactive lignocaine. Br J Anaesth 38:936–939, 1966.
24. Chabel C, Russell LL, Lee R. Tourniquet-induced limb ischemia: a neurophysiologic animal model. Anesthesiology 72:1038–1044, 1990.
25. Arthur GR, Feldman HS, Covino BG. Comparative pharmacokinetics of bupivacaine and ropivacaine, a new amide local anesthetic. Anesth Analg 67:1053–1058, 1988.
26. Arthur GR, Feldman HS, Norway SB, et al. Acute IV toxicity of LEA-103, a new local anesthetic, compared to lidocaine and bupivacaine in the awake dog [Abstract]. Anesthesiology 65(3A): A182, 1986.
27. Pedigo NW, Walmsley PN, Kasten GW, et al. Relative cardiotoxicity of the long-acting local anesthetics bupivacaine and ropivacaine in dogs [Abstract]. Anesth Analg 67:S166, 1988.
28. Feldman HS, Arthur GR, Covino BG. Comparative systemic toxicity of convulsant and supraconvulsant doses of intravenous ropivacaine, bupivacaine and lidocaine in the conscious dog. Anesth Analg 69:794–801, 1989.
29. Rudin DO, Fremont-Smith K, Beecher HK. Permeability of dura mater to epidural procaine in dogs. J Appl Physiol 3:388–398, 1951.
30. Bone JK, Beck JG. Epidural anesthesia in dogs. J Am Vet Med Assoc 128:236–238, 1956.
31. Tufvesson G. Local anaesthesia in veterinary medicine. Sodertalje, Sweden: Astra International, 1963:36–43.
32. Evers WH. Epidural anesthesia in the dog: a review of 224 cases with emphasis on cesarean section. Vet Med Small Anim Clin 63:1121–1124, 1968.
33. Klide AM, Soma LR. Epidural analgesia in the dog and cat. J Am Vet Med Assoc 153:165–173, 1968.
34. Persson F. Epidural analgesia in dogs with special reference to intra-arterial blood pressure. Acta Vet Scand 11:186–196, 1970.
35. Burfoot MF, Bromage PR. The effects of epinephrine on

mepivacaine absorption from the spinal epidural space. Anesthesiology 35:488–492, 1971.

36. Klide AM. Epidural anesthesia. In: Soma LR, ed. Textbook of veterinary anesthesia. Baltimore: Williams & Wilkins, 1971:450–467.

37. Lebeaux MI. Experimental epidural anaesthesia in the dog with lidocaine and bupivacaine. Br J Anaesth 45:549–555, 1973.

38. Morikawa K, Bonica JJ, Tucker GT, et al. Effect of acute hypovolaemia on lidocaine absorption and cardiovascular response following epidural block in dogs. Br J Anaesth 46:631–635, 1974.

39. Bradley RL, Withrow SJ, Heath RB, et al. Epidural anesthesia in the dog. Vet Surg 9:153–156, 1980.

40. Pandey SK, Dass LL, Bhargava MK, et al. Evaluation of lidocaine HCl as a spinal anesthetic in dogs. Indian Vet J 58:478–480, 1981.

41. Gerlach K, Bonath K, Ristic-Djuric Z, et al. Möglichkeiten der Langzeitanästhesie mit Bupivacaine und Langzeitanästhesie mit Morphine beim Hund mit Hilfe eines extraduralen Katheters. Fortschr Veterinärmed 37(15):237, 1983.

42. Greitz T, Andreen M, Irestedt L. Haemodynamics and oxygen consumption in the dog during high epidural block with special reference to the splanchnic region. Acta Anaesthesiol Scand 27:211–217, 1983.

43. Hally LE, Riedesel DH. Epidural anesthesia in the dog. Iowa State Vet 45:45–48, 1983.

44. Nolte JG, Watney CG, Hall LW. Cardiovascular effects of epidural blocks in dogs. J Small Anim Pract 24:17–21, 1983.

45. Dallman MJ, Mann FA. Epidural or spinal anesthesia for reduction of coxofemoral luxations in the dog. J Am Anim Hosp Assoc 21:485–488, 1985.

46. Feldman HS, Hurley RJ, Covino BG. LEA-103 (Ropivacaine) a new local anesthetic: experimental evaluation of spinal and epidural anesthesia in the dog, and sciatic nerve block in the rat [Abstract]. Anesthesiology 65(3A):A181, 1986.

47. Heath RB. The practicality of lumbosacral epidural analgesia. Sem Vet Med Surg Small Anim 1(3):245–248, 1986.

48. Heath RB, Broadstone RV, Wright M, et al. Using bupivacaine hydrochloride for lumbosacral epidural analgesia. Compend Small Anim Cont Educ #4, 11 (1):50–55, 1989.

49. Peters J, Kousoulis L, Arndt JO, et al. Effects of segmental thoracic extradural analgesia on sympathetic block in conscious dogs. Br J Anaesth 63:470–476, 1989.

50. Shibata K, Yamamoto Y, Murakami S. Effects of epidural anesthesia on cardiovascular response survival in experimental hemorrhagic shock in dogs. Anesthesiology 71:953–959, 1989.

51. Skarda RT. Local anesthesia in dogs and cats. In: Muir WW, Hubbell JAE, Skarda RT, eds. Handbook of veterinary anesthesia. Washington, DC: CV Mosby, 1989.

52. Mikat-Stevens M, Stevens R, Schubert A, et al. Deliberate injection of air into the canine epidural space: a radiographic study [abstract]. Anesth Analg 68:194, 1989.

53. Fletcher TF. Spinal cord and meninges. In: Evans HE, Christensen GC, eds. Millers anatomy of the dog, 2nd ed. Philadelphia: WB Saunders, 1979:947.

54. Liu P, Feldman HS, Covino BG. Comparative CNS and cardiovascular toxicity of various local anesthetic agents in awake dogs. Anesthesiology 181:55:A156, 1981.

55. Ravindran RS, Tasch MD, Baldwin SJ, et al. Subarachnoid injection of autologous blood in dogs is unassociated with neurologic deficits. Anesth Analg 60(8):603–604, 1981.

56. Sami HM, McNulty JA, Skaredoff MN, et al. The effect of spinal needle shape and bevel orientation on the size and shape of the dural defects: an SEM study in dogs. Anesthesiology 71(3A):A637, 1989.

57. Butterworth JF, Walker FO, Lysak SZ, et al. Pregnancy increases median nerve susceptibility to lidocaine. Anesthesiology 72:962–965, 1990.

58. Bromage PR. Continuous lumbar epidural analgesia for obstetrics. Can Med Assoc J 85:1136–1140, 1961.

59. Datta S, Lambert DH, Gregus J, et al. Differential sensitivities of mammalian nerve fibers during pregnancy. Anesth Analg 62:1070–1072, 1983.

60. Gianetti A, Cerimele D. Effect of steroid hormones on the matrix of the dermis of the rat. In: Balazs EA, ed. Chemistry and molecular biology of the intercellular matrix, vol. III. London: Academic Press, 1970:1821–1827.

61. Bonath KH, Gerlach K, Ristic-Djuric Z, et al. Einfluss der extraduralen Langzeitanästhesie mit Bupivacaine und Langzeitanalgesie mit Morphin auf Kreislauf und Atmung des Hundes. Fortschr Veterinärmed 37(15):237, 1983.

62. Feldman HS, Covino BG. Comparative motor-blocking effects of bupivacaine and ropivacaine, a new amino amide local anesthetic, in the rat and dog. Anesth Analg 67:1047–1052, 1988.

63. Usubiaga JE, Wikinski J, Wikinski R, et al. Transfer of local anesthetics to the subarachnoid space and mechanisms of epidural block. Anesthesiology 25:752–759, 1964.

64. Durant PAC, Yaksh TL. Distribution in cerebrospinal fluid, blood, and lymph of epidurally injected morphine and insulin in dogs. Anesth Analg 65:583–592, 1986.

65. Stanek B, Schwartz M, Zimpfer M, et al. Plasma concentrations of noradrenaline and adrenaline and plasma renin activity during extradural blockade in dogs. Br J Anaesth 52:305–311, 1980.

66. Peters J, Schlaghecke R, Thouet H, et al. Endogenous vasopressin supports blood pressure and prevents severe hypotension during epidural anesthesia in conscious dogs. Anesthesiology 73, 694 702, 1990.

67. Butterworth JF, Piccione W, Berrizbeitia LD, et al. Augmentation of venous return by adrenergic agonists during spinal anesthesia. Anesth Analg 65:612–616, 1986.

68. Warner DO, Brichant JF, Ritman EL, et al. Epidural anesthesia and intrathoracic blood volume. Anesth Analg 77:135–140, 1993.

69. Klassen GA, Bramwell RS, Bromage PR, et al. Effect of acute sympathectomy by epidural anesthesia on the canine coronary circulation. Anesthesiology 52:8–15, 1980.

70. Sessler DI, Ponte J. Shivering during epidural anesthesia. Anesthesiology 72:816–821, 1990.

71. Hammel HT, Wyndham CH, Hardy JD, et al. Heat production and heat loss in the dog at 8–36°C environmental temperature. Am J Physiol (Lond) 194:99–108, 1958.

72. Peters J, Breuksch E, Kousoulis L, et al. Regional skin temperature after total sympathetic blockade by epidural anaesthesia in conscious dogs. Brit J Anaesth 61:617–624, 1988.

73. Kehlet H. Epidural analgesia and the endocrine-metabolic response to surgery–updates and perspectives. Acta Anaesthesiol Scand 28:125–127, 1984.

74. Hole A, Unsgaard G, Breivik H. Monocyte functions are depressed during and after surgery under general anesthesia but not under epidural anesthesia. Acta Anaesthesiol Scand 26:301–307, 1982.

75. Hall LW, Clarke KW. Veterinary anesthesia, 8th ed. London: Baillière Tindall, 1983:336.

76. Lumb WV, Jones EW. Veterinary anesthesia, 2nd ed. Philadelphia: Lea & Febiger, 1984:407.

77. Goodger WJ, Levy W. Anesthetic management of cesarean section. Vet Clin North Am 3(1):85–99, 1973.

78. Probst CW, Webb AI. Cesarean section in the dog and cat: anesthetic and surgical techniques. In: Bojrab MJ, ed. Current techniques in small animal surgery. Philadelphia: Lea & Febiger 1983:346–351.

79. Yeager MP, Glass DD, Neff RK, et al. Epidural anesthesia and analgesia in high-risk surgical patients. Anesthesiology 66:729–736, 1987.

80. Bonath KH, Saleh AS. Long term pain treatment in the dog by peridural morphines. Proc 2nd Intl Cong Vet Anesth. Sacramento, CA: Veterinary Practice Publishing Company, 1985:161.

81. Hurley RJ. Continuous spinal anesthesia. Int Anesthesiol Clin 47:46–50, 1989.

82. Knorr-Henn S. Epidurale Morphinwirkung auf Hämodynamik und Atemfunktionen des Hundes [Dissertation]. Vet Med Faculty, Justus-Liebig-Universität, Giessen, Germany, 1986.

83. Westhues M, Fritsch R. Local anesthesia. In: Animal anesthesia. Edinburgh: Oliver and Boyd, 1964:114–119.

84. Thompson SE, Johnson JM. Analgesia in dogs after intercostal thoracotomy. A comparison of morphine, selective intercostal

nerve block, and interpleural regional analgesia with bupivacaine. Vet Surg 20(1):73–77, 1991.

85. Moore DC, Brindenbaugh LD, Thompson GE. Factors determining dosage of amide type local anesthetic drugs. Anesthesiology 47:263–268, 1977.

86. Tucker GT. Pharmacokinetics of local anaesthetics. Br J Anaesth 58:717–731, 1986.

87. Berg RJ, Orton EC. Pulmonary function in dogs after intercostal thoracotomy: comparison of morphine, oxymorphone, and selective intercostal nerve block. Am J Vet Res 47:471–474, 1986.

88. Kvalheim L, Reiestad F. Interpleural catheter in the management of postoperative pain. Anesthesiology 61:A231, 1984.

89. Reiestadt F, Strömskag KE, Kjell E. Interpleural catheter in the management of postoperative pain. A preliminary report. Reg Anesth 11(2):89–91, 1986.

90. Murphy DF. Interpleural analgesia. Br J Anaesth 71:426–434, 1993.

91. Strömskag KE, Reiestad F, Holmgvist EL, et al. Intrapleural administration of 0.25%, 0.375%, and 0.5% bupivacaine with epinephrine after cholecystectomy. Anesth Analg 67(5):430–434, 1988.

92. Rocco A, Reiestad F, Gudmon J, et al. Intrapleural administration of local anesthetics for pain relief in patients with multiple rib fractures. Reg Anesth 12:10–14, 1987.

93. Morrow, JS, Squier RC. Sympathetic blockade with interpleural analgesia [Abstract]. Anesthesiology 71(3A):A 662, 1989.

94. Sydow FW, Haindl H. Eine neue Technik der interpleuralen Blockade. Anaesthesist 39:280–282, 1990.

95. Symreng T, Gomez MN, Johnson B, et al. Intrapleural bupivacaine-technical considerations and intraoperative use. J Cardiothorac Anesth 3(2):139–143, 1989.

96. Riegler FX, Pelligrino DA,, Vade Boncouer TR. An animal model of intrapleural analgesia [Abstract]. Anesthesiology 69(3A):A 365, 1988.

97. Riegler FX, Vade Boncouer TR, Pelligrino DA. Interpleural anesthetics in the dog: differential somatic neural blockade. Anesthesiology 71:744–750, 1989.

98. Vade Boncouer TR, Pelligrino DA, Riegler FX, et al. Interpleural bupivacaine in the dog: distribution of effect and influence of injectate volume [Abstract]. Anesth Analg 68:S301, 1989.

99. Kowalski SE, Bradley BD, Greengrass RA, et al. Effects of interpleural bupivacaine (0.5%) on canine diaphragmatic function. Anesth Analg 75:400–404, 1992.

100. Waldman SD. Subcutaneous tunneled intrapleural catheters in the long-term relief of upper quadrant pain of malignant origin-description of a new technique and preliminary results. Reg Anesth 4(2S):54, 1989.

101. Aquilar JL, et al. Bilateral interpleural injection of local anesthetics. Reg Anesth 14(2):93–94, 1989.

102. Yaksh TL, Rudy TA. Analgesia mediated by a direct spinal action of narcotics. Science 192:1357–1358, 1976.

103. Cousins MG, Mather LE. Intrathecal and epidural administration of opioids. Anesthesiology 61(3):276–310, 1984.

104. Cousins MJ, Mather LE, Glynn CJ, et al. Selective spinal analgesia. Lancet 1:1141–1142, 1979.

105. Yaksh TL, Noueihed R. The physiology and pharmacology of spinal opioids. Annu Rev Pharmacol Toxicol 25:433–462, 1985.

106. Atchison SR, Durant PAC, Yahsh TL. Cardiorespiratory effects and kinetics of intrathecally injected D-ala2-D-leu5-enkephalin and morphine in unanesthetized dogs. Anesthesiology 65:609–616, 1986.

107. Covino BG. Epidural morphine provides postoperative pain relief in peripheral vascular and orthopedic surgical patients: a dose-response study. Anesth Analg 65:165–170, 1986.

108. Omote K, Nakagawa I, Kitahata LM, et al. The antinociceptive role of mu and delta opiate receptors and their interactions in the spinal dorsal horn of cats [Abstract]. Anesth Analg 68:S215, 1989.

109. Popilskis S, Kohn DI, Sanchez JA, et al. Comparison of epidural versus intramuscular oxymorphone analgesia after thoracotomy in dogs. Vet Surg 20(6):462–467, 1991.

110. Popilskis S, Kohn DF, Laurent L, et al. Efficacy of epidural morphine versus intravenous morphine for post-thoracotomy pain in dogs. J Vet Anaesth 20:21–25, 1993.

111. Williams LL, Boudrieau RJ, Clark G, et al. Evaluation of epidural morphine in dogs for pain relief after hindlimb orthopedic surgery [Abstract]. Vet Surg 22(1):89, 1993.

112. Valverde A, Dyson DH, Cockshutt JR, et al. Comparison of the hemodynamic effects of halothane alone and halothane combined with epidurally administered morphine for anesthesia in ventilated dogs. Am J Vet Res 52:505–509, 1991.

113. Valverde A, Dyson DH, McDonell WN. Use of epidural morphine in the dog for pain relief. Vet Comp Traumatol 2:55–58, 1989.

114. Pascoe PJ, Dyson DH. Postoperative analgesia following lateral thoracotomy: epidural morphine vs intercostal bupivacaine. Proc Annu Sci Mtg Am Coll Vet Anesthesiol, Las Vegas, Nevada, 1990:30.

115. Gourlay GK, Cherry DA, Plummer JL, et al. The influence of drug polarity on the absorption of opioid drugs into CSF and subsequent cephalad migration following lumbar epidural administration. Application to morphine and pethidine. Pain 31:297–305, 1987.

116. Pelligrino DA, Peterson RD, Albrecht RF. Cisternal CSF morphine levels and ventilatory depression following epidural administration of morphine sulfate in the awake dog [Abstract]. Anesth Analg 67:S167, 1988.

117. Valverde A, Dyson DH, Conlon P, et al. Cisternal CSF and serum concentrations of morphine following epidural administrations in the dog [Abstract]. Proc Vet Midwest Anesth Conf, University of Illinois, Champaign-Urbana, 1990:12.

118. Pybus DA, Torda TA. Dose-effect relationships of extradural morphine. Br J Anaesth 54:1259–1262, 1982.

119. Kafer ER, Brown JT, Scott D, et al. Biplanic depression of ventilating responses to CO_2 following epidural morphine. Anesthesiology 58:418–427, 1983.

120. Pelligrino DA, Peterson RD, Henderson SK, et al. Comparative ventilatory effects of intravenous versus fourth cerebroventricular infusions of morphine sulfate in unanesthetized dog. Anesthesiology 71:250–259, 1989.

121. Branson KR, Tranquilli WJ, Ko JCH, et al. Duration of analgesia induced by epidurally administered morphine and medetomidine in dogs [Abstract]. Vet Surg 22(1):88, 1993.

122. Greene SA, Keegan RD, Weil AB. Cardiovascular effects after epidural injection of xylazine in isoflurane-anesthetized dogs. Vet Surg 24:283–289, 1995.

123. Keegan RD, Greene SA. Cardiovascular effects of epidurally administered morphine and xylazine/morphine in isoflurane anesthetized dogs [Abstract]. Proc Annu Mtg Am Coll Vet Anesth, Washington, DC, 1993:29.

124. Du Pen SL, Peterson DG, Williams A, et al. Infection during chronic epidural catheterization: diagnosis and treatment. Anesthesiology 73:905–909, 1990.

125. Rawal N, Schott U, Dahlstrom B, et al. Influence of naloxon infusion on analgesia and respiratory depression following epidural morphine. Anesthesiology 66:194–201, 1986.

126. Dietz O. Die Anästhesie des Ganglion stellatum beim Hund. Zentralbl Veterinärmed 6(2):569–574, 1955.

127. Dietz O. Zur Grenzstrangblockade beim Tier. Arch Exp Veterinärmed 11:310–330, 349–385, 1957.

LOCAL AND REGIONAL ANESTHETIC AND ANALGESIC TECHNIQUES: HORSES

Introduction

Many diagnostic and surgical procedures are performed safely and humanely in the horse combining local anesthetic techniques with physical restraint and/or sedation. Sedation can be induced by drugs such as acepromazine, xylazine, or detomidine either alone or in combination with morphine or butorphanol, among others, to facilitate handling of fractious horses.

The techniques in performing nerve and joint blocks vary considerably, depending on such factors as operative size; nature; expected duration of surgery; size, temperament, and health of the patient; technical skill and personal preference of the veterinarian; and economics of time and material. Currently, the most common techniques in horses are surface (topical) anesthesia, infiltration (local anesthesia), and a considerable range of peripheral nerve blocks (regional anesthesia). Peripheral nerve blocks, intraarticular and intrabursal injections, and local infiltrations (ring block) are commonly used to aid diagnosis of equine lameness and as a means of providing analgesia to a surgery site. Peripheral nerve blocks, which are given at the end of an operation under general anesthesia, are helpful to control emergence excitement caused by pain in the recovery period. Major infiltrations (cervicothoracic ganglion block, sympathetic ganglion block) are used by a specialist to induce relief of vasoconstriction and pain. Similarly, central neural blockade techniques such as caudal epidural anesthesia, caudal subarachnoid anesthesia, segmental thoracolumbar epidural anesthesia, and thoracolumbar subarachnoid anesthesia are the province of the specialist. Caudal epidural administration of morphine can provide bilateral analgesia over various sacral and thoracic (S5 to T9) dermatomes, with slow onset (6 to 8 h) and long duration (17 to 19 h), and minimal sedation and cardiopulmonary effects in horses. Improper injection technique contributes to inadequate anesthesia and complications. Each technique has its own particular rate of onset and duration, which is probably related to the specific local anesthetic, neuroanatomy (thickness of the coverings of the nerve, arrangement of fibers within the mixed nerve, blood supply to the area of injection), and personal interpretation.

The equipment for performing local anesthesia should include sharp and sterile needles, syringes in good working condition, sterile catheters and stylets, and sterile anesthetic solution. Chances of infection must be minimized by surgically preparing the injection sites, especially puncture sites into joints and epidural and subarachnoid spaces. Desired anesthetic effects without complications can be obtained by using proper techniques, including aspiration before injection to avoid placing drug into the vascular system instead of the desired tissue and avoidance of inflamed areas.

Choice of Local Anesthetic

The most commonly used local anesthetic drugs in equine practice are 2% lidocaine (Xylocaine, Astra Pharmaceutical Products, Worcester, Mass.) or mepivacaine (Carbocaine-V, Winthrop Laboratories, New York, New York) hydrochloride solution, representing drugs of intermediate duration for 1 to 2 hours. In general, onset of anesthesia occurs most rapidly (within 3 to 5 min) during infiltration techniques and subarachnoid administration followed in order of increasing onset time by minor nerve blockade (5 to 10 min), major nerve blocks, and epidural anesthesia (10 to 20 min).(1) The addition of epinephrine at concentration of 5 μg/mL (1:200,000) to the local anesthetic solution improves the quality and prolongs the duration of regional and epidural anesthesia.

Nerve Blocks

REGIONAL ANESTHESIA OF THE HEAD

Although regional anesthesia of the head can be induced by various techniques, the most frequently desensitized nerves of the head are the supraorbital, infraorbital, mandibular alveolar, and auriculopalpebral; other techniques, which desensitize the maxillary (2, 3), mandibular (4), and ophthalmic nerves (6, 7), are not without dangers and seldom used.

Eyelids. Anesthesia of the eyelids requires sensory denervation of four individual branches of the trigeminal (fifth) cranial nerve: the supraorbital (or frontal), lacrimal, zygomatic, and infraorbital. Prevention of voluntary closure of the eyelids (palpebral akinesia) is achieved by desensitizing the dorsal and ventral branches of the palpebral nerve (auriculopalpebral nerve block). A 1.5- to 2.5-cm, 22- to 25-gauge needle is used to inject local anesthetic without epinephrine to each of the listed nerves (Fig. 16B–1).

Upper eyelid. The supraorbital (or frontal) nerve is the most commonly desensitized.(8, 9) The nerve emerges through the supraorbital foramen, which can be easily palpated with the index finger about 5 to 7 cm dorsal to the medial canthus and in the center of an imaginary triangle formed by grasping the supraorbital process of the frontal bone with the thumb and middle finger and sliding medially (Fig. 16B–2A). Approximately 2 mL of local anesthetic are injected subcutaneously over the foramen, 1 mL as the needle is inserted into the foramen and 2 mL as the needle is inserted to its full depth (2.5 cm) into the foramen (Fig. 16B–2B). Successful administration of local anesthetic desensitizes the forehead, including the middle two thirds of the upper eyelid and palpebral motor supply from the auriculopalpebral nerve (Fig. 16B–3A).

The lateral canthus and lateral aspect of the upper eyelid are desensitized by administering local anes-

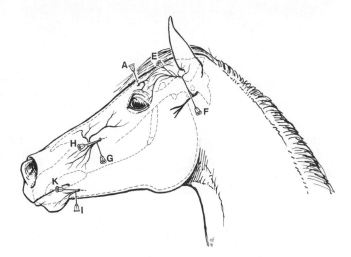

Fig. 16B–1. Sites for needle placement to desensitize the supraorbital (A), auriculopalpebral (E and F), infraorbital (G and H), mental (I), and alveolar mandibular (K) nerves.

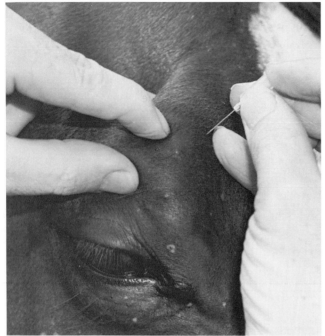

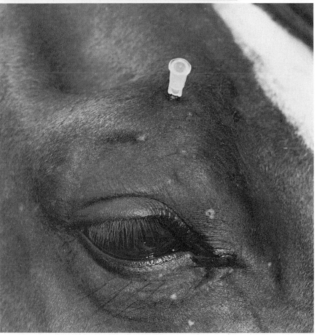

Fig. 16B–2. Palpation of the supraorbital nerve. A 2.5-cm, 25-gauge needle is inserted into the supraorbital foramen.

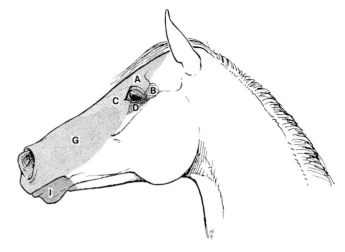

Fig. 16B–3. Area of skin desensitization after blocking the supraorbital (A), lacrimal (B), infratrochlear (C), zygomatic (D), infraorbital (G), and mental (I) nerves.

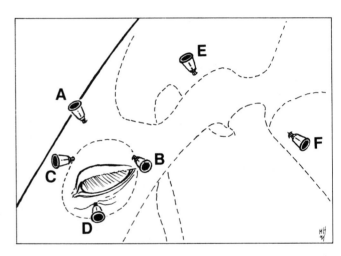

Fig. 16B–4. Needle placement to supraorbital (A), lacrimal (B), infratrochlear (C), zygomatic (D), and auriculopalpebral (E and F) nerves.

thetic to the lacrimal nerve.(9, 10) The needle is inserted percutaneously at the lateral canthus and directed medially along the dorsal rim of the orbit (Fig. 16B–4B). A deep injection of 2 to 3 mL of the anesthetic at this site also desensitizes the lacrimal gland, local connective tissue, and temporal angle of the orbit (Fig. 16B–3B).

Medial canthal anesthesia is achieved by inserting the needle through the bony notch or irregularity on the dorsal rim of the orbit near the medial canthus and injecting 2 to 3 mL of local anesthetic around the infratrochlear nerve (Fig. 16B–4C). This procedure also desensitizes the nictitans, lacrimal organs, and connective tissues (Fig. 16B–3C).(9, 10)

The lower two thirds of the lower eyelid, skin, and connective tissue are desensitized by placing the needle subcutaneously on the lateral aspect of the bony orbit and supraorbital portion of the zygomatic arch (the site where the rim begins to rise), and infiltrating the zygomatic nerve with 3 to 5 mL of the anesthetic (Figs. 16B–3D and 16B–4D).(9, 10)

Motor paralysis of the orbicularis oculi muscles. Desensitization of the auriculopalpebral nerve is most frequently used for examination of the eye and temporary relief of eyelid spasms, since voluntary closure of the eyelids (akinesia) is prevented. The eyelids remain sensitive. In combination with topical anesthesia, it is useful for removal of foreign bodies from the cornea and other ocular surgery. At least two injection sites have been suggested to paralyze the palpebral musculature: either the most dorsal point of the zygomatic arch (Fig. 16B–1E)(4) or the depression caudal to the mandible at the ventral edge of the temporal position of the zygomatic arch (Fig. 16B–1F).(10-12) In each location, the needle is placed subfascially and 5 mL of the local anesthetic are administered in a fan-shaped manner.

Upper lip and nose. Anesthesia of the upper lip and nose requires a 2.5-cm, 20-gauge needle and deposition of 5 mL of local anesthetic to the infraorbital nerve as it emerges from the infraorbital canal. (Fig. 16B–1G).(4, 8) After displacing the flat levator labii superioris muscle dorsally, the bony lip of the infraorbital foramen can be palpated by the index finger about half the distance and 2.5 cm dorsal to a line connecting the nasomaxillary notch and the rostral end of the facial crest. Successful perineural infiltration of the local anesthetic at that site results in anesthesia of the entire anterior half of the face from the foramen rostrally (Fig. 16B–3G).

Upper teeth and maxilla. If a 5.0-cm, 20-gauge spinal needle is inserted into the infraorbital foramen and is advanced into the infraorbital canal for a depth of up to 3.5 cm, (Fig. 16B–1H) the deposition of 5 mL of local anesthetic is adequate to desensitize the teeth as far as the first molar, the maxillary sinus, the roof of the nasal cavity, and the skin almost to the medial canthus of the eye.(13, 14) Although local anesthesia can be produced for premolars and maxilla, extraction of these teeth and trephination of the maxillary sinus is more easily accomplished using general anesthesia.

Lower lip. Anesthesia of the lower lip is induced by using a 2.5-cm, 22-gauge needle and successfully desensitizing the mental nerve rostrally to the mental foramen with 5 mL of local anesthetic. (Figs. 16B–1 and 16B–3I).(4, 12) The lateral border of the mental foramen is easily palpated at the horizontal ramus of the mandible in the middle of the interdental space, after displacing the tendon of the depressor labii inferioris muscle dorsally.

Lower incisors and premolars. A 7.5-cm, 20-gauge spinal needle is inserted into the mental foramen, and is advanced into the mandibular canal as far as possible in a ventromedial direction to inject 10 mL of local anesthetic to desensitize the mandibular alveolar nerve, thereby extending the area of anesthesia caudal as far as the third premolar. (Fig. 16B–1K).(4, 5, 8, 15) The technique is difficult, so extraction of teeth is better accomplished under general anesthesia.

REGIONAL ANESTHESIA OF THE FOOT

Regional anesthesia (peripheral nerve blocks)(1, 16-31), intraarticular injection(1, 31-47), and intrabursal injections(1, 48-50) and local infiltration (ring block) are used to provide intra- and postoperative anesthesia to a surgery site and aid in accurate diagnosis, prognosis, and especially recommendation and treatment of equine lameness.

All of these techniques for lameness diagnosis are seldom used, however. Instead, history, observation of the horse at rest (standing normally with all feet on the ground), particularly looking for exostosis or lumps, palpating areas that are inflamed, enlarged, or seam soar, using the hoof tester to determine painful areas and to determine if the horse goes more lame after a specific part of the leg has been manipulated, and observing the horse in motion are almost always used. In some cases the diagnosis is not obvious and nerve blocks and good-quality radiographs with adequate view are required to make a specific diagnosis. Rectal palpation of ovaries, uterus, aorta, iliacs, pelvis, kidney, and viscera of a female and palpation of the inguinal canal of a stallion or gelding are additional examinations in cases of difficult diagnosis of hindlimb lameness. Restraint is best achieved physically with a twitch applied to the horse's upper lip and a man picking up the front leg on the same side as the operator.

Sterile syringes, needles, and local anesthetic should be used for each injection to prevent infection. Subcutaneous injections require an alcohol prep as a minimum preparation. Show horse owners object to clipping and shaving of the site of needle penetration.(40) Intraarticular injections require a surgical scrub because of the risk of introducing contaminates; clipping the site may or may not be performed. Care must be taken not to put the fingers on the end of the needle hub or especially on the tip of the syringe because of risking any contamination. It is wise to use surgical gloves in some of the more complicated nerve and joint blocks to practice aseptic technique.

Nerve blocks and intraarticular injections are performed first on the most distal branches of nerve trunks and joints, and proceed proximally using a systematic approach. It is very uncommon to perform nerve blocks proximal to the carpus and tarsus. Proximal to the metacarpus, diagnostic anesthesia of the equine pectoral limb is not specific and is best accomplished by joint anesthesia.(19) All corresponding digital nerves can be blocked on the hind limb as similar to the front limb (Figs. 16B–5 and 16B–6). If the needle is inserted using a distal to proximal direction and is then attached to the syringe, it is less likely to break off if the horse makes a sudden movement. Adequate amounts of local anesthetic should be administered and enough time given for maximal effect. Postblock examination is best accomplished by using deep digital pressure, pressure exerted by hoof testers, manipulation, and testing skin sensation distal to the block by using a ballpoint pen for 1 to 2 seconds. Pressure from a blunt-tip instrument, such as a ballpoint pen, is preferable over a needle and avoids the production of numerous bleeding points.(25) The limb should be rubbed down and wrapped to prevent swelling and inflammation after the use of local anesthetic.

The failure or partial failure of local blocks may occur for several reasons, most common of which are incorrect

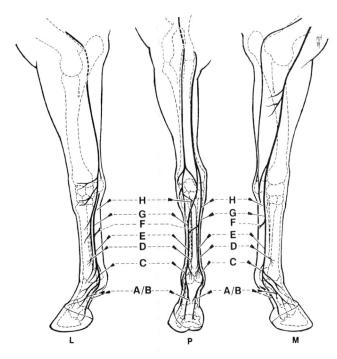

Fig. 16B–5. Needle placement for nerves of the distal part of the left thoracic limb of the horse, lateral (L), palmar (P), and medial (M) views: lateral and medial palmar digital nerves (A), dorsal branches (B), lateral and medial palmar digital nerves (base sesamoid) (C), lateral and medial palmar nerves (D and G), lateral and medial palmar metacarpal nerves (E), and communicating branch (F).

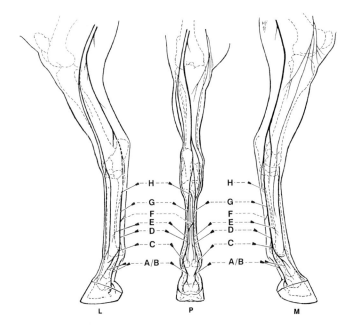

Fig. 16B–6. Needle placement for nerves of the distal part of the left pelvic limb of the horse, lateral (L), plantar (P), and medial (M) views: lateral and medial plantar digital nerves (A), dorsal branches (B), lateral and medial plantar digital nerves (base sesamoid) (C), lateral and medial plantar nerves (D and G), lateral and medial plantar metotarsal nerves (E), and communicating branch (F).

anatomic deposition, inadequate anesthetic volume, dilution or hemodilution of anesthetic agent, presence of fibrous connective tissue inhibiting diffusion of anesthetic agent, multiple sites of pain, and incorrect location of lameness.(47) Horses may become ataxic after nerve blockade in the limbs. This ataxia may lead to self-trauma because the horse may not know where the limbs are actually being placed.(30)

Digital nerves. The palmar (or plantar) digital nerve is desensitized with the leg either bearing weight or in an elevated position. It is palpated on the palmar (or plantar) aspect of the pastern medially and/or laterally midway between the coronary band and fetlock just palmar (or plantar) to the digital vein and artery (Figs. 16B–5A and 16B–6A). A 2.5-cm, 25-gauge needle is inserted in an anterior direction to a depth equal to the length of the needle and approximately 2 mL of local anesthetic are injected. Proper nerve blockade desensitizes the posterior one third of the foot including the navicular bursa 5 to 10 minutes after completing the injection (Fig. 16B–7A).

Anterior (or dorsal) digital nerve block. To block the dorsal or anterior digital nerve, which supplies sensory fibers to the anterior two thirds of the hoof, the needle is directed anteriorly to the site of the posterior digital nerve and is inserted to a depth equal to the length of the needle while infiltrating subcutaneously 3 to 5 mL of local anesthetic. (Figs. 16B–5B and 16B–6B) All

structures of the entire digit distal to the injection—including the phalanges P1, P2, and P3; the proximal and distal interphalangeal joints; the entire corium; the dorsal branches of the suspensory ligament; and the distal extensor tendon—become anesthetized.

Abaxial (basilar) sesamoidean nerve block. This block can be done at the anterior and posterior digital nerves at the abaxial surface of the proximal sesamoids, to give better analgesia of the pastern and proximal pastern joints. (Figs. 16B–5C and 16B–6C) Successful injections of 3 to 5 mL of local anesthetic subcutaneously at that site desensitize the entire foot distal to the injection, including the back of the pastern area and distal sesamoidean ligaments (Fig. 16B–7C).

Low palmar (or plantar) nerve block. This block is performed by injecting approximately 2 to 3 mL of local anesthetic at the following four points (four-point block) while the limb is bearing weight: the medial and lateral palmar nerves (Figs. 16B–5D and 16B–6D) and the medial and lateral palmar metacarpal (metatarsal) nerves (Figs. 16B–5E and 16B–6E) distal to the communicating branch of the medial and lateral palmar nerves (Figs. 16B–5F and 16B–6F). The injection is made between the flexor tendon and suspensory ligament (medial/lateral palmar nerve block) and between the suspensory ligament and the splint bone (medial/lateral palmar metacarpal [metatarsal] nerves). This procedure desensitizes almost all structures distal to the fetlock and fetlock joint except for a small area dorsal to the fetlock joint supplied by sensory fibers of the ulnar and

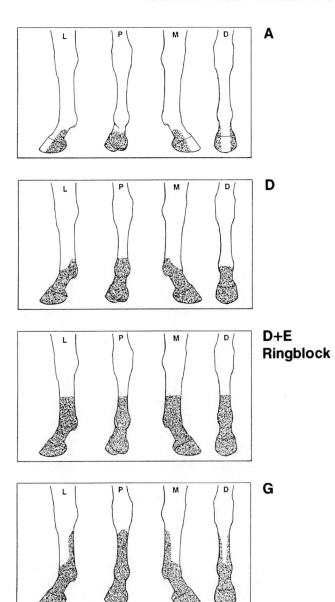

Fig. 16B–7. Desensitized subcutaneous area after A, C, D + E, and G blockade.

musculocutaneous nerves (Fig. 16B–7D).

High palmar (or plantar) nerve block. If the block is made proximal to the communicating branch of the medial and lateral palmar (or plantar) nerves (Figs. 16B–5F and 16B–6F), then it can be assured that the palmar metacarpal (or metatarsal) region, the fetlock and all of the digit are desensitized (Figs. 16B–5G and 16B–6G). A 3.75-cm, 22-gauge needle is placed subfascially into the groove between the suspensory ligament and deep flexor tendon on both the medial and lateral side approximately 5 cm distal to the carpometacarpal (carpometatarsal) joint, where 5 mL of the local anesthetic are injected.(51) The dorsal metacarpal (or metatarsal) region will still have sensation, but can be

desensitized by injecting the local anesthetic subcutaneously around the front of the cannon bone (ring block) (Fig. 16B–7E).

High suspensory block. Deposition of 5 mL of local anesthetic solution to the medial and lateral palmar metacarpal (or plantar metatarsal) nerves (Figs. 16B–5H and 16B–6H), which are subfascial between the superficial digital flexor tendon and suspensory ligament, desensitizes the interosseous muscle (suspensory ligament) and inferior check ligament, the caudal aspect of the metacarpus (metatarsus), and the adjacent splint bones. (Fig. 16B–7G)

Nerve blocks proximal to the carpus. It is very uncommon to perform higher nerve blocks than the high suspensory block on the forelimb; however, to induce anesthesia of the carpus and distal forelimb, three nerves must be desensitized: the median, ulnar, and branches of the musculocutaneous. The median nerve is desensitized on the medial aspect of the forelimb approximately 5 cm ventral to the elbow joint, by using a 3.75-cm, 20-gauge needle and injecting 10 mL of the anesthetic (Fig. 16B–8A). The ulnar nerve is desensitized by inserting a 2.5-cm, 22-gauge needle 10 cm proximal to the accessory carpal bone between the flexor carpi ulnaris and ulnaris lateralis muscles and injecting 5 mL of the anesthetic solution 1.5 cm deep beneath the fascia (Fig. 16B–8B). The medial cutaneous antebrachial nerve, a branch of the musculocutaneous nerve, is easily palpated just cranial to the cephalic vein at the anteromedial aspect of the forelimb half-way between the elbow and carpus. Approximately 10 mL of the anesthetic solution are deposited subcutaneously at that site, using a 2.5-cm, 22-gauge needle (Fig. 16B–8C).

Nerve blocks proximal to the tarsus. It is very uncommon to do any higher blocks than the high suspensory block in the hindlimb, but to complete anesthesia of the hindlimb from the tarsus distally, it is necessary to desensitize four nerves: the tibial, saphenous, superficial peroneal (superficial fibular), and deep peroneal (deep fibular). The tibial nerve is desensitized by injecting 15 to 20 mL of local anesthetic subfascially between the combined tendons of the gastrocnemius muscle and superficial flexor tendon, using a 2.5-cm, 22-gauge needle. Injection is best made on the medial aspect of the limb, approximately 10 cm proximal to the point of the tarsus, while the limb is partially flexed. Successful blockade desensitizes the posterior metatarsal region and most of the foot (Fig. 16B–9A). A ring block of the dorsal metatarsal region may be necessary to desensitize the anterolateral region. The saphenous nerve is desensitized by inserting a 2.5-cm, 22-gauge needle subcutaneously on the cranial or caudal aspect of the median saphenous vein, proximal to the tibiotarsal joint, and injecting 5 mL of the local anesthetic (Fig. 16B–9B). The medial aspect of the thigh and part of the metatarsal region will be anesthetized. The superficial and deep peroneal (fibular) nerves can be simultaneously desensitized by inserting a 3.75-cm, 22-gauge

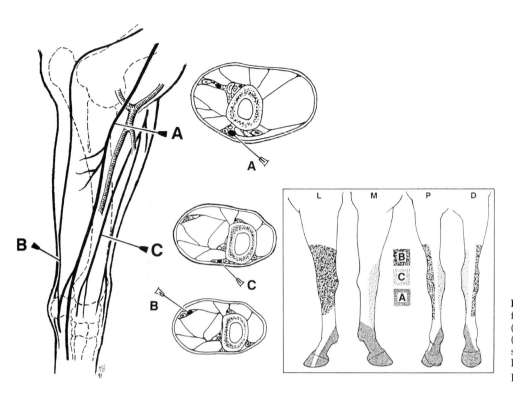

Fig. 16B–8. Needle placement for median nerve (A), ulnar nerve (B), and musculocutaneous nerve (C); crossections and desensitized subcutaneous areas of left forelimb; L, lateral; M, medial; P, palmar; D, dorsal aspect.

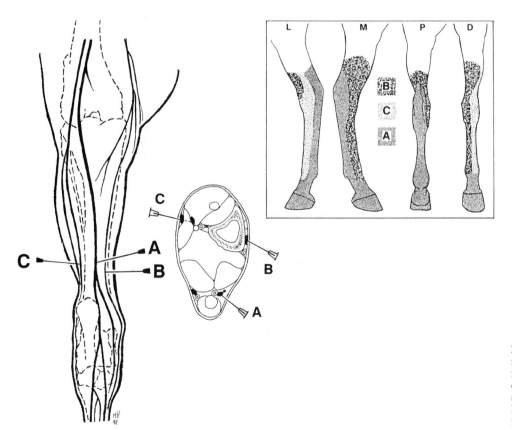

Fig. 16B–9. Needle placement for tibial nerve (A), saphenous nerve (B), and peroneal nerve (C); crossections and desensitized subcutaneous areas of left rearlimb; L, lateral; M, medial; P, plantar; D, dorsal aspects.

needle between the long and lateral digital extensor muscles approximately 10 cm proximal to the lateral malleolus of the tibia (Fig. 16B–9C). The superficial branch of the nerve is infiltrated subcutaneously with 10 mL of the local anesthetic. The needle is then advanced 2 to 3 cm to penetrate the deep fascia and to deposit 15 mL of the anesthetic around the deep branch. Anesthesia should include the anterolateral tarsal and metatarsal regions and the joint capsule of the tarsus.

Intraarticular Injections

Although arthrocentesis implies aspiration of synovial fluid, it allows for instillation of local anesthetic for the purpose of diagnostic anesthesia and use of therapeutic agents (e.g., saline flushes, antibiotics, hyaluronic acid and antiinflammatory drugs) as a therapy for certain diseases. The two most common local anesthetic agents used in intraarticular injections are mepivacaine and lidocaine hydrochloride solution. Mepivacaine appears to cause less irritation than lidocaine for use in intraarticular injections.(52) Proper restraint, either physical or chemical, is indicated, and each horse should be considered potentially fractious.

PODOTROCHLEAR (NAVICULAR) BURSA BLOCK

The procedure is best performed while the limb is weight bearing. Anesthesia of the podotrochlear (navicular) bursa is induced by inserting a 5- to 7.5-cm, 18-gauge spinal needle through the digital pad between the bulbs of the heel until it strikes the bone along the midline at a point approximately at the level of the coronary band (Fig. 16B–10A). The needle is then slightly withdrawn until very little synovial fluid is aspirated, and 3 to 5 mL of local anesthetic are injected.

COFFIN BLOCK

The distal interphalangeal (coffin) joint (P2-P3) is desensitized with 5 to 10 mL of local anesthetic. A 3.75-cm, 18- to 20-gauge needle is inserted 1.5 cm proximal to the coronet approximately 2 cm lateral to the vertical center of the pastern and is directed obliquely ventral to the tendon toward the extensor process (Fig. 16B–10B). Anesthesia of the podotrochlear (navicular) bursa depends upon diffusion of the local anesthetic through the suspensory ligament to the bursa, since the coffin joint and podotrochlear (navicular) bursa do not communicate. The combination of lidocaine HC1 (20 mg/mL), epinephrine (0.012 mg/mL), and sodium penicillin (800,000 IU) must not be injected into the coffin joint of horses. It can cause irreversible lameness based upon ossifying arthrodesis.(53)

PASTERN BLOCK

The proximal interphalangeal (pastern) joint (P1-P2) can be entered with ease by inserting a 3.75-cm, 20- to 22-gauge needle medially or laterally to the midline on the palpable epicondyles of P2, and injecting 5 to 8 mL of local anesthetic. The needle is directed vertically and is inserted for approximately 2.5 cm (Fig. 16B–10C).

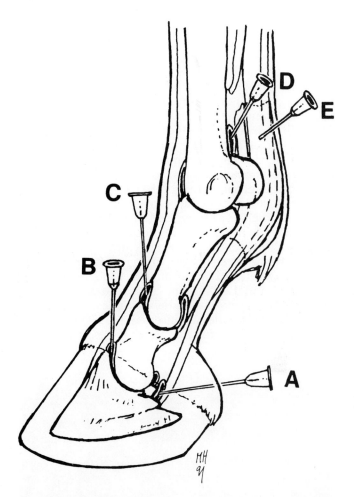

Fig. 16B–10. Needle placement into podotrochlear bursa (A), coffin joint (B), pastern joint (C), volar pouch of fetlock joint capsule (D), and digital flexor tendon sheath (E).

FETLOCK BLOCK

The metacarpophalangeal or metatarsophalangeal (fetlock) joint is one of the commonly and easily injected joints. A 3.75-cm, 20- to 22-gauge needle is inserted into the lateral pouch distal to the splint bone and dorsal to the annular ligament of the fetlock at a depth of approximately 0.5 to 1.5 cm (Fig. 16B–10D). When distended, this joint capsule may also be penetrated on the cranial surface of the joint. Approximately 8 mL of local anesthetic solution is injected.

DIGITAL FLEXOR TENDON SHEATH BLOCK

The digital flexor tendon sheath can be desensitized by inserting a 3.75-cm, 18- to 20-gauge needle to the distal end of the splint ("button") either medially or laterally cranial to the deep and superficial flexor tendons and caudal to the suspensory ligament and deposition of 10 mL of local anesthetic (Fig. 16B–10E).

CARPAL BLOCKS

The radiocarpal (antebrachial carpal) and intercarpal (middle carpal) joints are the two most commonly injected carpal joints. The carpometacarpal joint communicates with the middle (intercarpal) joint and therefore does not require separate entry.(51) In one commonly used technique, the carpus is flexed and a 3.75-cm, 20-gauge needle is inserted on either side of the palpable extensor carpi radialis tendon to deposit 5 to 10 mL of local anesthetic into each joint (Fig. 16B–11 and 12, A and B). In an alternative method, which is used by many racetrack practitioners in the standing horse, the needles are inserted perpendicularly through the skin on the posterolateral aspect of the radiocarpal and intercarpal joint spaces (Figs. 16B–12C and D). To locate the lateral site for penetration of the radiocarpal joint, the lateral digital extensor tendon and tendon of the ulnaris lateralis muscle are identified at the distal end of the ulna. These tendons narrow to form a depressed V anterior to the accessory carpal bone. The radiocarpal joint is then entered approximately 1 to 2 cm distal to this V (Fig. 16B–12C). The intercarpal joint is approximately 2 to 2.5 cm distal to the first injection site (Fig. 16B–12D). The needles are inserted 1 to 2 cm until the joint spaces are encountered. Advantages of this technique include minimal risk of injuring the articular surfaces of the bones and injecting local anesthetic into a larger space of a more stable position of the leg from a safe lateral approach.(43, 46)

CUBITAL (ELBOW) BLOCK

The cubital (elbow) joint is not a usual source of lameness, so it is rarely desensitized. A 5-cm, 18-gauge needle is inserted into the depression between the lateral epicondyle of the humerus and the lateral tuberosity of the radius at the anterior edge of the lateral collateral ligament (Fig. 16B–13A). Repeated flexion of the elbow joint greatly facilitates the identification of the palpable landmarks. The needle is directed obliquely in a caudomedial direction to reach the elbow joint at a depth of 3 to 4 cm; up to 20 mL of local anesthetic is required.

OLECRANON BURSA BLOCK

Olecranon bursa block is induced by inserting a 3.75-cm, 18-gauge needle from caudal of the olecranon, directing the needle obliquely from proximal to distal and injecting about 10 to 15 mL of the local anesthetic (Fig. 16B–13B).

BICIPITAL BURSA BLOCK

After the biceps brachii muscle is palpated, a 7.5-cm, 18-gauge spinal needle is inserted between the muscle and the proximal humerus from below and approximately 4 cm ventral and 2 cm posterior to the palpable anterior prominence of the lateral tuberosity of the humerus (Fig. 16B–13C). The needle is advanced up to 5 cm obliquely dorsomedial toward the opposite point of the shoulder to penetrate the bursa. At least 10 mL of local anesthetic is injected, and 20 minutes are given for maximal effect.

SHOULDER BLOCK

The scapula humeral (shoulder) joint can be difficult to enter because of its relative depth. Limb motion or muscle contraction must be prevented to avoid bending of a positioned needle. The tendon of the infraspinatus muscle can be palpated as a tense band extending from the scapula to the proximal humerus. A 7.5-cm to 12.5-cm, 18-gauge spinal needle is inserted just cranial to the tendon and between the palpable projections of the anterior and posterior parts of the lateral tuberosity of the humerus, and is directed to the opposite elbow (Fig. 16B–13D). Penetration from skin is up to 7.5 cm or until synovial fluid is aspirated. A volume of 30 mL or more of the anesthetic is deposited. The shoulder joint may communicate with the bicipital bursa in some horses; therefore, administration of local anesthetic into the shoulder joint may diffuse the anesthetic to the bicipital bursa and improve a lameness associated with that site.(44, 45)

CUNEAN BURSA BLOCK

The cunean bursa block is commonly done in standardbreds and less commonly in horses that are ridden.(48,

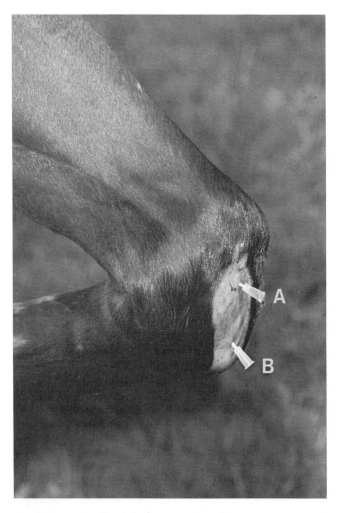

Fig. 16B–11. Needle placement into the radiocarpal joint (A) and intercarpal joint (B) of right forelimb.

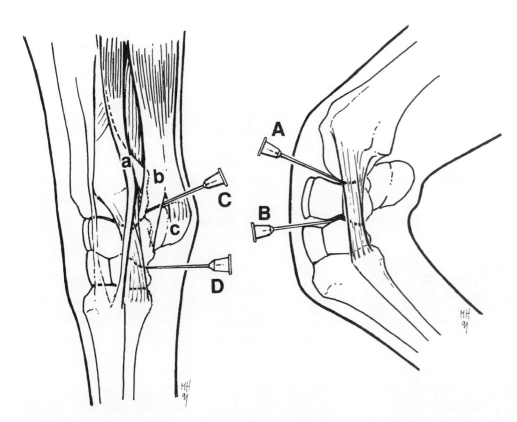

Fig. 16B–12. Needle placement into the radiocarpal (A and C) and intercarpal joints (B and D) of the left forelimb (a, lateral digital extensor tendon; b, tendon of ulnaris lateralis muscle; c, accessory carpal bone).

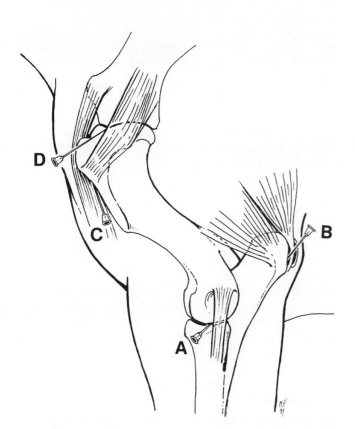

Fig. 16B–13. Needle placement into the elbow joint (A), olecranon bursa (B), bicipital bursa (C), and shoulder joint (D) of the left forelimb.

49) The cunean tendon is the tendon of the medial branch of the tibialis anterior muscle extending diagonally from anterior to posterior and inserting in the tarsal bone on the medial aspect of the tarsus (Fig. 16B–14A). A 2.5-cm, 22-gauge needle is inserted approximately 1.5 cm distal to the cunean tendon and is then advanced between the cunean tendon and the tarsal bone to penetrate the bursa from distally. This approach is safe, and should the horse move, it is less likely to break off the needle. At least 10 mL of local anesthetic are frequently required and administered as the needle enters the skin, coming up from distal under the tendon to fill the entire bursa after penetration (Fig. 16B–15). One way to test the block is to demonstrate increased intrabursal pressure by observing either the plunger of the syringe coming back after injection or the local anesthetic flowing forcefully from the needle after removal of the syringe. At least 20 minutes are required for maximum anesthetic effect.

TARSAL BLOCKS

Desensitizing the distal intertarsal and tarsometatarsal joints with local anesthetic improves lameness associated with early bone spavin. The tarsometatarsal joint is most easily entered by a 2.5-cm, 22-gauge needle on the posterior lateral aspect of the hock over the lateral head of the splint (metatarsal IV) (Fig. 16B–16). The intertarsal joint is entered by a 2.5-cm, 22-gauge needle at a right angle to the skin ventral to the cunean tendon on the medial aspect of the tarsus (Fig. 16B–14C). Approximately 6 mL of local anesthetic solution are injected into

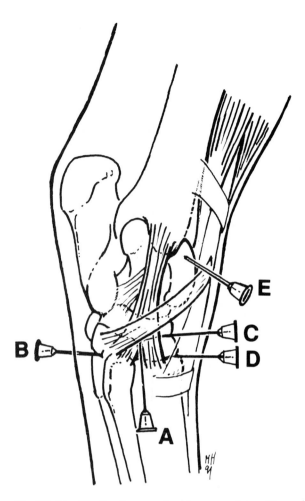

Fig. 16B–14. Needle placement into the cunean bursa (A), tarsometatarsal space (B and D), distal intertarsal space (C), and tibiotarsal space (E) of the left hock joint. Medial aspect.

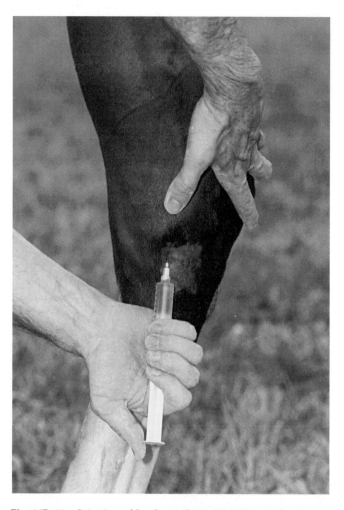

Fig. 16B–15. Injection of local anesthetic (10 mL) into the cunean bursa of the right rear limb. Medial aspect.

the intertarsal joint space with pressure. Considerable resistance will be encountered, even with the needle placed in the joint. Sometimes the needle must be turned to be sure that the bevel is not against bone and allows for injection of the anesthetic solution. In an alternative method, a 2.5-cm, 22-gauge needle can be placed into the tarsometatarsal joint approximately 2.5 cm distal to the intertarsal joint while injecting the local anesthetic (Fig. 16B–14D). Communication between the distal intertarsal and tarsometatarsal joints is variable, but can be demonstrated by placing one needle in each of the two joints and observing the local anesthetic to flow from one needle after the anesthetic is injected into the other needle.(36, 39) There is a great pressure in the distal joint and in order to get good dispersion of local anesthetic in both joints, both sites should be injected with local anesthetic solution.

TIBIOTARSAL BLOCK

One of the most common joints in which arthrodesis is done is the tibiotarsal (tarsocrural) joint. It is the easiest of all the equine joints to inject.(34) This joint is

penetrated with an 3.75-cm, 18-gauge needle at the craniomedial aspect 2 to 3 cm ventral to the medial malleolus of the tibia on either the medial or lateral side of the saphenous vein (Fig. 16B–14E). The capsule is thin, superficial, and easily observed and may also be distended caudomedially and craniolaterally in case of tarsal osteoarthrosis (bone spavin).(37) The needle is inserted in a slightly dorsal direction toward the anterior medial aspect of the hock to a depth of less than 2 cm. Approximately 15 mL of local anesthetic are injected after synovial fluid is recovered on aspiration. Complete anesthesia of the tibiotarsal joint has been achieved in healthy horses (250 to 680 kg) by intraarticular administration of 2 mL of 4% procaine HCl solution. The intraarticular concentration of procaine ranged from 3.7 to 5.4 mg procaine/mL at 1 hour after administration, which is above the anesthetic threshold concentration (0.2 mg/mL).(38)

STIFLE BLOCKS

The stifle (genual) joint is the largest joint in the hindlimb. It consists of the femoropatellar and femorotibial joint spaces, consisting of medial and lateral pouches. The medial femoropatellar pouch is the common site where the stifle joint is injected for diagnostic blocks. It is most easily entered dorsal to the tibial crest between the middle and medial patellar ligaments (Fig. 16B–17A). The medial femoropatellar pouch enclosing the femoropatellar joint communicates with the medial femorotibial pouch of the femorotibial joint in most horses. The communicating opening, however, can be obstructed in an inflamed stifle joint, necessitating the injection of local anesthetic or medication into each individual compartment.(21) Entering the medial pouch of the femorotibial joint is technically difficult, but it is accomplished between the medial patellar ligament and the medial collateral ligament approximately 4 cm dorsal to the proximal medial edge of the tibia (Fig. 16B–17B). The medial femorotibial pouch is chosen by some clinicians as the injection site because it is the area that is most likely to have injury and pain causing lameness. There is seldom an indication for injecting the lateral femorotibial pouch of the stifle joint because there is seldom injury in this area. The lateral femorotibial pouch can be entered between the lateral patellar ligament and the lateral collateral ligament (Fig. 16B–17C). In some cases (approximately 25%), a communicating opening between the femoropatellar pouch and the lateral

femorotibial pouch exists. A 5- to 7.5-cm, 18-gauge spinal needle is satisfactory for penetrating the joint capsule and injecting 30 to 40 mL of anesthetic into each pouch. To make the injection, it is best to feel around with the needle and insert it to a depth of 3 to 4 cm, until some resistance is encountered during penetration of the joint capsule. Additional resistance is felt as local anesthetic solution is injected. A few drops of joint fluid can be recovered after some local anesthetic has been administered, but seldom is joint fluid aspirated before the injection of local anesthetic. It is important to use a larger rather than a smaller amount of local anesthetic and give at least 20 minutes for maximal effect. Many horses will continue to improve until 60 minutes after the injection. Any improvement of lameness is significant, because few horses go entirely sound after injecting local anesthetic into the stifle joint. This is probably due to involvement of the medial collateral ligaments and/or cruciate

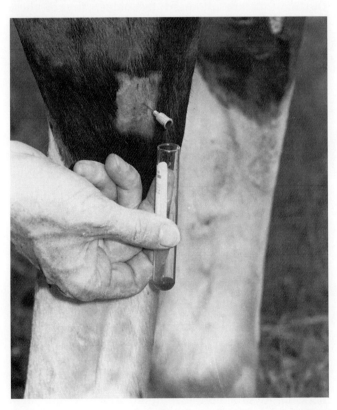

Fig. 16B–16. Collection of fluid from tarsometatarsal joint (left rear leg).

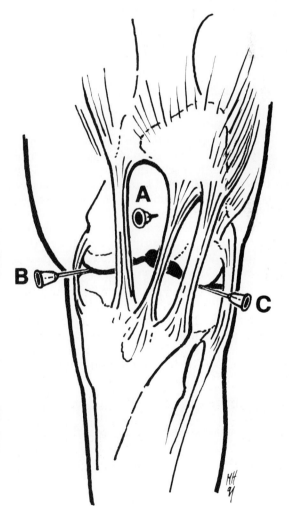

Fig. 16B–17. Needle placement into the femoropatellar pouch (A), medial femorotibial pouch (B), and lateral femorotibial pouch (C) of the stifle joint.

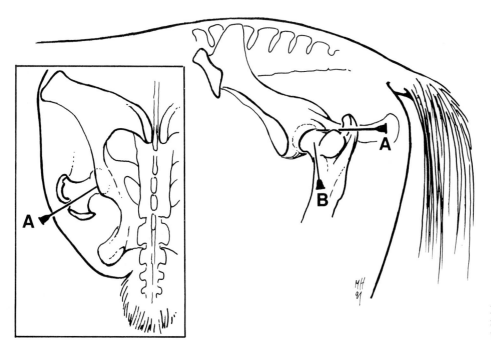

Fig. 16B–18. Needle placement into coxofemoral joint (A) and trochanteric bursa (B).

ligaments and structures adjacent to and not inside the joint capsule.

COXOFEMORAL BLOCK

The coxofemoral (hip) joint is the most difficult joint to enter, so several approaches have been described.(21, 34, 35, 42) The skin between the anterior and posterior eminences of the great trochanter of the femur is desensitized using a small amount of local anesthetic. A wide-bored needle (3.75-cm, 14-gauge) is first inserted at that site, through which a thinner (15-cm, 18-gauge) and more flexible needle is inserted. The needle is then advanced in an anteromedial direction along the femoral neck until the joint capsule is penetrated (Fig. 16B–18A). The deposition of 30 to 50 mL of local anesthetic is adequate, after synovial fluid is recovered on aspiration. Improvement of the lameness can be assessed after a minimum of 30 minutes has been given to reach maximal anesthetic effect.

TROCHANTERIC BURSA BLOCK

The trochanteric bursa is located on the lateral aspect of the hip between the anterior crest of the great trochanter of the femur and the middle gluteal muscle. The bursa is entered by a 7.5-cm, 18-gauge needle, which is inserted 3 to 5 cm ventral to the anterior crest of the great trochanter and is directed dorsally and medially (Fig. 16B–18B). Synovial fluid is recovered by using continuous suction of a syringe that is attached to the needle, then 10 to 15 mL of local anesthetic are injected.

Anesthesia for Laparotomy

At least four techniques for obtaining anesthesia of the paralumbar and abdominal wall in the standing horse have been described: (a) infiltration anesthesia, (b) paravertebral thoracolumbar anesthesia, (c) segmental dorsolumbar epidural anesthesia, and (d) segmental thoracolumbar subarachnoid anesthesia. Although infiltration of the incision line is the easiest and probably the most commonly used technique, any of these techniques may be used for abdominal surgeries such as exploratory laparotomy, intestinal biopsy, ovariectomy, cesarean section, embryo transfer, castration of stallions with abdominal cryptorchidism, and liver or kidney biopsy.

INFILTRATION ANESTHESIA

Simple infiltration of the incision line (line block) is commonly used in equine practice. A 2.5-cm, 20-gauge or smaller needle is used for multiple subcutaneous injections of 1 mL of local anesthetic for each centimeter of incision. This can be repeated until the entire length of the desired incision is blocked. Pain is minimized by slow and continuous injections as the needle is inserted at the edge of the desensitized skin. This technique assures that the horse senses only the initial needle penetration. The needle can be advanced in multiple directions to produce a fan-shaped area of desensitization. Usually 10 to 15 mL of anesthetic are adequate for the skin and subcutaneous line block, whereas 50 to 150 mL of the anesthetic may be required to desensitize the deeper layers of muscle and peritoneum, depending on the area to be desensitized. A 7.5- to 10-cm, 18-gauge needle is used for deep deposition of the anesthetic. Toxicity is not to be expected with doses of less than 250 mL of 2% lidocaine hydrochloride solution, which is equivalent to 5 g, for infiltration of the paralumbar fossa in adult horses (500 kg) for abdominal surgery,(2, 54) whereas intravenous bolus administration of smaller doses of lidocaine (up to 150 mL, 3 g/adult horse) causes convulsions. At least 15 minutes after infiltration are allowed for maximal anesthetic effects. The advantages of local infiltration anesthesia when compared to any other technique are the ease of performing the technique and that precise knowledge of nerve location is not necessary. The disadvantages include disruption of normal tissue architecture with excessive amount of fluid, hematoma, and trauma in that area; incomplete anesthesia (particularly of the peritoneum); incomplete muscle relaxation of the deeper layers of the abdominal wall; toxicity after injecting significant amounts of anesthetic solution into the peritoneal cavity; and increased cost and time required for long incisions (>20 cm) as would be required in a cesarean section.

PARAVERTEBRAL THORACOLUMBAR ANESTHESIA

If a long (>20 cm) incision of the skin, musculature, and peritoneum of the mid-flank region is required, paravertebral thoracolumbar anesthesia (paravertebral block) can be used as an alternative to infiltration anesthesia.(7, 55–57). This block is technically more difficult and less popular than other techniques, but can be accomplished in thin-muscled horses with palpable landmarks. The last thoracic (T18) and first and second lumbar (L1 and L2) spinal nerves are desensitized approximately 10 cm from the midline, after they have emerged from the intervertebral foramina and ramified into dorsal and ventral branches and their medial and lateral ramifications, respectively (Fig. 16B–19). Approximately 10 mL of local anesthetic is deposited to desensitize the lateral cutaneous branches of the dorsal spinal nerves T18, L1, and L2 subcutaneously at three sites: halfway between the last rib and distal end of the first lumbar transverse process (for T18), between the first and second transverse process (for L1), and between the second and third lumbar transverse process (for L2). The injection sites for desensitizing the spinal nerves are easily identified by locating the third lumbar transverse process, which lies on a line between the most caudal extension of the last rib and perpendicular to the long axis of the spinal vertebrae.(57) The distance between the injection sites ranges from 3 to 6 cm (Fig. 16B–20). After the skin is desensitized, a 7.5-cm, 18-gauge needle is inserted at each site to reach the

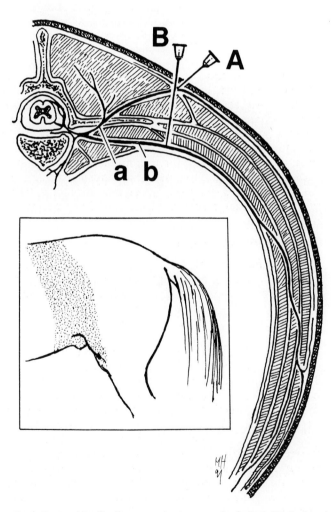

Fig. 16B–19. Needle placement for paravertebral nerve blockades: A cranial view of a transection of the first lumbar vertebra at the location of the intervertebral foramen: (A) subcutaneous infiltration, (B) retroperitoneal infusion (a, dorsal branch; b, ventral branch of L1 vertebral nerve). Inset, desensitized subcutaneous area after blockade of T18, L1, and L2 vertebral nerves.

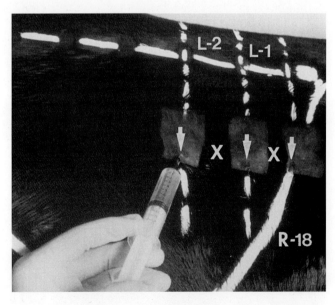

Fig. 16B–20. Right thoracolumbar area of a standing adult horse with injection sites (arrows) for distal paravertebral block (R18, last rib; L1 and L2, spinous processes of first and second lumbar vertebrae; X, lateral border of respective transverse processes). Dotted line transsects the corresponding interspaces between spinous and transverse processes. Subcutaneous injection of L2 is shown. (From Skarda R. Practical Regional Anesthesia. In: R.A. Mansmann, E.S. McAllister, and P.W. Pratt, eds. Edited by Equine Medicine, 3rd ed., vol. 1. Santa Barbara, CA, American Veterinary Publications, 1982:239.)

ventral branches of T18, L1, and L2. The needle is first advanced until the peritoneum is punctured, which is indicated by either a loss of resistance to needle insertion or a slight sucking sound as air enters the needle. The point of the needle is then withdrawn to a retroperitoneal position, where a second deposit of 15 mL of local anesthetic is placed (Fig. 16B–19B). The advantages of paravertebral anesthesia when compared to infiltration anesthesia include the use of small doses of anesthetic, a wide and uniform area of anesthesia and muscle relaxation, and absence of local anesthetic from the operative wound margin, thus minimizing edema, hematoma, and possible interference with healing. The disadvantages are difficulties in performing the technique. The fat and muscles in some horses almost put the transverse processes out of range of palpation, making the technique more time-consuming or unpractical. There is some bowing of the back toward the desensitized side, making it more difficult to close the incision and navigate. Inadvertent desensitization of the third lumbar spinal nerve, which carries motor fibers

to the femoral and ischial nerves, produces loss of motor control of the ipsilateral pelvic limb.

SEGMENTAL DORSOLUMBAR EPIDURAL ANESTHESIA

This technique is not routinely used in the horse because it is difficult to perform, requires a special catheter-stylet unit to catheterize the T18-L1 epidural space from the lumbosacral epidural space (Fig. 16B–21)(58), and is associated with the risk that the catheter will kink and curl at the lumbosacral epidural space with subsequent injection of local anesthetic to the femoral and ischial nerves, thereby producing loss of pelvic limb function and excitement.

SEGMENTAL THORACOLUMBAR SUBARACHNOID ANESTHESIA

Segmental thoracolumbar subarachnoid anesthesia is easier to master than segmental dorsolumbar epidural anesthesia. It produces the fastest and best-controlled surgical anesthesia of the flank in horses; however, special equipment and maintenance of aseptic technique are required.(59) A 17.5-cm, 17-gauge Huber-point Tuohy needle with stylet and with the bevel directed cranially is inserted into the subarachnoid space at the lumbosacral (L6-S1) intervertebral space (Fig. 16B–22A). This interspace is located 1 to 2 cm caudal of a line drawn between the cranial edge of each tuber sacral and the dorsal midline. Rectal palpation of the ventral lumbosacral eminence may be used to locate the L6-S1 intervertebral space.(59) The skin and lumbosacral fascia adjacent to the interspinous (L6-S1) ligaments are injected with 5 mL of 2% lidocaine hydrochloride solution to help minimize pain during the puncture procedure. Care must be taken not to inject the entire volume (5 mL) of local anesthetic into the subarachnoid space to prevent loss of motor control of the pelvic limbs. The needle is advanced along the median plane perpendicular to the spinal cord until it enters the subarachnoid space. The stylet is removed, and 2 to 3 mL of CSF is aspirated. A Formocath polyethylene catheter 100 cm long with a 0.095-cm outside diameter, reinforced with a stainless steel spring guide (0.052-cm outside diameter), is passed through the needle and advanced approximately 60 cm to the midthoracic area. First the needle is withdrawn over the catheter, then the spring guide is removed and the catheter is withdrawn a calculated distance to place its tip at T18-L1. Precise catheter positioning requires radiography for confirmation. A 23-gauge needle on a three-way stopcock is attached to the catheter, and 1.0 to 2.0 mL of spinal fluid (CSF) is removed. A small dose (1.5 to 2.0 mL) of a 2% mepivacaine hydrochloride solution is injected through the catheter at a rate of approximately 0.5 mL per minute. The previously collected CSF is used to remove the remaining local anesthetic from the catheter. Bilateral segmental anesthesia, extending from spinal cord segment T14 to L3, is maximal 5 to 10 minutes after injection and lasts for 30 to 60 minutes. Surgical anesthesia is easily maintained

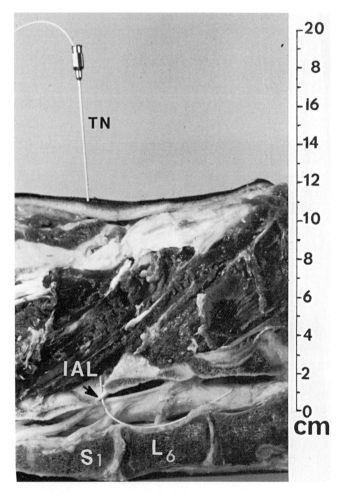

Fig. 16B–21. Lateral view of sagittal section of the sixth lumbar (L6) and first sacral (S1) vertebrae. A 17.5-cm, 17-gauge Huber-point Tuohy needle (TN) is in place for catheterization of the lumbar epidural space. The arrow indicates the interarcuate ligament (IAL).

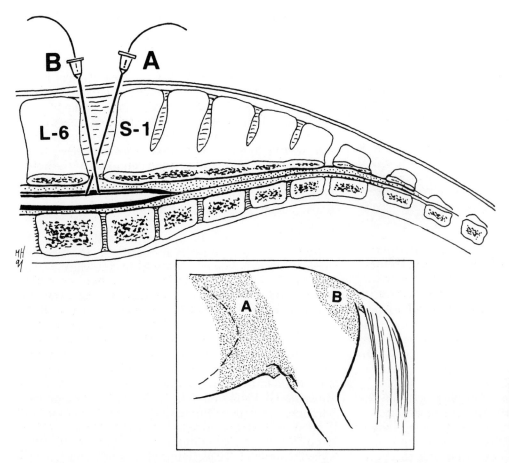

Fig. 16B–22. Needle and catheter placement for thoracolumbar subarachnoid anesthesia (A) and caudal subarachnoid anesthesia (B). Desensitized subcutaneous area after segmental (A) and caudal (B) blockade is stippled.

by fractional bolus administration of 0.5 mL of the anesthetic at 30-minute intervals or as needed (Fig. 16B–23). The duration of anesthesia is determined by the decline of the subarachnoid mepivacaine concentration owing to absorption of drug into the systemic circulation and not due to hydrolysis in CSF.(60)

The advantages of thoracolumbar subarachnoid anesthesia as compared with dorsolumbar epidural anesthesia include simplicity of needle and catheter placements, minimal dosage, deposition of the anesthetic at nerve roots, rapid onset of anesthesia, and minimal physiologic disturbance. The disadvantages include potential for traumatizing the conus medullaris, kinking and curling of the catheter in the subarachnoid space if the guidewire is recessed from the catheter tip, loss of motor control of the pelvic limbs and/or injecting the proper dose in a misplaced catheter, and meningitis after septic technique.

Caudal Anesthesia

Caudal epidural anesthesia, continuous caudal epidural anesthesia, and caudal subarachnoid anesthesia are possible techniques to produce regional anesthesia of the anus, perineum, rectum, vulva, vagina, urethra, and bladder in horses. Success in producing regional anesthesia of pelvic viscera and genitalia without losing locomotor function of the hind legs depends upon

cranial flow of local anesthetic to desensitize the caudal and the last three pairs of sacral nerves in the epidural space as they emerge either from the meninges (epidural technique) or the spinal cord (subarachnoid technique). In horses, the spinal cord and its meninges end in the midsacral region, and only the coccygeal nerves and the thin phylum terminale remain in the spinal canal.(61) The coccygeal nerves are not easily damaged at the site of needle penetration to produce caudal epidural blockade. Caudal subarachnoid blockade, however, requires the insertion of a spinal needle into the subarachnoid space at the lumbosacral intervertebral space and passing a catheter to the midsacral region; thus, potential trauma to the conus medullaris and nerve fibers by the needle or catheter exists. The neuroanatomy and results after sensory, motor and autonomic nerve blockade for spinal cord segments are summarized in Table 16B–1.(62, 63)

CAUDAL EPIDURAL ANESTHESIA

Caudal epidural anesthesia is routinely used in the horse because it is simple and inexpensive and requires no sophisticated equipment. The technique in horses was first described in 1925 (64); subsequently, many have reported its use for relieving pain and control of rectal tenesmus associated with irritation of the perineum, anus, rectum, and vagina during difficult labor,

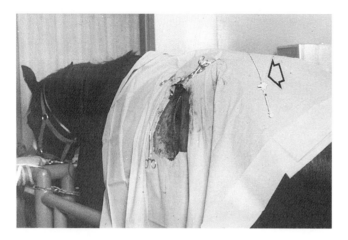

Fig. 16B–23. Ovariectomy (granulosa cell tumor) via left flank under segmental subarachnoid anesthesia (2 mL of 2% carbocaine HC1). The subarachnoid catheter is indicated by an arrow.

correction of uterine torsion, fetotomy, and various obstetric manipulations and surgical procedures such as amputation of the tail, rectovaginal fistula repairs, Caslick's closure (operation for pneumovagina), prolapsed rectum, urethrostomy, or anal, perineal, vulvar, and bladder procedures.(7, 65-81)

The injection site is the epidural space between the first and second coccygeal vertebrae. The first coccygeal interspace (Co1-Co2) is identified as the first obvious midline depression caudal to the sacrum. It can generally be felt with the finger as the first movable coccygeal articulation when the tail is raised and lowered. The sacrococcygeal joint in many horses is fused and generally intersects with the midline and a line drawn over the back joining the two coxofemoral joints. The Co1-Co2 interspace may be more difficult to palpate in obese or well-developed horses, but it generally lies at the most angular portion of the bend of the tail, approximately 5 cm cranial to the origin of the first tail hairs and the caudal fold of the tail. Correct needle placement requires the horse to be properly restrained and stand squarely with the croup symmetrical. In the standard technique, a 5- to 7.5-cm, 18-gauge spinal needle with fitted stylet is inserted through the disinfected skin in the center of the Co1-Co2 joint space while directing the needle at almost right angles to the general contour of the croup or ventrocranially at an angle of approximately 10° to vertical. The needle is inserted in a median plane until it contacts the floor of the vertebral canal and is then withdrawn for approximately 0.5 cm to avoid injection into the intervertebral disc or ligamentous floor of the canal (Fig. 16B–24A). Painful reaction to the epidural needle is minimized if 2 to 3 mL of a 2% lidocaine hydrochloride solution are injected subcutaneously and adjacent to the interspinous and interarcuate ligaments using a 2.5-cm, 25-gauge needle. A "popping" sensation is often detected as the interarcuate ligament is penetrated. A hissing sound may be heard upon penetration of the

epidural space, or confirmation can be made by injection of 3 to 5 mL of air or local anesthetic solution (test dose), and no blood upon aspiration.

In the alternative technique, the spinal needle is inserted at the caudal part of the first intercoccygeal depression and directed cranioventrally at almost 30° to the horizontal plane until its point glides along the floor of the neural canal (Fig. 16B–24B). The spinal needle can be inserted to its full length (5 to 7.5 cm). Depth from skin surface to the neural canal varies between 3 to 7.5 cm depending upon the size and condition of the horse. The alternative technique is useful in horses that have fibrous connective tissue from previous epidural injections, which limits the diffusion of local anesthetic agents.

The amount of anesthetic injection is determined by considering the type of local anesthetic, the size and conformation of the horse, the depth of needle insertion into the vertebral canal (the actual distance of the needle bevel to the spinal cord), and the extent of regional anesthesia required. A mature mare (450 kg) may require a total of 6 to 8 mL of a 2% lidocaine hydrochloride solution (0.26-0.35 mg/kg) to anesthetize the anus, perineum, rectum, vulva, vagina, urethra, and bladder. Other acceptable dosages to achieve caudal anesthesia in the standing horse are 10 to 12 mL of 2% procaine HC1 solution, 5 to 7 mL of 5% procaine HC1 solution, 5 to 7 mL of 2% mepivacaine HC1 solution, and 3 to 5 mL of 5% hexylcaine HC1 solution. When choosing an alpha$_2$-adrenoceptor agonist, 0.17 mg xylazine/kg(78) or 60 μg detomidine/kg(81) diluted in 10 mL of 0.9% NaC1 solution may be required to achieve similar anesthesia of pelvic viscera and genitalia without ataxia. Maximum effect should be manifest in 10 to 30 minutes. It is not advisable to redose during this time. If the needle is left in place and an injection cap is attached, additional amounts of local anesthetic or alpha$_2$-adrenoceptor agonist can be administered but should be regulated to keep the horse standing (Fig. 16B–25). The duration of anesthesia is dose related and lasts from 60 to 90 minutes for lidocaine (2%) and procaine (5%), 90 to 120 minutes for mepivacaine (2%), hexylcaine (5%), and detomidine (1%), and 180 to 240 minutes for xylazine (2%), respectively. Caudal epidurally administered local anesthetic solution and xylazine, when injected at recommended dosages, are without apparent side effects.(82, 83) In a recent study, cardiopulmonary and behavioral responses (pain, sedation, ataxia) to caudal (S5-Co1) epidural xylazine (0.25 mg/kg of body weight and expanded to a 6-mL volume with 0.9% NaC1) were determined in 8 adult mares (470 ± 19 kg).(84) Maximal dermatomal spread was variable and ranged from the first coccygeal to S3 spinal cord segments at 15 ± 6 minutes, and lasted for 165 to over 180 minutes after epidural administration of xylazine. Sedation and ataxia were minimal, and circulatory and respiratory variables, such as cardiac output, stroke, volume, mean right atrial pressure, mean pulmonary artery pressure, systemic and pulmonary vascular resistance,

Table 16B–1. Neuroanatomy and Action of Caudal Epidural Analgesia

Nerves	Ventral Branches	Spinal Cord Segment	Sensory	Motor	Parasympathetic	Sympathetic	Action
Caudal		Coccygeal	Most of the tail and skin between anus and tailroot	Coccygeal muscle			
Caudal rectal (hemorrhoidal)		S5	Anal region, tail folds, tail base	Coccygeus and levator ani externus muscle	Fibers in caudal rectal nerve		Straining in anorectal region due to excessive sympathetic stimulation
Middle rectal	Perineal nerve, caudal scrotal nerves, labial nerves	S4, S5	Perineum, posterior croup, scrotum along its caudal aspects, vulva without clitoris		Pelvic nerves, hypogastric plexus		Relaxation of bladder without sphincter, distal colon, rectum, sexual organs
Pudendal	Dorsal nerve of penis, deep perineal nerve	S4, S3, S2	Penis (corpus cavernosum and spongiosum); clitoris and vulva	Perineal muscles fascia of ischiorectal fossa, constrictor vulvae muscle		Retractor penis muscle	Prolapse of penis; relaxation of vulva and vagina
Caudal gluteal	Caudal cutaneous femoral nerve	S2, S1	Lateral and posterior surface of hip and thigh	Extension of hip			
Cranial gluteal		S1, L6, L5	Lateral aspect of thigh	Flexor and abductors of hip		Splanchnic lumbar nerves (in part)	Relaxation of bladder and sphincter of bladder, distal colon, rectum, sexual organs
Sciatic		S1, L6, L5	Middle to tibial region to foot	Flexor and abductors of hip; flexor of stifle (in part) and extensors of hock and digit			Ataxia, knuckling of hind fetlock

(From Skarda, R.T. Local and Regional Analgesia. In: Principles and Practice of Veterinary Anesthesia, edited by C.E. Short, Baltimore, Williams and Wilkins. 1987:105.) (63)

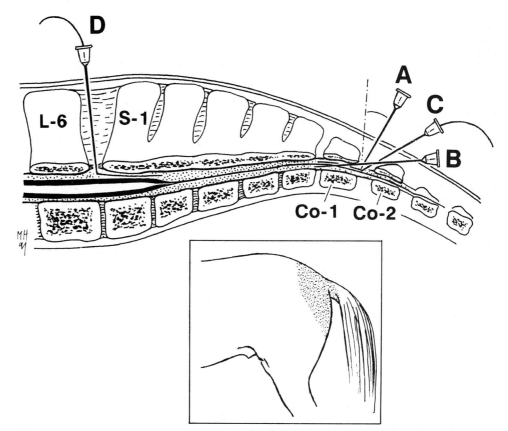

Fig. 16B–24. A and B, needle placement for caudal epidural anesthesia; C and D, catheter placement into sacral epidural space for continuous caudal epidural anesthesia (L6, sixth lumbar; S1, first sacral dorsal spinous process; Co1 and Co2, first and second coccygeal vertebrae). Desensitized subcutaneous area after caudal blockade is stippled.

oxygen consumption, core and rectal temperature, and arterial and mixed venous pH and gas tensions (P_{O_2}, P_{CO_2}) did not change significantly ($P < 0.05$) from baseline values in conscious, standing mares.(84) Recently, a mixture of lidocaine (0.22 mg/kg, 2% solution) and xylazine (0.17 mg/kg, 2% solution) was considered safe for inducing long-lasting caudal epidural anesthesia in healthy adult horses.(80) It resulted in rapid onset (5.3 min) and provided significantly longer duration (330 ± 6 min) of anesthesia of the perineum than either drug given alone (lidocaine 87 ± 7 min; xylazine 204 ± 13 min), thereby minimizing delay of obstetric and surgical procedures and minimizing the need for additional administration of drugs. Pulse and respiratory rate were not altered, ataxia was mild in some horses, the penis prolapsed in the males, and there was no sedation in horses after administration of the mixture of lidocaine/xylazine hydrochloride. Overdosing induces depression of CNS, respiratory, and cardiovascular activity; postural instability and/or recumbency; and excitement in conscious horses.

Detomidine induces selective caudal analgesia in mares along with sedation (Fig. 16B–26), mild ataxia, cardiopulmonary depression, and diuresis similar to the effects of intravenously or intramuscularly administered detomidine.(81) Detomidine-induced side effects were abolished by intravenously, epidurally, or subarachnoidally administered alpha$_2$-adrenoceptor antagonists, such as atipamezole (Fig. 16B–27), idazoxan,

yohimbine, and tolazoline.(85, 86) Should signs of rear limb ataxia or motor blockade with caudal epidural anesthesia develop, a tail-tie support is indicated until full hindlimb control is regained. General anesthesia may be necessary to completely immobilize an excited horse.

USE OF OTHER AGENTS

Epinephrine at concentration of 5 µg/mL (1:200,000) is occasionally incorporated or can be added to the local anesthetic solution to enhance the onset, prolong the duration, and improve the quality of epidural anesthesia. Carbonization of the base preparations of lidocaine increases pH and favors the anesthetic nonionic state and lipid solubility but does not demonstrate the theoretical expectation of increased diffusion and increases drug's effect in caudal epidural anesthesia in horses.(87)

Alcohol (ethyl alcohol) has been injected into the caudal epidural space in horses to induce denervation of coccygeal nerves and alter tail function, although its efficacy and safety for producing neurolysis in horses has not been reported. Axonal degeneration appears 20 minutes after injection and lasts for several months to 1 year, depending upon the completeness of neurolysis. Alcohol-induced alteration of tails in horses can be diagnosed by electromyography and used to prosecute owners and exhibitors of show-ring horses.(88) Inaccuracy of the technique and injection of excessive volumes of alcohol into the caudal epidural space result in painful paresthesias, neuritis, and paralysis of the bladder, rectum, and pelvic limb.

Caudal epidural morphine has been considered a reasonable alternative for relief of pain that is not responsive to other standard techniques (2 g phenylbutazone/450 kg body weight, IV q 12 h) in equine patients.(89) Pain, which originated from an open luxation of the fetlock joint and comminuted fracture of the first phalanx in a 10-months'-pregnant Thoroughbred mare (450 kg) was relieved approximately 30 minutes after injection of 50 mg morphine, diluted in 30 mL of 0.9% sodium chloride solution into the epidural space at the sacrococcygeal interspace. Analgesia lasted 8 to 16 hours, based upon the mare's normal behavior of prolonged period of standing, no sweating, normal appetite, and normal heart rate. Analgesia was easily maintained for 3 days by injecting additional morphine (0.2 mg/kg) into an epidural catheter (91.4 cm, 20 gauge) placed into the sacral epidural space, using a 8-cm, 16-gauge Tuohy needle.(89)

Recently, either 50 μg morphine/kg of body weight in 10 mL of 0.9% NaC1 solution (M50), 100 μg morphine/kg of body weight in 10 mL of 0.9% NaC1 solution (M100), or 10 mL of 0.9% NaC1 solution (control) was injected into the epidural space at the first coccygeal interspace (Co1-Co2) in 5 healthy horses (mean wt. 500 kg), in a crossover randomized blinded study.(90) Analgesia was assessed at hourly intervals for 24 hours by using deep pinprick and graduated electrical stimuli (up to 80 V max.) on perineal, lumbosacral and thoracic dermatomes. The onset of analgesia of dermatomes S1 to S5, L1 to L6, and other dermatomes (S5 to T9) occurred 8.0 ± 0.4 hours (mean ± SEM) after M50 and 6.3 ± 0.3 hours after M100 injection, respectively, and lasted 17.2 ± 0.6 hours (M50) and 19.1 ± 0.5 hours (M100). Indirect arterial blood pressure, heart rate, respiratory rate, and rectal temperature did not change significantly ($P > 0.05$) from controls. Perineal wheals were observed in 2 horses given M100 and 1 horse given M50. Serum morphine concentrations, measurable at 10 to 180 minutes after epidural administration, peaked at 40 minutes (M50, 17.3 ng/mL) and 10 minutes (M100, 48.5 ng/mL). Epidural morphine administration produced sedation and head drooping, with 100 μg/kg producing a more rapid onset, cranial spread and longer duration, than 50 μg/kg administration.(90)

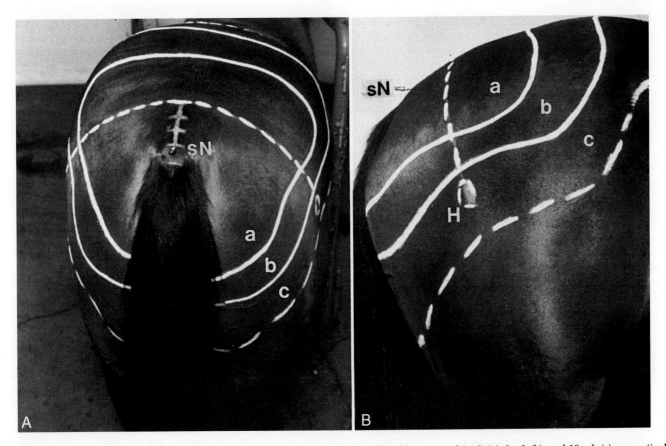

Fig. 16B–25. Desensitized skin area in a standing horse 20 minutes after epidural injection of 6 mL (a), 8 mL (b), and 10 mL (c), respectively, of 2% carbocaine via a 15-cm, 18-gauge spinal needle inserted at the third coccygeal interspace to its full length horizontally (SN = spinal needle with stylet; H, hip joint). Dorsocaudal (A) and lateral (B) aspects. (From Skarda, R. Practical Regional Anesthesia. In: R.A. Mansmann, E.S. McAllister, and P.W. Pratt, eds. Edited by Equine Medicine, 3rd ed., vol. 1. Santa Barbara, CA: American Veterinary Publications, 1982:243.)

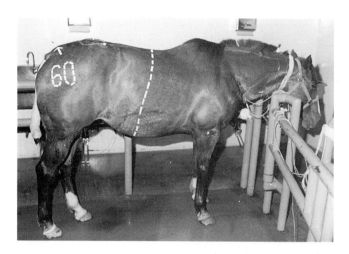

Fig. 16B–26. Desensitized skin area between T14 and coccyx and sedation in a standardbred mare (475 kg) at 60 minutes after administration of 2.9 mL of 1% detomidine hydrochloride solution, diluted to a 10-mL volume with sterile water, into the epidural space of the first coccygeal intervertebral space. The epidural needle is left in position and is indicated with a white arrow. A catheter is placed into the subarachnoid space at the lumbosacral intervertebral space for collection of CSF. (From Skarda, R, and Muir, W. In: Animal Pain. Edited by C.E. Short and A.V. Potzak, New York: Churchill Livingstone, 1992:295.)

Butorphanol (0.04 mg/kg), a widely used opiate in horses, has been added to lidocaine (0.25 mg/kg) for injection into the caudal epidural space of adult mares (mean wt. 500 kg), using a 8.75-cm, 18-gauge needle.(91) The addition of the opiate to the epidural local anesthetic prolonged cutaneous and visceral analgesia without affecting cardiorespiratory parameters such as heart rate, direct systemic arterial blood pressure, respiratory rate, blood gas tensions (Pao_2, $Paco_2$), and the central nervous system. The mares demonstrated an unusual way of walking (high steps with pointed hoof) in their hind limbs but ataxia and weakness were not evident.

CONTINUOUS CAUDAL EPIDURAL ANESTHESIA

Continuous caudal epidural analgesia is used in horses with extended surgery in the anal and perineal region, obstetric procedures, and relief of tenesmus. It can be simply achieved after aseptically placing a catheter into the epidural space using one of two methods described. In the simpler method, a 10.2-cm, 18-gauge thin-walled Tuohy needle with stylet is inserted on the midline into the Co1-Co2 interspace.(92) Pain from needle insertion is minimized if first a subcutaneous wheal of 2 to 3 mL of 2% lidocaine hydrochloride solution is made. Once through the skin, the needle, with the bevel pointed cranially, is directed at approximately 45° to vertical and is advanced until an abrupt reduction in resistance to needle passage is noted, indicating piercing through the interarcuate ligament and entry into the vertebral canal.

Injection of 5 mL of air or 2 to 3 mL of local anesthetic (test dose) should not encounter resistance. A commer-

cially available 91.8-cm, 20-gauge Teflon epidural catheter with graduated markings and stylet or a medical-grade vinyl tubing (0.036 cm outside diameter) is introduced into the needle and advanced cranially 2 to 4 cm beyond the tip of the needle (Fig. 16B–28A). The needle is removed fro n the catheter while the catheter is left in position. A catheter adapter (provided in the kit) or a three-way stopcock and 2.5-cm, 23-gauge needle is placed on the free end of the catheter for an injection port (Fig. 16B–29). Approximately 5 mL of anesthetic solution is then injected into the catheter over a period of 1 minute. Surgical anesthesia is easily maintained by fractional bolus administration of 3 mL of the anesthetic at 60-minute intervals or as needed.

In the alternative and more difficult method, a 19.5-cm, 17-gauge Huber point Tuohy needle with stylet and with the bevel directed caudally is aseptically inserted into the epidural space at the lumbosacral (L6-S1) intervertebral space.(92) A Formocath polyethylene catheter (0.095-cm outside diameter) reinforced with a stainless steel spring guide is introduced into the needle and advanced 10 to 20 cm, to place the catheter tip at the caudal position of the sacral (S3 to S5) epidural space in an adult horse (450 kg) (Fig. 16B–28B).

The route for repeated administration of small fractional doses of the anesthetic during surgery, while the tail is dorsally reflected for immobilization and surgical exposure, is the major advantage of the catheter technique when compared to the needle technique. In addition, the catheter tip is placed at the nerve roots of the pudendal and pelvic nerves, thus minimizing the dose of anesthetic required to produce caudal anesthesia. Fibrosis of the extradural space from repeated standard epidural blocks is avoided. The disadvantages of the catheter technique include greater cost of equipment, and complications from kinking and curling of the catheter and occlusion of the tip with fibrin. Optimal timing and amounts of repeated anesthetic doses, development of tachyphylaxis (acute tolerance to repeated injections), and augmented responses to long-term effects of repeated caudal epidural anesthesia in horses have not been reported.

CONTINUOUS CAUDAL SUBARACHNOID ANESTHESIA

Continuous caudal subarachnoid analgesia may be induced by repeated injections of local anesthetic solution or alpha-2-adrenoceptor agonists (xylazine, detomidine) given through a catheter introduced into the caudal subarachnoid space with a Tuohy needle (Fig. 16B–22B). The use of continuous caudal subarachnoid anesthesia in practice is limited owing to technical difficulty and potential trauma to the conus medullaris and nerve fibers by the needle or catheter, but it can be accomplished safely in horses while maintaining pelvic limb function with certain advantages when compared to epidural administration: subarachnoid administration of local anesthetics or alpha2-adrenoceptor agonists requires approximately three times less drug for a similar degree of caudal anesthesia, and the onset of

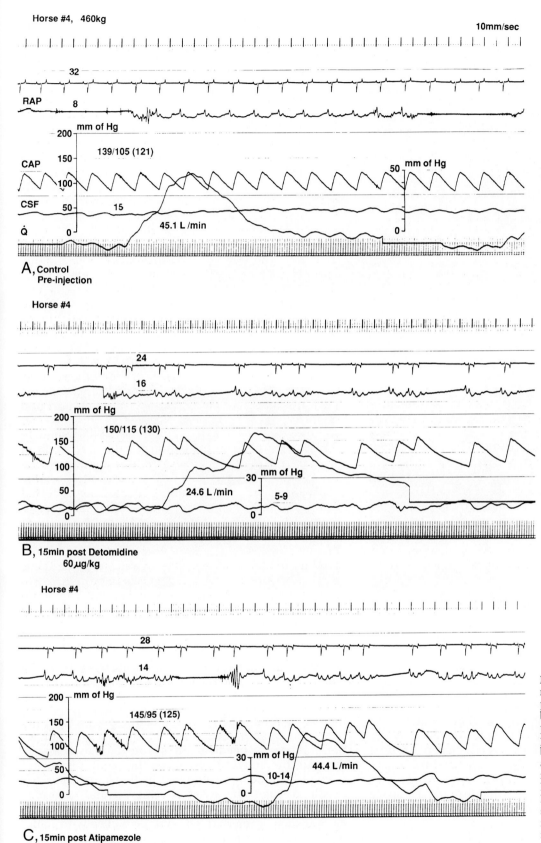

Horse #4, 460kg   10mm/sec

RAP

CAP

CSF

Q̇

A, Control
   Pre-injection

Horse #4

B, 15min post Detomidine
   60 μg/kg

Horse #4

C, 15min post Atipamezole
   120 μg/kg I.V.

Fig. 16B–27. (A), Recording (10 mm/s) of lead II ECG, right atrial pressure (RAP), carotid aterial blood pressure (CAP), spinal fluid pressure (CSF), and cardiac output (Q) (thermodilution curve) before (control) (A), at 15 minutes after caudal (Co1-2) epidural administration of 60 μg detomidine hydrochloride solution/kg (B), diluted to a 10-mL volume, using sterile water, and thereafter at 15 minutes after intravenous administration of 120 μg atipamezole/kg (C).

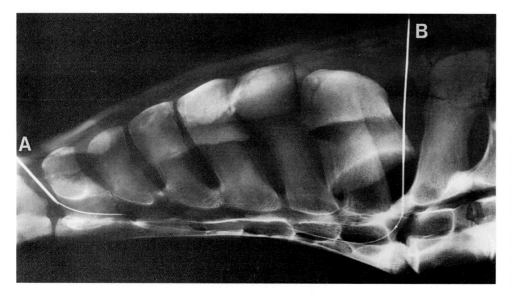

Fig. 16B–28. Lateral radiograph of the sixth lumbar to second coccygeal area. A, 10.2-cm, 18-gauge thin-walled Tuohy needle inserted at the Co1-Co2 interspace to insert a 20-gauge Teflon epidural catheter to the caudal (S5) sacral epidural space. B, 19.5-cm, 17-gauge Huber point Tuohy needle inserted at the lumbosacral (L6-S1) intervertebral space to insert a Formocath polyethylene catheter reinforced with a steel spring guide to the midsacral (S2-S3) epidural space.

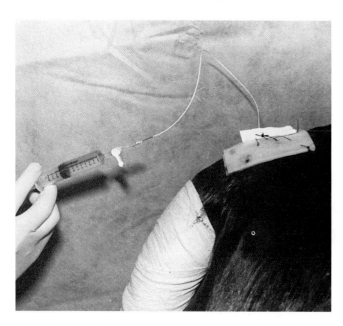

Fig. 16B–29. Epidural catheter is butterfly taped and sutured to the skin. The skin puncture site is covered with a sterile gauze which is also sutured to the skin.

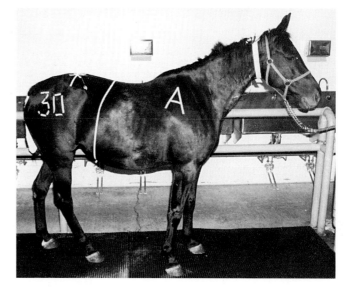

Fig. 16B–30. Desensitized skin area between T16 and coccyx in a horse (460 kg) at 30 minutes after administration of 1.4 mL of 1% detomidine hydrochloride solution into the subarachnoid space of the midsacral (S2-S3) intervertebral space. The subarachnoid catheter is butterfly taped and sutured to the skin at the lumbosacral junction, and is indicated with a white arrow. Sedation was reversed 5 minutes after intravenous administration of 40 µg atipamezole/kg.

anesthesia is twice as fast and the duration of action half as long as after epidural injection.(93)

The roots of the spinal nerves within the subarachnoid space are not covered by protective dural sheets and are more readily desensitized, making caudal subarachnoid analgesia the fastest and best-controlled surgical analgesia in horses. Also, incomplete or asymmetric analgesia due to septa within the epidural space or inadequate dispersal of the anesthetic due to epidural fat are avoided.

A 19.5-cm, 17-gauge Huber point-directional needle with a fitted stylet and with the bevel directed caudally is introduced through disinfected desensitized tissue at the lumbosacral (L6-S1) intervertebral space. Depth of needle penetration ranges from 11 to 14 cm in the adult horse. When the needle point is judged to have passed through the tough interarcuate ligament (ligament flavum), by noticing an abrupt reduction in resistance to needle passage, the stylet is removed and approximately 1 mL of 2% carbocaine hydrochloride solution or its equivalent is injected. The syringe is filled with 2 mL of air and attached to the needle, which is then advanced continuously until a second sudden loss of resistance to injection of air is noted, indicating that the

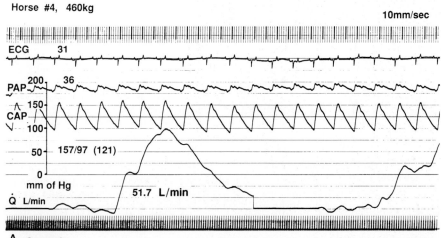

Horse #4, 460kg   10mm/sec

ECG   31

PAP   200   36
CAP   150
      100
       50   157/97 (121)
        0
      mm of Hg
Q L/min   51.7 L/min

A, Control

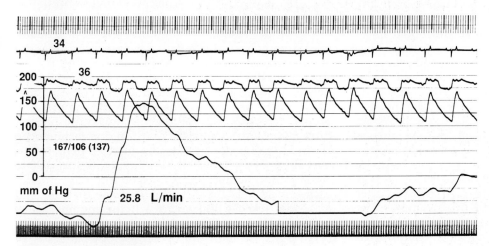

              34
      200   36
      150
      100
       50   167/106 (137)
        0
      mm of Hg   25.8   L/min

B, 10min post Detomidine
        30 µg/kg
        Subarachnoid S 1-2

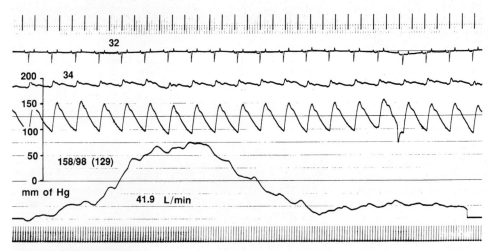

              32
      200   34
      150
      100
       50   158/98 (129)
        0
      mm of Hg   41.9   L/min

C, 10 min post Yohimbine
        50 µg/kg

Fig. 16B–31. Recording (10 mm/s) of lead II ECG, pulmonary artery pressure (PAP), carotid arterial blood pressure (CAP), and cardiac output (Q) (thermodilution curve) before (control) (A), and at 10 minutes after sacral (S1-S2) subarachnoid administration of 30 µg detomidine hydrochloride solution/kg (B), and thereafter at 10 minutes after intravenous administration of 50 µg yohimbine/kg (C).

dura has been penetrated. The subarachnoid space is then identified by free flow of spinal fluid (CSF) from the needle hub or aspiration of CSF. With full aseptic precaution, a 30-cm Formocath polyethylene catheter (0.062-cm outside diameter), reinforced with a stainless steel spring guide, is passed and advanced approximately 25 cm to the midsacral region. The catheter tip cannot be advanced beyond this point, which is usually the end of the subarachnoid space (Fig. 16B–22).

Not more than 1.5 to 2.0 mL of 2% mepivacaine hydrochloride is injected over a 3-minute period (0.5 mL/min) to give excellent bilateral caudal anesthesia from spinal cord segment S2 to coccyx within 5 to 10 minutes. Surgical anesthesia lasts for approximately 0.5 to 1.5 hours and is easily maintained by fractional bolus administration of 0.5 mL of the anesthetic at 30-minute intervals or as needed.(93) A similar pattern of local anesthetic spread (faster absorption of drug from the epidural space and similar maximum venous plasma concentrations after epidural and subarachnoid injections) has been reported in 7 adult mares (420 ± 17 kg) after midsacral epidural (S2-3 to S5-Co1) and subarachnoid (S2-3) administration of mepivacaine hydrochloride in aqueous solution (2%). An average dose of 91.4 ± 15.7 mg (4.6 ± 0.8 mL) mepivacaine HC1 was needed to induce caudal epidural analgesia extending from coccyx to S1 spinal cord segments at 15 to 25 minutes after injection, and analgesia lasted 80.0 ± 11.5 minutes. An average dose of 26.7 ± 5.4 mg (1.3 ± 0.3 mL) of mepivacaine HC1 was needed to induce caudal (coccyx to S1) subarachnoid analgesia at 5 to 10 minutes after injection, and analgesia lasted 67.4 ± 26.3 minutes. The venous plasma concentrations of mepivacaine determined during caudal epidural and subarachnoid analgesia did not produce measurable direct effects on heart rate, arterial blood pressure, pHa, and hematocrit.(94)

Detomidine hydrochloride (1% solution), when administered at a dose of 30 μg/kg into the midsacral subarachnoid space, induces analgesia that extends over dermatomes T15 to the coccyx 10 to 15 minutes after administration, and that lasts over 2 hours, along with minimal ataxia, cardiopulmonary depression, and marked sedation in standing horses.(81) Yohimbine (50 μg/kg BW, IV) or atipamezole (40 μg/kg BW, IV), a recently developed alpha₂-adrenoceptor antagonist, effectively reverses the subarachnoidally administered detomidine-induced sedation (Fig. 16B–30) and partially reverses the detomidine-induced analgesia, ataxia, and cardiopulmonary depression (Fig. 16B–31).(95)

There is likely to be further interest in the advantages obtained by using other adrenoceptor agonists, opioids, and combinations of local anesthetics with adrenoceptor agonists or opioids. An important component of analgesia produced by opiates and alpha₂-adrenoceptor agonists may be an inhibition of the release of neurotransmittors in the dorsal spinal cord (e.g., the tachykinin family of neuropeptides, including substance P [SP] and neurokinin [NKA]), from primary afferent terminals, thus preventing further propagation of nociceptive signals (Chapters 4 and 7). Only preservative free solutions should be administered into the subarachnoid space. Precise dosage (mg, mL, specific gravity) and catheter positioning and aseptic technique are necessary to avoid serious complications such as meningitis, sciatic nerve dysfunction, rear limb ataxia or motor blockade, recumbency, and cardiopulmonary depression or excitement in conscious horses.(96-98)

Anesthesia For Castration

One of the most commonly performed surgical procedures in general equine practice is castration of male horses. Regional anesthesia can be accomplished by injecting local anesthetic drug into the scrotum, testicle (99, 100), and spermatic cord (101, 102) of horses in either standing or laterally recumbent positions. Standing castrations are generally restricted to tractable yearlings and 2-year-olds, and even so it is mandatory to use proper restraint of the horse's head or sedation (e.g., tranquilizer- or sedative-narcotic combination) before surgery. The horse may be placed with its side against a wall and a twitch applied to its upper lip. The person holding the twitch and the operator should stand on the same side. The skin of the scrotum and prepuce are surgically prepared, and one of at least three popular techniques is used: In one technique, a 7.5-cm, 20-gauge needle is quickly inserted perpendicularly through the tensed skin of the scrotum and 20 to 30 mL of local anesthetic is injected into the center of each testicle (Fig. 16B–32). The local anesthetic should make the testicle firm and reach the inguinal canal within 90 seconds via lymph vessels for the blockade to begin.(99) Castration can be carried out painlessly in

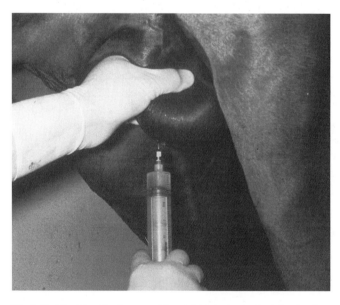

Fig. 16B–32. Needle placement for right intratesticular injection in a standing horse.

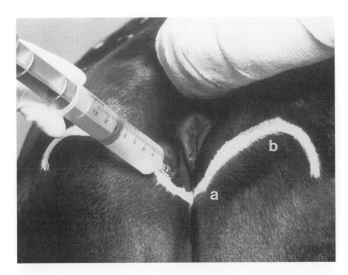

Fig. 16B–33. Topographic anatomy for perineal and pudendal nerve block. The palpable ischiatic arch (a) and ischiatic tuberosity (b) are marked. Infiltration of the left pudendal nerve with local anesthetic is shown. (From Skarda, R. Practical regional anesthesia. In: R.A. Mansmann, E.S. McAllister, and P.W. Pratt, eds. Edited by Equine Medicine, 3rd ed., vol. 1. Santa Barbara, CA: American Veterinary Publications, 1982:246.)

approximately 10 minutes after completion of the injection with no further use of the twitch. In a second method, percutaneous anesthesia of the spermatic cord is accomplished by inserting a 2.5-cm, 20-gauge needle into the cord as close to the external inguinal ring as possible, where 20 to 30 mL of local anesthetic is injected in a fan-shaped manner without perforating the skin, spermatic artery, and vein. The proposed incision line of the scrotal skin must also be infiltrated subcutaneously with 5 to 10 mL of the anesthetic because the scrotal skin is not desensitized after deposition of the anesthetic into the dartos or the substance of the testicle itself. The procedures are repeated to desensitize the opposite spermatic cord and scrotum. Infiltration of the spermatic cord is less effective than intratesticular infiltration for producing local anesthesia for castration. In a third method, a 15-cm, 18-gauge needle is inserted into the testicle and directed into the spermatic cord while 30 mL of the anesthetic are being injected. The incision sites of the scrotal skin are also infiltrated. Damage to the testes is unimportant as they are to be removed. Refractory horses are castrated in recumbent position under general anesthesia.(103)

Anesthesia of the Perineum

Regional anesthesia of the perineum allows perineal surgery, including urethrostomy, in the standing horse. Perineal anesthesia is accomplished by desensitizing the superficial and deep (subfascial) branches of the perineal nerves. These branches arise on both sides of the anus and pass ventrally over the ischial arch to the scrotum. A 2.5-cm, 22-gauge needle is inserted approximately 2.5 cm dorsal to the ischial arch and 2.5 cm lateral

to the anus, to deposit 5 mL of local anesthetic subcutaneously. A deeper subfascial deposit of 5 to 7 mL of the anesthetic is then made after directing the needle dorsally 0.5 to 1.0 cm. The procedure is repeated at the opposite site.(104)

Anesthesia of the Penis or Vulva

The penis or vulva is anesthetized by desensitizing the ventral branches of the pudendal nerve. First the perineal nerves are desensitized as described, then a 5-cm, 20-gauge needle is inserted at the same site as for perineal nerve anesthesia and is advanced toward the midline to strike the ischiatic arch. Approximately 10 to 20 mL of local anesthetic are deposited (Fig. 16B–33).(105) The procedure is repeated at the opposite site.

Therapeutic Local Analgesia

Infiltration of sympathetic nerves by local anesthetic solution effectively interrupts reflex spasm of local vasculature and pain. The two common sites, where the equine sympathetic nervous system is desensitized most effectively, are the cervicothoracic (stellate) gan-

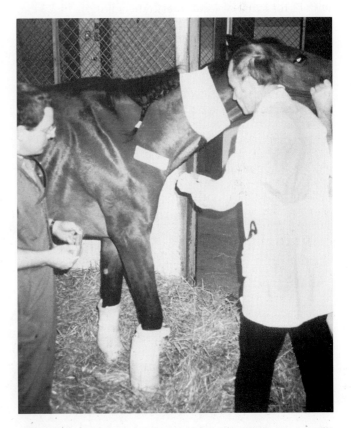

Fig. 16B–34. Restraint of a Thoroughbred mare (520 kg, 7 years old) during infiltration of the right side cervicothoracic ganglion (CTG) with 1 g = 100 mL 1% lidocaine hydrochloride solution. Plasma lidocaine concentrations were 0.5 and 0.35 μg/mL at 30 and 60 minutes after injection. Pain relief from fetlock arthrodesis after comminuted P1 fracture and secondary osteomyelitis was evident by more weight bearing and food uptake for at least 3 days after CTG-blockade.

glion and the paralumbar sympathetic ganglia. Sensory and motor interruption does not result unless the thoracic or lumbar somatic nerves have been desensitized by faulty technique.

CERVICOTHORACIC (STELLATE) GANGLION BLOCK

Infiltration of the cervicothoracic ganglion (CTG) in horses with local anesthetic solution is effective and therapeutically recommended for relief of vasoconstriction and pain in the head, neck, and front leg (Fig. 16B–34). It can be successfully accomplished in horses with a variety of skin, muscle, nerve, and joint and tendon sheath diseases.(106, 107) A single CTG blockade is effective in acute disorders, whereas two or three blockades are required for good results in chronic conditions of idiopathic shoulder lameness, radial nerve paralysis, and eczema of the head and neck.

The CTG is best reached from a cranial and paratracheal approach in a horse bearing equal weight with both thoracic limbs. The skin puncture site is 12 to 17 cm dorsal to the intermediate tubercle of the humerus in the jugular furrow dorsal to the jugular vein and carotid artery. This area is aseptically prepared and infiltrated with 2 to 3 mL of local anesthetic solution. A 25-cm, 16-gauge needle is inserted through the desensitized skin and advanced horizontally or 5° dorsomedially until it impinges on the transverse process or body of the seventh cervical vertebra, and 2 to 3 mL of the anesthetic are injected (Fig. 16B–35A). The depth of needle penetration ranges from 10 to 15 cm, depending upon the size of the musculus longus colli. The needle is first partially withdrawn and then reinserted more lateral and ventral, thereby bypassing the seventh cervical vertebrae and reaching the articulations of the first and second ribs (Fig. 16B–35B). The needle is then 15 to 20 cm from the surface of the skin.(108) After aspiration to be sure that the needle point has not entered a blood vessel, the pleural cavity or subarachnoid space, approximately 50 mL of 1% lidocaine HC1 in aqueous solution are injected with minimal resistance. This amount of anesthetic diffuses throughout the tissues surrounding the CTG. Additional 50 mL of lidocaine are injected during withdrawal of the needle for 5 to 10 cm to desensitize the sympathetic fibers between the CTG and the eighth cervical spinal nerve. Adequate sympathetic blockade is indicated by ipsilateral, increased subcutaneous temperature (up to 3.0° C) and profuse sweating of the head, neck, and thoracic limb; ipsilateral Horner's syndrome (e.g., ptosis, miosis, and enophthalmos) (Fig. 16B–36A); and ipsilateral paresis. These signs are present 10 to 15 minutes after injection and last for more than 75 minutes. Appearance

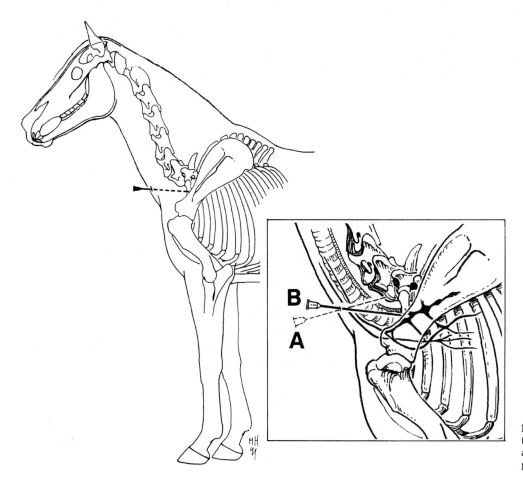

Fig. 16B–35. Needle placement to seventh cervical vertebra (A) and cervicothoracic (stellate) ganglion (left side).

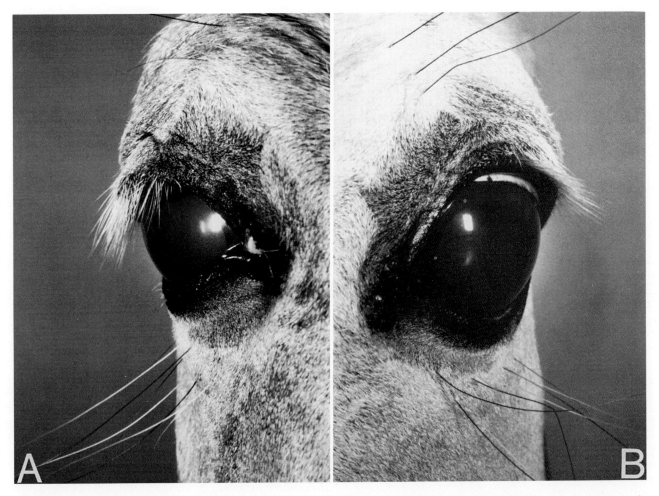

Fig. 16B–36. Horner's syndrome as evidence of sympathetic blockade to the head 15 minutes after infiltration of the right cervicothoracic ganglion with 100 mL 1% lidocaine. A, right eye with ptosis, miosis, and enophthalmos. B, left eye unaffected.

of Horner's syndrome with no increase in subcutaneous temperature of the thoracic limb indicates that the CTG blockade has not been effective and sympathetic nerve supply to the thoracic limb has not been interrupted for therapeutic purposes.

Increased skin temperature is related to increased blood flow (vasodilation) to muscle and cutaneous vascular beds and develops despite the cooling effect of profuse sweating. Factors responsible for sweating include blood supply and, hence, increased heat in the area, higher metabolism in sweat glands, and central stimulation caused by excitement of the horse. Horner's syndrome is caused by the interruption of the oculo-sympathetic pathway at the site of the CTG block and/or at the site of the ventral sympathetic roots between the eighth cervical and second thoracic spinal nerves.

Unilateral CTG blockade minimally changes heart rate, cardiac output, aortic blood pressure, and total peripheral resistance in conscious horses.(109) Maximal plasma concentrations of lidocaine after unilateral CTG blockade in adult horses were 0.4 to 1.3 μg/mL, indicating no toxic blood concentration.(109) Ipsilateral

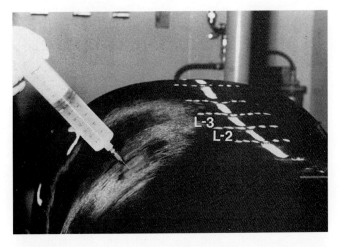

Fig. 16B–37. A 25 cm, 18-gauge needle in place for infiltration of the right lumbar sympathetic ganglia (L2 and L3, second and third lumbar spinous processes; dotted lines, palpable depression between spinous processes). (From Skarda, R. Practical Regional Anesthesia. In: R.A. Mansmann, E.S. McAllister, and P.W. Pratt, eds. Edited by Equine Medicine, 3rd ed., vol. 1. Santa Barbara, CA: American Veterinary Publications, 1982:248.)

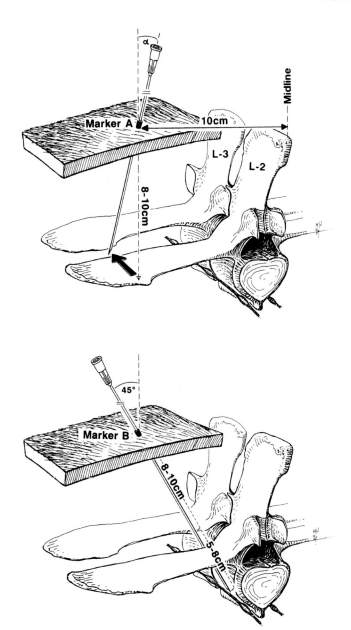

Fig. 16B–38. Needle placement to lumbar sympathetic ganglia. Marker A, needle tip at the L2 to L3 intertransverse space and marker B, right ganglionic chain.

laryngeal paralysis, decreased respiratory rates, and increased Pa_{CO_2} are indicative of vagal inhibition. However, induced hypoventilation in resting horses is not severe enough to induce significant respiratory acidosis or hypoxemia. Potential serious complications are transitory brachial plexus and recurrent laryngeal nerve paralysis and pneumothorax. Bilateral CTG blockade is contraindicated in horses.

PARAVERTEBRAL LUMBAR SYMPATHETIC GANGLION BLOCK

Infiltration of the lumbar sympathetic ganglia in horses with local anesthetic solution has been demonstrated as a therapeutic measure for myositis, periostitis, coxitis,

and paralysis of the fibular and penile nerves.(106, 107) Although any of the interspaces between the eighteenth thoracic and fourth lumbar vertebrae may be used as possible sites to reach the lumbar sympathetic ganglia, the ideal puncture site is between the transverse processes of the second and third lumbar (L2 and L3) vertebrae about 10 to 15 cm lateral to their spinous processes (Fig. 16B–37). This area is aseptically prepared and infiltrated with 2 to 3 mL of local anesthetic. A 25-cm, 18-gauge needle with a marker on the needle shaft is inserted through the desensitized skin and advanced until its tip contacts the transverse process of L2 or L3. The marker is used to note the depth of penetration (Fig. 16B–38A). The needle is partially withdrawn to the subcutaneous area and inserted at angle alpha and approximately 45° from vertical for a calculated distance, which equals the distance between the marker (skin puncture) and the needle point plus an additional 5 to 8 cm (Fig. 16B–38B). The needle is correctly placed if there is no air from the peritoneal cavity or blood from a blood vessel upon needle aspiration and no resistance to the injection of local anesthetic results. Approximately 100 mL of 1% lidocaine HC1 solution are slowly injected. This amount of anesthetic diffuses throughout the tissues surrounding the sympathetic trunk and two segments rostrally and caudally. Adequate sympathetic blockade is recognized by profuse sweating and increased (up to 2.5° C) subcutaneous temperature of the ipsilateral pelvic limb within 10 minutes after injection. Nonsedated horses tolerate unilateral lumbar sympathetic ganglionic blockade (ULSG-block) well. Hemodynamic and respiratory alterations induced by unilateral ULSG-blockade in horses are usually minor.(110) Potential complications include puncture of blood vessels resulting in hematoma, intravascular injection, abdominocentesis, and needle breakage.

References

1. Skarda RT. Local anesthetics and local anesthetic techniques in horses. In Muir WW, Hubbell JAE, eds. Equine anesthesia, monitoring and emergency therapy. St. Louis: CV Mosby, 1991: 215.
2. Hall LW. Wright's veterinary anaesthesia and analgesia, 7th ed. London: Balliere Tindall, 1971.
3. Skarda RT. Practical regional anesthesia. In: Mansmann RA, McAllister ES, Pratt PW, eds. Equine medicine and surgery, 3rd ed., vol. 1. Santa Barbara, CA: American Veterinary Publications, 1982: 229–238.
4. Wittman F, Morgenroth H. Untersuchungen über die Leitungsanästhesie des Nervus infraorbitalis und des Nervus mandibularis bei Zahn- und Kieferoperationen. Festschrift für Eugen Fröhner. Stuttgart; Verlag Von Ferdinand Enke, 1928: 384–399.
5. Bressou C, Cliza S. Contribution à l étude de l'anesthésie dentaire chez le cheval et chez le chien. Rec Med Vet 107:129–134, 1931.
6. Lichtenstern G. Die Verwendung von Tropakokain in der tierärztlichen Chirurgie mit besonderer Berücksichtigung hinsichtlich seiner Verwendbarkeit in der Augapfelinfiltration beim Pferde. Berl Münch Tierzärtl Wochenschr 55:337–359, 1911.
7. Skarda RT. Practical regional anesthesia. In Mansmann RA, McAllister ES, and Pratt PW, eds. Equine medicine, 3rd ed., vol. 1. Santa Barbara, CA; American Veterinary Publications, 1982: 239–245.

8. Bolz W. Ein weiterer Beitrag zur Leitungsanästhesie am Kopf des Pferdes. Berl Münch Tierzärtl Wochenschr 46:529–530, 1930.

9. Manning JP, and St. Clair LE. Palpebral frontal and zygomatic nerve blocks for examination of the equine eye. Vet Med 71:187–189, 1976.

10. Merideth RE, Wolf ED. Ophthalmic examination and therapeutic techniques in the horse. Compend Contin Educ 3(11):S426–433, 1981.

11. Rubin LF. Auriculopalpebral nerve block as an adjunct to the diagnosis and treatment of ocular inflammation in the horse. J Am Vet Med Assoc 144:1387–1388, 1964.

12. Lindsay WA, Hedberg EB. Performing facial nerve blocks, nasolacrimal catheterization, and paranasal sinus centesis in horses. Vet Med 86(1): 72–83, 1991.

13. Eeckhout AVP. Un procédé pratique pour obtenir l'anesthésie complète des dents molaires supérieures chez le cheval. Ann Med Vet 66:10–14, 1921.

14. Edwards JF. Regional anaesthesia of the head of the horse: an up-to-date survey. Vet Rec 10:873–975, 1930.

15. Schönberg F. Anatomische Grundlagen für die Leitungsanästhesie der Zahnnerven beim Pferde, Berl Münch Tierärztl Wochenschr 43:1–3, 1927.

16. Adams OR. Lameness in Horses, 3rd ed., Philadelphia: Lea & Febiger, 1974: 91–112.

17. Pohlmeyer K, Redecker R. Die für die Klinik bedeutsamen Nerven an den Gliedmassen des Pferdes einschliesslich möglicher Varianten. Dtsch Tierärztl Wochenschr 81:501–505, 537–541, 1974.

18. Zeller R. Die Lokalanästhesie bei der Lahmheitsuntersuchung, Berl Münch Tierärztl Wochenschr 91:166–171, 1978.

19. Derksen FJ. Diagnostic local anesthesia of the equine front limb. Equine Pract 2:41–47, 1980.

20. Gray BW, Engel HN, Rumph PF, et al. Clinical approach to determine the contribution of the palmar and palmar metacarpal nerves to the innervation of the equine fetlock joint. Am J Vet Res 41:940–943, 1980.

21. Wheat JD and Jones K. Selected techniques of regional anesthesia. Vet Clin North Am Large Anim Pract 3(1):223–246, 1981.

22. Worthman RP. Diagnostic anesthetic injections. In Mansmann RA, McAllister ES, and Pratt PW, eds. Equine medicine and surgery, 3rd ed. Santa Barbara, CA: American Veterinary Publications, 1982: 947–952.

23. Nyrop KA, Coffman JR, DeBowes RM, et al. The role of diagnostic nerve blocks in the equine lameness examination. Compend Contin Educ 5(12):669–676, 1983.

24. Colbern GT. The use of diagnostic nerve block procedures on horses. Compend Contin Educ 6(10):611–619, 1984.

25. Ordidge RM, Gerring EL. Regional analgesia of the distal limb. Equine Vet J 16(2):147–149, 1984.

26. Stashak TS. Diagnosis of lameness. In Stashak TS, ed. Adams' lameness in horses, Philadelphia: Lea & Febiger, 1986: 139–142, 659–661.

27. Gibson KT, Stashak TS. Effective techniques for localizing equine lameness. Vet Med 84(10):992–996, 1989.

28. Gibson KT, Stashak TS. Using perineural anesthesia to localize equine lameness. Vet Med 84(11):1082–1086, 1989.

29. Ford TS, Ross MW, Orsini PG. A comparison of methods for proximal palmar metacarpal analgesia in horses. Vet Surg 18(2):146–150, 1989.

30. Gaynor JS, Hubbell JAE. Perineural and spinal anesthesia. Vet Clin North Am Equine Pract 7(3):518, 1991.

31. Denoix MJM. Anesthésies semiologiques des régions proximales des membres. Swiss Vet 8(11a):12–22, 1991.

32. Van Pelt RW. Intra-articular injection of the equine carpus and fetlock. J Am Vet Med Assoc 140:1181–1190, 1962.

33. Tufvesson G. Local anaesthesia in veterinary medicine. Sodertalje, Sweden: Astra International, 1963.

34. Van Kruiningen HJ. Practical techniques for making injections into joints and bursae of the horse. J Am Vet Med Assoc 143:1079–1083, 1963.

35. Brown MP, Valko K. A technique for intra-articular injection of the equine tarso-metatarsal joint. Vet Med Small Anim Clin 75(2):265–270, 1980.

36. Gabel AA. Lameness caused by inflammation in the distal hock. Vet Clin North Am Large Anim Pract 2(1):101–123, 1980.

37. Lindsay WA, Tayler SD, Walters JW. Selective intra-articular anesthesia as an aid in the diagnosis of bone spavin. J Am Vet Med Assoc 178:297–300, 1981.

38. Wintzer HJ. Pharmacokinetics of procaine injected into the hock joint of the horse. Equine Vet J 13:68–69, 1981.

39. Sack WO, Orsini PG. Distal intertarsal and tarsometatarsal joints in the horse. Communication and injection sites. J Am Vet Med Assoc 179:355–359, 1981.

40. Byars TD, Brown C, Beisel D. Equine arthrocentesis. Equine Pract 4:28–39, 1982.

41. Gibson KT, Stashak TS. Employing intra-articular anesthesia to detect joint lesions in lame horses. Vet Med 84(11):1088–1092, 1989.

42. Moyer W. A guide to equine joint injection. Lawrenceville, NJ: Solvay Veterinary, Vet Learning Systems Co., 1986: 1–32.

43. Belling TH. A better approach to intracarpal injections. Vet Med 81(2):158–165, 1986.

44. Dyson S. Diagnostic technique in the investigation of shoulder lameness. Equine Vet J 18:25–28, 1986.

45. Dyson S. Problems associated with the interpretation of results of regional and intra-articular anaesthesia in the horse. Vet Rec 12:419–422, 1986.

46. Kiely RG, McMullan W. Lateral arthrocentesis of the equine carpus. Equine Pract 9:22–24, 1987.

47. Schmotzer WB, Trimm KI. Local anesthetic techniques for diagnosis of lameness. Vet Clin North Am Equine Pract 6(3):705, 1990.

48. Gabel AA. Diagnosis, relative incidence, and probable cause of cunean tendon bursitis-tarsitis of standardbred horses. J Am Vet Med Assoc 175:1079–1085, 1979.

49. Gabel AA. Treatment and prognosis for cunean tendon bursitis-tarsitis of standardbred horses. J Am Vet Med Assoc 175:1086–1088, 1979.

50. Lloyd KCK, Stover JM, Pascoe JR. A technique for catheterization of the equine antebrachiocarpal joint. Am J Vet Res 49:658–662, 1988.

51. Ford TS, Ross MW, Orsini PG. Communication and boundaries of the middle carpal and carpometacarpal joints in horses. Am J Vet Res 49:2161–2164, 1988.

52. Day TK, Skarda RT. The pharmacology of local anesthetics. Vet Clin North Am Equine Pract 7(3):498, 1991.

53. Rijkenhuizen ABM. Complications following the diagnostic anesthesia of the coffin joint in horses. In: Proceedings, 15th European Society of Vet Surg Congress. Bern, Switzerland: Klinik für Nutztiere und Pferde, 1984: 7–13.

54. Heavner JE. Local anesthetics. Vet Clin North Am Large Anim Pract 3:209–211, 1991.

55. Tillmann H. Zur Leitungsanästhesie bei Laparotomien am Pferd. Tierärztl Umschau 4:302–303, 1949.

56. Goncalves AP. Anesthesia paravertebral lombar no cavalo (Equus caballus) [dissertation]. Niteroi, Rio de Janeiro, Brazil, Faculdade de Veterinaria, Universidade Federal Fluminense, 1977.

57. Moon PF, Suter CM. Paravertebral thoracolumbar anaesthesia in 10 horses. Equine Vet J 25(4):304–308, 1993.

58. Skarda RT, Muir WW. Segmental epidural and subarachnoid analgesia in horses: a comparative study. Am Vet Res 44:1870–1876, 1983.

59. Skarda RT, Muir WW. Segmental thoracolumbar spinal (subarachnoid) analgesia in conscious horses. Am Vet Res 43:2121–2128, 1982.

60. Skarda RT, Muir WW, Ibrahim AL. Spinal fluid concentrations of mepivacaine in horses and procaine in cows after thoracolumbar subarachnoid analgesia. Am J Vet Res 46:1020–1024, 1985.

61. Hopkins GS. The correlation of anatomy and epidural analgesia in domestic animals. Cornell Vet 25:263–270, 1935.

62. Skarda RT. Local and regional analgesia. In: Short CE, ed. Principles and practice of veterinary anesthesia. Baltimore: Williams & Wilkins, 1987: 105.

63. Skarda RT. Local anesthetics and local anesthetic techniques in horses. In: Muir WW, Hubbell JAE, eds. Equine anesthesia, monitoring and emergency therapy. St. Louis: CV Mosby, 1991: 234.

64. Pape J, Pitzschk C. Versuche über extradurale Anästhesie beim Pferde. Arch Wiss Prakt Tierheilkd 52:558–571, 1925.
65. McLeod WM, Frank ER. A preliminary report regarding epidural anesthesia in equines and bovines. J Am Vet Med Assoc 72:327–335, 1927.
66. Cuillé J, Chelle P. L'anesthésie épidural chez les animaux domestiques. (Epidural anaesthesia in the domestic animal.) Rev Gen Med Vet 40:393–445, 1931.
67. Srnetz A. Ueber Lokalanästhesie mit Percain beim Pferde. Prager Arch Tiermed Vergl Pathol 11:207–211, 1931.
68. Brook GB. Spinal (epidural) anaesthesia in the domestic animals. Vet Rec 15:549–608, 1935.
69. Krukowski SM. Epidural anesthesia in the cow and horse. Vet Med (Chicago) 30:252–253, 1935.
70. Benesch F. Die Schmerzbetäubung in der Geburtshilfe und Gynäkologie der Haustiere. 13th World Vet Congress, Switzerland: Zürich-Interlaken, I:377–385, 1938.
71. Brown TG. Discussion. In: Anaesthesia in veterinary practice. Vet Rec 50:1617, 1938.
72. Byrne MJ. Epidural anaesthesia. In: Anaesthesia in veterinary practice. Vet Rec 50:1614, 1938.
73. Barone R, Chayer R. Essais d'interprétation anatomique des anesthésies rachidiennes (épidurales et sous-durales) chez le cheval et le boeuf. Rév Med Vet 101:27–43, 1950.
74. Heinze CD. Equine surgery: variations in technique: epidural anesthesia. Mod Vet Pract 49:39, 1968.
75. Heath EH, Myers VS. Topographic anatomy for caudal epidural anesthesia in the horse. Vet Med Small Anim Clin 67:1237–1239, 1972.
76. Slusher SH. Caudal epidural anesthesia in horses, Vet Med Small Anim Clin 76:1773–1775, 1981.
77. Greene SA, Thurmon JC. Epidural analgesia and sedation for selected equine surgeries. Equine Pract 7:14–19, 1985.
78. LeBlanc PH, Caron JP, Patterson JS, et al. Epidural injection of xylazine for perineal analgesia in horses. J Am Vet Med Assoc 193:1405–1408, 1988.
79. Fikes LW, Lin HC, Thurmon JC. A preliminary comparison of lidocaine and xylazine as epidural analgesics in ponies. Vet Surg 18(1):85–86, 1989.
80. Grubb TL, Riebold TW, and Huber MJ. Comparison of lidocaine, xylazine, and xylazine/lidocaine for caudal epidural analgesia in horses. J Am Vet Med Assoc 201:1187–1190, 1992.
81. Skarda RT, Muir WW. Caudal analgesia induced by epidural or subarachnoid administration of detomidine hydrochloride solution in mares. Am J Vet Res 55:670–680, 1994.
82. Le Blanc PH, Caron JP. Clinical use of epidural xylazine in the horse. Equine Vet J 22:180–181, 1990.
83. LeBlanc PH, Eberhart SW. Cardiopulmonary effects of epidurally administered xylazine in the horse. Equine Vet J 22:389–391, 1990.
84. Skarda RT, Muir WW. Cardiovascular effects of caudal epidurally administered xylazine or detomidine hydrochloride solution in mares: a comparative study [abstract]. In: Proc 5th Int Cong Vet Anesth, Guelph, Canada, 1994.
85. Skarda RT, Muir WW, Carpenter JA. Antagonistic effects of atipamezole on epidurally administered detomidine-induced sedation, analgesia, and cardiopulmonary depression in horses [abstract]. Proc Annu Sci Mtg Am Coll Vet Anesthesiol, Las Vegas, October 1990:9.
86. Skarda RT, Muir WW. Physiologic responses after caudal epidural administration of detomidine in horses and xylazine in cattle. In: Short CE, Poznak AV eds., (Animal pain.) New York: Churchill Livingstone, 1992: 292–302.
87. Schelling CG, Klein LV. Comparison of carbonated lidocaine and lidocaine hydrochloride for caudal epidural anesthesia in horses. Am J Vet Res 46:1375–1377, 1985.
88. Colter SB. Electromyographic detection and evaluation of tail alterations in show ring horses. Proc 6th Ann Vet Med Forum ACVIM 1988:421–423.
89. Valverde A, Little ChB, Dyson DH. Use of epidural morphine to relieve pain in a horse. Can Vet J 31:211–212, 1990.
90. Robinson EP, Moncada-Suiarez JR, Felice L. Epidural morphine analgesia in horses. Proc Annu Mtg Am Coll Vet Anesthesiol, Washington, DC, 1993:22.
91. Farny J, Blais D, Vaillancourt D, et al: Caudal epidural anesthesia with butorphanol in the mare. Proc 4th Intern Cong Vet Anaesth, Utrecht, The Netherlands, 1991:32.
92. Greene EM, Cooper RC. Continuous caudal epidural anesthesia in the horse. J Am Vet Med Assoc 184:971–974, 1984.
93. Skarda RT, Muir WW. Continuous caudal epidural and subarachnoid anesthesia in mares: a comparative study. Am Vet Res 44:2290–2298, 1983.
94. Skarda RT, Muir WW, Ibrahim AL. Plasma mepivacaine concentrations after caudal epidural and subarachnoid injection in the horse: comparative study. Am J Vet Res 45:1967–1971, 1984.
95. Skarda RT, Muir WW, Doerres-Phillips AJ. Antagonistic effects of atipamezole on subarachnoidally administered detomidine-induced sedation, analgesia, and cardiopulmonary depression in horses [abstract]. Proc 4th Intern Cong Vet Anaesth, Utrecht, The Netherlands, 1991:15.
96. Cuillé J, Sendrail M. Analgésie cocainique par voie rachidienne. Rev Vét 26:98–103, 1901.
97. Mettam AE. Surgical anaesthesia by the injection of cocaine into the lumbar subarachnoid space. Veterinarian (London) 74:115–121, 1901.
98. Saccani R. Cocainizzazione del midollo spinale negli animali domestici. Nuovo Ercolani 11:272–274, 1901.
99. Sarparanta L. Die Anwendung der Lokalbetäubung bei den Kastrationen, Finnish Vet 33:59–61, 1927.
100. Rieger H. Die testikuläre Injektion, Berl Munch Tierarztl Wochenschr 67:107–109, 1954.
101. Matyschtschuk J. Beitrag zur Kastration am stehenden Pferd. Wien Tierärztl Wochenschr 36:378–391, 1949.
102. Reed WD. Standing castration. Proc 14th Annu Mtg Am Assoc Equine Pract, Philadelphia, PA, 1968:239–240.
103. Wriedt WD, Schebitz H, and Böhm D. Zur Kastration des Hengstes. Berl Münch Tierärztl Wochenschr 92:41–42, 1979.
104. Magda JJ. Local anesthesia in operations on the male perineum in horses. Veterinariya 25:34–36, 1948.
105. Magda JJ. Leitungsanästhesie des Pferdepenis. Soviet Vet 16:96–98, 1940.
106. Dietz O. Zur Grenzstrangblockade beim Tier. Arch Exp Veterinarmed 11:310–330, 349–385, 1958.
107. Heidrich HD, Nöldner H. Ueber die Anwendung der Grenzstrang bzw. Stellatumblockade beim Pferd. Mh Vet Med 18:58–61, 1963.
108. Skarda RT, Muir WW, Swanson CR, et al. Cervicothoracic (stellate) ganglion block in conscious horses. Am J Vet Res 47(1):21–26, 1986.
109. Skarda RT, Muir WW, Couri D. Plasma lidocaine concentrations in conscious horses after cervicothoracic (stellate) ganglion block with 1% lidocaine HC1 solution. Am J Vet Res 48:1092–1097, 1987.
110. Skarda RT, Muir WW, Hubbell JA. Paravertebral lumbar sympathetic ganglion block in the horse. Proc 2nd Int Cong Vet Anesth. Sacramento, CA: Veterinary Practice Publishing Co. 1985:160.

LOCAL AND REGIONAL ANESTHETIC TECHNIQUES: RUMINANTS AND SWINE

Introduction

Local or regional analgesia is a preferred method in food animals owing to accepted practice and economic necessity. Many surgical procedures are performed safely and humanely using a combination of physical restraint, mild sedation or tranquilization, and local or regional anesthesia. The techniques should provide reversible loss of pain to a limited body area with minimal effects on the rest of the body. The standing position is optimal for a number of surgical procedures of ruminants, as it reduces the problems associated with bloat, salivation, recumbency-related regurgitation, and nerve or muscle damage (Chapter 20).(1-4)

Local or infiltration analgesia is achieved by injecting a local anesthetic solution into the tissues at a surgical site, whereas regional analgesia is induced after perineural injection of major nerves. The most commonly used techniques in ruminants are surface (topical) anesthesia, infiltration anesthesia, nerve block (conduction) anesthesia, epidural anesthesia, and intravenous regional anesthesia. Although local anesthetic drugs are routinely used, none has presently been approved by the Food and Drug Administration (FDA) for use in lactating dairy cows. Epidural morphine is safe and effective, and provides an alternative approach for treatment of pain after hind-limb orthopedic surgery.

Infiltration anesthesia, lumbosacral epidural anesthesia, and intratesticular injection are the most popular local anesthetic techniques in properly tranquilized pigs. The advantages of regional analgesia over general anesthesia include the need for minimal apparatus (e.g., syringe, needles, and drug) and little risk of toxic side effects. Several factors must be considered in the choice of a technique: (5)

1. The site, nature, and expected duration of surgery.
2. The species, temperament, and health of the patient.
3. Special requirements (such as minimum fetal depression during cesarean section).
4. The skill and experience of the veterinarian.
5. The economics of time and materials.

Local Anesthetics

A variety of local or regional anesthetic drugs can penetrate peripheral nerve barriers and provide reversible anesthesia with acceptable onset times and predictable duration.(6-8) The drugs vary as to the potency, toxicity, and cost, and none has been approved by the Food and Drug Administration (FDA) for use in lactating dairy cows, although such agents are commonly used (Table 16C–1). Lidocaine hydrochloride solution has become the single agent of choice because of its intermediate anesthetic duration of 90 to 180 minutes and the cost restrictions and limited space in a mobile practice vehicle.

The addition of a vasoconstrictor, such as epinephrine at concentrations of 5 to 20 µg per mL (1:200,000 to 1:50,000), is occasionally incorporated or can be added to the commercial local anesthetic solution to increase intensity, prolong anesthetic activity, and reduce the potential for toxicity.(9) These concentrations may be obtained by adding 0.1 mL of 1:1,000 (0.1 mg) epinephrine to 5 mL (1:50,000) and 20 mL (1:200,000) of local anesthetic solution. The use of local anesthetic drugs containing a vasoconstrictor often causes tissue necrosis along wound edges, especially in thin-skinned animals.

Adding hyaluronidase to lidocaine at a rate of 150 turbidity reducing units (TRUs) per 25 mL will hasten the time of onset of infiltration anesthesia and shorten duration of anesthesia owing to increased permeability of the tissues.(10) The necessity for its use, other than in combination with procaine hydrochloride solution (1%) has been questioned since the development of newer local anesthetics with improved spreading power. The

enzyme allows smaller volume of local anesthetic solutions to be used. The combination of local anesthetics, epinephrine, and hyaluronidase produces prolonged anesthesia due to reduced uptake while maintaining the spreading action of hyaluronidase combined with local anesthetics.(11) Accuracy in technique is still necessary because tissue fascial planes act as barriers. The greatest use of hyaluronidase is in ophthalmology (retrobulbar blocks) and local anesthetic nerve blocks for postoperative pain relief.

Regional Anesthesia of the Head

The most frequently desensitized nerves of the head are the auriculopalpebral, supraorbital, zygomaticotemporal (lacrimal), infraorbital, oculomotor, abducens, and trochlear nerve. Many of these nerves are maxillary and ophthalmic branches of the trigeminal (fifth) cranial nerve.

ANESTHESIA OF THE EYE AND RELAXATION OF THE GLOBE

The neuroanatomy of ocular structures is complex. The globe, conjunctiva, nictitans, and most of the eyelids are supplied by sensory fibers of the ophthalmic division of the trigeminal nerve. The extraocular muscles are supplied by motor fibers of the trochlear nerve (superficial oblique muscle), the abducens nerve (lateralis rectus and retractor oculi muscles), and the oculomotor nerve. The oculomotor, trochlear, ophthalmic and maxillary branches of the trigeminal and abducens nerves emerge from the foramen rotundum orbitale.

At present, topical and regional anesthetics are used to facilitate surgery of the eye and its associated structures. The eyelids (without anesthesia) are selectively paralyzed by desensitizing the auriculopalpebral branch of the facial nerve (akinesia). Anesthesia of the eye and orbit and immobilization of the globe are commonly achieved by retrobulbar injection of a local anesthetic or the Petersen technique (or its modification).(12)

For topical anesthesia, one or two drops of proparacaine hydrochloride (0.5%) solution are instilled in the eye. Pain associated with corneal disease is relieved in 30 seconds and for as long as 10 to 15 minutes.(13) In addition, blepharospasm due to superficial irritation of the cornea is relieved, so examination of the eye or minor surgery is greatly facilitated. The FDA has approved the use of proparacaine in food animals to induce topical anesthesia for cauterization of corneal ulcers, removal of foreign bodies and suture from the cornea, and measurements of intraocular pressure (tonometry) when glaucoma is suspected. Other ophthalmic anesthetic solution, such as xylocaine hydrochloride (4%) or tetracaine hydrochloride, is toxic to the corneal epithelium, suppressing mitosis and reducing protective blink reflexes, and should not be used for treatment of the eye.(14)

ANESTHESIA AND AKINESIA OF THE EYELIDS

The site for producing a linear subcutaneous infiltration (line block) is about 0.5 cm from the margin of the dorsal

Table 16C–1. Local Analgesics

Agent (Generic Name)	Trade Name	Chemical Name	Potency (Procaine = 1)	Toxicity (Procaine = 1)	Dosage	Stability	Comments
Procaine	Novocaine (Winthrop Sterns Inc., New York, NY)	Para-aminobenzoic acid ester of diethylaminoethanol	1:1	1:1	1–2% for infiltration and nerve block	Aqueous solutions are heat resistant, decomposed by bacteria	Hydrolyzed by liver and plasma esterase
Chloroprocaine	Nesacaine, (Astra Pharmaceutical Products Inc., Westboro, MA)	Para-amino-2-chlorobenzoic acid ester of B-diethyl amino ethanol	2.4:1	0.5:1	1–2% for infiltration and nerve block	Multiple autoclaving accelerates hydrolysis and impairs potency	Immediate onset of action; 2-h duration with epinephrine
Lidocaine	Xylocaine (Astra Pharmaceutical Products, Inc., Westboro, MA)	Diethylaminoacet-2,6-xylidide	2:1	0.5%, 1:1; 1%, 14:1; 2%, 1.5:1	0.5–2% for infiltration and nerve block; topically, 2–4%	Aqueous solutions are thermostable, multiple autoclaving possible	Excellent penetrability; rate of onset twice as fast as procaine; 2-h duration with epinephrine
Mepivacaine	Carbocaine (Winthrop Laboratories, New York, NY)	1-Methyl-2',6'-pipecoloxylidide monohydrochloride	2.5:1	Less toxic than lidocaine	1–2% for infiltration and nerve block	Resistant to acid and alkaline hydrolysis, multiple autoclaving possible	Absence of vasodilator effect makes addition of a vasoconstrictor unnecessary
Tetracaine	Pontocaine (Winthrop Laboratories, New York, NY)	Parabutyl amino benzoyl-dimethyl-amino-ethanol-HCl	12:1	10:1	0.1% for infiltration and nerve block; topically, 0.2%	Crystals and solutions should not be autoclaved	Slow onset of analgesia (5–10 min); 2-h duration; for eye instalation
Hexylcaine	Cyclaine (Merck, Sharpe and Dohme, West Point, PA)	1-Cyclo-hexamino 2-propylbenzoate	1–2:1	2–4:1	0.5–1% for infiltration; 2% for nerve block; 5% topically	Crystals and solutions are thermostable	Recommended for epidural and topical analgesia
Dibucaine	Nupercaine (CIBA Pharmaceutical Products, Summit, NJ)	α-Butyl-oxycinchoninic acid of diethylethylene-diamide	20:1	15:1	Topically, 0.1%	Thermostable but precipitation by alkalies	Slowly detoxified
Bupivacaine	Marcaine (Breon Laboratories Inc., New York, NY)	1-Butyl-2',6 pipecoloxylidide-HCl	8:1	Greater margin of safety than lidocaine	0.25% for infiltration; 0.5% for nerve block; 0.75% for epidural block	Stable compound	Intermediate onset, lasting 4–6 hrs

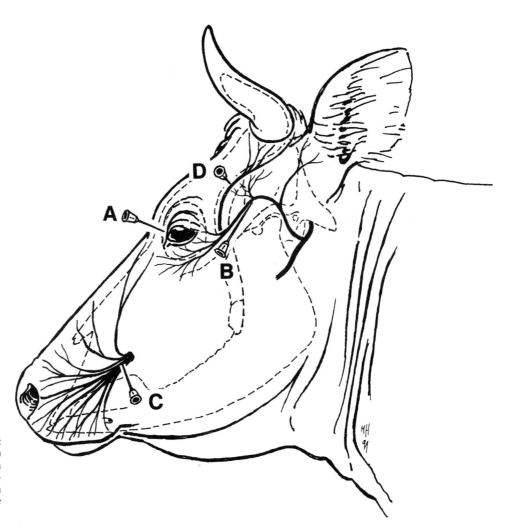

Fig. 16C–1. Needle placement for infiltration of the eyelids (A) and nerve blocks on the head in cattle: auriculopalpebral (B), infraorbital (C), and cornual branch of the zygomaticotemporal nerve (D).

and ventral eyelids in adult cattle. Approximately 10 mL of a 2% lidocaine hydrochloride solution are administered at multiple sites, 0.5 cm apart, using a 2.5-cm, 22- or 25-gauge needle (Fig. 16C–1A).

Paralysis of the eyelids (without analgesia) is commonly performed in cattle by selectively desensitizing the auriculopalpebral branch of the facial nerve (akinesia).(15) The nerve is sometimes palpable in a notch on the zygomatic arch, anterior to the base of the auricular muscles, where a 2.5-cm, 18-or 20-gauge needle is placed subcutaneously and 5 to 10 mL of the anesthetic is deposited (Fig. 16C–1B). The combination of topical anesthesia and auriculopalpebral akinesia is useful for removing foreign bodies from the cornea and conjunctival sac and for injecting medication into the bulbar subconjunctiva.

ANESTHESIA FOR ENUCLEATION

In doing a retrobulbar block for enucleation or to facilitate surgery and radiation therapy in cattle with squamous cell carcinoma at the cornea, a 15-cm, 18-gauge needle with a fairly large bend (approximately 25 cm diameter) is used in adult cattle. Head restraint

with a halter or nose grip is necessary. In small ruminants, a 3.75-cm, 22-gauge needle may be used.

The sites for lid penetration are at the superior, inferior, medial, or lateral orbital rim. The surgeon's index finger is used to deflect the globe and protect it from the needle point (Fig. 16C–2A). When using the medial canthus approach, the medial wall of the bony orbit is felt. The needle is then inserted in the fornix of the conjunctiva cranial to the nictitans dorsomedial to the operator's finger until the orbital apex is encountered (Fig. 16C–2B). Approximately 15 mL of a 2% lidocaine hydrochloride solution or equivalent are injected in small increments as the needle is advanced, thereby pushing initial structures from the needle point. Once the entire block is completed, the structures that will be desensitized include the optic nerve, the elevator palpebral muscles, the medial rectus, the dorsal rectus, the ventral rectus, and the inferior oblique muscle (all innervated by the oculomotor nerve), the superior oblique muscle (innervated by the fourth cranial nerve), the sensory part of the eye and adnexa (innervated by the fifth cranial nerve), the retractor oculi muscles, and lateral rectus muscle (innervated by the sixth cranial

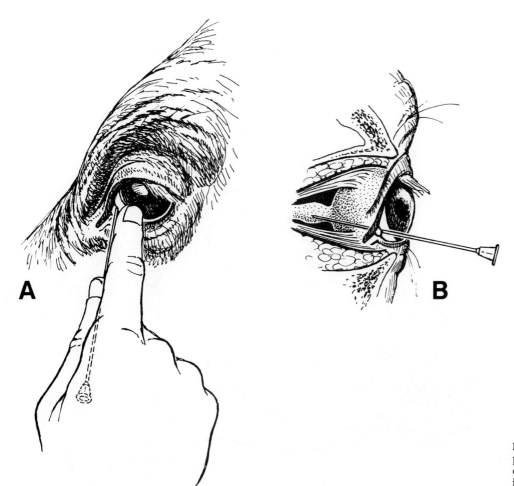

Fig. 16C–2. Retrobulbar needle placement through the medial canthus (A) to the orbital apex (B) in cattle.

nerve) and the orbicularis oculi muscles (innervated by the seventh cranial nerve) (Chapter 7). A satisfactory retrobulbar nerve block should then accomplish anesthesia for whatever procedure would be desired for the eye and eyelids and will allow for proptosing the eye for surgery on the cornea, enucleation, or exceneration (Chapter 24).

Adverse effects that may result from retrobulbar injections include orbital hemorrhage, direct pressure on the globe, penetration of the globe, damage to the optic nerve, initiation of the oculocardiac reflex, and injection into the optic nerve meninges. Damages to the globe may be serious for procedures other than enucleation. If the optic nerve or optic foramen is penetrated and local anesthetic is injected beneath the meningeal covering, epidural or subarachnoid anesthesia of the brain may result, which can be fatal. Risk of subarachnoid (CSF) injection is minimized by aspiration check.

In performing the Peterson block, the notch formed by the supraorbital process cranially, the zygomatic arch ventrally, and the coronoid of the mandible caudally, is identified. A 2.5-cm, 22-gauge needle is inserted at this notch and approximately 5 mL of a 2% lidocaine hydrochloride solution are injected subcutaneously. A 2.5-cm, 14-gauge needle (to serve as a cannula) is placed

through the desensitized skin as far anterior and ventral as possible in the notch. A straight or slightly curved 10- to 12-cm, 18-gauge needle is inserted into the cannula in a horizontal and slightly posterior direction until it encounters the coronoid process of the mandible at approximately 2.5 cm through the skin. The cow's head is fully extended with frontal and nasal bones parallel to the ground. The needle with no syringe attached (to feel the bony landmarks) is gently manipulated anteriorly until its point passes medially around the coronoid process. The needle is then advanced to the pterygopalatine fossa rostral to the solid bony plate that is in close proximity of the orbitorotundum foramen at a depth of 7.5 to 10 cm (Fig. 16C–3A). Penetration of the turbinates and nasopharynx must be avoided. Approximately 15 mL of the local anesthetic is injected under control of aspiration to ensure that the needle point has not entered the ventral maxillary artery. All the important nerves (oculomotor, trochlear, and abducens, and the three branches of the trigeminal nerve (ophthalmic, maxillary, and mandibular) that emerge from the foramen orbitorotundum are desensitized 10 to 15 minutes after completion of the injection (Fig. 16C–4).(16) A proper technique anesthetizes all the structures for sensory and motor function of the eye, except

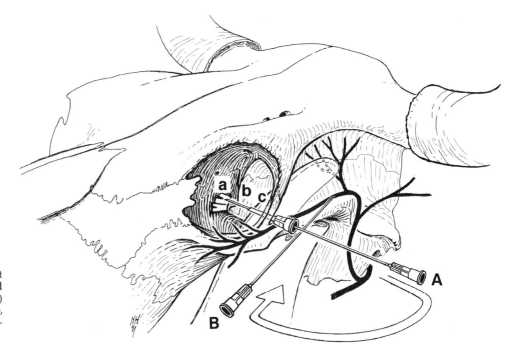

Fig. 16C–3. Needle placement for "Peterson" eye block (A) and auriculopalpebral nerve block (B) (a, foramen orbitorotundum; b, ptyerygoid crest; c, coronoid process).

for the eyelid. The lid block is accomplished by desensitizing the auriculopalpebral branch of the facial nerve, by withdrawing the needle to the subcutaneous tissue and reinserting it posteriorly for 5 to 7.5 cm lateral to the zygomatic arch, as an additional 5 to 10 mL of the anesthetic is injected (Fig. 16C–3B). If the upper lid is involved in the surgical procedure, a line of infiltration with 10 mL of the local anesthetic should be made subcutaneously approximately 2.5 cm from the margin of the lid (Fig. 16C–1A). The anesthetic is laid along its path while the needle is being advanced. Several different planes of anesthetic infiltration up the frontal crest are accomplished, so no matter where the nerve is coursing through that region, it should be desensitized by this fanning procedure.

As might be expected, some experience is required to strike a foramen that small at such great depth from the surface. To facilitate the Peterson procedure, a curved needle similar to that used for the retrobulbar block may be used. The concavity of the needle is kept caudal to facilitate the passage of the needle point rostral to the mandibular coronoid process. The needle is moved slightly back and forth, fanning across this area until some motor reaction and flinch of the animal's eye is determined.

When comparing the Peterson eye block and retrobulbar injection, it is apparent that the Peterson technique requires more skill to perform correctly but is safer and more effective if done properly. There is less edema and inflammation than when eyelids and orbit are infiltrated. In addition, the risk of orbital hemorrhage, direct pressure on the globe, penetration of the globe, damage to the optic nerve, or injection into the

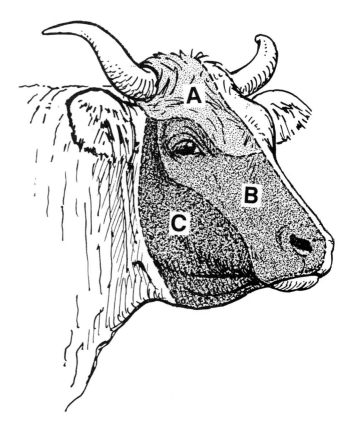

Fig. 16C–4. Cutaneous areas of the bovine head supplied by sensory fibers from the ophthalmic (A), maxillary (B), and mandibular (C) nerves.

optic nerve meninges is minimized with Peterson's technique.(17-19)

Both retrobulbar block and Peterson's technique prevent blinking for several hours. Antibiotic eye ointments of sterile saline solution should be applied to the cornea frequently during surgery and after orbital replacement of the globe to keep the cornea moist. Sunlight, dust, and wind in the eye must be avoided to prevent keratoconjunctivitis. Alternatively, the lids may be sutured together until motor activity of the lids returns. Local anesthetics in conventional concentrations should not produce nerve damage of clinical importance. Severe CNS toxicity in both procedures, however, may arise from penetration of the turbinates and injection of local anesthetic solution into the optic nerve meninges and nasopharynx. The clinical signs of local anesthetic CNS toxicity include hyperexcitability, lateral recumbency, opisthotonos, tonic clonic convulsions, respiratory arrest, and cardiac arrest.

NASAL ANESTHESIA

For repair of nasal lacerations in cattle and insertion of a nose ring in mature, ill-tempered bulls, nasal analgesia is required.(20) Bulls must be thoroughly restrained during the procedure, and if unruly, should be tranquilized before nasal analgesia is attempted. A 3.75-cm, 18-gauge needle is used for perineural injection of the infraorbital nerve at its point of emergence from the infraorbital canal. Difficult to palpate, the foramen is located rostral to the facial tuberosity on a line extending from the nasomaxillary notch to the second upper molar. Approximately 20 to 30 mL of a 2% lidocaine hydrochloride solution are injected along a line rostral to the infraorbital foramen and superficial to the maxilla (Fig. 16C–1C).

ANESTHESIA OF THE HORN

Anesthetic techniques for dehorning cattle (21-23) and goats (24, 25) and for disbudding young kids (26) have been described. Analgesia of the horn and base of the horn in cattle is achieved by desensitizing the cornual branch of the zygomaticotemporal (lacrimal) nerve, which is a portion of the ophthalmic division of the trigeminal nerve.(27, 28) The zygomaticotemporal nerve leaves the lacrimal nerve within the orbit and passes through the temporal fossa dorsal to the zygomatic process of the squamous temporal bone and around the lateral edge of the frontal bone dorsal to the temporal muscle. At first it lies deep, but on the upper third of the lateral temporal ridge it lies relatively superficial, 7 to 10 mm deep. The zygomaticotemporal nerve supplies sensory fibers to the horn and surrounding skin, particularly on its caudal aspect, and the skin of the ear. The nerve can usually be palpated halfway between the lateral canthus and the horn (bud) between the thin frontalis muscle and temporal muscle. A 2.5-cm, 20-gauge needle is inserted ventromedially close to the frontal bone approximately 2 to 3 cm in front of the base

of the horn, and 5 to 10 mL of a 2% lidocaine hydrochloride solution, depending on size, is injected (Fig. 16C–1D). Needle penetration is from 1.0 cm in small cattle to 2.5 cm in large bulls. The cornual artery and vein are close to the site of block; thus, aspiration ensures that the needle point is not inadvertently intravascular. Cornual anesthesia should result, unless anesthetic has been injected too deeply in the aponeurosis of the temporal muscle. With an adequately performed cornual nerve block, there is a blink response during infiltration and an ipsilateral lid droop because of blockade of some branches of the auriculopalpebral nerve. In exceptional cases (27) and in a fractured horn involving the frontal bone and sinuses (29), a large posterior branch of the sinuum frontalium nerve maintains sensitivity of the cornual process. This nerve can be desensitized by using the Peterson eye block technique. Adult cattle and bulls with well-developed horns require extensive subcutaneous infiltration of the caudal aspect of the horn base in order to desensitize the cutaneous branches of the second cervical nerve.(22, 30)

The horns and bases of the horns in goats are supplied by the cornual branches of the zygomaticotemporal (lacrimal) and infratrochlear nerves. The cornual branch of the zygomaticotemporal (lacrimal) nerve is desensitized by inserting a 2.5-cm, 22-gauge needle halfway between the lateral canthus of the eye and lateral base of the horn as close as possible to the caudal ridge of the supraorbital process and 1.0 to 1.5 cm deep, and injecting 2.0 to 3.0 mL of a 2% lidocaine hydrochloride solution in the adult goat (Fig. 16C–5A). A second injection is made halfway between the medial canthus of the eye and medial base of the horn to desensitize the cornual branch of the infratrochlear nerve. The needle is inserted dorsal and parallel to the dorsomedial margin of the orbit. The anesthetic is administered in a line, as this nerve is frequently branched (Fig. 16C–5B).

An elypsical ring block around the base of the entire horn should be laid for a cosmetic dehorning procedure to undermine tissue and bring it back for closure. Anesthesia of the nerve to the sinus mucosa and periosteum of the frontal sinus is impractical, since it arises deep within the orbit and enters the frontal bone without appearing superficial.(28) Sedation of the animal is required if the frontal sinus will be entered during horn removal.(25) To alleviate pain during disbudding of young kids between 7 and 14 days of age, 0.5 mL of a 2% lidocaine hydrochloride solution is injected subcutaneously around the horn base (ring block). A total dose of 10 mg/kg (0.5 mL of a 2% solution per kg or 1.0 mL of a 1% solution per kg) lidocaine must not be exceeded to minimize adverse reactions. Inadvertent rapid intravenous infusions produce the most dramatic and rapid onset of symptoms. Apparent signs of toxicity include excitation, lateral recumbency, muscular twitching, generalized tonic-clonic convulsions, and opisthotonos. Coma, respiratory arrest, and cardiac arrest occur

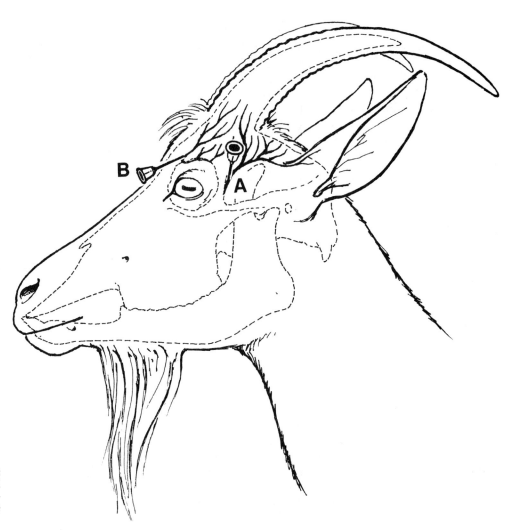

Fig. 16C–5. Needle placement for desensitizing the cornual branches of the zygomaticotemporal (A) and infratrochlear nerve (B) in the goat.

with high (>15 μg/mL) plasma concentrations of lidocaine.

Anesthesia for Laparotomy

At least six techniques for inducing anesthesia of the paralumbar fossa and abdominal wall in standing ruminants have been described: (a) infiltration, (b) proximal paravertebral thoracolumbar, (c) distal paravertebral thoracolumbar, (d) segmental dorsolumbar epidural, (e) continuous lumbar segmental epidural, and (f) thoracolumbar subarachnoid anesthesia. Any of these techniques may be used for surgeries such as rumenotomy, cecotomy, correction of gastrointestinal displacement, intestinal obstruction and volvulus, cesarean section, ovariectomy, liver or kidney biopsy, and others.(31, 32)

INFILTRATION ANESTHESIA

Line block. Simple infiltration of the incision line (line block) is the easiest and probably the most commonly used technique for producing analgesia of the flank in food animals. Multiple subcutaneous injections of 0.5 to 1.0 mL of a 2% lidocaine hydrochloride solution, 1.0 to 2.0 cm apart, are administered using a 2.5-cm, 20-gauge or smaller needle. Successive injections of 10 to 15 mL of the anesthetic are made slowly and continuously as the needle is inserted at the edge of the desensitized skin for the skin and subcutaneous line block. This is followed by inserting a 7.5- to 10-cm, 18-gauge needle through the desensitized skin and infiltrating the muscle layers and parietal peritoneum using 10 to 100 mL of the anesthetic, depending upon the area to be desensitized (Fig. 16C–6). Adult cattle (450 kg) safely tolerate 250 mL of a 2% lidocaine hydrochloride solution (5 g) for the line block, whereas in adult goats 10 mL of a 2% lidocaine hydrochloride solution (200 mg) should not be exceeded. It is common practice to dilute a 2% solution of the anesthetic with equal parts of sterile saline to make a 1% solution and decrease the total amount of drug by 50%. A 1% solution of lidocaine can also be used cautiously in goats. Fetal and newborn lambs should not be more sensitive to lidocaine toxicity than are adult sheep.(33)

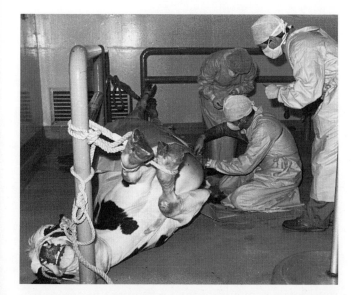

Fig. 16C–6. Restraint of a 5-year-old Holstein cow, weighing 600 kg, in dorsolateral recumbency for right ventral abomasopexis. Aproximately 25 mL of a 2% lidocaine hydrochloride solution desensitized a 15-cm abdominal incision line (From Skarda, R. Techniques of Local Analgesia in Ruminants and Swine. Vet Clin North Am Food Anim Pract 2(3):630, 1986.)

It remains advisable to limit the total dosage in small and young sheep and goats.

Inverted-7 or L block. Basically the inverted-7 or L block is a nonspecific regional analgesic technique in which up to 100 mL of a 2% lidocaine hydrochloride solution in adult cattle is injected into the tissues bordering the dorsocaudal aspect of the last rib and ventrolateral aspect of the lumbar transverse processes (Fig. 16C–7). All nerves entering the surgical field are desensitized 10 to 15 minutes after administration of the anesthetic. Deposition of the anesthetic away from the incision site minimizes edema, hematoma, and possible interference with healing. The disadvantages of the inverted-7 or L block are similar to local infiltration anesthesia (line block) and include incomplete analgesia and muscle relaxation of the deep layers of the abdominal wall (particularly of the peritoneum), toxicity after injecting significant amounts of the anesthetic solution into the peritoneal cavity, and increased cost owing to larger doses of anesthetic and longer time required.

PROXIMAL PARAVERTEBRAL THORACOLUMBAR ANESTHESIA

The proximal paravertebral anesthesia is a good alternative to the inverted-7 or line block. The dorsal and ventral branches of the last thoracic (T13) and first and second lumbar (L1 and L2) spinal nerves are desensitized as they emerge from the intervertebral foramina (Fig. 16C–8). The technique is also called the *Farquharson* (34), *Hall,* or *Cambridge technique.*(35) In addition, the third and fourth (L3 and L4) spinal nerves are desen-

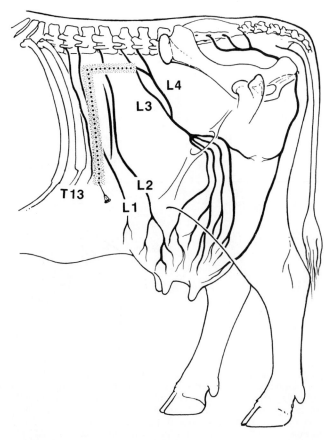

Fig. 16C–7. Regional analgesia of the bovine flank using inverted-L infiltration pattern. T_{13} to L_4, ventral branches of thirteenth thoracic and first to fourth lumbar vertebral nerves.

sitized, if analgesia of the caudalmost part of the paralumbar fossa for cesarean section or ipsilateral fore-teat and mammary gland is desired.(36) However, weakness of the pelvic limb may result by desensitizing the L3 and L4 nerves, which carry motor fibers to the femoral and ischial nerves.

In cattle, the skin overlying the spinal column on the side to be desensitized is clipped, surgically scrubbed, and disinfected. The skin at the most obvious parts of the transverse processes of L1, L2, and L3 at a point 2.5 to 5 cm from the dorsal midline is identified and desensitized by injecting 2 to 3 mL of a 2% lidocaine hydrochloride solution, using a short and comparatively fine needle (2.5 cm, 20 gauge). If the T13 and L1 transverse processes cannot be palpated, the distance between the more prominent transverse processes of L2 and L3 is measured to mark the anterior sites at which the needle is to be introduced to desensitize the nerves L1 and T13, respectively. The cranial aspect of the transverse processes will usually be on a same cross-sectional plane with the intervertebral foramina, thus palpation of the most cranial border of the transverse process of L2 is of value to locate the L1-L2 intervertebral

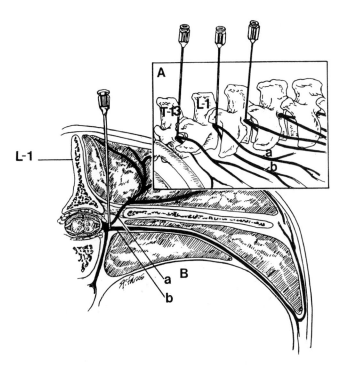

Fig. 16C–8. Needle placement for proximal paravertebral nerve block in cattle. A, left lateral aspect of thoraco-lumbar vertebrae T13 to L4 with needle tip placed at spinal nerves T_{13}, L_1, and L_2. B, cranial view of a transsection of the first lumbar vertebra at the location of the intervertebral foramen (a, dorsal branch; b, ventral branch of L1 vertebral nerve). (From Skarda, R. Techniques of Local Analgesia in Ruminants and Swine. Vet Clin North Am Food Anim Pract 2(3):631, 1986.)

foramen, from which the first lumbar (L1) spinal nerve emerges.

A 1.25-cm, 14-gauge needle (to serve as a cannula) is first inserted into the desensitized skin to minimize skin resistance during insertion of a stout 4.25- to 15-cm, 18-gauge spinal needle. The needle is passed ventrally until its point encounters the transverse process of L2 or the intertransverse (L1-L2) ligament. Small amounts (2 to 3 mL) of the anesthetic are injected as the needle is advanced to counteract spasm of the longissimus dorsi muscle and prevent bending of the long needle. When contact is made with bone, the needle is walked off the cranial edge of the transverse process of L2 and advanced approximately 1.0 cm to pass through the intertransverse fascia. The penetration of the intertransverse fascia can usually be felt. Approximately 10 to 15 mL of a 2% lidocaine hydrochloride solution are injected with little resistance to desensitize the ventral branch of L1. The needle is withdrawn 1.0 to 2.5 cm to above the fascia and dorsal surface of the transverse process. An additional 5 mL of the anesthetic is injected with slight resistance to desensitize the dorsal branch of L1. To desensitize T13 and L2, the needle is inserted cranial to the transverse processes of L1 and L3, its tip walked off the cranial edges of the transverse processes to a depth comparable to the previous injection site, and the nerves desensitized similarly to L1.

In sheep and goats, T13, L1, and L2 are desensitized similarly to the cattle method, but 2.5 to 3.0 cm off the midline and with less anesthetic (2 to 3 mL per site). Full anesthesia develops in approximately 10 minutes and lasts 90 minutes. Signs of successful nerve blockade include anesthesia of the skin, increased skin temperature due to hyperemia after paralysis of cutaneous vasomotor nerves, and scoliosis toward the desensitized side caused by paralysis of paravertebral muscles.

When compared with infiltration analgesia, proximal thoracolumbar paravertebral block offers a wide and uniform area of analgesia and muscle relaxation. Analgesia is developed from the thirteenth rib caudal to the tuber coxae and ventrally to the fold of the flank. There is no disruption of the incision site. Disruption occurs with an infiltration block when excessive amounts of anesthetic is injected into the tissues and multiple skin punctures with subsequent hemorrhage and trauma by the needle are made. With an infiltration block, a considerable amount of time is required to desensitize an area of approximately 45 cm, as would be required in an cesarean section. If an incision this long is necessary, a paravertebral nerve block could be done much more quickly and in a more professional and impressive manner. The technique relies on finding landmarks, but it is not at all difficult in thin bony cows with easily palpable transverse processes. The disadvantages of the thoracolumbar paravertebral nerve block are its technical difficulty, particularly in fat cattle and some beef cattle in which the lumbar transverse processes are out of range of palpation, arching up the spine owing to paralysis of back muscles, which are bowing out toward the area of incision after unilateral blockade, making the closure of the incision and navigation more difficult; the risk of penetrating vital structures such as the aorta and thoracic longitudinal vein on the left side and the caudal vena cava on the right side; and loss of motor control of the pelvic limb caused by caudal migration of the injection site to the femoral nerves.

DISTAL PARAVERTEBRAL THORACOLUMBAR ANESTHESIA

A lateral approach to the dorsal and ventral rami of spinal nerves T13, L1, and L2 in cattle has been utilized. The technique is also called the *Magda, Cakala,* or *Cornell technique.*(37) The skin is clipped and disinfected at the distal ends of the first lumbar (L1), second lumbar (L2), and fourth lumbar (L4) transverse processes, and 10 to 20 mL of a 2% lidocaine hydrochloride solution is injected in a fan-shaped infiltration pattern ventral to each transverse process, using a 7.5-cm, 18-gauge needle (Fig. 16C–9). The needle is withdrawn a short distance and reinserted slightly dorsal and caudal to the transverse process to inject additional 5 mL of the anesthetic and desensitize the cutaneous branch of the dorsolateral branches. The procedure is repeated for the second and fourth lumbar transverse processes.

Distal paravertebral anesthesia as compared with proximal paravertebral anesthesia offers the advantages of using more routinely sized needles, lack of scoliosis,

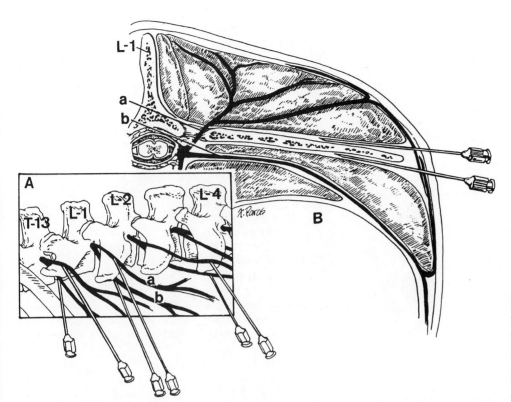

Fig. 16C–9. Needle placement for distal paravertebral nerve block in cattle to block dorsal (a) and ventral (b) rami of spinal nerves T_{13}, L_1, and L_2. (From Skarda, R. Techniques of Local Analgesia in Ruminants and Swine. Vet Clin North Am Food Anim Pract 2(3):633, 1986.)

lack of risk of penetrating a major blood vessel (e.g., the aorta or the posterior vena cava), minimal weakness in the pelvic limb, and minimal ataxia. On the other hand, the larger doses of the anesthetic needed and variations in efficiency, particularly if the nerves follow a variable anatomic pathway, are disadvantages of the technique.

SEGMENTAL DORSOLUMBAR EPIDURAL ANESTHESIA

Although not an easy technique to perform, injection of local anesthetic into the epidural space either between the first and second lumbar (L1 and L2) vertebrae or, less commonly, between the last thoracic (T13) and first lumbar (L1) vertebrae in cattle has been employed to desensitize a number of nerve roots as they emerge from the dura covering the spinal cord and produce a belt of anesthesia around the animal's trunk while maintaining control of the limbs (Fig. 16C–10). This type of spinal block may be referred to as *segmental dorsolumbar epidural anesthesia* or *Arthur block.*(38) The technique was first described in 1948 (39); subsequently, many have reported its use. Cattle must be thoroughly restrained during the procedure.

In the standard technique, the skin area caudal to the T13 or L1 spinous process and contralateral to the flank region to be desensitized is aseptically prepared, and 2.0 to 4.0 mL of a 2% lidocaine hydrochloride solution is injected subcutaneously and adjacent to the interspinous (T13-L1 or L1-L2) ligaments to minimize pain during the puncture procedure. The first lumbar (L1-L2) intervertebral space in cattle is located 1.5 to 2.0 cm caudal to an imaginary line drawn across the back from

the cranial edge of the transverse process of the second lumbar (L2) vertebrae. The dorsal lumbar processes and the depression between them can occasionally be palpated. A 1.25-cm, 14-gauge needle to facilitate penetration of a 11.25-cm, 18-gauge spinal needle with stylet is inserted at that site. The needle is advanced through the interosseus canal, which is formed by the arches of spinous processes T13 and L1, cranially and caudally, and the intervertebral articular processes laterally, until an abrupt reduction in needle passage is noted, indicating piercing through the interarcuate ligament and entry into the vertebral canal (Fig. 16C–11). The spinal needle is inserted for a distance of 8 to 12 cm while being directed ventrally and medially at an angle of 10 to 15° with the vertical, at which point the needle has reached the epidural space. The spinal needle can be inserted through the muscle with relative ease, but encounters a slight increase in resistance during the insertion process at the interspinous and interarcuate ligaments.

Withdrawal and redirection of the needle are necessary if the needle point impinges against the bony arches of T13 and L1 or L1 and L2, respectively. The needle is properly placed into the epidural space if no blood or cerebrospinal fluid (CSF) flows from the needle hub or is obtained upon aspiration. Sometimes a siffling sound is heard as air enters the needle immediately after penetration of the interarcuate ligament. Most often, the epidural space is identified by the loss-of-resistance method.(40) This means that first a marked resistance to injection of saline or air is encountered when the point of the needle enters the interarcuate

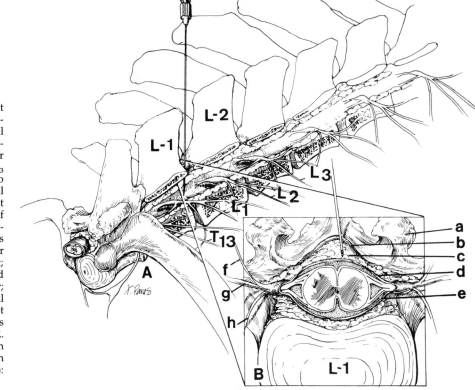

Fig. 16C–10. Needle placement for segmental dorsolumbar epidural analgesia in cattle. A, cranial and left lateral aspect of the thoracolumbar vertebrae and their associated spinal nerves T_{13} to L_3 with needle tip placed at the L1 to L2 intervertebral space. B, cranial view of a transection of the first lumbar vertebra at the location of the intervertebral foramen, showing the relation of the structures inside the spinal canal (a, articular process; b, interarcuate ligament; c, epidural space with fat and connective tissue; d, dura mater; e, arachnoid membrane; f, dorsal branch; g, ventral branch of first lumbar [L_1] spinal nerve; h, ramus communicans). (From Skarda, R. Techniques of Local Analgesia in Ruminants and Swine. Vet Clin North Am Food Anim Pract 2(3): 634, 1986.)

ligament and resistance completely disappears after the point of the needle has passed through the ligament. An alternative method is to place a few drops of saline or local anesthetic solution on the hub of the needle and observe the drops to be aspirated into the needle by the subatmospheric pressure of the epidural space (hanging-drop method).(41) If bleeding occurs, the stylet is placed into the needle and the needle is withdrawn after 2 to 3 minutes. If the dura is inadvertently punctured and CSF is obtained, segmental thoracolumbar subarachnoid anesthesia may be performed or the procedure terminated. After piercing through the interarcuate ligament, approximately 8 mL of either a 2% lidocaine hydrochloride solution or a 5% procaine hydrochloride solution in an average 500-kg cow are injected. This amount of anesthetic is sufficient to desensitize T13, L1, and L2 at 7 to 20 minutes after administration and for 45 to 120 minutes.(42) The needle must not be manipulated further but should be removed immediately after injection in order to avoid damage to the spinal cord and meninges (Fig. 16C–12).

Factors that influence epidural spread and duration of anesthesia include age, extradural fat, pregnancy, venous circulation, and variables that are under the direct control of the anesthetist such as positioning of the patient, choosing the site for epidural puncture, orientation of the needle bevel, and determining the volume. Although there is considerable disagreement among authors as to the ultimate mode of action of

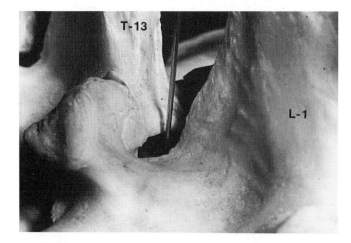

Fig. 16C–11. The spinal needle (11.25 cm, 18 gauge), is directed ventrally and medially of approximately 10° from vertical to enter the neural canal via intervertebral space which is surrounded by the bases of the spinous processes cranially and caudally and by the intervertebral articular processes laterally (T13, thirteenth thoracic; L1, first lumbar vertebra).

epidural anesthetics, spread of the anesthetic solution within the epidural space is the first event after injection. The epidural space at the thoracolumbar (T13-L1) or first lumbar (L1-L2) intervertebral space in cattle cannot be reached by the spinal needle if the interarcuate ligament is ossified due to old age (>8 years).(39, 42, 43)

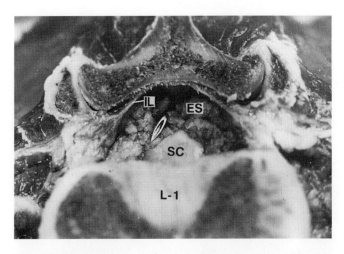

Fig. 16C–12. Cranial view of a transection of the first lumbar (L1) vertebra at the location of the intervertebral foramen of an adult cow, with needle tip placed for unilateral (right side) segmental dorsolumbar epidural anesthesia (ES, epidural space with fat and conective tissue; SC, spinal cord; L1, first lumbar vertebra).

The typical segmental blockade observed in the young may reflect a predominantly paravertebral site of action, whereas the widespread anesthesia produced by injection of small volumes in the elderly indicates a more intense action within the subarachnoid space. The dura becomes more permeable to local anesthetics with age owing to a progressive increase in the size and number of arachnoid villi, thereby providing a larger area through which local anesthetic can diffuse into the subarachnoid space. The epidural anesthetic dosages need to be reduced slightly in old patients. Similarly, migration of epidural anesthetics is enhanced by distension (engorgement) of epidural veins in full-term pregnancy and increased quantities of fat in obesity. Selective anesthesia on one side of the spinal column is achieved by placing the needle tip within the epidural space across the midline and injecting small volumes of the anesthetic to the nerve roots on the contralateral side (Fig. 16C–12). Bilateral anesthesia results from administering either a larger volume of the anesthetic or a regular dose through a needle with its tip placed within the epidural space in the median plane dorsal to the spinal cord, and desensitizing the nerve roots on both sides. The bevel of the spinal needle is directed cranially to limit the caudal flow of the anesthetic, thereby minimizing the risk of loss of motor control of the pelvic limbs.

The area of segmental anesthesia is a function of total mass (volume × concentration) of drug injected. Increasing the volume or concentration will increase the area of the blockade. In general, a single injection of a 2 or 3% lidocaine hydrochloride solution (10 mL), 4 or 5% procaine hydrochloride solution (10 mL), or a 2% tubocaine hydrochloride (10 to 15 mL) into the epidural space at the T13-L1 intervertebral space induced satisfactory anesthesia and relaxation of the abdominal wall and flank for operations such as rumenotomy and cesarean section, with the animal maintaining a standing position. Anesthesia develops approximately 10 minutes after injection and lasts approximately 2 hours. Onset and duration of anesthesia vary widely between drugs and are influenced by the size of the dose administered (Table 16C–1).

Segmental spread of anesthesia is improved by increasing the volume of the solution injected, whereas a more rapid onset of analgesia and motor blockade, greater frequency of adequate analgesia, greater depth of motor blockade, and longer duration of analgesia are obtained by increasing the concentration of the anesthetic.

The critical CSF concentration of local anesthetic required to eliminate response to deep needle prick stimulation at the thoracolumbar T13 to L1 dermatomes in 10 cows was approximately 200 μg of procaine/mL.(44) The subarachnoid threshold concentration of procaine was reached after repeated epidural injections, but not after a single administration, indicating that segmental lumbar epidural anesthesia in cattle may be primarily due to analgesia of dura-covered roots outside the epidural space (paravertebral site), and to be minimally, if at all, dependent upon desensitization of nerves within the subarachnoid space.(45)

Finally, segmental spread of anesthesia is improved by a fast injection, but the advantage of a larger segmental area of analgesia is offset by a shorter duration, increased occurrence of incomplete analgesia, and high frequency of the patient's discomfort upon injection, which is probably attributable to transient elevation of CSF pressure. The rate of injection should be slow, a volume of 10 mL being given over approximately 10 seconds.

Selective unilateral segmental (T13-L3) epidural anesthesia in adult nonpregnant cows is associated with decreases in mean systemic arterial blood pressure and total peripheral resistance, no changes in stroke volume, left ventricular stroke work, and left ventricular minute work, and increases in heart rate and cardiac output.(46) Increases in cardiac output are believed to be caused by an increase in heart rate secondary to the decreased vascular resistance. Respiratory rate; arterial and mixed venous pH, O_2, and CO_2 tensions; oxyhemoglobin saturation; oxygen content; oxygen transport; and oxygen uptake remain unaltered, indicating that the sympathetic blockade caused by thoracolumbar epidural injection is well tolerated by nonsedated healthy cows.(46)

The advantages of segmental dorsolumbar epidural anesthesia as compared to proximal and distal paravertebral anesthesia are the use of only one injection of a small quantity of anesthetic and uniform analgesia and relaxation of the skin, musculature, and parietal peritoneum. The disadvantages of segmental epidural anesthesia include difficulty in performing the technique, potential for trauma to the spinal cord or venous sinuses, and loss of motor control of the pelvic limbs; also, there is physiologic disturbance owing to overdose or subarachnoid injection.(47)

CONTINUOUS LUMBAR SEGMENTAL EPIDURAL ANESTHESIA

Continuous lumbar epidural anesthesia in cattle can be achieved by aseptically placing a catheter into the epidural space (Fig. 16C–13). A 10.2-cm, 18-gauge thin-walled Tuohy needle with stylet is inserted into the epidural space at the thoracolumbar (T13-L1) interspace as previously described. This space is identified with reference to the last rib (T13) and the cranial edge of the transverse process of the first lumbar (L1) vertebra.(48) A small quantity of local anesthetic solution (2.0–3.0 mL) is injected along the track of the needle. The distance from the skin to the thoracolumbar (T13-L1) epidural space may vary between 8.0 and 12.0 cm, depending upon size. Injection of 5 mL of air should not encounter resistance. If no CSF or blood flows from the needle, 1.0 mL of a 2% lidocaine hydrochloride solution is injected into the thoracolumbar epidural space during a 10-second period to avoid pain caused by impingement of the catheter and stylet at the spinal cord. After the bevel in the epidural space is directed caudally, a commercially available 91.8-cm, 20-gauge Teflon epidural catheter with graduated markings and stylet is introduced into the needle and advanced caudally 3.0 to 5.0 cm beyond the tip of the needle. The needle is removed from the catheter while the catheter is left in position and sutured to the skin at the site of emergence from the skin. Injection of approximately 6 mL of a 2% lidocaine hydrochloride solution or a 5% procaine hydrochloride solution at the anterior portion of the lumbar (L1 to L2) area should produce unilateral or bilateral anesthesia extending from spinal cord segments T12 to L4 of adult cows. Analgesia is achieved 10 to 20 minutes after completion of the injection and lasts 60 to 100 minutes.(48) A more caudal spread of epidural block can be expected with an injection of local anesthetic more caudal than L2. An overdose of local anesthetic (>6.0 mL) to the L2 area or a regular dose of anesthetic at a more caudal level than L2 should be avoided to prevent anesthesia of the femoral and sciatic nerves and thus loss of pelvic limb function.(48) The reason for unilateral analgesia could be attributable to placement of the epidural catheter at the nerve roots on one side, minimal circumferential dissipation (overflow) of local anesthetic around the dura mater spinalis, and lateral escape of the local anesthetic from the epidural space through patent intervertebral foramina.

In comparison to segmental epidural anesthesia, produced by injection of local anesthetic through a spinal needle, continuous segmental epidural anesthesia offers the advantages of providing a route for repeated small fractional maintenance doses of local anesthetic drug, making the extent of anesthesia more readily controlled and producing a lower frequency of accidental subarachnoid administration of local anesthetic. The disadvantages of the catheter technique include higher frequency of postanesthetic myositis, caused by the larger bore and blunter needle, higher frequency of unilateral blockade, unpredictability if

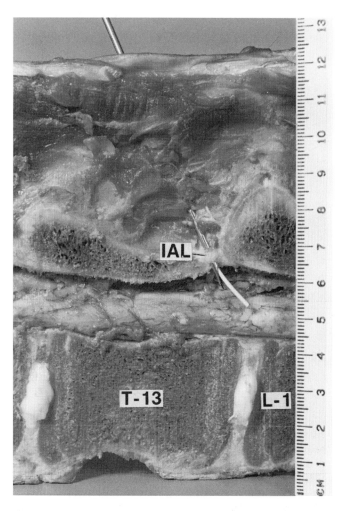

Fig. 16C–13. Paramedian sagittal section of the thoracolumbar area of an adult cow with needle placement for catheterization of the lumbar epidural space (T13, thirteenth thoracic; L1, first lumbar vertebra; IAL, interarcuate ligament).

ipsilateral or contralateral anesthesia develops, and lack of analgesia after passage of the catheter tip into the paravertebral space.

THORACOLUMBAR SUBARACHNOID ANESTHESIA

Thoracolumbar subarachnoid anesthesia in cattle is performed by aseptically introducing a catheter into the subarachnoid space at the lumbosacral (L6-S1) intervertebral space and advancing it to the thoracolumbar (T13-L1) intervertebral space (Fig. 16C–14).(48, 49-52) Although the dorsal subarachnoid space in cattle can be penetrated at the thoracolumbar (T13-L1) and first lumbar (L1-L2) intervertebral spaces, dura puncture at these sites is not recommended because of potential trauma to the spinal cord. Cattle must be well restrained in a stock to facilitate the catheterization procedure. The skin at the lumbosacral (L6-S1) intervertebral space and lumbosacral fascia adjacent to the interspinous (L6-S1) ligaments are injected with approximately 5 mL of a 2%

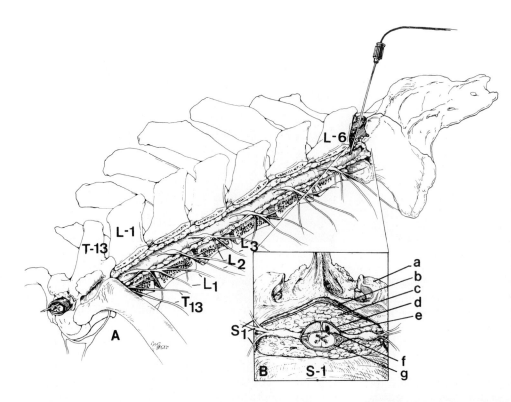

Fig. 16C–14. Needle and catheter placement for thoracolumbar subarachnoid analgesia in cattle. A, cranial and left lateral aspect of the bovine thoracolumbar and sacral vertebrae and their associated spinal nerves T_{13} to L_3 with needle tip placed at the lumbosacral intervertebral space. B, cranial view of a transection of the first sacral vertebra at the location of the intervertebral foramen, showing the relation of the structures inside the spinal canal (a, articular process; b, interarcuate ligament; c, epidural space with fat and connective tissue; d, dura mater; e, arachnoid membrane; f, subarachnoid space with cerebral spinal fluid and needle tip; g, pia mater). (From Skarda, R. Techniques of Local Analgesia in Ruminants and Swine. Vet Clin North Am Food Anim Pract 2(3): 635, 1986.)

lidocaine hydrochloride solution, using a 15-cm, 18-gauge spinal needle. The space is located 1.0 to 2.0 cm caudal of a line drawn between the cranial edge of each tuber sacrale and the dorsal midline.

A larger-bore (17.5-cm, 17-gauge) Huber-point Tuohy needle with stylet is inserted at the desensitized L6-S1 site and is advanced along the median plane perpendicular to the spinal cord until it enters the subarachnoid space. The bevel of the needle is directed cranially, the stylet removed, and 2 to 3 mL of CSF is aspirated. Occasionally it is necessary to make several minor adjustments before the needle is satisfactorily positioned into the subarachnoid space. Redirection of the needle is required if CSF cannot be obtained, and should be accomplished after almost complete withdrawal of the needle to prevent bending of the needle. Upon CSF aspiration, a Formocath polyethylene catheter 80 to 100 cm long with a 0.095-cm outside diameter, reinforced with a stainless steel spring guide (0.05-cm outside diameter), is passed through the needle (Fig. 16C–15) and advanced approximately 60 cm to the midthoracic area. Minimal resistance to catheter advancement and no movement of the patient indicate proper technique, without kinking and curling of the catheter and no trauma to the spinal nerve roots within the subarachnoid space. The needle is withdrawn over the catheter; then the spring guide is removed and a catheter adapter or a 23-gauge needle and three-way stopcock are attached to the catheter. The catheter is then gently withdrawn a calculated distance to place its tip at T13-L1.

The catheter must never be withdrawn after advancing it through the spinal needle as this could result in

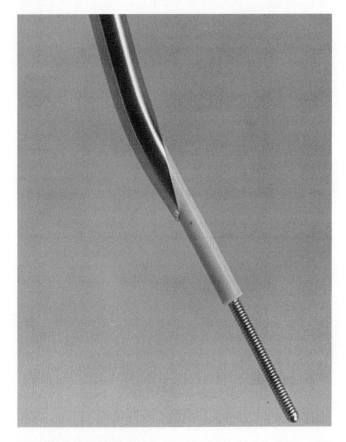

Fig. 16C–15. Tip of 17-gauge Huber-point Tuohy needle with Formocath polyethylene catheter (0.095-cm onside diameter), reinforced with a stainless steel spring guide (0.05-cm outside diameter).

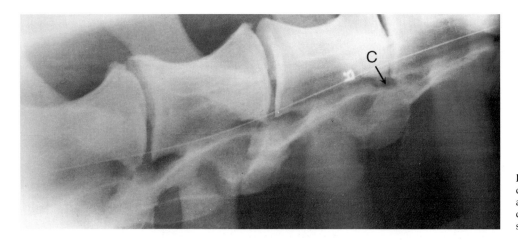

Fig. 16C–16. Radiograph of the caudal lumbar vertebrae of an adult Holstein cow (630 kg) with catheter (C) in subarachnoid space; a lateral oblique view.

shearing off the catheter within the subarachnoid space.(49, 52) The following measurements are made to place the catheter tip at the T13-L1 intervertebral space: (a) the total length of the catheter (T), (b) the distance BC between the skin surface (B) and the subarachnoid puncture site (C), and (c) the distance CD between the lumbosacral (C) and thoracolumbar (D) intervertebral space: $(T = AB + BC + CD)$. The length of the free end of the external catheter and the skin surface (AB) equals the total length of the catheter minus the distance from entering the skin to the tip of the subarachnoidally placed catheter: $AB = T - (BC + CD)$. The average distance between the palpable lumbosacral (L6-S1) and thoracolumbar (T13-L1) intervertebral spaces was 45.2 ± 4.1 cm in 18 adult cows (620 ± 54 kg).(49) Proper subarachnoid positioning of the catheter can be radiographically confirmed if the wireguide is left in position (Fig. 16C–16).

A small dose (1.5 to 2.0 mL) of a 2% lidocaine hydrochloride solution or a 5% procaine hydrochloride solution is injected at a rate of approximately 0.5 mL per minute. Surgical anesthesia extending from spinal cord segment T9 to L3 on one or both sides, is maximal 5 to 10 minutes after injection and lasts for 20 to 80 minutes.(49) The absorption of drug into the systemic circulation determines the decline of subarachnoid anesthetic concentration, and thus the duration of subarachnoid analgesia. The spinal fluid concentration necessary for analgesia is approximately 200 μg procaine/mL in calves (53) and adult cows (44, 47), and is easily maintained by fractional bolus administration of 0.5 mL of the anesthetic at 30-minute intervals or as needed.

When compared to dorsolumbar epidural analgesia, the advantages of thoracolumbar subarachnoid analgesia include simplicity of needle and catheter placements, anesthetic deposition at nerve roots (and thus minimal dosage), minimal physiologic disturbance, and small doses for maintenance of analgesia. A disadvantage of the catheter technique is the unpredictability of whether ipsilateral or contralateral analgesia develops. The cause for the one-sided block has not been investigated, but could be attributable to minimal circumferential dissipation (overflow) of local anesthetic around the pia mater spinalis after placement of the catheter at the ventral surface of the spinal cord, where it could be trapped between the trabecula and dorsal longitudinal ligament. Kinking and curling of the catheter are readily determined by lack of CSF aspiration and avoidance responses of cattle. Accidental vascular puncture and faulty catheter positioning make the technique ineffective for producing abdominal analgesia of the flank region. Thoracolumbar subarachnoid anesthesia may not be readily applicable for use in the field because it requires special equipment, precise dosage and catheter placement, and maintenance of sterility.

Anesthesia for Obstetric Procedures and Relief of Rectal Tenesmus

At least four techniques are advocated in ruminants for pain relief and muscle relaxation during obstetric manipulations and surgical procedures involving the tail, perineum, anus, rectum, vulva, vagina, prepuce, and skin and scrotum. These techniques are caudal epidural, continuous caudal epidural, sacral paravertebral anesthesia, and pudendal nerve blocks. Any of these techniques may be used for a number of surgical procedures such as suturing tears in the perineum and vulva, reconstruction of the perineum (Götze's operation), retraction of the uterine cervix, reduction of prolapsed uterus, ovariectomy, embryotomy, and others. These techniques may also be used as adjunctive treatments for controlling rectal tenesmus associated with irritation of the perineum, anus, rectum, and vagina. Proper techniques do not involve the femoral and ischial nerves, and thereby pelvic limb function is uninfluenced. The techniques are not effective in pigs.

CAUDAL EPIDURAL ANESTHESIA

Because this technique is simple and inexpensive, and requires no sophisticated equipment, it is routinely used in cows, sheep, and goats. Needle placement is either at the sacrococcygeal (S5-Co1) or more commonly at the first coccygeal (Co1-Co2) interspace, beyond the termination of the spinal cord and meninges (Fig. 16C–17).(54) Only the coccygeal nerves, the thin phylum terminale, the vasculature, and epidural fat and connective tissue remain in the spinal canal at the site of needle penetration, and these structures are not easily damaged when using aseptic technique.(55) The location of the Co1-Co2 interspace is easily identified by elevating and lowering the tail and palpating the depression and movement between the respective vertebrae. The Co1-Co2 interspace is larger and more easily penetrated than the S5-Co1 site. The S5-Co1 interspace may be ossified in older cows and is not so easily detectable in fat cows.(56)

The skin over the Co1-Co2 joint space is disinfected and desensitized with small amount (2 to 3 mL) of local anesthetic to ensure minimal movement during insertion of a 3.75- to 5-cm, 18-gauge needle. The epidural needle is inserted in a median plane until it contacts the floor of the vertebral canal while it is directed either at right angle to the general contour of the croup or ventrocranially at an angle of approximately 10° to vertical (Fig. 16C–18A). The needle is then withdrawn approximately 0.5 cm from the ligamentous floor or intervertebral disk to place its tip in the epidural space of the neural canal. Aspiration of a few drops of the anesthetic from the hub into the needle and minimal resistance to injection of the anesthetic indicate that the bevel is placed epidurally.

Production of caudal anesthesia depends upon the total dose (volume × concentration) of the anesthetic administered. When 1.0 mL of a 2% lidocaine hydrochloride solution per 100 kg of body weight is injected

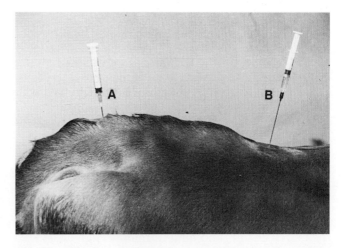

Fig. 16C–18. (A), A 3.75-cm, 18-gauge needle is placed into the epidural space at the first coccygeal (Co1-Co2) intervertebral space of a Jersey cow (460 kg). (B), A 15-cm, 20-gauge spinal needle is placed into the epidural space at the lumbosacral (L6-S1) intervertebral space.

at a rate of 1.0 mL per second, the area of anesthesia extends cranially to the middle of the sacrum and ventrally over the perineum to the inner aspect of the thigh. Proper techniques should desensitize the pelvic viscera and genitalia, and paralyze the tail and abolish abdominal contractions. However, locomotor function of the hind legs and uterine motility remain unaffected. Maximal anesthesia may require 10 to 20 minutes and can be expected to last 30 to 150 minutes. Although 2% lidocaine hydrochloride solution is now almost universally used, the addition of 0.125 mL 1:80,000 epinephrine per mL of anesthetic suppresses the tone and motility of the tail for more than 60 minutes.(57)

Adjusting the pH of 2% lidocaine hydrochloride solution from 6.3 to 6.9 by the addition of 1 mL of 8.4% $NaHCO_3$ solution (1 mEq) to 10 mL of lidocaine has little or no effect on the time of onset and duration of caudal epidural anesthesia in cattle.(58)

A significantly larger duration (up to 3 hours) of perineal anesthesia in cattle is observed when injecting 0.05 mg of xylazine/kg of body weight, diluted to a 5-mL volume with sterile water into the epidural space at the Co1-Co2 intervertebral space, than when lidocaine is injected.(59-61) However, side effects, such as sedation, mild ataxia and bradycardia, hypotension, respiratory acidosis, hypoxemia, and ruminal amotility are routinely observed in conscious standing cattle when xylazine is given epidurally.(60, 61) These side effects can be partially reversed by intravenous administration of tolazoline (0.3 mg/kg), an alpha2-adrenoceptor antagonist, while not diminishing desirable local (S3 to the coccyx) analgesic effects.(61) Care must be taken to limit the volume of xylazine and its rostral spread to the femoral and sciatic nerves. Xylazine appears to exhibit direct local anesthetic sensory and motor nerve blocking actions in addition to its spinal cord alpha2-adrenoceptor-mediated analgesic effects. Xylazine hydrochloride (0.05 mg/kg in 5 mL) diffuses from the

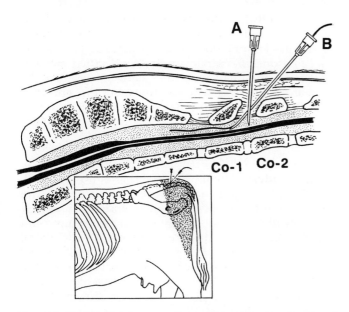

Fig. 16C–17. Needle placement for caudal epidural analgesia and catheterization of the sacral epidural space in cattle. Co1, first coccygeal; Co2, second coccygeal vertebra. Desensitized subcutaneous area after caudal blockade is stippled.

caudal epidural space into the cerebrospinal fluid (CSF) of adult cattle and can produce a degree of subarachnoid nerve root anesthesia.(62) At these doses, xylazine is detectable in bovine CSF at concentrations ranging from 0.2 to 5.1 μg xylazine/mL CSF. Xylazine is not detectable in bovine plasma, however (63), making it doubtful that its presence within the subarachnoid space after epidural administration is secondary to absorption of xylazine from the blood stream.

As might be expected, anesthesia, sedation, and ataxia is a dose-dependent phenomenon when injecting 60, 90, or 120 μg xylazine/kg diluted in 12 mL of 0.9% NaCl epidurally at the sacrococcygeal space in dairy cows (420 kg of body weight). Perineal analgesia lasts 90 to 220 minutes, depending upon the dose, and is limited to the tail, perineum, and hind extremity. High doses (120 μg/kg) extend analgesia to the udder without affecting the flank, along with marked sedation, sternal decubitus, ptyalism, and ptosis.(64) To the contrary, 60, 90, or 120 μg detomidine/kg of body weight diluted in 12 mL of 0.9% NaCl solution fails to produce any analgesia or sedation when it is injected into the epidural space of the sacrococcygeal interspace of dairy cows.(65)

Reducing the dose of xylazine to 0.03 mg/kg of body weight and adding a 2% lidocaine hydrochloride solution to a total volume of 5 mL per adult cow make the mixture of xylazine/lidocaine a more useful epidural anesthetic in cattle for surgical procedure at points more cranial than the perineal region, such as rumenotomy, cesarean section, correction of vaginal or uterine prolapse, repairs of perineal lacerations and rectovestibular fistulae, and removal of vaginal tumors.(66) The xylazine/lidocaine combination extends analgesia as far cranially as the T13 and L1 spinal segments, thereby covering the tail, perineum, udder, and flank areas. Surgical analgesia is attained in 3 to 4 minutes after drug administration and lasts for about 100 minutes with a moderate degree of ataxia occurring.(66)

Caudal epidural anesthesia in sheep and goats can be extremely useful for tail docking in lambs and intravaginal obstetric procedures. A 2.5- to 3.75-cm, 18-gauge needle is inserted epidurally at Co1-Co2 or S5-Co1 (Fig. 16C–19), and no more than 1.0 mL of a 2% lidocaine hydrochloride solution per 50 kg of body weight is injected.(67, 68) Careful aseptic precautions similar to the technique in cattle must be used.

Caudal epidural anesthesia in llamas is used on occasion. Either 2% lidocaine (0.22 mg/kg), or 10% xylazine (0.17 mg/kg) diluted with 2 mL/150 kg of sterile water, or the combination of 2% lidocaine (0.22 mg/kg) and 10% xylazine (0.17 mg/kg) into the epidural space at the sacrococcygeal (S5-Co1) junction in 6 healthy adult male llamas weighing 127 to 154 kg has been assessed (Chapter 20).(69) Time to onset of analgesia, as determined by lack of response to pin prick in the perineal area was not different ($P < 0.05$) between the lidocaine (3.2 ± 0.3 minutes) and lidocaine/xylazine (3.5 ± 0.6 minutes) groups, but both differed from xylazine alone (20.7 ± 3.4 minutes). Duration of anal-

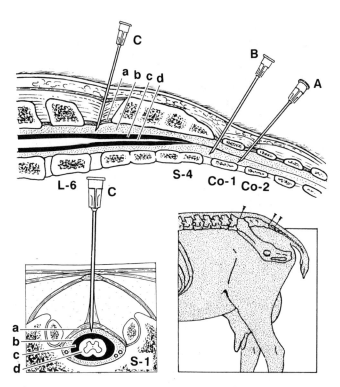

Fig. 16C–19. Needle placement for caudal epidural analgesia (A and B) and lumbosacral epidural analgesia (C) in the goat (L6, sixth lumbar; S4, fourth sacral; Co1, first coccygeal; Co2, second coccygeal vertebra). A cranial view of a transection of the first sacral vertebra at the location of the intervertebral foramen (a, interarcuate ligament; b, epidural space; c, subarachnoid space; d, spinal cord). Desensitized subcutaneous area after anterior epidural anesthesia is stippled.

gesia was different ($P > 0.05$) among all groups: lidocaine 71.0 ± 0.1 minutes; xylazine 186.9 ± 14.9 minutes; and lidocaine/xylazine 225.8 ± 25.4 minutes. Mild sedation was apparent in 4 llamas approximately 20 minutes after epidural xylazine and in 2 llamas after lidocaine/xylazine administration, and lasted approximately 30 minutes. Pulse rate and respiratory rate decreased over time with all drugs, but did not differ between groups, indicating that epidural lidocaine/xylazine administration can safely provide prolonged analgesia in llamas.(69)

CONTINUOUS CAUDAL EPIDURAL ANESTHESIA

Continuous caudal epidural analgesia is used in cattle and sheep with prolapse of the vagina and/or rectum, which provoke severe continuous straining. The technique in cattle is simply achieved by inserting a fine catheter into the epidural space at S5-Co1 or Co1-Co2 through a 7.5-cm, 16- or 17-gauge needle, which is either a thin-walled Huber-point directional needle or a Hustead needle.(70, 71) The skin and needle track are desensitized. After a stab incision on the midline is made to minimize resistance to the passage of the somewhat blunt needle, the spinal needle with stylet in place and bevel directed cranially, is advanced for 5.0 to 8.0 cm while being directed at approximately 45° to vertical, until an abrupt reduction in resistance to needle passage occurs. The stylet from the needle is removed and a test dose of 2.0 to 3.0 mL of anesthetic is injected with almost no resistance, assuring proper placement of the needle in the vertebral canal.

A 30-cm medical-grade vinyl epidural catheter (0.036 cm outside diameter) with gradual markings is introduced into the canal through the needle and advanced cranially 3.0 to 4.0 cm beyond the tip of the needle (Fig. 16C–17). The needle is then withdrawn leaving the catheter in position. Approximately 3 to 5 mL of a 2% lidocaine hydrochloride solution is injected into the catheter at 4- to 6-hour intervals or whenever the animal shows signs of straining. The catheter adapter or 23-gauge needle and three-way stopcock are placed on the free end of the catheter. The catheter can be used for many hours of infusion if it is secured at the skin puncture site with adhesive tape, which is sutured to the skin. The free end of the catheter is maintained sterile by protective sterile gauze (Fig. 16C–20).

Alcohol-epidural injection can be used for long-term demyelinization of nerve roots in sheep and goats. First, only 0.5 to 1.0 mL of a 2% lidocaine hydrochloride solution per 50 kg of body weight is injected epidurally at Co1-Co2 or S5-Co1 and the extent of caudal analgesia is noted to ensure that the level of rostral spread does not extend to the sciatic or femoral nerve roots. After full sensation has returned, a mixture of equal volumes of 70 to 95% ethyl or isopropyl alcohol and 2% lidocaine hydrochloride solution is injected at the same site, using a similar volume of the mixture and injection rate as the previous injection.

Analgesia of the pelvic and perineal area and paralysis of the tail should result and last from a few days to several months, depending upon the time required for remyelinization of the nerves.(72, 73) The alcohol technique is not practical in cattle because the prolonged flaccidity of the tail may lead to buildup of manure and urine in the perineal area with subsequent dermal excoriation and maggot infestation during fly season.(71) The problems of alcohol-epidural anesthesia in sheep and goats with docked tails are similar to but less serious than those in cattle. The chronic flaccid tail may possibly become inflamed, necrotic, and purulent, thus leading to a fly strike in the rectal area. Prolonged rear-limb paralysis may result from overdosing the alcohol-epidural anesthetic, thus demyelinating the sciatic and femoral nerve roots.

SACRAL PARAVERTEBRAL ANESTHESIA

Sacral paravertebral injection is advocated to relieve rectal tenesmus associated with rectal prolapse without sciatic nerve dysfunction. It is associated with minimal risk of the animal's lying down and maintenance of motor function of the tail.(73) Success of the technique depends upon blockade of the pelvic splanchnic nerve (medial hemorrhoidal nerve) and caudal rectal nerve (caudal hemorrhoidal nerve), which supply sensory

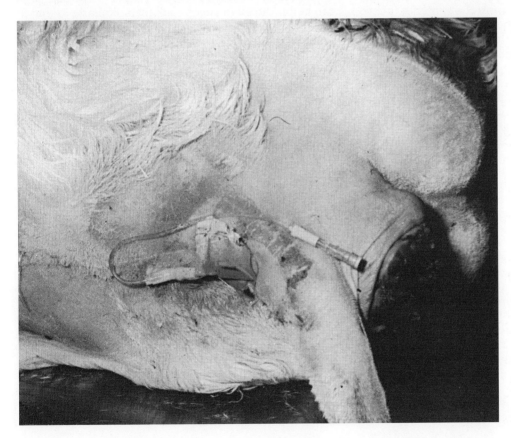

Fig. 16C–20. Epidural catheter with adapter in a calf with rectal prolapse.

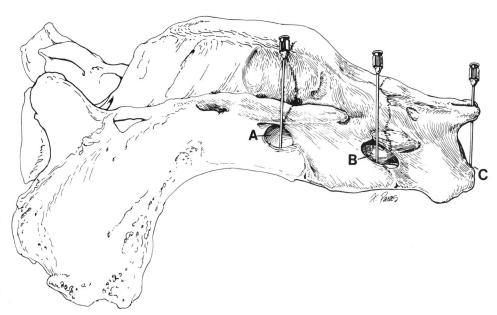

Fig. 16C–21. Needle placement for sacral paravertebral analgesia in cattle. Third (A), fourth (B), and fifth (C) sacral foramen. (From Skarda, R. Techniques of Local Analgesia in Ruminants and Swine. Vet Clin North Am Food Anim Pract 2(3):640, 1986.)

fibers to the anus, vulva, and vagina. The third, fourth, and fifth sacral (S3, S4, and S5) spinal nerves are major components of the pelvic splanchnic and caudal rectal nerves, and are desensitized at the emergence from the sacrum on both sides of the spine in cattle (74) and sheep.(75) In males, S3 supplies motor fibers to the retractor penis muscle and must not be desensitized in order to prevent preputial prolapse. With the animal in standing restraint and good control of anterior, posterior, and lateral movement, the skin of the dorsal sacral area is cleansed and disinfected. Hair removal is optional. The general anatomic site of sacral foramina S3, S4, and S5 is identified approximately 1.0 to 1.5 cm from the dorsal midline of the vertebral crest or usually just lateral to the border of the crest.

Nerve S5 is at the sacrococcygeal (S5-Co1) junction. Nerves S4 and S3 exit from the S4 and S3 foramina, 3.0 cm and 6.0 cm cranial to the S5 foramen in yearling-to-adult cattle. A 5.0- to 7.5-cm, 16- or 18-gauge needle, preferably with stylet, is inserted ventrally to a depth just beyond where it enters the foramen (Fig. 16C–21). A stab incision through the desensitized skin facilitates the insertion procedure of the needle. Five to 10 mL of a 2% lidocaine hydrochloride solution is injected into a 1.0-cm-diameter area within each dorsal foramen to desensitize both the dorsal and ventral rami of that nerve. Anesthesia of the anus, vulva, and vagina can be expected within 10 minutes after completion of injection and may last for approximately 2 hours. No unfavorable sequelae associated with urination and defecation should occur, because urinary bladder sphincter tone and motor function of the tail are maintained, although the motor function of the anal sphincter is slightly reduced.(73) Sensation to the clitoris is unaffected.

Long-term anesthesia (up to 5 weeks) of the sacral area, as determined by observing no avoidance re-

sponses to deep needle prick to skin and muscle, may result from the administration of 1.0 to 2.0 mL of 70 to 95% ethyl or isopropyl alcohol to S3, S4, and S5 without the unfavorable sequelae associated with alcohol-epidural anesthesia.(73) Caudal epidural analgesia with a 2% lidocaine hydrochloride solution greatly facilitates the subsequent alcohol paravertebral technique.

Bilateral sacral (S3, S4, and S5) paravertebral analgesia can be produced in sheep and goats similarly to that in cattle by using a 7.5-cm, 18-gauge needle, except that the volume of lidocaine, alcohol, and alcohol-anesthetic mixture is reduced to 1.0 to 2.0 mL per injection site.

The advantage of sacral paravertebral anesthesia when compared to epidural anesthesia is relief of straining without sciatic nerve dysfunction, thereby maintaining pelvic limb function and maintaining viability of the tail. The disadvantages are technical difficulty and paraphimosis in bulls if S3 is chronically desensitized with alcohol.(73)

DESENSITIZATION OF THE INTERNAL PUDENDAL (PUDIC) NERVES

This technique is used either in the standing male for penile analgesia and relaxation distal to the sigmoid flexure and examination of prolapsed penis (76) or in the standing female for relief of straining due to uterine prolapse or chronic vaginal prolapse.(77) The internal pudendal nerve block is useful in the surgical management of a number of surgical procedures including repair of uterovaginal prolapse; cervicovaginopexy; anorectal prolapse (rectopexy); ablation of anorectal, perianal, and intraanal tumors, polyps, and abscesses; and catheterization for dislodging urethral calculi.(78) The technique involves desensitizing the internal pudendal nerve fibers of the ventral branches (S3 and S4) and the anastomotic branch of the middle hemorrhoidal nerve (S3 and S4), using an ischiorectal fossa approach.

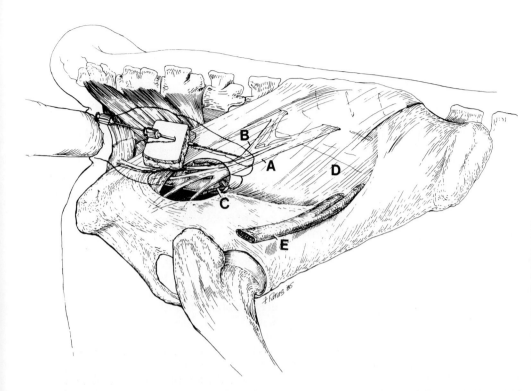

Fig. 16C–22. Needle placement to the internal pudendal nerve in cattle. The position of the hand palpating the internal pudendal nerve (A) on the right side is shown. (B), Caudal rectal nerve; (C), internal pudendal artery; (D), sacrosciatic ligament; (E), sciatic nerve. (From Skarda, R. Techniques of Local Analgesia in Ruminants and Swine. Vet Clin North Am Food Anim Pract 2(3): 641, 1986.)

With cattle restrained in a standing position, the lesser sciatic foramen is identified by rectal palpation as a soft circumscribed depression in the sacrosciatic ligament. The foramen is less than a hand's breadth (5 cm) cranial to the anus. The pulsation of the internal pudendal artery can be felt a finger's width ventral to the internal pudendal nerve in the fossa.

The skin over the ischiorectal fossa on both sides is disinfected and desensitized with 2.0 to 3.0 mL of a 2% lidocaine hydrochloride solution. A 1.25-cm, 14-gauge needle to serve as a cannula for a 8.25-cm, 18-gauge spinal needle is inserted through the desensitized skin. The longer needle is then inserted via cannula for a distance of approximately 5.0 to 7.0 cm in a slightly downward direction until it contacts the internal pudendal nerve at the deepest point of the ischiorectal fossa (Fig. 16C–22). The position of the needle point is verified by rectal digital control. Up to 25 mL of the local anesthetic solution (2 or 3% lidocaine hydrochloride) is injected around the nerve. The needle is then partially withdrawn and directed 2 to 3 cm more caudodorsally, where an additional 10 mL of the anesthetic is deposited at the cranial border of the foramen in order to desensitize the muscular branches and caudal rectal nerve (middle hemorrhoidal nerve).(76, 79) The position of the hands is reversed, and the procedure is repeated on the opposite side of the pelvis. Pudendal nerve block is effective after 30 minutes and should last for 2 to 4 hours. The addition of hyaluronidase (150 IU) and epinephrine (1:10,000) to the local anesthetic reduces the anesthetic required (20 mL) and increases the duration of anesthesia.(80) Success with the pudendal nerve block depends upon locating pelvic landmarks.

A relatively simple technique for approaching the internal pudendal nerve in sheep from the lateral side has been described.(81) A finger is placed into the rectum to locate the slitlike sciatic foramen. A 3.75-cm, 18-gauge needle is then inserted through the corresponding skin site while advancing its point to the foramen. Three to 5 mL of a 2% lidocaine hydrochloride solution are deposited at the foramen. The needle is withdrawn, and the injection site is massaged. The procedure is repeated on the opposite side while keeping the finger in the rectum.

When compared to caudal epidural anesthesia, the advantages of internal pudendal nerve desensitization are maintenance of sciatic nerve function and tail tone, and that the volume of local anesthetic needed to desensitize the nerve supply to the penis by the epidural technique invariably causes posterior paralysis. Ballooning of the vagina may also aid in retention after it is repositioned in the cow with prolapse.(77) The disadvantages of internal pudendal nerve block are lack of cervical analgesia and the necessity of identifying the injection sites by rectal palpation. The bull's penis should be protected from injury by replacing it into the prepuce and taping or purse-stringing the external preputial orifice.(23)

DESENSITIZATION OF THE DORSAL NERVE OF THE PENIS

The dorsal nerve of the penis as it passes over the ischial arch may be desensitized for penile anesthesia and relaxation as an alternative technique to the internal pudendal nerve block.(82) The skin adjacent to the penile body approximately 10 cm ventral to the anus and 2.5 cm from the midline is infiltrated with 2.0 to 3.0 mL of a 2% lidocaine hydrochloride solution, using a fine needle (22-to 25-gauge needle). A 4.0-cm, 20-gauge needle is then inserted through the desensitized skin and advanced for 5.0 to 7.0 cm to contact the pelvic floor. Aspiration assures that the needle tip is not placed into the dorsal artery of the penis. While the needle is withdrawn for approximately 1.0 cm, the region is infiltrated with 20 to 30 mL of 2% lidocaine hydrochloride solution. The procedure is repeated on the opposite side of the penis. Analgesia and paralysis of the penis are expected within 20 minutes and should last for 1 to 2 hours.

Anterior Epidural Anesthesia

INTRODUCTION TO TECHNIQUES

Anterior epidural anesthesia is advocated for all procedures caudal to the diaphragm. The anesthetic solution, dosed at 1.0 mL per 4.5 kg of body weight, is injected into the epidural space either at the lumbosacral (L6-S1) junction (lumbosacral epidural anesthesia) or at the sacrococcygeal (S5-Co1) or first intercoccygeal (Co1-Co2) space, using a larger volume of the anesthetic ranging from 40 mL to 150 mL in adult cattle and 5 mL to 25 mL in calves (high caudal epidural anesthesia). The site for needle placement at the lumbosacral site in lighter immature cattle, sheep, and goats is usually palpable as a depression on the midline caudal to a line joining the anterior border of the ilium on each side (Fig. 16C–19C), so injection is made at this site. The lumbosacral space in swine is the only practical injection site for inducing epidural anesthesia, making lumbosacral epidural block the most commonly used form of regional analgesia in swine. The sacrococcygeal or first intercoccygeal space is the injection site of choice in adult cattle and bulls for producing anterior block because the technique is relatively simple and trauma to the spinal cord and meninges are avoided. These structures end cranial to the site of injection, and the risk of injecting the local anesthetic into the subarachnoid space is almost nonexistent.

Proper techniques by either the lumbosacral or coccygeal approach should provide analgesia of the perineal region, the entire inguinal region, the flanks, and the abdominal wall up to the umbilicus. Cranial spread of the anesthetic affect the pelvic limb function by desensitizing the sixth lumbar (L6) and first and second sacral (S1 and S2) spinal nerves (sciatic supply), the fifth and sixth lumbar (L5 and L6) spinal nerves (obturator and femoral supply), and more cranial nerves. Depending upon the degree involved, the dysfunction of hind limbs ranges from mild ataxia to complete posterior paralysis. Injury (e.g., hip dislocation) during onset (ataxia) or recovery must be avoided and can be prevented if the animals are restrained in sternal recumbency with their hind legs roped together proximal to the tarsus until recovery is complete, as determined by normal tail function. A major

difficulty in producing anterior epidural anesthesia is the uncertainty of the precise extent of paralysis produced. Many factors have been shown to affect the cranial spread of the anesthetic within the epidural space. The major determinants are the size and age of the animal, the presence and size of abdominal mass (pregnancy), and other variables that can be controlled by the anesthetist, namely, positioning the patient, choosing the site of epidural puncture, orientation of the needle bevel, determining the volume and concentration of the anesthetic solution, and speed of injection.(47)

Increasing the dose (volume × concentration) increases the area of blockade. Increasing the volume will improve segmental spread, whereas increasing the concentration will provide a more rapid onset of analgesia and motor blockade, greater frequency of adequate anesthesia, greater depth of motor blockade, and longer duration of analgesia and motor blockade.(47) A greater area of epidural anesthesia may be achieved by a relatively fast injection. However, the advantage of a large segmental area of anesthesia is offset by the high frequency of patient discomfort upon injection because of transient elevation of CSF pressure and a relatively fast vascular and lymphatic absorption of the anesthetic, thereby reducing the duration and increasing the occurrence of incomplete block. Gravity has a more definite role in the spread of subarachnoid anesthesia than in epidural anesthesia; however, with both techniques a more rapid onset to maximal segmental analgesia, a longer duration of effect, and a more intensive motor blockade is achieved on the dependent side. Gravity also allows for perfect unilateral anesthesia in sheep and goats owing to preferential escape of the anesthetic solution toward the paravertebral region. The cephalic spread of anesthesia after epidural or subarachnoid injection of specifically prepared hyperbaric solutions is limited in the animal that is kept in a sitting position. Pregnant animals generally require a reduced dose per kilogram of body weight of the local anesthetic for satisfactory epidural and subarachnoid anesthesia. This may be attributable to decreased volume of the epidural space caused by distension of epidural veins (engorgement), increased sensitivity of neural tissue owing to hormonal changes, and a faulty overestimation of the lean body mass.

Migration of the anesthetic is enhanced by transmission of intraabdominal pressure (pregnancy) and respiratory-induced intrathoracic pressure. Elderly cattle (over 8 years) with progressively occluded intervertebral foramina may require a smaller volume of the anesthetic than younger cattle with open intervertebral foramina.(47)

LUMBOSACRAL EPIDURAL ANESTHESIA IN SWINE

The technique of epidural block is relatively easy to master in well-sedated pigs and is most commonly employed to facilitate cesarean section; repair of rectal, uterine, or vaginal prolapses; repair of umbilical, in-

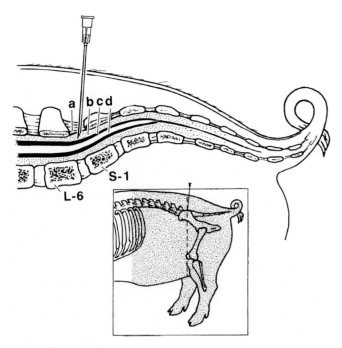

Fig. 16C–23. Needle placement for lumbosacral epidural anesthesia in the pig (L6, sixth lumbar; S1, first sacral vertebra; a, interarcuate ligament; b, epidural space; c, subarachnoid space; d, spinal cord). Desensitized subcutaneous area after epidural anesthesia is stippled.

guinal, or scrotal hernias; surgery of scirrhous cord; and surgery of the prepuce, penis, or rear limbs.(83-86) Epidural anesthesia, however, is contraindicated in pigs with known cardiovascular disease, bleeding disorders, and shock or toxemic syndromes, because of sympathetic blockade and consequent depression of blood pressure.(87) The use of sedatives that produce ataxia, partial recumbency, and hypotension should be avoided. A weighing crate, chute, or hog snare is generally necessary to properly restrain the pig. Chemical restraint is required in some instances. A small pig is restrained on its breast or side, whereas a large sow or boar is preferably injected in the standing position.

The site for the needle placement is on the midline immediately caudal to the spinous process of the last lumbar (L6) vertebra (Fig. 16C–23). The injection site is felt as a palpable depression a distance caudal to the transverse line between the cranial prominences of the wing of the ilium (iliac crest) on either side, 0.5 to 1.5 cm in pigs weighing 10 to 50 kg and 1.5 to 2.5 cm in pigs weighing 50 kg or more. In large pigs in which the iliac wings are not palpable, a vertical line through the patella may be used as a guide to locate the lumbosacral space 2.0 to 3.0 cm caudal to the vertical line.(86, 88, 89) The tissues over the space are thoroughly cleansed, disinfected, and infiltrated with 3 to 5 mL of a 2% lidocaine hydrochloride solution.

A 14-gauge needle can be used for support and guidance of the spinal needle. The appropriate spinal needles used vary between 6 to 8 cm, 20 gauge for pigs weighing 10 to 20 kg and 10 to 16 cm, 18 gauge for pigs weighing over 100 kg. The needle, preferentially with stylet and the bevel directed cranially is inserted at the lumbosacral space using an angle of approximately 20° caudal to the vertical. Penetration depends upon the size and condition of the pig, and may be up to 2 to 4 cm in pigs weighing between 10 and 20 kg and 4 to 10 cm in pigs weighing between 20 and 100 kg. For heavy boars and sows, a 10- to 15-cm spinal needle should be selected. The needle passes through a definite area of resistance as it encounters the interarcuate ligament. Penetration of the ligament by the needle tip is often felt as a slight "pop," and is associated with sudden movements indicating entrance into the vertebral canal. The lumbosacral aperture in the pig is relatively large (1.5 × 2.5 cm) and allows for some margin of error.(83, 90) The subarachnoid space containing CSF is comparatively small at the lumbosacral space, and is not easily penetrated at that site. The spinal cord ends anterior to the sixth lumbar (L6) vertebrae, and is unlikely to be traumatized by the needle.

The dose of anesthetic is calculated by either weight or length of the pig. Anesthesia caudal to the umbilicus can be expected after injecting 1.0 mL of a 2% lidocaine hydrochloride solution per 4.5 kg of body weight at a rate of approximately 1.0 mL per 2 to 3 seconds.(35) Anesthesia should occur within 10 minutes, and recovery should be complete at the end of the second hour. Similar results have been achieved by using a smaller dose, such as 1.0 mL per 7.5 kg for pigs weighing up to 50 kg and an additional 1.0 mL for every 10-kg increase in weight.(83, 89) Good results were obtained for laparotomy of pregnant sows at term using a 2% lidocaine hydrochloride solution with epinephrine (5 to 12.5 μg/mL) and calculating the dosage as 1.0 mL for the first 40 cm of back length as measured from the base of the tail to the occipital protuberance, and an additional 1.5 mL of 2% lidocaine for each additional 10 cm.(91, 92) Regardless of the weight or length, the dose should be adjusted to the condition of the pig and the surgical procedure (Fig. 16C–24). A maximum dose of 20 mL of 2% lidocaine is suggested as the upper limit: 4 mL per 100 kg, 6 mL per 200 kg, and 8 mL per 300 kg of body weight for standing castrations; 10 mL per 100 kg, 15 mL per 200 kg, and 20 mL per 300 kg of body weight for cesarean sections.(90)

The sedative, analgesic, and immobilizing effects of xylazine and detomidine, when injected into the lumbosacral (L6-S1) epidural space of pigs (31 ± 2 kg) using a rate of 1 mL each 2 to 3 seconds, have recently been evaluated and compared during a 2-hour test period.(93) Epidural xylazine (2 mg/kg in 5 mL 0.9% NaCl solution) induces immobilization and bilateral analgesia extending from the anus to the umbilicus within 5 minutes after completion of injection, and persists for at least 120 minutes. Epidural detomidine (500 μg/kg in 5 mL 0.9% NaCl solution) induces sedation and lateral recumbency but minimal analgesia caudal to the umbilicus, within 10 minutes after completion of injection. Atipamezole (200 μg/kg IV) immediately reverses

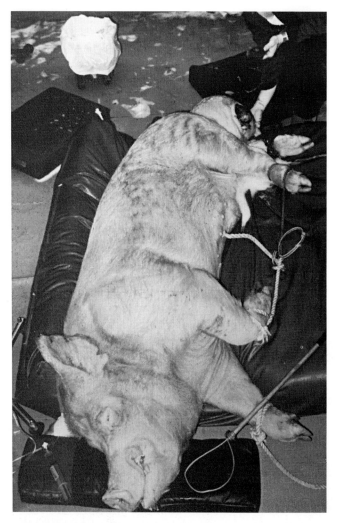

Fig. 16C–24. Restraint of a 3-year-old Yorkshire hog, weighing 325 kg, in lateral recumbency. Anesthesia and relaxation distal to the midthoracic region developed after injection of 20 mL of a 2% lidocaine hydrochloride solution into the epidural space at the lumbosacral intervertebral space. (From Skarda, R. Techniques of Local Analgesia in Ruminants and Swine. Vet Clin North Am Food Anim Pract 2(3):645, 1986.)

xylazine- and detomidine-induced sedation while xylazine-induced analgesia and hind-limb immobilization are not antagonized by atipamezole (Chapter 20).

In large sows undergoing elective cesarean sections, 1 mg/kg of 10% xylazine in 10 mL of 2% lidocaine injected at the lumbosacral space induces excellent analgesia extending from the anus to the umbilicus and produces rear-limb paralysis, as evidenced by a "dog sitting" posture, 5 to 8 minutes after completion of injection. The intravenous administration of 0.003 mL/kg of a Telazol mixture (50 mg/mL) with ketamine (50 mg/mL) and xylazine (50 mg/mL) immobilizes the forequarters. This mixture induces safe immobiliztion of sows. Palpebral and corneal reflexes are maintained

with only minimal changes in heart rate, respiratory rate, and mean arterial blood pressure. The rear limbs may be affected for as long as 7 to 8 hours after epidural injection with the xylazine/lidocaine mixture. Sows are usually able to walk normally 12 hours after completion of surgery. Piglets appeared healthy, without signs of sedation or tranquilization.(94)

The cardiopulmonary and analgesic effects of epidurally administered lidocaine (5 mg/kg of body weight), alfentanil (5 μg/kg), and xylazine (0.2 mg/kg) in pigs anesthetized with 1 to 1.2% end-tidal isoflurane anesthesia has been compared.(95) Lidocaine provides 45 to 60 minutes of analgesia and is associated with significant ($P < 0.05$) decreases in heart rate, respiratory rate, systolic arterial blood pressure, tidal volume, minute volume, core temperature, pHa, PaO_2 and TCO_2 and increases in pulmonary capillary wedge pressure and $PaCO_2$ and HCO_3^- concentration. Epidural alfentanil has no analgesic effect. Epidural xylazine provided 90 minutes of analgesia and decreased core temperature and tidal volume, offering the most desirable actions in isoflurane-anesthetized pigs.(95)

Epidural anesthesia is a good choice in swine with low morbidity and mortality, minimal CNS depression, and rapid recovery being its advantages. A rapid recovery is important for the sow on the farm if she is to nurse pigs or is to be sold for slaughter before other complications develop. A rapid recovery also allows a specific pathogen-free sow to leave the clinic as soon as the piglets do.(96) Epidural anesthesia can also be used with general anesthesia to reduce inhalant or injectable anesthetic requirements.(85)

Lumbosacral epidural anesthesia that extends anterior to the last rib is safe, although complications of major concern may arise from overdose. These include cardiovascular and respiratory collapse, transient loss of consciousness, tremors, convulsions, vomiting, and meningitis associated with septic technique.

ANTERIOR EPIDURAL AND SUBARACHNOID ANESTHESIA IN SMALL RUMINANTS

Anterior analgesia produced by epidural and subarachnoid spinal nerve blocks provide excellent conditions for cesarean section; intraabdominal, pelvic, or hind-limb surgery; and udder surgery in small ruminants. The technique may be accomplished by injecting local anesthetic into either the epidural or subarachnoid space at the lumbosacral intervertebral space.(97-100) With full aseptic precautions, a 6.0- to 7.0-cm, 20-gauge spinal needle with a fitted stylet is inserted on the midline in adult sheep and goats halfway between the last lumbar (L6) and first sacral (S1) vertebrae at approximately 90° to the skin (Fig. 16C–19C). The site for needle placement is usually palpable as a depression on the midline just caudal to a line joining the anterior border of the ilium on each side. Penetration of the interarcuate ligament is often associated with a sudden movement of the animal owing to pain or the lack of resistance either to further needle passage or to the injection of 5 mL of air, indicating that the vertebral space has been entered.

First, an attempt is made to aspirate CSF into a syringe. If CSF is not withdrawn, it can be assumed that the dura has not been punctured, and epidural injection is made with 1.0 mL of a 2% lidocaine hydrochloride solution per 4.5 kg of body weight. Posterior paralysis and anterior analgesia extending a fourth of the distance from the pubis to the umbilicus can be expected within 2 to 10 minutes, lasting as long as 2 hours. The dose of lidocaine recommended for epidural anesthesia in the sheep may vary from as low of 8 to 15 mL of 1.5% lidocaine hydrochloride solution with 1:100,000 epinephrine, depending on the size of the sheep (35), to 1.0 mL of 2% solution per 5.0 kg.(101)

If spinal fluid is aspirated into the syringe or drips from the hub after needle placement, it is obvious that the dorsal epidural space, the dura, and arachnoid meninges have been punctured and the subarachnoid space has been entered. Under these circumstances, half the epidural dose (0.5 mL per 4.5 kg) is injected at a rate of approximately 1.0 mL every 2 to 3 seconds. Posterior paralysis occurs in 1 to 3 minutes. Anesthesia may extend to the last rib, similar to epidural administration of 2% lidocaine but lasting 60 to 90 minutes (Fig. 16C–25). Serious side effects may result from injecting the full epidural dose into the subarachnoid space, thereby diffusing the anesthetic through lumbar, thoracic, cervical, and cranial subarachnoid spaces. Likewise, it is not safe to withdraw the needle from the subarachnoid to the epidural space and proceed with the epidural injection. A dura hole may be patent for many hours, and if spinal anesthesia is considered, a deliberate technique of subarachnoid injection using 1.5 to 2.0 mL of "Heavy Nupercaine" (1:200 Nupercaine in 6% glucose) in adult sheep is recommended.(35)

Gravity, not diffusion of drug in the cerebrospinal fluid, determines the spread of anesthesia. For bilateral anesthesia, the animal is placed on its back immediately after administration of the anesthetic and removal of the needle; for unilateral anesthesia, the animal is maintained in lateral decubitus with its affected side dependent. Although epidural and subarachnoid anesthesia in small ruminants are useful techniques and are easily performed, careful observation of the patients after injection and proper positioning must be considered to avoid complications and fatality.(102)

Complications may arise from faulty anterior epidural and subarachnoid anesthesia and lack of patient management. They are loss of consciousness, convulsions, respiratory paralysis, hypotension, and hypothermia after overdose (98), and possibly headache after dural puncture. Respiratory paralysis is caused by desensitization of motor nerves supplying the intercostal muscle and/or from desensitizing the phrenic nerves supplying the diaphragm. Animals with severe hypotension show signs of distress, collapse, tachycardia

or bradycardia, weak pulse, and shallow, rapid respiration. Therapy is comprised of rapid fluid infusion; raising the animal's hindquarters above the level of the heart to prevent pooling of blood in the hindquarters and to improve venous return, cardiac output, and arterial blood pressure; and supporting respiration by intubation, positive pressure ventilation and oxygen can be initiated. In addition, alpha$_1$-adrenergic agonists (e.g., methoxamine, metaraminol, ephedrine, and phenylephrine) have been recommended to constrict the epidurally or subarachnoidally induced dilation of vascular beds in splanchnic and pelvic viscera and muscles of the pelvic limbs. The routine use of metaraminol (5 mg intramuscularly) during epidural anesthesia in sheep has been advocated, and if hypotension is severe, 5- to 10-mg of methoxamine can be given intravenously.(35) The use of ephedrine in the pregnant ewe is advantageous because it preserves uterine blood flow.(103) Hypothermia is caused by the patient's inability to shiver. Heat lamps and warm blankets are useful in warming patients.

Postoperative analgesia in food animals has not been well studied and is often ignored. There is likely to be further interest in the use of alpha$_2$-adrenoceptor agonists and opioids by epidural and subarachnoid injection for this purpose.(104) For example, clonidine, an alpha$_2$-adrenoceptor agonist, when injected into the epidural space of sheep at a dose of 50 to 75 µg, induces sedation and dose-dependant antinociception to elec-

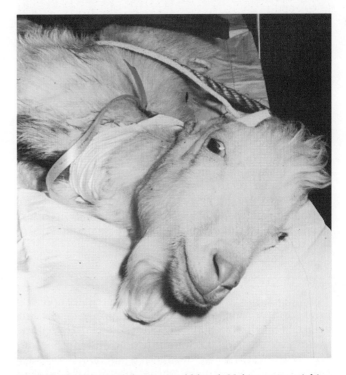

Fig. 16C–25. Restraint of an 8-year old female Nubian goat, weighing 80 kg, in lateral recumbency during lumbosacral epidural anesthesia (amputation of the right hind foot was performed).

tric stimulus applied to the flank of sheep, and does not cause hypotension, respiratory depression, or neurotoxicity.(105, 106)

In a more recent study, morphine (0.1 mg/kg) diluted in 0.9% NaCl solution (0.13 mL/kg) or the same volume of 0.9% NaCl solution was administered into the epidural space at the lumbosacral (L6-S1) junction in 10 halothane-anesthetized goats (21.4 ± 7.7 kg) after replacement of the anterior cruciate ligament with a patellar tendon autograft and immediately before discontinuation of halothane.(107) In general, goats that received epidural morphine were quieter and more sedate, vocalized less, were less likely to grind their teeth, and struggled less during recovery than goats in the control group. Respiratory depression or bloat did not occur during a 9-hour observation period. Heart rate, respiratory rate, arterial blood pressure, pHa, and $PaCO_2$ in goats receiving morphine did not differ significantly ($P < 0.05$) from those given saline, indicating that epidural morphine provides postoperative analgesia and sedation with minimal cardiopulmonary effects in goats.(107)

The opioid antagonist naloxone or alpha$_2$-adrenoceptor antagonist idazoxan has been injected subarachnoidally in sheep prior to the systemic administration of fentanyl or xylazine, respectively. The subarachnoid administration of the antagonists is associated with a 50% reduction in mechanical nociceptive threshold, indicating that spinal alpha$_2$ and mu receptors mediate analgesia produced by systemically administered analgesics.(108)

Teat and Udder Anesthesia of Cows

ANATOMY

The udder is supplied from fibers of the genitofemoral nerves, which have their origin from the third and fourth lumbar spinal cord segments.(109) Cranially, the skin and some glandular tissue of the forequarters are supplied by the ilioinguinal (L2) and iliohypogastric (L1) nerves. Caudally, the udder is supplied by the mammary branch of the pudendal nerve and distal branch of the perineal nerve, which originate from the second, third, and fourth sacral spinal cord segments (Fig. 16C–26). Secretion of the milk is under hormonal control, as there are no secretory nerves to the udder.

INTRODUCTION TO TECHNIQUES

Teat analgesia is required for repair of teat lacerations and injuries that most commonly affect the orifice. For this reason, local anesthesia (ring block, inverted-V block, teat cistern infusion, and intravenous regional anesthesia of the teat) is adequate for most surgical procedures, using either physical restraint or chemical tranquilization.(23, 31, 110) Xylazine on its own as a sedative and analgesic is very effective for minor procedures, but its use in advanced gestation

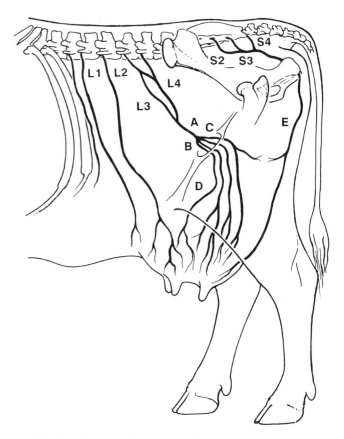

Fig. 16C–26. Schematic illustration of the nerve supply to the cow's udder. A, inguinal nerve; B, internal anterior; and C, posterior inguinal nerves; D, external inguinal nerve; E, perineal inguinal nerve. L$_1$ to L$_4$, ventral branches of the first to fourth lumbar vertebral nerves. S$_2$, S$_3$, S$_4$, ventral branches of the second, third, and fourth sacral vertebral nerves.

may be contraindicated. Standing restraint is advantageous because it prevents udder trauma; however, asepsis and safety to the operator must not be compromised. General anesthesia is rarely necessary for udder surgery except perhaps for udder amputation.

Paravertebral blockade of the first, second, and third lumbar (L1, L2, and L3) spinal nerves or segmental lumbar epidural block of these nerves may be used for surgical procedures of the fore-udder and fore-teats. Both techniques have been described as difficult, and they often result in cows lying down. Using the perineal nerve block in the standing ruminant, surgical procedures of the caudalmost teats and escutcheon areas of the udder may be performed. However, most surgical procedures of the caudal teats and body of the udder require high caudal epidural anesthesia or lumbosacral epidural anesthesia. Both techniques have been described, and there is no advantage to using one technique over the other in performing udder surgery. If high caudal epidural anesthesia is the method used for major udder surgery, up to 150 mL of a 2% lidocaine hydrochloride solution may be required to

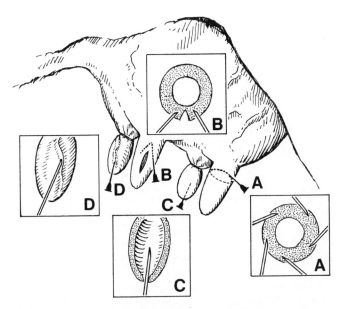

Fig. 16C–27. Needle placement for bovine ring block (A), inverted-V block (B), teat cistern infusion (C), and intravenous regional teat block (D).

extend the analgesia to L1 in adult cows. Analgesia can be expected within 10 to 15 minutes and lasts 60 to 90 minutes.

RING BLOCK OF THE TEAT

After thoroughly cleansing the entire teat and teat base, physical restraint (e.g., holding the nose, using a flank strap, rope around the legs, or dorsal tail elevation) is used. An elastic band may be applied firmly around the base of the teat to prevent diffusion of local anesthetic up into the udder. The tourniquet is not applied for removal of supernumerary teats. A 1.5-cm, 25-gauge needle is inserted subcutaneously transverse to the direction of the teat to deposit 4.0 to 6.0 mL of a 2% lidocaine hydrochloride solution in form of a peripheral ring block (Fig. 16C–27A). The solution is then massaged into the tissues. The technique provides adequate analgesia of the teat distal to the tourniquet within 10 minutes and lasts for approximately 2 hours. Minor procedures such as laceration repair, perforating fistula, nonperforating laceration, wart removal, teat removal in gangrenous mastitis, teat obstruction opening, and fistula and supernumerary teat removal are facilitated when using ring block. The technique is simple and inexpensive, and the cow remains standing. Potential complications are prevented by using aseptic technique and safety during infiltration.

INVERTED-V BLOCK OF THE TEAT

As an alternative to the ring block, a 1.5-cm, 25-gauge needle and 4.0 to 6.0 mL of the local anesthetic solution are used to infiltrate the skin and muscularis of the surgical site, using an inverted-V pattern (Fig. 16C–27B). Adequate analgesia for repairs of lacerations or fistulas

or wart removal in the standing cow is achieved by this technique. Again, physical restraint and tranquilization are required for aseptic technique and safety during infiltration.

TEAT CISTERN INFUSION

Infusion of the teat cistern with local anesthetic is recommended for procedures that require anesthesia of the mucous membrane lining of the cistern. Although the muscularis, subcutaneous layers, and skin are not desensitized by this technique, procedures such as removal of teat polyps, opening of contracted sphincters, and opening of the spider teats, may be facilitated. Combined with adequate physical restraint and chemical tranquilization, the cistern is milked out and the orifice thoroughly cleansed with alcohol. A narrow gauze bandage or suture is placed as high up on the teat as possible to act as a tourniquet, preventing milk entering the teat and diluting the anesthetic agent. To fill the teat, a teat cannula is introduced and approximately 10 mL of a 2% lidocaine hydrochloride solution is infused (Fig. 16C–27C). Anesthesia develops in 5 to 10 minutes; thereafter the remaining lidocaine is milked out and the tourniquet is removed.

INTRAVENOUS REGIONAL ANESTHESIA OF THE TEAT

This technique provides anesthesia of the entire teat distal to a preplaced tourniquet. The technique is best accomplished in a recumbent cow. A tourniquet is placed around the base of the teat as described for teat cistern infusion. Any superficial teat vein distal to the tourniquet may be used for injection of 5 to 7 mL of 2% lidocaine hydrochloride solution or its equivalent, using a 2.5-cm, 22- to 25-gauge needle (Fig. 16A–27D). Digital pressure and gentle massage are applied to the site of injection to prevent hematoma formation. Analgesia of the teat distal to the tourniquet occurs within 3 to 5 minutes and persists for the time the tourniquet is applied. Sensation returns to the teat 5 to 10 minutes after tourniquet removal. Restraint and aseptic technique are critical.

PERINEAL NERVE BLOCK

Desensitization of the perineal nerve facilitates repair of laceration and removal of supernumerary teats or warts in the caudalmost udder or escutcheon area.(109) The nerve is readily desensitized by injecting 5 to 7 mL of a 2% lidocaine hydrochloride solution into the subcutaneous and subfascial tissues at the ischial arch approximately 2 cm lateral to the midline on both sides.(111) The technique does not inhibit wound healing, but it is more difficult technically than local infiltration.

Anesthesia of the Foot

INTRODUCTION TO TECHNIQUES

Anesthesia of the foot may be induced by (a) infiltrating the tissues around the limb with local anesthetic solution (ring block); (b) injecting local anesthetic solution into an accessible superficial vein in an extremity isolated from circulation by placing a tourniquet on the animal's leg (intravenous regional anesthesia); (c) desensitizing specific nerves (regional analgesia, anesthesia of the brachial plexus, and epidural anesthesia); and (d) using general anesthesia in especially fractious animals or procedures requiring complete immobilization for asepsis and safety during operation.

RING BLOCK

Many practitioners consider the ring block or infiltration of local anesthetic from skin to bone, encircling the digit at the junction of the proximal and middle of the metatarsus or metacarpus, to be the most reliable way of anesthetizing the digit.(112) A 2.5-cm, 25-gauge needle may be used to inject approximately 15 mL of a 2% lidocaine hydrochloride solution at several sites: deep and superficial to the flexor tendons and in a partial circle around medially and laterally to the extensor tendons. The area between the anterior and posterior injection sites may be divided into thirds; the anesthetic may be injected at one third to two thirds of the distance between them. The technique does not require precise anatomic knowledge of the limb. The ring block increases the risk of inducing pyogenic bacteria from multiple injection sites, however, and is often only partially successful.

INTRAVENOUS REGIONAL ANESTHESIA

Intravenous regional anesthesia (IVRA) is a simple and safe method for producing analgesia of the digit in cattle, small ruminants, and pigs, substituting for the cumbersome local infiltration or nerve block procedures. It is ideal for digital surgery, in which the amount of bleeding at the surgical site must be decreased. In cattle, the technique involves placing either an elastic bandage, or a tourniquet of stout rubber tubing, or an inflatable cuff (inflation pressure > 200 mm Hg or 26.7 kPa) proximal (113, 114) or distal to the tarsus (114-116), proximal to the elbow (117-119), and proximal (113, 120) or distal to the carpus (116, 121) to obstruct the arterial inflow. In the pelvic limb, a rolled bandage is placed in the depression on either side of the limb between the Achilles tendon and the tibia to increase the pressure on the underlying vessels.(113-115)

IVRA is best performed on the leg of an animal that has been cast and restrained in lateral recumbency with the particular limb uppermost, but alternatively it can be induced in a raised leg of a sedated animal standing.(122) In the thoracic limb, the skin over the prominent common dorsal metacarpal vein, plantar metacarpal vein, or radial vein distal to the tourniquet is clipped, shaved, and disinfected (Fig. 16C–28A). The cranial branch of the lateral saphenous vein or lateral plantar digital vein is a suitable site for injection in the pelvic limb (Fig. 16C–28, B). A 2.5-cm to 3.75-cm, 20- or 22-gauge needle with syringe attached is inserted either in proximal or distal direction as close to the surgical site

as possible. In adult cattle, 30 mL of a 2% lidocaine hydrochloride solution (without epinephrine) is injected as rapidly as possible.(113-116, 120, 123) Smaller volumes (3 to 10 mL) of lidocaine are adequate for IVRA in small ruminants and pigs.(116)

The needle is removed from the vein, and digital pressure and gentle massage are applied to the site of injection to prevent development of subcutaneous hematoma. Anesthesia of the limb distal to the tourniquet develops after 5 minutes, is optimal in 10 minutes, and persists for the period the tourniquet is left in place. Analgesia occurs latest in the interdigital region. Ischemic necrosis, severe lameness, and edema are not expected to occur if the tourniquet is applied for less than 2 hours.(113, 114) Few surgical procedures require this length of time. Usually an operation has been completed in 10 to 30 minutes, when the tourniquet may be safely released. Sensation and motor function return to the leg within 10 minutes after tourniquet release and no signs of cardiovascular or CNS toxicity are likely.(113, 120, 124, 125) After tourniquet removal, partial analgesia may persist for an additional 30 minutes or more. Evidence of lidocaine toxicity has rarely been reported in cattle if the tourniquet has remained in place for 20 minutes or more. Maximal venous plasma concentration of lidocaine after tourniquet release was 1.5 μg/mL (125), which is less than that considered to be toxic.

A measurable concentration of lidocaine in jugular venous blood in buffalo calves (102 ± 9.4 kg) was demonstrated after infusion of 2% lidocaine hydrochloride solution (4 mg/kg body weight) into the dorsal digital vein, in spite of tourniquet occlusion.(126) The lidocaine concentration progressively rose after injection to 2.9 μg/mL and 3.67 μg/mL at 30 minutes and 60 minutes, and was further increased to 6.9 ± 0.9 μg/mL at 5 minutes after tourniquet release. There were no significant changes determined in heart rate, respiratory rate, rectal temperature, systolic, diastolic, mean arterial and central venous blood pressure, arterial pH, PO_2, PCO_2, and HCO_3^- concentration in buffalo calves, suggesting the safety of IVRA in these animals.(126) Salivation, tremors, and rapid pulse have occurred in cattle after early (<20 minutes) tourniquet removal. Lidocaine toxicity in cattle may occur if a large bolus of lidocaine hydrochloride (6 to 8 mg/kg) is injected into the systemic circulation, including CNS symptoms and signs such as convulsions and seizures, profuse salivation, and hypotension. Toxicity in early tourniquet removal is avoided if the tourniquet is loosened for 10 to 15 seconds and retightened for 2 to 3 minutes, and this procedure is repeated several times.(127) In cases of local sepsis in the distal limb in cattle, combined procedures of IVRA and antibiotics have been described.(128) It is advised, however, to limit the dose of sodium-penicillin to 100,000 IU dissolved in 15 to 20 mL of a 2% lidocaine hydrochloride solution in order to prevent thrombosis of the veins distal to the tourniquet.

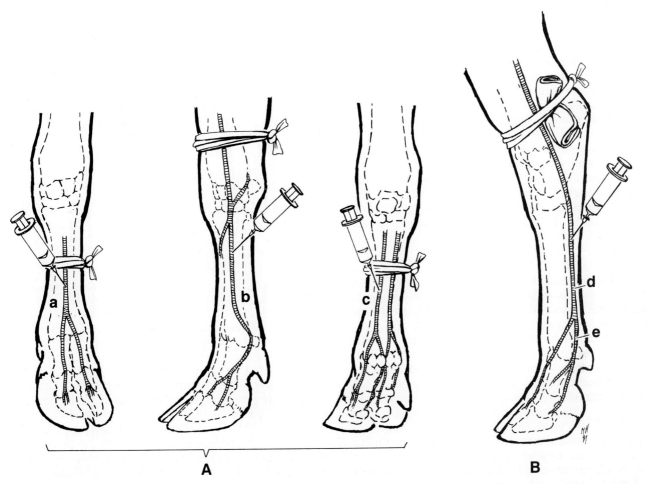

Fig. 16C–28. Tourniquet and needle placement for intravenous regional analgesia of the bovine forelimb (A) and rearlimb (B): (a) dorsal metacarpal vein (dorsal view); (b) radial vein (medial view); (c) plantar metacarpal vein (palmar view); (d) cranial branch of lateral saphenous vein; (e) lateral plantar digital vein.

Swelling of the forelimb and long-lasting (25 days) lameness in 18% of a group of water buffalo calves (85 to 100 kg of body weight) has been reported after IVRA, when 400,000 I.E. benzyl-penicillin was diluted in 12 to 15 mL of a 8 to 12% procaine-hydrochloride solution and injected into the radial vein distal to a tourniquet.(117) It is possible that microthrombosis of digital veins was produced in these animals by salt formation of procaine- and benzyl-penicillin.(129) In any case, animals should be carefully observed for changes in respiratory and pulse rates during the first 10 minutes after tourniquet release.

Advantages of IVRA when compared to ring block or regional nerve blocks are that it requires no precise anatomic knowledge of the limb, only a single injection is made, thereby reducing tissue trauma, contamination of fascial planes or tendon sheaths, and time required for producing digital analgesia. In addition, the amount of bleeding at the surgical site is decreased during application of the tourniquet. The disadvantages of IVRA are an approximately 7% inexplicable failure

rate with particular lack of analgesia in the interdigital area, even when the technique is performed correctly without hematoma formation at the puncture site.

Regional Anesthesia of the Thoracic Limb

BRACHIAL PLEXUS BLOCK

Anesthesia of the brachial plexus in cattle can be achieved by desensitizing the ventral roots of the sixth, seventh, and eighth cervical (C6, C7, and C8) and first and second thoracic (T1 and T2) spinal nerves as they pass over the lateral aspect of the middle third of the first rib, thereby inducing loss of sensation distal and including the elbow joint.(82) The skin puncture site is 12 to 14 cm cranial to the acromion of the scapula and lymph node. This area is surgically scrubbed and infiltrated with 2 to 3 mL of local anesthetic solution. The animal's head is held away from the side to be injected. A 16-cm, 18-gauge needle, preferably with stylet, is inserted through the desensitized area and pushed horizontally or 5° ventrocaudally until it impinges at the lateral surface of the first rib, where approximately 10 mL of a 1 or 2% lidocaine hydrochloride solution containing 1:200,000 epinephrine (to delay absorption and diminish the risk of toxicity) or equivalent are injected. The needle is first withdrawn 5 to 10 cm, then its tip is redirected 1.5 cm more distal to the first injection site, where an additional 10 mL of the anesthetic are deposited. Two to three more injections are made similarly, until a band of anesthetic 6 to 8 cm long has been injected along the rib and ventral to the initial site. The needle is correctly placed if there is no air, blood, or cerebrospinal fluid upon needle aspiration. Onset of analgesia and loss of motor power are gradual, with maximal effects achieved 15 to 20 minutes after injection and lasting 90 to 120 minutes.

DIGITAL NERVE BLOCK

The nerves in the digits of cattle are not easily located distal to the carpus and tarsus because of tense skin and subcutaneous fibrous tissue. However, desensitization of individual nerves can be accomplished.

To produce analgesia distal to the carpus, the median nerve, the ulnar nerve, the medial antebrachial nerve (a cutaneous branch of the musculocutaneous nerve), and the dorsal antebrachial nerve (a cutaneous branch of the radial nerve) must be desensitized.(8, 82, 130) Local infiltration of the skin and subcutis can be used effectively, where massive extensive muscle mass proximal to the carpus prohibits perineural injection.

The median nerve may be desensitized by injecting 10 to 20 mL of a 2% lidocaine hydrochloride solution beneath the fascia approximately 5 cm distal to the elbow anterior to the flexor carpi radialis muscle on the posterior radius. The nerve lies deep, but it can be palpated and perineurally infiltrated at that site, using a 5-cm, 18- to 20-gauge needle (Fig. 16C–29C).

The ulnar nerve can occasionally be palpated approximately 10 cm (a hand's breadth) above the accessory carpal bone at the posterolateral (volarlateral) surface of the radius. Approximately 5 mL of a 2% lidocaine hydrochloride solution is injected underneath the superficial fascia in a groove between the flexor carpi ulnaris and ulnaris lateralis muscle, using a 5-cm, 20-gauge needle (Fig. 16C–29B). The resulting median and ulnar nerve blocks desensitize the medial-posterior aspect of the metacarpus and posterior aspect of the digits.(82) The medial and dorsal antebrachial nerves supply sensory fibers to the medial and dorsal aspect of the carpus and, in conjunction with the median and ulnar nerves, the limb distal to the carpus. The cutaneous medial and dorsal antebrachial nerves may be desensitized anteriorly approximately 10 cm above the carpus by injection of 20 mL of a 2% lidocaine hydrochloride solution in a band 4 to 6 cm wide adjacent to the dorsal radius just anterior to the cephalic vein (Fig. 16C–29A).

Alternatively, it is possible to produce anesthesia from

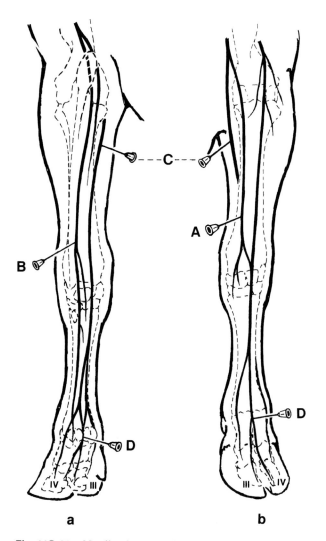

Fig. 16C–29. Needle placement for desensitizing the musculocutaneous (A), ulnar (B), median (C), and axial digital III and IV (D) nerves of the left forelimb in cattle (a, caudolateral; b, dorsomedial aspect).

the mid metacarpus distally, by desensitizing four nerves at the midmetacarpal area (four-point block): the dorsal metacarpal nerve (a superficial branch of the radial nerve), the medial palmar nerve (a continuation of the median nerve), and the dorsal and palmar branches of the ulnar nerve.(131) A 1.25-cm, 22-gauge needle may be used to inject 5 mL of a 2% lidocaine hydrochloride solution at each site. The point of the needle is directed proximally to prevent breaking of the needle in the event the animal should kick and pull the leg away. The dorsal metacarpal nerve is desensitized by subfascial injection of the anesthetic medial to the medial digital extensor tendon (Fig. 16C–30A). The medial palmar nerve is desensitized at the medial aspect of the superficial flexor tendon in the groove between the superficial flexor tendon and the suspensory ligament (Fig. 16C–30B). The dorsal branch and the lateral palmar branch of the ulnar nerve are desensitized by perineural infiltration on the lateral aspect of the limb

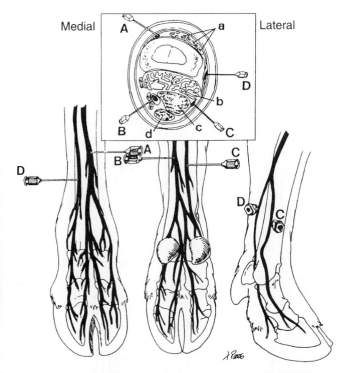

Medial / Lateral

Fig. 16C–30. Needle placement for midmetacarpal nerve blocks on the right forefoot in cattle: Dorsal metacarpal nerve (A), medial palmar nerve (B), lateral palmar branch of ulnar nerve (C), dorsal branch of ulnar nerve (D): d, dorsal aspect, p, palmar, l, lateral, and cross-sectional aspect. Insert: a, extensor tendons; b, interosseus ligament; c, deep digital flexor tendons; d, superficial digital extensor tendon. (From Skarda, R. Techniques of Local Analgesia in Ruminants and Swine. Vet Clin North Am Food Anim Pract 2(3):655, 1986.)

just anterior and posterior to the suspensory ligament (Fig. 16C–30C and D).

ANESTHESIA OF THE INTERDIGITAL REGION

For interdigital anesthesia of the front and hind foot, the branches of the medial dorsal and palmar (plantar) axial digital nerves must be desensitized. Using a 5-cm, 16- or 18-gauge needle, 5 to 10 mL of a 2% lidocaine hydrochloride solution are injected at a depth of 3.5 to 5 cm to infiltrate the soft region proximal to the junction of the claws on both the dorsal and volar aspects of the first phalanx (pastern) (Fig. 16C–29D).(23) This method should adequately desensitize all the dorsal and palmar (plantar) axial digital nerves for removal of interdigital fibromas (corns). Alternatively, it is possible to insert a 10-cm, 18-gauge needle at a 90° angle to the skin on the dorsum of the pastern and to infiltrate the middle of the interdigital space from a single injection site using 15 to 20 mL of the anesthetic solution.

Regional Anesthesia of the Pelvic Limb

Little emphasis upon nerve blocks of the pelvic limb in cattle has been given because IVRA and epidural anesthesia may be conveniently used for anesthesia of the hind legs. Regional anesthesia of the tarsus and

distally can be produced by desensitizing the common peroneal nerve and tibial nerve.(132) Both nerves are continuations of the sciatic nerve.(111) A 3- to 5-cm, 18- to 20-gauge needle with approximately 20 mL of a 2% lidocaine hydrochloride solution are used at each site, inducing anesthesia within 10 to 20 minutes. The common peroneal nerve is desensitized just caudal to the posterior edge of the lateral condyle of the tibia deep to the aponeurotic sheath of the biceps femoris muscle (Fig. 16C–31A). The tibia nerve is desensitized at a point approximately 10 cm above the tuber calcis between the gastrocnemius tendon and the deep digital flexor tendon on the medial aspect of the limb (Fig. 16C–31B). Alternatively, anesthesia distal to the tarsus is produced by desensitizing four nerves (four-point block): the lateral and medial plantar metatarsal nerves (both are continuations of the tibial nerve) and the superficial and deep branches of the peroneal nerve.(82, 130, 131, 133) The superficial peroneal nerve lies superficial to the extensor tendons, the deep peroneal nerve lies deep on the metatarsus; the lateral and medial plantar metatarsal nerves lie superficial in a fibrous sheath containing artery and vein lateral and medial to the flexor tendons, respectively. A 2.5-cm, 22-gauge needle with approximately 5 mL of a 2% lidocaine hydrochloride solution is used at each site, just above the middle of the junction between the proximal and middle third of the metatarsus.

The superficial peroneal nerve is desensitized subcutaneously on the dorsal surface of the metatarsal bone in the proximal third of the metatarsus (Fig. 16C–32A). The deep peroneal nerve is desensitized in the mid-metatarsal region beneath the extensor tendons (Fig. 16C–32B). Traditionally, the deep peroneal nerve is approached by placing a 22-gauge needle under the extensor tendons from the lateral side. Alternatively, a 2.5-cm, 25-gauge needle can be placed from dorsal through the extensor tendon, and using slow injection with considerable pressure. Penetration of the dorsal metatarsal artery must be avoided.

The medial and lateral plantar metatarsal nerves are desensitized approximately 5 cm above the fetlock in the groove between the suspensory ligament and flexor tendons on the medial and lateral aspect of the limb (Fig. 16C–32C and D). Adequate analgesia for claw-amputation can be expected after the four-point block. However, if sensation to the bulb of the heels after injection still remains, it is advisable to repeat the perineural infiltration not only of the lateral and medial plantar metatarsal nerves, but also of the deep peroneal nerve, which supplies sensory fibers to the interdigital area and bulb of the heels.

The advantages of specific nerve blocks in the foot as compared with general anesthesia are fewer complications associated with regional anesthesia and immediate ambulation of the animal after surgery. The most obvious disadvantage of regional anesthesia is that it requires a good knowledge of the anatomy of the region. Multiple injections are required for each region.

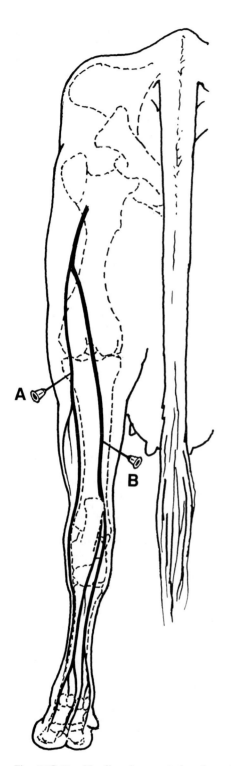

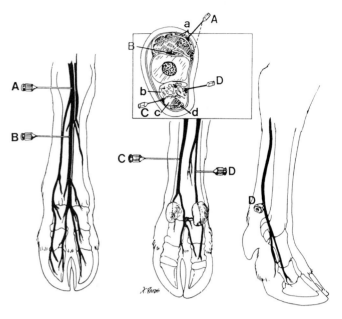

Fig. 16C–32. Needle placement for midmetatarsal nerve blocks on the right hind foot in cattle: superficial peroneal nerve (A), deep peroneal nerve (B), medial plantar metatarsal nerve (C), lateral plantar metatarsal nerve (D): d, dorsal, p, plantar, l, lateral aspect (a, extensor tendons; b, interosseus ligament; c, deep digital flexor tendon; d, superficial digital flexor tendon). (From Skarda, R. Techniques of Local Analgesia in Ruminants and Swine. Vet Clin North Am Food Anim Pract 2(3):657, 1986.)

of the local anesthetic into inflamed tissue, which is often painful, ineffective, and can cause the spread of infection or absorption of toxins.

INTRAARTICULAR ANESTHESIA

Arthrocentesis may be considered for diagnostic work in conjunction with examination of joint fluid, but intraarticular analgesia is seldom used.(134)

Anesthesia for Castration

Castration of bulls, sheep, goats, and pigs is one of the most commonly performed surgical procedures in general practice. The operation may be performed by using chemical restraint and regional anesthesia in either the standing or cast position, or using general anesthesia induced by intravenous or intratesticular injection of a barbiturate or dissociative (Chapter 20). The choice of method to be used largely depends upon the species and the opportunity to observe the animal following castration. Regional anesthesia can be induced by intratesticular injection of local anesthetic solution in all food animals.

The scrotum should be cleansed with a detergent antiseptic solution, and the proposed line of incision subcutaneously infiltrated with 3 to 5 mL of a 2% lidocaine hydrochloride solution. The anesthetic is injected as the skin is tensed over the testicle and is pulled on the needle.

Fig. 16C–31. Needle placement for desensitizing the common peroneal nerve (A) and tibial nerve (B) in cattle. Caudal aspect.

Analgesia is often incomplete, probably owing to anastomotic, collateral, or recurrent nerve branches.(133) General anesthesia may be advantageous in fractious animals that require complete immobilization. In addition, general anesthesia avoids the necessity of injection

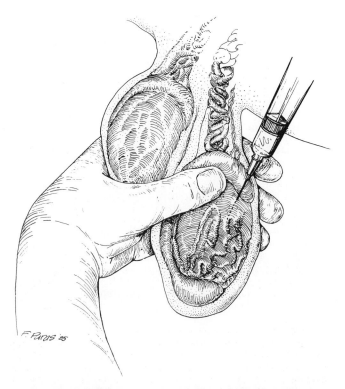

F. Puras '85

Fig. 16C–33. Needle placement for right testicular injection in a bull calf. (From Skarda, R. Techniques of Local Analgesia in Ruminants and Swine. Vet Clin North Am Food Anim Pract 2(3):659, 1986.)

In bulls and boars, a 3.75- to 7.5-cm, 16- to 18-gauge needle is first inserted through the skin below the tail of the epididymis and is then pushed quickly into the center of the testicle using an angle of approximately 30° from perpendicular without puncturing the side or bottom (Fig. 16C–33). Ten to 15 mL of the anesthetic per 200 kg of body weight are injected into the substance of each testicle. The anesthetic is said to quickly enter lymph vessels and to desensitize the sensory fibers in the spermatic cord.(135)

In bull calves, rams, and bucks, a smaller needle (2.5- to 3.75-cm, 20-gauge) is used to allow easy flow between 2 to 10 mL, depending on the size of the animal, of a 2% lidocaine hydrochloride solution to the center of the testicle and to minimize backflow through the needle tract. The bulk of the anesthetic quickly passes from the testes up the spermatic cord via the lymph vessels into the blood, so an excessive dose must be avoided or intoxication will occur. Intratesticular injection of 3 to 15 mL of a 2% lidocaine hydrochloride solution can be satisfactory for castration in male pigs up to approximately 5 months of age. Additionally, 2 to 5 mL of the anesthetic is injected subcutaneously beneath the scrotum as the needle is withdrawn. General anesthesia, however, is more suitable for older pigs.

INTRATESTICULAR INJECTION OF CHEM-CAST

A sclerosing agent (chem-cast) may be painlessly injected into the testes of bull calves weighing less than 70 kg in order to destroy the testicular tissue within 60 to 90 days without edema, hemorrhage, or unacceptable necrosis.(136) The recommended dose is 1.0 mL per testicle in calves weighing up to 45 kg and 1.5 mL per testicle in calves weighing 46 to 68 kg. As compared with surgical castration and mechanically crushing the cord (Burdizzo method), chemical castration is simple and fast; it lacks the high risk of infection associated with surgical castration, and it contributes to improved weight gain. There is no withdrawal time for nontesticular tissues obtained from calves treated with chemcast.(136)

Conclusion

Presently, sufficient clinical work has been done to establish the usefulness, safety, and limitations of local and regional anesthesia techniques in ruminants and swine. Generally speaking, the rational use of 2% lidocaine hydrochloride solution provides economic and good intraoperative analgesia with rapid recovery and minimal side effects.

References

1. Ames NK, Riebold TW. Anesthesia in cattle. Proc 11th Annu Conv Am Assoc Bovine Pract, 1978:75–77.
2. Thurmon JC, Benson GF. Anesthesia in ruminants and swine. In: Howard J, ed. Current veterinary therapy, food animal practice. Philadelphia: WB Saunders, 1981:58–89.
3. Trim CM. Sedation and general anesthesia in ruminants. Bovine Pract 16:137–144, 1981.
4. Cox VS, McGrath CJ, Jorgensen SE. The role of the downer cow syndrome. Am J Vet Res 43:26–31, 1982.
5. Skarda RT. Techniques of local analgesia in ruminants and swine. Vet Clin North Am Food Anim Pract. Philadelphia: WB Saunders, 2:621–663, 1986.
6. Booth NH. Local anesthetics. In: Jones LH, Booth NH, McDonald LE, eds. Veterinary pharmacology and therapeutics, 4th ed. Ames, IA: Iowa State University Press, 1977:417–436.
7. Heavner JE. Local anesthetics. Vet Clin North Am 3:209–221, 1981.
8. Lumb WV, Jones EW. Veterinary anesthesia, 2nd ed. Philadelphia: Lea & Febiger, 1984.
9. Link RP, Smith JC. Comparison of some local anesthetics in cattle. J Am Vet Med Assoc 129:306–309, 1956.
10. Moore DC. An evaluation of hyaluronidase in local and nerve block analgesia: a review of 519 cases. Anesthesiology 11:470–484, 1950.
11. Watson D. Hyaluronidase. Br Anaesth 71:422–425, 1993.
12. Hare WCD. A regional method for the complete anaesthetization and immobilization of the bovine eye and its associated structures. Can J Comp Med 21:228–234, 1957.
13. Rubin LF, Gelatt KN. Analgesia of the eye. In: Soma LR, ed. Veterinary anesthesia. Baltimore: Williams & Wilkins, 1971:489–499.
14. Cust RE. Anaesthesia and akinesia. In: Blogg JR, ed. The eye in veterinary practice. North Melbourne, Australia: VS Supplies, 1975:169–178.
15. Maksimovic B. Akinesie des M. orbicularis palpebrum bei Rindern. Vet Arch 20:75–78, 1950.
16. Schreiber J. Die anatomischen Grundlagen der Leitungsanästhesie beim Rind. I. Die Leitungsanästhesie der Kopfnerven. Wien Tierärztl Wochenschr 42:129–153, 1955.
17. Gibbons WJ. Local anesthesia in bovine practice. Mod Vet Pract 40:36–39, 1959.

18. Gabel AA. Practical technics for bovine anesthesia. Mod Vet Pract 45:39–44, 1964.
19. Elmore RG. Food-animal regional anesthesia. Bovine blocks: ocular. Vet Med Small Anim Clin 75:1760–1762, 1980.
20. Monke DR. Local nasal anesthesia in the bull. Vet Med Small Anim Clin 76:389–393, 1981.
21. Browne TG. The technique of nerve-blocking for dehorning cattle. Vet Rec 50:1336–1337, 1938.
22. Wheat JD. New landmark for cornual nerve block. Vet Med 45:29–30, 1950.
23. Elmore RG. Food-Animal regional anesthesia. Edwardsville, KS: Veterinary Medicine Publishing, 1981.
24. Vitums A. Nerve and arterial blood supply to the horns of the goat with reference to the sites of anesthesia for dehorning. J Am Vet Med Assoc 125:284–286, 1954.
25. Spoulding CE. Procedures for dehorning the dairy goat. Vet Med Small Anim Cin 72:228–230, 1977.
26. Baker JS. Dehorning goats. Bovine Pract 2:33–39, 1981.
27. Lauwers H, DeVos NR. The nerve-supply of the horn of the ox with regards to the course of the ophthalmic nerve. Vlaams Diergeneeskundig Tijdschrift 35:451–464, 1966.
28. Butler WF. Innervation of the horn region in domestic ruminants. Vet Rec 80:490–492, 1967.
29. Peterson DR. Nerve block of the eye and associated structures. J Am Vet Med Assoc 118:145–148, 1951.
30. Wallace CE. Cosmetic dehorning. In: Amstutz HE, ed. Bovine medicine and surgery, 2nd ed., vol. II. Santa Barbara, CA: American Veterinary Publications, 1980:1240.
31. Gibbons WJ, Catcott EJ, Smithcors JF, eds. Bovine medicine and surgery. Wheaton, IL: American Veterinary Publishing, 1970.
32. Oehme FW, Prier JE, eds. Textbook of large animal surgery. Baltimore: Williams & Wilkins, 1974.
33. Morishima HO, Pedersen H, Finster M, et al. Toxicity of lidocaine in adult, newborn, and fetal sheep. Anesthesiology 55:57–61, 1981.
34. Farquharson J. Paravertebral lumbar anesthesia in the bovine species. J Am Vet Med Assoc 97:54–57, 1940.
35. Hall LW, Clarke KW. Veterinary anaesthesia, 9th ed. Eastbourne, East Sussex: Balliere Tindall, 1991.
36. Arnold JP, Kitchell RL. Experimental studies of the innervation of the abdominal wall of cattle. Am J Vet Res 18:229–240, 1957.
37. Cakala S. A technique for the paravertebral lumbar block in cattle. Cornell Vet 51:64–67, 1961.
38. Arthur GH. Some notes on a preliminary trial of segmental epidural anesthesia of cattle. Vet Rec 68:254–256, 1956.
39. Buchholz JH. Beitrag zur extraduralen Anästhesie bei den Haustieren unter besonderer Berücksichtigung der Frage, ob die Injektionsstelle für die extradurale Anästhesie kranialwärts verschoben werden kann [Master's Thesis]. University of Giessen, Germany, 1948.
40. Dogliotti AM. A new method of block anesthesia. Segmental peridural spinal anesthesia. Amer J Surg 20:107–118, 1933.
41. Gutiérrez A. Anesthesia metamerica peridural. Rev Chir B Aires 11:665–685, 1932.
42. Skarda RT, Muir WW. Segmental lumbar epidural analgesia in cattle. Am J Vet Res 40:52–57, 1979.
43. Heeschen W. Erfahrungen mit der lumbalen Extraduralanästhesie (Segmentalanästhesie) bei Laparatomien am stehenden Rind. Dtsch Tierärztl Wochenschr 6:146–152, 1968.
44. Skarda RT, Muir WW, Ibrahim AL. Spinal fluid concentration of mepivacaine in horses and procaine in cows after thoracolumbar subarachnoid analgesia. Am J Vet Res 46:1020–1024, 1985.
45. Skarda RT, Yeary RA, Muir WW, et al. Appearance of procaine in spinal fluid during segmental epidural analgesia in cows. Am J Vet Res 42:639–646, 1981.
46. Skarda RT, Muir WW. Hemodynamic effects of unilateral segmental lumbar epidural analgesia in cattle. Am J Vet Res 40:645–650, 1979.
47. Skarda RT. Lumbar epidural and subarachnoid analgesia in cattle, horses, and humans: a comparative study. Habilitationsschrift, University of Zürich, Switzerland, 1984.
48. Skarda RT, Muir WW, Hubbell AEJ. Comparative study of continuous lumbar segmental epidural and subarachnoid analgesia in Holstein cows. Am J Vet Res 50:39–44, 1989.
49. Skarda RT, Muir WW. Segmental thoracolumbar subarachnoid analgesia in cows. Am J Vet Res 42L:632–638, 1981.
50. Skarda RT, Muir WW. Effects of segmental subarachnoid analgesia on arterial blood pressure, gas tensions and pH in adult conscious cows. Am J Vet Res 42:1747–1750, 1981.
51. McLeod WM, Frank ER. A preliminary report regarding epidural analgesia in equines and bovines. J Am Vet Med Assoc 72:327–335, 1928.
52. Skarda RT, Muir WW. Hemodynamic and respiratory effects of segmental subarachnoid analgesia in adult Holstein cows. Am J Vet Res 43:1343–1348, 1982.
53. Brown S. Fractional segmental spinal anesthesia in poor risk surgical patients. Report of 600 cases. Anesthesiology 13:416–428, 1952.
54. Numans SR, Havinga E. Die Wirkungsweise der Lokalanästhetika bei der Epiduralinjektion. Rec Trav Chim 62:497–502, 1943.
55. Hopkins GS. The correlation of anatomy and epidural analgesia in domestic animals. Cornell Vet 25:263–270, 1935.
56. Elmore RG. Food-animal regional anesthesia. Bovine blocks: Epidural. Vet Med Small Anim Clin 75:1017–1029, 1980.
57. Rülcker C. Lignocaine hydrochloride with and without adrenaline for epidural analgesia in cattle. Vet Rec 77:1180–1182, 1965.
58. Riebold TW, Hawkins JK, Crisman RO. Effect of buffered lidocaine on epidural anesthesia in cattle. In: Animal pain. CE Short, AV Poznak, eds. New York: Churchill Livingstone, 1992:303–306.
59. Caron JP, LeBlanc PH. Epidural analgesia in cattle using xylazine [Abstract]. Proc Am Coll Vet Anesth, San Francisco, 1988.
60. St. Jean, Skarda RT, Muir WW, et al. Caudal epidural analgesia induced by xylazine administration in cows. Am J Vet Res 51:1232–1236, 1990.
61. Skarda RT, St Jean G, Muir WW. Influence of tolazoline on caudal epidural administration of xylazine in cattle. Am J Vet Res 51:556–560, 1990.
62. Skarda RT, Muir WW. The physiologic responses after caudal epidural administration of xylazine in cattle and detomidine in horses. In: Animal pain. CE Short, AV Poznak, eds. New York: Churchill Livingstone, 1992:24034.
63. Skarda RT, Sams RA, St Jean G. Plasma and spinal fluid concentrations of xylazine in cattle after caudal epidural injection [Abstract]. Proc Annu Mtg Am Coll Vet Anesth, New Orleans, Louisiana 1989:37.
64. Gomez de Segura IA, Tendillo FJ, Marsico F, et al. Alpha-2 as a regional anaesthetic in the cow. Proc 4th Intl Cong Vet Anaesth, Utrecht, The Netherlands, 1991:111.
65. Gomez de Segura IA, Tendillo FJ, Marsico F, et al. Alpha-2 agonists for regional anaesthesia in the cow. J Vet Anaesth 20:32–33, 1993.
66. Nowrouzian I, Ghamsari SM. Field trials of xylazine/lidocaine HCL via epidural in cows. Proc 4th Intl Congr Vet Anaesth, Utrecht, The Netherlands, 1991:365.
67. Linzell JL. Some observations on general and regional anaesthesia in goats. In: Graham-Jones O, ed. Small animal anaesthesia. London: Pergamon Press, 1964.
68. Bradley WA. Epidural analgesia for taildocking in lambs. Vet Rec 79:787–788, 1966.
69. Grubb TL, Riebold TW, Huber MJ. Evaluation of lidocaine, xylazine, and a lidocaine/xylazine combination for epidural anesthesia in the Llama [Abstract]. Vet Surg 22(1):88, 1993.
70. Bierschwal CJ. A technic for continuous epidural anesthesia in the bovine. Vet Med 55:44–46, 1960.
71. Elmore RG. Food-animal regional anesthesia. Bovine blocks: continuous epidural analgesia. Vet Med Small Anim Clin 75:1174–1176, 1980.
72. Kuzucu EY, Derrick WS, Wilber SA. Control of intractable pain with subarachnoid alcohol block. J Am Med Assoc 195:541–544, 1966.

73. Noordsy JL. Sacral paravertebral alcohol nerve block as an aid in controlling chronic rectal tenesmus in cattle. Vet Med Small Anim Clin 77:797–801, 1982.

74. Adjanju JB. Alcohol block of the distal ventral sacral nerves of the bovine species as a method of controlling rectal tenesmus [Master's Thesis]. Manhattan, KS: Kansas State University, 1975.

75. Noordsy JL. Bovine surgery 1976. Proc 9th Intl Cong Cattle Dis, Paris, France, 1976:21–30.

76. Larson LL. The internal pudendal (pudic) nerve block for anesthesia of the penis and relaxation of the retractor penis muscle. J Am Vet Med Assoc 123:18–27, 1953.

77. Deshmukh SE, Deshpande KS. Internal pudendal nerve block in cows. Indian Vet J 57:73–75, 1980.

78. Misra SS. Studies on clinical use of pudic-nerve block in bovine. Proc 4th Intl Cong Vet Anaesth, Utrecht, The Netherlands, 1991:108.

79. Habel RE. A source of error in the bovine pudendal nerve block. J Am Vet Med Assoc 128:16–17, 1956.

80. Bhokre AP, Deshpande KS. Experimental study on effect of hyaluronidase in pudic nerve block in bovines. Indian Vet J 56:872–874, 1979.

81. McFarlane IS. The lateral approach to the pudendal nerve block in the bovine and ovine. J S Afr Vet Assoc 34:73–76, 1963.

82. Westhues M, Fritsch R. Animal Anesthesia, vol. 1. London: Oliver and Boyd, 1964:171–181.

83. Getty R. Epidural anesthesia in the hog–its technique and applications. Am Vet Med Assoc Sci Proc 100th Annu Mtg, New York, 1966:88–98.

84. Booth NH. Anesthesia in the pig. Fed Proc 28:1547–1552, 1969.

85. Runnels LJ. Practical anesthesia and analgesia for porcine surgery. Proc Am Assoc Swine Pract, March:80–87, 1976.

86. Elmore RG. Food-animal regional anesthesia. Porcine blocks: lumbosacral (epidural). Vet Med Small Anim Clin 76:387–388, 1981.

87. Benson GJ, Thurmon JC. Anesthesia of swine under field conditions. J Am Vet Med Assoc 174:594–596, 1979.

88. Anderson IL. Anaesthesia in the pig. Aust Vet J 49:474–477, 1973.

89. Trim CM. Epidural analgesia in swine. Vet Anesth 8:23–25, 1980.

90. Eibl K. Die Lumbalanästhesie in der täglichen Praxis bei Jungbullen und Schweinen. Münch Tierärztl Wochenschr 86:145–148, 1935.

91. Strande A. Epidural anaesthesia in young pigs: dosage in relation to the length of the vertebral column. Acta Vet Scand 9:41–49, 1968.

92. Farmstad T, Austad R, Knaevelsrud T. Epidural anesthesia of sows. Techniques and dosage for obstetric procedures. Nord Veterinaertidsskrift 102:363–369, 1990.

93. Ko JCH, Thurmon JC, Benson JG, et al. Evaluation of analgesia induced by epidural injection of detomidine and xylazine in swine. J Vet Anaesth 19:56–60, 1992.

94. Ko JCH, Thurmon JC, Benson JG, et al. A new drug combination for use in porcine cesarean sections. Vet Med Food Animal Practice 88(5):466–472, 1993.

95. Pera AM, Mascias A, Criado A, et al. Cardiopulmonary and analgesic effects of epidural lidocaine, alfentanil and xylazine in pigs anesthetized with isoflurane [Abstract]. Vet Surg 22(1):86, 1993.

96. Miniats OP, Jol D. Gnotobiotics pigs–derivation and rearing. Can J Comp Med 42:428–437, 1978.

97. Grono LR. Spinal anaesthesia in the sheep. Aust Vet J 42:58–59, 1966.

98. Hopcroft SC. Technique of epidural anaesthesia in experimental sheep. Aust Vet J 43:213–214, 1967.

99. Lebeaux M. Sheep: a model for testing spinal and epidural agents. Lab Anim Sci 25:629–633, 1975.

100. Nelson DR, Ott RS, Benson GJ, et al. Spinal analgesia and sedation of goats with lidocaine and xylazine. Vet Rec 105:278–280, 1979.

101. Gray PR. Anesthesia in goats and sheep. I. Local analgesia. Compend Contin Educ Pract Vet 8:33, 1986.

102. Clutton RE, Boyd C, Ward JL, et al. Fatal body positioning during epidural anesthesia in a ewe. Can Vet J 30:748–750, 1989.

103. Ralson DH, Shnider SM, de Lorimer AA. Effects of equipotent ephedrine, metaraminol, mephentermine, and methoxamine on uterine blood flow on the pregnant ewe. Anesthesiology 40:354–370, 1974.

104. Waterman AE, Livingston A, Bouchenafa O, et al. Analgesic actions of alpha 2 adrenergic agonist drugs administered intrathecally in conscious sheep [Abstract]. Proc 3rd Intl Cong Vet Anaesth, Brisbane, Australia, 1988.

105. Eisenach JC, Dewan DM, Rose JC, et al. Epidural clonidine produces antinociception, but not hypotension in sheep. Anesthesiology 66:496–501, 1987.

106. Eisenach JC, Grice SC. Epidural clonidine does not decrease blood pressure or spinal blood flow in awake sheep. Anesthesiology 68:335–340, 1988.

107. Pablo LS. Epidural morphine in goats after hindlimb orthopedic surgery. Vet Surg 22(4):307–310, 1993.

108. Waterman AE, Kyles AE, Livingston A. Spinal activity of analgesics in sheep [Abstract]. Proc 4th Intl Cong Vet Anaesth, Utrecht, The Netherlands, 1991:37.

109. St Clair LE. The nerve supply to the bovine mammary gland. Am J Vet Res 3:10–16, 1942.

110. Noordsy JL. Food animal surgery. Bonner Springs, KS: Veterinary Medical Publications, 1978.

111. Getty R. Sisson and Grossman's the anatomy of the domestic animals, 5th ed. Philadelphia: WB Saunders, 1975.

112. Greenough PR. Development of an approach to lameness examination in cattle. Vet Clin North Am Food Anim Pract 1:3–11, 1985.

113. Prentice DE, Wyn-Jones G, Jones RS, et al. Intravenous regional anaesthesia of the bovine foot. Vet Rec 94:293–295, 1974.

114. Estill CT. Intravenous local analgesia of the bovine lower leg. Vet Med Small Anim Clin 72:1499–1502, 1977.

115. Elmore RG. Food-animal regional anesthesia. Bovine blocks: intravenous limb block. Vet Med Small Anim Clin 75:1835–1836, 1980.

116. Knight AP. Intravenous regional anesthesia of the bovine foot. Bovine Pract 1:11, 14–15, 1980.

117. Manohar M, Kumar R, Tyagi RPS. Studies on the intravenous retrograde regional anaesthesia of the forelimb in buffalo calves. Br Vet J 127:401–407, 1971.

118. Kumar R, Manohar M, Tyagi RPS. The fate of intravascularly infused regional anesthesia: a radiographic investigation. J Am Vet Radiol Soc 14:87–92, 1973.

119. Tyagi RPS, Kumar R, Manohar M. Studies on intravenous retrograde regional anaesthesia for the forelimbs of ruminants. Aust Vet J 49:321–324, 1973.

120. Jones RS, Prentice DE. Some observations on intravenous anaesthesia of the bovine foot. Assoc Vet Anaesth Gr Br Ir Proc 5:13–17, 1974.

121. Fehlings K. Intravenöse regionale Anästhesie an der V. digitalis dorsalis communis III–eine brauchbare Möglichkeit zur Schmerzausschaltung bei Eingriffen an der Vorderzehe des Rindes. Dtsch Tierärztl Wochenschr 87:4–7, 1980.

122. Surborg H. Aspects of treatment of severe claw disease in a large animal practice. Bovine Pract 19:227–229, 1984.

123. Weaver AD. Intravenous local anesthesia of the lower limb in cattle. J Am Vet Med Assoc 160:55–57, 1972.

124. Antalovsky A. Technik der intravenösen Schmerzausschaltung im distalen Gliedmassenbereich beim Rind. Vet Med (Praha) 7:413–320, 1965.

125. Bogan JA, Weaver AD. Lidocaine concentrations associated with intravenous regional anesthesia of the distal limb of cattle. Am J Vet Res 39:1672–1673, 1978.

126. Gogoi SN, Nigam JM, Peshin PK, et al. Studies on intravenous regional analgesia of the hind limb in the bovine. J Vet Med Assoc 38:545–552, 1991.

127. Skarda RT. Local and regional anesthesia. In: CE Short, ed. Prin-

ciples and practice of veterinary anesthesia. Baltimore: Williams & Wilkins, 1987:91–133.

128. Steiner A, Ossent P, Mathis GA. Die intravenöse Stauungsanästhesie/Antibiose beim Rind–Indikationen, Technik, Komplikationen. Schweiz Arch Tierheilkd 132:227–237, 1990.

129. Kraus SJ, Green RL. Pseudoanaphylactic reactions with procaine penicillin. Cutis 17:765–767, 1976.

130. Taylor JA. The applied anatomy of the bovine foot. Vet Rec 72:1212–1215, 1960.

131. Raker CW. Regional analgesia of the bovine foot. J Am Vet Med Assoc 128:238–239, 1956.

132. Collin CW. A technic to produce analgesia of the hind digits of cattle. Vet Rec 75:833–834, 1963.

133. Jalaluddin AM, Rao SV. Diagnosis of lameness in the ox by means of nerve blocks. Indian Vet J 49:1246–1256, 1972.

134. Tufvesson G. Local Anesthesia in Veterinary Medicine. Stockholm: Astra International Publishing, 1963.

135. Rieger H. Die Testiculäre Injektion. Berl Münch Tierärztl Wochenschr 67:107–109, 1954.

136. Miller RE. An efficient and safe method of castration for the bovine by the intratesticular injection of Chem-Cast. Bovine Proc 15:156–159, 1983.

chapter 17

AIRWAY MANAGEMENT AND VENTILATION

Sandee M. Hartsfield

Introduction

Safe anesthesia includes establishment of a patent airway with assurance of adequate ventilation and oxygenation. If spontaneous ventilation is insufficient, the anesthetist should assist or control ventilation manually or mechanically. If hypoxemia develops, the anesthetist should provide supplemental oxygen; supplemental oxygen may be needed during the preanesthetic, induction, maintenance, and recovery phases of anesthesia.

Endotracheal Intubation

INDICATIONS

Indications for endotracheal intubation include maintenance of a patent airway, protection of the airway from foreign material, application of positive pressure ventilation, application of tracheal or bronchial suction, administration of oxygen, and delivery of inhalant anesthetics. Placement of an endotracheal tube also reduces anatomic dead space if the tube is of the correct size and correctly positioned. For maintenance of inhalant anesthesia, an endotracheal tube should create a seal with the trachea to prevent leakage of anesthetic gases into the environment. An endotracheal tube is basic for endotracheal intubation, but ancillary equipment may be required in certain species. Intubation can be accomplished through the oral cavity, nasal passages, an external pharyngotomy, or a tracheostomy.

ENDOTRACHEAL TUBES

Murphy-type and Cole-type endotracheal tubes are commonly used in veterinary anesthesia. Uniquely, the Murphy tube has an opening, called a *Murphy eye* or *side hole,* in the wall opposite the bevel (Fig. 17–1); this hole allows gas flow, even if the end hole is occluded.(1) Characteristics of cuffed Murphy endotracheal tubes designed primarily for human beings are diagramed in

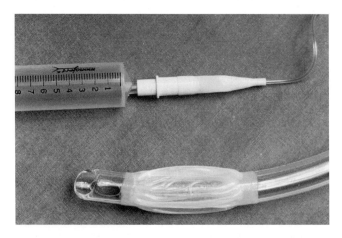

Fig. 17–1. A Murphy endotracheal tube characterized by a side hole ("Murphy eye") opposite the bevel at the distal end of the tube. The inflatable cuff, pilot balloon, self-sealing inflation valve, and syringe for inflation of the cuff are shown. The parts and characteristics of a Murphy tube are diagramed and labeled in Figure 17–2.

Figure 17–2; such tubes are used in most veterinary patients for which appropriate sizes are available.

Cole tubes are uncuffed and are characterized by a "shoulder" near the distal end (Figs. 17–3 and 17–4); the diameter of the patient end of the Cole tube is smaller than the remainder of the tube.(1) Only the smaller portion of the tube should fit into the larynx and trachea. Although fitting the sloping shoulder of the Cole tube against the arytenoid cartilages creates a seal (2), Dorsch and Dorsch indicate that the shoulder should not contact the larynx to avoid pressure against the laryngeal cartilages and to prevent laryngeal dilatation.(1) The diameter of the tube should be such that the laryngotracheal part of the tube creates a seal, which guards against egress of gas and aspiration of foreign material. An effective seal can be established in veterinary patients of various sizes.(2, 3)

Endotracheal tubes are made from polyvinyl chloride, rubber, silicone, and occasionally other plastic or rubberized materials. The most common tubes for human use are polyvinyl chloride (1), many of which are used in small animals. Some endotracheal tubes, designed specifically for veterinary patients, are made from silicone rubber (Fig. 17–5). In general, endotracheal tubes should be clear so that they can be inspected for cleanliness or obstructions before each use. Red rubber tubes have been advertised for veterinary patients; such tubes are opaque, prone to cracking, and difficult to clean and disinfect.

Cuffed endotracheal tubes (Fig. 17–6) designed for humans consist of a connector to fit the breathing system (15 mm o.d.), the tube itself, and a cuff system (inflating valve, inflating tube, and pilot balloon). Labels on these tubes may include the manufacturer's name, internal and external diameters in millimeters, markings in centimeters indicating the length of the tube from the patient (distal) end, and I.T., which indicates that the tube has been implantation tested. In addition, tubes labeled with either F29, or Z79 indicate that the tube material has been tested for tissue toxicity.(1, 4) The terms *oral* and/or *nasal* may appear beside the tube's sizes for internal and external diameters, respectively. Some endotracheal tubes have the size in French units (French size = external diameter in millimeters times pi), which indicates the outside diameter of the tube. Radiopaque markers are embedded in some endotracheal tubes.

Inflation of the cuff of an endotracheal tube applies pressure to the tracheal mucosa. The perfusion pressure of the tracheal mucosa ranges from 25 to 35 mm Hg. A cuff pressure on the tracheal wall of 20 to 25 mm Hg will usually not interfere with tracheal mucosal blood flow.(5) Greater pressures in the cuff can lead to ischemic injury, mucosal damage, and ultimately tracheal strictures in serious cases. Therefore, the design of contemporary human endotracheal tubes includes a high-volume, low-pressure cuff that creates a good seal between the tracheal mucosa and the cuff wall when the cuff is properly inflated. The intent of the high-

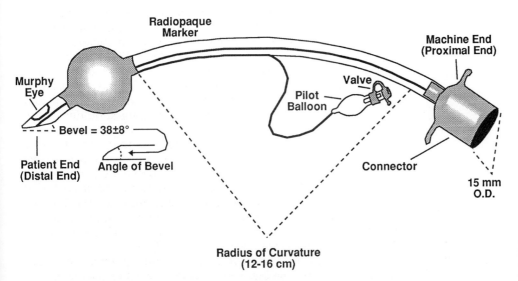

Fig. 17–2. Diagram illustrating the parts and desirable characteristics (e.g., radius of curvature and angle of the bevel) of a Murphy endotracheal tube.(1)

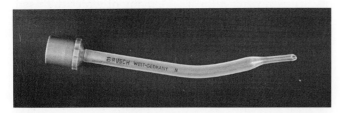

Fig. 17–3. A 10-French Cole endotracheal tube appropriate for small veterinary patients. Note the smaller diameter of the laryngotracheal portion of the tube (distal end of the tube, right side of the photograph).

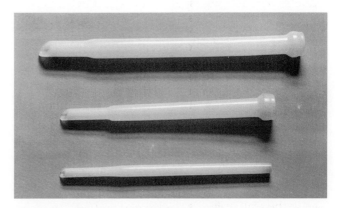

Fig. 17–4. Three sizes of Cole endotracheal tubes appropriate for large veterinary patients. Note the smaller diameter of the laryngotracheal portion of each tube (distal ends of the tubes, left side of the photograph). The proximal ends of the top two tubes are designed to fit the outside diameter of a Y-piece of a circle breathing system for large animals.

volume nonelastic cuff is to distribute the low-pressure seal over a relatively large area of the tracheal mucosa.(4) A cuff should be inflated with the smallest amount of air that will provide effective protection of the airway. A general recommendation is that pressure on the lateral wall of the trachea exerted by the cuff be maintained between 25 and 34 cm of H_2O.(1) Generally, a leak should occur around the cuff when pressure equal to approximately 25 cm of H_2O is applied to the airway (end-expiration).

Armored or reinforced endotracheal tubes (Fig. 17–7) are specially designed with helical wire or plastic implanted within the wall of the tube to prevent kinking of the tube and obstruction of the airway when the patient's head and neck are flexed. Such tubes are useful for ophthalmic surgery, cervical spinal taps, myelograms, oral surgery, and head and neck surgery. Armored tubes have thicker walls than standard tubes, causing them to have smaller internal diameters than standard tubes of equivalent external size.(4) Therefore, resistance to gas flow is increased, and reinforced tubes should not be used unnecessarily. Typically, these tubes are very flexible and more difficult to insert than standard polyvinyl chloride tubes. A stylet or guide tube will facilitate insertion of an armored tube into the larynx, but a stiff stylet should not extend past the distal end of the endotracheal tube.

Endotracheal intubation through a tracheostomy is sometimes necessary to provide a patent airway. Cuffed tracheostomy tubes with 15-mm-o.d. connectors (Fig. 17–8) are available for human use. However, standard endotracheal tubes for both large and small animals may be placed via tracheostomy to facilitate general anesthesia (Fig. 17–9). Endotracheal tubes are also recommended for intubation by external pharyngotomy (Fig. 17–10).(6)

Normally, endotracheal intubation is accomplished in anesthetized patients. Forced intubation in awake or lightly anesthetized patients should be avoided unless dictated by special circumstances. Traumatic intubation can produce laryngeal edema, laryngeal spasm, hemorrhage, and vagal stimulation leading to bradycardia and other arrhythmias. Direct application of a local anesthetic (e.g., lidocaine, Fig. 17–11) to the larynx may prevent laryngeal spasms in susceptible animals (e.g., cats, swine). The local anesthetic can be sprayed into the larynx, applied with a cotton swab, or squirted from a syringe and hypodermic needle. When using a syringe, the hypodermic needle must be firmly attached to prevent its dislodgement and entrance in to the larynx. The total dose of local anesthetic should not approach a toxic dose, based on the patient's species and body weight. In very small patients, spraying local anesthetic onto the larynx can easily exceed a toxic dose.

Endotracheal and tracheostomy tubes should be cleaned thoroughly after use. The tubes should be gently scrubbed with a soft brush, rinsed, dried, and sterilized or disinfected. If ethylene oxide is not available, chemical disinfectants can be used; glutaraldehyde has been recommended.(7) After disinfection, tubes should be rinsed thoroughly, according to recommendations for use of the disinfectant, and dried. If tubes are inadequately rinsed, tissue reactions to the disinfectant can occur. Ethylene oxide sterilization should be done according to the manufacturer's recommendations for the product and its sterilization equipment. Endotra-

cheal tubes should be clean and dry before they are sterilized with ethylene oxide. Appropriate aeration time should be allowed between sterilizing a tube and its use in a patient, typically 48 hours at 120° F in an aeration chamber or 14 days if no aeration chamber is available. Failure to allow sufficient aeration time can cause serious respiratory complications.(8) Most endotracheal or tracheostomy tubes should not be autoclaved; however, silicone rubber tubes can be steam autoclaved.(7, 9)

Laryngoscopy is required for endotracheal intubation of some species. Often, the laryngoscope's light source is the main benefit of laryngoscopy, but the blade can be used to manipulate the tongue, soft palate, and epiglottis to view the glottis (Fig. 17–12). Useful blades include the Miller, the McIntosh, and the Bizarri-Guiffrida (Figs. 17–13 and 17–14), and other blades are available. Different lengths of blades are needed for various species. As examples, very short blades designed for human infants are useful in rabbits, and blades up to 205 mm designed for human adults are appropriate for large dogs. Specially designed, very long (350 to 450 mm) blades can be purchased for veterinary use, and may be needed in llamas, cattle, swine, and other species (Chapters 20, 21, 23).

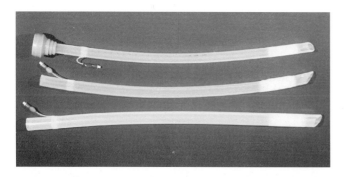

Fig. 17–5. Silicone rubber endotracheal tubes designed for veterinary use. The proximal end of the top tube has been fitted with a connector that will conform to the outside diameter of a Y-piece of a circle breathing system for large animals.

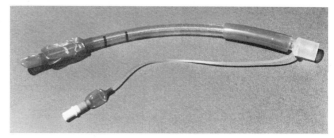

Fig. 17–7. An armored endotracheal tube with a spiral wire embedded in the wall of the tube. The endotracheal tube connector, bite guard near the proximal end of the tube, inflatable cuff, pilot balloon, inflation line, and self-sealing inflation valve are present.

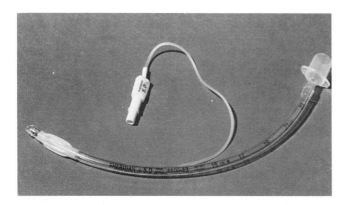

Fig. 17–6. A Murphy endotracheal tube designed for human beings, but commonly used for small animals. Numbers and markings indicate the internal (5.0 mm) and external (8.0 mm) diameters, the length (13, 15, 17, 19, 21, and 23 cm) of the tube from the patient end, the manufacturer (Sheridan), and an indication of tissue toxicity testing (Z79). The internal diameter (5.0 mm) and manufacturer are also shown on the pilot balloon.

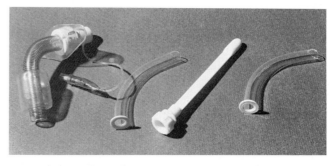

Fig. 17–8. A cuffed tracheostomy tube (left) designed for human beings but applicable to veterinary patients. From left to right are the cuffed tracheostomy tube with inflation line and pilot balloon, a removable lumen for the tube, an obturator to facilitate insertion of the tube, and another removable lumen.

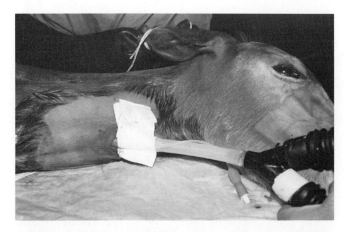

Fig. 17–9. A silicone rubber endotracheal tube placed through a tracheostomy site to facilitate inhalant anesthesia for oral and nasal surgery in a foal.

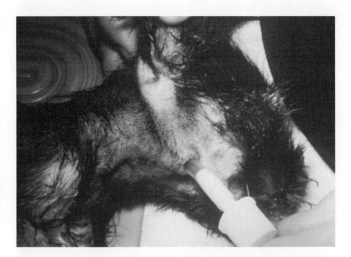

Fig. 17–10. An endotracheal tube placed by external pharyngotomy in a small dog to facilitate oropharyngeal surgery. (From Hartsfield, S.M. Alternate Methods of Endotracheal Intubation in Small Animals/ Emphasis on Patients with Oropharyngeal Pathology. Tex Vet Med J 47:25, 1985.)

Techniques of Endotracheal Intubation

DOGS

For most dogs, an endotracheal tube and adequate lighting are the only necessities for intubation of the trachea. However, a laryngoscope, a stylet to stiffen the endotracheal tube, a guide tube (Fig. 17–15), sterile water-soluble lubricant, a mouth speculum, and local anesthetic may be desirable and even necessary under certain circumstances.

Sizes of endotracheal tubes for canine patients range from 1.5 mm to approximately 15 mm i.d.(2) It is difficult, if not impossible, to find cuffed tubes smaller than 3.0 mm i.d. There are breed differences that preclude generalizations about the choice of tube diameter based on the patient's body weight or some other arbitrary guide. For example, a 25-kg English bulldog usually accepts only about a 7.5-mm i.d.

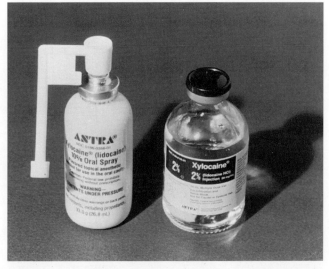

Fig. 17–11. Lidocaine as a spray (left) or as a liquid (applied with a cotton swab or delivered by squirting it with a syringe and needle) can be applied topically to the larynx to facilitate endotracheal intubation in various species. With either method of delivery, the anesthetist should keep the total dose of lidocaine less than the toxic dose for the patient and species involved.

endotracheal tube, but a 25-kg mixed breed dog may easily accept a 10-mm tube. Most tubes designed for human beings are too long for dogs and should be cut at the proximal end to fit the patient; the connector should be positioned at the level of the dog's incisors, and the distal end should be located in the trachea near the thoracic inlet (Fig. 17–16).

After induction of anesthesia, the dog is positioned in sternal recumbency for intubation. An assistant holds the dog's head with one hand, placing the finger and thumb behind the maxillary canine teeth and pulling the lips upward to create the best field of view. With the other hand, the assistant opens the dog's mouth widely and extends its tongue. The assistant should not put pressure under the dog's neck because the view of the larynx will be obstructed by the soft palate. With a good light source, most dogs can be intubated without a laryngoscope. If an assistant is unavailable, an oral speculum will keep the dog's mouth open during intubation. In small patients, dogs with oral or pharyngeal lesions, and brachycephalic dogs, a laryngoscope facilitates intubation and should always be available if difficulty should arise. The endotracheal tube should be secured to prevent its dislocation during anesthesia. Using a piece of rolled gauze, the tube can be tied to the maxilla (Fig. 17–17), the mandible, or behind the head depending on the breed, the type of surgery, the presence and condition of the canine teeth, and the anesthetist's preference.

Extubation should be done when the dog's oral and pharyngeal reflexes have returned. The tube should be pulled directly between the upper and lower incisor teeth. If a tube is allowed to deviate laterally, the dog

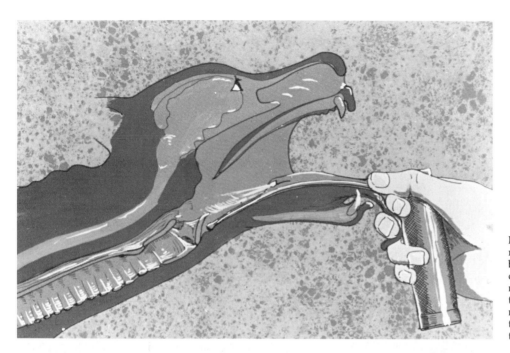

Fig. 17–12. Diagram of the correct positioning of a laryngoscope blade for maximum visualization of the larynx. Note that the dog's mouth is opened widely, the tongue is extended from the mouth maximally, and the tip of the laryngoscope blade is positioned at the base of the epiglottis.

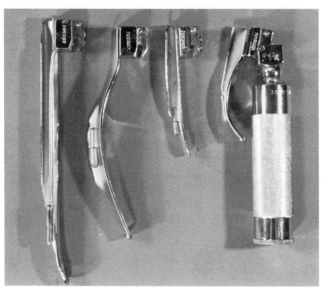

Fig. 17–13. From left to right, an adult Miller laryngoscope blade, an adult Bizarri-Guiffrida blade, a pediatric Miller blade, and a pediatric Bizarri-Guiffrida blade on a laryngoscope handle. The Bizarri-Guiffrida blades allow the maximum field of view without the interference of a flange.

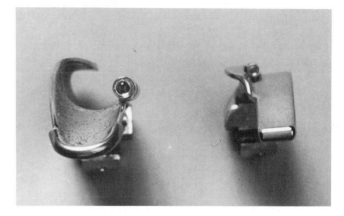

Fig. 17–14. End-on view of Miller (left) and Bizarri-Guiffrida (right) laryngoscope blades. The Bizarri-Guiffrida blade allows maximum space for passage of the endotracheal tube and the Miller blade provides a flange to elevate redundant tissue (e.g., soft palate).

may shear the tube. This damages tubes and creates the potential for aspiration or ingestion of a part of the tube (Chapter 20).

CATS

The primary equipment required for feline intubation are an endotracheal tube and a light source. However, a laryngoscope, a stylet to stiffen the endotracheal tube, a guide tube (canine polyethylene urinary catheter), sterile water-soluble lubricant, a mouth speculum, and local anesthetic may be useful. If a wire stylet is used to stiffen the tube, the stylet should not extend past the distal end of the tube to avoid injury to the trachea.(2) Inadequate depth of anesthesia is probably the most common reason for difficult intubation.

Sizes of endotracheal tubes for domestic cats range from 1.5 mm to approximately 5.5 mm i.d.; most adult cats readily accept 4.0- to 4.5-mm-i.d. tubes, a range that provides optimal internal diameter with minimal difficulty in intubation. It is difficult to find cuffed tubes smaller than 3.0 mm i.d., and such sizes may be needed for small kittens. One option is to use small Cole tubes. Since most endotracheal tubes designed for human beings are too long for cats, the tube should be cut at the proximal end to fit the patient. The proximal end of the tube should be positioned at the level of the cat's incisors, and the distal end should be located in the trachea near the thoracic inlet.

After induction of anesthesia, the cat should be positioned in sternal recumbency. Although not necessary in every case, local anesthetic (lidocaine, 0.5%) applied to the larynx may desensitize the arytenoid cartilages and the epiglottis to facilitate intubation and prevent laryngospasm. An assistant holds the head with one hand, placing a finger and thumb behind the cat's maxillary canine teeth and pulling the lips upward to create the best field of view (Figs. 17–18 and 17–19). With the other hand, the assistant extends the cat's tongue. If the tongue is not protruding from the mouth, the laryngoscope blade can be used to manipulate the tongue so that the assistant can grasp it. Neither the anesthetist nor the assistant should put their fingers into a lightly anesthetized cat's mouth. The assistant should not put pressure under the cat's neck because the view of the larynx may be obstructed by the soft palate. As in dogs, with a good light source, most cats

can be intubated without the aid of a laryngoscope. However, a laryngoscope is often helpful. The blade should not touch the arytenoid cartilages or the epiglottis (Fig. 17–19), since such stimulation may cause active closure of the glottis. A laryngoscope should always be available for a difficult intubation (e.g., oral or pharyngeal lesions). If an assistant is unavailable, an oral speculum will keep the cat's mouth open while intubation is accomplished. The routine use of a guide tube (5- to 8-French canine urinary catheter) that extends past the cuffed end of the endotracheal tube (Fig. 17–18) for a distance of 2 or 3 cm makes feline intubation very easy. As the endotracheal tube is advanced toward the glottis, rotating it from 0° to 90° or greater will facilitate its passage. Rolled gauze can be used to secure the tube behind the cat's head with a simple bow knot. In cats, the tube should be tied for rapid removal at recovery (Chapter 20).

Extubation should be done when the cat's oral and pharyngeal reflexes have returned. The tube should be pulled directly between the upper and lower incisor teeth. If a tube is allowed to move laterally, the cat may shear the tube (Fig. 17–20), which creates the potential for aspiration or ingestion of part of the tube.

HORSES

Blind passage of the endotracheal tube in horses can be aided by a mouth speculum. For routine intubation, polyvinyl chloride (PVC) connectors (10 cm long, variable diameters) for PVC pipe make economic, effective specula that can be placed between the horse's upper and lower incisors to protect the tube. The connectors can be wrapped with adhesive tape to increase friction between the teeth and the speculum.(7) Other supplies that may be useful for equine intubation under certain conditions include a guide tube (equine stomach tube), sterile water-soluble lubricant, local anesthetic, and a fiber-optic endoscope (Chapter 20).

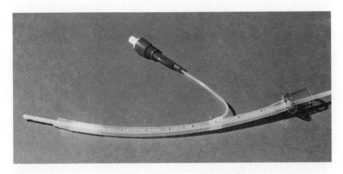

Fig. 17–15. Photograph of a silicone rubber endotracheal tube with a 10-French canine polyethylene urinary catheter preplaced for use as a guide tube. The guide tube will pass easily through the larynx and into the cranial part of the trachea to facilitate passage of the endotracheal tube.

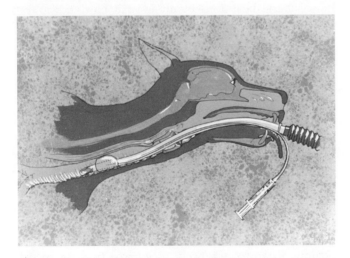

Fig. 17–16. Diagram illustrating correct placement of an endotracheal tube in a dog. Note that the connector is located near the incisor teeth to minimize mechanical dead space and that the cuffed end of the tube is in the cervical trachea near the thoracic inlet.

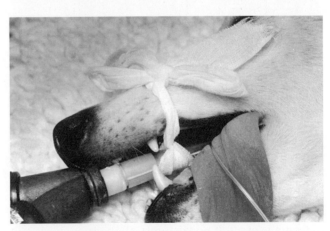

Fig. 17–17. An endotracheal tube secured to the dog's maxilla with a piece of rolled gauze. Note that the gauze is tied tightly around the tube without constricting the lumen, that the connector is at the level of the incisor teeth, and that the gauze is positioned immediately caudal to the maxillary canine teeth and tied in a bow.

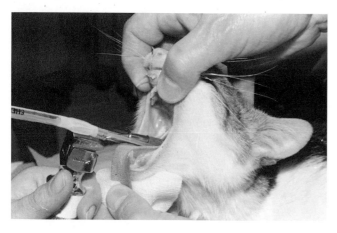

Fig. 17–18. Ilustration of an excellent method of positioning a cat for endotracheal intubation. Note the secure grip on the maxilla with the index finger and thumb caudal to the canine teeth. The tongue is extended, maximizing the field of view.

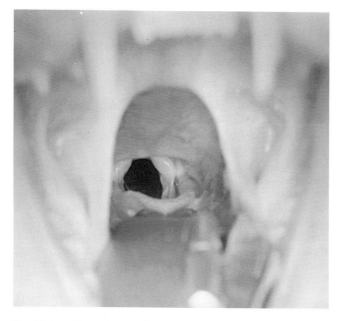

Fig. 17–19. View of a cat's glottis using the restraint and positioning depicted in Figure 17–18. The laryngoscope blade is placed on the tongue with the tip just ventral to the epiglottis.

To assure an appropriate range of sizes of endotracheal tubes for equine patients (miniature horses to draft horses), tubes as small as 7 mm i.d. and as large as 30 mm i.d. should be available. Larger sizes (e.g., 35 mm i.d.) have been recommended for large Thoroughbred and draft horses.(10) Tube size varies with the size of the patient and with the location of the tube (oral versus nasal intubation). Modern 26-mm-i.d. silicone rubber cuffed endotracheal tubes are appropriate for a high percentage of adult horses, with 30-mm tubes indicated for very large horses. In general, a tube that is passed nasally should be about two sizes smaller than a tube that is passed orally.(9)

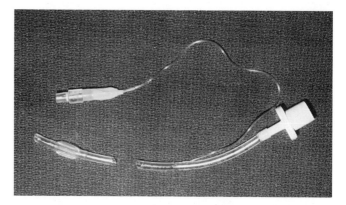

Fig. 17–20. A 4-mm-i.d. endotracheal tube sheared during extubation of a cat at the time of recovery from anesthesia. Aspiration or ingestion of the smaller piece is possible.

In preparation for oropharyngeal intubation, the horse's mouth should be flushed with water to remove any debris that may be retained in the oropharynx including the cheek pouches. Horses are positioned in lateral recumbency for intubation with a lubricated endotracheal tube. A sterile water-soluble lubricant should be used; lubricants containing local anesthetic are unnecessary and may irritate airway tissues.(7, 11) The mouth speculum is placed between the upper and lower incisors, the head and neck are extended, and the endotracheal tube is advanced into the pharynx until the tip of the tube touches the larynx. In some patients, the tube enters the larynx without any interference. However, several attempts (a series of 10- to 15-cm advancements and retractions of the tube, with rotation of the tube from 0° to 90° or greater as it approaches the glottis) may be necessary for intubation, even in normal horses. Although the technique is somewhat of an art, intubation can be facilitated by positioning the head and neck maximally extended in a straight line with the horse's back (best done by an assistant), extending the tongue during intubation, and holding the endotracheal tube so that the proximal end is curved below the mandible during attempts at intubation. In general, an endotracheal tube of proper size passes into the larynx with little if any resistance once correct positioning and technique have been established.

For a difficult intubation, an equine stomach (guide tube) may be passed into the larynx and trachea over which the endotracheal tube can be manipulated through the larynx and into the trachea. In some instances (e.g., laryngeal or pharyngeal abnormalities), equine intubation may be successful only after visualizing the glottis with a fiber-optic endoscope; this allows adjustments in the position of the endotracheal tube or a guide tube as it approaches the glottis.

A properly positioned endotracheal tube is usually obvious to an experienced anesthetist because of the absence of resistance as the tube enters the larynx and trachea. Air flow into and out of the tube during spontaneous ventilation can be used to verify tube placement. Some veterinarians advocate compression of the thorax to create air flow from a properly placed tube, but this technique may not be foolproof. Finally, water may condense on the inner surface of the tube during exhalation if the tube is placed properly (Chapter 20).

SWINE

Endotracheal intubation of swine is relatively difficult for several reasons (12): The distance from the tip of the snout to the larynx is comparatively long, the mouth does not open widely, the larynx is rather loosely attached and mobile, and the larynx is relatively small and slopes ventrally, creating a sharp angle for passing an endotracheal tube (Fig. 17–21). In addition, laryngospasm is rather easily induced in lightly anesthetized pigs. An endotracheal tube, a laryngoscope, 2% lidocaine in a syringe, sterile water-soluble lubricant, and a guide tube should be available for intubation of swine.

Compared to other domestic species, swine have small laryngeal and tracheal diameters. Endotracheal tube sizes from 3 mm i.d. in piglets to 16 mm i.d. in larger swine may be needed. Mature sows and boars may accept even larger tubes. After induction of anesthesia, the pig is placed in sternal recumbency, an assistant holds the head with a small rope or piece of rolled gauze passed through the mouth, and the pig's tongue is extended. A mouth speculum can be employed if necessary. Using the appropriate length of blade, the pig's larynx is visualized with the aid of a laryngoscope; this usually requires some manipulation to position the blade for a good view of the glottis, especially in large swine with a narrow pharynx and excessive tissue in the area of the soft palate. Lidocaine can be squirted onto the larynx for desensitization. The guide tube (usually two 10-French canine urinary catheters in tandem) is passed through the larynx and into the trachea; manipulation of the guide tube through the larynx should be done without excessive force, and best results are obtained by passing the guide tube along the dorsal aspect of the larynx to the midcervical trachea. Then, a well-lubricated endotracheal tube is directed over the guide tube, through the larynx, and into the trachea; firm, gentle advancement of the tube with a simultaneous twisting motion (0° to greater than 90°) is helpful. The tube should be positioned with the connector at the level of the tip of the snout, and the distal end should be near the thoracic inlet. The cuff should be inflated with the minimum amount of air that will create a seal. The tube can be secured to the snout with adhesive tape or behind the ears with rolled gauze.

Miniature pet pigs are intubated using the same equipment (smaller sizes) and method just described, but gentle technique should be emphasized. Laryngospasm, laryngeal edema, and death have been associated with traumatic intubation in miniature pigs (Chapter 20).(13)

CATTLE

The primary implements for endotracheal intubation in adult cattle are an endotracheal tube, a mouth speculum (e.g., Bayer dental wedge, Guenther mouth speculum, Weingart mouth speculum, or Drinkwater mouth gag), and a equine stomach tube (two to three times longer than the endotracheal tube) for use as a guide. For smaller cattle, a long laryngoscope blade (e.g., 14, 16, or 18 inches) may be necessary for passage of a guide tube. Sizes of endotracheal tubes ranging from 18 to 30 mm i.d. may be needed for adult cattle.

After induction of anesthesia, a mouth speculum is positioned to hold the mouth open; this helps to prevent damage to the endotracheal tube cuff and to the anesthetist's hand and arm during intubation. The tongue is extended from the mouth, and the cow's head and neck should be extended. The anesthetist passes one hand through the mouth and palpates the epiglottis and glottis. The anesthetist passes the guide tube into the pharynx and then slides the tube through the glottis, assuring its proper placement by palpation as the tube enters the larynx. The guide tube is advanced until its tip is in the midcervical trachea. After the arm is removed from the mouth, the endotracheal tube is advanced over the guide tube and into the larynx and trachea. Rotation of the tube from 0° to greater than 90° as the tube approaches the arytenoid cartilages will help to advance the endotracheal tube into the trachea. The cuff should be inflated immediately to decrease the likelihood of aspiration of regurgitated rumen contents. Should active or passive regurgitation of large quantities of ruminal content occur just before or simultaneously with endotracheal intubation, external pressure applied over the esophagus will halt the flow of ruminal contents. Alternatively, the endotracheal tube can be quickly passed into the esophagus and the cuff inflated, permitting the regurgitant to flow through the

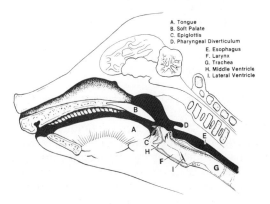

A. Tongue
B. Soft Palate
C. Epiglottis
D. Pharyngeal Diverticulum
E. Esophagus
F. Larynx
G. Trachea
H. Middle Ventricle
I. Lateral Ventricle

Fig. 17–21. Sagittal section of a pig's head. The diagram illustrates the irregular course that an endotracheal tube must travel as it moves through the mouth, pharynx, larynx, and cranial trachea. (From Lumb, W.V., and Jones, E.W. Oxygen Administration and Artificial Respiration. In: Veterinary Anesthesia, 2nd ed. Philadelphia: Lea & Febiger, 1984:145.)

endotracheal tube beyond the pharynx and out of the mouth, preventing its aspiration into the lungs. A properly positioned endotracheal tube in a cow is shown in Figure 17–22.

Bovine intubation can be accomplished without a guide tube. The endotracheal tube is passed beside or under the anesthetist's arm and palpated as it enters the larynx.(12) Alternately, the anesthetist can take the tube into the cow's mouth, cupping the distal end of the tube in his hand.(14) The disadvantage of either method is that the size of the endotracheal tube that can be readily passed is limited, especially if the anesthetist has a large arm (Chapter 20).

SMALL RUMINANTS

Equipment required for endotracheal intubation in small ruminants includes an endotracheal tube, a laryngoscope, and a guide tube. Endotracheal intubation in small ruminants (sheep, goats, calves, cattle less than about 250 kg, deer, exotic ruminants) is best accomplished by direct visualization of the larynx with an illuminated laryngoscope. Sternal recumbency facilitates the procedure, but intubation can be achieved during lateral recumbency. After induction of anesthesia, an assistant holds the head while the anesthetist extends the tongue. The anesthetist passes the laryngoscope blade over the base of the tongue to visualize the glottis, and then passes a guide tube (e.g., a small equine stomach tube in calves or a polyethylene catheter in sheep or goats) into the larynx and into the trachea to about the midcervical area. The laryngoscope is removed, and the endotracheal tube is passed over the guide tube and into the trachea. The cuff is inflated immediately to decrease the likelihood of aspiration of regurgitated rumen contents. The use of a metal rod has been advocated as a guide tube.(14) Excessive force with a metal guide tube increases the risk of damaging the larynx or trachea and is not recommended.

NASOTRACHEAL INTUBATION

Nasotracheal intubation is commonly used in foals for the administration of inhalant anesthetics during induction.(9) The technique can also be used in calves and adult horses, and has been described in llamas.(15)

The characteristics of an ideal nasotracheal tube include a tube with minimal curvature and with extra length (55 cm). The tube should be made of inert material (e.g., silicone rubber), and should have relatively thin walls for maximum internal diameter. The tube should resist kinking. Low-volume, high-pressure cuffs may be less traumatic during placement, but high-volume, low-pressure cuffs may be best for longer periods of anesthesia. Tubes as small as 7 mm i.d. may be required for neonatal foals. In general, in any given patient a nasotracheal tube should be one to two sizes smaller than the appropriately sized orotracheal tube.(9) Once induction is completed using a nasotracheal tube, the nasotracheal tube can be removed and

replaced with an appropriately sized orotracheal tube to decrease resistance to gas flow.

Nasotracheal intubation (Figs. 17–23 to 17–26) involves passage of a properly sized endotracheal tube through the nostril (Fig. 17–23), ventral nasal meatus, and larynx and into the trachea. Lidocaine gel (10%) is a good lubricant for the tube and should be applied to the nostril and rostral portion of the nasal passage before advancing the tube in awake animals. A sterile water-soluble lubricant without lidocaine is appropriate for anesthetized patients. With the head and neck extended, the tube is advanced into the pharynx and passed into the larynx on inspiration. Air moves freely through a correctly placed tube during spontaneous ventilation. The tube should be secured to prevent its dislocation. Taping the tube to the muzzle is appropriate (Fig. 17–26).

For uncooperative foals and calves, sedation may facilitate nasotracheal intubation. Some awake patients

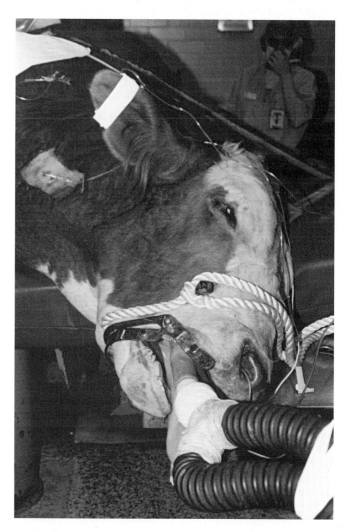

Fig. 17–22. A 26-mm-i.d. silicone rubber endotracheal tube placed in a cow. The tube was passed with the Weingart mouth speculum in place as shown.

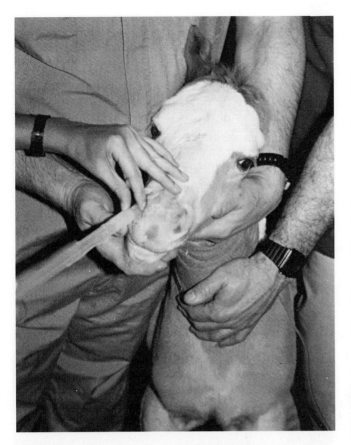

Fig. 17–23. Restraint of an untranquilized foal for nasotracheal intubation. A lubricated tube is directed through the ventral meatus.

cough and close the glottis in response to the tube contacting the larynx. With the nasotracheal tube positioned with the cuffed end near the larynx, lidocaine solution (2%) can be flooded onto the larynx via the tube (Fig. 17–24). This desensitizes the larynx and eases intubation.

Extubation following nasotracheal intubation should be done carefully. After deflation of the cuff, the tube should be withdrawn slowly and deliberately, with the patient's head restrained to avoid any sudden, jerky motions. Rapid, rough extubation may cause unnecessary nasal hemorrhage.

RABBITS AND OTHER LABORATORY ANIMALS

Intubation techniques for rabbits and other small laboratory animals have been described.(16) Most techniques for intubation of small laboratory animals include the use of a laryngoscope or a modified otoscope to expose the glottis, a catheter or stylet to serve as a guide tube, a small-diameter lubricated endotracheal tube, and lidocaine to desensitize the larynx before passing the endotracheal tube. In my experience with laboratory rabbits weighing about 3.0 kg, 3.5-mm (i.d.), 14-cm (length) endotracheal tubes are appropriate.(17)

The rabbit has been described as "probably the most difficult animal to anesthetize."(18) Undoubtedly, problems with airway management influenced that descrip-

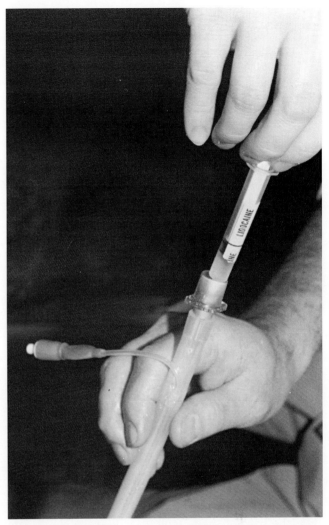

Fig. 17–24. Lidocaine (2%) being injected through the endotracheal tube, the distal end of which is near the foal's glottis. The lidocaine should desensitize the epiglottis and arytenoid cartilages to facilitate passage of the tube through the glottis.

tion. However, the technique for endotracheal intubation in rabbits can be mastered with practice when using proper equipment. Guide tube technique causes minimal trauma during intubation and allows selection of the largest suitable endotracheal tube. Endotracheal intubation in rabbits requires gentle manipulations. Rough technique invariably leads to trauma to the tongue, pharynx, larynx, or trachea. Trauma with associated edema and hemorrhage can result in lethal complications.

Rabbits should be intubated in sternal recumbency with the head and neck extended and the fleshy tongue gently withdrawn from the mouth (Figs. 17–27 to 17–30). The rabbit's head can be held with a piece of rolled gauze placed caudal to the maxillary incisors. A size-0 Miller laryngoscope blade (75 mm long) is used to expose the glottis; the blade is carefully manipulated lateral to the maxillary incisors, into the mouth, and

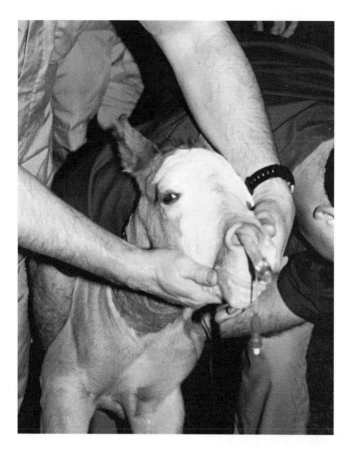

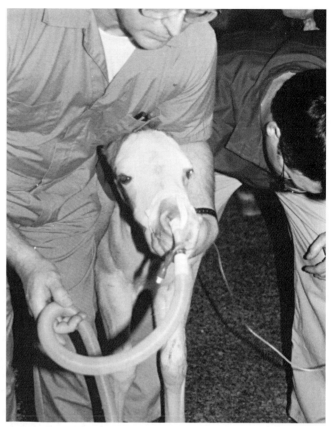

Fig. 17–25. A nasotracheal tube positioned in the trachea, ready to be secured to the patient. The proximal end of the tube extends a few centimeters from the nostril to facilitate taping (see Figure 17–26).

Fig. 17–26. A nasotracheal tube secured to a foal's muzzle. The cuff has been inflated, and an adult Bain breathing system has been connected to the endotracheal tube to facilitate induction of anesthesia with isoflurane in oxygen.

over the base of the tongue to expose the soft palate, epiglottis and glottis. All are very fine, but distinct anatomic structures. The epiglottis may be positioned behind the soft palate. The anesthetist should definitively identify the glottis before proceeding. Then, a guide tube (a 5- to 8-French canine urinary catheter) can be passed through the larynx and into the mid-cervical trachea, about 2 cm past the glottis (Fig. 17–27). The guide tube should not be forced because the trachea is easily torn, which can eventually lead to subcutaneous emphysema, pneumothorax, pneumomediastinum, pneumoabdomen, and death. The endotracheal tube is passed over the guide tube, through the larynx, and into the trachea. If resistance to passing the endotracheal tube through the glottis is apparent, less than 0.5 mL of 2% lidocaine can be flushed through the endotracheal tube to the larynx. The lidocaine desensitizes the larynx, and intubation usually proceeds uneventfully. The cuff should be inflated minimally, the pilot balloon should remain soft, and a leak around the cuff should occur at an inspiratory pressure of about 15 cm of H_2O. The tube should be secured with rolled gauze behind the rabbit's ears. Alternatively, in large rabbits, a blind approach to

endotracheal intubation is often successful when the head and neck are maximally extended and the endotracheal tube is advanced into the remiglottis. Intubation of the trachea is expedited at this point by listening for air movement through the tube while gently advancing it beyond the larynx into the trachea (Chapter 21).

BIRDS AND REPTILES

Endotracheal intubation in birds and reptiles that are commonly presented for anesthesia is relatively easy. The glottis is usually located on the midline at the base of the tongue and is readily apparent when the patient's mouth is opened. Appropriately sized endotracheal tubes should be selected, and if cuffed tubes are used, the cuff should not be inflated excessively to avoid damage to the tracheal rings. Owing to the small size of some birds and reptiles and the propensity for mucus to collect in the distal end of the tube, the anesthetist should be careful to assure a patent airway at all times. The use of lubricating jelly can also result in the obstruction of air flow through small endotracheal tubes (Chapter 20).

Special Techniques for Endotracheal Intubation

The common techniques for endotracheal intubation may fail if oropharyngeal pathology is present (Fig. 17–31) or if movement of the temporomandibular joint is impaired. In such patients, "blind" intubation can be performed successfully on occasion. With the patient's head and neck extended, the larynx can be manipulated externally with one hand while the other hand maneuvers the tube through the larynx and into the trachea.

However, the technique may be traumatic or fail completely. Other options for intubation are available.

GUIDE TUBE TECHNIQUE FOR ENDOTRACHEAL INTUBATION

In some patients, a laryngoscope blade will allow exposure and illumination of the glottis by diverting the obstruction to one side, permitting direct placement of the endotracheal tube into the larynx. However, it may

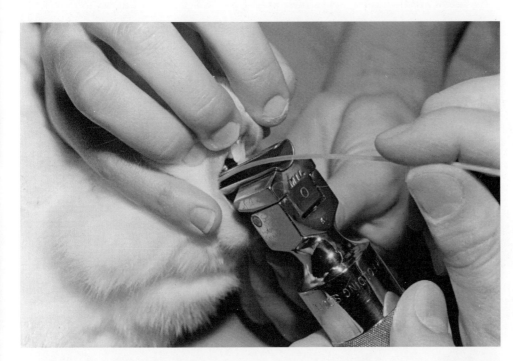

Fig. 17–27. Endotracheal intubation in a rabbit. The rabbit is positioned in sternal recumbency, the glottis has been exposed with a size 0 Miller blade, and the anesthetist is passing a 7-French canine urinary catheter to serve as a guide tube for intubation.

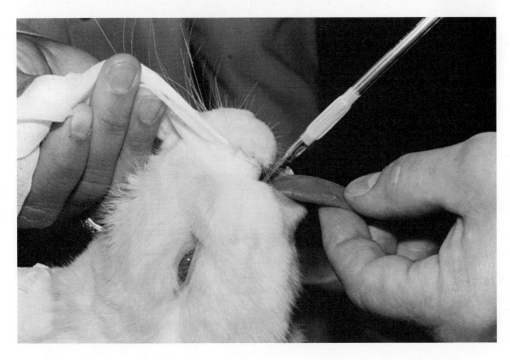

Fig. 17–28. Endotracheal intubation in a rabbit. The endotracheal tube is advanced over the guide tube (distal end of the guide tube located 2 cm caudal to the cricoid cartilage) and into the mouth.

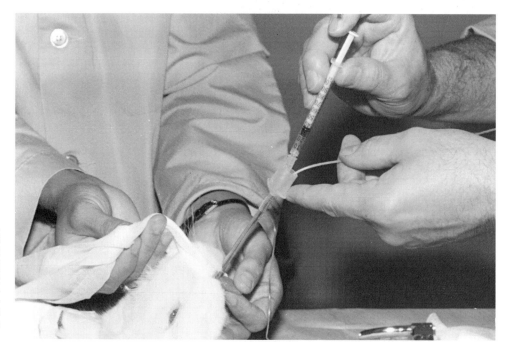

Fig. 17–29. Endotracheal intubation in a rabbit. The distal end of the endotracheal tube is located just rostral to the glottis, the tip of the guide tube is in the cervical trachea, and lidocaine is flushed through the lumen of the endotracheal tube to desensitize the larynx before advancement of the endotracheal tube.

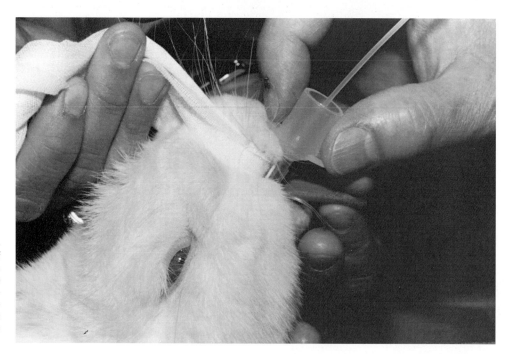

Fig. 17–30. Endotracheal intubation in a rabbit. The distal end of the endotracheal tube has been advanced through the larynx to its final position in the midcervical trachea. The anesthetist is preparing to extract the guide tube and secure the endotracheal tube behind the rabbit's ears.

be easier to pass a small-diameter guide tube (e.g., a canine urinary catheter), rather than an endotracheal tube, through the glottis. Guide tube technique has been previously described for various species, and it can be beneficial in dogs and cats with oropharyngeal pathology.(19) Once the tip of the guide tube is situated about half the distance from the cricoid cartilage to the thoracic inlet, the endotracheal tube can be passed into place (Fig. 17–32). Then, the guide tube is removed, and the endotracheal tube is secured as appropriate for the species involved.

RETROGRADE INTUBATION TECHNIQUE

If direct visualization of at least a portion of the glottis is impossible, other techniques of intubation have been advocated.(19, 20) One method, use of a retrograde guide tube or wire, involves passing a hypodermic needle through the skin of the neck and into the trachea at the junction of the second and third tracheal rings. In human beings, the needle is passed through the cricothyroid membrane. A guide wire is then maneuvered through the needle cranially into the larynx, pharynx, and oral cavity until it can be used as a guide for passage of an endotracheal tube (Fig. 17–33). After the tip of the endotracheal tube is within the larynx, the needle and the guide tube are removed, and the endotracheal tube is manipulated into its final position with the cuffed end near the thoracic inlet. The cuff should be located caudal to the puncture site of the hypodermic needle to avoid forcing gases subcutaneously or into the mediastinum during positive pressure ventilation. Subcutaneous emphysema and pneumothorax are possible complications with this technique.

ENDOTRACHEAL INTUBATION THROUGH LATERAL PHARYNGOTOMY

Endotracheal intubation by external pharyngotomy has been described.(6) The technique has been advocated for selected canine and feline patients requiring oropharyngeal surgery or orthopedic procedures involving the mandible or maxilla. The major advantages are improved visualization within the operative field during oropharyngeal surgery and normal dental occlusion to aid in the proper reduction of mandibular or maxillary fractures.

The basics of tube placement involve passage of a correctly sized, cuffed endotracheal tube in a routine fashion. With the patient sufficiently anesthetized, a skin incision is made near the angle of the mandible. Then, hemostats are bluntly passed through the skin incision into the caudal part of the pharynx. After removing the endotracheal tube adapter, the adapter end of the tube is grasped and pulled from the pharynx, through the subcutaneous tissue, and through the skin incision. The endotracheal tube adapter is replaced, and the tube is reconnected to the breathing system for maintenance. A correctly placed tube should be secured to the skin with tape and several sutures.

ENDOTRACHEAL INTUBATION USING A FIBER-OPTIC ENDOSCOPE

Laryngoscopy with a flexible fiber-optic endoscope can be useful for intubation in patients with abnormal anatomy or disease processes involving the pharynx or head and neck. Depending on the species and the specific conditions, the endoscope can be placed inside the endotracheal tube to directly guide intubation, passed orally beside the endotracheal tube, or advanced through the nasal passage to view the endotracheal tube entering the glottis. The technique can be particularly advantageous in horses with abnormal oropharyngeal, laryngeal, and/or nasal anatomy, and can be helpful in small laboratory species that are difficult to intubate. The technique is applicable to any species in which intubation is impaired by anatomic abnormalities or disease. The technique is illustrated in a normal cat in Figures 17–34 to 17–36.

ENDOTRACHEAL INTUBATION BY TRACHEOSTOMY

A temporary tracheostomy can be chosen for airway management in lieu of the techniques suggested earlier for difficult cases. In some patients, the only reasonable option for intubation is tracheostomy, and some patients with airway disease arrive in the induction room with a tracheostomy tube in place. For anesthesia, intubation of the trachea through the tracheostomy site gives all of the advantages of oral intubation or intubation by pharyngotomy. However, tracheostomy has been associated with infection, granulomas, tracheal stricture, cartilage damage, hemorrhage, pneumotho-

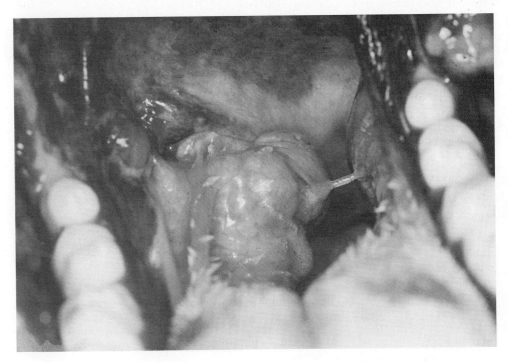

Fig. 17–31. A pharyngeal tumor in a dog obstructing the larynx and inhibiting passage of an endotracheal tube. Intubation was accomplished by using a laryngoscope blade to expose the glottis enough for a guide tube to enter the larynx, followed by passage of the endotracheal tube over the guide tube. (From Hartsfield, S.M. Alternate Methods of Endotracheal Intubation in Small Animals/Emphasis on Patients with Oropharyngeal Pathology. Tex Vet Med J 47:25, 1985.)

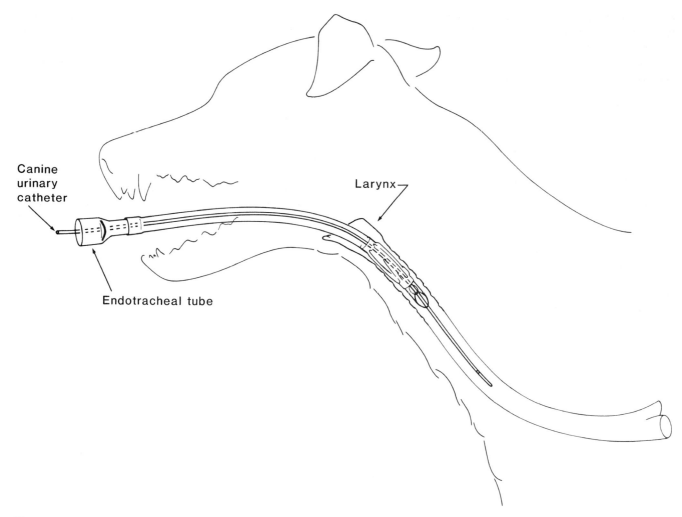

Canine urinary catheter

Larynx

Endotracheal tube

Fig. 17–32. Diagram illustrating passage of an endotracheal tube into the trachea using a guide tube. (From Hartsfield, S.M. Alternate Methods of Endotracheal Intubation in Small Animals/Emphasis on Patients with Oropharyngeal Pathology. Tex Vet Med J 47:25, 1985.)

rax, tracheocutaneous or tracheoesophageal fistula, aspiration, dysphagia, and tracheal malacia; thus, tracheostomy should not be considered to be innocuous.(21) Intubation via tracheostomy is generally reserved for patients requiring pre- or postoperative tracheostomy for airway management. A tracheostomy tube with a replaceable lumen (Fig. 17–8) should be used if available, but standard endotracheal tubes can be used satisfactorily (Fig. 17–9). Care of the tube is very important. Neglected tubes that are not cleaned regularly can become obstructed by mucus that dries within the lumen of the tube (Figs. 17–37 and 17–38).

CHANGING ENDOTRACHEAL TUBES IN AN ANESTHETIZED PATIENT

Changing endotracheal tubes during a surgical or diagnostic procedure in an anesthetized animal is occasionally required owing to a failing cuff or simply the need for a different size or length of tube. The patient positioned and draped for surgery is generally not ideally situated for intubation. Changing the tube with guide tube technique is probably the easiest, most

efficient way to accomplish the procedure.(19, 22) Depending on the size of the patient and the endotracheal tube, a canine urinary catheter (8- to 10-French), two such canine urinary catheters in tandem, or an equine stomach tube makes an excellent guide tube.

To change endotracheal tubes, the guide tube is inserted through the original endotracheal tube to the area of the midcervical trachea. Next, the endotracheal tube cuff is deflated and the endotracheal tube is pulled over the guide tube without removing the guide tube from the trachea. Then, the new endotracheal tube is maneuvered through the larynx and into the trachea using the guide tube to direct its passage. The cuff of the new tube is inflated to protect the airway, and the new tube is secured in the manner appropriate for the specific species.

Extubation of the Trachea

Extubation is performed after patients regain the ability to swallow and protect their airways. When the cuff is deflated, the endotracheal tube is removed slowly and deliberately, taking care to avoid damage to the patient's tissues with the endotracheal tube and damage to the cuff as the tube passes the teeth. After extubation, protection of the airway from foreign material and maintenance of a patent airway remain important. The type of surgical or diagnostic procedure, the species and breed of animal, and preexisting conditions affect these considerations.

The anesthetist should be certain that no foreign material remains in the oropharynx before beginning the process of extubation. In dogs and cats, the pharynx should be inspected visually, and any debris should be removed. Specifically, surgery of the mouth and pharynx, dental procedures, and endoscopy promote the accumulation of blood, fluids, lubricants, tartar, or other materials. Animals anesthetized for gastrointestinal surgery are prone to passive movement of fluid into the pharynx; two examples are dogs with gastric dilation and volvulus (GDV), and horses with colic. Nasogastric or orogastric tubes commonly used in these procedures may promote flow of gastric contents into the pharynx during surgery or when the tube is removed. With either species, the head should be positioned to allow drainage of fluid from the pharynx and mouth before the cuff of the endotracheal tube is deflated. In patients that have had fluid in the pharynx during surgery, removing the endotracheal tube with the cuff inflated may be prudent.

Assuring a patent airway after extubation is essential, especially in patients with small-diameter upper airways (e.g., kittens, piglets, rabbits, small brachycephalic dogs). A number of factors can be responsible for postextubation problems. Edema of the upper airway including the larynx and nasal passages, laryngeal spasm, interference with the integrity of the airway by the soft palate, and laryngeal paralysis are all possible causes of obstructive problems. The anesthetist should be prepared to manage the airway at the time of extubation, knowing that these complications can impair ventilation and oxygenation. In some instances of postextubation airway obstruction, reanesthetizing the patient and reintubation may be the only feasible options.

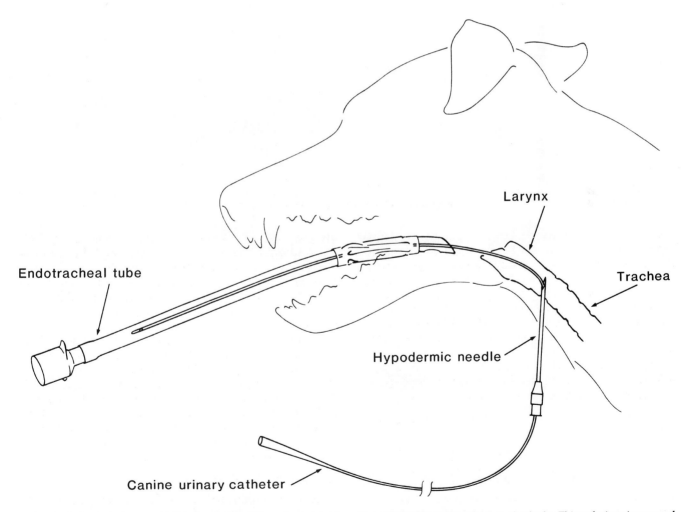

Fig. 17–33. Diagram illustrating the placement and use of a retrograde guide tube for passage of an endotracheal tube. This technique is reserved for patients that cannot be intubated by other methods. (From Hartsfield, S.M. Alternate Methods of Endotracheal Intubation in Small Animals/Emphasis on Patients with Oropharyngeal Pathology. Tex Vet Med J 47:25, 1985.)

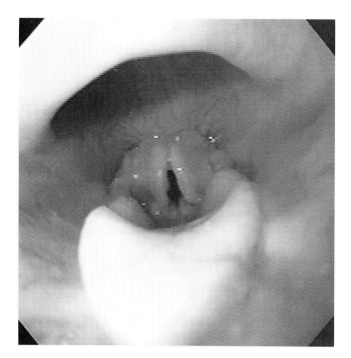

Fig. 17–34. Epiglottis, arytenoid cartilages, and glottis of a cat, as viewed through a fiber-optic endoscope.

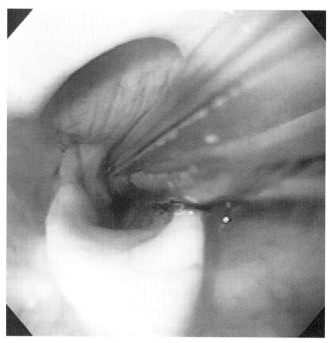

Fig. 17–36. An endotracheal tube passing into the larynx of a cat as viewed through a fiber-optic endoscope. Although not generally necessary for intubation in the cat, this technique is effective in other species.

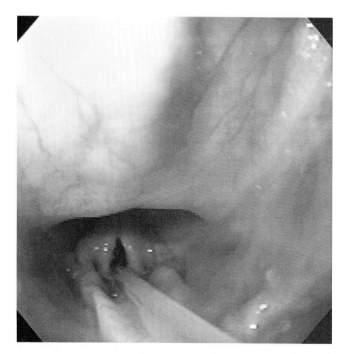

Fig. 17–35. A polyethylene guide tube (8-French) passing through the glottis and into the larynx and trachea of a cat as viewed through a fiber-optic endoscope. Although not generally necessary for intubation in the cat, this technique is effective in other species.

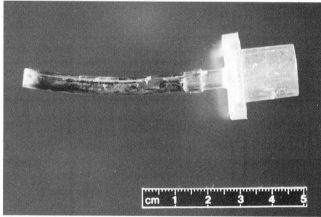

Fig. 17–37. An endotracheal tube that had been placed through a tracheostomy to maintain an airway in a cat during transport of the cat to a referral center. On presentation, the cat was dyspneic and cyanotic. The tube was filled with dried mucus, and the extent of the occlusion of the lumen is illustrated more dramatically in Figure 17–38. The tube had not been changed or cleaned for several hours.

Techniques for Administration of Oxygen

Supplemental oxygen is used in anesthetized and critical patients to increase the partial pressure of oxygen in arterial blood (PaO_2) and to promote delivery of oxygen to the tissues. When a patient is breathing room air, values for PaO_2 that are less than 80 mm Hg indicate the potential for hypoxemia. If the PaO_2 decreases to less than 60 mm Hg, supplemental oxygen is indicated (Chapter 15).(23) Although ventilation is a factor in maintaining oxygenation, the fraction of oxygen in inspired gases (F_IO_2) plays a significant role in establishing the PaO_2. As a rule, the PaO_2 equals approximately five times the F_IO_2 if there are no major abnormalities in the matching of pulmonary ventilation and perfusion. Supplemental oxygen may be the only effective way of correcting hypoxemia in animals with diffusion abnormalities and ventilation-perfusion mismatching. Supplemental oxygen may not significantly affect PaO_2 in patients with pulmonary or cardiac shunts (Chapter 6).

Several techniques can be used to administer oxygen to anesthetized and critically ill patients. The effectiveness of oxygen supplementation is assessed by evaluation of the patient's clinical responses (e.g., improvement in mucous membrane color and character of ventilation), by measuring the F_IO_2, and by monitoring of PaO_2, SaO_2, and SpO_2. Although PaO_2 and SaO_2 data are reliable, they require periodic arterial blood sampling and the use of an acid-base, blood-gas analyzer. The SpO_2 can be conveniently measured by pulse oximetry. Pulse oximetry is a practical method for noninvasive, moment-to-moment estimation of the saturation of hemoglobin with oxygen in anesthetized, recovering, and critically ill patients (Chapter 15).(24, 25)

MASKS FOR DELIVERY OF SUPPLEMENTAL OXYGEN

Masks for delivery of oxygen to veterinary patients are useful for preoxygenation immediately before induction of anesthesia and for emergency situations in awake patients. The use of masks for oxygenation requires constant attention, and some patients will not accept a mask unless they are sedated. Both factors limit the effectiveness of masks in awake patients. Indeed, some patients object to a mask so vigorously that the increase in oxygen consumption associated with restraint may nullify the benefits of a greater F_IO_2.

The flow rates generally recommended for increasing F_IO_2 when using masks are variable among species. For example, flow rates of 10 to 15 L/min of supplemental

oxygen have been recommended to increase the inspired oxygen concentration to approximately 35 to 60% in adult horses.(26) Flow rates for smaller patients including dogs and cats usually range from 3 to 5 L/min. With a tight-fitting mask, higher flow rates of oxygen will produce greater F_IO_2 values and less rebreathing of expired CO_2.

A mask should be used with a breathing system with a reservoir that is capable of meeting the patient's tidal volume demands or with a valved system that allows room air to be entrained. As an example, a dog with a tidal volume of 300 mL and an inspiratory time of 1 second has a peak inspiratory gas flow of approximately 18 L/min, which exceeds the practical flow rate for oxygen during masking. High inspiratory flow rates can be provided if the mask is attached to a circle breathing system with a reservoir bag. In addition, a breathing system has an overflow (pop-off) valve that prevents the buildup of excessive pressure with a tight-fitting mask.

NASAL INSUFFLATION OF OXYGEN

Insufflation involves delivery of oxygen into the patient's airway at relatively high flow rates (Fig. 17–39); the patient inspires both oxygen and room air, the relative proportions of each being determined primarily by the oxygen flow rate and the rate of gas flow during inspiration.

Insufflation can be accomplished by a variety of methods. For horses recovering from anesthesia, oxygen may be delivered from a flowmeter through a delivery tube and into an orotracheal, nasotracheal, or tracheostomy tube. For most awake veterinary patients, oxygen is insufflated through a nasal catheter, the tip of which is positioned in the nasopharynx. The catheter is usually made of soft rubber, and the tube should have several fenestrations to prevent jetting lesions from developing in the nasopharyngeal mucosa.(27) For awake small animals, instilling 2% lidocaine into the nasal passage with the patient's head and neck extended and held upward may facilitate passage of the

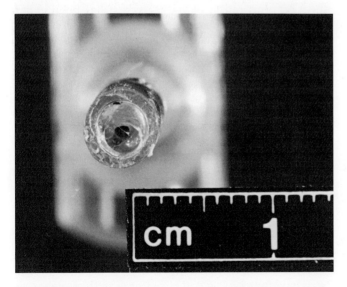

Fig. 17–38. End-on view of the endotracheal tube shown in Figure 17–37 showing that the lumen was almost occluded. The cat was dyspneic prior to removal of the tube from the tracheostomy site. The tube had not been changed or cleaned for several hours.

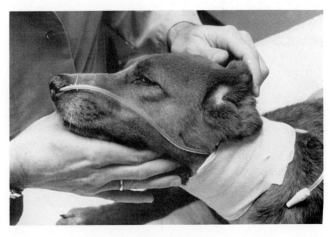

Fig. 17–39. A nasal catheter for administration of oxygen in a dog. The tube is secured to the muzzle with suture.

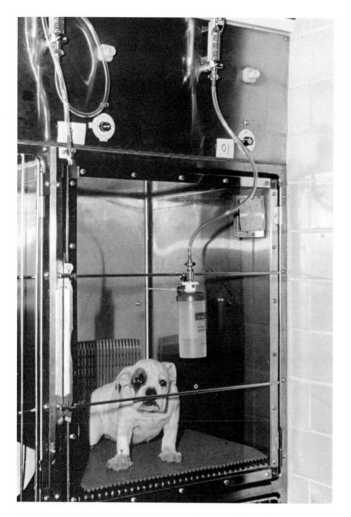

Fig. 17–40. A standard stainless steel cage with a plexiglass door facilitating administration of humidified oxygen to an English bulldog. Although very high concentrations of oxygen are unlikely to be achieved, patients with respiratory distress often show clinical improvement.

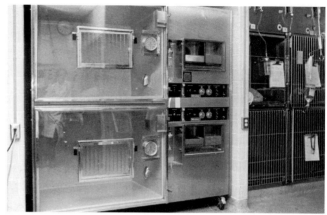

Fig. 17–41. Two commercial oxygen cages designed for small veterinary patients. The cages are capable of controlling environmental temperature, delivering oxygen, and absorbing carbon dioxide from expired gases.

tube. Placement involves insertion of the rubber catheter into the nasal passage and the nasopharynx, the distance being approximately the same as from the tip of the nose to the medial canthus of the eye. The external portion of the catheter is secured to the patient's head with tissue adhesive, tape, and/or sutures. A flexible length of tubing supplies oxygen from a flowmeter and allows the patient some freedom for movement in a cage or stall. Changing the catheter to the opposite nasal passage every 24 to 48 hours has been recommended to prevent pressure necrosis, jet lesions, and accumulation of mucus.(27)

The flow rate requirements for oxygen during insufflation are quite variable, the patient's ventilation and the desired F_IO_2 being two important factors. Following anesthesia, adult horses require a minimum of 15 L/min of oxygen flow to improve the partial pressure of oxygen in arterial blood, and proportionally lower flows are suitable for smaller horses and foals (e.g., 5 L/min) (Chapter 20).(26) In small animals, flow rates of 1 to 7

L/min are typically used for the administration of nasal oxygen. Approximate flow rates for dogs and cats to achieve rather specific ranges for F_IO_2 have been suggested.(27, 28) In dogs, various flow rates of 100% oxygen administered intranasally were studied, and flow rates of 50, 100, 150, and 200 $mL \cdot kg^{-1} \cdot min^{-1}$ produced inspired oxygen concentrations measured at the tracheal bifurcation of 28, 37, 40, and 47%.(29) To prevent mucosal drying with prolonged insufflation, oxygen should be flowed through a bubble-type humidifier.

TRACHEAL INSUFFLATION OF OXYGEN

An intratracheal catheter placed percutaneously into the trachea through the cricothyroid membrane or between tracheal rings near the larynx can be used to insufflate oxygen to a compromised patient. Intratracheal administration of 100% oxygen has been evaluated in dogs, and flow rates of 10, 25, 50, 100, 150, 200, and 250 $mL \cdot kg^{-1} \cdot min^{-1}$ produced inspired oxygen concentrations at the tracheal bifurcation of 25, 32, 47, 67, 70, 78, and 86%, respectively.(30) The technique for tracheal insufflation has been described for small animals.(27, 30) The catheter should be placed aseptically, should be of the over-the-needle type, relatively large bore, should have several smooth fenestrations to prevent jet lesions, and ultimately positioned with the tip near the bronchial bifurcation. Oxygen should be humidified, and flow rates approximate those used for nasal insufflation.

OXYGEN CAGES

Oxygen cages (Figs. 17–40 and 17–41) specifically designed for small animals are commercially available but expensive. These cages regulate oxygen flow, control humidity and temperature, and eliminate carbon dioxide from exhaled gases. For small animals, flow rates of oxygen, cage temperature, and cage humidity have been recommended to be less than 10 L/min, approximately 22° C, and 40 to 50%, respectively.(27)

With these flow rates, most oxygen cages produce an environmental oxygen concentration of about 40 to 50%.(27) Oxygen concentrations of 30 to 40% generally are adequate for patients with moderate pulmonary disease.(23) Oxygen cages are not practical for large horses (26), and even in smaller animals, the effectiveness of an oxygen cage diminishes as body size increases. Because of this, nasal insufflation of oxygen has supplanted oxygen cages in many instances, even for smaller dogs and cats.

Smaller patients can be managed relatively easily in oxygen cages, but temperature and humidity are more difficult to control with larger dogs. A major disadvantage of an oxygen cage is that the animal must be removed from the cage for examination and treatment, requiring the patient to breathe room air or oxygen by mask during this period. Clinically, some dogs and cats with serious ventilatory compromise respond very well to an oxygen-enriched environment as initial therapy; the increase in F_IO_2 is associated with decreased ventilatory effort, and the patient stabilizes and becomes more manageable prior to further examination and treatment.

OXYGEN TOXICITY

Oxygen toxicity develops with prolonged exposure to high oxygen concentrations.(31, 32) Oxygen toxicity leads to the deterioration of pulmonary function, pulmonary edema, and death. The length of time that a patient's PaO_2 is elevated may be more predictive of oxygen toxicity than the duration of exposure to a high F_IO_2.(32) There is significant species and individual variability in susceptibility to oxygen toxicity.(27, 32) In humans, the guideline is that 100% oxygen should not be administered for more than 12 hours.(31) In dogs, microscopic and early pulmonary effects of oxygen toxicity develop within 24 hours of exposure to 100% oxygen.(27) In general, a patient should not be deprived of a high concentration of oxygen if a high F_IO_2 is required to maintain an adequate PaO_2; it has been stated that the brain softens (due to hypoxemia) before the lungs harden (owing to changes induced by prolonged exposure to high oxygen tensions).(33) As guidelines for prolonged administration of oxygen, 40 to 50% oxygen is generally safe, but higher inspired concentrations should be used if necessary to maintain the patient's PaO_2 at approximately 90 to 100 mm Hg to ensure hemoglobin saturation with oxygen.

Mechanical Ventilation

Essentially all anesthetized patients hypoventilate; they do not maintain $PaCO_2$ values near 40 mm Hg because of abnormal alveolar ventilation. While controlled ventilation is not necessary for all anesthetized patients, various circumstances may compel the anesthetist to employ intermittent positive pressure ventilation (IPPV). The absolute indication for mechanical ventilation is apnea.(34) However, IPPV should be instituted if hypoventilation becomes significant, if neuromuscular blocking drugs are employed, or if intrathoracic surgery is performed. General anesthesia for longer than 90 minutes may constitute a reason for IPPV.(36) In addition, IPPV may be needed to facilitate inhalant anesthesia. Hypoventilating animals may not absorb enough anesthetic to maintain surgical anesthesia. IPPV will enhance alveolar ventilation and increase the uptake of the inhalants. This may help in eliminating the oscillations between deep and light anesthesia associated with depression of spontaneous ventilation.

Maintaining relatively normal carbon dioxide tensions in arterial blood is the primary goal of mechanical ventilation in anesthetized patients. Normal values for $PaCO_2$ are generally in the range of 35 to 45 mm Hg for most species. However, controversy exists about the routine use of IPPV in anesthetized patients, particularly anesthetized horses, simply to keep $PaCO_2$ near 40 mm Hg. Because IPPV is associated with reduced cardiovascular function and moderate increases in $PaCO_2$ are associated with improvement in some cardiovascular variables, IPPV for every anesthetized patient is neither universally accepted nor universally practiced. Also, the definition of an acceptable degree of hypercapnia in an anesthetized animal is not without debate. For spontaneously breathing horses, a range of 60 to 80 mm Hg of $PaCO_2$ has been suggested as perhaps safer than controlled ventilation with its potentially adverse effects on cardiovascular function (36). Others have recommended IPPV for horses only when $PaCO_2$ values exceeded 60 (37) or 70 mm Hg.(26, 37) However, employing IPPV in anesthetized animals, including horses and other species, to maintain $PaCO_2$ values between 35 and 50 mm Hg remains common practice. For a more definitive answer to this debate large-scale clinical trials with various size horses and anesthetic-surgical conditions need to be completed.

The direct cardiovascular effects of CO_2 include dilation of peripheral arterioles and myocardial depression. Indirectly, CO_2 evokes sympathoadrenal responses, which cause elevation of blood pressure, tachycardia, and increased myocardial contractility.(38) Moderate (60 to 70 mm Hg) to high (75 to 85 mm Hg) increases in $PaCO_2$ in spontaneously breathing and mechanically ventilated, lightly anesthetized horses were associated with augmented cardiovascular function compared to horses with normal carbon dioxide tensions; these hemodynamic effects were accompanied by increases in circulating catecholamines.(39) Therefore, normal arterial carbon dioxide tensions may correlate with lower values for blood pressure, myocardial contractility, and cardiac output in anesthetized animals. Spontaneously breathing anesthetized animals may maintain cardiovascular function better than anesthetized animals in which ventilation is controlled. Inotropic drugs may be necessary to maintain cardiovascular function during surgical anesthesia in mechanically ventilated horses. Nevertheless, there are good reasons to maintain $PaCO_2$ values within reasonable limits in anesthetized animals.

Inhalant anesthetics (e.g., halothane) and epidural or spinal anesthesia reduce the circulatory responses to

CO_2.(38, 40) In addition, hypercapnia has been associated with increases in vagal tone and slowing of heart rate.(41) Indeed, hypercapnia has long been related to enhanced vagal responsiveness, bradycardia, and even cardiac arrest. It used to be said that "hypercarbia does not stimulate vagal activity directly, but it 'sets the stage' for cardiac arrest if such a stimulus is present." (42) It is known that carbon dioxide produces narcosis in the dog, the degree of which depends on the $PaCO_2$ value; narcosis progressively increases with $PaCO_2$ values above 95 mm Hg to result in complete anesthesia at 245 mm Hg.(43) Hypercapnia and the associated increases in circulating catecholamines have been linked to the development of cardiac arrhythmias, especially when the heart has been sensitized by halogenated inhalant anesthetics.(44) In human pediatric patients whose airways were managed by masks, hypercapnia was associated with an increased incidence of arrhythmias.(45) The authors noted that light anesthesia or combination of factors such as hypercapnia and halothane might have been as important as hypercapnia alone in the production of arrhythmias in these children. Thus, there is a negative side to uncontrolled hypercapnia that should be considered for the anesthetized patient, and the veterinarian or anesthesiologist should weigh the advantages against the disadvantages in the management of their patient during anesthesia.

Mechanical ventilation affects cardiovascular function (Fig. 17–42). The depression of cardiovascular function may be significant. When ventilation is controlled and negative pressures are not generated during inspiration, venous return is not enhanced. Indeed, IPPV may physically impede venous return to the right side of the heart, leading to decreases in stroke volume, cardiac output, and arterial blood pressure. In the anesthetized, mechanically ventilated horse, a reduction in blood pressure and damping of the pressure waveform is not uncommon, especially in a critically ill patient with a marginal blood volume. The negative effects of mechanical ventilation on cardiovascular function can be exacerbated by prolonging inspiratory time, holding positive pressure in the lungs at the end of inspiration, retarding exhalation, applying positive pressure during the expiratory phase, and employing an excessively rapid respiratory rate. Some of these effects are illustrated in Figure 17–42. Fortunately, these negative effects can be overcome in many cases by the appropriate expansion of extracellular fluid volume and, if necessary, the administration of inotropic drugs.

Guidelines for mechanical ventilation usually include values for inspiratory time, respiratory rate, inspiratory to expiratory time ratio, and tidal volume. Some variations exist because of differences in body size, species, physical condition of the lungs and thorax, and existing disease processes.

Normal tidal volume is generally considered to range between 10 and 20 mL per kg of body weight.(46) A good working guideline for tidal volume in the domes-

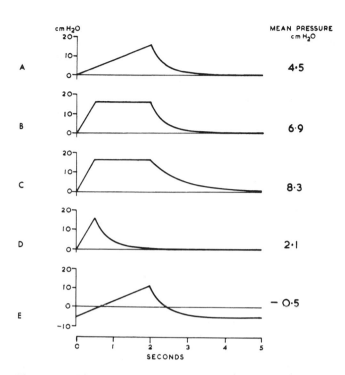

Fig. 17–42. Diagrams illustrating the mean pressure in the lungs in relation to positive pressure ventilation. The effects of a long inspiratory time (A), an inspiratory plateau or holding pressure at the end of inspiration (B), an inspiratory plateau with retarded expiration (C), a rapid inspiration (D), and a slow inspiration with a negative expiratory phase (E) are shown. Lower mean pressure is most desirable from the standpoint of cardiovascular function, and D illustrates the most desirable type of ventilation although the inspiratory time depicted is shorter than normally used clinically. (From Mushin, W.W., et al. Automatic Ventilation of the Lungs, 2nd ed. Philadelphia: FA Davis, 1969. Used in Lumb, W.V., and Jones, E.W. Oxygen Administration and Artificial Respiration. In: Veterinary Anesthesia, 2nd ed. Philadelphia: Lea & Febiger, 1984.)

tic species is approximately 10 mL/kg (Chapters 6 and 15).(47) For IPPV, the tidal volume set on a mechanical ventilator is usually increased above the normal spontaneous tidal volume to compensate for pressure-mediated increases in the volume of the breathing system and airways. Increasing the tidal volume (bellows volume) by 2.2 to 4.4 mL/kg has been recommended.(35) Settings for tidal volume, 15 mL/kg in large animals and 20 mL/kg in small animals, have been suggested.(47) Use of small tidal volumes may result in atelectasis, which may only be recognized grossly during thoracotomy, or during blood-gas analysis because atelectasis contributes to mismatching of pulmonary ventilation and perfusion leading to decreased PaO_2. The tidal volume should be delivered to the patient over a relatively short period of time to avoid maintaining positive intrathoracic pressure. Inspiratory time should be approximately 1 to 1.5 seconds in small animals and 1.5 to 3 seconds in large animals.

The inspiratory time compared to time during the entire expiratory phase is termed the *I:E ratio*. That fraction should be 1:2 (I:E) or less for mechanical ventilation in all patients. Ratios that approach 1:1

result in a long duration of positive intrathoracic pressure, which interferes with cardiovascular function. If a patient's respiratory rate is 10 breaths/min and the inspiratory time is 1.5 seconds, the I:E ratio will be 1:3. In general, the exact value of the I:E ratio is not important as long as the ratio is less than 1:2. With some ventilators that incorporate specific, unchangeable I:E ratios, the options for controlling respiratory rate may be limited.

Tidal volume and inspiratory time affect the development of peak inspiratory pressure. In general, 15 to 30 cm of H_2O will expand the lung.(47) Fifteen to 20 cm of H_2O and 20 to 30 cm of H_2O have been recommended as peak inspiratory pressures for mechanical ventilation of small animal species with normal lungs and large animal species with normal lungs, respectively.(35) Excessive or sustained pressure during IPPV can cause volotrauma, leading to disruption of the alveolar membrane, to the development of interstitial air, and ultimately to tracking of air to the mediastinum, pleural space, or abdomen.(48) A guideline for peak inspiratory pressure is 30 cm of H_2O. Special attention to peak pressure is important for animals that have experienced lung trauma (e.g., diaphragmatic hernia).(49)

The appropriate respiratory rate for mechanical ventilation varies with the species and the tidal volume selected. The following recommendations have been published: dogs, 8 to 14 breaths/min; cats, 10 to 14 breaths/min; horse and cow, 6 to 10 breaths/min; and small ruminants and pigs, 8 to 12 breaths/min.(47) In patients requiring smaller than usual tidal volumes, to avoid excessive inspiratory pressures (e.g., diaphragmatic hernia, gastrointestinal distension including GDV), respiratory rates should be increased to maintain the appropriate minute ventilation.

When controlled ventilation is discontinued at the end of anesthesia, the return of spontaneous ventilation may be impaired. If $PaCO_2$ is low, spontaneous ventilation may not resume. Part of the management of controlled ventilation should be maintenance of relatively normal carbon dioxide tensions, and hypocarbia should be avoided. The residual effects of opioids, anesthetics, and adjunctive drugs (e.g., neuromuscular blocking drugs) at the end of anesthesia may contribute to a delayed return to spontaneous ventilation (Chapter 13). Complicating factors associated with general anesthesia or surgery (e.g., hypothermia or hypovolemia) may slow the animal's return to consciousness and spontaneous ventilation. In general, the arterial tension of carbon dioxide must increase to stimulate the animal to breathe spontaneously, or the patient must regain a level of consciousness that promotes spontaneous ventilation. Before attempting to discontinue controlled ventilation, the anesthetist should ascertain that depth of anesthesia is decreasing, that the effects of muscle-relaxing drugs have subsided or have been antagonized, and that cardiovascular function is relatively normal. Then, the animal can be weaned from controlled ventilation.

The patient should continue to receive supplemental oxygen until spontaneous ventilation is relatively normal. Reducing the rate of controlled ventilation usually increases $PaCO_2$ enough to stimulate spontaneous breathing when the animal is regaining consciousness. Generally, the patient is mechanically or manually ventilated at a rate of one to four breaths per minute until spontaneous ventilation resumes. In many cases, animals begin to breathe spontaneously after the vaporizer has been turned off and most of the inhalant anesthetic has been eliminated, even though controlled ventilation has not been stopped. Some patients require some type of external stimulus to begin breathing (e.g., pinching the skin between the toes in a dog). After the animal begins to breathe spontaneously, assisted ventilation and supplemental oxygen should be provided until the respiratory rate and tidal volume begin to normalize.

Anesthesia Ventilators

Anesthesia ventilators provide for mechanical ventilation of patients being maintained with inhalant anesthetics. Simply, an anesthesia ventilator is a reservoir bag (a bellows or concertina bag) in a closed container (bellows housing) that can substitute for the reservoir bag of an anesthesia breathing system. Within limits, the ventilator has the capability of driving its bellows to produce a specific tidal volume or a specific inspiratory pressure at a preselected rate. The anesthesia ventilator performs the same job as the anesthetist who periodically squeezes the circle system's reservoir bag to ventilate the patient. Some anesthesia ventilators are stand-alone units that are attached to an anesthesia machine when needed, whereas other ventilators are manufactured as an integral part of the anesthesia machine. Most anesthesia ventilators designed for human beings are appropriate for veterinary patients weighing less than approximately 140 kg. Ventilators specifically designed for large animals are needed for patients weighing more than 140 kg. Admittedly, these guidelines for body weight and selection of a ventilator are somewhat arbitrary.

CLASSIFICATION

The power source, drive mechanism, cycling mechanism, and type of bellows have been used to classify anesthesia ventilators.(50) The power source may be electricity, compressed gas, or both. The drive mechanism is commonly compressed gas, even when electric controls are used. Anesthesia ventilators are usually double-circuit units (Fig. 17–43). Double circuit refers to two gas sources: (a) the driving gas circuit (outside of the bellows), which compresses the bellows, and (b) the patient gas circuit (inside the bellows), which originates at the anesthesia machine and provides oxygen and anesthetic to the breathing system and patient. Specific ventilators for veterinary applications are classified in Table 17–1.

Anesthesia ventilators are typically, though not always, time cycled.(50) Fluidic timing devices were

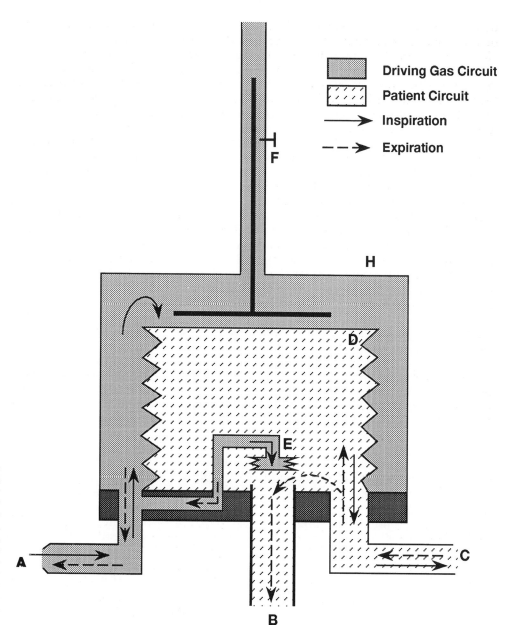

Fig. 17–43. Diagram of a generic, double-circuit ventilator. Driving gas enters at A, leading to compression of the bellows and forcing gas in the patient circuit toward the breathing system and the patient's respiratory system (C). Overflow gas from the patient circuit exits through the pop-off valve (E) and flows into the scavenger system (B). Item F is the tidal volume adjustment, D is the bellows, and H is the bellows housing.

common in the late 1970s, and fluidic-controlled ventilators remain in use. Newer electronic ventilators incorporate solid-state timing circuitry and are classified as time cycled and electronically controlled. A pressure cycling mechanism may be present in some ventilators, and some have been described as volume cycled. In most cases, a timing mechanism plays a major role in a ventilator's function, and volume or pressure limits may affect the change in the respiratory cycle from inspiration to expiration.

The direction that the bellows moves during expiration, either ascending or descending, also helps to characterize anesthesia ventilators. Newer anesthesia ventilators usually have ascending bellows. The ascending bellows is considered safer because it will not fill

if a disconnection occurs in the breathing circuit.(50) The ascending bellows falls to the bottom of the bellows housing during a disconnection, giving an immediate visual indication that ventilatory failure has occurred. Ascending bellows are incorporated into modern electronic ventilators. Ventilators with descending bellows may continue to cycle even with a complete disconnection of the ventilator from the breathing system.

The terms *tidal-volume preset, volume preset,* and *volume-constant* have been used to describe anesthesia ventilators; these terms have been included in operations manuals and other descriptive literature authored both by manufacturers and by medical personnel. The implication is that the ventilator delivers exactly the tidal volume selected despite the total inspiratory time or the amount of inspiratory pressure that develops. However, the tidal volume that actually reaches the patient's lungs may vary from the setting on the ventilator. Variations are related to the compliance of the breathing system, leaks in the system, and the entry of fresh gases into the breathing system. Although the terms *tidal-volume preset*, *volume preset*, and *volume-constant* may be practical, the user should understand the unknown influences on the quantity of gas actually delivered to the patient.

In addition, ventilators may be called *pressure preset*, indicating that inspiration continues until a selected pressure is reached, no matter what tidal volume is achieved. The amount of gas delivered to the patient depends on a number of factors including the resistance and compliance of the breathing system and the patient's respiratory system. Although inspiratory pressure may not vary over time, the tidal volume may change as compliance of the respiratory system changes.

Even though ventilators have been classified as *volume limited* and *pressure limited*, and *pressure cycled*, *time cycled*, and *volume cycled*, these terms may be somewhat misleading or confusing because the mechanism that actually causes the change from expiration to inspiration is most often a timing mechanism. Indeed, the change from one phase of ventilation to the other may involve more than one mechanism, including volume, pressure, and/or time. Some ventilators may utilize different cycling mechanisms depending on the mode of operation.(50) A pressure-limited ventilator is one that delivers gas to the patient during inspiration until a preset pressure develops in the bellows, at which point the expiratory phase begins. The disadvantage of pressure-limited ventilation is that the tidal volume delivered to the patient may decrease if respiratory compliance decreases during ventilation. A volume-limited ventilator delivers a preset tidal volume (within the limits discussed earlier) without regard for the maximum inspiratory pressure (up to the preset maximum pressure for the ventilator). Inspiratory pressure may increase if compliance decreases during mechanical ventilation. Most anesthesia ventilators have a maximum pressure limit during inspiration for the safety of the patient, and that pressure limit varies with the model of the ventilator. Ventilators that are used as volume-limited units may truly be limited by time rather than by volume, and that fact becomes apparent if the inspiratory flow rate is too slow.

TERMINOLOGY OF MECHANICAL VENTILATION

Several abbreviations are used in the medical literature to describe various types of ventilation. Common abbreviations are included and discussed in the following paragraphs.

Table 17–1. Classification and Characteristics of Anesthesia Ventilators

Ventilator	Power Source	Drive Mechanism	Cycling Mechanism	Bellows*	Type of Ventilation
Drager SAV (SA)	Pneumatic	Pneumatic	Time-Fluidic	Ascend	Control
Hallowell EMC 2000 (SA)	Pneumatic and Electronic	Pneumatic	Time-Electronic	Ascend	Control
Mallard 2400 V (SA)	Pneumatic and Electronic	Pneumatic	Time-Electronic	Ascend	Control
Metomatic (Ohio)-SA	Pneumatic	Pneumatic	Time-Fluidic	Descend	Assist/Control
Ohmeda 7000 (SA)	Pneumatic and Electronic	Pneumatic	Time-Electronic	Ascend	Control
ADS 1000 (SA)	Pneumatic and Electronic	Pneumatic	Time-Electronic	None	Control
SAV 75 (SA)	Pneumatic	Pneumatic	Time-Pressure	Ascend	Assist/Control
Drager AV (LA)	Pneumatic and Electronic	Pneumatic	Time-Fluidic	Descend	Control
Narkovet:E Electronic LA Control Center	Pneumatic and Electronic	Pneumatic	Time-Electronic	Descend	Control
LAVC 2000 (LA)	Pneumatic	Pneumatic	Time-Pressure	Descend	Assist/Control
Mallard 2800 (LA)	Pneumatic and Electronic	Pneumatic	Time-Electronic	Ascend	Control

LA, large animal, and SA, small animal, indicate the primary use of the ventilator.
*Bellows—described in reference to the direction of movement during expiration.

IPPV (intermittent positive pressure ventilation).
With IPPV, airway pressure is maintained above ambient pressure during inspiration, and airway pressure falls to ambient pressure to allow passive expiration.(48) *Conventional positive pressure ventilation* (CPPV), also called *control mode ventilation* (CMV), is a form of IPPV in which a ventilator delivers a preset tidal volume at a preset frequency.(51) Assist-control mode ventilation (AMV) provides a preset tidal volume from the ventilator in response to patient-initiated attempts to inspire; a preset frequency of ventilation is delivered by the ventilator if the patient fails to initiate breathing.(51) The term *IPPB (intermittent positive pressure breathing)* is synonymous with IPPV.

PEEP (positive end expiratory pressure). With PEEP, airway pressure at end-expiration is maintained above ambient pressure. The term *PEEP* is applied when positive pressure is maintained between inspirations that are delivered by a ventilator.(51) The term *ZEEP,* for *zero end-expiratory pressure,* has been used in studies comparing the effects of PEEP to the effects of ZEEP.(52) In addition, some ventilators can create negative pressure to assist expiration or to speed the egress of gases during the expiratory phase. This has been termed *NEEP* or *negative end expiratory pressure.*

CPAP (continuous positive airway pressure). When airway pressure is maintained above ambient pressure during spontaneous breathing, the term *CPAP* is applied instead of PEEP.(51)

IMV (intermittent mandatory ventilation). This method of ventilation is used for ventilatory support and for weaning of patients from ventilators. The technique allows the patient to breathe spontaneously, but it inserts mechanical breaths at a preset tidal volume and frequency.(51, 52) Most veterinary anesthesia ventilators are not designed for delivering this form of ventilation, and IMV is provided by critical care ventilators for human beings. The periodic sigh that the anesthetist provides manually during spontaneous ventilation to expand the lung and decrease collapsed alveoli in anesthetized animals has been termed *IMV.*(26)

The terms *assisted ventilation* and *controlled ventilation* are common in the veterinary literature. Assisted ventilation can be performed manually by the anesthetist, who synchronizes his or her compression of the breathing bag with the patient's spontaneous breathing to augment the tidal volume.(53) With a mechanical ventilator, assisted ventilation is basically patient-initiated ventilation, with the ventilator delivering the preselected tidal volume. Since the patient determines the frequency of ventilation, it also determines minute volume.(54) Some veterinary ventilators are capable of providing assisted ventilation, delivering a tidal volume from the bellows when the patient creates negative pressure during an attempt to breathe.(55)

During *controlled ventilation* as defined earlier for CMV, inspiration is initiated by the ventilator and a preset respiratory rate is maintained. The ventilator sets frequency, tidal volume, and minute volume. Controlled ventilation is necessary in any situation that renders the patient unable to initiate an adequate number of breaths. Essentially all anesthesia ventilators will operate in this mode, and some operate only in this mode. Controlled ventilation can be provided manually by the anesthetist using the reservoir bag of the breathing system to establish both rate and tidal volume, and thus minute volume, for the patient.(53)

The term *assisted-controlled ventilation* has been defined as assisted ventilation (patient-controlled rate with ventilator-controlled tidal volume) with a preset minimum acceptable respiratory rate; if the patient-initiated rate falls below the preset rate, the ventilator will cycle at the minimum preset rate. This mode is similar to AMV as defined earlier. Assisted-controlled ventilation has been suggested for the transition period between spontaneous and controlled ventilation.

GUIDELINES FOR USE

The controls on most anesthesia ventilators include settings for tidal volume, inspiratory time, inspiratory pressure, respiratory rate, and I:E ratio (either adjustable or preset). Other controls may be present, but the four listed are basic. The following guidelines have already been discussed but will again be briefly reviewed. The setting for tidal volume is usually between 10 and 20 mL/kg, and the inspiratory pressure is normally between 12 and 30 cm of H_2O. In small patients, the respiratory rate should be set between 8 and 12 breaths per minute, while the respiratory rate for large animals should be set between 6 to 10 breaths per minute. In setting the ventilator, inspiratory time should be short in comparison to expiratory time so that positive interpleural pressure will minimally interfere with venous return and cardiac output. Inspiratory time should be 1 to 1.5 seconds in small animals and preferably less than 3 seconds in large animals. Therefore, the I:E ratio should be 1:2 or less (e.g., 1:3 or 1:4) depending on the respiratory rate.

VENTILATORS FOR SMALL ANIMALS

Although not all-inclusive, the following discussion describes ventilators that are appropriate for small animal patients. Some of these ventilators were designed specifically to support anesthetized veterinary patients; others were designed for human use, but are applicable to veterinary patients. The classification, principles of operation, and other points about the general function of each ventilator are included. Before operating a ventilator, the user should consult the operation manuals and follow all preuse evaluation procedures recommended by the manufacturer.

Drager SAV Small Animal Ventilator. The Drager SAV Small Animal Ventilator (Fig. 17–44) was marketed as an optional component for the Drager Narkovet 2 Anesthesia Machine, but was available on a mobile stand (universal pole) specifically designed for the ventilator.(56) Presently, the ventilator is not being

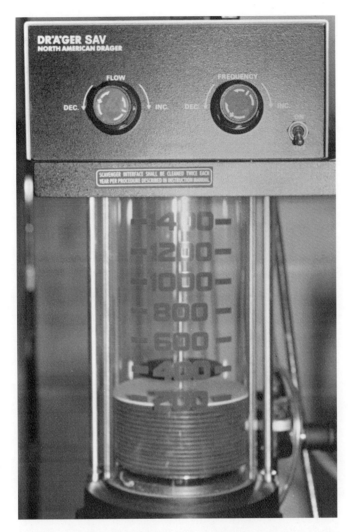

Fig. 17-44. Drager SAV Small Animal Ventilator (front view). The ascending bellows and the bellows housing with the tidal volume marked in milliliters are shown in the lower portion of the photograph, and the inspiratory flow control knob (left), the frequency control knob (center, right), and the power switch (far right) are shown in the upper portion of the photograph.

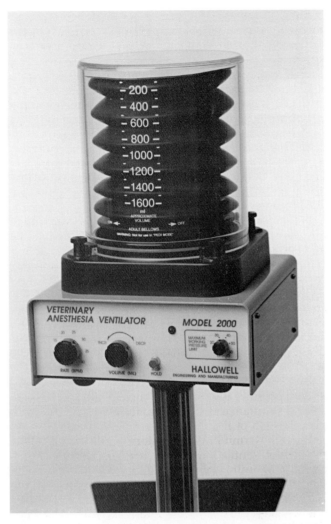

Fig. 17-45. Hallowell EMC Model 2000 Small Animal Veterinary Anesthesia Ventilator (front view). The bellows shown is the medium sized bellows for tidal volumes between 300 and 1600 mL, and the basic control knobs and alarm indicator light are on the front panel. (Photograph courtesy of W. Stetson Hallowell.)

manufactured, but these ventilators remain in use for veterinary anesthesia. The SAV is classified as a double-circuit, tidal-volume-preset, time-cycled ventilator with an ascending bellows; it is pneumatically powered and has fluidic circuitry. The pressure of the driving gas should be between 40 and 60 psi. The controls include a power ("on-off") switch, a tidal-volume adjustment rod to set the attached plate within the bellows housing to the selected tidal volume (200 to 1600 mL), a frequency control knob (10 to 30 breaths per minute), and an inspiratory flow knob, which controls rate of flow into the bellows housing to drive the bellows. The inspiratory flow knob should be set so that the bellows is fully compressed at the end of the inspiratory phase; however, the bellows should not be deformed at the end of inspiration. Deformation of the bellows at the end of inspiration may be indicative

of an increase in tidal volume by as much as 100 mL. The inspiratory flow control setting affects the peak pressure that is achieved on inspiration and the inspiratory time. Higher inspiratory flows produce shorter inspiratory times and tend to produce higher peak inspiratory pressures. The inspiratory to expiratory time phase ratio is preset to 1:2. This ventilator provides only controlled ventilation. The ventilator relief valve behind the bellows chamber compensates for the continuous entry of fresh gases into the breathing system. Because the ventilator uses an ascending bellows, the effect of gravity on the bellows maintains positive end-expiratory pressure of approximately 2 cm of H_2O.

Before using the ventilator, the proper connections to the gas supply and scavenger system should be made and the appropriate preuse checkout procedures should be done. Assuming that the anesthesia machine, breathing system, and ventilator are functional, the following is a reasonable step-by-step approach to the operation of this ventilator with a circle breathing system:

1. The tidal-volume adjustment rod is set appropriately for the patient.
2. Corrugated tubing from the ventilator's breathing hose terminal is connected to the circle system's bag mount.
3. The circle system's pop-off (APL) valve is closed.
4. The ventilator's power switch is turned on.
5. The frequency of ventilation is adjusted to approximately the desired number of breaths per minute.
6. The inspiratory flow control knob is adjusted to produce the desired inspiratory time to deliver the preset tidal volume.
7. Frequency of ventilation and inspiratory flow may need to be readjusted to achieve the desired rate of breathing and inspiratory time.

Hallowell EMC Model 2000 Small Animal Veterinary Anesthesia Ventilator. The Hallowell EMC Model 2000 Small Animal Veterinary Anesthesia Ventilator (Fig. 17–45) is designed for use with standard small animal anesthesia machines and breathing systems, and the connections to the breathing system, scavenger, and driving gas are shown in Figure 17–46.(57) This ventilator is classified as double circuit and time cycled with an ascending bellows; it is pneumatically and electrically powered. The ventilator is essentially volume constant within the practical limits described earlier. The ventilator is pneumatically driven and electronically controlled (by an electrically activated solenoid valve that allows gas pressure to be supplied to the volume control during the inspiratory phase of the ventilatory cycle). The ventilator's power switch is incorporated into the respiratory rate control. Therefore, the ventilator is on when the rate selector is turned from the off position to the desired frequency of respiration (6 to 40 breaths per minute). The pressure of the driving gas supply (either oxygen, nitrogen, or clean dry air) should be regulated between 30 to 60 psi and be capable of supplying 100 L/min at 30 psi. This high flow is necessary only for larger patients.

The control module of the ventilator has the following adjustable components: the on-off and respiratory rate control knob, a volume control knob, an inspiratory hold pushbutton, and a maximum working pressure limit (MWPL) selector. The inspiratory to expiratory time phase ratio is preset at 1:2. However, this ventilator is available with an optional adjustable I:E ratio in the range of 1:1.5 to 1:4, enabling the user to minimize the inspiratory time when ventilating at a lower frequency of ventilation. The volume control is a variable orifice metering valve that regulates the driving gas flow, which compresses the bellows. Basically, the volume control is used to set minute volume. It regulates the inspiratory flow rate directly, and a higher inspiratory flow rate at any given respiratory rate will produce a greater tidal volume. The inspiratory hold pushbutton

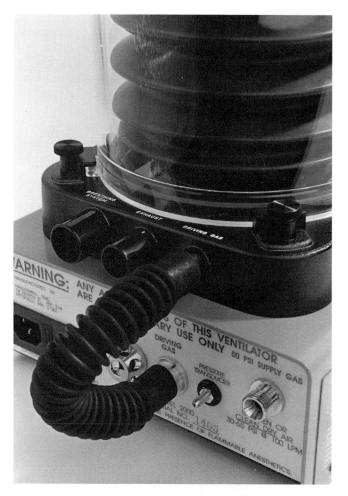

Fig. 17–46. Hallowell EMC Model 2000 Small Animal Veterinary Anesthesia Ventilator (rear view). Note the connectors on the bellows housing for the breathing system, scavenger system (exhaust), and driving gas. The port for connecting the pressure transducer to the breathing system, the DISS connector for the driving gas supply, and the electric connector (left) are present. (Photograph courtesy of W. Stetson Hallowell.)

interrupts the ventilatory cycle and prevents discharge of gas from the bellows housing until the button is released or the MWPL is reached. The MWPL can be set between 10 and 60 cm of H_2O. If the MWPL is reached at any time, the inspiratory phase of ventilation is terminated and exhalation is allowed. Low breathing system pressure will be detected if pressure at the end of inspiration is less than 5 cm of H_2O, and a red warning light will illuminate and an alarm will sound indicating the possibility of a disconnection of the patient circuit from the ventilator. This ventilator provides for controlled ventilation; assisted ventilation is not an option.

Three sizes of interchangeable bellows and bellows housings are available to allow various sizes of patients to be ventilated effectively (Fig. 17–47). With the proper bellows, the manufacturer indicates that tidal volumes as small as 20 mL and as large as 3 L can be delivered and that the patient can effectively breathe spontaneously from the bellows when the ventilator is not in operation. The ventilator relief valve compensates for the continuous entry of fresh gas into the breathing system, and the resistance of the relief valve creates a positive end-expiratory pressure between 2 and 3 cm of H_2O.

Before using the ventilator, connections to the gas supply and scavenger system should be made and the appropriate preuse checkout procedures should be done. Assuming proper function of the anesthesia machine, breathing system, and ventilator, the following is a reasonable operational approach for this ventilator with a circle breathing system:

1. The MWPL selector (Fig. 17–45) is set to the desired maximum pressure (safety limit), and the pressure transducer (Fig. 17–46) is connected to the breathing system according to the manufacturer's recommendations.

2. Corrugated tubing from the ventilator's breathing system connector is attached to the circle system's bag mount, and the ventilator is attached to the scavenger system.

3. The circle system's APL (pop-off) valve is closed.

4. The ventilator's volume control is adjusted to the minimum setting.

5. The ventilator's power-rate switch is turned on, and the desired frequency of ventilation is set.

6. The volume control knob is adjusted to produce a flow of gas during inspiration that results in the desired tidal volume and/or peak inspiratory pressure.

7. During maintenance, the minute volume is adjusted with the volume control, and the rate control can be used to adjust the size of each tidal volume.

Mallard Medical Model 2400V Anesthesia Ventilator.
The Mallard Medical Model 2400V Anesthesia Ventilator (58) (Fig. 17–48) was originally designed to allow continuous mechanical ventilation of anesthetized pediatric and adult human patients. It is sold to veterinarians as a standalone unit for use with a breathing system and anesthesia machine. Classified as a double-circuit ventilator, it has electric and pneumatic power sources. The ventilator is controlled by a microprocessor, and the manufacturer describes the ventilator as electronically time cycled and volume limited. The tidal volume is selected by limiting the upward expansion of the bellows; tidal volume is adjusted by moving a cylinder within the bellows housing to coincide with the desired setting in milliliters, and the cylinder within

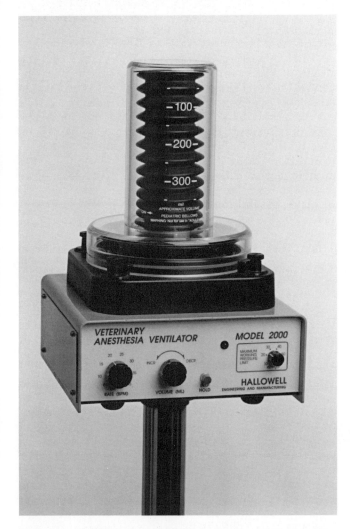

Fig. 17–47. Hallowell EMC Model 2000 Small Animal Veterinary Anesthesia Ventilator (front view). The bellows shown is the smallest bellows for tidal volumes between 0 and 300 mL. The basic control knobs and alarm indicator light are on the front panel. (Photograph courtesy of W. Stetson Hallowell.)

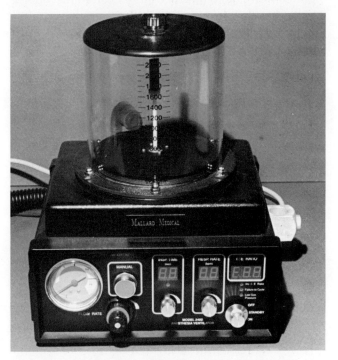

Fig. 17–48. Mallard 2400V Small Animal Anesthesia Ventilator. The bellows is collapsed on the floor of the bellows housing. The tidal volume control is set at approximately 1600 mL. The control knobs on the console are described in the text.

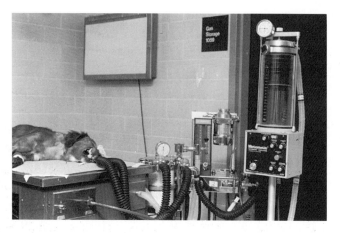

Fig. 17–49. Metomatic Veterinary Ventilator. The ventilator's bellows is connected by a corrugated breathing tube to the reservoir bag port of the circle breathing system to allow controlled ventilation. Anesthesia was maintained with halothane in oxygen in this dog.

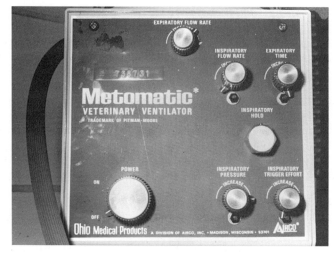

Fig. 17–50. Control panel of a Metomatic Veterinary Ventilator. The function of the various controls of this ventilator are discussed in the text.

the bellows housing is secured by a control knob (nut) located on the top center of the housing. This ventilator employs an ascending bellows. The bellows is pneumatically driven, and the ventilator operates at a pressure of 50 ± 10 psi.

The controls are positioned on a console, which is located below the bellows housing. A master on/standby/off switch is present in the right lower corner of the console's front panel; the standby mode allows preselection of respiratory rate and inspiratory time, and the I:E ratio is computed and displayed digitally on light emitting diode (LED) displays before mechanical ventilation is initiated. Respiratory rate and inspiratory time are controlled by ten-turn potentiometers to allow selection of 2 to 80 breaths per minute (respiratory rate) and 0.1 to 3.0 seconds (inspiratory time), respectively. The I:E ratio display shows the relationship of inspiratory time to expiratory time, giving inspiratory time a value of 1. A black control knob located in the left lower portion of the front panel allows adjustment of inspiratory flow rate (10 to 100 L/min), and a display gauge near the control knob indicates if the flow being used is low, medium, or high. A green pushbutton is located in the front center portion of the control console; this button will activate inspiration as long as the button is pushed in. This button can be used to maintain mechanical ventilation in the event of a power failure and can be used to sigh the patient.

Two sizes of bellows are available. The adult bellows provides tidal volumes ranging from 200 to 2200 mL; the pediatric bellows produces volumes ranging from 50 to 300 mL. An exhalation valve assembly is located on the back of the control console. This valve is closed pneumatically during the inspiratory phase of ventilation, and it opens automatically during the expiratory phase. Excess gas from the patient circuit exits through this valve to prevent the buildup of excessive pressure. The port (19 mm) of this valve should be attached to a scavenger system for elimination of waste gases from

the working environment. With an ascending bellows, positive end-expiratory pressure (PEEP), usually 2 or 3 cm of H_2O, will be present. In addition, PEEP of up to 20 cm of H_2O can be added to the system with the control knob of the optional PEEP valve. There is also an adjustable overpressure relief valve within the console that is preset to 80 cm of H_2O, and this limits the maximum pressure that can be developed in the patient breathing circuit. Externally, this pressure can be adjusted from 20 to 100 cm of H_2O. This ventilator has audible alarms if the ventilator fails to cycle or if an electric power failure occurs. In addition, the LED displays will indicate selection of an inverse I:E ratio, failure of the ventilator to cycle, and low supply gas pressure (<30 psi).

Before using the ventilator, the proper connections to the gas supply and scavenger system should be made and the appropriate preuse checkout procedures should be done. Assuming proper function of the anesthesia machine, breathing system, and ventilator, the following is a reasonable operational approach for this ventilator with a circle breathing system:

1. Prior to clinical applications, refer to the operations manual for instructions and conduct performance verification procedures.
2. Select the appropriate control settings for the tidal volume by limiting the upward expansion of the bellows.
3. Place the master switch in the standby mode, and dial the desired settings for the respiratory rate and the inspiratory time, based on the patient's needs.
4. Set the inspiratory flow control to the desired rate of flow–low, medium, or high, depending on the needs of the patient.
5. Connect the corrugated tubing from the ventilator's bellows to the circle system's bag mount, and attach the ventilator to the scavenger system.

6. Close the circle system's APL (pop-off) valve.
7. Set the master switch to the on position.
8. The ventilator should cycle according to the selected settings, and only minor adjustments should be necessary (i.e., slight alterations in inspiratory time).

Metomatic Veterinary Ventilator. The Metomatic Veterinary Ventilator is shown in Figures 17–49 and 17–50. This unit was designed to ventilate anesthetized small animals being maintained with circle breathing systems. The ventilator is no longer being manufactured, but many units are still in operation in veterinary hospitals.

This ventilator is classified as double circuit and time cycled with fluidic circuitry and a descending bellows. Within the limits of the definitions, it can be used as a volume-preset ventilator or as a pressure-limited ventilator. The ventilator is powered pneumatically and will function properly with an oxygen supply pressure of 45 to 55 psi.

Controls (Fig. 17–50) for this ventilator are as follows (59, 60): power switch ("on-off"), tidal-volume control, inspiratory flow rate control, expiratory time control, expiratory flow rate control, inspiratory hold pushbutton, and inspiratory trigger effort control. The power switch controls a valve that supplies pneumatic power (oxygen at 50 psi) to the ventilator. The tidal-volume control adjusts the bellows from 0 to 1400 mL. The inspiratory flow rate control regulates the rate of delivery of gas from the bellows to the patient during inspiration and is adjustable from 20 to 70 L/min. The inspiratory pressure control sets the maximum pressure that can be delivered to the patient circuit during inspiration, up to 40 cm of H_2O; pressure is adjustable from 10 to 40 cm of H_2O. The expiratory time control adjusts the time between the end of one inspiratory phase of respiration and the beginning of the next and can be varied from less than 1 to at least 12 seconds; essentially, it is a setting for respiratory rate although rate is influenced to some degree by other controls. The expiratory flow rate control allows variation in the rate at which the bellows descends to the fully extended position and is adjustable from 15 to 100 L/min. The inspiratory hold pushbutton allows the initiation of inspiration at any point during the respiratory cycle by depressing and immediately releasing the button. If the pushbutton is depressed and held, inspiration will be initiated and the bellows will remain at the end-inspiratory position until the button is released. The inspiratory trigger effort control sets the sensitivity of the ventilator to the negative pressure resulting from the patient's inspiratory effort. The setting can be low, which would require only a slight negative pressure to initiate a cycle, or high, which prevents the patient from triggering inspiration; the setting is adjustable from −0.5 to −5.0 cm of H_2O. Many of these ventilators were equipped with a patient circuit pressure gauge (manometer) mounted on top of the bellows housing. This ventilator can be set to provide controlled or assisted ventilation.

The ventilator provides a relief valve (pop-off valve) to allow the escape of excess gases that are delivered to the patient circuit. Generally, the pressure in the patient circuit returns to zero at end-expiration, since a descending bellows is employed.

Four modes of ventilation can be employed with this ventilator:

1. **Controller, Volume Controlled and Pressure Limited.** The rate and pattern of respiration are controlled by the ventilator. The selected tidal volume is delivered as long as inspiratory pressure does not exceed 40 cm of H_2O. If the pressure limit is reached before the entire tidal volume is delivered, inspiration will cease.
2. **Controller, Pressure Controlled and Volume Limited.** The rate of ventilation is controlled by the ventilator. The ventilator delivers gas to the patient until the preset pressure limit is reached or until the contents of the bellows is fully discharged. Since tidal volume is affected by pressure, changes in airway resistance and compliance of the lungs can alter tidal volume.
3. **Assistor/Controller, Volume Controlled and Pressure Limited.** The respiratory cycle is initiated by any spontaneous inspiratory effort on the part of the patient. The minimum frequency of ventilation is set by the ventilator, and if the patient fails to initiate the preset number of breaths, the ventilator will cycle at the minimum frequency. The preset tidal volume is delivered unless the inspiratory pressure reaches 40 cm of H_2O, at which point inspiration will cease.
4. **Assistor/Controller, Pressure Controlled and Volume Limited.** The respiratory cycle is initiated by spontaneous inspiratory efforts, and the minimum frequency is set by the ventilator. The patient may initiate a faster rate of respiration. The ventilator delivers gas to the patient until a preset pressure is reached or until the bellows is fully discharged. The tidal volume will be affected significantly by changes in compliance of the lung and airway resistance.

When using the Metomatic ventilator the first mode (controller, volume controlled and pressure limited) is most frequently used. Before using the ventilator, the proper connections to the gas supply and scavenger system should be made and the appropriate preuse check-out procedures should be done. Assuming that the anesthesia machine, breathing system, and ventilator are functional, the following is a step-by-step approach to the operation of the ventilator with a circle breathing system:

1. Select the desired tidal volume.
2. Set the inspiratory trigger effort control to a high setting, but not to the maximum.
3. Turn the inspiratory pressure control to a high setting (the maximum setting or high enough to assure that the bellows will deliver a complete tidal volume).

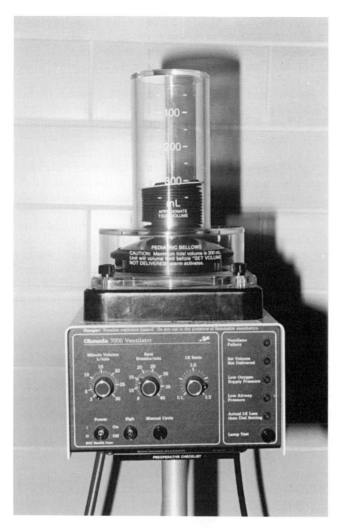

Fig. 17–51. Ohmeda 7000 Ventilator. The control module is shown with six controls on the left two thirds of the panel and six warning indicators on the right two thirds of the panel. This ventilator is equipped with a pediatric bellows (0 to 300 mL for tidal volume) assembly.

4. Set the inspiratory flow rate control to a midrange setting. After the ventilator is in use, this control will be reset to deliver the tidal volume in approximately 1 to 1.5 seconds.
5. Set the expiratory flow rate to a midrange setting. Refinements in this setting can be done after the ventilator is in use, usually employing a setting that will not impede ventilation.
6. Set the expiratory time control to a midrange setting. This control should be reset to allow the appropriate frequency of ventilation after the ventilator is in use.
7. Connect the corrugated tube from the ventilator's bellows to the circle system's reservoir bag port.
8. Close the APL (pop-off) valve of the circle.
9. Turn the power switch to the on position.
10. Observe the character and rate of ventilation, and make refinements in the adjustments of the

various controls. Usually, inspiratory flow rate is adjusted first, followed by frequency or expiratory time, and expiratory flow rate.

Ohmeda 7000 Electronic Anesthesia Ventilator. The Ohmeda 7000 (Fig. 17–51) is a double-circuit ventilator with an ascending bellows that is pneumatically driven and electronically controlled with a preset minute volume. It is specifically designed as an anesthesia ventilator and can be fitted with either an adult or a pediatric bellows, and its application in human anesthesia has been described.(50, 54, 61) This ventilator and upgraded models are available for use in human beings (54) and are readily applicable to small animal anesthesia. The control module (Fig. 17–51) has six controls including the minute volume dial (2 to 30 L/min with the adult bellows and 2 to 12 L/min with the pediatric bellows), the respiratory rate dial (6 to 40 breaths per minute), the I:E ratio dial (1:1, 1:2, 1:3), power switch (on, off), sigh switch (to provide a "sigh" equal to 150% of the tidal volume once every 64 breaths), and a manual cycle button (used to manually initiate a ventilatory cycle only during the expiratory phase). The scale on the bellows housing ranges from 100 to 1600 mL on the adult bellows and from 0 to 300 mL on the pediatric bellows. The bellows assembly exhaust port is 19 mm o.d., the connection to the anesthesia machine is 22 mm, and there is a high-pressure (50-psi) DISS fitting for an oxygen line for the driving gas circuit. The control module of the ventilator computes tidal volume, inspiratory time, expiratory time, and inspiratory flow based on the settings of the various control dials. The bellows should be fully distended (starts at the zero mark on the bellows housing scale) before the beginning of inspiration.

The driving gas supply is oxygen at 50 psi, which is reduced to 38 psi by a precision regulator within the ventilator; the gas line with the reduced pressure connects to a manifold of five solenoids. Electronic controls regulate the solenoid valves to deliver flows in 2-L/min increments from 4 to 60 L/min. Based on control settings, a precise volume of gas (equal to the tidal volume) is delivered to the bellows chamber to drive the bellows during the inspiratory phase, which forces gas from the bellows into the patient circuit. Flow stops when the full tidal volume has been delivered. A high-pressure relief valve opens at a pressure of 65 cm of water if such pressures should occur. During the expiratory phase, gas from the patient circuit (flowmeters of the anesthesia machine) enters the bellows. The ventilator relief opens when the bellows is fully distended and a pressure of 2.5 cm of water has been exceeded; excess gas from the patient circuit is vented into the scavenger system.

The manufacturer recommends a bellows assembly leak test. With the ventilator attached to a circle breathing system with the breathing system's pop-off valve closed, the Y-piece occluded, all fresh gas flow off, and the bellows filled from the anesthesia machine's oxygen flush valve, the bellows should drop no more than 100 mL per minute. If a significant leak is present, the ventilator should not be used until the leak is corrected. If the anesthesia machine, breathing system, and ventilator are all in proper working order as indicated by preuse checkout procedures, the following guidelines are appropriate for use of the ventilator:

1. Properly connect the electric and pneumatic power sources for the ventilator.
2. Using the control dials, set the desired values for minute volume, respiratory rate (frequency), and I:E ratio.
3. Make the appropriate connections from the ventilator bellows to the circle system's reservoir bag port and to the scavenger system.
4. Close the APL (pop-off) valve of the circle system.
5. Be sure that the bellows is completely filled with oxygen/anesthetic mixture.
6. Switch the power control to the on position.
7. Make final adjustments in minute volume and respiratory rate to meet the needs of the patient.

The next generation of ventilators from Ohmeda, the 7800 series of ventilators, is the most advanced group of ventilators from that manufacturer. The 7800 is available as a standalone unit and potentially could be applied to small animal patients. The ventilator is classified as electronically controlled, pneumatically driven, and tidal-volume preset, and can accurately deliver tidal volumes of 50 to 1500 mL. A major difference between the 7000 and the 7800 is that tidal volume, rather than minute ventilation, is selected by the operator, which appears to be a significant advantage.(61)

Vet-Tec SAV-75 Anesthesia Ventilator. The Model SAV-75 Ventilator is designed for use in small animal anesthesia.(62) The bellows is designed to ascend on expiration and is pneumatically driven by a Bird ventilator. Used without a bellows, Bird ventilators are classed as single-circuit ventilators, but the SAV-75 performs as a double-circuit unit. This ventilator can be used for ventilation in assist, control, or assist-control modes. When the system is operating, the Bird ventilator supplies gas to pressurize the space between the bellows and the bellows housing (canister) to force the bellows downward, which delivers gases from the bellows through the interface hose (corrugated breathing tube) to the breathing system. The controls on the Bird ventilator include inspiratory pressure, inspiratory flow rate, expiratory time (apnea control), and inspiratory sensitivity. In addition, a manometer, a hand timer (push-pull mechanism), and a DISS connector for the source of pneumatic power are prominent features of the ventilator. Inspiratory pressure can be varied to a maximum of 60 cm of H_2O, inspiratory sensitivity from -0.5 to -5.0 cm of H_2O, expiratory time to produce 4 to 60 controlled breaths per minute, and inspiratory flow to a maximum of 70 L/min. Safety relief occurs on inspiration if a pressure of 65 cm of H_2O is developed. The pneumatic power source should be delivered to the ventilator inlet at 50 psi. The bellows can deliver a tidal volume of up to 2000 mL. Inspiration can be started or stopped by use of the hand timer. The Bird ventilator is time cycled unless the push-pull manual cycling rod is pulled out causing the ventilator to be pressure cycled.(55) Figure 17–52 shows a typical Bird ventilator.

Before using the SAV-75 ventilator for controlling ventilation during anesthesia, the power supply and scavenger system should be connected, and the appropriate preuse checkout procedures should be done for all equipment. Assuming proper function of the anesthesia machine, breathing system, and ventilator, the following is a reasonable operational approach for the ventilator with a circle breathing system in the control mode:

1. Set the inspiratory sensitivity control to a high setting to eliminate the possibility of patient-initiated ventilation.

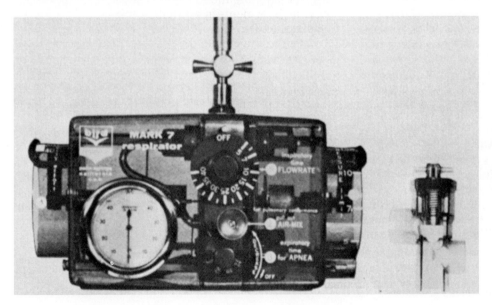

Fig. 17–52. A Bird Mark 7 Ventilator and expiratory-valve assembly. The inspiratory sensitivity control is on the left end of the ventilator, the inspiratory pressure limit is on the right end, the driving gas inlet is on the top, and the manometer, inspiratory flow control, air-mix selector, and expiratory time control are on the front panel of the ventilator. (From Lumb, W.V., and Jones, E.W. Oxygen Administration and Artificial Respiration. In: Veterinary Anesthesia, 2nd ed. Philadelphia: Lea & Febiger, 1984.)

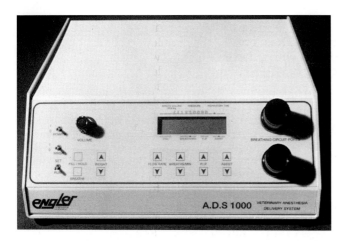

Fig. 17–53. ADS 1000 Veterinary Anesthesia Delivery System and Critical Care Ventilator. The ports for the breathing hoses are located on the right side of the ventilator, and the controls for the ventilator are located on the front panel of the console.

2. Set the inspiratory pressure control to the range of 15 to 20 cm of H_2O, and readjust the setting to achieve the desired tidal volume after Steps 5 and 6 have been completed.
3. Connect the corrugated hose (interface hose) from the ventilator's bellows to the reservoir bag port of the circle system.
4. Close the APL (pop-off) valve of the circle system. At this point, the bellows may need to be filled by increasing the flow of oxygen to the patient circuit (oxygen flowmeter of the anesthesia machine).
5. Turn the inspiratory flow control on to start the ventilator, and set the flow control to deliver a tidal volume in approximately 1 to 1.5 seconds.
6. Set the expiratory time control to establish a respiratory rate appropriate for the patient, often 8 to 12 breaths per minute.
7. For final settings, the operator should understand that there are interactions between the controls on a Bird ventilator (e.g., changing inspiratory flow may affect respiratory rate).

ADS 1000 Veterinary Anesthesia Delivery System and Critical Care Ventilator. The ADS 1000 Veterinary Anesthesia Delivery System and Critical Care Ventilator is a microprocessor-controlled ventilator that is marketed either for use with a vaporizer or for patients not requiring an anesthetic (e.g., critical care patients).(63) The ventilator-anesthesia system (Fig. 17–53) functions as a nonrebreathing circuit, does not incorporate a bellows assembly, and does not include a canister for chemical absorbent to eliminate carbon dioxide. It is not intended for connection to another breathing system. Based on the patient's body weight, the microprocessor determines the values for the various ventilatory parameters to be provided by the ventilator.

This ventilator fits into the single-circuit class and is powered electrically and pneumatically. According to

the operations manual, the ventilator must be supplied with oxygen at a pressure of 50 psi for the display to accurately report the minute volume per kilogram of body weight for the patient. Little published information other than testimonials is available about the clinical effectiveness of this ventilator system, but in vitro performance with a test lung has been studied.(64) The performance of the ventilator system in vitro changed across the range of body weights (1 to 20 kg) included in the study. Overventilation occurred at body weights less than 4 kg, and underventilation was evident at body weights greater than 8 kg. The authors concluded that the ventilator was capable of supporting ventilation but the displayed parameters did not always accurately reflect the actual performance of the ventilator.

The front panel of the ventilator has the following controls and components (Fig. 17–53): power switch, mask-mode switch, set-run switch, weight selection buttons, fill-hold button, breathe button, display for various ventilatory parameters with adjustments for these parameters below the display, and two ports for attachment of corrugated breathing tubes. Before attempting to use the ventilator, the operator should read the entire manual supplied by the manufacturer. The following is a summary of the manufacturer's guidelines for operating the ventilator, but is not intended to replace or supplant the manual supplied for the ventilator:

1. Connect the green oxygen hose on the back of the ventilator to an oxygen source (50 psi).
2. Attach the breathing tubes to the breathing circuit ports on the front of the ventilator.
3. Connect the scavenger out port on the back of the ventilator to the hospital scavenger system.
4. Connect the electric cord to the 120-VAC–1.5-amp port on the back of the ventilator to an electric outlet.
5. Attach the vaporizer connectors to the appropriate ports on the back of the ventilator.
6. Allow the ventilator to complete the self-diagnostic test described in the operator's manual. The test will help to determine failure of the safety pop-off valve, inadequate oxygen supply, and the presence of leaks.
7. After diagnostics are complete, the mask function should be off and the set-run switch should be in the "set" position. The display will then show settings for a 20-kg patient (minute volume of 24 L/min, 9 breaths/min, peak inspiratory pressure of 15 cm of H_2O, and the assist mode in the off position).
8. Using the weight up or weight down button, enter the correct weight of the patient in kilograms into the display, and the ventilator will automatically set the ventilatory parameters based on the patient's weight. Ventilation will be completely controlled (the default setting for "assist" is off).
9. Then, the patient should be anesthetized and

intubated with a cuffed endotracheal tube, the Y-piece connecting the breathing tubes should be attached to the endotracheal tube connector, and the vaporizer should be set appropriately. The ventilator's set-run switch should be set to "run." Controlled ventilation should begin.

SPECIFIC VENTILATORS FOR LARGE ANIMALS

Although not all-inclusive, the following discussion includes descriptions of ventilators that are appropriate for use during anesthesia in large animal patients. Classification, principles of operation, and function are discussed.

Drager AV Large Animal Anesthesia Ventilator. The Drager AV Anesthesia Ventilator (Fig. 17–54) is included as a part of the Narkovet-E Large Animal Anesthesia Machine; the entire system is called the Narkovet-E Large Animal Anesthesia Control Center. The ventilator was not marketed as a stand-alone unit for large animal anesthesia. Although they are no longer being manufactured, some of these ventilator–anesthesia machine combinations remain in use in veterinary hospitals. The ventilator is powered pneumatically, generally at a

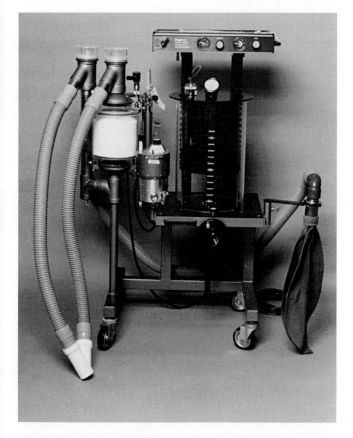

Fig. 17–54. Narkovet-E Large Animal Anesthesia Control Center. The ventilator's bellows and the bellows housing with tidal volume markings (4 to 15 L) are shown with the large animal circle system on the left and the reservoir bag for the circle breathing system on the right. The controls for the ventilator are on the panel above the bellows housing at the top of the unit.

pressure of 50 psi.(65) It is classed as double circuit, tidal-volume preset, time cycled, and pneumatically driven with a descending bellows, and it utilizes fluidic circuitry. The controls include an on-off switch, a tidal-volume control with a scale of 4 to 15 liters on the bellows housing, frequency control (6 to 18 breaths per minute), and a flow-control knob that determines inspiratory flow (a combination of flow and maximum pressure being delivered to the bellows compartment); the manufacturer recommended that the flow setting be adjusted so that the bellows always reached the upper stop. The inspiratory to expiratory time ratio of 1:2 is preset.

Before using the ventilator, the proper connections to the gas supply and scavenger system and the appropriate preuse checkout procedures should be done. The instruction manual for the ventilator included a standard preuse check for the ventilator.(65) The following is a logical approach to the operation of the ventilator with a circle breathing system:

1. Connect the compressed air supply hose to the ventilator.
2. Adjust the tidal-volume control to the appropriate setting for the patient, and be sure that the self-locking mechanism is engaged to prevent inadvertent movement of the bellows stop plate during use.
3. Attach the corrugated breathing hose from the bellows to the bag port of the circle system.
4. Close the APL valve (pop-off) on the circle system.
5. Turn the power supply switch to the on setting.
6. Adjust the frequency control knob to the desired respiratory rate.
7. Adjust the flow control knob so that the bellows reaches the upper stop at end-inspiration. If the bellows does not return to its original position during expiration (usually indicative of a leak in the patient circuit), the bellows can be filled using a higher flow from the oxygen flowmeter, and the leak should be corrected.

Narkovet E: Electronic Large Animal Control Center. The Narkovet E: Electronic Large Animal Control Center is a combination of Drager's Narkovet E-2 Large Animal Anesthesia System (anesthesia machine and circle breathing system) with a Drager AV-E ventilator (Figs. 17–55 to 17–57); the ventilator is not available as a stand-alone unit for large animals and is no longer being manufactured, but machines are still in use. The unit is classified as a double-circuit, tidal-volume-preset, time-cycled ventilator with a descending bellows; it is electronically controlled and pneumatically driven. It is powered electrically (120 VAC) and pneumatically (40 to 60 psi with oxygen, but air is an option).(66) The controls (Figs. 17–55 and 17–56) include an on-off switch, a self-locking knob located below the bellows assembly to control the tidal volume (4 to 15 L), a thumbwheel controller-indicator switch to adjust the respiratory rate (frequency control from 1 to 30 breaths/min), flow control setting to determine the inspiratory

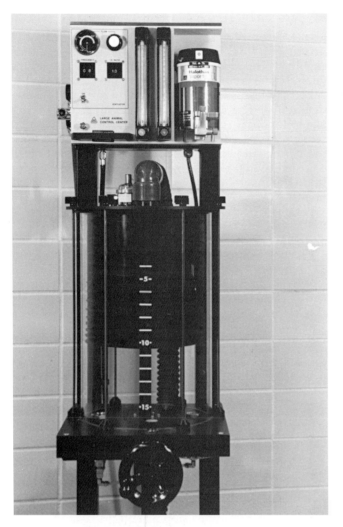

Fig. 17–55. Narkovet E: Electronic Large Animal Control Center. The bellows and bellows housing with markings for tidal volume (4 to 15 L), the corrugated breathing hose from the bellows to the circle system (behind the bellows housing), and the self-locking knob or wheel (lower center) for selection of tidal volume are shown. In addition, the controls for the ventilator and anesthesia machine (upper part of the photograph) are included and are shown in detail in Figure 17–56.

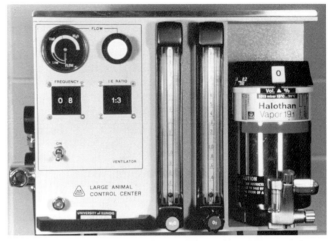

Fig. 17–56. Narkovet E: Electronic Large Animal Control Center. The control panel for the ventilator is shown on the left side of the photograph. The power switch in the off position is directly under the thumbwheel controller-indicator switch for frequency (respiratory rate) selection on the left of the panel. The thumbwheel controller-indicator switch for I:E ratio selection is on the right of the panel with the inspiratory flow control directly above it. Some of the basic parts of the anesthesia machine, including the flowmeters (center of the photograph) for oxygen and nitrous oxide, the halothane vaporizer, and the flush valve (lower left), are present.

flow rate, and the inspiratory-expiratory phase time ratio control (a thumbwheel indicator-controller to adjust the I:E ratio in increments of 0.5 from 1:1 to 1:4.5). The manufacturer recommends that the flow control knob be adjusted so that the bellows always reaches the upper stop on inspiration. The ventilator provides for controlled ventilation; assisted ventilation is not an option.

Before using the ventilator, the proper connections to the gas supply and scavenger system should be made and the appropriate preuse checkout procedures should be done. The instruction manual for the ventilator included a standard preuse check for the ventilator. The following is a step-by-step approach to the operation of the ventilator with a circle breathing system:

1. Connect the supply gas (oxygen hose) to the anesthesia machine and ventilator.
2. Adjust the tidal-volume control to the appropriate setting for the patient, and be sure that the self-locking mechanism is engaged to prevent inadvertent movement of the bellows stop plate.
3. Select the desired frequency of ventilation.
4. Select the desired I:E ratio.
5. Attach the corrugated breathing hose from the bellows to the reservoir bag port of the circle system.
6. Close the APL (pop-off) valve on the circle system.
7. Turn the power supply switch to the on setting.
8. Adjust the flow control knob so that the bellows reaches the upper stop at end-inspiration. If the bellows does not return to its original location during expiration, it can be filled by increasing the flow from the oxygen flowmeter.

Mallard Medical Rachel Model 2800 Anesthesia Ventilator. The Mallard Medical Rachel Model 2800 Large Animal Anesthesia Ventilator (Fig. 17–58) is a microprocessor-based, electronic control system that facilitates controlled ventilation in large animals being maintained on circle breathing systems.(58, 67) The ventilator is designed to interface with currently available large animal circle systems. The stand for the ventilator and the bellows is designed for the attachment of a circle breathing system and at least two vaporizers for inhalant anesthetics, and it has shelves to accommodate physiologic monitoring devices.

Most of the functional considerations for the Model 2800 are similar to those for the Model 2400V. The control console for the 2800 is located above the bellows housing, instead of below the housing as it is in the 2400V, and LED displays are employed as they are in the 2400V. The ventilator is controlled by a microprocessor, but the pneumatics have been modified for generation of greater inspiratory flows, which are adjustable from 10 to 600 L/min. The bellows is inverted and ascends during expiration, and two sizes of bellows are available, 3 L and 21 L, allowing the selection of appropriate tidal volumes for patients with a wide range of body weights. Like other ventilators with inverted bellows, the Model 2800 produces PEEP because of the effect of gravity on the bellows. However, the amount of PEEP is controlled by a pneumatic vacuum pump on the 2800; the pump creates negative pressure between the bellows and the bellows housing during the expiratory phase of ventilation and functions to reduce the level of PEEP according to the adjustments made by the operator. An ambient end-expiratory pressure may be achieved.

Before using the ventilator, the proper connections to the gas and electric power supplies and the scavenger system should be made, and the appropriate preuse check-out procedures should be done for all equipment. The following is a reasonable operational approach for the Model 2800 ventilator with a circle breathing system:

1. Place the master switch in the standby mode, and dial the desired settings for respiratory rate and inspiratory time, according to the patient's needs.
2. Set the inspiratory flow control to the desired rate of flow–low, medium, or high, depending on the patient's needs (typically in the high range for large animals).

3. Connect corrugated tubing from the ventilator's bellows to the circle system's bag mount and the ventilator exhalation port to the scavenger system.
4. Close the circle system's APL (pop-off) valve, and release the ventilator's bellows. Assure that the bellows is fully inflated and positioned at zero.
5. Turn the master switch to the on position, and inspiration should begin.
6. If the bellows does not return to zero during the expiratory phase, the bellows can be filled with flow from the oxygen flowmeter. Alternately, the bellows can be filled with the flush valve, but the anesthetic concentration in the breathing circuit will be reduced any time this is done.
7. The inspiratory time can be adjusted to produce the appropriate tidal volume for the patient.
8. Finally, the PEEP control is adjusted to set the desired end-expiratory pressure.

Vet-Tec Model LAVC-3000 Large Animal Anesthesia Ventilator. The Model LAVC-3000 is a large animal anesthesia ventilator designed for use in equine and bovine practices.(68) A similar ventilator in combination

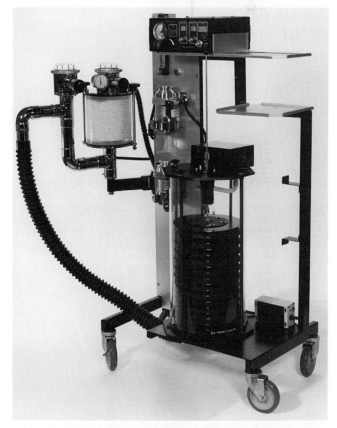

Fig. 17–58. Mallard Medical Rachel Model 2800 Large Animal Anesthesia Ventilator. The ventilator with a Matrx circle system attached (left side) is shown. The corrugated breathing hose that exits the bellows below the bellows housing is attached to the reservoir bag port of the circle system. The control console for the ventilator is located at the top of the photograph. The controls for the 2800 are similar to those shown in Figure 17–48 for the Model 2400V.

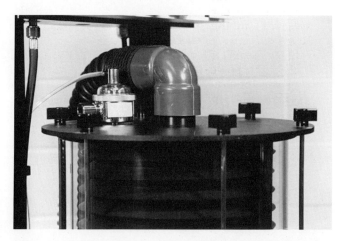

Fig. 17–57. Narkovet E: Electronic Large Animal Control Center. The top of the bellows and the bellows housing are shown with an elbow connecting the bellows to the corrugated breathing tube, which attaches to the reservoir port of the circle breathing system. To the left of the elbow is the overflow valve from the bellows, which is connected to the scavenger system when the ventilator is in use. The clear, small-diameter tubing attaching to the pop-off valve is part of the mechanism for closing the pop-off valve during the inspiratory phase of controlled ventilation.

with a large animal anesthesia machine (Model LAVC-2000 Large Animal Anesthesia Machine and Ventilator; Fig. 17–59) is also available. The ventilator system has been described as a "bag-in-a-barrel powered by a Bird ventilator."(35) The LAVC-2000 and the LAVC-3000 systems can be converted to a 5-liter system for use in foals by adding a 5000-mL bellows and a canister (bellows housing) insert (Fig. 17–60). Numerous variations of these ventilator–anesthesia machine combinations are possible, since the manufacturer will customize the unit upon request. The bellows in this ventilator system is driven by a modified Bird Mark 7 ventilator (Fig. 17–61). Used without a bellows, the Bird Mark 7 is classed as a single-circuit ventilator, but the LAVC ventilator system is a double-circuit unit and has been classified as a pressure-preset ventilator.(35) The ventilator has been produced with a descending bellows, but newer literature from the manufacturer indicates the availability of an inverted bellows. The Bird ventilator is pneumatically powered. This ventilator system can be used for ventilation in assist, control, or assist-control modes. When the system is operating, the Bird ventilator supplies gas to pressurize the space between the bellows and the bellows housing (canister) to force the bellows in an upward motion delivering gases from the bellows, through the interface hose, to the breathing system.

The controls on a Bird Mark 7 (Figs. 17–52 and 17–61) include inspiratory pressure, inspiratory flow rate, expiratory time (apnea control), and inspiratory sensitivity. In addition, a manometer, a hand timer (push-pull mechanism), and a DISS connector for the source of pneumatic power are prominent features of the ventilator. With the modified Bird Mark 7, inspiratory pressure can be varied from 5 to 65 cm of H_2O, inspiratory sensitivity from -0.5 to -5 cm of H_2O, expiratory time from 5 to 15 seconds, and inspiratory flow from 0 to over 450 L/min. The pneumatic power source should be delivered to the inlet of the ventilator at 50 psi. The bellows can deliver a tidal volume of up to 20 liters. Inspiration can be started or stopped by use of the hand timer. The Bird Mark 7 is a time-cycled ventilator unless the push-pull manual cycling rod is pulled out, which causes the ventilator to be pressure cycled.(55)

Before using the Model LAV-3000 ventilator for controlling ventilation during anesthesia, the power supply and scavenger system should be connected and the appropriate preuse checkout procedures should be done for all equipment. The following is a reasonable

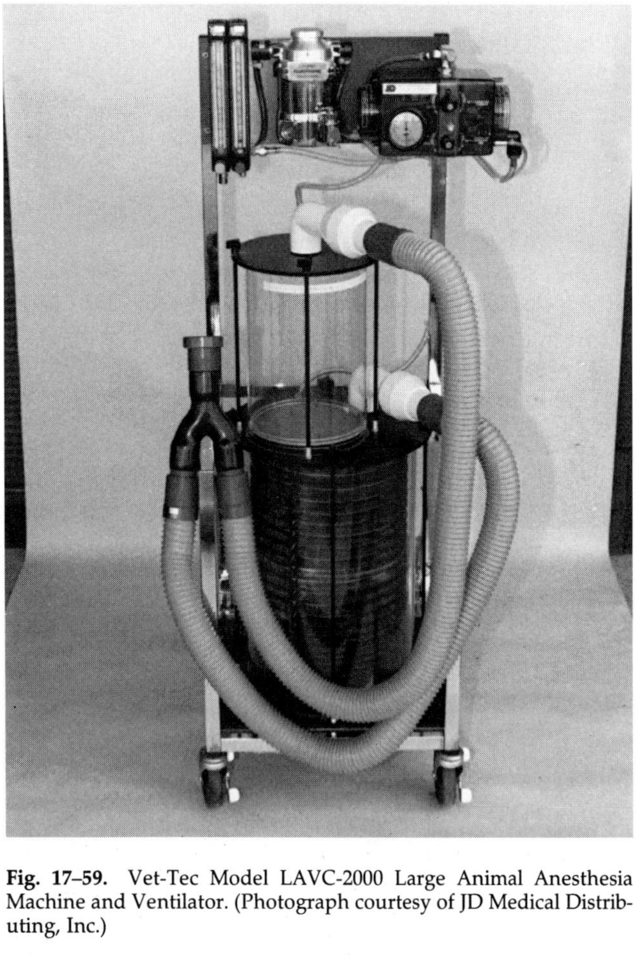

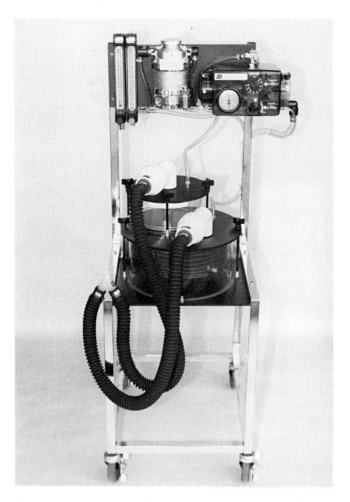

Fig. 17–59. Vet-Tec Model LAVC-2000 Large Animal Anesthesia Machine and Ventilator. (Photograph courtesy of JD Medical Distributing, Inc.)

Fig. 17–60. Model CAV-2500 Foal Anesthesia Machine and Ventilator. (Photograph courtesy of JD Medical Distributing, Inc.)

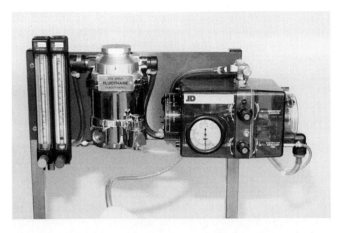

Fig. 17–61. Bird Mark 7 Ventilator and Anesthesia Machine controls (flowmeters and vaporizer) for a Vet Tec LAVC 2000 Large Animal Anesthesia Machine and Ventilator. (Photograph courtesy of JD Medical Distributing, Inc.)

operational approach for the ventilator with a circle breathing system in the control mode:

1. Set the inspiratory sensitivity control to a high setting to eliminate the possibility of patient-initiated ventilation.
2. Set the inspiratory pressure control to the range of 20 to 30 cm of H_2O, and readjust the setting to achieve the desired tidal volume after Steps 5 and 6 have been completed.
3. Connect the corrugated hose (interface hose) from the bellows to the reservoir bag port of the circle system.
4. Close the APL (pop-off) valve of the circle system. Then, the bellows may need to be filled by increasing the flow of oxygen to the patient circuit (oxygen flowmeter on the anesthesia machine).
5. Turn the inspiratory flow control on to start the ventilator, and set the flow control to deliver a tidal volume in approximately 1.5 to 3 seconds.
6. Set the expiratory time control to establish a respiratory rate appropriate for the patient, often 7 to 10 breaths per minute.
7. For final settings, the operator should understand that there are interactions between the controls on a Bird ventilator (e.g., changing inspiratory flow may affect respiratory rate, and vice versa).

Hazards Associated With the Use of Ventilators

During anesthesia, the use of a ventilator allows the anesthetist to concentrate on monitoring and supportive procedures. If the anesthetist is preoccupied with manually controlling or assisting ventilation, monitoring and support may be neglected. A good example is the use of a mechanical ventilator in anesthesia for equine colic surgery. However, there is some loss of contact between the anesthetist and the patient when a ventilator is used, especially in regard to respiratory function. Without a "hand on the reservoir bag," the anesthetist may miss such developments as disconnections in the patient circuit, variations in respiratory

resistance and compliance, and changes in the rate of spontaneous ventilation. In addition, a ventilator, because of its sounds and regularity, may lull the anesthetist into believing that ventilation is adequate when, in fact, it is not.(61) Ventilators are mechanical and may malfunction, and many veterinary ventilators are not equipped with the alarm systems that are now required for human ventilators. Finally, ventilators add a source of possible contamination to the breathing system.(61)

The hazards of mechanical ventilation are usually associated with malfunctions and failure of the equipment or inappropriate or inadvertently altered control settings. The operator should select a ventilator capable of meeting the respiratory requirements for the patient. Ventilators designed specifically for small animals or human beings are not necessarily appropriate for large animals. A ventilator must be able to generate an adequate inspiratory flow rate and tidal volume if it is to be safe for use in large animals. General hazards associated with ventilators include hypoventilation, hyperventilation, excessive airway pressure, negative pressure during expiration, and failure of alarms if the ventilator is so equipped. Hypoventilation can be associated with power failure, dysfunction of the ventilator, cycling failure, inadequate design for the patient, leak of driving gas, loss of breathing system gas, incorrect settings, and obstruction to flow.(61)

Respiratory Assist Devices

Several types and brands of respiratory assist devices are available. Some are completely manual in operation (resuscitation bags with one-way valves); some use compressed gas (oxygen) to assist ventilation (demand valves). The mechanics of these devices have been reviewed.(61)

MANUAL RESUSCITATORS

A manual resuscitator is appropriate for application of IPPV to small veterinary patients. Several brands of resuscitators are available (Figs. 17–62 and 17–63). The basic components of a manual resuscitator are a compressible self-reexpanding bag, a bag refill valve, and a nonrebreathing valve.(69) Some resuscitators can be attached to a source of oxygen to enrich the oxygen content of inspired gases (Fig. 17–63). Manual resuscitators can be fitted with a reservoir to serve as a source of oxygen when the oxygen flow to the resuscitator does not meet the filling demands of the resuscitator. The addition of such a reservoir makes the resuscitator more cumbersome to use.(69)

DEMAND VALVES

A demand valve can be used to deliver intermittent positive pressure ventilation. The demand valve is set to deliver oxygen when the patient begins to inspire (creating a negative inspiratory pressure) until exhalation starts or until a certain preset pressure is reached.(69) Expiration is passive through the valve outlet. The outlet may be restrictive to expiration in large patients. The device can be disconnected from the endotracheal tube after inspiration to decrease the resistance to exhalation if the demand valve must be used for an extended time.(26) A demand valve can be triggered manually to deliver oxygen to the patient as long as the activation button is held or until the preset pressure limit is reached. Alternately compressing and releasing the control button allows application of IPPV. A demand valve with the capacity for a high inspiratory flow rate is most desirable for use in large animals; demand valves generating low inspiratory flows will cause an excessively long inspiratory time in patients requiring a large tidal volume (Chapter 20).

Demand valves are available from various manufacturers. The Hudson Demand Valve (Fig. 17–64) has been described for use in horses.(70) It delivers approximately 200 L/min if the oxygen supply pressure is 50 psi and greater than 275 L/min if the supply pressure is 80 psi. This valve will accept a standard

connector for an endotracheal tube (15 mm), and an adapter will allow attachment of the demand valve to a large animal endotracheal tube connector (Fig. 17–64). The equine demand valve sold by J.D. Medical (Phoenix, Arizona) functions at an inlet pressure of 50 to 75 psi. This demand valve is available with various lengths of supply gas hose and several sizes of adapters for endotracheal tubes (Fig. 17–65). The Elder CPR/Demand Valve (Fig. 17–66) is intended to provide 100% oxygen to breathing or apneic patients.(71) The unit operates on a regulated inlet supply of oxygen at pressures between 40 and 80 psi. There is a variable pressure limit of 60 cm of H_2O. Variable pressure (0 to 60 cm of H_2O $\pm$ 5 cm of H_2O) can be delivered to the patient depending on the amount of pressure that

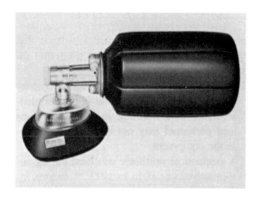

Fig. 17–62. A Hope Resuscitator (Ohio Medical Products, Madison, Wisconsin). This unit is fitted to a mask, but can be attached to an endotracheal tube to support ventilation. (From Lumb, W.V., and Jones, E.W. Oxygen Administration and Artificial Respiration. In: Veterinary Anesthesia, 2nd ed. Philadelphia: Lea & Febiger, 1984.)

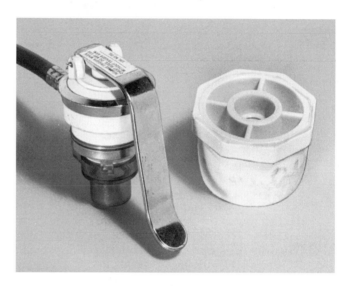

Fig. 17–64. The Hudson Demand Valve (left) with an adapter for attachment to a large animal endotracheal tube connector.

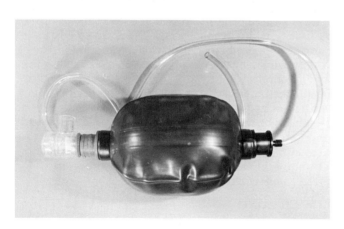

Fig. 17–63. A manual resuscitation bag. Plastic tubing, which may be connected to an oxygen flowmeter, is attached to the bag refill valve to facilitate the addition of oxygen to inspired gases. The components of the resuscitation bag include the clear elbow (left), which is a nonrebreathing valve, the black self-inflating bag, and a refill valve (black apparatus on the right end of the bag). The nonrebreathing valve may be connected to a mask or to an endotracheal tube.

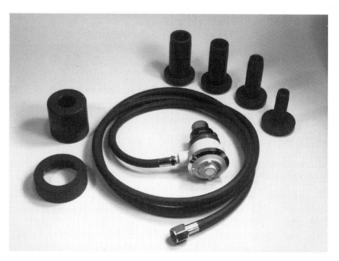

Fig. 17–65. The JD Medical Demand Valve. The demand valve is available with different lengths of high-pressure hose to supply oxygen and with several sizes of endotracheal tube adapters. (Photograph courtesy of JD Medical Distributing, Inc.)

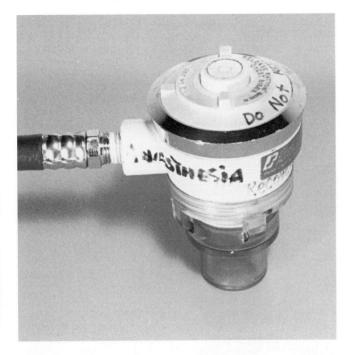

Fig. 17–66. The Elder CPR/Demand Valve. The oxygen inlet is shown with high-pressure oxygen hose connected. The clear plastic connector at the bottom of the photograph will fit endotracheal tube connectors, and the button in the top center of the demand valve activates and controls the flow of oxygen.

is placed on the manual control button. Two models of this demand valve allow the choice of two set flow rates, 40 L/min at 40 psi and 160 L/min at 40 psi. The inlet for the valve is a DISS male oxygen fitting, and the outlet is 15 mm i.d. for attachment to an endotracheal tube connector and 22 mm o.d. for accepting a standard adult mask. This demand valve is easily adapted to fit both large and small animal endotracheal tubes with an adapter similar to the one shown in Figure 17–64.

References

1. Dorsch JA, Dorsch SE. Tracheal tubes. In: Understanding anesthesia equipment. 3rd ed. Baltimore: Williams & Wilkins, 1994:439.
2. Sawyer DC. Canine and feline endotracheal intubation and laryngoscopy. Compend Contin Educ Pract Vet 11:973, 1984.
3. Heath RB. Complications associated with general anesthesia of the horse. Vet Clin North Am Large Anim Pract 3:45, 1981.
4. Smith TC. Anesthesia breathing systems. In: Ehrenworth J, Eisenkraft JB, eds. Anesthesia equipment, principles and applications. St. Louis: Mosby, 1993:89.
5. Guyton DC. Endotracheal and tracheotomy tube cuff design: influence on tracheal damage. Crit Care Updates 1:1, 1990.
6. Hartsfield SM, et al. Endotracheal intubation by pharyngotomy. J Am Anim Hosp Assoc 13:71, 1977.
7. Shawley RV, Bednarski RM. Endotracheal intubation in the horse. In: Muir WW III, Hubbell JAE, eds. Equine anesthesia. St. Louis: CV Mosby, 1991:310.
8. Trim CM, Simpson ST. Complications following ethylene oxide sterilization. J Am Anim Hosp Assoc 18:507, 1982.
9. Webb AI. Nasal intubation in the foal. J Am Vet Med Assoc 185:48, 1984.
10. Soma LR. Intubation of the trachea. In: Textbook of veterinary anesthesia. Baltimore: Williams & Wilkins, 1971:229.
11. Loeser EA, et al. The influence of endotracheal tube cuff design and cuff lubrication on postoperative sore throat. Anesthesiology 58:376, 1983.
12. Thurmon JC, Benson GJ. Anesthesia in ruminants and swine. In: Howard JL, ed. Current veterinary therapy, food animal practice 2. Philadelphia: WB Saunders, 1986:51.
13. Ko JCH, et al. Problems encountered when anesthetizing potbellied pigs. Vet Med 88:435, 1993.
14. Hubbell JAE, Hull BL, Muir III WW. Perianesthetic considerations in cattle. Compend Contin Educ Pract Vet 8:F92, 1986.
15. Riebold TW, et al. Orotracheal and nasotracheal intubation in llamas. J Am Vet Med Assoc 204:779, 1994.
16. Sedgewick C, Jahn S. Techniques for endotracheal intubation and inhalation anesthesia for laboratory animals. Calif Vet 34:27, 1980.
17. Boothe HW, Hartsfield SM. Use of the laboratory rabbit in the small animal student surgery laboratory. J Vet Med Educ 17:16, 1990.
18. Hughes HC. Anesthesia of laboratory animals. Lab Anim 10:40, 1981.
19. Hartsfield SM. Alternate methods of endotracheal intubation in small animals/emphasis on patients with oropharyngeal pathology. Tex Vet Med J 47:25, 1985.
20. Borland LM, Swan DM, Leff S. Difficult pediatric endotracheal intubation: a new approach to the retrograde technique. Anesthesiology 55:557, 1981.
21. Hedlund CS. Tracheostomy. Prob Vet Med 3:198, 1991.
22. Millen JE, Glauser FL. A rapid, simple technique for changing endotracheal tubes. Anesth Analg 57:735, 1978.
23. Haskins SC. Standards and techniques of equipment utilization. In: Sattler FP, Knowles R, Whittick WG, eds. Veterinary critical care. Philadelphia: Lea & Febiger, 1981:60.
24. Fairman NB. Evaluation of pulse oximetry as a continuous monitoring technique in critically ill dogs in the small animal intensive care unit. J Vet Emerg Crit Care 2:50, 1992.
25. White GA, et al. Pulse oximetry for estimation of oxygenation in dogs with experimental pneumothorax. J Vet Emerg Crit Care 4:69, 1994.
26. Hubbell JAE. Oxygen supplementation and ventilatory assist devices. In: Muir WW III, Hubbell JAE, eds. Equine anesthesia, monitoring and emergency therapy. St. Louis: Mosby, 1991:401.
27. Court MH. Respiratory support of the critically ill small animal patient. In: Murtaugh RJ, Kaplan PM, eds. Veterinary emergency and critical care medicine. St. Louis: Mosby, 1992:575.
28. Mann FA, et al. Comparison on intranasal and intratracheal oxygen administration in healthy awake dogs. Am J Vet Res 53:856, 1992.
29. Fitzpatrick RK, Crowe DT. Nasal oxygen administration in dogs and cats: experimental and clinical investigations. J Am Anim Hosp Assoc 22:293, 1986.
30. Haskins SC. Physical therapeutics for respiratory disease. Semin Vet Med Surg Small Animal 1:276, 1986.
31. Benumof JL. Respiratory physiology and respiratory function during anesthesia. In: Miller RD, ed. Anesthesia, 2nd ed. New York: Churchill Livingstone, 1986:1115.
32. Nunn JF. Hyperoxia and oxygen toxicity. In: Nunn JF, ed. Applied respiratory physiology, 3rd ed. London: Butterworth, 1987:478.
33. Winter PM. Pulmonary oxygen toxicity. In: Refresher Courses in Anesthesiology–American Society of Anesthesiologists. Philadelphia: JB Lippincott, 1974:163.
34. Steffey EP. Mechanical ventilation of the anesthetized horse. Vet Clin North Am Large Anim Pract 3:97, 1981.
35. Muir WW III, Hubbell JAE, Skarda RT, Bednarski RM. Ventilation and mechanical assist devices. In: Handbook of veterinary anesthesia, 2nd ed. St. Louis: CV Mosby, 1995:209.
36. Thurmon JC. General clinical considerations for anesthesia of the horse. Vet Clin North Am Equine Pract 6:485, 1990.
37. Hodgson DS, Dunlop CE. General anesthesia for horses with specific problems. Vet Clin North Am Equine Pract 6:625, 1990.

38. Cullen DJ, Eger EI II. Cardiovascular effects of carbon dioxide in man. Anesthesiology 41:345, 1974.
39. Wagner AE, Bednarski RM, Muir WW III. Hemodynamic effects of carbon dioxide during intermittent positive-pressure ventilation in horses. Am J Vet Res 12:1922, 1990.
40. Shibata K, Futagami A, Take Y, Kobayashi T. Epidural anesthesia modifies the cardiovascular response to marked hypercapnia in dogs. Anesthesiology 81:1454, 1994.
41. Horwitz LD, Bishop BS, Stone HL. Effects of hypercapnia on the cardiovascular system of conscious dogs. J Appl Physiol 25:346, 1968.
42. Price HL. Effects of carbon dioxide on the cardiovascular system. Anesthesiology 21:652, 1960.
43. Eisele JH, Eger EI II, Muallem M. Narcotic properties of carbon dioxide in the dog. Anesthesiology 28:856, 1967.
44. Smith TC, Gross JB, Wollman H. The therapeutic gases, oxygen, carbon dioxide, helium, and water vapor. In: Gilman AG, Goodman LS, Rail TW, Murad F. Goodman and Gilman's the pharmacological basis of therapeutics, 6th ed. New York: Macmillan, 1985:322.
45. Rolf N, Cote CJ. Persistent cardiac arrhythmias in pediatric patients: effects of age, expired carbon dioxide values, depth of anesthesia, and airway management. Anesth Analg 73:720, 1991.
46. Haskins SC. Monitoring the anesthetized patient. In: Short CE, ed. Principles and practice of veterinary anesthesia. Baltimore: Williams & Wilkins, 1987:455.
47. Shawley RV. Controlled ventilation and pulmonary function. In: Short CE, ed. Principles and practice of veterinary anesthesia. Baltimore: Williams & Wilkins, 1987:419.
48. Nunn JF. Artificial ventilation. In: Applied respiratory physiology, 3rd ed. London: Butterworth, 1987:392.
49. Bednarski RM. Diaphragmatic hernia: anesthetic considerations. Sem Vet Med Surg Small Animal 1:256, 1986.
50. Andrews JJ. Inhaled anesthetic delivery systems. In: Miller RD, ed. Anesthesia, 3rd ed. New York: Churchill Livingstone, 1991:171.
51. Sassoon CSH, Mahutte CK, Light RW. Ventilator modes: old and new. Crit Care Clin 6:605, 1990.
52. Wilson RS. Techniques of ventilatory control: indications and complications. Refresher Courses in Anesthesiology–American Society of Anesthesiology 13:221, 1985.
53. Soma LR. Anesthetic management. In: Soma LR, ed. Textbook of veterinary anesthesia. Baltimore: Williams & Wilkins, 1971:287.
54. Grogono AW, Travis JT. Anesthesia ventilators. In: Ehrenworth J, Eisenkraft JB, eds. Anesthesia equipment, principles and application. St. Louis: CV Mosby, 1993:140.
55. Mushin WW, et al. The Bird ventilators. In: Automatic ventilation of the lungs, 3rd ed. Oxford: Blackwell Scientific Publications, 1980:373.
56. Operator's Instruction Manual, Narkovet 2 Small Animal Anesthesia Machine. Telford, PA: North American Drager, 1988:6.
57. Hallowell EMC Model 2000 Small Animal Veterinary Anesthesia Ventilator–Functional Description. Pittsfield, MA: Hallowell Engineering and Manufacturing Corporation, 1993:1.
58. Operator's Manual and Service Instructions, Mallard Medical Model 2400V Anesthesia Ventilator. Irvine, CA: Mallard Medical, Inc., 1991.
59. Soma LR. Controlled Ventilation of the Veterinary Patient. Washington Crossing, NJ: Pitman-Moore, Inc., 1973.
60. Operation Maintenance, Metomatic Veterinary Ventilator. Madison, WI: Ohio Medical Products, pp. 1–23.
61. Dorsch JA, Dorsch SE. Anesthesia ventilators. In: Understanding anesthesia equipment, 3rd ed. Baltimore: Williams & Wilkins, 1994:255.
62. Vet-Tec SAV-75 Small Animal Anesthesia Ventilator. Phoenix, AZ: JD Medical Distributing, Inc, 1990.
63. ADS 1000 Veterinary Anesthesia Delivery System and Critical Care Ventilator Operations Manual. Hialeah, FL: Engler Engineering Corporation, 1994.
64. Faudskar L, Raffee M, Randall D. In vitro performance evaluation of the ADS 1000 veterinary ventilator [Abstract]. J Vet Emerg Crit Care 4:107, 1994.
65. Instruction Manual, Drager AV Anesthesia Ventilator. Telford, PA: North American Drager, 1982.
66. Instruction Manual, Drager AV-E Anesthesia Ventilator. Telford, PA: North American Drager, 1981.
67. Personal communication. R Pearson, Mallard Medical, Irvine, California, 1995.
68. Vet-Tec LAVC-2000 Large Animal Anesthesia Machine and Ventilator–Product Information Brochure. Phoenix, AZ: JD Medical Distributing, Inc, 1990.
69. Dorsch JA, Dorsch SE. Manual resuscitators. In: Understanding anesthesia equipment, 3rd ed. Baltimore: Williams & Wilkins, 1994:225.
70. Riebold TW, Goble DO, Geiser DR. Clinical techniques for equine anesthesia. In: Large Animal Anesthesia. Ames, IA: Iowa State University Press, 1982:41.33
71. Elder CPR/Demand Valve Product Information Brochure. Irvine, CA: Life Support Products, Inc., 1990.

section VI

ACID-BASE PHYSIOLOGY AND FLUID THERAPY

chapter 18

ACID-BASE BALANCE: TRADITIONAL AND MODIFIED APPROACHES

W.W. Muir, H.S.A. deMorais

Introduction

Probably the most fundamental and important principle of physiology is homeostasis: the maintenance of constant conditions through dynamic equilibrium of the internal environment of the body. One of the many processes that maintains homeostasis is the regulation of *acid-base balance,* a term introduced by L. J. Henderson (1909). Central to all schemes of acid-base balance is the understanding that normal oxygen-dependent metabolism of food (carbohydrates, lipids, and proteins) results in the predictable production of work, heat, and waste. Indeed, normal metabolic processes are responsible for the production of thousands of mmoles of carbon dioxide (CO_2; volatile acid) and potentially hundreds of mEq of nonvolatile hydrogen ions (fixed acid) daily. Individual differences in the amount of CO_2 and H^+ produced are influenced by diet, cellular basal metabolic rate, and body temperature. Animals consuming high protein diets, for example, produce CO_2 and excess

quantities of H^+ precursors, whereas animals consuming diets high in plant material produce CO_2 and excess quantities of bicarbonate ion (HCO_3^-) precursors. The CO_2 that is produced is combined with water and is catalyzed by carbonic anhydrase (CA) to form carbonic acid (H_2CO_3). The formation of carbonic acid from CO_2 and H_2O (CO_2 hydration equation; Eq. 18–1) and the subsequent generation of H^+ and HCO_3^- (Eq. 18–2) serves as the focal point for almost all discussions of acid-base balance because (a) Henderson's studies highlighted that large quantities of CO_2 are produced by all metabolizing cells, (b) CO_2 is in equilibrium with H^+ and HCO_3^- ion, and (c) in the 1950s the plasma CO_2 content was the only relevant acid-base quantity that could be conveniently determined.

$$CO_2 + H_2O \rightarrow H_2CO_3 \qquad (18\text{--}1)$$

$$H_2CO_3 \rightleftarrows H^+ + HCO_3^- \qquad (18\text{--}2)$$

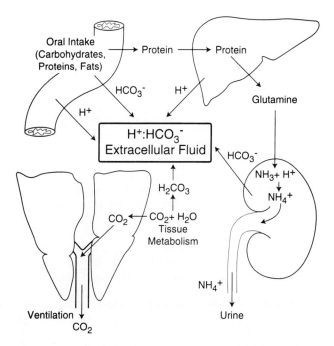

Fig. 18–1. Integration of the gut, liver, lung and kidney in acid-base balance.

Combining Equations 18–1 and 18–2 yields

$$CO_2 + H_2O \overset{ca}{\rightleftarrows} H_2CO_3 \rightleftarrows H^+ + HCO_3^- \quad (18\text{--}3)$$

Although current understanding and appreciation for the many processes responsible for acid-base homeostasis has expanded considerably since Henderson's introduction of the term *acid-base balance*, the central importance of H^+ regulation to cell function and animal health cannot be overemphasized. This led A. B. Hastings (1961) to state: "Tiny though it is, I suppose no constituent of living matter has so much power to influence biological behavior."

Acid-base homeostasis ($[H^+]$ regulation) involves the integrated normal activity of the lungs, kidney and liver (Figure 18–1). The lung removes CO_2, the kidneys remove H^+ as fixed acid, and the liver metabolizes protein, generating 1 mmol H^+/kg body weight daily. Following is a review of basic principles of acid-base balance and their integration into both the traditional and independent-variable (Stewart) approach to understanding and interpreting acid-base abnormalities in animals. Other more specific texts should be consulted for a more comprehensive review of the subject.(1-8)

Acids, Bases, pH, pK, and the Henderson-Hasselbalch Equation

Most formal definitions of acids or bases when applied to biologic solutions universalize the Bronsted-Lowery concept, which classifies acids as proton donors and bases as proton acceptors. A more appro-

priate working definition, however, may be that acids are substances that increase H^+ concentration ($[H^+]$), a term used synonymously with *protons* in aqueous solutions. The strength of an acid and resultant acidity of a solution is determined by its activity coefficient, a factor influenced by temperature that determines the degree of dissociation. Since, by definition, a base is a H^+ (proton) acceptor, each acid dissociates into H^+ and a potential H^+ acceptor or conjugate base. For example, H_2CO_3 in aqueous solution dissociates into H^+ and its conjugate base HCO_3^-. Substances that are strong acids have weak conjugate bases and vice versa. Interestingly, water, the most abundant solvent in the body, can function as both an acid (H_3O^+; proton donor) or a base (H_2O; proton acceptor) depending upon local conditions ($H^+ + H_2O \rightleftarrows H_3O^+$). At normal pH (7.40) and temperature (37–38° C) water is the most abundant base in the body.

Emphasis in acid-base physiology is placed upon the formation of acids and therefore H^+ production because the end product of oral intake, tissue metabolism, and many pathophysiologic disease processes is the production and release of hydrogen ion. Sorensen (1909) developed the concept of pH ($-\log_{10}[H^+]$) in order to simplify the notation necessary to describe the large changes of $[H^+]$ observed in nature and chemical experiments. This notation, although cumbersome mathematically and somewhat misleading because of nonlinearity, converts $[H^+]$ to pH by the formula (Figure 18–2)

$$pH = -\log_{10}[H^+] = \log_{10}(1/[H^+]) \quad (18\text{-}4)$$

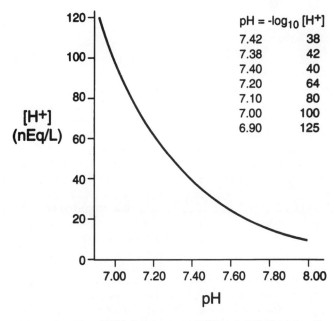

Fig. 18–2. The relationship between $[H^+]$ and pH. Note that the relationship is exponential and not linear.

Regardless of the relatively narrow range (20–150 nEq/L) over which changes in $[H^+]$ occur in biologic fluids, the concept of pH persists and is routinely reported on most pH and blood gas machines. Conversion formulas for pH to $[H^+]$ have been developed:

$$pH > 7.40 \quad [H^+] = (pH_m - 7.40)\,(40)\,(0.8) \quad (18\text{--}4a)$$

$$pH < 7.40 \quad [H^+] = (7.40 - pH_m)\,(40)\,(1.25) \quad (18\text{--}4b)$$

where pH_m is the measured pH. The development of the pH concept by Sorensen combined with the theory of acid-base balance proposed by Henderson (1909) and the introduction of methods to measure pH in blood by Hasselbalch (1912) led to the development of the Henderson-Hasselbalch equation and the characterization of acid-base disturbances as being either respiratory or nonrespiratory (metabolic) in origin. Application of the law of mass action to body fluids produces many potential equilibrium equations that could be used to explain acid-base balance. The reasons why the carbonic acid equilibrium equation (Eqs. 18–1 and 18–2) was chosen to describe acid-base balance are (a) historical (method of assay development) factors, (b) the finding that other than water, HCO_3^- is the major base in the extracellular fluid and H_2CO_3 the major acid, and (c) that the carbonic acid equation incorporates both volatile and nonvolatile substances. The law of mass action states that the rate (velocity) of a reaction is proportional to the concentration of the reactants and the dissociation constant (K) for the reaction. The rate of dissociation (r) for an acid can be characterized by

$$[HA] \rightarrow [H^+] + [A^-] \quad (18\text{--}5)$$

Using the dissociation constant K_1,

$$r_1 = K_1\,[HA] \quad (18\text{--}6)$$

Similarly,

$$[H^+] + [A^-] \rightarrow [HA] \quad (18\text{--}7)$$

and

$$r_2 = K_2\,[H^+]\,[A^-] \quad (18\text{--}8)$$

which at equilibrium results in $r_1 = r_2$, or

$$\frac{K_2}{K_1} = K_a = \frac{[H^+][A^-]}{[HA]} \quad (18\text{--}9)$$

Where K_a is the dissociation constant for the acid HA. Applying this law to carbonic acid, Henderson derived

$$[H^+] = \frac{K_a[CO_2]}{HCO_3^-} \quad (18\text{--}10)$$

Henderson used the concentration of dissolved molecular CO_2 instead of H_2CO_3 because H_2CO_3 could not be measured. Hasselbalch then introduced PCO_2 into Henderson's equation and put the equation into logarithmic form, producing the now universally applied Henderson-Hasselbalch equation:

$$pH = pK_a + \log_{10}\left\{\frac{[HCO_3^-]}{[s \times PCO_2]}\right\} \quad (18\text{--}11)$$

Where pH is $-\log_{10}[H^+]$, pK_a is $= \log_{10}K_a$, and s is the solubility of CO_2. This equation is frequently rewritten for explanatory purposes as

$$pH = pK_a + \log\left(\frac{[base]}{[acid]}\right) = \frac{kidney\ function}{lung\ function} \quad (18\text{--}12)$$

Henderson deliberately applied the law of mass action to the equilibrium of carbonic acid. The Henderson-Hasselbalch Equation indicates the amount of H^+ (protons) available to react with bases. Since acids and bases are charged particles, the application of this equation to biologic fluids assumes that

1. Mass is conserved: The concentration of all substances can be accounted for as the sum of the concentrations of dissociated and undisassociated forms.
2. All dissociation constants for all incompletely dissociated substances (weak acids or bases) are satisfied.
3. Electroneutrality is preserved: All positive charges must equal all negative charges.

These assumptions have particular relevance to the application of acid-base principles and to the interpretation of acid-base imbalance and are the basis for always integrating electrolyte (Na^+, K^+, Cl^-, etc.) abnormalities into the evaluation of acid-base balance.

Body Buffering Systems

The body uses three principle mechanisms to minimize or buffer changes in H^+.(6, 7) *Chemical buffers* act within seconds to resist or reduce changes in $[H^+]$ and are the first line of defense against changes in pH. The *respiratory system* responds within minutes to resist changes in $[H^+]$ by regulating the partial pressure of carbon dioxide (physiologic buffering) and eliminating excess CO_2 molecules caused by an increase in H^+ production (chemical buffering).

$$\uparrow H^+ + HCO_3^- \rightarrow H_2CO_3 \rightarrow H_2O + \quad (18\text{--}13)$$
$$CO_2\ (increased\ minute\ volume)$$

Finally, H^+ that are produced by nonrespiratory mechanisms (metabolic or nonrespiratory acidosis) are excreted by the *kidney* in the urine over a period of hours or days (Fig. 18–3).

CHEMICAL BUFFERS

These are compounds that minimize changes in the $[H^+]$ or the pH of a solution when an acid or base is added. A buffer solution consists of a weak acid and its conjugate base and is most effective when the pH is within 1.0 pH units of its dissociation constant (pK_a) (Table 18–1). Alterations in blood, interstitial, and intracellular $[H^+]$ are immediately modified by chemical buffer systems. The ratio of the anion $[A^-]$ form of the buffer to its conjugate acid [HA] is a function of its dissociation constant (pK_a) and the $[H^+]$. For weak acids as [H^+] increases [A^-] decreases and [HA] increases by equal amounts, keeping the total amount of A_{tot}(A_{tot} = HA + A^-) the same. The principle chemical buffers for excess H^+ production are the bicarbonate (HCO_3^-/H_2CO_3), phosphate (HPO_4^-/ H_2PO_4), and protein (Prot$^-$/H Prot) buffer systems. Bone can contribute calcium carbonate and calcium phosphate to the extracellular fluid, thereby increasing the buffering capacity. Indeed, bone may account for up to 40% of the buffering of an acute acid load. Functionally, anytime there is an increase in [H^+] in the body, the anion form of the buffer (HCO_3^-, HPO_4^-, Prot$^-$) accepts the excess proton, converting the buffer to its conjugate acid (H_2CO_3, H_2PO_4, H Prot). Because the body can have only one [H^+], the ratio of the acid to salt forms of the various buffer pairs in solution can always be predicted by the Henderson-Hasselbalch equation (isohydric principle), providing their concentration and their dissociation constant (pK_a) are known. Knowledge of the behavior of one buffer pair predicts the behavior of all the other buffer pairs in solution. The HCO_3^-/H_2CO_3 buffer pair is most frequently used to determine acid-base status in clinical practice because it is the most prominent chemical buffer in the extracellular fluid. Another important reason why the HCO_3^-/H_2CO_3 buffer pair is used to express acid-base status is that in

the presence of carbonic anhydrase, carbonic acid forms CO_2, which is eliminated by alveolar ventilation. Thus, the body can be considered an "open" system.

Approximately 60% of the body's chemical buffering capacity is accomplished by intracellular phosphates and proteins. Inorganic and organic (ATP, ADP, 2,3-DPG) phosphates possess pK_a values that range from 6.0 to 7.5, making them ideal chemical buffers over a wide range of potential intracellular pH values. Inorganic phosphate (pK_a 6.8) is the major buffer in urine because renal tubular pH (6.0-7.0) includes the pK_a of the HPO4$^-$/H_2PO_4 buffer pair.

Intracellular pH regulation depends upon the activity of two cell membrane ion transport systems, the Na^+-H^+ antiporter and the Cl^--HCO_3^- antiporter (chloride pump), and intracellular proteins. Proteins are by far the most important intracellular buffers. Hemoglobin contributes approximately 80% of the nonbicar-

Table 18–1. pK$_a$ Values of Important Chemical Buffers *

Compound	pK$_a$
Carbonic acid (pK$_a$)	3.6
Lactic acid	3.9
3-Hydroxybutyric acid	4.7
Creatinine	5.0
Organic phosphates	6.0–7.5
Carbonic acid (pK$_a$)	6.1
Imidazole group of histidine	6.4–6.7
Oxygenated hemoglobin	6.7
Phosphate$^-$	6.8
α-Amino (amino terminal)	7.4–7.9
Deoxygenated hemoglobin	7.9
Ammonium	9.2
Bicarbonate	9.8

*Compounds with pK$_a$ values in the range of 6.4–8.4 are most useful as buffers in biologic systems. The pK$_a$ values for the imidazole group of histidine and for α-amino (amino-terminal) groups are for those side groups in proteins. The pK$_a$ range for organic phosphates refers to such intracellular compounds as ATP, ADP, 2,3-DPG, etc.

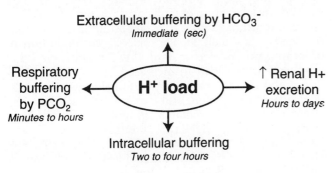

Fig. 18–3. Rate of response of the different buffering mechanisms in the body.

Table 18–2. Major Body Buffers

	pK$_a$	Compartment pH	Basis of Effectiveness	Weakness
ECF				
HCO$_3^-$	6.1	7.4	• CO$_2$ removal by the lungs • Quantity	• Distance of pH from pK • Depends on lungs
ICF*				
Imidazole	Close to 7	7.0	• Exceedingly large quantity	• Changes charge on ICF proteins†
HCO$_3^-$	6.1	7.0	• Relatively large quantity	• Depends on lungs for CO$_2$ removal
Urine				
Phosphate	6.8	5–7	• pK higher than urine pH	• Little capacity to increase excretion rate

*Although ICF creatine phosphate is not a buffer, during acidemia it is hydrolyzed, rendering it capable of H^+ binding.
†This change in charge on ICF proteins can have important effects on enzyme activities, transporters, and ICF volume.
Key: ECF = Extracellular fluid; ICF = Intracellular fluid.

bonate buffering capacity of whole blood and with other intracellular proteins is responsible for three fourths of the chemical buffering power of the body. The most important intracellular protein dissociable groups is the imidazole ring of histidine (pK_a 6.4–6.7). The alpha-amino groups of proteins (pK_a 7.4–7.9) play a secondary but important role in intracellular buffering. Plasma proteins, particularly albumin, also contain histidine and alpha-amino groups, and collectively are responsible for 20% of the nonbicarbonate buffering capacity of whole blood (Table 18–2).

RESPIRATORY SYSTEM

The respiratory system offers an alternative route by which [H^+] can be regulated by varying the partial pressure of carbon dioxide (PCO_2; Figure 18–1). Chemoreceptors throughout the body, but particularly those located in the medulla and carotid body, monitor changes in [H^+] and PCO_2 and adjust breathing (tidal volume and frequency) in order to maintain a normal [H^+]. The association of H^+ with HCO_3^- and the subsequent formation of CO_2 and H_2O is an example of chemical buffering (closed system), and the elimination of CO_2 by the lung (open system) constitutes a physiologic buffering mechanism. Changes in blood CO_2 also have important consequences for hemoglobin affinity for oxygen and its buffering capacity. Increases in PCO_2 increase blood [H^+] and decrease hemoglobin affinity for oxygen (Bohr effect) (Chapter 6). This change in the oxygen affinity of hemoglobin is advantageous in tissues, allowing hemoglobin to release more oxygen for metabolism. Unoxygenated hemoglobin in turn can transport more carbon dioxide in the form of hemoglobin contained carbamino compounds (H^+ Prot) to the lungs (Haldane effect). It is important to realize that anytime there is a change in the partial pressure of carbon dioxide there is a relatively much greater change in [H^+] than [HCO_3^-], since [HCO_3^-] is measured in mEq/L and [H^+] in nEq/L. Maintenance of [H^+] within a narrow range is vital to normal tissue enzyme activity.

THE KIDNEY

The synthesis of new HCO_3^- and excretion of excess H^+ emphasizes the role of the kidneys as both a chemical and physiologic buffer system (Fig. 18–1). Although relatively slow (hours, days), compared to the lungs (minutes) and chemical buffering (seconds), the kidney serves as the principal means by which acids that are produced by metabolic processes (not owing to CO_2 production but rather fixed acids) are ultimately eliminated (Fig. 18–3). All hydrogen ions produced by metabolic processes are excreted in the urine in combination with weak anions (titratable acidity), primarily phosphate and ammonium salts. The term *titratable acidity* may be considered synonymous with *urinary phosphate concentration* but actually represents all weak acids including creatinine and urate. Net acid excretion by the kidney includes the titratable acidity and ammonium minus the HCO_3^- eliminated in the urine. Ammonium ($NH4^+$) is produced in the proximal tu-

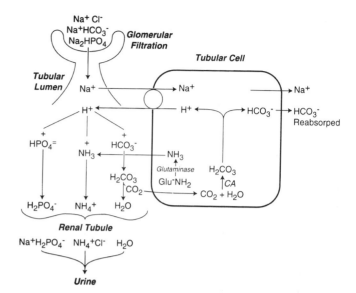

Fig. 18–4. Reabsorption and regeneration of HCO_3^- in the renal tubules. Bicarbonate reabsorption in the proximal tubule coincides with H^+ secretion. Bicarbonate regeneration in the renal tubules coincides with titration of phosphate by H^+ and ammonium formation.

bule primarily from glutamine metabolism to alpha-ketoglutarate and NH_3, a process that simultaneously generates HCO_3^-. Increases in H^+ production can increase the rate of ammonium salt excretion by five times during severe metabolic acidosis (Fig. 18–4).

It is important to note that potassium loss from cells can lead to intracellular H^+ or Na^+ accumulation in order to maintain electric neutrality. This effect in renal tubular cells can lead to increased H^+ excretion (aciduria) and HCO_3^- reabsorption (alkalemia and "paradoxical aciduria"). Renal tubular cell acidosis may also augment glutamine metabolism and NH_3 production, leading to enhanced NH_4^+ excretion. Alkalemia and paradoxical aciduria is known to occur in humans, rats and ruminants. Its importance in dogs and cats is questionable. Hyperkalemia has the opposite effects.

Temperature Effects on Acid-Base Balance

Increases and more routinely decreases in body temperature are frequently encountered in patients subjected to anesthesia and surgery. Increases in body temperature may be associated with stress, increases in skeletal muscle activity (inadequate relaxation), systemic disease, and/or infectious and genetic disorders (malignant hyperthermia) (Chapters 11 and 20). Decreases in body temperature are much more common than increases during anesthesia and surgery. Hypothermia may be much more profound in smaller patients ($<$8–10 kg) because of their larger body surface area to body mass ratio and is exaggerated by cleaning solutions (water, alcohol), cold exposure (steel tables), illness (shock), drugs that cause vasodilation (phenothiazine, barbiturates, isoflurane), and toxicity. Changes in body temperature affect the [H^+] of all body fluids. Increases in body temperature decrease pH and vice

Table 18–3. Effect of Temperature upon PO_2, PCO_2 and pH

Temp °C	PO_2	PCO_2	pH
39	90	44	7.37
37	80	40	7.40
30	54	30	7.50

versa such that blood pH changes by 0.015 to 0.02 units /°C. Changes in pH with body temperature are expected because of known temperature-induced changes on dissociation constants (pK_a) and the solubility of carbon dioxide in blood. For example, as body temperature decreases, the pK_a and blood solubility of CO_2 increase, producing an increase in pH and decrease in PCO_2 (Table 18–3). These temperature-dependent changes in both intra- and extracellular pH are believed to be important in maintaining an $OH^-:H^+$ (relative alkalinity) ratio of 16:1 throughout the body. A constant relative alkalinity of 16:1 for OH^- and H^+ is known to be optimal for cellular enzyme systems to function normally. The most important of the dissociable groups responsible for maintenance of a constant ratio between $[H^+]$ and $[OH^-]$ is the imidazole ring of the histidine residues of hemoglobin. Indeed, the fractional dissociation of imidazole-histidine remains constant as temperature changes and varies with pH during isothermal conditions. This regulation of the functional imidazole-histidine dissociation in order to maintain acid-base balance is termed *alpha-stat* (α-stat) *regulation* in contrast to *pH stat regulation*, in which pH values are maintained constant (Table 18–4).(7, 9)

Both the alpha-stat and pH-stat concepts of acid-base balance have been used clinically when interpreting pH and blood gases in patients with body temperatures greater or lower than normal.(7, 9) Proponents of the pH-stat hypothesis argue that it is important to maintain a constant pH of 7.40 and PCO_2 of 40 mm Hg at any temperature, whereas proponents of the alpha-stat strategy attempt to keep a constant ratio of $[H^+]$ to $[OH^-]$ of 1:16. Proponents of the pH-stat strategy realize that if the pH and PCO_2 were kept constant at pH of 7.40 and PCO_2 of 40 mm Hg during hypothermia, the patient would be acidotic, but they argue that pH-stat-oriented therapy reduces morbidity. Proponents of alpha-stat-oriented therapy argue similarly and point out that blood flow to vital organs, particularly cerebral blood flow, becomes pressure dependent with pH-stat management. A great deal more research is required to resolve the current controversies regarding the potential benefits of either strategy. From a practical standpoint, however, pH and PCO_2 need not be corrected for temperature. Measuring a blood sample taken from a hypothermic patient at 37 or 38° C (the temperature at which most blood gas machines are calibrated) permits appropriate therapeutic decisions and eliminates the need to know the patient's precise body temperature for interpretation of acid-base abnormalities (Chapter 15).

Clinical Acid-Base Terminology

Descriptions of acid-base balance and acid-base abnormalities have been based upon familiarity with the Bronsted-Lowery definition of an acid and base, the Henderson-Hasselbalch equation, and standard medical terms describing body fluids or fluid compartments. The terms *acidosis* and *alkalosis*, for example, are used to describe the abnormal or pathologic (osis) accumulation of acid $[H^+]$ or alkali $[OH^-]$ in the body.(5) The terms *acidemia* and *alkalemia* are used to describe whether the blood pH is acid or alkaline respectively. The Henderson-Hasselbalch equation characterizes all acid-base disturbances as being either respiratory or metabolic because of the body's production and elimination of volatile (dissolved CO_2; H_2CO_3) and nonvolatile or fixed (lactic and phosphoric) acids, respectively. Therefore, only four primary acid-base abnormalities are possible: respiratory acidosis, metabolic acidosis, respiratory alkalosis, metabolic alkalosis (Table 18–5). Clinically, the terms *respiratory* and *metabolic* have been used to imply the involvement of the lung and kidney in acid-base regulation:

$$pH = \frac{HCO_3^-}{PaCO_2} = \frac{\text{kidney function (fixed acids)}}{\text{lung function (volatile acids)}}$$

The term *nonrespiratory* frequently replaces *metabolic* in many discussions of acid-base imbalance because the term *metabolic* is not totally descriptive and is somewhat misleading (because it implies that all fixed acids are produced by cellular metabolism). The term *nonrespira-*

Table 18–4. Comparison of pH-Stat and α-Stat Acid Base Regulation

Concept	Purpose	Total CO_2	pH and $PaCO_2$ Maintenance	Intracellular State	Alpha-Imidazole and Buffering	Enzyme Structure and Function
pH-stat	Constant pH	Increases	Normal corrected values	Acidotic (excess H^+)	Excess (+) charge, buffering decreased	Altered and activity decreased
Alpha-stat	Constant OH^-/H^+	Constant	Normal uncorrected values	Neutral ($H^+ = OH^-$)	Constant net charge, buffering constant	Normal and activity maximal

tory incorporates all mechanisms responsible for acid-base imbalance other than the production of carbon dioxide and carbonic acid (H_2CO_3). These mechanisms include alterations in the PCO_2, concentrations of strong (fully dissociated) ions and strong ion difference (SID), nonvolatile plasma buffers (primarily serum proteins; A_{tot}), and the ionic strength (dissociation constants; pK_a) of the solution (Fig. 18–5). The four factors used to describe these changes in $[H^+]$ are collectively referred to as *independent variables* (PCO_2, SID, A_{tot}, pK_a) because each of them is regulated or changed independent of the others.(10-12) It should be noted, however, that changes in temperature can affect all the independent variables, a consideration that has special importance during surgery and anesthesia.

Primary abnormalities in acid-base balance can arise from disturbances in any one or several of the independent variables. Simple acid-base abnormalities are said to occur only when one independent variable is responsible for the acid-base disturbance. Mixed acid-base abnormalities are caused by disturbances in two or more of the independent variables. Mixed acid-base abnormalities may be additive (respiratory and nonres-piratory acidosis) or offsetting (respiratory alkalosis and metabolic acidosis) with regard to their ability to influence $[H^+]$ measured as pH. Offsetting mixed acid-base abnormalities occur when two primary acid-base abnormalities produce opposite effects on plasma $[H^+]$. Patients with offsetting mixed acid-base abnormalities have both acidosis and alkalosis but do not necessarily demonstrate acidemia or alkalemia since blood pH may be normal. Some observations that should lead to suspicions of a mixed acid-base disturbance when evaluating blood gas results are (2, 13, 14)

1. the presence of a normal pH with abnormal PCO_2 and/or $[HCO_3^-]$;
2. a pH change in a direction opposite that predicted for the known primary disorder; and
3. PCO_2 and $[HCO_3^-]$ changing in opposite directions.

Mixed acid-base disorders can be classified based on the origin of the primary disturbances as mixed respiratory disturbances, mixed nonrespiratory and respiratory disturbances, mixed nonrespiratory disturbances, and triple disorders. They also can be classified based on

Table 18–5. Characteristics of Primary Acid-Base Disturbances

Disorder	pH	$[H^+]$	Primary Disturbance	Compensatory Response
Nonrespiratory acidosis	↓	↑	↓$[HCO_3^-]$	↓PCO_2
Nonrespiratory alkalosis	↑	↓	↑$[HCO_3^-]$	↑PCO_2
Respiratory acidosis	↓	↑	↑$[PCO_2]$	↑$[HCO_3^-]$
Respiratory alkalosis	↑	↓	↓$[PCO_2]$	↓$[HCO_3^-]$

Nonrespiratory is used in preference to metabolic.

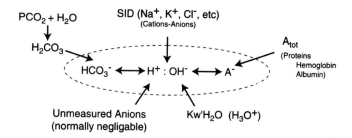

Fig. 18–5. The influence of independent variables on acid-base balance. The dependent variables (H^+ and OH^-) are enclosed by the dashed line.

Table 18–6. Classification of Mixed Acid-Base Disorders

Classification	Effect on the pH
Mixed respiratory disorders	
Acute and chronic respiratory acidosis	Additive
Acute and chronic respiratory alkalosis	Additive
Mixed respiratory and nonrespiratory disorders	
Respiratory acidosis and nonrespiratory acidosis	Additive
Respiratory acidosis and nonrespiratory alkalosis	Offsetting
Respiratory alkalosis and nonrespiratory acidosis	Offsetting
Respiratory alkalosis and nonrespiratory alkalosis	Additive
Mixed nonrespiratory disorders	
Nonrespiratory acidosis and nonrespiratory alkalosis	Offsetting
Normal plus high anion gap nonrespiratory acidosis	Additive
Mixed high anion gap nonrespiratory acidosis	Additive
Mixed normal anion gap nonrespiratory acidosis	Additive
Triple disorders	
Nonrespiratory acidosis, nonrespiratory alkalosis, and respiratory acidosis	Final pH is function of relative dominance of acidifying and alkalinizing processes
Nonrespiratory acidosis, nonrespiratory alkalosis, and respiratory alkalosis	

Table 18–7. Expected Compensatory Responses in Primary Acid-Base Disorders

Disorder	Primary Change	Expected Range of Compensation
Nonrespiratory acidosis	$\downarrow [HCO_3^-]$	PCO_2 = last 2 digits of pH × 100 $\Delta PCO_2 = 1 - 1.13\ (\Delta[HCO_3^-])$ $PCO_2 = [HCO_3^-] + 15$ $PCO_2 = 0.7\ [HCO_3^-] \pm 3$ (Dogs)
Nonrespiratory alkalosis	$\uparrow [HCO_3^-]$	PCO_2: variable increase PCO_2 = increases of 0.6 mm Hg for each new mEq/L increase in $[HCO_3^-]$ $PCO_2 = [HCO_3^-] \pm 3$ (Dogs)
Respiratory acidosis		
Acute	$\uparrow PCO_2$	Acute $[HCO_3^-]$ increases 1 mEq/L and pH decreases 0.05 units for every 10 mm Hg increase in PCO_2 $[HCO_3^-] = 0.15\ PCO_2 \pm 2$ (Dogs)
Chronic	$\uparrow PCO_2$	$[HCO_3^-]$ increases 3.5 mEq/L and pH decreases 0.07 units for every 10 mm Hg increase in PCO_2 $[HCO_3^-] = 0.35\ PCO_2 \pm 2$ (Dogs)
Respiratory alkalosis		
Acute	$\downarrow PCO_2$	$[HCO_3^-]$ falls 2 mEq/L and pH increases 0.1 units for each 10 mm Hg fall in PCO_2 $[HCO_3^-] = 0.25\ PCO_2 \pm 2$ (Dogs)
Chronic	$\downarrow PCO_2$	$[HCO_3^-]$ falls 5 mEq/L and pH increases 0.15 units for each 10 mm Hg fall in PCO_2 $[HCO_3^-] = 0.55\ PCO_2 \pm 2$ (Dogs)

their effect on the patient's pH in additive combinations, offsetting combinations, and triple disorders (Table 18–6).(2) In additive combinations, both primary disorders tend to change pH in the same direction (e.g., respiratory acidosis and nonrespiratory acidosis), whereas in offsetting combinations, the primary disorders tend to change the pH in opposite directions (e.g., respiratory alkalosis and nonrespiratory acidosis). The final pH reflects the dominant of the two offsetting disorders in offsetting combinations.(2) Detailed reviews of mixed acid-based disorders in domestic animals have been presented elsewhere.(2, 13-15)

Secondary or compensatory (adaptive) acid-base changes frequently occur in response to most primary acid-base abnormalities and aid in "buffering" or minimizing changes in plasma $[H^+]$. Respiratory acid-base abnormalities, for example, are generally compensated for by controlled, oppositely directed changes in nonrespiratory function. In simple acid-base abnormalities such as primary respiratory acidosis caused by hypoventilation, the kidney compensates by producing nonrespiratory alkalosis.

Respiratory compensation in metabolic acid-base disorders is obtained by changing alveolar ventilation and therefore changing CO_2 excretion by the lungs. Nonrespiratory acidosis is characterized by an increase in $[H^+]$, a decrease in blood $[HCO_3^-]$ and pH, and a decrease in PCO_2 caused by secondary hyperventilation, whereas nonrespiratory alkalosis is characterized by a decrease in $[H^+]$, increase in blood $[HCO_3^-]$ and pH, and an increase in PCO_2 owing to compensatory hypoventilation.

In respiratory acid-base disorders, the compensation occurs in two phases. The first phase consists of titration by nonbicarbonate buffers, and the second phase reflects renal compensation of the acid-base disorder, by increasing or decreasing HCO_3^- and Cl^- excretion in the urine. Respiratory acidosis is characterized by increased PCO_2, increased $[H^+]$, decreased pH, and a compensatory increase in blood $[HCO_3^-]$. Carbon dioxide accumulation is caused by alveolar hypoventilation. Renal compensation occurs by titration of nonbicarbonate buffers, increase in net acid and Cl^- excretion, and increase in HCO_3^- reabsorption by the kidneys.(6, 14) Respiratory alkalosis is characterized by decreased PCO_2, decreased $[H^+]$, increased pH, and a compensatory decrease in blood $[HCO_3^-]$. The initial compensation in respiratory alkalosis is caused by release of H^+ ions from nonbicarbonate buffers within cells. The second phase is mediated by a compensatory decrease in net acid excretion by the kidneys.(14)

When analyzing secondary changes in a given acid-base disorder, it is important to remember that

1. with the exception of chronic respiratory alkalosis, compensation does not return the pH to normal,
2. overcompensation does not occur, and
3. sufficient time must elapse for compensation to reach a steady state, at which time the expected compensation can be estimated using the formulas in Table 18–7.

Care should be exercised when dealing with cats because they may not be able to compensate for nonrespiratory acidosis as well as dogs.

Table 18–8. Simple Primary Nonrespiratory Acid-Base Disorders*

Nonrespiratory Disorder	$Na^+ - Cl^-$†	AG†	TCO_2	Respiratory Compensation	Biochemical Profile
Alkaloses					
Hypoalbuminemia	N	N, ⇓	⇑	No	⇓ Albumin
Hypochloremia	⇑	N	⇑	No	⇓ [Cl⁻] corrected
Concentration	⇑	N	⇑	Yes	⇑ [Na⁺]
Acidoses					
Hyperalbuminemia	N	N, ⇑	⇓	No	⇑ Albumin
Hyperphosphatemia	N	N, ⇑	⇓	No	⇑ Inorganic phosphate
Hyperchloremia	⇓	N	⇓	Yes	⇑ [Cl⁻] corrected
Dilution	⇓	N	⇓	Yes	⇓ [Na⁺]
Organic	N	⇑	⇓	Yes	Specific assays required

*$Na^+ - Cl^-$ difference between sodium and chloride concentration; AG, anion gap; TCO_2, total CO_2; ⇑, increase; N, normal; ⇓, decrease; see text for limitations in using $Na^+ - Cl^-$ difference and AG.

† From de Morais, H.S.A., and Muir, W.W. Strong Ions and Acid-Base Disorders. In: Kirk's Current Veterinary Therapy XII, 12th ed. Edited by J.D. Bonagura and R.W. Kirk. Philadelphia, WB Saunders, 1995:121–127.(12)

The question that often arises when analyzing simple acid-base abnormalities that demonstrate both respiratory acidosis and nonrespiratory alkalosis is which is primary and which is secondary or compensatory. The answer is not always obvious, although simple primary acid-base abnormalities change pH in the direction of the primary disorder. For example, a patient with respiratory acidosis and compensatory nonrespiratory alkalosis would have an acid pH (e.g., 7.35). Mixed respiratory and nonrespiratory acid-base abnormalities are much more difficult to decipher, and like simple acid-base abnormalities must be carefully evaluated in the context of the patient's signs, symptoms, and other available diagnostic information.

Because nonrespiratory acidosis is so frequently associated with disease processes in animals, indices of acid-base balance have evolved that permit the quantitative evaluation of the nonrespiratory component of acid-base abnormalities. The standard bicarbonate is the concentration of bicarbonate in plasma after the whole blood sample has been equilibrated to a PCO_2 of 40 mm Hg at 38° C. This index quantifies the nonrespiratory component of any acid-base abnormality, since differences in the standard bicarbonate from normal (approx. 25 mEq/L) cannot be caused by changes in PCO_2, which is held constant at 40 mm Hg at 38° C. Similarly, the base excess quantitates the number of mEq/L of acid or base required to titrate 1 liter of blood to pH 7.40 while the PCO_2 is held constant at 40 mm Hg at 38° C. Both the standard bicarbonate and base excess (or deficit) can be determined from nomograms. The base excess has a normal value of zero (±3) and is changed only by nonvolatile acids thereby indicating nonrespiratory acidosis. The numerical magnitude of the base excess is a guide to therapy:

$$\text{Base } (Na^+HCO_3^-) \text{ needed} \qquad (18\text{–}14)$$
$$= (0.3) \times (BE) \times (\text{body weight in kg})$$

where 0.3 = % body weight that is extracellular water.

Anion Gap

The anion gap (AG) is a useful tool to assess mixed acid-base disorders.(10, 11, 14) Chemically, there is no anion gap because electroneutrality must be maintained and the "anion gap" actually is the difference between the unmeasured anions (UA^-) and unmeasured cations (UC^+). Following the electroneutrality law,

$$([Na^+] + [K^+] + [UC^+]) - ([Cl^-] + \qquad (18\text{–}15)$$
$$[HCO_3^-] + [UA^-]) = 0$$

or when applied clinically,

$$AG = ([Na^+] + [K^+]) - ([Cl^-] + \qquad (18\text{–}16)$$
$$[HCO_3^-]) = [UA^-] - [UC^+]$$

Based on Equation 18–15, every time there is a decrease in $[HCO_3^-]$, either $[Cl^-]$ or $[UA^-]$ must increase to maintain electroneutrality. When titrated HCO_3^- is replaced by Cl^- in nonrespiratory acidosis, the difference ($[UA^-] - [UC^+]$; and consequently the AG) will remain the same (called *hyperchloremic* or *normal AG acidosis*). When titrated HCO_3^- is replaced by UA^-, the difference ($[UA^-] - [UC^+]$; i.e., the AG) will increase while $[Cl^-]$ remains the same (called *normochloremic* or *high AG acidosis*).(2, 15)

Negatively charged proteins, phosphates, sulfates, and organic acids (e.g., lactate, beta-hydroxybutyrate, acetoacetate, citrate) constitute the UA^-.(16) Usually an increase in AG implies an accumulation of organic acids in the body.(17) An increase in AG also occurs in alkalemia caused by an increase in the net negative charge on serum proteins or in situations where concomitant nonrespiratory alkalosis or respiratory alkalosis overrides a high-AG nonrespiratory acidosis.(18, 19) Hypoalbuminemia probably is the only important cause of a decrease in AG, and each decrease in albumin concentration by 1 g/dL has been associated with a decrease of 3 mEq/L in the AG.

The AG concept has some limitations. The summation of $[Cl^-]$ and $[HCO_3^-]$ is not acceptable based on principles of chemistry.(20) Each of these anions has a different activity coefficient partially because they are present in extracellular fluid at concentrations that differ by a factor of more than 5 (i.e., $[Cl^-]$ = 110 mEq/L vs $[HCO_3^-]$ = 21 mEq/L).(20) Regardless, this simplification of the anion gap is helpful clinically (Table 18–8). The AG also can change because of excessive exposure of serum to air, resulting in changes of 6.5 ± 2.3 mEq/L after 2 hours.(21) These changes are more pronounced in patients with respiratory acidosis.(20)

$[NA^+] - [CL^-]$ Difference

Plasma Cl^- and HCO_3^- concentrations have a tendency to change in the opposite direction in nonrespiratory alkalosis and hyperchloremic acidosis, whereas sodium concentration tends to remain normal in acid-base disturbances unless the primary disorder also affects water balance. The difference between sodium and chloride concentrations ($[Na^+] - [Cl^-]$) is therefore useful in the assessment of those nonrespiratory disturbances not associated with an increase in unmeasured anions. The $[Na^+] - [Cl^-]$ is approximately 35 mEq/L. If $[Na^+]$ is normal, an increase in this value is caused by hypochloremia and is an indication of metabolic alkalosis, whereas a decrease in the $[Na^+] - [Cl^-]$ gradient is an indication of hyperchloremic acidosis.(8) This difference, used in association with the AG, is useful in identifying the presence of a mixed metabolic process (Table 18–9).

Strong Ion Difference

A new theory of acid-base regulation has been proposed.(8) According to this theory $[HCO_3^-]$ and pH ($[H^+]$) are dependent on PCO_2, the total concentration of plasma weak nonvolatile acids ($[A_{tot}]$, composed mostly of albumin and inorganic phosphates), and the difference between the strong cations and the strong anions (called the *strong ion difference* or SID) (Fig. 18–5).(4, 8) As was previously pointed out, strong ions are substances that are completely dissociated in plasma at body pH. The most important strong ions in plasma are Na^+, K^+, Ca^{2+}, Mg^{2+}, Cl^-, lactate, beta-hydroxybutyrate, acetoacetate, and SO_4^{2-}. The influence of strong ions on pH and $[HCO_3^-]$ can always be expressed in terms of the SID. An increase in SID correlates with nonrespiratory alkalosis, whereas a decrease in SID correlates with nonrespiratory acidosis. Body homeostatic mechanisms indirectly regulate $[H^+]$ (and pH) and $[HCO_3^-]$ by changing PCO_2 (by changes in alveolar ventilation relative to carbon dioxide elimination rate) and SID (by differential reabsorption of Na^+ and Cl^- in the kidneys). Although changes in $[A_{tot}]$ will change $[HCO_3^-]$ and $[H^+]$, control of albumin production and inorganic phosphate concentration is not primarily directed at acid-base homeostasis.

Simple acid-base disturbances occur when abnormalities in one of the principal determinants of $[H^+]$ (e.g., PCO_2, SID, or $[A_{tot}]$) is present.(3, 11, 12) A simple acid-base disturbance includes both the primary process and the compensatory response. That is, if a sustained primary disturbance occurs in PCO_2, a compensatory change of regulated magnitude normally occurs in the SID and vice versa. If the primary disturbance results from a change in $[A_{tot}]$, however, renal or ventilatory compensation does not occur.(3)

Clinical Disturbances

A new classification of primary acid-base disorders has been developed.(3, 4) This classification provides a mechanistic view of the causative disturbances and integrates serum electrolytes and albumin concentration into the interpretation of acid-base status.

DISORDERS OF PCO_2

Primary respiratory disturbances result from increases (respiratory acidosis) or decreases (respiratory alkalosis) in PCO_2. Carbon dioxide tension can be changed by alveolar ventilation, which has a profound effect on $[HCO_3^-]$ and $[H^+]$. Approximately 50% of daily variability of $[HCO_3^-]$ in normal dogs can be attributed to changes in PCO_2 alone. Because arterial PCO_2 ($PaCO_2$) is inversely proportional to the alveolar ventilation, measurement of $PaCO_2$ provides the clinician with direct information about the adequacy of alveolar ventilation. Respiratory acidosis is therefore caused by and synonymous with hypoventilation, whereas respi-

Table 18–9. Relative Changes in $[Na^+]_o$ and $[Cl^-]_o$ as an Index of Disorders in Hydration or Acid-Base Balance or Both

a. Proportionate change in $[Na^+]_o$ and $[Cl^-]_o$ are always due to the disturbances of hydration alone.
   Dehydration
      $[Na^+]_o$ ↑ and $[Cl^-]_o$ ↑
   Overhydration
      $[Na^+]_o$ ↓ and $[Cl^-]_o$ ↓
b. Changes in $[Cl^-]_o$ without any change in $[Na^+]_o$ is always due to disturbances of acid-base alone.
   Respiratory acidosis or nonrespiratory alkalosis
      $[Na^+]_o$ and $[Cl^-]_o$ ↓
   Respiratory alkalosis or hypercholemic acidosis
      $[Na^+]_o$ and $[Cl^-]_o$ ↑
c. Disproportionate changes in $[Na^+]_o$ and $[Cl^-]_o$ are due to disturbances in both hydration and acid-base balance.
   Dehydration plus respiratory acidosis or nonrespiratory alkalosis
      $[Na^+]_o$ ↑ and $[Cl^-]_o$
   Overhydration plus respiratory alkalosis or hyperchloremic acidosis
      $[Na^+]_o$ ↓ and $[Cl^-]_o$
   Dehydration plus respiratory acidosis or nonrespiratory alkalosis
      $[Na^+]_o$ ↑ and $[Cl^-]_o$ ↓
   Overhydration plus respiratory acidosis or nonrespiratory alkalosis
      $[Na^+]_o$ ↓ and $[Cl^-]$ ↓↓
   Dehydration plus respiratory acidosis or nonrespiratory alkalosis
      $[Na^+]_o$ ↑↑ and $[Cl^-]_o$ ↑

(Modified from Emmett, M., and Seldin, D.W. Evaluation of Acid-Base Disorders from Plasma Composition. In: The Regulation of Acid-Base Balance. Edited by D.W. Seldin and G. Giebisch. New York: Raven Press, 1989:259.) (2)

ratory alkalosis is caused by and synonymous with hyperventilation (Chapter 6). The principal disorders associated with respiratory acidosis are airway obstruction, respiratory center depression (e.g., drugs, neurologic disorders), cardiopulmonary arrest ($PaCO_2$ may be below normal during cardiopulmonary resuscitation), neuromuscular diseases, diaphragmatic hernia, chest wall trauma, and inadequate mechanical ventilation. Therapy of respiratory acidosis should be directed toward the elimination of the underlying cause of alveolar hypoventilation. Ventilatory assistance should be provided when necessary. Respiratory acidosis is not an indication for bicarbonate therapy. Administration of $NaHCO_3$ will decrease $[H^+]$ and decrease ventilatory drive, thus worsening hypoxemia and hypercapnia. It is not usually possible to remove the underlying cause of hypercapnia in patients with chronic pulmonary disease, but appropriate treatment of the underlying disease should be attempted.

The principal causes of respiratory alkalosis are hypoxia, low cardiac-output, severe anemia, pulmonary disease (stimulation of peripheral reflexes, e.g., pneumonia), CNS-mediated hyperventilation (e.g., drugs, CNS inflammation or tumor, liver disease, fear, pain), and overzealous mechanical ventilation. Hypocapnia itself is not a major threat to the well-being of patients with respiratory alkalosis. The arterial pH in chronic primary respiratory alkalosis is usually normal or slightly alkalemic owing to efficient renal compensation in this setting. Therapy of the underlying disease responsible for hypocapnia should be the primary focus in patients with respiratory alkalosis.

Increases in alveolar-arterial oxygen difference. The alveolar-arterial oxygen difference [$P(A-a)O_2$ gradient] may be useful in differentiating intrinsic pulmonary disease from extrapulmonary disease in animals with hypoxemia. The (A-a) gradient estimates the difference between the PO_2 in the alveoli (P_AO_2) and the arterial blood (PaO_2). It can be calculated clinically as (A-a) gradient = $(150 - 1.25 \cdot PaCO_2) - PaO_2$. In normal animals at sea level, the $P(A-a)O_2$ gradient should be less than 15 mm Hg, although values up to 25 mm Hg had been considered normal.

Hypoxia can be caused by hypoventilation, decreased partial pressure of inspired O_2 (P_IO_2), diffusion impairment, ventilation/perfusion mismatch, and right-to-left shunts (Chapter 6). The $P(A-a)O_2$ gradient will be

Table 18–10.   Disorders of SID

Free Water Abnormalities
Increase in $[Na^+]$	$\Rightarrow$ Concentration alkalosis
Decrease in $[Na^+]$	$\Rightarrow$ Dilution acidosis

Chloride abnormalities
Decrease in $[Cl^-]$ corrected	$\Rightarrow$ Hypochloremic alkalosis
Increase in $[Cl^-]$ corrected	$\Rightarrow$ Hyperchloremic acidosis

Unmeasured strong anions abnormalities
Increase in $[XA^-]$	$\Rightarrow$ Organic acidosis

$[XA^-]$, unidentified strong anions

Table 18–11.   Principal Causes of Free Water Abnormalities

Concentration Alkalosis ($\Uparrow [Na^+]$)
  Pure water deficit
    Primary hypodipsia
    Diabetes Insipidus
    Fever
    Inadequate access to water
    High environmental temperature
  Hypotonic fluid loss
    Vomiting
    Peritonitis
    Pancreatitis
    Nonoliguric renal failure
    Postobstructive diuresis
  Sodium gain
    Salt poisoning
    Hypertonic fluid administration (e.g., hypertonic saline, $NaHCO_3$)
    Hyperaldosteronism
    Hyperadrenocorticism
Dilution Acidosis ($\Downarrow [Na^+]$)
  Severe liver disease
  Nephrotic syndrome
  Advanced renal failure
  Congestive heart failure
  Psychogenic polydipsia
  Excessive sweating in horses
  Hypotonic fluid administration (e.g., 0.45% NaCl solution)
  Vomiting
  Diarrhea
  Uroabdomen
  Hypoadrenocorticism
  Diuretic Administration

(Adapted from de Morais, H.S.A., and Muir, W.W. Strong ions and acid-base disorders. In: Kirk's Current Veterinary Therapy XII, 12th ed. Edited by J.D. Bonagura and R.W. Kirk. Philadelphia, WB Saunders, 1995:121–127.) (12)

normal in patients with hypoventilation or decreased P_IO_2 (e.g., residence at high altitude) because they have normal lung function. Patients with hypoventilation have an increase in PCO_2, whereas patients breathing air with a low P_IO_2 have a lower than normal PCO_2 (hyperventilating). The $P(A-a)O_2$ gradient is increased in patients with diffusion impairment (rarely recognized in veterinary medicine), ventilation/perfusion mismatch, and right-to-left shunt. Administration of 100% O_2 will usually correct hypoxemia in patients with ventilation/perfusion mismatch, but not in patients with significant right-to-left shunt.

DISORDERS OF [A_{tot}]

Albumin and inorganic phosphate are nonvolatile weak acids and collectively are the major contributors to [A_{tot}] (Fig. 18–5). Consequently, changes in their concentrations will change [H^+]. Hypoalbuminemia will tend to decrease [A_{tot}] and cause a nonrespiratory alkalosis. Although less common, an increase in albumin concentration can cause nonrespiratory acidosis owing to an increase in [A_{tot}]. Phosphate is the second most important component of [A_{tot}] and is normally present in plasma at a low concentration. Severe hyperphosphatemia can cause a large increase in [A_{tot}], which can result in nonrespiratory acidosis. The treatment for hyperphosphatemic acidosis, hyperalbuminemic acidosis, and hypoalbuminemic alkalosis should be directed at the underlying cause.

DISORDERS OF SID

Changes in SID usually are recognized by changes in [HCO_3^-] or base excess (BE). A decrease in SID is associated with nonrespiratory acidosis, whereas an increase in SID is associated with nonrespiratory alkalosis. There are three general mechanisms by which SID can change (Table 18–10): (a) changing the free water content of plasma, (b) changing the Cl^- concentration, and (c) increasing the concentration of unidentified strong anions (XA^-).

Free water abnormalities. Changing the water content of the various body fluid compartments will dilute or concentrate both strong anions and cations. Consequently, SID will change by the same proportion. Changes in free water can be identified by evaluating the [Na^+]. An increase in SID caused by increases in [Na^+] results in concentration alkalosis, whereas a decrease in SID caused by decreases in [Na^+] results in dilution acidosis. It has been suggested that changes in extracellular fluid (ECF) volume alone lead to acid-base disturbances. However, change in ECF volume by itself does not change SID, PCO_2, or [A_{tot}] and therefore cannot change acid-base status.(4) The so-called contraction alkalosis believed to be caused by a decrease in ECF volume is increased by a decrease in [Cl^-].(10, 22) The principal causes of concentration alkalosis and dilution acidosis are listed in Table 18–11.

Therapy for dilution acidosis and concentration alkalosis should be directed at treating the underlying cause responsible for changing [Na^+]. If necessary, [Na^+] and osmolality should be corrected.(1) Nonrespiratory acidosis should be treated only in patients with severe acidemia (pH <7.2).

Isonatremic chloride abnormalities. If there is no change in the water content of plasma, plasma [Na^+] will be normal. Other strong cations (e.g., K^+) are regulated for purposes other than acid-base balance, and their concentration never changes sufficiently to substantially affect SID.(4) Consequently, SID changes only as a result of changes in strong anions when water content is normal. If [Na^+] remains constant, changes in [Cl^-] can substantially increase or decrease SID. Evaluation of [Cl^-] must be considered in conjunction with measurement of [Na^+] because [Cl^-] can change for reasons other than a change in water balance. Patient [Cl^-] is therefore "corrected" for changes in [Na^+], applying a formula developed for use in humans (23) and adapted for use in small (11) and large (24) animals:

$$[Cl^-] \text{ corrected} = \frac{[Cl^-] \times [Na^+] \text{ normal}}{[Na^+]} \quad (18-17)$$

where [Cl^-] and [Na^+] are the patient Cl^- and Na^+ concentrations. The normal [Na^+] is the normal Na^+ concentration for the species being evaluated. Suggested values for [Na^+] in dogs are 146 (11) and 147 mEq/L (24), whereas for cats they range from 150 (24) to 156 mEq/L.(11) In large animals, normal [Na^+] is approximately 136 mEq/L in horses and 144 mEq/L in cattle.(24) Normal [Cl^-] is approximately 107 to 113 mEq/L for dogs (10), 117 to 123 mEq/L for cats (10), 97 to 103 mEq/L for horses (24), and 101 to 107 mEq/L for cattle.(24) These values may vary for different laboratories and different analyzers. An increase or decrease in corrected [Cl^-] indicates that Cl^- is responsible at least in part for the changes in SID. An increase in corrected [Cl^-] (i.e., an increase in [Cl^-] relative to [Na^+]) results in a hyperchloremic nonrespiratory acidosis, whereas a decrease in corrected [Cl^-] (i.e., a decrease in [Cl^-] relative to [Na^+]) results in hypochloremic nonrespiratory alkalosis. A [Cl^-] corrected to normal in the presence of abnormal observed [Cl^-] indicates that SID changes are caused by dilution acidosis or concentration alkalosis.

The principal causes of hyperchloremic acidosis and hypochloremic alkalosis are shown in Table 18–12. Treatment of hyperchloremic acidosis should be directed at correction of the underlying disease. Admin-

Table 18–12. Principal Chloride Disorders

Hypochloremic alkalosis* ($\Downarrow$ [Cl^-] corrected)
  Excessive loss of chloride relative to sodium
    Vomiting of stomach contents
    Gastric reflux in horses with ileus
    Abomasum torsion (ruminants)
    Vagal indigestion with internal vomiting (ruminants)
    Therapy with thiazides or loop diuretics
    Hyperadrenocorticism
  Excessive gain of sodium relative to chloride
    $NaHCO_3$ therapy
Hyperchloremic acidosis† ($\Uparrow$ [Cl^-] corrected)
  Excessive loss of sodium relative to chloride
    Diarrhea
  Excessive gain of chloride relative to sodium
    Fluid therapy (e.g., 0.9% $NaCl$, KCl supplemental fluids)
    Salt poisoning
    Total parenteral nutrition
    NH_4Cl or KCl therapy
  Chloride retention
    Renal failure
    Renal tubular acidosis
    Hypoadrenocorticism
    Diabetes mellitus
    Drug induced (e.g., acetazolamide, spironolactone)

*Chronic respiratory acidosis will cause a compensatory decrease in corrected [Cl^-].

†Chronic respiratory alkalosis will cause a compensatory increase in corrected [Cl^-].

(Adapted from de Morais, H.S.A., and Muir, W.W. Strong Ions and Acid-Base Disorders. In: Kirk's Current Veterinary Therapy XII, 12th ed. Edited by J.D. Bonagura and R.W. Kirk. Philadelphia, WB Saunders, 1995:121–127.) (12)

istration of $NaHCO_3$, when needed, will tend to correct hyperchloremic acidosis because this solution has an SID greater than plasma.

Hypochloremic alkalosis can be caused by excessive loss of Cl^- relative to Na^+ or by administration of substances containing more Na^+ than Cl^- compared to ECF (e.g., $NaHCO_3$). The former can occur following the administration of diuretics that cause Cl^- wasting (e.g., furosemide) or when the lost fluid has a low or negative SID, as in the case of vomiting of stomach contents. Chloride administration is essential in the treatment of hypochloremic alkalosis. Renal Cl^- conservation is ordinarily enhanced in hypochloremic states and renal Cl^- ion reabsorption does not return to normal until plasma Cl^- concentration is restored to normal or near normal.(22) In cases where expansion of extracellular volume is desired, intravenous infusion of 0.9% NaCl is the treatment of choice. This solution has an SID of 0 and will decrease plasma SID.(4) If hypokalemia is present, KCl should be added to the fluid (Chapter 19). When volume expansion is not necessary, Cl^- can be administered using salts without Na^+ (e.g., NH_4Cl, KCl, $CaCl_2$, $MgCl_2$). These salts will correct the alkalosis because Cl^- is given together with cations that are regulated within narrow limits for purposes not related to acid-base balance.(4)

Isonatremic organic acid abnormalities. Accumulation of metabolically produced organic anions (e.g., lactate, acetoacetate, citrate, beta-hydroxybutyrate) or addition of exogenous organic anions (e.g., salicylate, glycolate from ethylene glycol poisoning, and formate from methanol poisoning) will cause nonrespiratory acidosis because these strong anions decrease SID. Addition of some inorganic strong anions (e.g., SO_4^{2-} during renal failure) will resemble organic acidosis because these substances decrease SID without changing electrolytes.(1,11) The most frequently encountered causes for organic acidosis are shown in Table 18–13.

Table 18–13. Principal Disorders of the Unidentified Strong Anions in Organic Acidosis ($\Uparrow$ [XA^-])

Disorder	Strong Anions Decreasing SID
Uremic acidosis	SO_4^{2-} and other anions of renal failure
Diabetic ketoacidosis, ketosis, pregnancy toxemia	Acetoacetate, β-hydroxybutyrate
Lactic acidosis	Lactate
Salicylate intoxication	Salicylate
Ethylene glycol toxicity	Glycolate
Methanol toxicity	Formate

[XA^-], unidentified strong anions
(Adapted from de Morais, H.S.A., and Muir, W.W. Strong Ions and Acid-Base Disorders. In: Kirk's Current Veterinary Therapy XII, 12th ed. Edited by J.D. Bonagura and R.W. Kirk. Philadelphia, WB Saunders, 1995:121–127.) (12)

Treatment of organic acidosis should be directed toward the primary disorder and stabilization of the patient.(1) Sodium bicarbonate should be used cautiously because metabolism of accumulated organic anions will normalize SID and increase [HCO_3^-]. The initial goal in patients with severe organic acidosis is to raise systemic pH to 7.2.

Estimation of Strong Anions (XA^-) Concentration

Organic acidoses increase the AG whereas hyperchloremic acidosis does not. The AG is used clinically to estimate the concentration of "unmeasured anions" (UA^-). Unfortunately, UA^- includes the strong (XA^-) and weak (variable charges of albumin and phosphates) unmeasured anions. The AG is therefore influenced by the concentration of plasma proteins, and changes in albumin concentration significantly change AG.(4) Hyperphosphatemia may also increase the AG. The AG will change secondarily to changes in PCO_2, SID, or [A_{tot}].(3) Thus, changes in AG do not always reflect a stoichiometric change in UA^- even in the presence of organic acidosis. Two mathematic models have been developed for estimation of XA^- in human beings.(16, 23) One of these models has been used in evaluating acid-base disorders in veterinary medicine.(10, 11, 24) Both models, however, still need to be validated in domestic animals. The history (e.g., ingestion of ethylene glycol); the clinical condition (e.g., shock); increases in serum creatinine concentration, BUN, or serum glucose; and the presence of ketonuria may help in establishing a diagnosis of organic acidosis. The measurement of plasma lactate concentration may be attempted in patients with suspected lactic acidosis.

Evaluations of Acid-Base Balance

A stepwise approach should be followed in all animals with suspected acid-base disorders.(1) After obtaining the samples, the first step is to determine the pH and the nature of the primary disorder from the blood gas result. The possibility of a mixed respiratory and nonrespiratory acid-base disorder should be assessed by calculating the expected compensation (Table 18–7). If a nonrespiratory acid-base disorder is present, it should be determined if it is caused by a change in [A_{tot}], SID, XA^- or a combination of these factors. Unfortunately, evaluation of changes in SID caused by increases in [XA^-] is not straightforward. An increase in [XA^-] may be suspected in acidotic patients with diseases known to be associated with organic acidosis (e.g., renal failure, diabetic ketoacidosis). Measurement of lactate concentration permits the quantification of one of the many XA^-. When blood gas results are not available, the biochemical profile may help in determining the nonrespiratory abnormalities present (Tables 18–8 and 18–14).(12, 24)

Two quantitative clinical approaches for assessment of nonrespiratory acid-base disturbances have been proposed, one based on the use of BE and the other

Table 18–14. Estimation of Changes in Base Excess Caused by Changes in SID and [A$_{tot}$]

Changes in [A$_{tot}$]:

Changes in albumin concentration

ΔAlbumin (mEq/L) = 3.7 × ([Alb]normal − [Alb]patient)

or if total protein (TP) is used instead of albumin,

ΔTP (mEq/L) = 3.0 × ([TP]normal − [TP]patient)

Changes in phosphate ([Pi] in mmol/L)

([Pi] = Phosphate in mg/dL × 10/30.97)

ΔPhosphate (mEq/L) = (1.6 × [Pi]patient) + (0.2 × [Pi]patient)

Changes in SID:

Changes in free water

ΔFree water (mEq/L) = Z([Na$^+$]patient − [Na$^+$]normal)

Changes in chloride concentration

ΔCl$^-$ (mEq/L) = [Cl$^-$]normal − [Cl$^-$] corrected

Changes in unidentified anions

ΔXA$^-$ (mEq/L) = BE − (Δ Free water + Δ Cl$^-$ + Δ Albumin + Δ Phosphate)

[Alb]normal, = normal albumin concentration; [Alb]patient, = patient albumin concentration is g/dL; [TP]normal, = normal total protein concentration; [TP]patient, = patient total protein concentration in g/dL; [Pi]patient, = patient phosphate concentration in mmol/L; Z, = 0.25 for dogs and cats and 0.3 for horses and cows; [Na$^+$] normal, = normal [Na$^+$]; [Na$^+$]patient, = patient sodium concentration in mEq/L; [Cl$^-$] normal, = normal [Cl$^-$] concentration; [Cl$^-$]corrected, = patient [Cl$^-$] in mEq/L after corrected for changes in free water; XA$^-$, = unidentified strong anions; BE, = patient base excess.

(Adapted from de Morais, H.S.A., and Muir, W.W. Strong Ions and Acid-Base Disorders. In: Kirk's Current Veterinary Therapy XII, 12th ed. Edited by J.D. Bonagura and R.W. Kirk. Philadelphia, WB Saunders, 1995:121–127. [12] Data for horses and cows from Whitechair, K.J., Haskins, S.C. Whitechair, J.G., and Pascoe, P.J. Clinical Applications of Quantitative Acid-Base Chemistry. J Vet Intern Med 9:1–11, 1995. [24])

based on a mathematical relationship to estimate SID. Base excess has been used to assess changes in the nonrespiratory component because *SID* is synonymous with *buffer base*. Base excess is a measurement of the deviation of buffer base (and therefore SID) from normal values. It should be pointed out, however, that Siggaard-Andersen studied blood, not plasma, and protein was not considered an acid-base variable. The BE has been used clinically for decades to assess the nonrespiratory acid-base status in humans.(3, 4) Formulas to estimate changes in base excess due to changes in SID and [A$_{tot}$] are presented in Table 18–14. These formulas are helpful in understanding complex acid-base disorders in domestic animals.(11, 24) Recently, a new mathematical approach has been developed to evaluate nonrespiratory acid-base disorders.(16) The

XA$^-$ obtained using this mathematic model is not constrained by the limitations mentioned earlier for the AG and UA$^-$. Despite being very promising for assessment of nonrespiratory acid-base disorders, this model and the BE model were developed using protein behavior of human albumin. However, calculation of SID$_{eff}$ in this model is not simple and may be clinically impractical.(16)

References

1. Dibartola SP. In: Dibartola SP, ed. Fluid therapy in small animal practice. Philadelphia: WB Saunders, 1992:216–275.
2. Emmet M, Narins RG. Mixed acid-base disorders. In: Maxwell MH, Kleeman CR, Narins RG, eds. Clinical disorders of fluid and electrolyte metabolism. New York: McGraw-Hill, 1987:743–758.
3. Fencl V, Leith DE. Stewart's quantitative acid-base chemistry: applications in biology and medicine. Respir Physiol 91:1, 1993.
4. Fencl V, Rossing TH. Acid-base disorders in critical care medicine. Annu Rev Med 40:17, 1989.
5. Jones NL. Blood gases and acid-base physiology. New York: Thieme Medical Publishers, 1987.
6. Rose BD. Clinical physiology of acid-base and electrolyte disorders, 3rd ed. New York: McGraw-Hill, 1989.
7. Seldin DW, Giebisch G. The regulation of acid-base balance. New York: Raven Press, 1989.
8. Stewart PA. How to understand acid-base. A quantitative acid-base primer for biology and medicine. New York: Elsevier, 1981.
9. Nattie EE. The alphastat hypothesis in respiratory control and acid-base balance. J Appl Physiol 69(4):1201–1207, 1990.
10. de Morais HSA. Chloride ion in small animal practice: the forgotten ion. J Vet Emerg Crit Care 2:11, 1992.
11. de Morais HSA. A Non-traditional approach to acid-base disorders. In: DiBartola SP, ed. Fluid therapy in small animal practice. Philadelphia: WB Saunders, 1992:297.
12. de Morais HSA, Muir WW. Strong ions and acid-base disorders. In: Bonagura JD, Kirk RW, eds. Kirk's current veterinary therapy xii, 12th ed. Philadelphia: WB Saunders, 1995:121–127.
13. Bia M, Thier SO. Mixed acid-base disturbances: a clinical approach. Med Clin North Am 65:347–361, 1981.
14. de Morais HSA, DiBartola SP. Mixed acid-base disorders. Parts I and II. Clinical approach. Compend Contin Educ Pract Vet Part I, 15:1619–1626, 1993; Part II, 16:477–488, 1994.
15. Adams LG, Polzin DJ. Mixed acid-base disorders. Vet Clin North Am Small Anim Pract 19:307–326, 1989.
16. Figge J, Mydosh T, Fencl V. Serum proteins and acid-base equilibria: a follow-up. J Lab Clin Med 120:713, 1992.
17. Narins RG, Emmet M. Simple and mixed acid-base disorders: a practical approach. Medicine 56:38–54, 1980.
18. Gabow PA. Disorders associated with high altered gap. Kidney Int 27:472–483, 1985.
19. Goodkin DA, Krishna GG, Narins RG. The role of the anion gap in detecting and managing mixed metabolic acid-base disorders. Clin Endocrin Metab 13:333–349, 1984.
20. Natelson S. On the significance of the expression "anion-gap." Clin Chem 29:283–284, 1988.
21. Nanji A, Blank D. Spurious increases in the anion gap due to exposure of serum to air. N Engl J Med 307:190, 1982.
22. Galla JH, Gifford JD, Luke RG, Rome L. Adaptations to chloride-depletion alkalosis. Am J Physiol 261:R771, 1991.
23. Leith DE. The new acid-base: power and simplicity. Proc 9th ACVIM Forum, 1991:611–617.
24. Whitehair KJ, Haskins SC, Whitehair JG, Pascoe PJ. Clinical applications of quantitative acid-base chemistry. J Vet Intern Med 9:1–11, 1995.

chapter 19

FLUID AND ELECTROLYTE THERAPY

David C. Seeler

Body Fluid and Electrolyte Composition

At birth, total body water is in excess of 75% of the body weight. Maturational changes result in reductions of total body water content to 60 to 66% of the adult's body weight.(1-5) Lower water content can be anticipated to exist in the obese patient. Total body water is comprised of intracellular and extracellular compartments. The intracellular fluid volume increases slightly with age, and in the mature animal it is equivalent to approximately 40% of body weight. The volume of the extracellular fluid compartment decreases with maturation and accounts for 20% of the weight of the adult animal.(2) The extracellular fluid compartment is further divided into the interstitial, plasma or intravascular, and transcellular fluid compartments. The volume of water in the interstitial compartment accounts for 15% of the mature animal's weight. Plasma water volume constitutes 5% of the body weight and approximately 50% of the total blood volume (Table 19–1). The transcellular fluid compartment consists of joint and CSF fluid in addition to water located within the eye and pleural, peritoneal, and pericardial spaces. Transcellular water volume approximates 1.0 to 3.0% of body weight.

Constituents of the various fluid compartments are listed in Table 19–2. Chemical substances that dissociate in solution to form electrically charged particles or ions are referred to as *electrolytes*. Their concentrations in solution are generally expressed in millimoles per liter (mmol/L) or as milliequivalents per liter (mEq/L). Sodium is the most important extracellular cation, while chloride and bicarbonate are the primary extracellular anions. Together, these ions form more than 90% of the total solute within the extracellular fluid compartment.(6-8) Plasma proteins, which at a vascular pH of 7.4 have a net negative charge, play a key role in the maintenance of intravascular fluid volume (Chapter 18). The primary intracellular ions are potassium, magnesium, and phosphate. Cytoplasmic proteins play a role in the maintenance of intracellular electric neutrality. Despite the fact that the cell membrane is freely permeable to sodium and potassium, the sodium-potassium pump maintains a concentration gradient for each cation across the cell membrane. Thus, sodium salts serve as an osmotic skeleton for the extracellular fluid volume while potassium salts serve the same function intracellularly. In addition to maintaining electric neutrality, ionic concentration differences on either side of the semipermeable cell membrane perform a key role in the normal physiologic function of excitable cells.

Table 19–1. Approximate Vascular Fluid Volumes (mL/kg) in Mature Animals of Domestic Species

Species	Plasma Volume	Total Blood Volume
Bovine	38	57–60
Canine	50	88
Caprine	53	70
Equine		
Thoroughbred	61	100
Other		72
Feline	47	68
Ovine	50	60
Porcine	47	50

Table 19–2. Electrolyte Distribution Across Fluid Compartments (mEq/L)

Ion	Plasma	Interstitial	Intracellular
Na^+	142	145	13
K^+	5	4	155
Ca^{2+}	5	3	2
Mg^{2+}	2	2	35
Cl^-	106	115	2
HCO_3^-	24	30	10
Phosphates	2	2	113
Sulfates	1	1	20
Organic Acids	5	5	0
Protein	16	1	60

Movement of body water throughout and between compartments occurs by osmosis. Osmosis describes the process by which the net movement of water occurs owing to concentration gradients across a semipermeable membrane. The pressure required to prevent water movement across semipermeable membranes is defined as the osmotic pressure. Osmotic pressure is dependent upon the number of nondiffusible, nondifferentiable particles such as ions or molecules in solution and not their mass. In order to express the concentration of these particles in terms of their numbers, a unit called the osmol is used. One osmol is equivalent to one gram mol of nondiffusible and nonionizable substance. Osmolality refers to the osmolal concentration of a solution when the concentration is expressed in osmols per kilogram of water. In contrast, osmolarity refers to the concentration of a solution when expressed in osmols per liter of water. Both terms are often used interchangeably in respect to discussions of fluid balance and therapy. One milliosmol per liter exerts an osmotic pressure of 19.3 mm Hg.

Total body water is determined by the number of osmotically active agents in both compartments.(9) Water distribution across the intracellular and extracellular compartments depends upon osmotic equilibrium between the two compartments. In excess of 80% of the osmolality of the extracellular fluid compartment is determined by sodium and its associated anions.(10) As a result, sodium regulation plays a major role in extracellular fluid osmolality and extracellular fluid volume. The various cardiovascular, renal, and neurohormonal mechanisms that function in an integrated fashion in order to maintain and preserve sodium and water homeostasis are discussed in detail elsewhere (Chapter 5).(11, 12) Fifty percent of the intracellular fluid compartment's osmolality is determined by potassium, while the remainder is exerted by other intracellular constituents. Disturbances in osmolality of either compartment results in a rapid shift in water balance in order that equilibrium between the two compartments is reestablished. For example, increases in extracellular osmolality, owing to either pure water loss or the gain of osmotically active agents, result in water movement from the intracellular compartment into the extracellular fluid space until an osmotic equilibrium is reached. Plasma electrolyte and osmolality values for the various domestic species are listed in Table 19–3.

Within the extracellular fluid space, plasma water communicates directly with water in the interstitial space at the level of the capillary beds. The direction and magnitude of water movement between the interstitial and intravascular spaces are determined by the algebraic sum of hydrostatic and osmotic forces in each compartment as originally described by Starling (Chapter 5).(13, 14) The capillary walls are freely permeable to sodium, chloride, and glucose. As a result, these substances are osmotically inactive across capillary membranes. However, plasma proteins are limited in their ability to cross capillary membranes. Blood or plasma volume is ultimately maintained by the colloid osmotic pressure or plasma oncotic pressure exerted by plasma proteins. Colloid osmotic pressure is approximately 23 mm Hg and results in a plasma osmolarity of 1.5 mOsm/L greater than that found in the interstitial or intracellular fluid spaces.(7) Despite that, the net forces in the capillary beds lead to a net filtration of a small amount of fluid into the interstitial space. This loss is balanced by fluid return to the intravascular space through the lymphatic system.(9, 13)

Alterations in volume or composition of either the extracellular or intracellular fluid compartments are readily assessed if a number of basic principles are followed. It is important to remember that the osmolalities of both compartments are at equilibrium except for a brief period of time (minutes) after a change in one of the compartments occurs. Fluids are defined as isotonic, hypotonic, or hypertonic based on their effect on erythrocyte size or volume. Isotonic solutions exert no volume changes on erythrocytes, while hypotonic solutions increase erythrocyte size and hypertonic solutions decrease erythrocyte size. Administration of isotonic solutions to the intravascular space does not alter the osmolality of the extracellular fluid. As a result, there is no net osmotic effect and only the volume of the extracellular fluid compartment is expanded. Parenteral administration of hypotonic solutions, however, re-

Table 19–3. Fluid and Electrolyte Panel: Normal Values for Chemistry and Hematologic Data at the Atlantic Veterinary College

	Units*	Canine	Feline	Bovine	Equine	Porcine	Ovine
Sodium	mmol/L	144–162	150–160	135–151	135–148	140–150	143–151
Potassium	mmol/L	3.6–6.0	4.0–5.8	3.9–5.9	3.0–5.0	4.7–7.1	4.6–7.0
Chloride	mmol/L	106–126	118–128	96–110	98–110	100–105	102–116
Calcium	mmol/L	2.24–3.04	2.23–2.80	2.11–2.75	2.80–3.44	1.80–2.90	2.30–2.86
Phosphorus	mmol/L	0.82–1.87	1.03–1.92	1.08–2.76	1.00–1.80	1.30–3.55	0.82–2.66
Magnesium	mmol/L	0.70–1.16	0.74–1.12	0.80–1.32	0.74–1.02	0.78–1.60	0.9–1.26
Urea	mmol/L	3.0–10.5	5.0–11.0	3.0–7.5	3.5–7.0	3.0–8.5	2.0–10.0
Creatinine	μmol/L	60–140	90–180	67–175	110–170	90–240	69–105
Glucose	mmol/L	3.3–5.6	3.3–5.6	1.8–3.8	3.6–5.6	3.6–5.3	1.2–3.6
Total protein	g/L	51–72	68–80	66–78	60–77	34–60	61–81
Albumin	g/L	22–38	22–38	23–43	25–36	18–22	27–39
A/G ratio	–	0.60–1.50	0.60–1.50	0.66–1.30	0.60–1.50	0.60–1.50	0.54–1.22
Hemoglobin	g/L	120–180	80–150	80–150	110–190	100–160	80–160
Hematocrit	L/L	0.37–0.55	0.24–0.45	0.24–0.46	0.32–0.52	0.32–0.50	0.24–0.50
RBC	$\times 10^{12}$/L	5.5–8.5	5.0–10.0	5.0–10.0	6.5–12.5	5.0–8.0	8.0–16.0
Reticulocytes	%	0–1.5%	0–1%	0%	0%	0–1%	0%
Platelets	$\times 10^9$/L	200–900	300–700	100–800	100–600	310–510	250–750
Calculated Osmolality	mOsm/Kg	280–320	280–320	274–306	280–320	280–320	283–307
Anion gap	mmol/L	14–26	13–26	14–26	10–25	10–25	12–24

*Factors used to convert SI units to conventional units are located in Table 9–6.

duces extracellular fluid osmolality and results in the osmotic movement of water into the intracellular compartment. Similarly, hypertonic solutions increase the osmolality of extracellular fluids, which results in a fluid shift out of the intracellular compartment.

Second, the number of osmotically active agents in either compartment remains constant unless one of the substances moves from one to the other compartment or is added or lost from either of the compartments. In this instance, sodium or potassium imbalances and acid-base or metabolic disorders can result in compositional changes that impact upon fluid balance between compartments.

Composition of Parenteral Solutions

CRYSTALLOID PREPARATIONS

The term *crystalloid solution* refers to any solution of crystalline solids that are dissolved in water such as sodium-based electrolyte solutions or solutions of dextrose in water. If the electrolyte composition of the prepared solution approximates that of extracellular fluid, then the parenteral fluid is referred to as a *balanced electrolyte solution*. Multiple or balanced electrolyte solutions are formulated based on the concept that the amount of water and electrolytes that a patient retains is dependent upon intact regulatory mechanisms in the body, not on the amount of water and electrolytes received. Commercial preparations are available as inexpensive sterile nonpyrogenic isotonic, hypotonic, or hypertonic solutions. The composition of each solution varies according to its intended purpose.

Parenteral fluids provide water, electrolytes, and in some instances alkalinizing agents or a source of calories, or both. Solutions that are polyelectrolytic have value in maintaining or replenishing electrolytes. Those preparations that contain lactate, acetate, or gluconate produce an alkalinizing effect when the anion is metabolized to carbon dioxide and water.

Maintenance Solutions. Daily water loss includes the insensible loss of water through evaporation from the respiratory system and skin as well as sensible losses in which there is an associated obligatory loss of electrolytes. For many domestic species and birds, the daily maintenance water requirement ranges from 40 to 60 mL · kg^{-1} · day^{-1}.(15-20) The daily requirement for nonlactating dairy cows and lactating cows has been estimated at 29 L/day and 56 L/day respectively.(21) The net daily loss of sodium in small animals ranges from 35 to 50 mmol/L (35 to 50 mEq/L) while daily potassium losses are 20 to 30 mmol/L (20 to 30 mEq/L).(15) Maintenance solutions are designed to meet the water and electrolyte requirements of patients that are not taking in amounts sufficient to meet their daily losses.

In order to meet these specific daily requirements, maintenance solutions have lower sodium and chloride concentrations and an increased potassium concentration when compared to extracellular fluid. If the concentration of potassium in the parenteral solution is less than 20 mmol/L (20 mEq/L), then the maintenance fluid may be supplemented with additional potassium chloride to that level. Hypotonic preparations or solutions that contain dextrose provide free water. Isotonic salt solutions provide osmolar water, not free water. In the case of solutions containing dextrose, free water is not available until the dextrose has been metabolized. Maintenance fluids are generally administered over a 24-hour period. These solutions should not be used in situations where large volumes might be infused rapidly. This could result in significant electrolyte abnormalities in the extracellular fluid of the patient caused by the electrolyte composition of maintenance solutions.

Replacement Solutions. The composition of isotonic, balanced electrolyte solutions such as Lactated Ringer's USP closely approximates that of extracellular fluid. These solutions may be administered rapidly, in large volumes, in order to reexpand the extracellular fluid volume without inducing changes in its electrolytic composition. Because they are isotonic, their use does not induce fluid shifts between the intracellular and extracellular compartments, yet balanced electrolyte solutions will rapidly equilibrate across the intravascular and interstitial fluid compartments. As a result, only 25% of the administered volume remains within the intravascular space. This must be considered when using replacement fluids to replenish intravascular losses. It is necessary to administer a volume equivalent to at least three times the volume of blood lost in order to replace the vascular deficit. Many of the preparations that are presently available contain lactate, acetate, or gluconate, which serve as alkalinizing agents. Acid-base considerations in acute patient care situations are discussed in Chapters 18 and 24.

Replacement solutions are commonly utilized as maintenance fluids. In this situation, normal renal function should be present in order to ensure that electrolytes in excess of daily requirements are eliminated. Long-term management of a patient's maintenance requirements with a replacement solution may result in hypokalemia. In this instance, replacement solutions should be supplemented with potassium chloride to provide a final potassium concentration of 20 mmol/L (20 mEq/L). Replacement fluids that have been supplemented with potassium chloride should not be used in clinical situations where large volumes may be infused rapidly.

Other Parenteral Solutions. **Isotonic and Hypotonic Saline.** Isotonic saline is prepared as a 0.9% solution that contains 154 mmol/L (154 mEq/L) each of sodium and chloride ions and has an osmolarity of 308 mOsm/L. Isotonic saline is often referred to as *normal* or *physiologic saline.* However, only the sodium ion concentration of the preparation matches that of extracellular fluid. The use of 0.9% sodium chloride solutions has been advocated for maintenance and replacement purposes. Isotonic saline does not meet the patient's free water and electrolyte needs for maintenance purposes. Isotonic saline is used for rapid expansion of the extracellular fluid volume. Similar to other crystalloid solutions, intravenously administered saline solutions rapidly distribute throughout the extracellular fluid space.

However, their composition does not match that of extracellular fluid, and excessive use of isotonic saline for replacement purposes could result in the unnecessary dilution of other extracellular electrolytes and buffers. Isotonic saline may also be used for the correction of hyponatremia or nonrespiratory alkalemia.

Hypotonic saline solutions are available in a number of strengths. Commercial preparations of 0.45% saline are hypotonic (osmolarity of 154 mOsm/L) and may be used as a hydrating solution. Hypotonic saline preparations may be used for maintenance purposes, particularly when they are supplemented with dextrose and potassium chloride. When 2.5% dextrose is added to 0.45% saline the resultant solution is isotonic. Upon metabolism of the dextrose, free water is made available for distribution across all compartments.

Hypertonic Saline. Traditionally, solutions of 3 and 5% saline have been used in the treatment of patients with severe hyponatremia where rapid sodium replacement is considered necessary. More recently, hypertonic saline solutions have been used with success in the management of severe shock, particularly hemorrhagic shock.(22-27) The infusion of small volumes of hypertonic saline enables the clinician to treat critically ill or moribund patients rapidly. Hypertonic saline solutions of 7.5%, although not commercially available, are commonly utilized for this purpose. The osmolarity of 7.5% saline is 2400 mOsm/L. In order to prepare 7.5% saline it is necessary to purchase 5% saline in 500-mL bags and 23.4% saline in 30 mL bottles (American Reagent Labs, Shirley, New York; Lyphomed Canada Inc., Markham, Ontario). Remove 120 mL of 5% saline from the 500-mL bag and inject 60 mL of the 23.4% saline solution into the bag to make a 7.5% solution.(22)

The administration of 4 to 6 mL/kg of 7.5% saline results in the rapid restoration of hemodynamic parameters with subsequent improvements in tissue perfusion.(15, 23, 28, 29) One study suggests that in dogs, an infusion rate of $2 \text{ mL} \cdot \text{kg}^{-1} \cdot \text{min}^{-1}$ should be used in order to reduce the possibility of inducing an acute hypotension.(30) In conscious horses, 5 mL/kg of 7.5% saline was infused at rates of 80 mL/min and no adverse effects were noted.(31) Since relatively small volumes are infused, the clinician need not worry about fluid overload or the development of interstitial edema in the patient. However, hypertonic saline solutions should not be used in situations where hemorrhage is not controlled or if the patient is hypernatremic or significantly dehydrated.(22, 32, 33)

The mechanisms by which hypertonic saline exerts its physiologic effects are subject to debate.(28, 34, 35) Overall changes include improved cardiac output and aortic blood pressure, reduced peripheral vascular resistance, an increase in plasma volume with hemodilution, and an increase in interstitial fluid volume. These overall improvements in cardiovascular function and tissue perfusion are the result of direct and indirect effects of the hypertonic saline solution.(16, 25, 26, 30, 32, 34, 35) Upon administration, hypertonic saline equilibrates rapidly throughout the extracellular fluid space. Because of the increase in extracellular fluid osmolality caused by the hypertonic solution, water moves out of the intracellular fluid compartment. As a result, the extracellular fluid compartment volume is expanded. Solutions of 7.5% saline, when infused intravenously into dogs, increase plasma volume 2 to 4 mL for each mL of solution administered.(30) Maximum vascular volume expansion occurs within 30 minutes of the administration of the hypertonic saline solution. These fluid shifts result in an intracellular water debt and an eventual decrease in total body water because of obligatory water loss in association with natriuresis.(34, 36, 37)

To maximize the beneficial effects of hypertonic saline it is advisable to administer the solution intravenously. This is to ensure that the maximum possible concentration of the solution passes through the pulmonary circulation.(25, 34) It has been postulated that the sodium administered in hypertonic solution stimulates pulmonary osmoreceptors or chemoreceptors and activates a pulmonary vagal reflex. Subsequent to this, it is suggested that there is selective activation of sympathetic pathways to the vascular system.(35) This activity may result in venoconstriction of capacitance vessels leading to increased cardiac filling pressures and selective precapillary vasoconstriction in skin and muscle, which redistributes blood volume within the vascular space. These proposed mechanisms are subject to debate.(28, 30, 37) Vasodilation occurs in some vascular beds because of the direct hyperosmotic effect of the solution. This reduces total peripheral resistance and enhances perfusion of vital organs.(25, 30, 35)

Concern has been expressed that the hemodynamic effects of 7.5% hypertonic saline are not sustained.(23, 25, 32, 36, 37) The duration of effect in cats was found to be approximately 60 minutes or less in one study, while another study found improved hemodynamic function over a period of at least 180 minutes.(38) This concern has led to a number of studies that examined the feasibility of prolonging the beneficial effects of hypertonic saline by adding hyperoncotic preparations such as dextran 70 to the mixture.(34, 36, 37, 39-45) Regardless of the eventual outcome of these and similar studies, it is advisable to use hypertonic saline solutions in the initial resuscitative management of the moribund patient and to follow up with more traditional therapeutic measures.

Dextrose Solutions. Dextrose solutions are commercially available in a wide range of concentrations ranging from 2.5 to 50% dextrose in water. Five percent dextrose in water contains 50 grams dextrose monohydrate per liter of water and exerts an osmolarity of 252 mOsm/L. Dextrose solutions provide a source of free water for total body distribution once the carbohydrate is metabolized. An additional 0.6 mL of water is made available for each gram of dextrose that is metabolized. Because the volume of water administered distributes across all fluid compartments, dextrose solutions are not

effective for use as plasma volume expanders. However, they are effective in replenishing primary total body water deficits (e.g., dehydration).

Five percent dextrose solutions contain 171 Calories per liter, which is not capable of meeting the energy requirements of domestic animal species. Hypertonic dextrose solutions are generally utilized for the purpose of caloric supplementation of parenteral maintenance fluids.(46) Long-term infusions of 5% dextrose or the infusion of hypertonic dextrose solutions may result in the development of thrombophlebitis. Care should be taken to ensure that hypertonic preparations in particular are infused via the caudal or cranial vena cava.(46) The administration rate of dextrose solutions should be carefully regulated in order that the glucose concentration in the glomerular filtrate does not exceed the capacity of the renal tubules to reabsorb the carbohydrate, resulting in a glucose-induced osmotic diuresis.

Alkalinizing Agents. **Sodium Bicarbonate.** Sodium bicarbonate solution is a preparation of sodium bicarbonate ($NaHCO_3$) in sterile water for injection. Solutions contain 5.0%, 7.5% and 8.4% sodium bicarbonate in 50-mL ampules or vials and 500-mL bottles. Sodium bicarbonate solution is administered intravenously, either in another parenteral solution or undiluted in emergencies. An isotonic solution results when a 50-mL vial of 7.5% sodium bicarbonate is added to 200 mL of water for injection; with a 50-mL vial of 8.5% solution, 224 mL of sterile water are required.

Sodium bicarbonate is indicated in the treatment of metabolic acidosis. Sodium bicarbonate is also indicated in barbiturate intoxication to facilitate dissociation of barbiturate-protein complex. Overcorrection of the bicarbonate deficit produces metabolic alkalosis with a rise in blood pH. From a clinical standpoint, alkalosis is seldom encountered. However, administration of sodium bicarbonate is generally contraindicated in patients losing chloride through vomiting or in those with hypokalemia. Because sodium bicarbonate produces sodium retention, it should be used with caution in patients with congestive heart failure or other conditions causing edema.

The dose of sodium bicarbonate is determined by the base deficit of blood and the clinical symptoms of the patient. Quantitative estimation of the bicarbonate dose may be calculated from the formula: Base deficit $\times$ 0.3 $\times$ body weight (kg) = mEq of $NaHCO_3$(Chapter 18). The factor 0.3 $\times$ body weight is an approximation of the acute volume of distribution of infused HCO_3^- and approximates the volume of the extracellular fluid compartment. Distribution to interstitial fluid requires approximately 30 minutes to be 98% complete. Although the factor 0.6 has been utilized in the formula, the use of 0.6 $\times$ body weight assumes that the volume of HCO_3^- distribution is total body water. About 18 hours are required for completion. When the 0.6 factor is used, the dose of HCO_3^- may be too high and, if given, must be administered slowly. The amount of

HCO_3^- needed to correct base deficit in metabolic acidosis varies widely depending upon the cause of the acidosis and variations in distribution of HCO_3^- into intracellular spaces. Overtreatment should be avoided. Acid-base measurements should be made frequently, since changes with anesthesia and disease processes are dynamic. Usually half the calculated dose is administered and a second base deficit determination made. Should alkalosis result from sodium bicarbonate administration, the use of bicarbonate should be discontinued, and the patient should be treated according to the degree of alkalosis. Sodium chloride injection (0.9%) intravenously is usually sufficient to correct plasma chloride. If the alkalosis is severe enough to be accompanied by hyperirritability or tetany, intravenous ammonium chloride (NH_4Cl) may be given as a 1/6 molar solution (167 mEq/L). Calcium gluconate may also be useful in controlling tetany.

To correct for the acidity inherent in ACD-preserved blood, the contents of 1 ampule added to 250 mL of sterile water for injection may be given for every 2 units (1000 mL) of blood administered.

Intravenous sodium bicarbonate administration leads to increased CO_2 levels in blood and cerebrospinal fluid (CSF). Because plasma HCO_3^- enters the CSF slowly, a paradoxical acidosis in the brain may result. General depression of the central nervous system, including the medullary centers, may develop, reducing respiratory drive. Adequate ventilation of the patient is thus mandatory to prevent these adverse side effects.

Hypertonic sodium bicarbonate (7.5% = 1500 mOsm/L) has been shown to cause hyperosmolality of blood when given in large quantities for acute cardiac resuscitation. Experimental and clinical observations indicate that increases in plasma osmolality to levels exceeding 350 mOsm are potentially fatal. Detrimental effects of alkalemia include an increase in the affinity of hemoglobin for oxygen and an unfavorable effect on oxygen release. Routine measurement of plasma osmolality, in addition to acid-base determinations, is recommended prior to administration of additional doses of alkali. Another detrimental effect is prolongation of thrombin clotting and prothrombin times.

Tromethamine (THAM). Tromethamine (Fig. 19–1) is an organic amine buffer used for correction of severe systemic acidosis, such as that which occurs during shock, cardiac operations with extracorporeal circulation, cardiac arrest, and massive transfusions of ACD blood. Given intravenously, it acts as an amine proton acceptor, attracting hydrogen ions to form salts that are then excreted by the kidneys. There is no increase in CO_2 levels when tromethamine is administered.

Tromethamine also acts as an osmotic diuretic, increasing urine flow, urine pH, excretion of electrolytes, fixed acids, and carbon dioxide. Approximately 30% of tromethamine at a pH of 7.4 is not ionized and is capable of penetrating cells to combine with intracellular acid ions. About 70% is ionized and is effective in the extracellular fluid.

Tromethamine is contraindicated in anuria and uremia. Large doses may depress respiration owing to pH change and CO_2 reduction with subsequent increase in blood lactate. Rapid infusion may produce ECG changes similar to those of hyperkalemia. Hypoglycemia may also occur. For these reasons, blood pH, P_{CO_2}, bicarbonate, glucose, and electrolyte determinations should be performed during administration of large quantities of this drug. The coagulation time is increased in dogs.

Tromethamine is supplied in 500-mL bottles containing 18 g (150 mEq) of tromethamine and approximately 3 g (50 mEq) of acetic acid. The pH of the formulation is approximately 8.6. The approximate intravenous dose may be estimated from the buffer base deficit.

Tromethamine (ml, of 0.3 M) required
= body weight (kg) × base deficit (mEq/L) × 1.1.

In treatment of cardiac arrest, tromethamine solution should be given at the same time that other standard resuscitative measures, including cardiac massage, are being applied. Doses ranging from approximately 3.5 to 6.0 mL/kg have been administered intravenously. Additional amounts may be required to control the systemic acidosis which persists after the cardiac arrest is reversed. The intravenous lethal dose of tromethamine in the dog is 500 mg/kg when given at $50 \ mg \cdot kg^{-1} \cdot min.^{-1}$

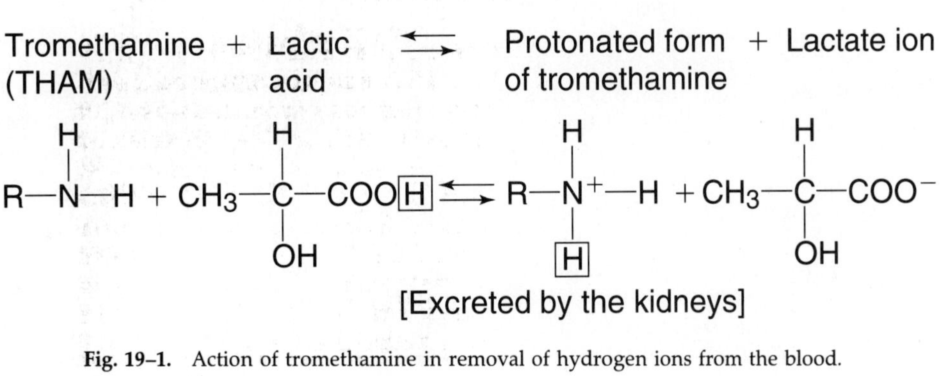

Fig. 19–1. Action of tromethamine in removal of hydrogen ions from the blood.

COLLOID PREPARATIONS

Solutions that are in effect a suspension of large molecular weight particles are termed colloids. If the average molecular weight of the particles in solution exceeds 50,000, they will tend to remain within the vascular compartment. This results in an increase in intravascular colloid osmotic pressure, which not only limits further water movement out of the intravascular space but may also result in water movement from the interstitial to intravascular space. Because of these properties, colloid preparations are effective when used for vascular volume expansion. Colloids are also used in acute hypoproteinemic states where plasma albumin levels are less than 15 g/L (1.5 g/dL) or total serum protein levels are less than 35 g/L (3.5 g/dL) in order to ensure that an effective vascular volume is maintained.

Natural colloids include plasma, albumin preparations, and whole blood. Artificial colloids include dextran, gelatin preparations, and hydroxyethyl starch. The effectiveness of the artificial colloids is determined by their physiochemical characteristics such as average molecular weight, colloid content, and biodegradability. Artificial colloids exert a vascular effect similar to that of plasma. They are more expensive than plasma, but under certain circumstances, such as during intraoperative procedures in large animals, they may be more readily available.

Plasma. Plasma proteins play a predominant role in establishing plasma oncotic pressure, which is ultimately responsible for maintaining vascular volume at the level of the capillary beds. The albumin fraction of total serum protein ranges from 35 to 50% (Table 19–3), and albumin accounts for 75% of the plasma oncotic pressure exerted by plasma proteins. Reductions in serum albumin levels to 15 g/L (1.5 g/dL) or total serum protein levels to 35 g/L (3.5 g/dL) or lower results in a net water loss from the vascular compartment to the interstitial space. If untreated, vascular volume diminishes and interstitial edema occurs.

Plasma is harvested from whole blood and either used as fresh plasma for the treatment of coagulopathies or stored at −70° C as fresh frozen plasma.(47) Each gram of albumin will retain approximately 17 to 18 mL of water within the vascular space. In the perioperative period, plasma is commonly utilized to treat vascular volume deficits or hypoproteinemia. Plasma must be gradually warmed to 37° C prior to being administered. Plasma should not be thawed using temperatures in excess of 37° C. A blood administration set with an in-line filter is used when plasma is infused intravenously. It has been recommended that for dogs, the recipient should receive 28 to 33 mL/kg of plasma in order to administer one gram per kilogram of albumin when the protein concentration of plasma of the donor is 30 to 35 g/L.(47) Alternatively, one may estimate the total protein deficit by multiplying the plasma protein deficit by the estimated plasma volume of the patient. Care should be taken to ensure that there are no allergic reactions to the transfusion and that the patient is not volume overloaded.

Whole blood. Patients who are severely anemic or who have had a significant decrease in their pack cell volume from normal (Table 19–3) are candidates for whole blood transfusion or the administration of packed red cells if plasma protein levels are normal. Acute blood loss in the perioperative period in excess of 10 to 15% of the patient's blood volume should be replaced with whole blood. Chronic reductions in the hematocrit to 15% in the healthy nonexercising animal does not necessarily result in clinical signs of oxygen debt. However, when one considers the cardiopulmonary effects of most anesthetic agents, it is advisable to maintain a hematocrit of at least 25% in the surgical patient.(48) This helps ensure that there is adequate oxygen delivery to the peripheral tissues in the perioperative period where excitement may occur.(49, 50)

Whole blood is collected from donors in an anticoagulant such as acid citrate dextrose (ACD), citrate phosphate dextrose (CPD), citrate phosphate dextrose adenine (CPAA-1), sodium citrate, or heparin. Once blood has been collected, plasma may be harvested and stored separately if desired. Whole blood and packed red cells are stored at 1 to 6° C.(51) Details in regard to the collection and storage of whole blood or blood components may be obtained elsewhere.(51-56)

The duration of storage that is considered acceptable in terms of red cell viability is dependent upon the anticoagulant used and the use of appropriate storage procedures.(52) Transfused red cell viability of previously stored blood 24 hours after the transfusion should exceed 70%. Nonviable transfused red cells are removed from circulation within 24 hours. Whole blood or packed cells that are properly stored in ACD may be used up to 21 days after collection, while CPD and CPAA-1 maintains adequate red cell viability for up to 30 and 35 days respectively. Storage of red blood cells results in dramatic reductions in 2,3-DPG, which shifts the oxygen hemoglobin dissociation curve to the left.(52) Left shifts of the oxygen hemoglobin dissociation curve decreases oxygen availability to the peripheral tissues. In man, 2,3-DPG returns to 50% of normal levels within 24 hours of transfusion. If oxygen delivery to peripheral tissues is of significant concern to the clinician in the perioperative period, then consideration should be given to utilizing freshly collected blood or blood that has been stored for a minimum period of time in CPD or CPAA-1.

The number and type of clinically significant blood groups with respect to transfusion reactions varies among the domestic animal species (Table 19–4). Normal red blood cell viability or circulation half-life also varies significantly among the various species (Table 19–5). Where possible, all donors should be typed and all potential transfusion recipients should be typed and crossmatched with the donor.(47, 55, 57) Canine blood donors should be DEA 1.1, 1.2, and 7 negative.(54) In cats there are significant variations between breeds as to the predominant blood group, and naturally occurring isoagglutinins exist.(57, 58) As a result, it has been recommended that all feline donors and recipients be

Table 19–4. Major Blood Groups of Domestic Animal Species

Species	Number of Major Groups	Clinically Significant Groups
Bovine	12	B, J
Canine	7	DEA 1.1, 1.2, 7
Caprine	5	?
Equine	9	A, C, Q
Feline	2	A, B
Ovine	7	B, R
Porcine	16	?

Table 19–5. Red Blood Cell Survival Times

Species	Days
Bovine	140–160
Canine	110–120
Caprine	125
Equine	140–150
Feline	75–80
Ovine	64–94
Porcine	75–95

typed, donors of each blood group be available, and a crossmatch be performed on the first transfusion.(57)

If donors are not typed, as is often the case, then a crossmatch should be carried out on fresh blood collected from the donor and recipient. This procedure enables the clinician to determine if the recipient has been previously sensitized or if the recipient has naturally occurring isoantibodies to the donor's red blood cells. A minor crossmatch would indicate if the donor has antibodies against the recipient's red blood cells. It should be noted that the crossmatch procedures test only for isoagglutinins. In cattle and horses isohemolysins play a major role in transfusion reactions.(56, 59, 60) As a result, the crossmatch procedure in these species may not provide an adequate indication of the potential for a transfusion reaction and alternative tests may be necessary.

Whole blood and packed red cells, like plasma, must be rewarmed slowly to 37° C prior to being transfused into the patient. Temperatures in excess of 37° C should not be used to rewarm whole blood or blood products. Infusion warmers (Figure 19–2) may be utilized to maintain blood or blood products at that temperature. Packed red cells may be diluted with 0.9% saline in order to facilitate the transfusion process by reducing the viscosity of the suspension. Under no circumstances should rewarmed whole blood, or red cells, be rerefrigerated if unused. Intravenous administration sets used for transfusion purposes should contain inline filters with a pore size of 80 microns so that cellular debris and blood clots are not transfused into the patient. In cats, where blood is often collected into a syringe, syringe filters (Hemo-nate Filter, Gesco International, San Antonio, Texas) may be used to accomplish the same

purpose. All blood transfusions should be administered through a separate intravenous access and other therapeutic agents should not be administered to the patient via the blood administration set.

The volume of blood to be administered may be set empirically at 10 to 40 mL/kg in dogs and 5 to 20 mL/kg in cats or calculated.(61) In species where the blood volume approximates 7% of total body weight, the following formulas may be utilized to calculate the required volume of whole blood or packed red cells for transfusion purposes. If the hematocrit of the donor's blood is 40%, then administration of 17.5 mL/kg will raise the recipient's hematocrit by 1%. Similarly, if the hematocrit of the packed cell solution is 70%, then administration of 1.0 mL/kg will raise the recipient's hematocrit by 1%.(62) Alternatively, in small animals the following formulas may be used: (47, 63)

For cats:

$$\text{mL of blood required} = BW_{kg} \times 70 \left[\frac{\left(\begin{array}{c} \text{Desired PCV} \\ - \text{Patient PCV} \end{array} \right)}{\text{Donor PCV}} \right]$$

For dogs:

$$\text{mL of blood required} = BW_{kg} \times 90 \left[\frac{\left(\begin{array}{c} \text{Desired PCV} \\ - \text{Patient PCV} \end{array} \right)}{\text{Donor PCV}} \right]$$

Whole blood or suspensions of packed red cells may be administered at rates of 5 to 10 mL per hour. In critical situations, where rapid restoration of blood volume is of concern, administration rates of 22 $mL \cdot kg^{-1} \cdot h^{-1}$ in small animals and rates of 20 to 40 $mL \cdot kg^{-1} \cdot h^{-1}$ in large animals have been suggested.(56) The patient must be continuously monitored for clinical signs that suggest that there is an

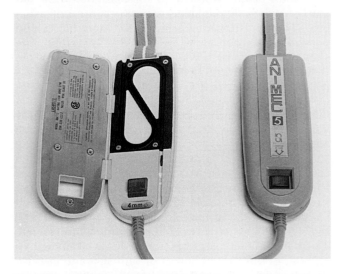

Fig. 19–2. Infusion warmers are available in two sizes, which can accommodate intravenous fluid or blood administration sets. Their use is indicated when infusing solutions that have been refrigerated or stored at temperatures below 37° C.

adverse reaction by the patient to the transfusion. Adverse reactions may occur owing to prior bacterial contamination of the donor's blood, allergic or immunologic reactions to the transfusion itself, circulatory overload, or citrate-induced hypocalcemia. The nature of the observed clinical signs of transfusion reaction varies. In some species, hemolysis as opposed to agglutination occurs. Clinical signs may include tachycardia, dysrhythmias, hypotension, tachypnea, dyspnea, tremors, emesis, wheals, urticaria, transient fever, hemoglobinemia, and hemoglobinuria.(53, 55-57, 63) It is important to remember that a number of these clinical signs may not occur in the anesthetized patient. Therefore, any unexpected changes in the clinical status of an anesthetized patient that is receiving a transfusion must be critically evaluated. If a transfusion reaction is suspected, then the transfusion must be terminated and supportive therapy instituted. Sepsis, circulatory overload, and hypocalcemia are detected by careful monitoring of the anesthetized patient and treated accordingly.

Dextran. Dextrans are low to average molecular weight polysaccharides that are produced as a result of bacterial enzymatic action on sucrose. Dextran 40 is a low molecular weight polysaccharide with an average molecular weight of 40,000 and a molecular weight range of 10,000 to 70,000. Dextran 70 and Dextran 75 consist of glucose polymers with an average molecular weight of 70,000 and 75,000 respectively. Both preparations have a molecular weight range of 20,000 to 200,000, and as a result their clinical effects are similar. Polymers with a molecular weight less than 50,000 are eliminated from the circulation by glomerular filtration and renal excretion. Polysaccharides with a molecular weight in excess of 50,000 are eventually stored in the reticuloendothelial system and subsequently metabolized.

Dextran solutions are used for plasma volume expansion when hematogenous products are not available. They are not a substitute for whole blood and possess no oxygen carrying capacity. Therefore, care should be exercised when dextran is used in the treatment of severe hemorrhage in order that the patient's hematocrit not be reduced to critical levels. Dextran may be used in situations where hypoproteinemia has been induced by the infusion of a large volume of a crystalloid solution and plasma is not available.

Dextran 70 and 75 are slightly hyperoncotic when compared to plasma. As a result, they induce a water shift from the interstitial fluid space into the vascular system of approximately 20 to 25 mL/g. Dextran 70 and 75 increase the plasma volume by an amount that is slightly in excess of the colloidal volume administered. The maximum increase in plasma volume occurs within an hour of the termination of the infusion and lasts for up to 6 hours. The duration of effect is dependent upon the volume infused and rate of clearance from the vascular system.

Dextran 40 is used for vascular volume expansion. The 10% solution is significantly hyperoncotic when compared to plasma. For this reason, dextran 40 should be administered with an equal volume of a crystalloid solution in order to minimize fluid shifts from the interstitial space. The improvement in vascular volume that results from the administration of dextran 40 is equivalent to twice that of the volume infused. The peak volume effect occurs quickly but is short in duration, lasting only 2 to 3 hours. Fifty percent of the administered dose of dextran 40 is excreted within 3 hours, and 75% is excreted within 24 hours. Low molecular weight dextran has been advocated for the treatment of impaired microcirculation or capillary sludging during low-flow states induced by hypovolemia or shock. The ability of dextran 40 to enhance blood flow in the microcirculation is attributed to (a) volume expansion and subsequent hemodilution, (b) maintenance of red cell electronegativity, (c) coating of red blood cells and platelets, (d) decreased blood fibrinogen levels, (e) subsequent reductions in blood viscosity, and (f) an increased suspension stability of blood.

The primary concerns with respect to the use of dextran solutions relates to the potential for allergic reactions or interference with the normal hemostatic mechanisms of blood. The recommended dose for dextran 40, 70, or 75 is 10 mL to 20 mL $\cdot$ kg^{-1} $\cdot$ day^{-1} in order to reduce the possibility of an adverse reaction in the patient. Infusion rates of 5 mL $\cdot$ kg^{-1} $\cdot$ h^{-1} may be utilized in noncritical situations. However, rates of up to 20 mL $\cdot$ kg^{-1} $\cdot$ h^{-1} have been recommended in situations where the vascular volume must be restored quickly.(64) This rate of infusion induced minimal hemostatic abnormalities in clinically normal animals, but the authors caution that bleeding may be precipitated in dogs with deficiencies in hemostatic function.(64)

Hydroxyethyl Starch. Hydroxyethyl starch or hetastarch is a synthetic polymer that is synthesized from a waxy starch composed primarily of amylopectin. Hydroxyethyl ether groups are introduced into the glucose units of the starch in order to retard degradation of the compound by serum amylase. Commercially available preparations are sterile, nonpyrogenic solutions of 6% hetastarch in 0.9% saline. The oncotic pressure of the solution is 30 mm Hg, and it has an osmolarity of 310 mOsm/L. The average molecular weight of hetastarch is 69,000, and the molecular weight of the polymers ranges from 10,000 to 1,000,000. The smaller particles are eliminated through glomerular filtration and renal excretion. Approximately 40% of the hetastarch is excreted in urine within 24 hours in patients with normal renal function.(65) The larger molecules are slowly degraded by serum amylase until they are small enough to be excreted or taken up into the reticuloendothelial system. This results in a sustained ability of hetastarch to maintain vascular volume expansion as compared to dextran preparations.

Hetastarch may be used for the same purposes as dextran solutions. The colloidal properties of hetastarch are similar to that of albumin. One gram of hetastarch results in a fluid shift into the vascular space of approximately 14 mL of water from the interstitial space.(65) The infusion of hetastarch results in a plasma volume expansion only slightly in excess of the volume infused. The volume expansion effect lasts from 3 to 24 hours. Hetastarch should not be used in normovolemic patients due to the potential for volume overload. Other complications associated with the infusion of hetastarch solutions include anaphylactoid reactions and coagulopathies.(15, 65) A dose of 10 to 20 mL $\cdot$ kg^{-1} $\cdot$ day^{-1} of 6% hetastarch has been recommended for administration to dogs.(15)

Considerations For Fluid Therapy

Perioperative recognition and management of fluid and electrolyte disturbances are important components of the anesthetic management of the surgical patient. Patients that are presented for anesthesia and surgical or diagnostic procedures vary in size, age, metabolic requirements, and physical condition in addition to the nature of the ongoing disease process (Chapter 2). The anesthesiologist must consider each patient's current fluid and electrolyte status in addition to changes that are anticipated to occur during the immediate perioperative period.

In all but the most critical of emergencies, clinically significant fluid and electrolyte imbalances in the patient should be identified, assessed, and corrected prior to the induction of anesthesia. Many anesthetic protocols require that patients be kept off food and water for varying periods of time preoperatively. The use of NPO orders results in varying degrees of total body water deficits that should be taken into account by the anesthesiologist during the anesthetic procedure. Furthermore, anesthetic agents and many surgical procedures have a significant effect upon the cardiovascular stability of the patient. There is a net loss of vascular volume during the surgical procedure caused by hemorrhage, redistribution and sequestration of fluids into traumatized tissues at the surgical site, and increased losses owing to evaporation from the surgical site as well as from the respiratory system. Postoperatively, fluid and electrolyte imbalances may continue to occur, requiring that the patient be continuously assessed and treated.

PREOPERATIVE CONSIDERATIONS

A thorough history should be obtained from the owner. This should provide the clinician with information relating to the type, volume, and duration of fluid losses that have been experienced by the patient. This information, in conjunction with a detailed physical examination, should enable the clinician to assess the degree of dehydration and the type of electrolyte disturbance that might exist in the patient. The degree of dehydration can be estimated by assessing the patient's skin turgor and correlating that information with the other clinical findings. Age, nutritional status of the animal, and individual variations make assessment of skin turgor difficult. In small animals, skin turgor is tested by pinching a skin fold over the torso and twisting it while the animal is in lateral recumbency. Skin turgor is tested in large animals by pinching and twisting the skin of the upper eyelid or neck. Skin turgor can also be used to determine the hydration status of avian patients.(66) Total body water deficit in liters is calculated in terms of percentage of body weight measured in kilograms. A patient that is estimated to be 10% dehydrated has lost a volume of water in liters equivalent to 10% of the animal's weight.

Patients with a history of water loss but that have no obvious clinical signs associated with dehydration are assumed to be less than 5% dehydrated. The skin tent persists for less than 2 seconds in these animals. An animal is assumed to be 6 to 8% dehydrated if on clinical examination the eyes are mildly sunken in their orbits, the mucous membranes are sticky to dry, and the skin tent persists for more than three seconds. Clinical signs are very pronounced when the animal is 10 to 12% dehydrated. The eyes will be deeply sunken into the orbits, with as much as a 2- to 4-mm gap between the eyeball and bony orbit. The mucous membranes are dry and possibly cold to the touch. The skin tent and twist will persist indefinitely. Animals that are dehydrated in excess of 15% are often moribund.

The initial clinical assessment is confirmed by collecting baseline samples from the patient for laboratory analysis. This data provides a confirmation of the diagnosis and a reference point for subsequent therapeutic measures. The information also ensures that the clinician is later able to assess the patient's response to therapy. Analysis of whole blood, plasma, and serum samples enables the clinician to determine hematologic values, plasma osmolality, serum electrolyte concentrations, and serum glucose, urea or creatinine values. The measured parameters are then evaluated in relation to the patient's current condition and to expected normal values of each (Table 19–3). Table 19–6 lists the conversion factors required to convert from SI to conventional units.

Hematocrit and total protein values are commonly utilized to determine the degree of hemoconcentration or hemodilution that exists in the patient. Total protein levels may represent a more effective index of plasma volume variations than packed cell volume. Normally, hematocrit values vary widely in some species, while in others the spleen plays a major role in altering packed cell volume.(20, 67) The hematocrit should not be permitted to decrease below 20 to 25% in the anesthesia candidate. Normovolemic reductions in packed cell volume to 20% in dogs results in a reduced capacity of blood to deliver oxygen to peripheral tissues.(48, 50, 68) Stable surgical patients will tolerate normovolemic reductions in hematocrit to 25% if cardiac output is maintained and arterial oxygenation is ensured in the

Table 19–6. Conversion of System International Units to Conventional Units

Constituent	SI Unit	×	Factor	=	Conventional Unit
Sodium	mmol/L		1		mEq/L
Potassium	mmol/L		1		mEq/L
Chloride	mmol/L		1		mEq/L
Calcium	mmol/L		4.0080		mg/dL
Magnesium	mmol/L		2.4307		mg/dL
Phosphorus	mmol/L		3.0969		mg/dL
Creatinine	μmol/L		0.0113		mg/dL
Glucose	mmol/L		18.0148		mg/dL
Urea nitrogen	mmol/L		2.8011		mg/dL
Hematocrit	L/L		100		mL/dL, %
Hemoglobin	g/L		0.1		g/dL
Protein	g/L		0.1		g/dL
Albumin	g/L		0.1		g/dL

perioperative period. Further reductions in hematocrit increases the potential for inadequate oxygen delivery to peripheral tissues of the anesthetized patient. This is of particular importance to the patient with hemodynamic instability. Polycythemia, on the other hand, increases blood viscosity and reduces capillary flow, which can result in a reduced oxygen delivery capacity of blood with respect to peripheral tissues.(50) Patients, particularly large animal patients, with packed cell volumes in excess of 50% should be treated with fluids in order that the hematocrit is restored to more normal levels.(67)

Serum protein levels should be maintained above 35 g/L (3.5 g/dL) and albumin levels above 15 g/L (1.5 g/dL) in order to ensure that interstitial edema does not develop. It has been recommended that in large animals, fluid therapy is indicated if total serum protein exceeds 80 to 100 g/L (8.0 to 10 mg/dL).(67)

Measurement of serum electrolytes enables the clinician to calculate or measure plasma osmolality and determine if there are significant life-threatening compositional changes within the extracellular fluid. Plasma osmolality may be calculated as follows:

SI Units:

$$\text{mOsm/L} = 1.86\,(Na^+ + K^+) + \text{Glucose} + \text{BUN} + 9$$

Conventional Units:

$$\text{mOsm/L} = 1.86\,(Na^+ + K^+)$$
$$+ \left(\frac{\text{Glucose}}{18}\right) + \left(\frac{\text{BUN}}{2.8}\right) + 9$$

Differences between measured and calculated plasma osmolality indicate the presence of unmeasured osmotically active substances in plasma. Plasma osmolality may also aid in the assessment of the degree of dehydration of the patient. The fluid deficit in liters may be calculated as follows: (69)

$$\text{Fluid deficit (L)} = (0.6)\,BW_{kg}\left[\frac{(\text{mOsm plasma} - 300)}{300}\right]$$

Urine should be collected and its specific gravity, osmolality, and pH determined. In addition, the sample should be tested for the presence of protein, red blood cells, and glucose.

Once the clinician has assessed the patient's fluid and electrolyte status, a plan for therapeutic intervention, if required, is initiated. Selection of the appropriate fluid for replacement purposes is dependent upon the nature of the disease process and the composition of the fluid lost from the patient. The following criteria have been utilized in determining the appropriate therapeutic intervention: (a) volume deficit; (b) packed cell volume and total serum protein concentration; (c) plasma osmolality; (d) electrolyte concentrations; (e) acid-base status; (f) caloric requirements–water-soluble vitamins, carbohydrates, and amino acids–and (g) trace element concentrations.(70) In those situations where it is necessary to correct fluid and electrolyte deficits prior to surgery, consideration is given to the replacement of previous and continuing losses as well as the provision of maintenance requirements if the animal is not currently ingesting food or water. It is preferable to replenish total body water and correct electrolyte deficits over a 24- to 48-hour period. The patient may be stabilized over the first 2 to 4 hours, with 50% of the estimated deficit being corrected during that time period. Seventy-five percent of the deficit may be corrected within 24 hours in addition to the replacement of concurrent losses and the administration of maintenance requirements. The remainder of the deficit, in conjunction with maintenance requirements, may be administered over the next 24 hours. Continuing losses should be estimated and replaced, if necessary, over this time period as well.

In critically ill or moribund patients, vascular and interstitial volume deficits must be corrected as rapidly as is necessary to ensure the survival of the patient. In the treatment of shock, fluid administration rates of 90 mL · kg^{-1} · h^{-1} in the dog and 50 to 60 mL · kg^{-1} · h^{-1} in cats have been recommended for the first hour. In subsequent hours, where appropriate, reductions in fluid administration rates to 10 to 12 mL $\cdot$ kg^{-1} $\cdot$ h^{-1} in dogs and 5 to 6 mL $\cdot$ kg^{-1} $\cdot$ h^{-1} in cats have been suggested.[71] In large animal species, administration rates of 60 mL $\cdot$ kg^{-1} $\cdot$ h^{-1} (equine); 80 mL $\cdot$ kg^{-1} $\cdot$ h^{-1} (calves) and 40 mL $\cdot$ kg^{-1} $\cdot$ h^{-1} (cattle) may be used in the initial stages of shock therapy.[20, 72, 73]

FLUID ADMINISTRATION

Fluids may be administered orally, subcutaneously, or directly into the vascular space by the intravenous or intraosseous routes. Oral administration of fluids is recommended unless the animal is in critical condition or has severe gastrointestinal disease. Isotonic, nonirritating maintenance solutions may be administered subcutaneously if time and the clinical condition of the patient permit. In critically ill patients, where rapid response to therapy is desired, fluids and electrolytes should be administered directly into the intravascular compartment. Fluids that are administered intravenously, particularly if administered rapidly or in large volumes, should be warmed to 37° C before they are infused or transfused. Infusion warmers are available to facilitate warming of intravenous fluids or whole blood to 37° C (Figure 19–2)

Venipuncture, for fluid administration purposes, may be accomplished with intravenous butterfly sets or catheters. Butterfly infusion sets are not suitable for unsupervised fluid therapy procedures because of the potential for extravascular infusion of fluids. Similarly, they should not be used routinely for perioperative venous access of the surgical patient, since they cannot be relied upon to remain intravascular. Short-term venous access for anesthetic procedures and fluid or drug administration is best accomplished with the use of over the needle-type catheters. Angiocath (Deseret Medical Inc., Sandy, Utah) intravenous catheters are available in sizes of 24 gauge × 1.9 cm to 10 gauge × 7.6 cm and are made of Teflon. More recently, Insyte catheters have been made available that are constructed of Vialon (Deseret Medical Inc., Sandy, Utah). These catheters have increased wall strength, which would facilitate their passage through the tough skin of some domestic and exotic animal species. Catheters made of Vialon have been associated with a 46% lower incidence of thrombophlebitis when compared to catheters made from Teflon.[74] Another product, the Streamline IV catheter (Menlo Care Inc., Menlo Park, California) is also available. This catheter is made of an elastomeric hydrogel that undergoes hydration and enlargement after being placed intravenously. One study demonstrated an increase in flow through a 20-gauge catheter of 26% within 1 hour of its intravenous placement.[75] The 20-gauge catheter expanded in size to approximate an 18-gauge catheter in this study.[75] Such products may be of value in establishing an intravenous access quickly when larger catheters may not be easily placed. Through the needle-type intravenous catheters (I-Cath, Delmed Inc., New Brunswick, New Jersey) are ideal for long-term fluid therapy, although similar catheter styles

and lengths are available as over-the-needle catheter placement units (E-Z Cath, Deseret Medical Inc., Sandy, Utah). The length of these intravenous placement units ensures that they are less likely to be dislodged from the intravenous space. This is of concern, particularly in the large animal patient.

Selection of the venous access site depends upon the species involved, the physical condition of the patient, the volume and type of fluid to be administered, the rate of fluid administration, and the accessibility of a peripheral or central vein. The jugular and saphenous veins may be catheterized in most species. The cephalic vein is commonly used in small animal patients, and the auricular vein may be used in some large animal species. The saphenous or jugular vein may be used in larger birds, while the cutaneous ulnar vein may be used in the small avian patient.[76, 77] In situations where large volumes are to be infused quickly, the jugular vein is often the best choice. Catheterization of the jugular vein enables the clinician to administer fluids, monitor central venous pressure and collect blood samples for laboratory analysis. There is a reduced chance of thrombophlebitis occurring if dextrose or hypertonic solutions are infused into the jugular vein. Infusions of dextrose or hypertonic solutions into smaller peripheral veins increase the risk that the patient will develop thrombophlebitis.

All catheters should be placed and maintained in an aseptic manner. Details in regard to appropriate catheter placement and maintenance techniques may be found elsewhere.[20, 78-80] Phlebitis that occurs after short-term catheter placements, such as that which occurs in the perioperative period, is most often the result of excessive trauma to the vein upon catheter placement. Thrombophlebitis is of concern when catheters are placed for long-term intravenous therapy.[20, 80-82] Appropriate techniques should be used to minimize the possibility of contaminating the catheter, intravenous administration set, or parenteral solution. Administration sets and bandages should be changed every 24 hours. The catheter site is inspected daily for signs of phlebitis, and the catheter replaced every 48 to 72 hours (or earlier if signs of thrombophlebitis are present). It is important to remove the catheter as soon as the patient no longer requires intravenous support, and the catheter site should be observed for 1 or 2 days afterward to ensure that phlebitis does not develop.

The rate at which fluids may be administered is determined by factors such as (a) viscosity of the fluid, (b) internal diameter of the catheter and intravenous administration system, (c) length of the intravenous administration system, and (d) the height at which the fluid reservoir is hung above the patient.[83] Of these, the internal diameter of the catheter and the fluid administration set are the most important factors in determining the maximum rate of flow through the system. In situations where rapid administration of fluid is required, large bore catheters should be used. A 20-gauge catheter will only permit up to 75 mL/min to flow into the cephalic vein of a canine patient with a

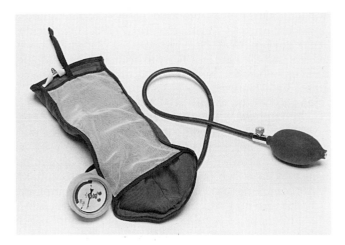

Fig. 19–3. Pressure infusers may be utilized in order to increase the rate with which fluids may be administered intravenously. They are available in a number of sizes that can accommodate up to a 5-liter crystalloid solution bag (Viaflex, Baxter Corp, Toronto, Ontario).

gravity feed of 1.75 meters. However, if an 18-gauge catheter is used, the flow rate would increase from 75 to 114 mL/min using a gravity feed of 1.0 to 1.75 meters.(83) Similarly, increasing catheter size to a 16-gauge device increases flow to 160 to 210 mL/min.(20, 83) Further increases in flow of up to 21% may be obtained by using a blood administration set as opposed to a traditional intravenous fluid administration set. In large animals, flow rates can be improved upon dramatically by modifying a Y Type TUR/Bladder Irrigation Set (Baxter Corp., Toronto, Ontario) to end in a standard Luer Lock connector. Further increases in fluid administration rates can be obtained by using Pressure Infusor sets (Fig. 19–3), which can accommodate a 1-liter (Pressure Infusor, Baxter Corp., Toronto, Ontario) or a 5-liter fluid bag (Disposable Pressure Infusor, Biomedical Dynamics, Minneapolis, Minnesota). Further increases in fluid administration rates may be accomplished, if necessary, by using mechanized intravenous fluid pumps and multiple intravenous catheter sites.

The intraosseous space provides an alternative route for the parenteral administration of fluids and therapeutic agents into the vascular space. This method of fluid administration should be used whenever an intravenous access cannot be established for the treatment of the critically ill patient. Therapeutic agents and fluids that are administered into the intraosseous space rapidly attain the systemic circulation via the bone marrow.(84, 85) In small animals, the intraosseous space may be accessed through the tibial tuberosity, the trochanteric fossa of the femur or the flat medial surface of the proximal tibia just distal to the tibial tuberosity. In the avian species, the distal end of the ulna is cannulated since pneumatic bone must be avoided. The details with respect to cannula placement, maintenance and use of intraosseous administration techniques in small animals has been described.(86)

ASSESSMENT

Once the fluid therapy regimen is initiated, the clinician should continue to reevaluate the patient in order to determine its response to therapy. Serial measurements of weight and laboratory values in conjunction with frequent physical examinations enable the clinician to alter the therapeutic regimen according to the patient's changing status. Additional data may be obtained with respect to the patient's status and response to therapy through monitoring systemic blood pressure, central venous pressure, the electrocardiogram and volume of urine production. These parameters are commonly monitored by the veterinarian in the perioperative period and are discussed in detail in Chapters 5 and 15.

INTRAOPERATIVE CONSIDERATIONS

The most common changes that occur during the intraoperative period are alterations to the volume or composition of the extracellular fluid. These alterations occur as the result of evaporative losses of free water, sequestration of plasma water into traumatized tissues, and hemorrhage.

Maintenance deficits in the anesthetized patient occur in the preoperative period owing to NPO orders and continue throughout the intraoperative and recovery periods. Consideration should be given to the fact that intraoperative losses of free water by evaporation may, in fact, be in excess of values commonly estimated for routine maintenance purposes. The perioperative free water deficit can be estimated to be at least 2.0 to 2.5 mL/kg for each hour that the animal is not eating or drinking. Ideally, free water deficits should be replaced using a hypotonic solution, 5% dextrose in water, or a maintenance solution. However, replacement solutions, such as lactated Ringer's, are often used for this purpose in order to simplify the intraoperative fluid therapy regimen.

In addition, third space losses occur as the result of translocation of plasma water into surgically traumatized tissues. The degree to which the vascular volume is reduced is directly related to the extent of the surgical trauma to the patient. These losses lead to hemoconcentration and in some instances may be estimated as follows:

$$\text{Plasma deficit (mL)} = \text{Normal blood volume} - \left[\frac{\left(\begin{array}{c} \text{Normal blood volume} \\ \times \text{ Initial PCV} \end{array} \right)}{\text{Measured PCV}} \right]$$

Third space losses are replaced with a balanced electrolyte solution using an administration rate of up to $2 \; \text{mL} \cdot \text{kg}^{-1} \cdot \text{h}^{-1}$ for superficial procedures, 3 to 5 $\text{mL} \cdot \text{kg}^{-1} \cdot \text{h}^{-1}$ for mildly traumatic procedures, 5 to 10 $\text{mL} \cdot \text{kg}^{-1} \cdot \text{h}^{-1}$ for moderately traumatic surgeries, and up to 15 $\text{mL} \cdot \text{kg}^{-1} \cdot \text{h}^{-1}$ for severely traumatic procedures. In the avian species intraoperative fluid administration rates of 10 $\text{mL} \cdot \text{kg}^{-1} \cdot \text{h}^{-1}$ for the first 2 hours and 5 to 8 mL · kg^{-1} · h^{-1} for subsequent hours have been recommended.(17) This volume of fluid is administered in addition to that which is being administered for maintenance purposes to the surgical patient.

Acute, intraoperative losses of blood in excess of 15% of total blood volume in the normal patient or 10% in the critically ill patient should be replaced with whole blood or packed red cells. Artificial blood solutions, although costly and not readily available, may be of value in instances where whole blood or packed red cells are not available.(87) An excellent review of artificial blood is recommended to the reader for additional information on whole blood substitutes.(88) Losses that do not exceed these limits may be replaced with balanced electrolyte or replacement solutions. As already mentioned, crystalloid solutions equilibrate across the extracellular fluid space and it is necessary to administer a volume of fluid that is equivalent to three times the volume of blood that has been lost from the vascular space. Whole blood losses are replaced as they occur with the appropriate volume of colloid or balanced electrolyte solution.

Finally, consideration must also be given to the administration of fluids in order to maintain cardiovascular stability and organ perfusion, which might be altered due to the hemodynamic effects of the anesthetic protocol. The total volume of fluid that is administered to the patient in the perioperative period should be adjusted to ensure that vital signs such as blood pressure and urine production are maintained above critical levels.

The administration of large volumes of replacement fluids can lead to hemodilution and the interstitial accumulation of fluids. Although some degree of hemodilution may be beneficial, the hematocrit should be maintained at approximately 25% and total serum protein levels should not be permitted to decrease below 35 g/L (3.5 g/dL).(48) It has been suggested that hypertonic saline and dextran 70 solutions may be of value for the intraoperative management of hemorrhagic episodes in order to maintain hemodynamic function and reduce the possibility of inducing a fluid volume overload in the patient.(39)

Continual assessment of the patient is necessary in order to maintain cardiovascular stability postoperatively. If continuing blood losses are not of concern, then the clinician's attention should be directed toward continuing third space losses and maintenance requirements. Care should be exercised when administering crystalloid solutions in the postoperative period. Overt fluid overloading of the patient may not be readily apparent until 24 to 72 hours after the surgical procedure. Postsurgical alterations in aldosterone and ADH activity result in reduced free water clearance in the postoperative period. Once the neurohormonal responses to the surgical procedure abates, third space fluid and the fluid that has accumulated to excess in the interstitial space is mobilized and returned to the vascular space. This can result in a volume overload that might be detrimental to the critically ill patient (e.g., pulmonary edema).(32)

Electrolyte Disturbances

Compositional changes in the extracellular fluid during the perioperative period may result from previous or ongoing disease processes or they may be iatrogenic in origin. Clinically significant disturbances in electrolyte balance should be corrected preoperatively. Acute, life-threatening, intraoperative alterations of serum sodium, calcium, or magnesium concentrations are uncommon unless iatrogenically induced.

SODIUM

Sodium is the osmolar skeleton of extracellular fluid. Alterations in sodium balance may occur as the result of depletion or retention of water or sodium or both. Sodium regulation and diseases that result in sodium imbalances are discussed elsewhere (Chapter 18).(11,15,89)

Hyponatremia exists when serum sodium concentrations are less than 136 mmol/L (136 mEq/L). Clinical signs relating to neurologic dysfunction occur when sodium concentrations are less than 120 mmol/L (120 mEq/L) and become marked when serum sodium is less than 110 mmol/L (110 mEq/L). Clinical signs that might be observed include anorexia, lethargy, weakness, vomiting, muscle cramping, myoclonus, seizures, and coma. The EKG may reveal a widened QRS complex with an elevated ST segment and a nonrespiratory dilutional acidosis may develop (Chapter 18). Ventricular tachycardia or fibrillation can occur when serum sodium levels are less than 100 mmol/L (100 mEq/L). Severe hyponatremia may be corrected with the careful administration of 3% saline over 24 hours. It has been recommended that the amount of sodium to be administered during this time period be calculated as follows: (15)

$$\text{mmol Na}^+ = 0.2\, BW_{kg}\, (\text{Normal } [Na^+] - \text{Patient's } [Na^+])$$

In less severe situations, free water restriction, correction of the underlying cause, and intravenous administration of 0.9% saline may be considered.

Hypernatremia occurs most commonly owing to water loss in excess of the loss of sodium in small animal patients. Those animals that do not have free access to water are prone to develop hypernatremia if they have increased water losses such as would occur from heat prostration or burns, and so forth. Salt poisoning occurs commonly in cattle and swine.(89) Serum sodium concentrations above 156 mmol/L (156 mEq/L) in dogs and 160 mmol/L (160 mEq/L) in cats and large animal species constitute hypernatremia. Severe hypernatremia may result in nonrespiratory concentration alkalosis. Clinical signs include lethargy, confusion, muscle weakness, myoclonus, seizures, and coma. The severity of the clinical signs depends upon the rate of onset and the degree of hypernatremia. Treatment is dependent upon the initial cause of the hypernatremia and the chronicity of the electrolyte imbalance. Significant sodium imbalances should be medically managed and corrected prior to any anesthetic or surgical procedure. Details in regard to the medical management of hypernatremic states are readily available from a number of sources.(11,15,89)

CALCIUM

Calcium plays a major role in the physiology of neuromuscular function, cell membrane permeability, muscle contraction, and hemostasis (Chapters 5 and 13). With respect to total body content, up to 99% of calcium is located within bone. Total serum calcium consists of an ionized portion, a protein-bound portion, and a portion that is bound to divalent anions such as phosphate and bicarbonate. Close to 50% of total serum calcium is bound to proteins, primarily albumin. Although the ionized portion (40%) is the physiologic active fraction, it is rarely measured. Serum ionized calcium levels are pH dependent, with alkalemia reducing and acidemia increasing ionized serum calcium levels. In dogs, formulas have been developed to adjust calcium measurements to account for alterations in serum protein or albumin concentrations.(90) In cats, at least one study has recommended that similar adjustments not be made.(91)

Symptomatic hypocalcemia can occur due to hypoparathyroidism and eclampsia in small animals or parturient paresis in large animal species. Intraoperative hypocalcemia, induced by the administration of large volumes of citrated whole blood, reduces ventricular function and systemic blood pressure.(92) Hypocalcemia exists when serum calcium levels are less than 1.75 mmol/L (7 mg/dL) in small animals and 2.0 mmol/L (8 mg/dL) in large animals. Hypoalbuminemia may induce a hypocalcemia in small animals of 1.75 to 2.0 mmol/L (7 to 8 mg/dL). Serum calcium concentrations below 1.62 mmol/L (6.5 mg/dL) are generally the result of a metabolic disorder. Small animals that present with hypocalcemia may show clinical signs of restlessness, muscle fasciculations, tetany, or convulsions. The EKG may show prolonged QT and ST segments due to prolonged myocardial action potentials. Recently calved, mature cows with parturient paresis often have serum calcium levels less than 1.25 mmol/L (5 mg/dL). These cows become recumbent when serum calcium levels are less than 1.5 mmol/L (6 mg/dL). Serum calcium levels less than 1.0 mmol/L (4 mg/dL) are fatal.

Hypercalcemia can result from hyperparathyroidism or malignancies in small animals, whereas in large animals it is often iatrogenic in origin–in many instances the result of excessive dietary supplementation. Hypercalcemia has been reported to occur in horses with chronic renal failure.(89) Hemoconcentration results in increased serum albumin levels. This may increase serum calcium levels to 3.2 mmol/L (13 mg/dL). Serum calcium concentrations in excess of 3 mmol/L (12 mg/dL) in the dog and 2.74 mmol/L (11 mg/dL) in the cat are indicative of hypercalcemia. Clinical signs include anorexia, vomiting, and gastrointestinal dysfunction. Generalized locomotor weakness may also be evident. Bradycardia, a prolonged PR interval, and a shortened ST segment may be observed. Rapid increases in serum calcium levels in excess of 3.74 mmol/L (15 mg/dL) may result in vagal stimulation and severe bradycardia, while severe but less acute increases may result in ventricular dysrhythmias.(93, 94)

Acute, intraoperative hypocalcemic episodes that are iatrogenic in origin may be treated with 10% calcium chloride or gluconate. Ten percent calcium chloride contains 1.4 mEq/mL calcium, and calcium gluconate contains 0.45 mEq calcium per mL. The dose to be administered depends on the severity of the situation and ranges from 5 to 15 mg/kg administered over a period of 1 hour. The EKG should be observed for evidence of calcium toxicity during the infusion, and additional laboratory data should be assessed prior to administering subsequent doses of calcium.

POTASSIUM

Potassium is the primary intracellular cation. At least 90% of the total body potassium content is located within the intracellular compartment. Extracellular fluid potassium content represents approximately 2% of total body potassium. As a result, serum potassium concentration often does not accurately represent the extent or severity of a potassium disorder, particularly in chronic disease processes. Potassium is highly labile, and serum levels are altered significantly in the presence of acidemia, alkalemia, or extracellular fluid osmolality changes, or as the result of alterations in serum insulin, glucagon or catecholamine concentration. Changes in extracellular fluid pH result in rapid and significant alteration in the potassium concentration of extracellular fluid. Acute reductions in $PaCO_2$ of 10 mm Hg have been shown to increase plasma pH by 0.1 unit and decrease plasma potassium by 0.4 mmol/L (0.4 mEq/L).(95) Intraoperative ventilatory or metabolic acid-base disturbances are common, particularly in patients that are critically ill. It is incumbent upon the anesthesiologist to monitor for, and respond to, significant alterations in plasma potassium levels before they become life threatening.

Hypokalemia results from reductions in dietary intake or increased losses through the urinary or gastrointestinal systems. Increased losses through the urinary system can be the result of osmotic diuresis, chronic steroid therapy, or the use of loop or thiazide diuretics. Alkalemia will result in a reduction of serum potassium levels as extracellular potassium moves intracellularly in exchange for hydrogen ions. The degree to which clinical signs become apparent depends upon the rapidity by which the electrolyte alteration occurs, and the chronicity of the disease process. An acute reduction in serum potassium levels to less than 3.0 mmol/L (3 mEq/L) results in clinical signs. These may include reduced gastrointestinal motility and generalized muscle weakness. Rapid reductions in extracellular potassium levels disrupt the normal intracellular to extracellular potassium ratio and lead to hyperpolarization of myocardial cells. The EKG demonstrates evidence of prolonged repolarization times with a prolonged PR, QRS, and QT intervals, depression of the ST segment, and a flattened or inverted T wave. Severe cardiac manifestations of hypokalemia include sinus bradycardia, heart block and AV dissociation. Clinical signs may not be apparent until potassium concentration approaches 2.5 mmol/L (2.5 mEq/L) in chronic conditions.

Patients in which serum potassium levels have been acutely reduced to below 3.0 mmol/L (3 mEq/L) should have their serum potassium levels corrected, if at all possible, prior to inducing anesthesia. Moderate to severe reductions in serum potassium levels (2.5 mEq/L) may require the intravenous administration of potassium chloride. It is important that the clinician assess the patient's cardiac and renal function and that the fluid volume and acid-base status of the patient be determined. Volume deficits and acid-base disturbances should be corrected early on in order to ensure adequate renal perfusion and to enable the clinician to determine plasma potassium levels in a more normalized situation with respect to the patient's acid-base status. Potassium chloride may be infused at a rate of 0.5 mmol·kg^{-1}·h^{-1} (0.5 mEq·kg^{-1}·h^{-1}) to a maximum daily dose of 2 to 3 mmol/kg (2 to 3 mEq/kg). It is necessary to continually monitor the patient's status during this period. In addition to serial potassium determinations, the patient should be monitored with an EKG so that the clinician can detect the early signs of potassium toxicity.

In situations where the potassium imbalance is the result of a chronic disease process, anesthesia and surgery should be delayed if possible and the imbalance corrected and medically managed over a period of 3 to 5 days. In this situation, the goal is to replenish the total body potassium deficit without inducing clinical signs of potassium toxicity. This may be accomplished through the oral administration of potassium supplements or the parenteral administration of a maintenance solution in which the potassium level has been adjusted to at least 20 to 30 mmol/L (20 to 30 mEq/L). Again, it is imperative to continually assess the patient's status and alter the therapeutic regimen accordingly.

If the surgical procedure cannot be delayed, then it may be prudent not to correct serum potassium levels that have been reduced to values between 2.5 to 3.0 mmol/L (2.5 to 3.0 mEq/L) as a result of a chronic process. Rapid corrections of plasma potassium concentration in this instance may acutely disturb the intracellular to extracellular potassium ratio and induce alterations in cell membrane stability. In humans, chronic reductions of serum potassium concentration to

2.6 mmol/L (2.6 mEq/L) were not associated with, or predictive of, intraoperative dysrhythmias. Instead, intraoperative dysrhythmias are better correlated with the incidence of preoperative dysrhythmias.(96)

Hyperkalemia is not as common in large animals as compared to small animals but does occur with acidemia. In small animals, increases in plasma potassium levels in excess of 6.5 mmol/L (6.5 mEq/L) may be iatrogenic in nature or occur as the result of renal failure, urethral obstruction, hypoadrenocorticism, or acidemia. Postoperatively, increased plasma potassium levels may occur owing to increased tissue catabolism or acidemia. In most instances, there is no total body excess of potassium and the increase in potassium content is limited to the extracellular fluid compartment.

Increases in extracellular fluid potassium concentrations decrease the magnitude of cell membrane polarization, which subsequently enhances membrane excitability. Clinical signs become apparent once plasma potassium concentration exceeds 6.5 mmol/L (6.5 mEq/L). Myocardial contractility decreases and bradycardia develops. As plasma potassium concentration approach 8 mmol/L, the EKG will show peaked T waves and a decrease in the amplitude of the P wave. Plasma potassium concentrations in excess of 8 mmol/L have a significant effect on myocardial activity. There is a prolongation of the PR interval, and the P wave may be absent. As the potassium level increases, the QRS complex widens until it assumes a sine wave appearance and AV dissociation occurs. Eventually, asystole or ventricular fibrillation ensues. Patients with plasma potassium concentration in excess of 6.5 mmol/L (6.5 mEq/L) should not be anesthetized unless the patient's life is immediately threatened by some other process.

Severe potassium-induced cardiotoxicity may be initially antagonized by the intravenous administration of 10% calcium chloride or gluconate at a dose of 0.2 to 0.3 mEq/kg. If the dysrhythmias persist, the dose may be repeated in 5 minutes. Additional doses of calcium salts are unlikely to be of benefit. Calcium helps restore cell membrane potentials, and although its effect will last only 10 to 20 minutes, this will provide time for the clinician to institute other therapeutic measures. Acute, intraoperative decreases in plasma potassium concentration may also be accomplished by instituting controlled ventilation of the patient to rapidly reverse respiratory acidosis.(95)

Fluid volume deficits and acid-base disturbances should be assessed and corrected. Five percent dextrose or 0.9% saline may be utilized to correct the fluid deficit, promote diuresis, and functionally dilute the extracellular potassium. Dextrose solutions not only provide free water for volume replacement purposes but also enhance the cellular uptake of potassium as part of the normal mechanisms of glucose metabolism. In situations where plasma potassium levels are significantly increased, glucose may be administered at a dose of 0.5 to 1.0 g/kg in order to enhance the intracellular movement of potassium. The effect of this therapeutic measure should last for a few hours. The effect of glucose on serum potassium concentration may be facilitated by administering 1 unit of regular insulin for every 2 g dextrose administered. Correction of acidemia will result in an intracellular shift of potassium in exchange for hydrogen ions. Considerations for therapeutic measures in acid-base disturbances are discussed in Chapters 6 and 18. Patients should be continually assessed and care taken to ensure that the therapeutic measures undertaken do not result in hypokalemia or other functional disturbances.

References

1. Spurlock SL, Furr M. Fluid therapy. In: Koterba AM, Drummond WH, Kosch PC, eds. Equine clinical neonatology. Philadelphia: Lea & Febiger, 1990.
2. Carlson GP. Fluid, electrolyte and acid-base balance. In: Kaneko JJ, ed. Clinical biochemistry of domestic animals, 4th ed. Boston: Academic Press, 1989.
3. Ruckebusch Y, Phaneuf, L-P, Dunlop R, eds. Physiology of small and large animals. Philadelphia: BC Decker, 1991.
4. Carlson GP. Blood chemistry, body fluids and hematology. In: Gillespie JR, Robinson N, eds. Equine exercise physiology 2. Davis, CA: ICEEP Publications, 1987.
5. Wagstaff AJ, Maclean I, Michell AR, Holmes PH. Plasma and extracellular volume in calves: comparison between isotopic and cold techniques. Res Vet Sci 53:271, 1992.
6. Turner DAB. Fluid, electrolyte and acid-base balance. In: Aitkenhead AR, Smith G, eds. Textbook of anaesthesia, 2nd ed. New York: Churchill Livingstone, 1990.
7. Stoelting RK. Pharmacology and physiology in anesthetic practice. Philadelphia: JB Lippincott, 1987.
8. Saxton CR, Seldin DW. Clinical interpretation of laboratory values. In: Kokko JP, Tannen RL, eds. Fluids and electrolytes. Philadelphia: WB Saunders, 1986.
9. Rose BD. Clinical physiology of acid-base and electrolyte disorders, 2nd ed. New York: McGraw-Hill, 1984.
10. Walker, V. Fluid balance disorders in neurosurgical patients: Physiological basis and definitions. Acta Neurochir Suppl (Wien) 47:95, 1980.
11. Scott RC. Disorders of sodium metabolism. In: Schaer M, ed. Fluid and electrolyte balance, Vet Clin N Am: small animal practice. Philadelphia: WB Saunders, 1982.
12. Hardy RM. Disorders of water metabolism. In: Schaer M, ed. Fluid and electrolyte balance, Vet Clin N Am: small animal practice. Philadelphia: WB Saunders, 1982.
13. Goudsouzian N, Karamanian A. Physiology for the anesthesiologist, 2nd ed. Norwalk, CT: Appleton-Century-Crafts, 1984.
14. Guyton AC, Barber BJ, Moffatt DS. Theory of interstitial pressures. In: Hargens AR, ed. Tissue pressure and composition. Baltimore: Williams & Wilkins, 1981.
15. Garvey MS. Fluid and electrolyte balance in critical patients. In: Kirby R, Stamp GL, eds. Critical care, veterinary clinics of north america: small animal practice. Philadelphia: WB Saunders, 1989.
16. Schaer M. General principles of fluid therapy in small animal medicine. In: Schaer M, ed. Fluid and electrolyte disorders, veterinary clinics of north america: small animal practice. Philadelphia: WB Saunders, 1989.
17. Ritchie BW. Fluid therapy in avian patients. Vet Med Rep 2:316, 1990.
18. Rose RJ. A physiological approach to fluid and electrolyte therapy in the horse. Equine Vet J 13:7, 1981.
19. Barragry TB. Some aspects of fluid and electrolyte imbalances in animals. Ir Vet J Aug: 153, 1974.
20. Tremblay RRM. Intravenous fluid therapy in calves. In: Roussel AJ, ed. Fluid and electrolyte therapy, Vet Clin N Am: food animal practice. Philadelphia: WB Saunders, 1990.
21. Reece WO. Physiology of domestic animals. Philadelphia: Lea & Febiger, 1991.
22. Gibbons G. Hypertonic solutions in the treatment of shock. Proceedings of the Eighth Annual Veterinary Medical Forum. Madison, WI: Omnipress, 1990.
23. Prough DS, et al. Hypertonic/hyperoncotic fluid resuscitation after hemorrhagic shock in dogs. Anesth Analg 73:738, 1991.
24. Zoran DL, et al. Evaluation of hemostatic analytes after use of hypertonic saline solutions combined with colloids for resuscitation of dogs with hypovolemia. Am J Vet Res 53:1791, 1992.
25. Muir WW, Sally J. Small volume resuscitation with hypertonic saline solution in hypovolemic cats. Am J Vet Res 50:1883, 1989.
26. Schmall LM, Muir WW, Robertson JT. Haemodynamic effects of small volume hypertonic saline in experimentally induced haemorrhagic shock. Equine Vet J 22:273, 1990.
27. Schmall LM, Muir WW, Robertson JT. Haematological, serum electrolyte and blood gas effects of small volume hypertonic saline in experimentally induced haemorrhagic shock. Equine Vet J 22:278, 1990.
28. Muir WW. Small volume resuscitation using hypertonic saline. Cornell Vet 80:7, 1990.
29. Hinchcliff KW, Schmall LM, McKeever KH, Fenger CK. Effect of hypertonic saline administration on blood and plasma volume of normal horses. Proceedings of the Ninth Annual Veterinary Medical Forum. Madison, WI: Omnipress, 1991.
30. Kien ND, Kramer GC, White DA. Acute hypotension caused by rapid hypertonic saline infusion in anesthetized dogs. Anesth Analg 73:597, 1991.
31. Bertone JJ, Shoemaker KE. Effect of hypertonic and isotonic saline solutions on plasma constituents of conscious horses. Am J Vet Res 53:1844, 1992.
32. Shackford SR. Hypertonic saline and dextran for intraoperative fluid therapy: more for less. Crit Care Med 20:160, 1992.
33. Rabinovici R, Krausz MM, Feuerstein G. Control of bleeding is essential for a successful treatment of hemorrhagic shock with 7.5 percent sodium chloride solution. Surg Gynecol Obstet 173: 98,1991.
34. Muir WW. Comparative aspects of hypertonic saline resuscitation. Proceedings of The Seventh Annual Veterinary Medical Forum. Madison, WI: Omnipress, 1989.
35. Rocha e Silva M, Velasco IT. Hypertonic saline resuscitation: the neural component. Prog Clin Biol Res 299:303, 1989.
36. Gala GJ, Lilly MP, Thomas SE, Gann DS. Interaction of sodium and volume in fluid resuscitation after hemorrhage. J Trauma 31:545, 1991.
37. Kramer GC, English TP, Gunther RA, Holcraft JW. Physiological mechanisms of fluid resuscitation with hyperosmotic/hyperoncotic solutions. Prog Clin Biol Res 299:311, 1989.
38. Rocha e Silva M, et al. Hypertonic resuscitation from severe hemorrhagic shock: patterns of regional circulation. Circ Shock 19:165, 1986.
39. Pascual JMS, et al. Resuscitation of intraoperative hypovolemia: a comparison of normal saline and hyperosmotic/hyperoncotic solutions in swine. Crit Care Med 20:200, 1992.
40. Allen DA, Schertel ER, Muir WW, Valentine AK. Hypertonic saline/dextran resuscitation of dogs with experimentally induced gastric dilatation–volvulus shock. Am J Vet Res 52:92, 1991.
41. Horton JW, Walker PB. Small volume hypertonic saline dextran resuscitation from canine endotoxic shock. Ann Surg 214:64, 1991.
42. Moon PF, Snyder JR, Haskins SC, Perron PR. Effects of a highly concentrated hypertonic saline-dextran volume expander on cardiopulmonary function in anesthetized horses. Am J Vet Res 52:1611, 1991.
43. Kramer GC, et al. Small-volume resuscitation with hypertonic saline dextran solution. Surgery 100:239, 1986.
44. Okrasinski EB, Krahwinkel DJ, Sanders WL. Treatment of dogs in hemorrhagic shock by intraosseous infusion of hypertonic saline and dextran. Vet Surg 21:20, 1992.
45. Anaya C, Drace C, Myers T, Kramer GC. Less net volume loading with hypertonic saline dextran resuscitation of intraoperative hypovolemia. Anesthesiology 75:A1122, 1991.

46. Remillard RL, Thatcher CO. Parenteral nutritional support in the small animal patient. In: Kirby R, Stamp GL, eds. Critical care, veterinary clinics of north america: small animal practice. Philadelphia: WB Saunders, 1989.

47. Wolfsheimer KJ. Fluid therapy in the critically ill patient. In: Schaer M, ed. Fluid and electrolyte disorders, veterinary clinics of north america: small animal practice. Philadelphia: WB Saunders, 1989.

48. Sunder-Plassmann L, et al. The physiological significance of acutely induced hemodilution. Proceedings of the Sixth European Conference on Microcirculation, 1970. Basel: S Karger, 1971.

49. Messmer K, Kreimeier U, Intaglietta M. Present state of intentional hemodilution. Eur Surg Res 18:254, 1986.

50. Messmer K. Hemodilution. In: Burke JL, ed. A physiologic approach to critical care, Surg Clin N Am. Philadelphia: WB Saunders, 1975.

51. Cotter SM. Blood banking. I–Collection and storage. In: Proceedings of the Sixth Annual Veterinary Medical Forum. Madison, WI: Omnipress, 1988.

52. Ou D, Mahaffey E, Smith JE. Effect of storage on oxygen dissociation of canine blood. J Am Vet Med Assoc 167:56, 1975.

53. Cotter SM. Blood banking. II–Indications and side effects. Proceedings of the Sixth Annual Veterinary Medical Forum. Madison, WI: Omnipress, 1988.

54. Pichler ME, Turnwald GH. Blood transfusion in the dog and cat. Part I. Physiology, collection, storage, and indications for whole blood therapy. Compend Cont Educ Pract Vet 7:64, 1985.

55. Turnwald GH. Blood transfusions in dogs and cats. Part II. Administration, adverse effects, and component therapy. Compend Cont Educ Pract Vet 7:115, 1985.

56. Hunt E, Moore JS. Use of blood and blood products. In: Roussel AJ, ed. Fluid and electrolyte therapy, Vet Clin N Am: food animal practice. Philadelphia. WB Saunders, 1990.

57. Giger U, Bucheler J. Transfusion of type-A and type-B blood to cats. J Am Vet Med Assoc 198:411, 1991.

58. Giger U, Kilrain CG, Filippich LJ, Bell K. Frequencies of feline blood groups in the United States. J Am Vet Med Assoc 195:1230, 1989.

59. Kallfelz FA, Whitlock RH, Schultz RD. Survival of ^{59}Fe-labelled erythrocytes in cross-transfused equine blood. Am J Vet Res 39:617, 1978.

60. Stormont CJ. Blood groups in animals. J Am Vet Med Assoc 181:1120, 1982.

61. Kirk RW, Bistner SI, Ford RB, eds. Handbook of veterinary procedures & emergency treatment. Philadelphia: WB Saunders, 1990.

62. Cassady JF, Patel RI, Epstein BS. Calculations for predicting blood transfusion needs. Anesthesia 59:491, 1983.

63. Hammer AS, Couto CG. Disorders of hemostasis and principles of transfusion therapy. In: Allen DG, ed. Small animal medicine. Philadelphia: JB Lippincott, 1991.

64. Concannon KT, Haskins SC, Feldman BF. Hemostatic defects associated with two infusion rates of dextran 70 in dogs. Am J Vet Res 53:1369, 1992.

65. Fritsch R. A review of plasma substitutes. Proc Assoc Vet Anaesth Gr Br Ir 10:170, 1982.

66. Murray MJ. Use of subcutaneous fluids in the avian patient. J Assoc Avian Vet 3:194, 1989.

67. Blood DC, Radostits OM, eds. Veterinary medicine: a textbook of the diseases of cattle, sheep, pigs, goats and horses, 7th ed. Philadelphia: Balliere Tindall, 1989.

68. Messmer K. Compensatory mechanisms for acute dilutional anemia. Bibl Haematol 47:31, 1981.

69. Genetzky RM, Loparco FV, Ledet AE. Clinical pathologic alterations in horses during a water deprivation test. Am J Vet Res 48:1007, 1987.

70. Haskins SC. Fluid and electrolyte therapy. Compend Cont Educ Pract Vet 6:244, 1984.

71. Goodwin, J-K, Schaer M. Septic shock. In: Kirby R, Stamp GL, eds. Critical care, veterinary clinics of north america: small animal practice. Philadelphia: WB Saunders, 1989.

72. Roussel AJ. Fluid therapy in mature cattle. In: Roussel AJ, ed. Fluid and electrolyte therapy, veterinary clinics of north america: food animal practice. Philadelphia: WB Saunders, 1990.

73. McDonell WN. General anesthesia for equine gastrointestinal and obstetric procedures. In: Steffey EP, ed. Equine anesthesia, veterinary clinics of north america: large animal practice. Philadelphia: WB Saunders, 1981.

74. Gaukroger PB, Roberts JG, Manners TA. Infusion thrombophlebitis: a prospective comparison of 645 Vialon and Teflon cannulae in anaesthetic and postoperative use. Anaesth Intensive Care 16:265, 1988.

75. Jones BR, Scheller MS. Flow increases with an enlarging intravenous catheter. J Clin Anesth 4:120, 1992.

76. Abou-Madi N. Avian Fluid Therapy. Proceedings of the Ninth Annual Veterinary Medical Forum. Madison, WI: Omnipress, 1991.

77. Redig PT. Fluid therapy and acid-base balance in the critically ill avian patient. Proceedings of the International Conference on Avian Medicine. Toronto: Am Assoc Avian Vet, 1984.

78. Crow SE, Walshaw SO. Manual of clinical procedures in the dog and cat. Philadelphia: JB Lippincott, 1987.

79. Bayly WM, Vale BH. Intravenous catheterization and associated problems in the horse. Compend Cont Educ Pract Vet 4:S227, 1982.

80. Spurlock SL, Spurlock GH, Parker G, Ward MV. Long-term jugular vein catheterization in horses. J Am Vet Med Assoc 196:425, 1990.

81. Deem DA. Complications associated with the use of intravenous catheters in large animals. Calif Vet 6:19, 1981.

82. Spurlock SL, Spurlock GH. Risk factors of catheter related complications. Compend Cont Educ Pract Vet 12:241, 1990.

83. Fulton RB, Hauptman JG. In vitro and in vivo rates of fluid flow through catheters in peripheral veins of dogs. J Am Vet Med Assoc 198:1622, 1991.

84. Aeschbacher G, Webb AI. Intraosseous infusion during cardiopulmonary resuscitation. Vet Surg 20:159, 1991.

85. Hoelzer MF. Recent advances in intravenous therapy. Emerg Med Clin North Am 4:487, 1986.

86. Otto CM, Crow DT. Intraosseous resuscitation techniques and applications. In: Kirk RW, Bonagura JD, eds. Current veterinary therapy xi, small animal practice. Philadelphia: WB Saunders, 1992.

87. Cotter SM, Rentko VT. Blood substitutes. Proceedings of the Ninth Annual Veterinary Medical Forum. Madison, WI: Omnipress, 1991.

88. Gould SA, Sehgal LR, Sehgal HL, Moss GS. Artificial blood: current status of hemoglobin solutions. Crit Care Clin 8:293, 1992.

89. George LW. Diseases of the nervous system. In: Smith BP, ed. Large animal internal medicine. Philadelphia: CV Mosby, 1990.

90. Meuten DJ, Chew DJ, Capen CC, Kociba GJ. Relationship of serum total calcium to albumin and total protein in dogs. J Am Vet Med Assoc 180:63, 1982.

91. Flanders JA, Scarlett JM, Blue JT, Neth S. Adjustment of total serum calcium concentration for binding to albumin and protein in cats: 291 cases (1986–1987). J Am Vet Med Assoc 194:1609, 1989.

92. Cote CJ, Drop LJ, Daniels AL. Treatment of citrate-induced hypocalcemia in dogs: comparative response to calcium chloride and calcium gluconate. Anesth Analg 64:203, 1985.

93. Armstrong J, Meuten DJ. Parathyroid disease and calcium metabolism. In: Ettinger SJ, ed. Textbook of veterinary internal medicine, diseases of the dog and cat, 3rd ed. Philadelphia: WB Saunders, 1989.

94. Yates DJ, Hunt E. Disorders of calcium metabolism. In: Smith BP, ed. Large animal internal medicine. Philadelphia: CV Mosby, 1990.

95. Muir WW, Wagner AE, Buchanan C. Effects of acute hyperventilation on serum potassium in the dog. Vet Surg 19:83, 1990.

96. Vitez TS, Soper LE, Wong KC, Soper P. Chronic hypokalemia and intraoperative dysrhythmias. Anesthesia 63:130, 1985.

section *VII*

ANESTHESIA AND IMMOBILIZATION OF SPECIFIC SPECIES

chapter **20**A

DOGS AND CATS

Richard M. Bednarski

Introduction

The selection of a particular anesthetic drug or anesthetic regimen is predicated upon the patient's physical status and temperament, the type of procedure for which anesthesia is being considered, the familiarity of the anesthetist with the anesthetic drugs, the type of facility and available equipment, the personnel available for assistance, and the cost of anesthetic drugs (Chapter 2). There is no single best method for anesthetizing dogs or cats, and familiarity with just one anesthetic technique at best limits the veterinarian's ability to perform the myriad of surgical and diagnostic procedures commonly performed in a modern veterinary practice. A debilitated dog or cat undergoing extensive repair of a fractured limb will require a different anesthetic regimen than one undergoing routine neutering, one requiring short-term restraint for radiography or ultrasonography, or the geriatric patient requiring extensive dental manipulations. Some breeds respond atypically to routine administration of an anesthetic drug. The sight hounds tolerate less thiobarbiturate than comparably sized mixed-breed dogs.(1)

This is due to a lack of body fat, which slows thiobarbiturate redistribution as well as their atypical hepatic metabolism of the barbiturates (see Chapter 9).(2) Therefore, the anesthetist must be familiar with an alternative to the thiobarbiturates for short-term chemical restraint. As a general rule, when formulating an anesthetic plan it is best to consider using relatively low doses of several different drugs rather than a large dose of a single drug. For example, xylazine is a good sedative, muscle relaxant, and analgesic, but if it is used alone to produce sufficient immobilization for a major surgical procedure, the large dose required would produce significant and unacceptable cardiopulmonary depression. The apnea resulting from a large bolus of thiobarbiturate can be eliminated or its duration shortened by prior administration of a tranquilizer such as acepromazine, which allows for the administration of a lower barbiturate dose.

The one thing that should not vary among anesthetic procedures is the degree of vigilance associated with monitoring the anesthetized dog or cat. Early warning of impending anesthetic difficulty is the single most

591

important factor responsible for decreasing anesthetic related morbidity and mortality (Chapter 2).

Preanesthetic Considerations

A thorough history and physical examination are the most important components of the preanesthetic evaluation. Even young, seemingly healthy, animals presented for routine neutering require a history and physical examination. These animals may have never been previously examined by a veterinarian, and congenital disorders, severe parasitism, or heartworm disease may be discovered.

SIGNALMENT

The importance of identifying breed idiosyncrasies to certain anesthetic drugs was emphasized earlier. Most breed-related anesthesia problems are anecdotally reported. Anesthesiologists are often queried about "sensitivity to anesthesia" in a variety of dog and cat breeds, including, but not limited to, soft-coated wheaten terriers, the Chinese shar pei, collies, the Belgian breeds, and among cats, the Maine coon. All breeds have been successfully anesthetized using standard anesthetic regimens. Other than the sensitivity of sight hounds to barbiturates, brachycephalic breeds and their associated airway problems can present anesthetic challenges. Toy breeds require special attention to maintenance of body heat. Furthermore, a toy breed will require a relatively greater drug dose per kilogram than a giant breed. Generally there is no sex-related difference in the response to anesthesia. However, a history of the estrous cycle will identify recent estrus and its associated enlarged and vascularized uterus. This would potentially cause concern regarding blood loss during an ovariohysterectomy. These patients should have an intravenous cannula inserted for crystalloid administration. Age is an important anesthetic consideration. Generally the very young (less than 11 weeks) and the aged (more than 80% of the expected life span) do not metabolize anesthetic drugs as well as the young, healthy patient (Chapter 24). Healthy geriatric patients should receive sedatives, hypnotics, and tranquilizers at 15 to 30% of the dose given to a comparable young healthy animal. Geriatric dogs and cats should receive intravenous fluids perioperatively to maintain optimal perfusion of the vital organs (Chapter 19).

HISTORY

In addition to questions concerning organ system function (Table 20A–1) the owner should be queried regarding any previous anesthetic episodes and past and current medication history (Chapter 3) including history of heartworm prophylaxis. The duration since the last feeding should be noted.

PHYSICAL EXAMINATION

The preanesthetic physical examination should be thorough, with all body systems considered (Table 20A–2). Any abnormality discovered by physical exami-

Table 20A–1.   Signalment and History, Including Questions of Organ System Function

A. Signalment
  1. Age
  2. Breed
  3. Sex
B. Body weight
C. Duration of ongoing complaint
D. Concurrent medications
  1. Organophosphates
  2. H$_2$ blockers
  3. Antibiotics: Aminoglycosides, chloramphenicol
  4. Cardiac glycosides
  5. Phenobarbital
  6. NSAIDs
  7. Calcium channel blockers
  8. Beta blockers
E. Signs of organ system disease
  1. Diarrhea
  2. Vomiting
  3. Polyuria-polydipsia
  4. Seizures, personality change
  5. Exercise intolerance
  6. Coughing, stridor
  7. Weight loss, loss of body condition
F. Previous anesthesia and allergies
G. Duration since last meal

Table 20A–2.   Preanesthesia Physical Examination

A. Body weight and body condition
  1. Obesity
  2. Cachexia
  3. Dehydration
B. Cardiopulmonary
  1. Heart rate and rhythm
  2. Auscultation
      Heart sounds and murmurs
      Breath sounds
  3. Capillary refill time
  4. Mucous membrane color
      Pallor
      Cyanosis
  5. Pulse character
C. CNS and special senses
  1. Temperament
  2. Seizure, coma, stupor
  3. Vision, hearing
D. Gastrointestinal
  1. Parasites
  2. Abdominal palpation
E. Hepatic
  1. Icterus
  2. Abnormal bleeding
F. Renal
  1. Palpate kidneys and bladder
G. Integument
  1. Tumors
  2. Flea infestation
H. Musculoskeletal
  1. Lameness
  2. Fractures

nation or suggested by the medical history should be followed with appropriate laboratory or other suitable diagnostic testing. The assessment of the animal's temperament is critical. The vicious or aggressive dog will require a different approach to anesthesia than the quiet relaxed individual.

LABORATORY EVALUATION

The minimum laboratory data required for young healthy dogs are hematocrit (packed cell volume) and plasma protein. These tests are easily, quickly, and inexpensively performed. Packed cell volume is an indicator of hemoglobin concentration. Hemoglobin (g/dL) is approximated by PCV/3. Middle–aged to older animals should have a blood dipstick test performed for BUN. If the results are out of the normal range, a more accurate test for BUN should be performed. Other laboratory tests should be performed if the history or physical examination suggests organ system disease.

Physical Status

Patients should be classified according to relative anesthetic risk. A convenient system of classification has been adapted from the American Society of Anesthesiologists (Chapter 2).(3) Physical status I and II patients are those with less risk for anesthetic complications. Physical statuses III through V indicate relatively greater anesthetic risk. However, this is not to imply that category I and II patients are at no risk from unanticipated anesthetic mishaps.

I. Normal healthy patient
II. Incapacitating systemic disease (e.g., obesity, simple fractures)
III. Severe systemic disease not incapacitating (e.g., compensated renal insufficiency, stable congestive heart failure, controlled diabetes mellitus, cesarean section)
IV. Severe systemic disease that is a constant threat to life (e.g., gastric dilation, volvulus)
V. Moribund, not expected to live 24 hours irrespective of intervention (e.g., severe uncompensated systemic disturbance).

Patient Preparation

FASTING

Healthy dogs and cats should receive no food for at least 6 hours prior to being anesthetized. Water should be allowed free choice until just prior to anesthesia. Dogs and cats less than 8 weeks old and those weighing less than 2 kg should not be fasted longer than 1 or 2 hours (Chapter 24). They should also receive dextrose containing intravenous fluids during any prolonged anesthesia (greater than 15 minutes).

PATIENT STABILIZATION

When possible, life-threatening disturbances should be corrected prior to anesthesia (Table 20A–3). This may not be possible, however, and anesthesia should never

Table 20A–3. A List of Conditions that Should be Corrected Prior to Anesthesia

A. Severe dehydration
B. Anemia or hypoproteinemia
   PCV < 20 with acute blood loss
   Albumin < 2.0 g/dL
C. Acid-base and electrolyte disturbances
   pH < 7.2
   Potassium < 2.5–3.0 or >6.0
D. Pneumothorax
E. Cyanosis
F. Oliguria or anuria
G. Congestive heart failure
H. Severe, life-threatening cardiac arrhythmias

be delayed if immediate surgical or medical intervention is the only way to save the patient's life.

VENOUS ACCESS

Advantages to inserting an intravenous catheter into a peripheral vein include these: tissue-toxic drugs such as the thiobarbiturates can be administered without fear of perivascular administration, intravenous fluid administration is facilitated, and the circulation is immediately accessible for administration of emergency drugs. The most common site for catheter insertion is the cephalic vein. The lateral and medial saphenous veins are also easily accessible. The jugular vein can also be used. Typically an over-the-needle style of catheter, which is relatively inexpensive, is most suitable. A 20-gauge, 2-inch catheter is suitable for most dogs and cats weighing more than 2 kg, and a 22-gauge, 1.25-inch catheter is suitable for those that are smaller. An 18-gauge catheter can be used in medium to large dogs if more rapid fluid administration is needed.

INTRAVENOUS FLUIDS

The purpose of perianesthetic administration of intravenous fluids is to maintain vascular volume, which is decreased as a result of anesthetic drugs, blood loss, and insensible fluid loss. For routine use a balanced electrolyte solution such as lactated Ringer's solution is most suitable, as most fluid loss during anesthesia is isotonic. The patient's disease process may warrant the use of other fluids such as normal saline, fluids containing dextrose, or a colloid solution such as whole blood, plasma, or a plasma expander (Chapters 18 and 19). Routine crystalloid administration rate is 10 mL $\cdot$ kg^{-1} $\cdot$ h^{-1}. This rate can be decreased to 5 mL $\cdot$ kg^{-1} $\cdot$ h^{-1} for the second and subsequent hours of anesthesia if the surgical procedure is associated with minimal blood loss. A rate of 20 mL $\cdot$ kg^{-1} $\cdot$ h^{-1} is suitable if mild dehydration is present.

Several styles of fluid administration sets are available. An administration set with a 10 drop/mL drip chamber is most convenient for patients weighing greater than 5 kg. For smaller patients a 60 drop/mL drip chamber allows a more precise estimation of proper fluid rate. It is convenient to calculate the number of drops/min necessary to deliver the calculated hourly fluid amount. An example follows using a 10 drop/mL drip set in a 25 kg dog at a rate of $10 \text{ mL} \cdot \text{kg}^{-1} \cdot \text{h}^{-1}$.

$$25 \text{ Kg} \times 10 \text{ mL/kg/h} = 250 \text{ mL/h}$$

$$250 \text{ mL/h} \times 10 \text{ drops/mL} = 2500 \text{ drops/h}$$

$$2500 \text{ drops/h/60 min} = 42 \text{ drops/min}$$

A danger of perioperative fluid administration to very small animals is inadvertently administering too much fluid by improperly adjusting the drip rate. This problem can be minimized by attaching a measured volume administration set to the fluid line.

The Anesthetic Plan

Several things should be considered when selecting an anesthetic plan (Table 20A–4). In general terms the anesthetic technique will be one relying primarily on local anesthesia, injectable anesthesia, or inhalation anesthesia. These techniques can overlap. For example, inhalation anesthesia is usually initiated with injectable anesthetics, and local anesthesia is usually accompanied by mild to strong sedation. Local anesthetic techniques are used more frequently in dogs than in cats. Those techniques most commonly used include lumbosacral epidural blocks, local infiltration or "line" blocks, and Bier blocks. Refer to Chapter 16 for further information. The remainder of the discussion regarding the choice of anesthetic drugs assumes the reader has reviewed and has a familiarity with the pharmacology of the

Table 20A–4. Considerations for Selecting an Anesthetic Plan

A. Procedure to be performed
   Duration
      <15 minutes
      15 minutes to 1 hour
      >1 hour
   Type of procedure
      Minor medical or surgical
      Major invasive surgery
      Anticipated post surgical pain
B. Available assistance and equipment
   Assistance
      Ventilatory assist or control
      Restraint
   Equipment
      Anesthetic machine
      Type of inhalation anesthetic
C. Temperament of the patient
   Quiet, relaxed, calm
   Nervous, excitable
   Vicious
   Moribund, comatose
D. Physical status
   ASA category I–V
E. Breed
   Sight hounds
   Brachycephalic
   Toy breeds

various anesthetic drugs (Section 3). Although the drug combinations described are suitable for a variety of patients the reader should refer to the appropriate sections for management of patients with organ system dysfunction and other special situations (Chapters 23 and 24).

LESS THAN 15 MINUTES

Several drugs are available for short-term restraint (Tables 20A–5 to 20A–8). The thiobarbiturates are relatively inexpensive and are suitable for short-term restraint of most healthy dogs and cats. The disadvantage to their use is that full recovery usually takes up to an hour and can be associated with ataxia and disorientation. These effects are reduced when the thiobarbiturate is preceded by a tranquilizer such as acepromazine. Another disadvantage is that they must be administered intravenously, a problem with fractious or uncooperative animals. Alternatives to the thiobarbiturates include propofol, etomidate, and the combination of diazepam and ketamine. These are more expensive than the thiobarbiturates, and the duration after one bolus dose is shorter, generally less than 10 minutes. Preceding these drugs with a sedative or tranquilizer such as acepromazine, xylazine, or diazepam decreases their dosage and improves the quality of recovery.(4, 5)

Neuroleptanalgesic combinations are suitable for short-term restraint for mildly invasive procedures or those procedures not requiring general anesthesia. An advantage is that one or both components of neuroleptanalgesia are reversible, allowing rapid return to preanesthetic mentation (Table 20A–9).

The relatively cumbersome nature of inhalation anesthesia makes it less suitable for very short procedures. The rapid induction and recovery associated with isoflurane, however, make it the most suitable of the commonly available inhalants for short-term restraint (Chapter 11).

FIFTEEN MINUTES TO ONE HOUR

For procedures of intermediate duration, the drugs described earlier can be used and redosed to effect. Typically one third to one half of the original dose is administered to prolong the anesthetic effect. The thiobarbiturates should not be repeatedly redosed, however. Although their initial duration of action primarily depends on redistribution away from the brain to other tissues such as muscle, when these tissues are saturated, metabolism ultimately is responsible for awakening. Again, inhalation anesthesia is also appropriate for procedures of intermediate duration.

GREATER THAN ONE HOUR

Procedures of long duration are best managed with inhalation anesthesia. Awakening from halothane and isoflurane anesthesia is predictably rapid. Even sick and debilitated patients recover from prolonged periods of inhalation anesthesia relatively quickly.

Table 20A–5. Sedatives and Tranquilizers

Drug	Dosage (mg/kg)*	Comments
Acepromazine	0.025–0.2 IV, IM, SQ (3–4 mg maximum)	Mild to moderate sedation of 1- to 2-h duration
Xylazine	0.3–2.2 IV, IM	Moderate to deep sedation, analgesia; 20 min to 1 h
Medetomidine	Dogs 0.01–0.05 IV, IM Cats 0.05–0.12 IV, IM	Similar effects to xylazine but 1- to 3-h duration
Diazepam	0.2–0.4, IV, IM	Most useful when combined with other sedatives, opioids, or ketamine; Avoid IM in cats and small dogs
Midazolam	0.1–0.3 IV, IM, SQ	Similar to diazepam but also useful IM or SC

*Generally the low end of the dosage range is used IV and in sick or debilitated patients.

Table 20A–6. Opioids and Neuroleptanalgesia

Drug(s)	Dosage (mg/kg)*	Comments
Oxymorphone	0.05–0.1 IV, IM, SQ	Excitement when used alone in young healthy dogs; duration of analgesia is 1–4 h
Morphine	0.2–0.6 IM, SQ	Mild sedation when used alone; duration of analgesia is 1–4 h
Butorphanol	0.2–0.4 IV, IM, SQ	Minimal sedation when used alone; duration of analgesia is 1–3 h
Fentanyl/Droperidol (Innovar-Vet)	1 mL per 10–30 kg, IV, IM	Excellent for aggressive dogs; dose-dependent sedation (30 min–1 h)
Acepromazine/Oxymorphone	0.05/0.05–0.1 IV, IM	Can be combined in same syringe; sedation lasts 15 min–1 h
Acepromazine/Butorphanol	0.05/0.2 IV, IM	Can be combined in same syringe; sedation lasts 15 min–1 h
Acepromazine/Buprenorphine	0.03/0.01 IV	Moderate sedation for 2–3 h
Midazolam/Oxymorphone	0.1–0.2/0.05–0.1 IV, IM	Can be combined in same syringe; sedation lasts 15–40 min
Midazolam/Butorphanol	0.1–0.2/0.2 IV, IM	Can be combined in same syringe; sedation lasts 15–40 min
Xylazine/Oxymorphone	0.4–0.6/0.05–0.1 IV, IM	Both drugs are reversible; sedation lasts 30–40 min
Xylazine/Butorphanol	0.4–0.6/0.2–0.4 IV, IM	Both drugs are reversible; sedation lasts 30–40 min

*Use low end of opioid dosage in cats.

Table 20A–7. Cyclohexylamines and Cyclohexylamine Combinations

Drug(s)	Dosage (mg/kg)	Comments
Ketamine	2.0–10.0 IV, IM	Not useful alone in dogs. Useful restraint in cats lasts 5–30 min
Ketamine/Diazepam and Ketamine/Midazolam	5.5/0.20 IV	Diazepam and midazolam are equally effective in this combination; useful restraint lasts 5–10 min; poor muscle relaxation and analgesia
Ketamine/Xylazine	10.0/0.7–1.0	Useful restraint lasts 20–40 min
Ketamine/Acepromazine	10.0/0.2	Useful restraint lasts 20–30 min
Tiletamine/Zolazepam (Telazol)	2.0–8.0 IV, IM	Limited shelf-life after reconstitution; useful restraint for 20 min to 1 h

Table 20A–8. Injectable Anesthetic Drugs and Drug Combinations*

Drug	Dosage (mg/kg)	Comments
Thiamylal	6.0–15.0 IV	Use lower dosage after premedication
Thiopental	8.0–20.0 IV	Use lower dosage after premedication
Methohexital	3.0–8.0 IV	Muscle rigidity; best if preceded by a tranquilizer or sedative; 3–5 min duration
Etomidate	0.5–2.0 IV	Duration 5–10 min; myoclonus, gagging/retching
Propofol	4.0–6.0 IV 0.4–0.8 mg/kg/min	Duration 5–10 min after single bolus dose; apnea for several minutes with rapid injection
Xylazine/Midazolam/Butorphanol	0.4/1.0/0.1 IV	Effects of all 3 drugs are reversible; duration 30–40 min

*Injectable combinations using ketamine are listed in Table 20A–7.

Table 20A–9. Antagonists of Various Classes of Anesthetic Drugs

Drug	Dosage (mg/kg)
Alpha₂	
Yohimbine	0.1 IV, IM
Atipamezole	0.04–0.5 IM
Benzodiazepine	
Flumazenil	0.2–5.0 IV
Opioid	
Naloxone	0.003–0.01 IV, IM

Table 20A–10. Suggestions for Premedication in Dogs and Cats

Dogs	Premedication
Young normal healthy:	Acepromazine Xylazine Acepromazine/Oxymorphone Acepromazine/Butorphanol
Aggressive/vicious:	Innovar-Vet Acepromazine/Oxymorphone Telazol
Geriatric:	Acepromazine Diazepam Midazolam/Oxymorphone Midazolam/Butorphanol
Painful procedures:	Acepromazine/Oxymorphone Acepromazine/Butorphanol Midazolam/Oxymorphone Midazolam/Butorphanol
Cats	Acepromazine/Oxymorphone Ketamine Ketamine/Acepromazine Xylazine

All can be given IM or SQ except diazepam, which should be given IV immediately preceding the induction drug.

Premedication

Inhalation anesthesia can be initiated without premedication; however, premedication with a sedative, tranquilizer, or other injectable drug (Table 20A–5 and 20A–6) is recommended. Preanesthetic drugs aid in restraint, reduce apprehension, decrease the quantity of potentially more dangerous drugs used to produce general anesthesia, facilitate induction, enhance analgesia, and reduce autonomic reflex activity (Chapter 8). Drugs for premedication are usually administered intramuscularly or subcutaneously 15 to 20 minutes before induction. The choice of premedication depends on species, temperament, physical status, the procedure to be performed, and personal preference (Table 20A–10). For procedures associated with significant postoperative pain, premedication should include an analgesic such as an opioid or alpha₂-agonist. Less postoperative analgesics are needed when analgesia is provided before initiation of a painful stimulus (preemptive analgesia) (Chapter 4).(6)

Induction

Induction is most easily accomplished with an ultrashort-acting barbiturate or other equally short-acting drug (Table 20A–8). Advantages to this method of induction include rapid loss of consciousness and ability to quickly intubate. Alternatives to this rapid induction include chamber or mask induction, or opioid induction. These techniques can be useful in special circumstances but for routine use their disadvantages outweigh their advantages.(7, 8)

CHAMBER/MASK

A disadvantage to chamber and mask induction is the associated waste gas pollution (Chapter 14). Another disadvantage to chamber/mask induction in nonpremedicated healthy animals is the struggling and associated stress during the induction phase. Mask induction is most easily accomplished in moribund animals, tractable dogs, and those that have been adequately sedated. Chamber induction is most useful in cats or tiny dogs. Isoflurane and halothane are most suitable because they produce a relatively rapid induction. Relatively high oxygen flow rates (4 L/min for chamber, 3 L/min for mask) and vaporizer settings (4% halothane or isoflurane in healthy animals) are used. The use of nitrous oxide is not necessary during chamber or mask induction. During chamber induction, once the animal loses its righting reflex and is unresponsive when the chamber is tilted from side to side, the animal is removed from the chamber and induction is continued using an appropriately sized mask. Mask induction is begun by exposing the animal to the mask and oxygen. The inhalation concentration is slowly increased to 4%. This is accomplished with a nonrebreathing or rebreathing circuit by gradually increasing the vaporizer setting from 0 to 4% over 2 to 3 minutes. The vaporizer can be initially set to 4% if a circle system is used, since the concentration within the circle gradually increases with time.

OPIOID

A disadvantage to opioid induction is the attendant relatively slow loss of consciousness. Advantages include good cardiovascular stability and the attenuation of the stress response associated with anesthesia and surgery. Opioid induction works best in debilitated dogs and is not recommended in cats or young healthy dogs that are not well sedated. Low doses of oxymorphone or fentanyl (Table 20A–6) are alternated with low doses of diazepam or midazolam (Table 20A–5) until the dog can be intubated.

Maintenance

The maintenance phase of anesthesia begins when unconsciousness is induced and continues through the time the patient is disconnected from the anesthesia breathing circuit. After the loss of consciousness a properly sized cuffed endotracheal tube or alternative airway is inserted (Chapter 17). Adequate cardiovascular function is verified and the anesthetic vaporizer turned on. The initial and subsequent anesthetic vaporizer settings (Table 20A–11) vary with the condition of the patient, the type of vaporizer used, the type of breathing circuit used, and the fresh gas flow rate (Chapter 14). The relatively high fresh gas flow rate and vaporizer setting that are initially used after induction

are decreased to maintenance settings when the palpebral reflex disappears and the heart rate begins to decrease. The vaporizer setting is adjusted according to signs of anesthetic depth. The most useful signs of anesthetic depth in the dog and cat include muscle tone (assessed by opening the mouth its full extent), heart and respiratory rates, and systemic blood pressure. All but systemic blood pressure are easily and inexpensively monitored and should be performed routinely (Chapters 2 and 15). An anesthetic record should be maintained and should include notation of patient status, the anesthetic drugs used including dose and effect, the duration of the surgery, and notation of significant perioperative events. Ideally, heart rate, respiratory rate, blood pressure, and any other monitored variables should be recorded at regular intervals. Recording this data at regular intervals creates a visual aid that assists in determining the change in patient status over the course of the anesthetic episode. For example, a decrease in heart rate and blood pressure during a 15-minute interval could signal increasing anesthetic depth and should signal a decrease in vaporizer setting. This change with time is easily observed on the anesthetic record but may not be noticed without the visual prompt of the record (Chapter 2).

Recovery

Recovery begins when the procedure for which the patient has been anesthetized is finished and the anesthetic drugs have been discontinued. Monitoring patient status should occur regularly during recovery until the patient is alert and extubated, and heart rate, respiratory rate, and body temperature have returned to normal. Young healthy animals undergoing routine procedures need not receive supplemental oxygen during recovery unless nitrous oxide was used. If nitrous oxide was used, the breathing circuit should be repeatedly flushed with oxygen and the patient should be allowed to breathe an oxygen enriched gas mixture for the first 5 to 10 minutes. This helps prevent diffusion hypoxia (Chapter 11). Sick or debilitated dogs or cats benefit from supplemental oxygen during recovery, particularly if shivering is present, as shivering significantly increases oxygen consumption. The endotracheal tube cuff should be deflated and the gauze se-curing the tube should be untied when the patient is disconnected from the anesthetic machine. This permits extubation in the event that the patient rapidly awakens and begins chewing. Similarly, if an esophageal stethoscope was used it should be removed at this time. Dogs and cats should be extubated as soon as the swallowing reflex occurs, unless there is some specific contraindication to removing the endotracheal tube at this time (Chapters 23 and 24). Dogs and cats should never be unobserved if the endotracheal tube is still in place. Recovery should occur in a well-ventilated room, since the inhalation anesthetics are exhaled at that time.

Table 20A–11. Vaporizer Settings*

Drug	Induction Phase	Maintenance Phase
Vaporizer out of Circle†		
Isoflurane	3–4	1.5–3.0
Halothane	3	1.0–2.0
Methoxyflurane	3	0.5–1.5
Enflurane	4–5	2.5–4.0
Vaporizer in Circle‡		
Isoflurane	2/3 open	1/8–1/2 open
Halothane	2/3 open	1/8–1/2 open
Methoxyflurane	2/3 to full open	1/8–1/2 open

*Listed vaporizer settings assume a fresh gas flow of 1–2 L/min during the induction phase and a fresh gas flow of 10 mL/kg/min during the maintenance phase. Low-flow system vaporizer settings are typically 1 to 2% higher.

†Numbers listed are %.

‡Vaporizer in circle refers to the Stephens vaporizer or the Ohio 8 vaporizer. The wick in these vaporizers is used only for methoxyflurane.

Occasionally a dog or cat will awaken from anesthesia disoriented and will vocalize, paddle, and appear incoherent. This is most often caused by emergence delirium or pain. Emergence delirium occurs most frequently in nonpremedicated animals and in particular those awakening rapidly from anesthesia. With emergence delirium the dog or cat will usually become quiet and more comfortable within a short time, usually within 10 minutes. A quiet reassuring voice and restraint are all that is usually necessary to guide the animal through this period of excitement. Occasionally a low dose of acepromazine (0.05 mg/kg IV) is necessary to quiet the animal. If the apparent excitement is due to post operative pain the animal should receive a systemic analgesic or some other analgesic technique (Chapters 4, 16, 24).

Some loss of body heat is unavoidable during anesthesia and surgery, and the patient should be warmed during recovery.(9) Devices are available for patient warming. These include circulating warm water heating blankets, infrared heat lamps, incubators, and circulating warm air blankets. Electric heating pads should never be used, since they have been associated with severe burns.(10) These burns usually are manifest from several days to a week after contact with the heating pad. The burn pattern often traces the pattern of the heating wire within the blanket. Care must be used with heat lamps, since they also have produced thermal burns by being placed too close to unprotected skin. An advantage of using warm water heating blankets is that temperature is uniform over their entire surface and their maximum temperature is well below 105° F, the maximum safe patient heating-source interface.(10) Warming will be hastened if the patient is cocooned within the warm water heating blanket. Incubators are convenient for warming small dogs and cats, and if needed, supplemental oxygen can also be introduced through the incubator during the warming period. Circulating warm air blankets that cocoon the patient are the most effective devices for postoperative warming.(11)

References

1. Robinson EP, Sams RA, Muir WW. Barbiturate anesthesia in greyhound and mixed-breed dogs: comparative cardiopulmonary effects, anesthetic effects, and recovery rates. Am J Vet Res 47:2105, 1986.
2. Sams RA, Muir WW. Effects of phenobarbital on thiopental pharmacokinetics in greyhounds. Am J Vet Res 49:245, 1988.
3. Dripps RD, Lamont A, Eckenhoff JE. The role of anesthesia in surgical mortality. J Am Med Assoc 178:261, 1961.
4. Smith JA, Gaynor JS, Bednarski RM, Muir WW. Adverse effects of administration of propofol with various preanesthetic regimens in dogs. J Am Vet Med Assoc 202:1111, 1993.
5. Heard DJ, Webb AI, Daniels AA. Effect of acepromazine on the anesthetic requirement of halothane in the dog. Am J Vet Res 47:2113, 1986.
6. Woolf CF, Chong M. Preemptive analgesia–treating postoperative pain by preventing the establishment of central sensitization. Anesth Analg 77:362, 1993.
7. Bednarski RM. Precautions when using opioid agonists for induction of anesthesia. Vet Clin North Am Small Anim Pract 22:273, 1992.
8. Harvey RC. Precautions when using mask induction. Vet Clin North Am Small Anim Pract 22:310, 1992.
9. Imrie MM, Hall GM. Body temperature and anaesthesia. Br J Anaesth 64:346, 1990.
10. Swaim SF, Lee AH, Hughes KS. Heating pads and thermal burns in small animals. J Am Anim Hosp Assoc 25:156, 1989.
11. Hynson J, Sessler DI. Comparison of intraoperative warming devices. Anesth Analg 72:S118, 1991.

chapter 20 B

HORSES

John A. E. Hubbell

Introduction

Anesthesia in adult horses is complicated by a relatively unique set of problems associated with their temperament, large body mass, and thoracoabdominal anatomy. Thus, although an understanding of the pharmacology of the drugs used is essential for safe anesthetic practice, the knowledge base must not stop there. Prolonged recumbency is an unnatural position for the horse. This, coupled with the horse's seeming desire to escape unfamiliar situations by running, makes induction and recovery from anesthesia difficult. In addition, the potential for inadequate muscle blood flow and deleterious changes in cardiopulmonary function associated with lateral and dorsal recumbency must be understood. Thus, although the science of anesthesia in horses has progressed rapidly, the skill and art of the anesthetist remains a significant component of good practice. The pharmacology of the various drugs used in the horse is discussed in Chapters 8 to 13. This chapter will focus on practical aspects of handling horses and the use of specific drugs, alone and in combination.

Physical Restraint

Prior to the development of appropriate sedatives, tranquilizers, and other anesthetics, physical restraint was a primary method by which practitioners accomplished the treatment and the completion of some surgical and diagnostic techniques. With the advent of useful anesthetics the reliance on physical restraint has diminished, but the techniques remain an integral part of safe equine practice. Physical restraint may be as innocuous as taking hold of a horse's halter or picking up a leg to limit patient movement. Historically, the limits of physical restraint have been left to the discretion of the handler and veterinarian. Currently, techniques such as casting horses without tranquilization have been and should continue to be reexamined as to their humaneness. In most situations, some level of physical restraint is combined with appropriate drugs to induce a tractable patient. The method of physical restraint should be based on (a) the age, size, and temperament of the horse; (b) the physical status; (c) the number and training of available personnel; and (d) the duration and nature of the procedure (Chapter 2).

Methods of Drug Delivery

Anesthetics are administered to horses by topical, oral, subcutaneous, intramuscular, epidural, intravenous, and inhalant routes. The effective application of topical anesthetics is probably limited to the eye and mucous membranes (Chapter 12). Oral formulations for tranquilization can be mixed with feed but are somewhat unpredictable because the potential for limited consumption and absorption makes it difficult to predict the timing and magnitude of the effects produced.

Intramuscular injection is more effective than subcutaneous injection. Sedatives and tranquilizers are often administered intramuscularly because of ease of administration, longer duration of action, and a decrease in the intensity of deleterious side effects when compared to intravenous administration. Disadvantages of intramuscular administration of drugs include delayed onset of action, decreased intensity of effect, and (because a larger quantity of drug is required) increased cost. Epidural injection of drugs that induce analgesia can be used for analgesia. Drugs used by the epidural route include the local anesthetics, alpha$_2$-agonists, and opioids (Chapter 16). The intravenous route is preferred by most veterinary practitioners. Sedatives, tranquilizers, and injectable anesthetics (barbiturates, ketamine) can be administered intravenously. Intravenous injection induces rapid onset of action, higher peak intensity of effect, shorter durations of action, and a greater ability to titrate the desired effect by repeated administration. Inhalation anesthesia (e.g., halothane or isoflurane) requires the constant administration of drug that is delivered in oxygen (Chapter 11).

Equipment

The equipment required for the delivery of anesthetic to the equine patient varies from a syringe and needle to expensive inhalation anesthetic systems equipped with ventilators (Chapter 17). Most equine anesthesia is performed as short-term anesthesia in the field. In this setting the ability to supplement the inspired oxygen concentration of the patient is usually limited. In the absence of the ability to supplement inspired oxygen, time of recumbency should be limited to 1 hour. Oxygen supplementation benefits all anesthetized patients. Methods of supplementing oxygen in the field include the use of insufflation and the use of a demand valve (Fig. 20B–1). Insufflation is performed by inserting a tube into the horse's nose. Oxygen can be supplied in a small tank equipped with a pressure reducing valve and flowmeter. Flow should be set at a minimum of 15 L/min in order to be effective.(1) A size E oxygen cylinder contains approximately 650 liters of oxygen when full, so it can supply 40 to 45 minutes of oxygen. If apnea occurs, the flow rate can be increased and a breath can be delivered by occluding the nostrils until the thoracic wall rises appropriately, then releasing the nostrils to allow exhalation. Alternatively, a demand valve can be used. A demand valve delivers oxygen by one of two mechanisms. When the horse inhales the demand valve is triggered and delivers oxygen at high flow rates. The increased airway pressure generated by exhalation shuts the demand valve off. In the absence of ventilation, the demand valve can be triggered by the operator by pushing a button. The button is released upon appropriate chest excursion, the flow stops, and the patient exhales. A demand valve can be used with a tube that is inserted in the nostril and advanced in the airway (if the nostrils are occluded) but is best used in combination with an appropriately placed endotracheal tube.

Oxygenation should be maximized if extended anesthesia is contemplated. The best way to provide optimal oxygenation is to use an anesthetic machine in combination with an endotracheal tube that allows the airway to be sealed. Anesthetic machines for adult horses provide for the delivery of high oxygen concentrations (greater than 95%) whether or not inhalation anesthetics are being used. Oxygen flow rates to maintain high inspired oxygen concentrations are dependent on the horse's metabolic rate but are in the range of 2 to 5 L/min in the adult horse.

As previously stated, endotracheal tubes are helpful both in the field and in more sophisticated settings

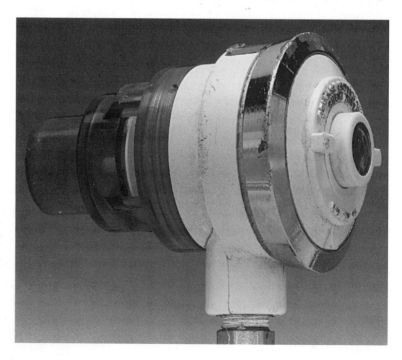

Fig. 20B–1. The demand valve (Hudson Demand Valve, Temecula, California) delivers oxygen at high flow rates (approximately 200 L/min) when the horse inspires. Alternatively, a tidal volume can be delivered by depressing a triggering button and watching the chest rise until a normal excursion has been completed. Although the valve does allow expiration to occur through its mechanism, respiratory resistance may be excessive, particularly in larger horses. In this instance, disconnect the demand valve to allow exhalation.

where inhalation anesthetics are employed. To be effective, endotracheal tubes should seal the airway. This is usually done by inflating a cuff. Alternatively, Cole endotracheal tubes utilize a tapered tip to seal the airway by producing a snug fit within the larynx (Chapter 17).

Endotracheal tubes are usually placed orally. The use of a bite block, easily made with 2-inch polyvinyl chloride pipe, will extend the life of the tube (Fig. 20B–2). Endotracheal tubes can also be placed via the ventral meatus of the nasal cavity. This route is particularly useful for intraoral surgery. Somewhat smaller endotracheal tubes should be used. Prior to anesthesia, the halter should be checked to make sure that it is appropriately applied and sufficiently strong to withstand the forces generated during induction and recovery.

Safe anesthesia in the horse depends on maintaining relatively light levels of anesthesia, which is sometimes

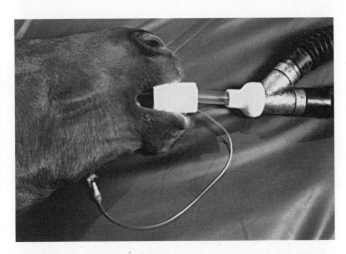

Fig. 20B–2. An inexpensive bite block for intubation of adult horses can be fashioned from 2-inch polyvinylchloride pipe. The endotracheal tube is advanced through the pipe. The pipe can be wrapped to reduce the chance of its inadvertently slipping out of the mouth.

difficult to assess. Should movement occur, control is important until additional anesthetic can be administered. The use of a chest rope (Fig. 20B–3) and casting harness or hobble system allows control of movement. A hobble system is easily devised by using a 35- to 40-foot length of 1-inch cotton rope. Soft, larger diameter rope is preferred because the chance for a rope burn is minimized.

Some anesthetic techniques require only drugs, needles, syringes, and the ability to effect a venipuncture. The placement of an intravenous catheter increases the safety of anesthesia by assuring venous access, ensuring (with proper placement) that medications are given intravenously, and reducing the number of venipunctures to one. Anesthetic agents, particularly the thiobarbiturates and to a lesser extent guaifenesin, are irritating and can cause tissue destruction when administered extravascularly. The relative guarantee of venous access is important when administering anesthetic agents because of the dilemmas faced when an anesthetic agent is administered to no apparent effect. The lack of effect could be caused by perivascular injection of the drug, administration of an inadequate dose, or an idiosyncratic reaction of the patient. The presence of a properly placed catheter gives assurance that the drug was administered intravascularly and allows for administration of additional drug if required. Useful catheter sizes for horses are 10 to 14 gauge for adult horses and 14 to 20 gauge for foals. The jugular vein is the usual site for catheterization. In the absence of patent jugular veins, the median, cephalic, lateral thoracic, or saphenous veins can be used. In those settings where inhalation anesthesia of horses for durations of greater than 1 hour is routine and frequent, additional equipment is required. The maintenance of adequate arterial blood pressure in the horse has been shown to correlate with a reduced number of post anesthetic complications. Arterial blood pressure can be measured inexpensively using an aneroid manometer following aseptic placement of a catheter (18 to 22

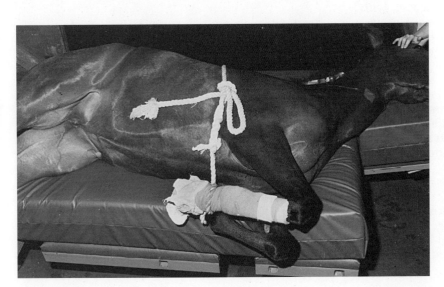

Fig. 20B–3. One-inch cotton rope is used to position and restrain the front legs of anesthetized horses. A "Tom Fool" knot is used to create a pair of hobbles. The hobbles are placed around the front legs just below the fetlocks and the free end of the rope is passed around the horse's chest. The rope is also useful if adjustments in body position must be made. The positioning of the legs reduces the weight placed on the forearms and shoulders by flexing the front legs. The hobbles should not be used as a replacement for appropriate levels of anesthesia.

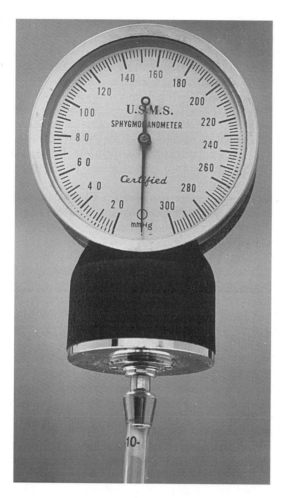

Fig. 20B–4. Aneroid manometers can be used to estimate mean arterial blood pressure in anesthetized horses. A length of noncompliant tubing and a three-way stopcock are adapted to the manometer. Following placement of a catheter into a peripheral artery, the manometer assembly is attached. The upward deflection of the needle is an indication of mean arterial blood pressure.

gauge) in a peripheral artery. Aneroid manometers allow estimation of mean arterial blood pressure (Fig. 20B–4).(2) At more expense, some oscilloscopes with blood pressure amplifiers allow measurement of systolic, mean, and diastolic blood pressures and may automatically display these values digitally. The maintenance of a mean arterial blood pressure greater than 60 to 70 mm Hg is associated with a reduction in postoperative complications, so the use of such devices and the correction of hypotension appears prudent.(3, 4) Appropriate padding helps to prevent pressure injury to muscle tissues. Commercially available foam rubber pads, air mattresses, and water mattresses can be used for this purpose.

Preparation of the Patient

A physical examination should be performed prior to the administration of any anesthetic drug. If the horse is only to be tranquilized, a brief physical examination should emphasize the cardiovascular and respiratory systems. If recumbency is to be induced, a more complete physical examination should be performed. A thorough evaluation of the respiratory system is warranted. Physical signs of respiratory disease include cough, discharge at the nostrils or eyes, submandibular lymph node enlargement, fever, and increases in respiratory rate. Auscultation should be performed over both sides of the thorax. Occlusion of the nostrils or the use of a plastic rebreathing bag in order to stimulate deep breathing allows a better evaluation of breath sounds. Palpation of the trachea and larynx may elicit a cough. Incipient respiratory disease can be further evaluated by performing a white blood cell count. White blood cell counts in excess of 12,000 to 14,000 cells/mL are cause for further evaluation. Serum fibrinogen levels can also be used as an index of systemic inflammation. Horses with respiratory infections should be allowed 3 weeks to recover prior to elective procedures. Many horses present with subclinical respiratory disease. General anesthesia has been associated with depression of immune function. A horse with subclinical respiratory disease could develop overt disease following anesthesia.

Respiratory stridor is another cause for concern. Most anesthetics cause relaxation of the muscles of the upper airway, particularly the nostrils. Relaxation of these muscles may allow the nostrils to sag inward on inhalation, partially occluding the airway. A tracheostomy should be performed prior to the induction of anesthesia if there is severe upper airway obstruction or if the nasal cavity will be occluded as part of the surgery. For example, surgical techniques for removal of the nasal septum and ethmoid hematomas require the placement of a absorbent pack in the nasal cavity in order to effect hemostasis. A tracheostomy is required

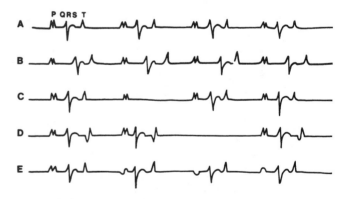

Fig. 20B–5. Normal physiologic cardiac rhythm variations in the horse. A, Normal sinus rhythm, base-apex lead. B, First-degree heart block. Note the extended P-R intervals. C, Second-degree heart block. Note the P wave not followed by a QRS complex. This arrhythmia should resolve with exercise. D, Sinus arrest or sinoatrial block. Note the lack of depolarization at regular intervals. The T-wave configuration is a normal variation. D, Sinus arrest or sinoatrial block. Note the lack of depolarization at regular intervals. The T-wave configuration is a normal variation. This arrhythmia should resolve with exercise. E, Wandering pacemaker. The P wave takes on variable configurations. (Reprinted with permission from Hubbell, J.A.E., Robertson, J.T., Muir, W.W., and Gabel, A.A. Perianesthetic considerations in the horse. Compend Contin Educ Pract Vet 6:S401, 1984.)

because horses are obligate nasal breathers.

The cardiovascular system is evaluated clinically by auscultating for heart sounds, palpating peripheral pulses, evaluating the color of mucous membranes, and assessing capillary refill time and skin turgor. Physical signs of cardiovascular abnormalities may include lack of exercise tolerance, distension of the jugular veins with and without jugular pulses, and pallor. Cardiac auscultation must be performed in a quiet environment. Heart rate should be determined and the presence or absence of pauses noted. Pauses should disappear if the horse is exercised briefly. Further evaluation of occasional pauses can be done with an electrocardiogram. Common physiologic rhythm variations in the horse include first-degree heart block, second-degree heart block, sinus arrest or sinoatrial block, and variably configured P waves (Fig. 20B–5). The most common arrhythmia of clinical significance in the horse is atrial flutter or fibrillation. A presumptive diagnosis of atrial flutter can be made by auscultating heart sounds of various intensities that occur at irregular rates. The palpation of pulses of varying strengths occurring at irregular intervals provides more evidence. The diagnosis of atrial fibrillation can be confirmed with an electrocardiogram (Fig. 20B–6). Atrial and ventricular premature contractions are occasionally observed in horses prior to surgery. Atrial premature contractions seem to have little significance. Premature ventricular contractions, particularly if they occur at a rate faster than three per minute, should be evaluated further. Cardiac murmurs in the horse can be difficult to

evaluate. Most soft systolic murmurs (grade III out of V or less) are interpreted as innocent flow murmurs in the absence of other signs of cardiac disease. Potential sources of significant murmurs in horses include ventricular septal defects, mitral valve insufficiency, and aortic insufficiency.

Neuromuscular function, in particular the presence or absence of ataxia, should be evaluated in order to anticipate possible problems with recovery from anesthesia. Other pertinent factors would include a history of "tying up" (rhabdomyolysis) or hyperkalemic periodic paralysis.

Following a complete physical and history, ancillary tests and procedures should be applied as indicated by the physical status and history. The determination of packed cell volume and plasma total protein is easy and inexpensive, and it provides baseline information about the oxygen carrying capacity and hydration status of the patient (Chapter 19).

Some surgical procedures, such as ovariectomy, are facilitated if food is withheld for 24 to 48 hours prior to anesthesia. A prolonged fast does not seem to be necessary for other procedures. Gastric emptying occurs rapidly in the horse; thus, a 4- to 6-hour period of withholding food should be adequate. Access to water should be maintained. It has been suggested that horses anesthetized at altitude benefit from a longer period without food because of their propensity for gas distension. The shoes should be removed or at least covered to decrease the chance that the horse will lacerate itself on recovery. Before induction the horse's

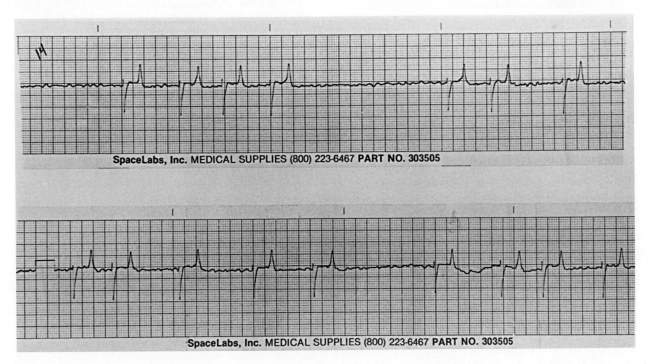

Fig. 20B–6. Electrocardiogram (25 mm/s) from a 4-year-old Standardbred mare with atrial fibrillation. Note the lack of discernible P waves, the undulating baseline (fibrillation or flutter waves) and the irregularly spaced QRS complexes. Atrial fibrillation is the most common arrhythmia of significance seen in horses. Conversion to normal sinus rhythm should be attempted prior to anesthesia.

mouth should be rinsed to remove foreign material.

Standing Chemical Restraint

A wide variety of agents have been used to produce chemical restraint in the standing horse. Current practice has evolved to the point where three groups of agents are commonly used: phenothiazines, alpha$_2$-agonists, and opioids. Butyrophenone tranquilizers were reported to be effective in horses, but more recent reports suggest significant undesirable side effects that prevent their recommendation.(5, 6) Diazepam is used as a muscle relaxant in the horse, but the level of sedation produced is not profound enough to be useful for restraint.(7) Chloral hydrate is a sedative-hypnotic that was widely used for sedation and anesthesia prior to the availability of inhalation anesthetics. The best use of chloral hydrate was for augmentation of the effects of other sedatives and tranquilizers in particularly obstreperous horses. Chloral hydrate is given intravenously and produces severe tissue necrosis if given perivascularly. Chloral hydrate is not currently available in pharmaceutical preparations suitable for horses.

Phenothiazine tranquilizers produce calming and a relaxed state from which the horse can be aroused. The pharmacology of phenothiazine tranquilizers is discussed in Chapter 8. Phenothiazine tranquilizers are administered orally, intramuscularly, and intravenously to horses. The two drugs that are in common use are promazine and acepromazine. Phenothiazines produce tranquilization by blocking the action of neurotransmitters both centrally and peripherally. As in other species, hypotension caused by alpha-adrenergic blockade can be produced. Hypotension is of particular concern in nervous or excitable horses or horses that have sustained blood loss or are dehydrated. The respiratory effects of phenothiazines are minimal and are generally limited to decreases in respiratory rate. Persistent penile paralysis (priapism) is reported after phenothiazine administration to horses. The mechanism of the effect is unknown. Priapism is uncommon but remains a consideration. Treatment of priapism should include support of the penis in order to prevent or reduce swelling. A recent report of two cases suggests that benztropine mesylate may be effective in resolving priapism.(8) Eight milligrams of benztropine were given to two adult horses, and the priapism resolved within 10 minutes.(8) Benztropine is used in the treatment of Parkinson disease and is believed to have central anticholinergic effects.

Promazine is available in a granular form for oral administration to horses. Typically, the granules are mixed with a small quantity of feed and offered to the animal. The effects of the drugs begin to appear approximately 45 minutes after ingestion, with peak tranquilization at 1 to 2 hours. The dose is 3 to 7 grams of granules per kg of body weight, which approximates 1 to 2 mg of promazine per kg. Promazine granules have some utility as a calming agent in horses that cannot be restrained for parenteral injection. Promazine granules can also be used a an aid to training if repeated injections are impossible or undesirable. Problems with the use of promazine granules include difficulty in predicting the effect from an administered dose, the long time interval until peak effect, and the less than profound level of sedation/tranquilization that is produced. The lack of predictability is tempered by the fact that the drug has a relatively wide margin of safety. More frequently, less than the desired level of tranquilization is produced. This fact, coupled with the long lag period to full effect (45 minutes to 2 hours) makes the judgment of whether or not to administer additional drug difficult. When used as a training aid, readministration of an increased dose on subsequent days is possible. The delayed onset of effect makes the drug impractical in most practice settings. In particularly difficult animals, the drug could be left with the attendant to be administered 1 hour before the veterinarian is to arrive. Finally, the less than profound sedation/tranquilization reduces the drug's utility. If a horse is given granules because it cannot be restrained for an injection, it is unlikely that the level of tranquilization will be profound.

Acepromazine is available as a 1% solution (10 mg/mL) for parenteral injection. The onset of effect of acepromazine occurs within 15 to 30 minutes of administration. The duration of tranquilization following acepromazine depends on the dose but may persist for 6 to 10 hours. Acepromazine produces calming with minimal muscle relaxation or ataxia. Acepromazine does not produce analgesia but may potentiate other drugs such as the opioids that are analgesics. Acepromazine will not transform an aggressive horse into a docile one but will reduce the animal's awareness and response to external stimuli. Increasing the dose does not ensure more pronounced effects, as approximately 30 to 40% of horses administered acepromazine do not attain the desired effect. Acepromazine is used as an aid to training, to produce standing restraint, and prior to transportation because it is long acting, inexpensive, and does not produce severe ataxia. The most reliable indication that the horse has been sedated with acepromazine is extrusion of the penis from the sheath.(9) Other signs include some drooping of the eyelids and slight protrusion of the third eyelid. Contraindications to the use of acepromazine would include the previously mentioned blood loss or shocklike state because of acepromazine's alpha$_1$ blocking effects. The resulting hypotension is particularly prone to occur after intravenous administration of acepromazine and can result in fainting and recumbency. Treatment includes the intravenous administration of large volumes of polyionic fluids. Known bleeding disorders are another contraindication to acepromazine because phenothiazines inhibit platelet function.

Alpha$_2$-adrenoceptor agonists produce sedation, analgesia, and muscle relaxation when administered intravenously or intramuscularly to horses. The pharmacology of alpha$_2$-agonists is discussed in Chapter 8. The two alpha$_2$-adrenoceptor agonists currently available for equine use in the United States are xylazine and detomidine. The effects of the drugs are similar, but detomidine is approximately 80 to 100 times more potent than xylazine and has a duration of action twice as long. Alpha$_2$-agonists are used for the temporary relief of colic pain, as adjuncts to general anesthesia, and alone and in combination with other drugs for standing chemical restraint (Chapter 10). Xylazine has also been administered epidurally to produce regional analgesia (Chapter 16).(10) The alpha$_2$ agonists reach peak effect in 3 to 5 minutes after intravenous administration and within 10 to 15 minutes of intramuscular administration. Sedation with alpha$_2$ agonists is characterized by profound depression, with the horse assuming a "head down" posture (Fig. 20B–7). The horse may attempt to head press. The eyelids and lips droop, and the horse may sway due to the muscle relaxation and ataxia produced. The muscles of the nostrils relax. This may lead to snoring or potentially obstruction in predisposed horses. Normal horses rarely become recumbent following alpha$_2$-agonist administration, but they may be difficult to move because of ataxia and muscle relaxation. Alpha$_2$-agonists may have more pronounced effects in foals, so the dose should be reduced. As in other species, the administration of alpha$_2$-agonists is characterized by decreases in cardiac output, primarily caused by decreases in heart rate. Alpha$_2$-agonists may induce or exacerbate first- and second-degree atrioventricular blockade. Respiration is depressed, but the effect is usually not apparent unless other drugs are coadministered or anesthesia is induced. The frequency and volume of urination is increased following administration of alpha$_2$-agonists. In adult horses, serum glucose levels increase and serum insulin levels decrease.(11) The effects of alpha$_2$-agonists can be antagonized by the administration of yohimbine or tolazoline.(12)

Alpha$_2$-agonists are frequently used in the horse with abdominal pain to facilitate evaluation and for pain relief. By repeated evaluation, alpha$_2$-agonists are the most effective available drugs for the treatment of colic pain.(13, 14) The use of alpha$_2$-agonists is controversial, however, because in addition to relieving colic pain, they cause decreases in intestinal propulsive activity. Thus, although the pain is controlled, the resolution of the cause of the abdominal pain may be slowed. The duration of the reduction in propulsive activity approximates the duration of sedation. A rational approach is to administer small doses of alpha$_2$-agonists intravenously and frequently reevaluate the patient, then readminister the drug as necessary. Xylazine may be more useful in this setting than detomidine because of its shorter duration of action, prompting more frequent reevaluation.

Opioids have been used to produce analgesia and augment chemical restraint in the horse. Because of their ability to cause nervousness and excitability, opioids are most frequently used in combination with sedatives and tranquilizers to produce standing chemical restraint. Butorphanol, a synthetic opioid agonist-antagonist, is approved for use in the horse for treatment of abdominal pain. Butorphanol is less apt to cause excitement than opioid agonists but can cause nervousness and ataxia at higher doses. Both the analgesia and nervousness produced by opioid agonists and agonists-antagonists can be reversed by the opioid antagonist, naloxone (Chapter 8). Caution should be used however, because the duration of effect of some opioid agonists, such as morphine, may be longer than the duration of effect of the antagonist. This could lead to renarcotization (resumed excitement) 4 to 6 hours after narcotic administration. Such excitement responds to the administration of additional antagonist or a tranquilizer. The clinical use of opioids is discussed in "Standing Chemical Restraint." A myriad of potential combinations can be used to produce standing chemical restraint, but most combine a sedative-tranquilizer with an opioid.

Acepromazine-xylazine, the combination of acepro-

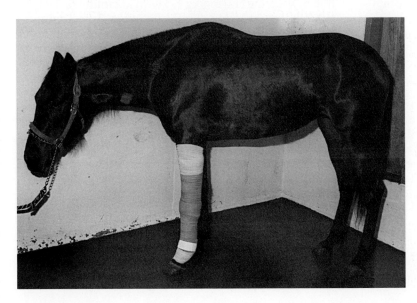

Fig. 20B–7. The assumed posture of a horse tranquilized with xylazine. Note the head down posture and the slight drooping of the eyelids. The horse was administered 150 mg of xylazine intravenously to facilitate clipping and surgical preparation for arthroscopy of the carpus. With larger doses of xylazine, significant muscle relaxation and ataxia can be produced.

mazine and xylazine, has been used to produce improved tranquilization with some reduction of the deleterious side effects.(15) Reduced doses of both drugs are used, typically 0.02 to 0.03 mg/kg of acepromazine and 0.2 to 0.5 mg/kg of xylazine. The drugs can be combined in the same syringe and are usually given intravenously. The reduced dose of xylazine produces less ataxia and less of a "head down" posture than would be seen with xylazine alone (given in a higher dose). Thus the horse stands more squarely on all four feet. The combination produces faster onset and longer duration of action than either agent given alone. The suppliers of xylazine caution against its coadministration with tranquilizers.

Sedative/tranquilizer-butorphanol. The combination of xylazine and butorphanol has been investigated.(16) When combined, the dose of xylazine is usually reduced because butorphanol provides some analgesia with few deleterious cardiovascular side effects. Because of the reduced dose of xylazine, the horse is usually less ataxic. Occasionally, horses twitch and jerk their heads after being given this combination. Head pressing may occur. The drugs can be given in combination in the same syringe. The analgesia produced is not sufficient to perform a skin incision, so local anesthetic blockade may need to be used. Butorphanol has also been used in combination with detomidine.(17)

Sedative/tranquilizer-morphine. The combination of xylazine and morphine has been used to produce standing chemical restraint for surgery.(18) Morphine should not be given until the horse is fully sedate because of the potential for excitement. Within 5 minutes of morphine administration the horse assumes a head down, sawhorse position. The placement of a nose twitch and elevation of the head may be helpful in stabilizing the patient on all four feet. Although analgesia is produced, the horses remain sensitive to touch, so the technique is usually combined with local blockade. Both drugs are potentially reversible with either yohimbine (xylazine) or naloxone (morphine). Occasionally, renarcotization (excitement or nervousness) occurs following administration of the combination, owing to the long half-life of morphine in the horse. The excitement can be abated by administration of a narcotic antagonist or simply by tranquilizing the patient.

Intravenous Anesthesia

A number of combinations have been used to produce anesthesia in the horse. The most commonly used agents include the thiobarbiturates, ketamine, and guaifenesin in combination. It is paramount that a horse be calmed prior to the induction of anesthesia. The administration of appropriate doses of preanesthetic agents, primarily phenothiazines and alpha$_2$ agonists, not only produces a calm, sedate patient, but in addition allows for a reduced dose of anesthetic. The maxim "Never anesthetize an excited horse" should serve as a warning. Intravenous anesthesia is commonly used because of the ambulatory nature of equine practice. Although all anesthetized horses benefit from oxygen

supplementation, intravenous anesthesia can be safely produced in healthy horses for periods of 60 minutes without oxygen supplementation.

Thiobarbiturates can be used to produce short- or long-term intravenous anesthesia in the horse (Chapter 9). The horse should be sedated prior to thiobarbiturate administration because this allows for a reduction of dose. The dose can be further reduced if guaifenesin is administered prior to or in combination with the barbiturates (discussed later). Induction of anesthesia with thiobarbiturates in unpremedicated horses is often stormy. Induction and recovery can be smoothed by prior administration of a sedative or tranquilizer. The larger the dose of thiobarbiturate, the more likely that apnea will occur. Anesthesia from a single barbiturate bolus lasts approximately 15 to 20 minutes, with recovery occurring within 45 to 60 minutes. More than one attempt to stand may be required and there may be a period of ataxia. Recovery is usually acceptable if the total intravenous dose of thiobarbiturate is less than 7 mg/kg. The use of thiobarbiturates as the *sole* anesthetic agent has been largely supplanted by other techniques, although they are frequently used in combination with other agents (guaifenesin) or to induce anesthesia that is maintained with inhalant agents.

Cyclohexamine anesthetics (ketamine, tiletamine) produce a state that has been called *dissociative anesthesia* and is characterized by comparatively good cardiopulmonary support and short duration. Heart rate, arterial blood pressure, and cardiac output are well maintained. Although respiration is depressed, with a characteristic apneustic breathing pattern, apnea is infrequent. The main complication of cyclohexamine anesthesia is poor to inadequate skeletal muscle relaxation. Cyclohexamine anesthetics should *not* be given to horses unless a profound degree of skeletal muscle relaxation is present. Skeletal muscle relaxation is usually produced by the administration of either an alpha$_2$-agonist or guaifenesin. The most frequently used technique for the production of intravenous anesthesia is the combination of xylazine (1.0 mg/kg IV) with ketamine (2.2 mg/kg IV).(19) The xylazine should be given 3 to 5 minutes prior to ketamine to ensure the that horse is sedate and muscle relaxation is evident. The horse becomes recumbent within 90 to 120 seconds of ketamine administration, is anesthetized for approximately 15 to 20 minutes, and stands within 30 to 45 minutes after induction. Horses that are not completely sedated prior to ketamine administration may not lie down or may stay recumbent for only a short time.(20) The recoveries from xylazine-ketamine anesthesia are generally smooth, with the horse requiring a single attempt to stand. Diazepam has been added to the combination in order to improve skeletal muscle relaxation.(21) Xylazine-ketamine anesthesia can be extended by re-administering half of the original dose of each agent, by administering boluses of thiobarbiturates (thiopental 1.0 mg/kg IV), or by the administration of guaifenesin.(22) The combination of xylazine (1.0 mg/kg IV) with a commercially available cyclohexamine combination of tiletamine and zolazepam (Telazol, 1.0–1.5 mg/kg IV) produces somewhat longer-term anesthesia (25 to 35 min) with improved muscle relaxation and greater respiratory depression.(23) Zolazepam is a benzodiazepine tranquilizer (similar to diazepam) that produces skeletal muscle relaxation. The recoveries from xylazine-tiletamine-zolazepam anesthesia are not as smooth as those following xylazine-ketamine anesthesia. Either xylazine-ketamine or xylazine-tiletamine-zolazepam can be used for induction of anesthesia prior to the administration of inhalant agents. Neither ketamine nor tiletamine-zolazepam are approved for use in the horse (Chapter 10).

Guaifenesin is a centrally acting skeletal muscle relaxant that produces mild sedation and variable analgesia. Guaifenesin is intravenously administered in 5, 10, and 15% concentrations given to effect (50 to 100 mg/kg). Higher concentrations of guaifenesin are difficult to use and may be associated with hemolysis.(24) Guaifenesin should *not* be given alone, as it does not provide sufficient analgesia for surgery. Guaifenesin is usually administered in combination with agents that produce analgesia (xylazine, ketamine) or a hypnotic state (thiobarbiturates). Guaifenesin is incorporated in many anesthetic techniques because it allows a reduction in these other drugs that produce greater cardiopulmonary depression. Guaifenesin produces profound skeletal muscle relaxation with comparatively minimal depression of arterial blood pressure and cardiac output (Chapter 13). Diaphragmatic function is minimally depressed but arterial pH and blood gases are affected when recumbency is produced. Horses should be sedated prior to the beginning guaifenesin infusion. Guaifenesin can be mixed with thiobarbiturates (thiopental 0.2 to 0.3%, 2–3 g in 1 L of guaifenesin), allowing a reduction in the dose of thiobarbiturate required. The combination is administered rapidly, to effect. Once recumbency has been produced, the rate of administration is slowed or stopped, depending on the depth of anesthesia required. The induction dose produces a duration of anesthesia of 15 to 25 minutes. If longer periods are required, additional guaifenesin-thiopental can be administered. Alternatively, guaifenesin can be administered to effect (buckling of the knees, lowering of the head) followed by a bolus of thiobarbiturate (thiopental 3–4 mg/kg) or ketamine (1.5–2.2 mg/kg). This latter technique allows for more accurate prediction of when recumbency will occur.

The combination of xylazine, guaifenesin, and ketamine has been used to produce anesthesia in the horse or as a method of extending the anesthesia produced by other techniques.(25) The combination is formulated by combining 500 mg of xylazine, 2000 mg of ketamine and 50 g of guaifenesin in 1 liter of sterile water. Anesthesia is usually induced by administering xylazine, then ketamine, as described earlier, but may be induced by administering the combination to effect (approximately 1–2 mL/kg) followed by an infusion of 2.2 mL · kg^{-1} · h^{-1} for maintenance. This combination provides useful anesthesia with good muscle relax-

ation. Respiratory depression and bradycardia are primary concerns and should be monitored carefully. Additionally, the appearance of the eyeball helps in determining if the horse is appropriately anesthetized. The patient should have a brisk palpebral reflex, occasional nystagmus should be present, and the eye should appear wet, evidence of tear production. Recovery from anesthesia is generally good.

Inhalation Anesthesia

Inhalation anesthetics are frequently used for maintenance of general anesthesia in the horse. Inhalation anesthetics are occasionally used for induction of anesthesia in the foal following nasotracheal intubation, but adult horses are more safely induced with an intravenous technique. Halothane and isoflurane are the two inhalant anesthetic agents that are commonly used clinically. Nitrous oxide is not recommended because of the difficulties in maintaining adequate oxygenation in the recumbent horse. Nitrous oxide diffuses into closed gas spaces (intestinal gas) and enlarges them, predisposing the horse to bloat (Chapter 11). Inhalation anesthetics are usually delivered in oxygen via a sealed airway, thus optimizing the inspired concentration of oxygen. The administration of inhalation anesthetic agents to horses requires specifically designed large animal anesthetic machines and precision, out-of-the-circle vaporizers (Chapter 17). Inhalation anesthesia is preferred over intravenous anesthesia for horses that are anesthetized for greater than 45 minutes and for horses that have cardiovascular or respiratory compromise. Because the inhalation anesthetic agents are continuously administered, their administration requires more vigilant monitoring of anesthetic depth and cardiopulmonary function than short-term techniques that utilize a single delivery of drug. Monitoring the effects of inhalation anesthesia in the horse involves evaluation of eye reflexes as well as measuring the effect of the drugs on heart and respiratory rate and arterial blood pressure. The anesthetic states produced by halothane and isoflurane are very similar.(26) Both drugs are cardiopulmonary depressants. Cardiac output may be somewhat better maintained with isoflurane but arterial blood pressure may be lower. Respiratory depression is comparable, but horses breathing isoflurane may breathe more slowly. Horses receiving isoflurane will recover from anesthesia more rapidly than those receiving halothane owing to the lower solubility coefficients of isoflurane (Chapter 11). This may alter the management of the latter part of the anesthetic period in that the administration of isoflurane may have to be continued longer in order to assure that the horse does not attempt to rise too quickly.

Monitoring

Monitoring is the key to safe anesthetic practice. Documentation, through the development of an anesthetic record, of the physical status of the patient and the drugs administered, and periodic evaluations of the drug's cardiopulmonary effects are necessary, not only for the production of safe anesthesia but also for the veterinarian's protection should complications arise that result in examination of the methods used (Chapters 2 and 15). For short-term anesthesia physical methods of monitoring (no equipment required) usually suffice. The skills required for physical monitoring of anesthesia parallel those skills required to perform a physical exam. The eye is of particular interest. During surgical levels of anesthesia, horses have a dull palpebral reflex (eyes close slowly when the eyelashes are stimulated) and a strong corneal reflex (eyes close rapidly when pressure is applied to the cornea). Nystagmus can be present, but it is usually slow and the eye stays moist, evidence of some tear formation. Spontaneous blinking or rapid nystagmus are signs of light planes of anesthesia. Eye signs are not helpful during anesthesia with the cyclohexamine anesthetics (ketamine, tiletamine) because these agents cause rapid nystagmus, blinking, and tearing, irrespective of the anesthetic plane (Chapter 2). For longer anesthetic periods, particularly those where hypotension or respiratory depression are expected, technologic methods, particularly measurement of arterial blood pressure, should be applied. The maintenance of mean arterial blood pressure at levels greater than 60 mm of Hg has been identified as a critical factor in the prevention of postanesthetic myopathies in horses.(3, 4) The preferred method of measurement of arterial blood pressure is the use of an intraarterial catheter and a measuring device that indicates pressure in mm Hg. Such devices are discussed in Chapter 15.

Anesthetized horses hypoventilate to varying degrees. The compromises produced by hypoventilation are generally well tolerated during short anesthetic periods (less than 45 minutes). The compromises become more critical as anesthesia lengthens. Horses anesthetized for greater than 45 to 60 minutes benefit from oxygen supplementation and may benefit from assistance of ventilation (Chapters 6 and 17). In the absence of arterial blood gas analysis, oxygen should be supplemented during prolonged anesthesia. Arterial blood gas analysis can help identify those horses that are hypoventilating and direct therapy toward intervention.

Recovery

Recovery is a critical phase of equine anesthesia but in many ways the least controllable. As the horse awakens from anesthesia, it may try to rise prematurely and subsequently fall, creating excitement. This excitement may lead to further attempts to stand with poor results. Ideally, horses regain consciousness within 10 to 20 minutes of anesthetic discontinuation, roll to sternal recumbency for a brief period, then rise. Most horses return to standing within an hour of discontinuation. Attempts to speed the recovery process usually cause the horse to have a prolonged period of unsteadiness once it stands. Recovery should only be prompted if the

horse had cardiopulmonary embarrassment while anesthetized. In this instance, rolling the horse into sternal recumbency during recovery improves oxygenation. Insufflation or the use of a demand valve can also support oxygenation. Horses that try to rise too quickly can be sedated with small doses of intravenous xylazine (0.2 mg/kg). Laryngospasm is infrequent in the horse. Some anesthetists prefer to leave the endotracheal tube in place until the horse is standing. Others remove the endotracheal tube when the horse begins to swallow (in lateral recumbency). It is important that the horse swallow when the endotracheal tube is removed so that the soft palate is replaced in its normal position under the epiglottis. Occasionally, particularly following dorsal recumbency, snoring occurs due to edema of the nasal passage.

Smooth recoveries are facilitated by placing the horse in a quiet, darkened environment. Good footing is important. As the horse tries to stand, it needs to be able to plant its feet and not have them slip. The horse can be aided to its feet by attaching head and tail ropes. In stalls specifically designed for recovery, strong metal rings can be attached to opposite walls. The head and tail ropes can be passed through the rings (Fig. 20B–8), removing the supporting personnel from the immediate area of the horse.

Horses that fail to rise within 90 minutes of the end of anesthesia should be evaluated further. Potential causes include weakness, rhabdomyolysis, or neurogenic paralysis. Weakness may occur due to residual tranquilization or electrolyte abnormalities (hypocalcemia or hyperkalemia). Rhabdomyolysis and neurogenic paralysis are difficult to differentiate. Horses often

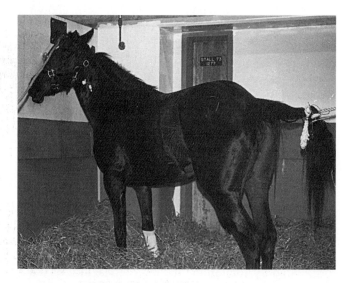

Fig. 20B–8. Head and tail ropes are used to assist the recovery from anesthesia. The ropes are run through strong rings that are attached to opposite walls of the recovery stall. This allows some support and control of the horse's movements once it stands without placing assisting personnel in a position where they might get injured. The horse needs to move its head to balance itself as it stands, so the head rope should not be pulled until the animal is standing.

attempt to stand but cannot or stand on three legs if a single limb is affected. Orthopedic injury should be ruled out. The treatment of rhabdomyolysis and neurogenic paralysis is similar and essentially supportive.(27) Intravenous fluids are indicated to promote perfusion and assure urine formation to minimize the chances for myoglobinuric renal failure. Acepromazine in small doses can be given to calm the horse and to promote peripheral perfusion. Small doses of diazepam (0.02–0.04 mg/kg IV) can reduce muscle cramping. The muscle relaxant dantrolene and nonsteroidal antiinflammatory agents have also been advocated. Unaffected weight-bearing limbs should be wrapped with support bandages. Horses that have a single limb affected usually can stand and have a good prognosis for recovery. Prolonged recumbency worsens the prognosis. Early aggressive treatment is required for a successful outcome.

Perianesthetic Supportive Care

Horses that have undergone blood loss or are in shock should be aggressively treated with intravenous fluids prior to induction of anesthesia. Horses anesthetized for greater than 30 minutes benefit from intravenous fluid administration in order to help maintain perfusion and promote urine output. As previously stated, the maintenance of mean arterial blood pressures of greater than 60 to 70 mm Hg is critical. Horses with mean arterial blood pressures below 60 mm Hg should be evaluated for excessive anesthetic depth and fluid administration rate increased. If the arterial blood pressure does not increase, the administration of vasopressors should be considered. Dobutamine is a useful agent that increases arterial blood pressure, primarily by increasing cardiac contractility.(28) Dobutamine is given by infusion at a dose of 1 to 5 $\mu g \cdot kg^{-1} \cdot min^{-1}$. Arterial blood pressure should increase within 5 to 10 minutes. Other agents that have been advocated include dopamine, ephedrine, epinephrine, phenylephrine, and methoxamine (Chapters 5 and 23).

Horses are prone to hypoventilation and hypoxemia when anesthetized. Horses placed in dorsal recumbency are particularly susceptible because of increases in ventilation/perfusion mismatches and the development of shunts (Chapter 6). Arterial partial pressures of carbon dioxide in the range of 55 to 75 mm Hg are common in anesthetized horses. Horses in dorsal recumbency may have arterial partial pressures of oxygen as low as 40 to 50 mm Hg. Arterial blood gas analysis, if available, allows evaluation of both ventilation and oxygenation. In the absence of arterial blood gas analysis, anesthetized horses should have their ventilation assisted or controlled if anesthesia extends for greater than 45 minutes (Chapter 17).

References

1. Mason DE, Muir WW, Wade W. Arterial blood gas tensions in horses during recovery from anesthesia. J Am Med Vet Assoc 190:989, 1987.
2. Riebold TW, Evans TE. Blood pressure measurements in the anesthetized horse. Comparison of four methods. Vet Surg 14:332, 1985.
3. Klein L, et al. Panel on anesthetic related myopathy. Proc Am Assoc Equine Practitioners 23:89, 1978.
4. Grandy JL, et al. Arterial hypotension and the development of postanesthetic myopathy in halothane anesthetized horses. Am J Vet Res 48:192, 1987.
5. Lees P, Serrano L. Effects of azaperone on cardiovascular and respiratory functions in the horse. Br J Pharmacol 56:263, 1976.
6. Dodman NH, Waterman E. Paradoxical excitement following the intravenous administration of azaperone in the horse. Equine Vet J 11:33, 1979.
7. Muir WW, et al. Pharmacodynamic and pharmacokinetic properties of diazepam in horses. Am J Vet Res 43:1756, 1982.
8. Wilson DV, Nickels FA, Williams MA. Pharmacologic treatment of priapism in two horses. J Am Vet Med Assoc 199:1183, 1991.
9. Ballard S, et al. The pharmacokinetics, pharmacologic responses, and behavioral effects of acepromazine in the horse. J Vet Pharmacol Ther 5:21, 1982.
10. LeBlanc P, et al. Epidural injection of xylazine for perineal analgesia in horses. J Am Vet Med Assoc 193:1405, 1988.
11. Tranquilli WJ, Thurmon JC, Benson GJ, et al. Hyperglycemia and hypoinsulinemia during xylazine-ketamine anesthesia in Thoroughbred horses. Am J Vet Res 45:11, 1984.
12. Gross ME, Tranquilli WJ. Use of alpha-2 adrenergic receptor antagonists. J Am Vet Med Assoc 195:378, 1989.
13. Kalpravidh M, et al. Effects of butorphanol, morphine, and xylazine in ponies. Am J Vet Res 45:211, 1984.
14. Muir WW, Robertson JT. Visceral analgesia: effects of xylazine, butorphanol, meperidine, and pentazocine in horses. Am J Vet Res 38:195, 1985.
15. Muir WW, Skarda RT, Sheehan WC. Hemodynamic and respiratory effects of a xylazine-acetylpromazine drug combination in horses. Am J Vet Res 30:1518, 1979.
16. Robertson JT, Muir WW. A new analgesic drug combination in the horse. Am J Vet Res 44:1667, 1983.
17. Clarke KW, Paton BS. Combine use of detomidine with opiates in the horse. Equine Vet J 20:331, 1988.
18. Muir WW, Skarda RT, Sheehan WC. Hemodynamic and respiratory effects of xylazine-morphine sulfate in horses. Am J Vet Res 40:1417, 1979.
19. Muir WW, Skarda RT, Milne DW. Evaluation of xylazine and ketamine hydrochloride for anesthesia in horses. Am J Vet Res 38:195, 1977.
20. Trim CM, Adams JG, Hovda LR. Failure of ketamine to induce anesthesia in two horses. J Am Vet Med Assoc 190:201, 1987.
21. Butera ST, et al. Diazepam/xylazine/ketamine combination for short term anesthesia in the horse. Vet Med Small Anim Clin 73:490, 1978.
22. McCarty JE, Trim CM, Ferguson, D. Prolongation of anesthesia with xylazine, ketamine, and guaifenesin in horses: 64 cases (1986–1989). J Am Vet Med Assoc 197:1646, 1990.
23. Hubbell JAE, Bednarski RM, Muir WW. Xylazine and tiletamine-zolazepam anesthesia in horses. Am J Vet Res 50:737, 1989.
24. Grandy JL, McDonell WN. Evaluation of concentrated solutions of guaifenesin for equine anesthesia. J Am Vet Med Assoc 176:619, 1980.
25. Greene SA, Thurmon JC, Tranquilli WJ, Benson GJ. Cardiopulmonary effects of continuous intravenous infusion of guaifenesin, ketamine, and xylazine in horses. Am J Vet Res 47:2364, 1986.
26. Steffey EP, Howland, D. Comparison of circulatory and respiratory effects of isoflurane and halothane anesthesia in horses. Am J Vet Res 41:821, 1980.
27. Hennig GE, Court MH. Equine postanesthetic myopathy: an update. Compend Contin Educ Pract Vet 13:1709, 1991.
28. Swanson CR, et al. Hemodynamic responses in halothane-anesthetized horses given infusions of dopamine or dobutamine. Am J Vet Res 46:365, 1985.

chapter 20c

RUMINANTS

Thomas W. Riebold

Introduction

As in other species, sedation and anesthesia are required in ruminants for surgical or diagnostic procedures. The decision to induce general anesthesia may be influenced by the ruminant's anatomic and physiologic characteristics. Ruminants usually accept physical restraint well, and that, in conjunction with local or regional anesthesia, is often sufficient to allow completion of many procedures. Other diagnostic and surgical procedures that are more complex require general anesthesia.

In addition to techniques for cattle, goats, and sheep, anesthetic techniques for South American camelids, primarily llamas and alpacas, are discussed. South American camelids do not accept restraint quite as well as domestic ruminants and more often require sedation in addition to physical restraint and local or regional anesthesia. Although they have some unique species characteristics regarding anesthesia, many of the principles and techniques used in domestic ruminant and equine anesthesia also apply to South American cam-

elids. Except for differences in size, anesthetic management of alpacas and llamas is similar.

Preanesthetic Preparation

Considerations for preanesthetic preparation include fasting, assessment of hematologic and blood chemistry values, venous catheterization, and estimation of body weight (Chapter 2). Domestic ruminants have a multicompartmental stomach with a large rumen that does not empty completely. South American camelids have a stomach divided into three compartments.(1) Each species, therefore, is susceptible to complications associated with recumbency and anesthesia: tympany, regurgitation, and aspiration pneumonia. It is recommended that calves, sheep, goats, and camelids be fasted for 12 to 18 hours and deprived of water for 8 to 12 hours. Adult cattle should be fasted 18 to 24 hours and deprived of water for 12 to 18 hours. In nonelective cases, this is often not possible and precautions should be taken to avoid aspiration of gastric fluid and ingesta. Fasting neonates is not advisable because hypoglycemia may result. Fasting and water deprivation will decrease the likelihood of tympany and regurgitation by decreasing the volume of fermentable ingesta. It also may produce bradycardia in cattle.(2) Additionally, pulmonary functional residual capacity may be better preserved in the fasted anesthetized ruminant.(3) Although gas accumulation in the first compartment of anesthetized camelids does not appear to occur, these precautions are recommended to decrease the incidence of regurgitation. Even with these precautions, some ruminants will become tympanitic and others will regurgitate.

Hematologic and blood chemistry values may be determined before anesthesia. Results should be compared to reference values.(4) Venipuncture and catheterization of the jugular vein are often performed prior to anesthesia. Sixteen-gauge catheters are appropriate for adult camelids, calves, and large goats and sheep. Eighteen-gauge catheters are appropriate for juvenile camelids, sheep, and goats. Adult cattle require 12- to 14-gauge catheters. Physical restraint during venipuncture or catheterization varies and can consist of a handler holding the animal's halter or use of head gates and chutes for adult cattle and llamas. If the camelid is fractious, grasping an ear may be helpful. Turning the head to either side may hinder venipuncture and catheter placement in goats and camelids. Infiltration of a local anesthetic at the site of catheterization is recommended.

Camelids do not have a jugular groove. The jugular vein lies deep to the sternomandibularis and brachiocephalicus muscles, ventral to the cervical vertebral transverse processes, and superficial to the carotid artery and vagosympathetic trunk within the carotid sheath for most of its length.(5-7) Beginning at a point about 15 cm caudal to the ramus of the mandible, the rostral course of the jugular vein is separated from the carotid artery by the omohyoideus muscle. The bifurcation of the jugular vein is located at the intersection of a line drawn caudally along the ventral aspect of the body of the mandible and another line connecting the base of the ear and the lateral aspect of the cervical transverse processes. Venipuncture or catheterization can be performed at the bifurcation or at any point caudal to it. Because of the close proximity of the carotid artery to the jugular vein, one must ascertain that the vein has been catheterized and not the artery. After occlusion of the vessel, one will be unable to see the jugular vein distend; however, the vein can be palpated, particularly rostrally, and more easily in females and altered males because their skin is thinner. On occasion, one will be able to see the jugular vein distend on crias and juvenile camelids. Camelids can have 4 or 5 jugular venous valves that prevent flow of venous blood into the head when the head is lowered during grazing.(5) Contact with jugular venous valves may prevent catheterization; a site caudal to the point where the valve was contacted should be used.

Finally, body weight must be determined by weighing the animal for accurate drug administration. It is easy to overestimate the body weight of camelids because they are fairly tall and have a long haircoat that obscures their body condition. Adult male llamas usually weigh 140 to 175 kg, occasionally reaching or exceeding 200 kg. Adult female llamas usually weigh 100 to 150 kg but may occasionally exceed 200 kg. Adult male alpacas usually weigh 60 to 100 kg, and adult female alpacas usually weigh 50 to 80 kg. Body weight of crias and small juveniles may be determined on a bathroom scale.

Anticholinergics are usually not administered to domestic ruminants prior to induction of anesthesia. They do not consistently decrease salivary secretions unless used in high doses and repeated frequently. Anticholinergics, while decreasing the volume of secretions, make them more viscous and difficult to clear from the trachea. Usual doses of atropine to prevent bradycardia in domestic ruminants (0.06–0.1 mg/kg IV) do not prevent salivation during anesthesia. Camelids are prone to increased vagal discharge during intubation or painful stimuli during surgery. Atropine (0.02 mg/kg IV or 0.04 mg/kg IM) is recommended to prevent bradyarrhythmia and will also decrease salivary secretions.(8) Glycopyrrolate (0.005–0.01 mg/kg IM or 0.002–0.005 mg/kg IV) may be substituted for atropine.(9)

Sedation/Restraint

Drugs used to induce tranquilization and/or sedation in ruminants include acepromazine, the alpha$_2$-agonists, xylazine, detomidine, medetomidine, and romifidine; pentobarbital, chloral hydrate, and diazepam.

Acepromazine is the most commonly used phenothiazine-derivative tranquilizer in veterinary anesthesia. It is not commonly used in ruminants but can be used in a manner similar to its use in horses. In general, though, lowered doses of acepromazine are required for cattle than horses. Usual doses of acepromazine are 0.03 to 0.05 mg/kg intravenously and 0.05 to 0.1 mg/kg in sheep and goats.(10) It may increase the risk of regurgitation during anesthesia.(10) Injection of acepromazine should not be made in the coccygeal vein. Close proximity of the coccygeal artery makes the risk of inadvertent intraarterial injection possible, with subsequent loss of the tail.(11) Acepromazine can also cause prolapse of the penis with the potential for trauma. Acepromazine is contraindicated in debilitated and hypovolemic patients.

Xylazine and detomidine provide sedation by activation of central alpha$_2$-adrenoceptors. Xylazine is often used to provide sedation or, in higher doses, restraint (recumbency and light planes of general anesthesia) in ruminants. There appears to be some variation in response between species and within a species. Xylazine is a more potent drug in ruminants than in horses.(12) Some investigators feel that goats are more sensitive to xylazine than sheep (10), with cattle appearing to be of intermediate sensitivity when compared to sheep and goats. South American camelids appear to be intermediate between cattle and horses in sensitivity to xylazine and alpacas appear to be less sensitive to xylazine than llamas. Hereford cattle are more sensitive to xylazine than Holstein cattle (13), and anecdotal evidence indicates that Brahmans are the most sensitive of cattle breeds.(14) Stressful environmental conditions appear to cause a pronounced or prolonged response to xylazine in cattle.(15) There is also variation in the analgesic effects of xylazine among breeds of sheep.(16, 17) Detomidine has been used to a lesser extent in the United States but is also effective for providing sedation and/or analgesia in domestic ruminants.(18-20)

Sedation following use of alpha$_2$-adrenoceptors can be reversed with alpha$_2$-adrenoceptor antagonists (tolazoline, idazoxan, atipamezole, or yohimbine). The recommended dose of yohimbine is 0.12 mg/kg IV, although there is some variability in response to its administration in cattle (21, 22) and this dose is ineffective in sheep.(23) Higher doses of yohimbine (1.0 mg/kg IV) will reverse xylazine sedation in sheep.(24) Tolazoline can be given at doses of 0.5–2.0 mg/kg IV.(22) Higher doses of tolazoline are usually given to small ruminants, and the dose rate is decreased as body weight increases. Tolazoline given at 2.0 mg/kg IV will cause hyperesthesia in unsedated cattle.(25) Idazoxan can be given at a dose of 0.05 mg/kg IV to sheep (23) and calves.(26) The dose of atipamezole is 20 to 60 μg/kg IV.(27) Tolazoline is available for human use but it as well as idazoxan and atipamezole are not as yet commercially available for veterinary use. Doxapram, an analeptic, can be used to enhance CNS stimulation after yohimbine or tolazoline administration. Doxapram (1.0 mg/kg IV) is an effective stimulant in cattle (28) but is ineffective in llamas at 2.0 mg/kg IV for reversing xylazine sedation.(29)

Although complete data are not available on the cardiovascular and respiratory effects of xylazine in camelids, xylazine causes bradycardia (29), as it does in other species (13, 30–32), and probably has little effect initially on blood pressure followed by hypotension. Poorly trained or berserk male camelids tend to be less responsive, whereas debilitated individuals are more responsive to sedative doses of xylazine. As in other species, xylazine also induces hyperglycemia and hypoinsulinemia in cattle and sheep.(33–38) Additionally, xylazine causes hypoxemia, hypercarbia, and increased urine production (10, 13, 39), and can cause pulmonary edema.(40) Xylazine also has an oxytocin-like effect in pregnant cattle (41) and sheep.(42) Detomidine does not have this effect on the gravid uterus in cattle (19) and may be the drug of choice for sedation in pregnant ruminants.

The degree of sedation or restraint produced by xylazine depends on the amount given and the animal's temperament. Low doses (0.015–0.025 mg/kg IV or IM) will provide sedation without recumbency in domestic ruminants. Higher doses (0.1–0.2 mg/kg IV) provide sedation without recumbency in camelids. Detomidine

is given at 2.5–10.0 μg/kg IV in cattle (18) and at 10.0–20.0 μg/kg in sheep (10) to provide standing sedation of approximately 30 to 60 minutes' duration. Higher doses of detomidine (30 μg/kg IV) will produce recumbency in sheep and are equivalent to xylazine at 0.15 mg/kg IV, medetomidine at 10 μg/kg IV, or romifidine at 50 μg/kg IV.(20)

Higher doses of xylazine (goats, 0.05 mg/kg IV or 0.1 mg/kg IM [10, 43]; sheep, 0.1–0.2 mg/kg IV or 0.2–0.3 mg/kg IM; [10, 43]; cattle, 0.1 mg/kg IV or 0.2 mg/kg IM [14]) will provide recumbency and seemingly light planes of general anesthesia for approximately 1 hour. Xylazine (0.3–0.4 mg/kg IV) usually induces 20 to 30 minutes of recumbency in llamas.(5-8) Alpacas may require an increased dose to achieve the same result. Higher doses in all species can be expected to induce longer periods of recumbency.

Pentobarbital (2 mg/kg IV) has been used in cattle for standing sedation and tranquilization.(44) Caution must be exercised to avoid administering enough to cause excitement. Pentobarbital provides moderate sedation for 30 minutes and mild sedation for an additional 60 minutes. Chloral hydrate or chloral hydrate/magnesium sulfate solutions can be used to sedate ruminants.(14) These drugs must be injected intravenously in order to avoid tissue necrosis. Diazepam (0.25–0.5 mg/kg IV) will provide 30 minutes' sedation without analgesia in sheep and goats.(10, 43) It is recommended that diazepam be given slowly intravenously. Butorphanol, an opioid agonist-antagonist, can be used to provide sedation and analgesia in camelids and domestic ruminants. It is given at 0.1–0.2 mg/kg IM in camelids (45) and at 0.05–0.5 mg/kg IM in sheep and goats.(10, 46, 47) No behavioral effects are seen with butorphanol given at 0.05 mg/kg IV in sheep.(47) Ataxia occurs following butorphanol administration at a dose of 0.4 mg/kg IV, and excitement can occur following butorphanol at 0.1–0.2 mg/kg IV in sheep.(47)

Combinations of xylazine and butorphanol have be used in camelids and domestic ruminants to provide neuroleptanalgesia. Doses are 0.01–0.02 mg/kg IV of each drug given separately in domestic ruminants (48) and 0.2 mg/kg IV of each drug in camelids.(49) Duration of action is approximately 1 hour.

Induction

Ruminants are not commonly sedated prior to induction of anesthesia. Physical restraint can be used in lieu of sedatives prior to induction. Because ruminants seldom experience emergence delirium, sedation during the recovery period is not required. In some instances, though, sedation is required to make handling of the animal, primarily adult bulls, safer during the induction period. Sedation will lengthen the recovery period from general anesthesia (18) and increase the likelihood of regurgitation.(10)

General anesthesia can be induced by either injectable or inhalation techniques. Available drugs include thiobarbiturates, ketamine, guaifenesin, tiletamine-zolazepam (Telazol), propofol, pentobarbital, halothane, and isoflurane (Chapters 9 and 10).

Small ruminants, weighing less than 50 to 100 kg, can be induced by mask with halothane or isoflurane. Larger animals can be induced with either intravenous or intramuscular techniques. Mask induction with halothane or isoflurane can also be performed in small or debilitated camelids, or camelids immobilized with xylazine-ketamine or Telazol. Mask induction in healthy untranquilized adult camelids is usually not attempted because application of the mask may provoke spitting. Addition of nitrous oxide (50% of total flow) to the inspired gas mixture will increase the speed of induction. During induction, halothane or isoflurane is administered at 3% when the patient weighs less than 25 kg. Higher concentrations are used with larger patients.

BARBITURATES/THIOBARBITURATES

The thiobarbiturates, thiamylal and thiopental, have been used extensively in veterinary anesthesia, alone and in combination with guaifenesin. Used separately, they quickly induce anesthesia. Muscle relaxation is relatively poor but still sufficient to accomplish intubation. The acid-base status and physical status of the patient affect the actions of these drugs. Acidemia increases the nonionized fraction (the active portion) of the drug, thus increasing its activity and decreasing the dose required (Chapter 9).(50) In addition, the heart, brain, and other vital organs receive a larger portion of cardiac output when patients are in shock.(51) Because patients in shock are often acidemic, altered kinetics and hemodynamics can result in relative overdose (Chapter 2).

Recovery from induction doses of thiobarbiturates is based upon redistribution of the drug from the brain to other tissues in the body. Metabolism of the agent continues for some time following recovery until final elimination occurs. Maintenance of anesthesia with thiobarbiturates is not recommended because saturation of tissues with thiobarbiturate causes recovery to be dependent on metabolism and recovery will be prolonged. Concurrent use of nonsteroidal antiinflammatory drugs is contraindicated because they will displace the thiobarbiturates from protein and delay recovery.(52)

Thiamylal is given at 6–10 mg/kg IV in unsedated animals and will provide approximately 10 to 15 minutes of anesthesia. Camelids may require additional thiamylal for tracheal intubation. Thiopental is administered in similar fashion, although in slightly higher doses, usually 25 to 30%.

Formerly, pentobarbital was used to anesthetize domestic ruminants but is no longer commonly used. The dose is 20–25 mg/kg IV, half given rapidly and the remainder to effect. In an anesthetic dose, pentobarbital causes profound respiratory depression and is not an effective analgesic. Sheep appear to metabolize pentobarbital more readily than other species.(10) Recovery in domestic ruminants is usually prolonged, and today other anesthetic techniques are more appropriate.

KETAMINE

Ketamine stimulates the limbic system, causing dysphoria, hallucinations, and excitement in addition to tonic-clonic muscle activity when used alone in the horse. These same effects occur in ruminants, although perhaps not to the same extent as in the horse. It also provides mild cardiovascular stimulation and is safer than the thiobarbiturates. Although ketamine does not eliminate the swallowing reflex in ruminants, tracheal intubation can be accomplished.

Although ketamine will induce immobilization and incomplete analgesia when given alone, it is usually combined with a sedative or tranquilizer (Chapter 10). Most commonly xylazine or diazepam is recommended for use in combination with ketamine, although the availability of detomidine offers another alternative. Xylazine (0.1–0.2 mg/kg IM) can be given followed by ketamine (10–15 mg/kg IM) in small domestic ruminants.(10, 43, 53) In goats, it is preferable to use the lower dose of xylazine followed by ketamine.(10, 43) Anesthesia usually lasts about 45 minutes and can be prolonged by injection of 3–5 mg/kg IM of ketamine. The longer duration of action of xylazine when compared to ketamine obviates the need for readministration of xylazine in most cases. Alternatively, xylazine (0.03–0.05 mg/kg IV) followed by ketamine (5 mg/kg IV) or xylazine (goats, 0.1 mg/kg IM; sheep, 0.2 mg/kg IM) followed by ketamine (5 mg/kg IV) can be used to provide anesthesia of 15 to 20 minutes' duration.(10) Adult cattle can by anesthetized with xylazine (0.1–0.2 mg/kg IV) followed by ketamine (2.0 mg/kg IV).(54) The lower dose of xylazine is used when cattle weigh more than 600 kg.(54) Duration of anesthesia is approximately 20 to 30 minutes; anesthesia can be prolonged for 10 to 15 minutes with additional ketamine (0.75–1.25 mg/kg IV) administration. When evaluated in sheep, xylazine (0.1 mg/kg IV) and ketamine (7.5 mg/kg IV) provided anesthesia of 25 minutes' duration and caused a decrease in cardiac output, mean arterial pressure, and peripheral vascular resistance.(55) Diazepam (0.1 mg/kg IV) followed immediately by ketamine (4.5 mg/kg IV) can be used in domestic ruminants. Muscle relaxation is usually adequate for tracheal intubation although the swallowing reflex may not be completely obtunded with this mixture. Anesthesia usually is of 10 to 15 minutes' duration following diazepam-ketamine, with recumbency of up to 30 minutes. Higher doses of diazepam (0.25–0.5 mg/kg IV) with ketamine (4.0–7.5 mg/kg IV) have also been used in sheep and provide anesthesia of the same duration (10, 43, 55) Investigations into the cardiopulmonary effects of diazepam (0.375 mg/kg IV) and ketamine (7.5 mg/kg IV) in sheep have shown a decrease in cardiac output and an increase in peripheral vascular resistance without affecting arterial pressure.(55) Medetomidine has been combined with ketamine to provide anesthesia in calves. Because medetomidine (20 μg/kg IV) is much more potent that xylazine, very low doses of ketamine (0.5 mg/kg IV) can be used.(27) However, use of a local anesthetic at the surgical site may be required when ketamine is used at this dose.(27) Reversal of anesthesia can be achieved with alpha₂-adrenoceptor antagonists without causing excitement.

Xylazine (0.25–0.35 mg/kg IM) and ketamine (6.0–10.0 mg/kg IM, 15 minutes later) usually provide 30 to 60 minutes of restraint in camelids.(5, 8) Use of xylazine (0.44 mg/kg IM) and ketamine (4.0 mg/kg IM) administered simultaneously usually provides restraint of 15 to 20 minutes' duration.(7) Depth of anesthesia varies with the amount given and the camelid's temperament, but is usually sufficient for minor procedures such as suturing lacerations, draining abscesses, or cast application. When this combination provides insufficient analgesia, supplemental local anesthesia may be required to allow completion of surgery. Tracheal intubation may not be possible. However, this combination does immobilize the animal, facilitating venipuncture and administration of additional anesthetic agent or application of a face mask to increase the depth of anesthesia. If desired, xylazine (0.25 mg/kg IV) and ketamine (3.0–5.0 mg/kg IV) may be administered 5 minutes apart to obtain a more uniform response and sufficient depth of anesthesia for tracheal intubation.(5) Diazepam (0.1 mg/kg IV) and ketamine (4.5 mg/kg IV) as used for domestic ruminants produces recumbency of approximately 20 minutes' duration but does not reliably provide enough muscle relaxation for tracheal intubation.

GUAIFENESIN

Guaifenesin is a centrally acting skeletal muscle relaxant exerting its effect at the internuncial neurons in the spinal cord and at polysynaptic nerve endings (Chapter 13).(56) It induces recumbency in domestic ruminants and camelids but is not recommended alone because it provides little if any analgesia.(57) Addition of ketamine or a thiobarbiturate to guaifenesin improves induction quality and decreases the volume required for induction. Muscle relaxation is improved when compared to inductions with ketamine or the thiobarbiturates given alone. Typically, 5% guaifenesin solutions are used. Hemolysis can occur with 10% guaifenesin solutions. (58) Commonly these solutions are given rapidly intravenously to effect in either tranquilized or untranquilized patients. The calculated dose is 2.0 mL/kg. The amount of ketamine added to guaifenesin varies but is usually 1.0 to 2.0 mg/mL. The amount of thiobarbiturate added to guaifenesin ranges from 2.0 to 4.0 mg/mL. For convenience, guaifenesin-based mixtures may be injected with large syringes rather than administered by infusion to camelids and small ruminants.

Following induction, guaifenesin-based solutions can be infused to effect and maintain anesthesia. If desired, xylazine can also be added to ketamine-guaifenesin solutions for induction and maintenance of anesthesia in cattle (54, 59) and sheep.(60) Final concentrations within the mixture are guaifenesin (50 mg/mL), ketamine (1–2 mg/mL), and xylazine (0.1 mg/mL). This solution is infused at 0.5–1 mL/kg IV for induction. Anesthesia is maintained by infusion of the mixture at 1.5 mL·kg^{-1}·h^{-1} for calves (59) and at 2 mL·kg^{-1}·h^{-1} for adult cattle (54) and sheep (60), although the final administration rate will vary with patient requirements. If the procedure requires more than 2 mL/kg of the guaifenesin-ketamine-xylazine mixture to allow completion of the surgical procedure, the amount of xylazine added should be decreased by 50% because its duration of action is longer than the other two agents (Chapter 10).(48)

TILETAMINE-ZOLAZEPAM

Telazol is a proprietary combination of equal parts of tiletamine and zolazepam and is FDA approved for use as an anesthetic agent in cats and dogs. It consists of tiletamine, a dissociative anesthetic agent similar to, but more potent than, ketamine; and zolazepam, a benzodiazepine sedative similar to diazepam. When used alone, tiletamine induces poor muscle relaxation and causes excitement during recovery. The addition of zolazepam to tiletamine modifies these effects. As with ketamine, the swallowing reflex remains but is obtunded. Like ketamine, this combination provides slight cardiovascular stimulation, causing an increase in heart rate.(61) Elimination of tiletamine and zolazepam is not uniform with variation occurring in each drug's clearance among species. Differential clearance of the two drugs can affect recovery quality.(61)

In many respects Telazol is similar to ketamine premixed with diazepam. When used alone in the horse, it provides unsatisfactory anesthesia.(62) Muscle relaxation is poor, and recovery is characterized by excitement. However, when combined with a sedative such as xylazine, it can be successfully used in the horse. Because of the differences in temperament between horses and domestic ruminants and camelids, Telazol can be used successfully with or without xylazine. However, adding xylazine to Telazol will lengthen the duration of effect and enhance muscle relaxation.

Telazol given at 4.0 mg/kg IV in untranquilized calves causes minimal cardiovascular effects while providing anesthesia of 45 to 60 minutes' duration.(63) Xylazine (0.1 mg/kg IM) followed immediately by Telazol (4.0 mg/kg IM) produces onset of anesthesia within 3 minutes and duration of anesthesia of approximately 1 hour.(64) Calves are able to stand approximately 130 minutes following injection. Increasing xylazine to 0.2 mg/kg IM increased duration of anesthesia and recumbency, and the incidence of apnea.(64) This drug mixture can also be administered intravenously when xylazine is given at 0.05 mg/kg IV followed by Telazol at 1.0 mg/kg IV.(54)

When Telazol is given at a dose of 12.0 mg/kg IV to sheep it provides approximately 2.5 hours of surgical anesthesia with a total recumbency time of 3.2

hours.(65) More recent investigations have shown that Telazol at 12 mg/kg or 24 mg/kg IV causes cardiopulmonary depression with anesthesia of approximately 40 minutes.(66) Rather than using these relatively large doses, it may be more appropriate to decrease the initial amount of Telazol to 2.0–4.0 mg/kg IV and administer additional Telazol as needed to prolong anesthesia. This method may allow greater flexibility in duration of anesthesia and recumbency. Butorphanol (0.5 mg/kg IV) combined with Telazol (12 mg/kg IV) given either simultaneously or 10 minutes apart induces about 25 to 50 minutes of anesthesia in sheep but is accompanied by cardiopulmonary depression.(67)

Telazol at a dose of 4.0 mg/kg IM provides up to 2 hours of restraint in camelids.(68) Length of recumbency is unaffected by administration of flumazenil, indicating that the duration of action is more influenced by tiletamine rather than zolazepam.(68) Cardiovascular function is preserved, although hypercarbia and hypoxemia occur in some animals. Airway reflexes are maintained. Local anesthesia may be required in some instances when surgical procedures are performed.(68) In a limited number of camelids, Telazol (2.0 mg/kg IV) provided 15 to 20 minutes of restraint and 25 to 35 minutes of recumbency. The depth of anesthesia is adequate to intubate the animals nasally, but muscle relaxation is poor and oral intubation difficult.

PROPOFOL

Propofol is a nonbarbiturate, nonsteroidal hypnotic agent (Chapter 9). It can be used to provide brief periods (5–10 minutes) of anesthesia. The dose is 4.0–6.0 mg/kg IV for induction.(10, 69–71) Constant infusion can be used to maintain a light plane of anesthesia. Induction is smooth, as is recovery. If propofol is injected rapidly, apnea may occur, although slow administration will usually prevent that complication. Economic considerations will dictate its use in domestic ruminants.

Maintenance

Tracheal intubation is recommended in ruminants and camelids because it provides a secure airway and prevents aspiration of salivary and ruminal contents if

passive regurgitation occurs. Several techniques can be used to accomplish intubation. Adult cattle can be intubated blindly or with digital palpation. Blind intubation is successful about 50% of the time. Following insertion of a mouth speculum, the animal's head and neck are hyperextended to make the orotracheal axis approach 180°. An endotracheal tube of appropriate size is inserted and manipulated into the larynx (Table 20C–1). When that technique is unsuccessful, a hand should be inserted into the mouth with the tube. After the epiglottis is located and depressed, a finger can be placed between the arytenoid cartilages and the tube inserted. If desired, an equine nasogastric tube can be inserted into the larynx serving as a guide for the endotracheal tube. Often adult cattle are intubated by palpation for maintenance of inhalation anesthesia. During intubation, the operator's hand is placed in the oropharynx and guides the endotracheal tube into the larynx. Depending on the size of the animal and the individual's arm, airway obstruction can occur. It is important that intubation be accomplished promptly. If the technique requires more than a minute, the hand and arm should be withdrawn from the oral cavity to allow the animal to ventilate before continuing intubation.

When blind orotracheal intubation is unsuccessful in calves or other small ruminants, a laryngoscope with a 250- to 350-mm blade is required for laryngoscopy. Visibility of the larynx is improved by hyperextending the head and neck to make the orotracheal axis approach 180° (Fig. 20C–1). Using suction or gauze on a sponge forceps to swab the pharynx will improve visibility. Attempting intubation or swabbing the oropharynx when the anesthetic plane is insufficient will often provoke active regurgitation. With adequate depth of anesthesia, this reflex is eliminated. The epiglottis is depressed allowing visibility of the larynx. The endotracheal tube should be placed in the oral pharynx and inserted into the larynx during inspiration. If desired, a guide tube (e.g., a 1-meter, 0.5-cm stylet

Table 20C–1.	Sizes of Endotracheal Tubes Needed for Ruminants and Camelids of Various Body Weights
Body Weight (kg)	Endotracheal Tube Size (mm i.d.)
< 30	4–7
30–40	8–10
60–80	10–12
100	12
200–300	14–16
300–400	16–22
400–600	22–26
> 600	26

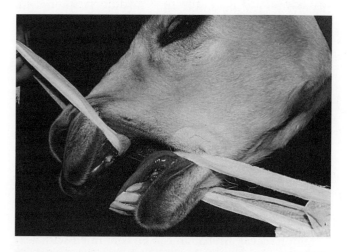

Fig. 20C–1. Use of two gauze loops to open a llama's mouth and fix the tongue in place during intubation.

[72] or a large male dog urinary catheter) can be inserted through the endotracheal tube. The guide tube should be three times the length of the endotracheal tube. The endotracheal tube is then passed over the guide tube and into the trachea.

Blind oral intubation is more difficult in sheep and goats, and intubation is best performed under laryngoscopy. To perform blind oral intubation, the animal's head and neck are extended following placement of the endotracheal tube in the oral pharynx. The larynx can be palpated and the tube directed into the larynx.(43) Members of both of these species have active laryngeal reflexes that may be obtunded by topical application of 2% lidocaine. This can be performed with an adjustable pattern plant sprayer (73) and with a syringe. Cetacaine is not recommended because overdosage can easily occur or because benzocaine-based local anesthetics can cause methemoglobinemia (Chapter 12).(74) After desensitization of the larynx, intubation can be performed with the same technique that one would use in calves. Oral intubation is performed in camelids similar to domestic ruminants. Oral blind intubation is usually unsuccessful, and laryngoscopy with a 250- to 350-mm laryngoscope is recommended.

Nasotracheal intubation is also possible in sheep (18) and camelids (75), although it requires an endotracheal tube one size smaller than that used orally. Camelids are prone to epistaxis, and use of a lubricant that contains phenylephrine is recommended. Blind nasal intubation is technically easier than blind oral intubation; but nasal intubation under laryngoscopic control is technically more difficult than orotracheal intubation. Even though nasotracheal intubation can be more difficult, it offers the option of recovering the animal with the endotracheal tube in place as a method of preventing airway obstruction during recovery. The endotracheal tube is advanced through the external nares into the ventral meatus with slow gentle pressure. An obstruction encountered at approximately 10 cm in adults is usually caused by placement of the tube in the middle meatus. If an obstruction is encountered more caudally, approximately 25 cm in adults, the tube is likely in the nasopharyngeal diverticulum.(75) In either case the tube should be withdrawn and redirected. If the endotracheal tube cannot be redirected past the nasopharyngeal diverticulum, placement of a prebent stylet into the tube to direct its tip ventrally is usually effective.

After the endotracheal tube has been advanced into the nasopharynx, the camelid's head and neck should be extended and the tube manipulated into the larynx. If the tube will not enter the larynx, placing a prebent stylet in the endotracheal tube to direct the tube tip ventrally into the larynx instead of the esophagus is helpful. Although visibility of the larynx is somewhat limited, oral laryngoscopy will aid intubation and confirm correct placement of the tube.

Endotracheal intubation can be confirmed with several techniques. Initially they include visualization of the endotracheal tube passing into the larynx. When transparent endotracheal tubes are used, water vapor condensation will appear and clear during each breath. One can feel gas being expelled from the tube during exhalation, and when the endotracheal tube is connected to the anesthesia machine, observation of synchrony between movement of the rebreathing bag and the thorax will be noted. Finally, if a CO_2 analyzer is available, CO_2 will be noted in exhaled gas.

Anesthesia in ruminants can be maintained with halothane, isoflurane, or methoxyflurane. Halothane and isoflurane are preferred. Although methoxyflurane can be used in small domestic ruminants and camelids, induction and recovery are prolonged. Liver failure has been reported in goats subjected to halothane anesthesia.(76) Flunixin meglumine should not be used immediately before or after methoxyflurane anesthesia in dogs, as renal failure can result.(77) It would appear that one should avoid the combination of these drugs in ruminants.

Conventional small animal anesthetic machines can be used to anesthetize ruminants weighing less than 60 kg. Conventional human anesthetic machines or small animal machines with expanded soda lime canisters are adequate for animals not exceeding 200 kg. Oxygen flow rates of 20 mL $\cdot$ kg^{-1} $\cdot$ min^{-1} during induction and 12 mL $\cdot$ kg^{-1} $\cdot$ min^{-1} during maintenance with minimal flow rates of 1 L/minute are adequate. Anesthesia is usually maintained with halothane at 1.5 to 2.5% or isoflurane at 1.5 to 3% for camelids. Because domestic ruminants have a respiratory pattern characterized by rapid respiratory rate and small tidal volume, higher vaporizer settings (e.g., halothane 2–3%) may be required to maintain anesthesia in spontaneously breathing patients.

Supportive Therapy

Supportive therapy is an important part of anesthetic practice. As veterinarians become more familiar with use of the anesthetic drugs, longer and more involved surgical procedures are attempted. As duration and difficulty increase, the likelihood of complications can also increase. Attention to supportive therapy in anesthetized ruminants and camelids can decrease the incidence of complications and improve outcome. Supportive therapy includes patient positioning, fluid administration, mechanical ventilation, cardiovascular support, and good monitoring techniques (Chapters 2, 15, and 19).

PATIENT POSITIONING

Improper positioning and padding of anesthetized horses have been implicated as one of the causes of postanesthetic myopathy-neuropathy.(78) A similar situation may occur in adult cattle. Postanesthetic myopathy does not appear to occur in goats, sheep, and South American camelids. Anesthetized ruminants should be positioned on a smooth, flat, padded surface. Adult cattle require either water beds, dunnage bags, or 4-inch-high density foam pads. Pads of 2-inch thickness are sufficient for sheep, goats, and South American

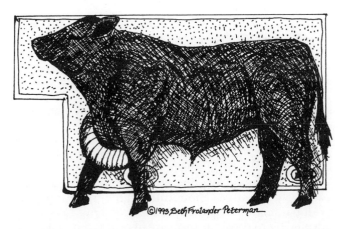

Fig. 20C–2. Cattle positioned in lateral recumbency should be placed on padding with an inner tube placed over the dependent foreleg and that leg drawn cranial. Support should be placed under the nondependent foreleg and hind leg so they are parallel to the table.

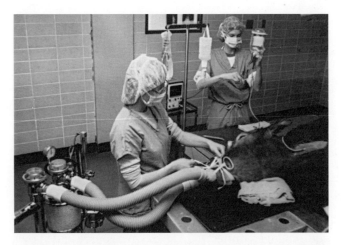

Fig. 20C–3. Position of the head and neck is slightly extended and elevated at the pharynx to help drain secretions and regurgitant material from the larynx-endotracheal tube interface within the oral cavity. The endotracheal tube is secured with tape or gauze to the Y piece of the rebreathing circuit and to the dental wedge that is left in place during anesthesia.

camelids. Patients positioned in dorsal recumbency should be balanced squarely on their back with both gluteal areas bearing equal weight. The forelegs should be flexed and relaxed, and the hind legs relaxed and flexed. External support should be placed under the maxilla to prevent hyperextension of the neck.

Adult cattle in lateral recumbency should have an automobile inner tube (valve stem pointed down) placed under the shoulder of the dependent foreleg to help minimize pressure on the radial nerve as it traverses the musculospiral groove of the humerus. The point of the elbow should be positioned at 5 o'clock in the inner tube for cattle in right lateral recumbency or at 7 o'clock for cattle in left lateral recumbency. The dependent foreleg is drawn anteriorly so that the weight of the thorax rests on the triceps rather than on the humerus. Alternatively, the lower forelimb could be inserted through an inner tube and that limb pulled cranial.(48) Nonelastic tape covering the portion of the inner tube not under the shoulder will prevent over-expansion of that section of inner tube and collapse of the inner tube under the shoulder to help ensure that shoulder support remains (Fig. 20C–2). The other three legs are positioned perpendicular to the body with the uppermost legs elevated and parallel to the table surface. Support of these legs will improve venous drainage and prevent injury to the brachial plexus. The head and neck are maintained in a slightly extended position with the head resting on a pad or Turkish towel (Fig. 20C–3). If possible the patient's head should be positioned so that salivary secretions and gastric contents, if regurgitation occurs, will drain from the mouth and not wick between the animal's head and the pad and contact the eye. The dependent eye should be closed prior to placing the head on the padding and bland ocular ointment instilled in the other eye. Camelids have prominent eyes, and special attention should be given to the dependent eye to avoid injury. Use of circulating warm water heating blankets should be considered to prevent hypothermia in juvenile cattle,

sheep, camelids, and goats. Adults aren't as likely to become hypothermic, and use of warm water heating blankets isn't required.

FLUID ADMINISTRATION

Fluid administration during anesthesia is important to correct preexisting dehydration if present, provide volume to offset anesthesia-related vasodilation, and provide maintenance needs. A balanced electrolyte solution is preferred. Lactated Ringer's, Normosol-R, or equivalents are most commonly used and are administered rapidly ($10–25 \text{ mL} \cdot \text{kg}^{-1} \cdot \text{h}^{-1}$) in hypotensive patients. After hypotension is corrected, fluid administration may be slowed to 4 to $6 \text{ mL} \cdot \text{kg}^{-1} \cdot \text{h}^{-1}$ (Chapter 19). Although ruminants salivate copiously while anesthetized, replacement of HCO_3^- is usually not required. Other fluid (e.g., saline) may be given when indicated. To increase fluid delivery rate when needed, two administration sets can be connected to one catheter with a Y-connector, multiple catheters can be placed, or a peristaltic pump may be used. For convenience, fluids packaged in 3- or 5-liter bags can be used for large volume administration. When administering large volumes of fluid, serial determinations of hematocrit and plasma total solids should be performed to prevent hemodilution and pulmonary edema. Hematocrit should remain above 25% and plasma total solids above 4 g/dL. Plasma or whole blood transfusion should be considered for hypoproteinemic or anemic individuals. Sodium bicarbonate is indicated for correction of nonrespiratory acidemia as determined by blood gas analysis or total CO_2 determination.

RESPIRATORY SUPPORTIVE THERAPY

Although anesthetized South American camelids ventilate well, domestic ruminants tend to hypoventilate while anesthetized. Mechanical ventilation should be considered when the procedure will exceed 1.5 hours and is indicated to prevent hypoventilation in individuals that will not maintain sufficient alveolar ventilation. To minimize the effects of mechanical ventilation on the cardiovascular system, inspiratory time should be 2 or 3 seconds, inspiratory pressure 20 to 30 cm H_2O, tidal volume 13 to 22 mL/kg, and respiratory rate 6 to 10 breaths/minute (Chapter 17). Hypocarbia can occur and can cause bradycardia in ruminants. In the absence of blood gas analysis in ruminants during controlled ventilation, minute volume should be decreased if unexplained bradycardia occurs.

During intravenous anesthesia ruminants also benefit from supplemental oxygen. If the animal is intubated, it could be connected to a demand valve. This piece of equipment is connected to an oxygen source and allows the patient to breathe spontaneously.(79) Compression of a button on the demand valve allows the anesthetist to "sigh" the patient. Because demand valves are designed for humans, there is an increase in the work of breathing associated with their use in large animals.(80) Insufflation (5 L/min for small ruminants, 15 L/min for adult cattle) with oxygen can also be done in intubated ruminants. A flowmeter is connected to an oxygen source and tubing. The tubing is inserted into the endotracheal tube.(81)

CARDIOVASCULAR SUPPORTIVE THERAPY

Mean arterial pressure ($\overline{AP}$) of at least 75 mm Hg or systolic pressure of 100 mm Hg and diastolic pressure of 60 mm Hg should be maintained in sheep, goats, and South American camelids. Systolic pressure (120 to 150 mm Hg), diastolic pressure (80 to 110 mm Hg), and mean arterial pressure (90 to 120 mm Hg) values in anesthetized cattle are greater than those in awake cattle.(82) Hypotension in anesthetized ruminants can occur and may be corrected by adjusting anesthetic depth. When movement occurs before hypotension is corrected, therapy is indicated to restore blood pressure and minimize the incidence of complications. Vasopressors can be used to correct hypotension. However, expansion of vascular volume with rapid fluid administration and use of drugs that improve cardiac output are better alternatives. When hypotension without bradycardia occurs, inotropes are preferred to increase stroke volume and cardiac output. Calcium borogluconate (23% solution) increases myocardial contractility and is given as a slow intravenous infusion (0.5–1.0 mL $\cdot$ kg^{-1} $\cdot$ h^{-1}) to effect. Often calcium administration can be discontinued after $\overline{AP}$ returns to normal values. Calcium borogluconate administration can cause bradycardia, necessitating use of a chronotrope if hypotension persists. Ephedrine, a mixed alpha- and beta-sympathomimetic drug, can be used at 0.02–0.06 mg/kg IV to increase $\overline{AP}$ through an increase in cardiac contractility.(83) Lack of response at low doses can indicate excessive depth of anesthesia. Dobutamine, a synthetic beta catecholamine, can be used to improve cardiac output. At low doses it increases myocardial contractility, and at higher doses it can increase heart rate.(84) Overdosing causes tachycardia and arrhythmias. Dobutamine is recommended over dopamine because improvement in hemodynamics occurs with smaller increases in heart rate.(85) It is administered at 1.0–2.0 μg $\cdot$ kg^{-1} $\cdot$ min^{-1} IV to effect.(84) To prepare a solution for infusion, 62.5 mg (5.0 mL) of dobutamine is added to 250 mL of saline. Initially, a 454-kg cow would receive 1.0–2.0 μg $\cdot$ kg^{-1} $\cdot$ min^{-1} (0.5–1.0 mg/min) corresponding to 2–4 mL/min of this solution. Using a standard IV set (15 drops/mL), 0.5 to 1 drop/second is the recommended infusion rate. It is preferable to place a separate 20-gauge venous catheter for gravity infusion of dobutamine so that adjustment of flow rate is not affected by hydrostatic pressure of concurrently administered intravenous fluids. Use of a fluid pump to administer the drug is recommended for both convenience and consistency. IVAC-type infusion pumps can be used with this preparation, or syringe pumps containing dobutamine diluted to 1 mg/mL with saline can be used. After correction of hypotension, the infusion rate can often be decreased for maintenance but not completely discontinued, as hypotension can recur.

MONITORING

As with any species, good anesthetic technique requires monitoring to allow drug administration to meet the animal's requirements and prevent excessive insult to the cardiovascular, respiratory, central nervous, and musculoskeletal systems, thereby decreasing the risk of complications. Monitoring includes those techniques that require the tactile, visual, and hearing skills of the anesthetist, and sophisticated techniques that require instrumentation. Attention is directed to three organ systems: the cardiovascular, respiratory, and central nervous systems. Ideally, one would monitor variables that respond rapidly to changes in anesthetic depth and allow the anesthetist sufficient time to make alterations in anesthetic administration before the anesthetic plane becomes either excessive or insufficient. Although monitoring is done constantly, most variables are recorded at 5-minute intervals. In many instances, monitoring equipment is used to aid in the evaluation of physiologic responses to anesthesia and, therefore, anesthetic depth. Use of these instruments can make the evaluation more precise and make administration of anesthetic drugs and selection of ancillary drugs more rational (Chapters 2 and 15).

Variables that can be used to monitor the cardiovascular system are heart rate, pulse pressure (pulse strength), color of mucous membranes, and capillary refill time. In healthy anesthetized adult cattle, the heart rate is usually 70 to 90 beats/minute. Animals that have received an anticholinergic will have an increased heart rate. Normal heart rate for calves, sheep, and goats varies with age. Juveniles will have a heart rate of 90 to 130 beats/minute, decreasing as they mature. Normal heart rate for adult anesthetized camelids following an anticholinergic is 80 to 100 beats/minute. For anesthetized juvenile camelids following an anticholinergic, it is 100 to 125 beats/minute. Heart rate may exceed normal range at the beginning of anesthesia due to excitement associated with induction or hypotension, but, most often, it returns to the normal range within 10 to 20 minutes. In compromised patients heart rate begins to approach the normal range during anesthesia as oxygen administration, fluid administration, analgesia and cardiovascular support drugs exert their effects. Heart rate usually decreases as depth of anesthesia increases, although this response can be masked by prior administration of anticholinergics.

Pulse pressure can be ascertained at several locations, should be full and bounding, and may decrease with excessive anesthetic depth. The common digital, caudal auricular, radial, and saphenous arteries are commonly palpated. The facial artery can be palpated in young calves, but it becomes more difficult to do so as the animal ages. Because most anesthetic agents depress the cardiovascular system and overdosage causes the heart to function less effectively as a pump, diminished pulse pressure should be indicative of anesthetic overdosage. Pulse pressure should be strong and palpated at different locations for comparison. Noting the amount of turgor present in the vessel during diastole can give an indication of diastolic pressure. If the vessel is easily collapsed by digital pressure during diastole, then diastolic pressure, and therefore, systolic pressure and AP can be assumed to be low even though pulse pressure may feel adequate.

Mucous membranes should be pink, although the mucous membranes of some ruminants and camelids are pigmented, making assessment difficult. The presence of cyanosis must also be noted, although animals breathing oxygen and an inhalation agent may be apneic for several minutes before cyanosis occurs. Because at least 5 g/dL of reduced hemoglobin is required before cyanosis can be detected, severely anemic animals may not show this sign. Flushed mucous membranes are associated with vasodilation. Vasodilation can be caused by hypercarbia, halothane, alpha-adrenergic antagonists, or histamine release, or may be associated with postural hypostatic congestion.(86) Brick-red mucous membranes are associated with endotoxic shock. Following digital compression to blanch an area of the gum, capillary refill should occur in 1 or 2 seconds.

Both of these variables give an indication of tissue perfusion. Excessive depth of anesthesia will cause the color of the mucous membranes to become pale and capillary refill time to increase. By combining data from these variables, one can qualitatively assess adequacy of blood pressure. For example, if the animal has normal heart rate, strong pulse pressure, pink mucous membranes, and short capillary refill time, and the peripheral arteries are not easily collapsed by digital pressure during diastole, then one can assume that blood pressure is in the normal range. Conversely, if pulse

pressure is weak, mucous membranes are pale, capillary refill time is prolonged, and peripheral arteries are easily occluded by digital pressure, then the animal's blood pressure is below normal and either the depth of anesthesia is excessive and/or cardiovascular support drugs are needed.

The respiratory system is evaluated by monitoring respiratory rate and tidal volume. Spontaneous breathing rates are usually 20 to 30 breaths/minute in adult cattle; calves, sheep, and goats usually have respiratory rates of 20 to 40 breaths/minute. Awake cattle have a decreased tidal volume when compared to horses.(87) That relationship persists in anesthetized cattle and other domestic ruminants in that they have a decreased tidal volume when compared to other species. Tidal volume is estimated by observing the amount of emptying of the rebreathing bag during inspiration. Increasing the depth of anesthesia can usually be expected to cause a decrease in tidal volume and eventually respiratory rate. Normal values for respiratory rate in anesthetized camelids are 15 to 30 breaths/ minute (adults) and 20 to 35 breaths/minute (juveniles). Camelids tend to ventilate well when allowed to do so spontaneously as judged by blood gas and respiratory gas analysis when anesthetized with either halothane or isoflurane if xylazine is not part of the anesthetic protocol.

The central nervous system can be monitored by observation of ocular reflexes. The palpebral reflex disappears with minimal depth of anesthesia in cattle, sheep, and goats, and is usually of no value during anesthesia. Rotation of the globe will occur as anesthetic depth changes in cattle (Fig. 20C–4). The eyeball is normally centered between the palpebra in lateral recumbency. As anesthesia is induced the eyeball rotates ventrally, with the cornea being partially obscured by the lower eyelid. As depth of anesthesia is increased, the cornea becomes completely hidden by the lower eyelid; this sign indicates stage III, plane 2–3 anesthesia (Chapter 2). A further increase in anesthesia is accompanied by dorsal rotation of the eyeball. Dorsal movement is complete when the cornea is centered between the palpebra; this sign indicates deep surgical anesthesia with profound muscle relaxation. During recovery, eyeball rotation occurs in reverse order to that occurring during induction.(88) Rotation of the globe does not occur in response to changes in depth of anesthesia in goats, sheep, or South American camelids. Usually the palpebral reflex of the dorsal eyelid of camelids remains during surgical anesthesia. However, if the camelid can move its ventral eyelid without tactile stimulation, anesthetic depth is decreasing and eventually limb movement will occur.(8) Nystagmus usually does not occur during anesthesia of domestic ruminants or camelids. When it does occur, it cannot be correlated with changes in depth of anesthesia. The corneal reflex should be present.

Response to pain from the surgical procedure can also be used to estimate depth of anesthesia. In some

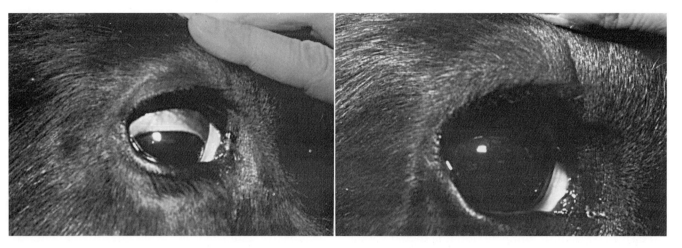

Fig. 20C–4.   Ocular rotation in the animal on the right indicates either insufficient or excessive depth of anesthesia. Ocular rotation in the animal on the left indicates surgical anesthesia. (See Fig 2.2 for additional explanation on eye movement in cattle.)

instances camelids may respond by showing more active palpebral reflex. Purposeful movement in all species indicates insufficient depth of anesthesia. In all species an increase in arterial pressure associated with the surgical procedure indicates adequate anesthesia if purposeful movement does not occur.

Electrocardiography (ECG) is used with either standard limb leads (I, II, III) or a dipole lead for detection of cardiac rate and rhythm disturbances. The lead that has the largest amplitude should be selected. A recorder is optional and useful as it allows one to record an ECG at the beginning of the case for future reference. Most ECG units emit an audible tone whenever a QRS complex is detected. The anesthetist should learn to always listen to the audible rhythm in the background during the case, especially during distractions. Because an ECG gives no information regarding blood pressure or pulse strength, emphasis should also be placed on monitoring pulse and arterial pressure instead of relying solely on the ECG.

Arterial pressure provides an accurate variable for assessing depth of anesthesia. In most instances, changes in depth of anesthesia become evident quickly through increases or decreases in blood pressure before changes in other variables are noted. Additionally, it is a more definitive variable than monitoring pulse pressure alone. Monitoring pulse pressure determines the difference between systolic and diastolic pressure. An animal with systolic and diastolic pressures of 120/90 mm Hg will have pulse pressure similar to that of another with pressures of 90/60 mm Hg. However, a large difference in $\overline{AP}$ or perfusion pressure exists. The former case will have $\overline{AP}$ of about 100 mm Hg, while the latter case will have $\overline{AP}$ of about 70 mm Hg. Since animals with low $\overline{AP}$ during anesthesia are more at risk for developing complications, identification of this situation is important. Normal values for systolic and diastolic pressure are 120–150/80–110 mm Hg in cattle and 90–120/60–80 mm Hg in the other species. Normal values for $\overline{AP}$ are 90–120 mm Hg in cattle and 75–100

mm Hg in the other species. However, if camelids are aroused by painful stimuli, mean arterial pressure may approach 150 mm Hg.

Arterial pressure can be monitored either indirectly or directly. Indirect methods of determining arterial pressure require the use of various infrasonic and ultrasonic devices to detect blood flow in peripheral arteries. The Doppler and Dinamap devices can be used with cuffs wrapped around the tail of cattle and limbs of sheep and goats (14), or around the tail or limbs of South American camelids.(7) Cuff diameter should be 40% of limb or tail circumference.(89) Direct methods require catheterization of an artery and use of a pressure transducer and amplifier or an aneroid manometer to determine pressure values. A transducer system determines systolic, diastolic, and mean arterial pressures. An aneroid manometer can be substituted for the pressure transducer and amplifier, but only $\overline{AP}$ can be obtained.(90) However, changes in $\overline{AP}$ do occur rapidly in response to changes in anesthetic stage, and use of this system allows the anesthetist to make appropriate responses (Chapter 15).

Percutaneous arterial catheterization is easily performed in most ruminants and is relatively free of complications.(90, 91) The caudal auricular, saphenous, and common digital arteries are most commonly catheterized using over-the-needle Teflon catheters. Passage of this type of catheter through the unbroken skin will damage the catheter, making arterial placement difficult. Thus incising the skin or piercing it with a slightly larger needle at the catheterization site is recommended.(91) A skin incision is usually not necessary when the caudal auricular artery is catheterized, because the skin is relatively thin in that location and the artery is often inadvertently hit because the skin is relatively immobile in that area. For adults, 3- to 5-cm, 18- to 20-gauge catheters are used with 2.5- to 3-cm, 20- to 22-gauge catheters being used in juveniles. An extension set with a two-way stopcock is used to connect the arterial catheter to a syringe containing heparinized (2.0 units/mL) saline and a piece of non-compliant tubing attached to the pressure transducer or aneroid manometer. Following removal of the arterial catheter, digital pressure is maintained at the site for at least 5 minutes to prevent hematoma formation. If desired, a pressure bandage can be used.

Central venous pressure can be determined to assess venous return, myocardial function, and the need for fluid replacement. This variable, along with serial determinations of hematocrit, plasma total solids, and urine production is a good method for evaluating fluid replacement but often gives little information regarding changes in depth of anesthesia. Normal values are 5 to 10 cm H_2O.

Normal values for arterial blood gas analysis are similar to those of other species. Respiratory gas analysis to determine end-tidal CO_2 and anesthetic agent concentration can be performed. Because domestic ruminants have a respiratory pattern characterized by small tidal volume, end-expired gas is not sufficiently representative of alveolar gas and an accurate assessment of blood gas tension cannot be obtained with capnography. End-tidal gas monitors more accurately reflect blood gas tensions when controlled ventilation is used.

Recovery

Ruminants recover well from general anesthesia and seldom experience emergence delirium or make premature attempts to stand. When an alpha$_2$-agonist is used as part of the anesthetic regimen, an antagonist can be used to hasten recovery.(27, 92, 93)

Extubation of domestic ruminants should not occur until the laryngeal reflex has returned. Extubation of orally intubated camelids should not occur until the animal is able to cough and trying to actively expel the endotracheal tube. Precautions should be taken to prevent the camelid from damaging or aspirating the endotracheal tube. If the patient has regurgitated, the buccal cavity and pharynx should be lavaged to prevent aspiration of the material. In these instances, the endotracheal tube should be withdrawn with the cuff inflated in an attempt to remove any material that may have located in the trachea. Because llamas are obligate nasal breathers (75), gas exchange must be confirmed after extubation; airway obstruction can commonly occur during the transition from oral endotracheal intubation to nasal breathing. The endotracheal tube of nasally intubated camelids can be removed after they stand. Although ruminants recover well from general anesthesia with minimal assistance, an attendant should be available.

Complications

INTRAOPERATIVE COMPLICATIONS

Fortunately, major complications do not occur often during or following well-planned anesthesia in ruminants. However, one must be vigilant so that unexpected occurrence of a complication can be recognized

and effectively treated. As is the case in anesthesia of other species, complications are most effectively treated by prevention, so emphasis should be placed on formation and implementation of a rational anesthetic regimen.

Airway obstruction. Airway obstruction can be caused by several factors during ruminant anesthesia. If left untreated, it causes dyspnea, hypoxemia, hypercarbia, apnea, and eventually cardiac arrest. Animals with an airway obstruction have a characteristic pattern to their respiratory excursions. The thorax expands partially and then remains static during inspiration, collapsing quickly during expiration. Because of the obstruction, limited expansion of the thoracic cavity occurs, along with negative thoracic pressure during inspiration. Negative pressure causes rapid recoil of the thorax during expiration. Lack of gas exchange from the nares or endotracheal tube will confirm airway obstruction.

Airway obstruction can occur following regurgitation in ruminants. In lightly anesthetized ruminants, active regurgitation can occur during intubation (8, 54) and passive regurgitation can occur at any time during anesthesia owing to relaxation of the cardia. Because rumen contents contain more solid material than do gastric contents of monogastric animals, there is greater potential for ingesta to obstruct the larynx, while the more fluid portion will drain from the mouth. Patients that are not intubated are most at risk, but intubated animals that have regurgitated during anesthesia are at risk following extubation. Treatment involves removal of ingesta from the buccal cavity or buccal lavage prior to extubation. If the cause is active regurgitation, depth of anesthesia should be rapidly increased and the airway established to prevent aspiration.

Partial or complete airway obstruction in intubated animals can occur following kinking or collapse of the endotracheal tube or esophageal placement of the endotracheal tube. Improper positioning of the head can result in kinking of the endotracheal tube, as can malposition of anesthetic equipment. Collapse can occur following overinflation of the cuff: The trachea limits expansion of the cuff, and as the pressure increases, the wall of the endotracheal tube begins to buckle. Diffusion of nitrous oxide into the cuff during the anesthetic procedure can also cause collapse of the tube.(94) In each of these instances, absence of movement or diminished movement of the rebreathing bag of the anesthetic machine would be noted along with increased resistance to gas flow during manual compression of the rebreathing bag. Correction of the underlying cause is indicated.

Following esophageal placement of the endotracheal tube, movement of the rebreathing bag does not usually occur. In addition, esophageal intubation may provoke regurgitation.(54) Following confirmation of improper endotracheal tube placement, the tube should be removed and placed in the trachea.

Dorsal displacement of the soft palate occurs with some degree of frequency in equine anesthesia. The soft palate remains dorsal to the epiglottis hindering airflow into the larynx. Although this condition is usually not a problem in domestic ruminants, it can be a problem in llamas, as they are obligate nasal breathers.(75) It can occur at any time in nonintubated llamas, but more often occurs following extubation. This condition can be corrected by inducing the animal to swallow, causing the soft palate to resume its normal position. Animals sometimes correct themselves; however, if the anesthetic plane is sufficient to abolish deglutition, the problem is much more severe because the animal cannot correct itself, causing impaired ventilation and the possibility of apnea and cardiac arrest. Passage of a small stomach tube into the oropharynx will stimulate swallowing. If the animal cannot swallow, it should be reintubated and remain so until the anesthetic plane decreases to the point where the animal can swallow.

Apnea. Apnea can have several causes. It can occur secondary to airway obstruction or to hypercarbia and hypoxemia caused by hypoventilation. Hypoxemia often occurs in anesthetized animals breathing room air or can be caused by ventilation–perfusion inequality or right–to–left shunts (Chapter 6).(54) In addition, ruminal tympany and the volume of ingesta and viscera in ruminants hinders diaphragmatic function, increasing the degree of hypoventilation and decreasing functional residual capacity.(95) Overdosage with xylazine, barbiturates, or other anesthetics also cause apnea. Because ruminants have very low levels of pseudocholinesterase, metabolism of succinylcholine is slow, causing prolonged effects of the drug.(96) This drug is contraindicated in ruminants except in very narrow circumstances, and can be used only in conjunction with mechanical ventilation. Other unusual causes of apnea are anterior migration of local anesthetic in the epidural space blocking innervation to the diaphragm and intercostal muscles, and neuromuscular blockade caused by interaction of anesthetics and aminoglycoside antibiotics (Chapters 13 and 16).(97)

No matter what the cause of respiratory arrest, symptomatic therapy must be instituted until the cause can be identified and corrected. The most effective treatment is tracheal intubation and controlled ventilation (preferably with oxygen, but room air or compressed air could be used). In anesthetized animals receiving inhalation anesthesia, alternate compression and release of the rebreathing bag will provide ventilatory support. Mechanical ventilators can also be used to provide support in this instance. A demand valve can be used to provide controlled ventilation by intermittent compression and release of a button. This piece of equipment is small, portable, and capable of generating sufficient gas flow to effectively ventilate adult horses and ruminants.(79) An E cylinder of oxygen will last about 15 minutes when used on 500-kg cattle, with the demand valve becoming progressively less efficient as the cylinder empties. Because it is capable of generating high gas flow, caution should be exercised when using the demand valve on small patients to decrease the risk of volotrauma and pneumothorax.

Another method of intermittent positive pressure ventilation (IPPV) involves the use of an oxygen cylinder and nasogastric tube.(81) After connection of the tube to the cylinder, the cylinder is opened until gas flow is felt about 18 inches from the tube tip. The tube is passed into the endotracheal tube, and by alternately occluding the endotracheal tube around the smaller tube and releasing it, IPPV can be delivered. This method isn't as efficient as the others. When dealing with small domestic ruminants or camelids (< 100 kg), an Ambu bag can be used to ventilate the animal when connected to the endotracheal tube.(54) Periodic compression and release of the bag will ventilate the animal. With all techniques, the inspiratory phase should be ended following observation of adequate thoracic expansion. Symptomatic therapy can include the use of an analeptic, doxapram (0.5–1.0 mg/kg IV).

During controlled ventilation, attempts should be made to identify the cause of apnea. When a specific antagonist such as naloxone, tolazoline (22, 93), or yohimbine (21, 22, 29, 92); or a drug such as doxapram (28), which has antagonistlike action, is available and indicated, it should be used. If ruminal tympany is severe enough to cause apnea, the rumen should be decompressed, preferably by passage of a stomach tube, but if that isn't possible, the rumen should be trocarized with a 12-gauge needle. When specific therapy is unavailable, controlled ventilation and other supportive therapy (IV fluids, heating blankets, etc.) should be continued until the animal recovers. If the animal shows signs of arousal without spontaneous ventilation, hypocarbia may be the cause and the respiratory rate should be lowered to allow sufficient carbon dioxide accumulation to initiate spontaneous ventilation.

Cardiac arrhythmias. Cardiac arrhythmias usually do not occur in anesthetized food animals. When they do occur, the most likely arrhythmia is premature ventricular contraction (PVC). They can occur following induction of anesthesia with the thiobarbiturates and are often coupled with a normal beat, giving rise to the term *bigeminal rhythm.*(98) Usually they are transitory and disappear without treatment. Other arrhythmias that may be seen following thiobarbiturate induction are sinus tachycardia, ventricular tachycardia, multifocal ventricular tachycardia, and ventricular fibrillation.(98)

Following the induction period, PVCs are most commonly caused by hypoxemia and/or hypercarbia and traumatic myocarditis. An occasional solitary PVC is usually of little concern, but runs of three or more consecutive PVCs are serious in that cardiac output drops dramatically because the heart does not have time to fill adequately between beats. Therefore, coronary perfusion decreases, increasing the irritability of the focus of the PVC and the likelihood of ventricular fibrillation.

Presumptive diagnosis of PVCs can be made by palpation of a peripheral artery and noting the change in the sequence or rhythm of pulsations or by auscultation and noting the change in rhythm of heart sounds.

Diagnosis can be confirmed by ECG. Therapy is directed at controlling the irritable focus, usually by the administration of lidocaine, followed by identification and correction of the underlying cause. Causes of hypoxemia/hypercarbia are hypoventilation, exhausted soda lime, and inadequate F_IO_2. Lidocaine (1–2 mg/kg IV) is administered as a bolus.(99) If the arrhythmia persists after one or two lidocaine treatments, a slow infusion of lidocaine (40–60 $\mu g \cdot kg^{-1} \cdot min^{-1}$ IV) should be instituted.(99)

Atrial fibrillation can occur in cattle as a sequela to metabolic derangement caused by another problem. Most often, it occurs secondary to gastrointestinal obstruction. Atrial fibrillation usually resolves in these cases following correction of the primary problem. Because cattle are amenable to physical restraint and local anesthesia, corrective surgery can be performed without general anesthesia. Diagnosis can be confirmed with electrocardiography.

The oculocardiac reflex is a well-recognized reflex in dogs, cats, and horses (Chapter 24).(98–100) It is mediated by the trigeminal and vagus nerves, and initiated by traction or pressure on the globe during surgery. Bradycardia is the usual response, but cardiac arrest can occur. Whenever major ophthalmic surgery (e.g., enucleation) is planned, the possibility of arrhythmias or bradycardia caused by surgical manipulations exists. Discontinuation of the surgical manipulations allowing normal heart rate rhythm to return followed by resumption of surgery with less traumatic technique is usually sufficient to correct the problem. If bradyarrhythmia persists or returns despite gentle tissue handling, atropine or glycopyrrolate should be administered. Vagal discharge secondary to manipulation of the viscera can also cause bradyarrhythmia. It is treated similar to the oculocardiac reflex. Sinus bradyarrhythmia (<30 beats/minute) or sinus arrest can also occur during painful stimuli in camelids, and atropine or glycopyrrolate may be required if none was given prior to induction.

Other complications. Circulatory collapse can occur from dehydration, hemorrhage, inappropriate use of vasodilators, overdose of anesthetic agents, hypoxemia, and endotoxic shock. The problem is recognized by deterioration of variables used to assess cardiovascular performance. Decrease in pulse pressure, hypotension ($\overline{AP}$ < 80 mm Hg in cattle and $\overline{AP}$ < 60 mm Hg in camelids, sheep, and goats), increased gingival perfusion time, pale mucous membranes, and either bradycardia or tachycardia would be noted. Supportive therapy is instituted consisting of rapid administration of intravenous fluids, reduction or cessation of anesthetic administration, and use of positive inotropic agents to improve cardiac output.(83–85) Examples of inotropic drugs include calcium borogluconate, calcium chloride, dobutamine, and dopamine. If severe bradycardia is present (HR < 70 beats/minute for small domestic ruminants, HR < 50 beats/minute for adult cattle) use of a chronotrope is indicated. If possible,

specific therapy should be implemented to correct the cause (e.g., whole blood transfusion, increased ventilation, or increased F_IO_2.

Hypothermia can occur during food animal anesthesia as the anesthetic agents interfere with heat regulation.(18) In adult cattle and camelids this is usually of little consequence. Because of their large body mass to surface area ratio, body temperature seldom decreases by more than 0.5° C during anesthesia if no major body cavities are opened. Even if a body cavity is opened, temperature usually decreases by less than 3° C. However, hypothermia can become a significant clinical problem in smaller ruminants and camelids during prolonged surgery, causing a decrease in anesthetic requirement and should be suspected whenever recovery is delayed.(18) Warm water recirculating blankets placed under the animal will help maintain normal body temperature. At the least, towels should be placed between the animal and surgery table.

Although anesthetized camelids do not appear to become tympanitic, ruminal tympany often occurs during anesthesia of domestic ruminants owing to fermentation of ingesta and the animal's inability to eructate. As tympany develops, more pressure is placed on the diaphragm, decreasing functional residual capacity and impeding ventilation.(95) In addition, tympany increases the risk of regurgitation. Therapy involves passage of a stomach tube to decompress the rumen. On occasion, one will be unable to pass the stomach tube into the rumen. In these difficult cases, placing the animal in sternal recumbency will aid the procedure. When that is not possible, the rumen can be decompressed with a 12-gauge needle inserted through the abdominal wall. Fortunately, ruminal tympany is usually of the nonfrothy type and decompression is easily accomplished. External pressure placed on the rumen will help expel gas from the orogastric tube. Ruminal tympany can also occur during the use of nitrous oxide, as it tends to accumulate in gas-filled viscus.(98) Discontinuation of nitrous oxide administration along with decompression of the rumen is recommended.

Connective tissue is not as fibrous in ruminants' lungs, and therefore excessive airway pressure can cause pneumothorax and emphysema more easily than in the horse.(101) Signs include dyspnea and increased resistance to inspiration because of tension pneumothorax. It is treated by placement of a chest tube and aspiration of the gas. It is much easier to prevent than treat. Do not use excessive airway pressure (>30 cm H_2O) when "sighing" the animal or using controlled ventilation.

Intracarotid injections seldom occur in cattle because of the depth that the carotid artery lies in the neck. However, in small ruminants and especially in camelids, an inexperienced individual could inadvertently inject a tranquilizer or anesthetic agent intracarotidly. Severe sequelae can result from the irritating effects of the drugs on the cerebral circulation. At the least, seizures can occur and quite possibly death. If seizures do occur, they must be controlled with an anticonvulsant. Because the sequelae can be so severe, every effort must be made to avoid intracarotid injection.(102)

POSTOPERATIVE COMPLICATIONS

Thrombophlebitis can occur following perivascular injection of irritating compounds, although usually not with the frequency or severity that occurs in horses. When performing intravenous injections, a needle or catheter of sufficient size and length should be placed in the jugular vein and secured. Its placement should be verified before and after each injection. If perivascular injection has occurred, early recognition is essential if treatment is to prevent massive tissue damage. Following recognition, the area should be infiltrated with normal saline to dilute the injected drug, 2% lidocaine to relax venospasm and enhance absorption, and a corticosteroid to decrease inflammation. Once the inflammatory process has started, symptomatic therapy is indicated. Hydrotherapy can be used to minimize swelling, or a cold hydrocolloidal pack can be incorporated in a bandage around the animal's neck. After the area begins to drain, hydrotherapy should continue. Depending on the severity of the lesion, surgical debridement and ligation of the jugular vein may be required to prevent exsanguination should the vessel wall erode. Injections in the mammary veins of cows should be performed with caution, as abscesses can occur.

Corneal ulcers can occur following anesthesia. If an ulcer does occur, as evidenced by photophobia, lacrimation, and fluorescein staining, routine treatment should be instituted.(103)

Food animals and camelids tend to recover well from general anesthesia without the emergence delirium that can occur in equine anesthesia. Consequently, long bone fractures and cervical fractures seldom occur during recovery. Should they occur, therapy is based upon severity of the fracture and the economic value of the animal.

Aspiration pneumonia can occur following regurgitation of rumen or gastric contents and subsequent inhalation of the material. If active regurgitation occurs, the animal may inhale the material deeply into the pulmonary tree, initiating bronchospasm and physical obstruction of the airways. Signs include dyspnea and, depending on severity, cyanosis. Aminophylline can be used for bronchodilation at 11 mg/kg IV over 20 minutes along with oxygen.(104) If the patient survives the initial insult, pneumonia is certain. Broad spectrum antibiotics are indicated. Silent or passive regurgitation can occur with the same results, except that there usually isn't as much particulate material in the regurgitant. Similar treatment is instituted. Because of the potential severity of this complication, emphasis must be placed on prevention. Tracheal intubation is recommended. If this is not possible, the occiput should be elevated to encourage fluids to drain from the mouth and not into the trachea (Fig. 20C–3).(18)

Postoperative myopathy-neuropathy can occur in cattle but doesn't seem to occur as often as in horses. It does not seem to be a problem in calves, sheep, goats, or camelids. The problem is recognized by muscle weakness and inability to stand. Therapy is symptomatic, with intravenous fluids to maintain hydration, acid-base status, and electrolytes, and analgesics, nonsteroidal antiinflammatory agents, and vitamin E-selenium compounds as indicated. Slinging the animal may be helpful but can increase muscle damage. The problem may take several days to resolve and can be life threatening. Again, it is better to prevent the problem by positioning the anesthetized animal properly and avoiding excessive depth of anesthesia.

In conclusion, provision of general anesthesia to domestic ruminants and South American camelids to allow completion of complex diagnostic and surgical procedures can be very rewarding. Although each species may exhibit some characteristics unique to itself, the variety of challenges encountered while anesthetizing ruminants provides the opportunity to expand the science and art of anesthesia while improving the humaneness of patient care.

References

1. Vallenas A, Cummings JF, Munnell JF. A gross study of the compartmentalized stomach of two new-world camelids, the llama and guanaco. J Morph 143:399–424, 1971.
2. Bednarski RM, McGuirk SM. Bradycardia associated with fasting in cattle [Abstract]. Vet Surg 15:458, 1986.
3. Tranquilli WJ. Techniques of inhalation anesthesia in ruminants and swine. Vet Clin North Am Food Anim Pract 2:593–619, 1986.
4. Lassen ED, Pearson EG, Long PO, et al. Serum biochemical values in llamas: reference values. Am J Vet Res 47:2278–2280, 1986.
5. Fowler ME. In: Medicine and Surgery of the South American Camelid. Ames, IA: Iowa State University Press, 1989, pp 35–63.
6. Amsel SI, Kainer RA, Johnson LW. Choosing the best site to perform venipuncture in a llama. Vet Med 82:535–536, 1987.
7. Heath RB. Llama anesthetic programs. Vet Clin North Am Food Anim Pract 5:71–80, 1989.
8. Riebold TW, Kaneps AJ, Schmotzer WB. Anesthesia in the llama. Vet Surg 18:400–404, 1989.
9. Short CE. Preanesthetic medications in ruminants and swine. Vet Clin North Am Food Anim Pract 2:553–566, 1986.
10. Taylor PM. Anaesthesia in sheep and goats. Practice 13:31–36, 1991.
11. Thurmon JC. College of Veterinary Medicine. University of Illinois. Personal communication, 1970.
12. Greene SA, Thurmon JC. Xylazine–a review of its pharmacology and use in veterinary medicine. J Vet Pharmacol Ther 11:295–313, 1988.
13. Raptopoulos D, Weaver BMQ. Observations following intravenous xylazine administration in steers. Vet Rec 114:567–569, 1984.
14. Trim CM. Special anesthesia considerations in the ruminant. In: Short CE, ed. Principles and practice of veterinary anesthesia. Baltimore: Williams & Wilkins, 285–300, 1987.
15. Fayed AH, Abdalla EB, Anderson RR, et al. Effect of xylazine in heifers under thermoneutral or heat stress conditions. Am J Vet Res 50:151–153, 1989.
16. Ley S, Waterman A, Livingston A. Variation in the analgesic effects of xylazine in different breeds of sheep. Vet Rec 126:508, 1990.

17. O'Hair KC, McNeil JS, Phillips YY. Effects of xylazine in adult sheep. Lab Anim Sci 36:563, 1986.
18. Hall LW, Clarke KW. In: Veterinary anaesthesia, 9th ed. Philadelphia: Balliere Tindall, 1991.
19. Jedruch J, Gajewski Z. The effect of detomidine hydrochloride Domosedan® on the electrical activity of the uterus in cows. Acta Vet Scand Suppl 82:192–198, 1986.
20. Celly, CS, McDonell WN, Black WD, Young S. Comparative cardiopulmonary effects of four α-2 adrenoceptor agonists in sheep [Abstract]. Vet Surg 22:545–546, 1993.
21. Kitzman JV, Booth NH, Hatch RC, Wallner B. Antagonism of xylazine sedation by 4-aminopyridine and yohimbine in cattle. Am J Vet Res 43, 2165–2169, 1982.
22. Thurmon JC, Lin HC, Tranquilli WJ, et al. A comparison of yohimbine and tolazoline as antagonist xylazine sedation in calves [Abstract]. Vet Surg 18:170–171, 1989.
23. Hsu WH, Hanson CE, Hembrough FB, Schaffer DD. Effects of idazoxan, tolazoline, and yohimbine on xylazine-induced respiratory changes and central nervous system depression in ewes. Am J Vet Res 50:1570–1573.
24. Ko, JCH, McGrath CJ, Jacobson JD. Effects of atipamezole and yohimbine on medetomidine-induced central nervous system depression and cardiorespiratory changes in lambs [Abstract]. Vet Surg 23:79, 1994.
25. Ruckenbusch Y, Toutain PL. Specific antagonism of xylazine effects on reticulo-rumen motor function in cattle. Vet Med Rev 5(1):3–12, 1984.
26. Doherty TJ, Ballinger JA, McDonell WN, et al. Antagonism of xylazine-induced sedation by idazoxan in calves. Can J Vet Res 51:244–248, 1987.
27. Raekallio M, Kivalo M, Jalanka, Vaisio O. Medetomidine/ ketamine sedation in calves and its reversal with atipamezole. J Vet Anaesth 18:45–47, 1991.
28. Zahner JM, Hatch RC, Wilson RC, et al. Antagonism of xylazine sedation in steers by doxapram and 4-aminopyridine. Am J Vet Res 45:2546–2551, 1984.
29. Riebold TW, Kaneps AJ, Schmotzer WB. Reversal of xylazine-induced sedation in llamas using doxapram or 4-aminopyridine and yohimbine. J Am Vet Med Assoc 189:1059–1061, 1986.
30. Aouad JI, Wright EM, Shaner TW. Anesthesia evaluation on ketamine and xylazine in calves. Bov Pract 2:22–31, 1981.
31. Campbell KB, Klavano PA, Richardson P, Alexander JE. Hemodynamic effects of xylazine in the calf. Am J Vet Res 40:1777–1780, 1979.
32. Freire ACT, Gontijo RM, Pessoa JM, Souza R. Effect of xylazine on the electrocardiogram of the sheep. Br Vet J 137:590–595, 1981.
33. Symonds HW. The effect of xylazine upon hepatic glucose production and blood flow rate in the lactating dairy cow. Vet Rec 99:234–236, 1976.
34. Symonds HW, Mallison CB. The effect of xylazine and xylazine followed by insulin on blood glucose and insulin in the dairy cow. Vet Rec 102:27–29, 1978.
35. Eichner RD, Prior RL, Kvasnicka WG. Xylazine induced hyperglycemia in beef cattle. Am J Vet Res 40:127–129, 1979.
36. Brockman RP. Effect of xylazine on plasma glucose, glucagon and insulin concentration in sheep. Res Vet Sci 30:383–384, 1981.
37. Muggaberg J, Brockman RP. Effect of adrenergic drugs on glucose and plasma glucagon and insulin response to xylazine in sheep. Res Vet Sci 33:118–120, 1982.
38. Thurmon JC, Nelson DR, Hartsfield SM, Rumore CA. Effects of xylazine hydrochloride on urine in cattle. Aust Vet J 54:178–180, 1978.
39. Hopkins TJ. The clinical pharmacology of xylazine in cattle. Aust Vet J 48:109–112, 1972.
40. Uggla A, Lindqvist Å. Acute pulmonary oedema as adverse reaction to the use of xylazine in sheep. Vet Rec 113:42, 1983.
41. LeBlanc MM, Hubbell JAE, Smith HC. The effect of xylazine hydrochloride on intrauterine pressure in the cow and the mare. Proc Annu Mtg Soc Theriogenol, Denver, Colo 1984:211–220.
42. Jansen CAM, Lowe KC, Nathanielsz PW. The effects of xylazine on uterine activity, fetal and maternal oxygenation, cardiovas-cular function, and fetal breathing. Am J Obstet Gynecol 148:386, 1984.
43. Gray PR. Anesthesia in goats and sheep. II. General anesthesia. Compend Cont Educ Pract Vet 8:S127–S135, 1986.
44. Valverde A, Doherty TJ, Dyson D, Valliant AE. Evaluation of pentobarbital as a drug for standing sedation in cattle. Vet Surg 18:235–238, 1989.
45. Barrington GM, Meyer TF, Parish SM. Standing castration of the llama using butorphanol tartrate and local anesthesia. Equine Pract 15:35–39, 1993.
46. O'Hair KC, Dodd KT, Phillips YY, Beattie RJ. Cardiopulmonary effects of nalbuphine hydrochloride and butorphanol tartrate in sheep. Lab Anim Sci 38:58–61, 1988.
47. Waterman AE, Livingston A, Amin A. Analgesic activity and respiratory effects of burorphanol in sheep. Res Vet Sci 51:19–23, 1991.
48. Thurmon JC. College of Veterinary Medicine. University of Illinois. Personal communication. 1993.
49. MJ Huber. College of Veterinary Medicine. Oregon State University. Personal communication. 1993.
50. Rouse S. Pharmacodynamics of thiobarbiturates. Veterinary Anesthesia 5:22–26, 1978.
51. Pascoe PJ. Emergency care medicine. In: Short CE, ed. Principles and practice of veterinary anesthesia. Baltimore: Williams & Wilkins, 1987:558–598.
52. Chaplin MD, Roszkowski AP, Richards RK. Displacement of thiopental from plasma proteins by nonsteroidal anti-inflammatory agents. Proc Society for Experimental Biology and Medicine 143:667–671, 1973.
53. Blaze CA, Holland RE, Grant AL. Gas exchange during xylazine-ketamine anesthesia in neonatal calves. Vet Surg 17:155–159, 1988.
54. Thurmon JC, Benson GJ. Anesthesia in ruminants and swine. In: Howard JC, ed. Current veterinary therapy, food animal practice, 3rd ed. Philadelphia: WB Saunders, 1993:58–76.
55. Coulson NM. The cardiorespiratory effects of diazepam/ ketamine and xylazine/ketamine anesthetic combinations in sheep. Lab Anim Sci 39:591–597, 1989.
56. Grandy JL, McDonell WN. Evaluation of concentrated solutions of guaifenesin for equine anesthesia. J Am Vet Med Assoc 176:619–622, 1980.
57. Thurmon JC. Injectable anesthetic agents and techniques in ruminants and swine. Vet Clin N Am Food Anim Pract 2:567–592, 1986.
58. Wall R, Muir WW. Hemolytic potential of guaifenesin cattle. Cornell Vet 80:209–216, 1990.
59. Thurmon JC, Benson GJ, Tranquilli WJ, Olson WA. Cardiovascular effects of intravenous infusion of guaifenesin, ketamine, and xylazine in Holstein calves [Abstract]. Vet Surg 15:463, 1986.
60. Lin, HC, Tyler JW, Welles EG, et al. Effects of anesthesia induced and maintained by continuous intravenous administration of guaifenesin, ketamine, and xylazine in spontaneously breathing sheep. Am J Vet Res 54:1913–1916, 1993.
61. Tracy CH, Short CE, Clark BC. Comparing the effects of intravenous and intramuscular administration of Telazol. Vet Med 83:104–111, 1988.
62. Hubbell JAE, Muir WW. Xylazine and tiletamine-zolazepam anesthesia in horses. Am J Vet Res 50:737–742, 1989.
63. Lin HC, Thurmon JC, Benson GJ, et al. The hemodynamic response of calves to tiletamine-zolazepam anesthesia. Vet Surg 18:328–334, 1989.
64. Thurmon JC, Lin HC, Benson GJ, et al. Combining Telazol and xylazine for anesthesia in calves. Vet Med 84:824–830, 1989.
65. Conner GH, Coppock RW, Beck CC. Laboratory use of CI-744, a cataleptoid anesthetic, in sheep. Vet Med Small Anim Clin 69:479–482, 1974.
66. Lagutchik MS, Januszkiewicz AJ, Dodd KT, Martin DG. Cardiopulmonary effects of a tiletamine-zolazepam combination in sheep. Am J Vet Res 52:1441–1447, 1991.
67. Howard BW, Lagutchik MS, Januszkiewicz AJ, Martin DG. The cardiovascular response of sheep to tiletamine-zolazepam and butorphanol tartrate anesthesia. Vet Surg 19:461–467, 1990.

68. Klein LV, Tomasic M, Olsen K. Evaluation of Telazol in llamas [Abstract]. Vet Surg 19:316–317, 1990.
69. Waterman AE. Use of propofol in sheep. Vet Rec 122:260, 1988.
70. Nolan AM, Reid J, Welsh E. The use of propofol as an induction agent in goats [Abstract]. J Vet Anaesth 18:53–54, 1991.
71. Handel IG, Weaver BMQ, Staddon GE, Cruz Madorran JI. Observation on the pharmacokinetics of propofol in sheep. Proc 4th Internat Cong Vet Anes, Utrecht, The Netherlands, 1991: 143–154.
72. Hubbell JAE, Hull BL, Muir WW. Perianesthetic considerations in cattle. Compend Cont Educ Pract Vet 8:F92–F102, 1986.
73. Kinyon GE. A new device for topical anesthesia. Anesthesiology 56:154, 1982.
74. Lagutchik MS, Mundie TG, Martin DG. Methemoglobinemia induced by a benzocaine-based topically administered anesthetic in eight sheep. J Am Vet Med Assoc 201:1407–1410, 1992.
75. Riebold TW, Engel HN, Grubb TL, et al. Anatomical considerations during intubation of the llama: the presence of a nasopharyngeal diverticulum. J Am Vet Med Assoc 204:779–783, 1994.
76. O'Brien TD, Raffe MR, Cox VS, et al. Hepatic necrosis following halothane anesthesia in goats. J Am Vet Med Assoc 189:1591–1595 1986.
77. Mathews K, Doherty T, Dyson D, et al. Nephrotoxicity in dogs associated with methoxyflurane anesthesia and flunixin meglumine analgesia [Abstract]. Can Vet J 31:766–771, 1990.
78. White NA. Postanesthetic recumbency myopathy in horses. Compend Cont Educ Pract Vet 4:S44–S52, 1982.
79. Riebold TW, Evans AT, Robinson NE. Evaluation of the demand valve for resuscitation of horses. J Am Vet Med Assoc 176:1736–1742, 1980.
80. Watney GCG, Watkins SB, Hall LW. Effects of a demand valve on pulmonary ventilation in spontaneously breathing, anaesthetized horses. Vet Rec 117:358–362, 1985.
81. Gabel AA, Heath RB, Ross JN, et al. Hypoxia–its prevention in inhalation anesthesia in horses. Proc Am Assoc Equine Pract 12:179–196, 1966.
82. Matthews NS, Gleed RD, Short CE. Cardiopulmonary effects of general anesthesia in adult cattle. Mod Vet Pract 67:618–620, 1986.
83. Grandy JL, Hodgson DS, Dunlop CI, et al. Cardiopulmonary effects of ephedrine in halothane anesthetized horses. J Vet Pharmacol Ther 12:389–396, 1989.
84. Daunt DA. Supportive therapy in the anesthetized horse. Vet Clin North Am Equine Pract 6:557–574, 1990.
85. Tranquilli WJ, Greene SA. Cardiovascular medications and the autonomic nervous system. In: Short CE, ed. Principles and practice of veterinary anesthesia. Baltimore: Williams & Wilkins, 1987:426–454.
86. Manley SV. Monitoring the anesthetized horse. Vet Clin North Am Large Anim Pract 3:111–134, 1981.
87. Gallivan GJ, McDonell WN, Forrest JB. Comparative ventilation and gas exchange in the horse and cow. Res Vet Sci 46:331–336, 1989.
88. Thurmon JC, Romack FE, Garner HE. Excursion of the bovine eyeball during gaseous anesthesia. Vet Med Small Anim Clin 63:967–970, 1968.
89. Grandy JL, Hodgson DS. Anesthetic considerations for emergency equine abdominal surgery. Vet Clin North Am Equine Pract 4:63–78, 1988.
90. Riebold TW, Evans AT. Comparison of simultaneous blood pressure determinations by four methods in the anesthetized horse. Vet Surg 14:332–337, 1985.
91. Riebold TW, Brunson DB, Lott RA, Evans AT. Percutaneous arterial catheterization in the horse. Vet Med Small Anim Clin 75:1736–1742, 1980.
92. Kruse-Elliott KT, Riebold TW, Swanson CR. Reversal of xylazine-ketamine anesthesia in goats [Abstract]. Vet Surg 16:321, 1987.
93. Young DB, Shawley RV, Barron SJ. Tolazoline reversal of xylazine-ketamine anesthesia in calves [Abstract]. Vet Surg 18:171, 1988.
94. Ward, CS. Anaesthetic equipment: physical principles and maintenance. London: Balliere Tindall, 1985.
95. Masewe VA, Gillespie JR, Berry JD. Influence of ruminal insufflation on pulmonary function and diaphragmatic electromyography in cattle. Am J Vet Res 40:26–31, 1979.
96. Tavernor WD. Muscle relaxants. In: Soma LR, ed. Veterinary anesthesia. Baltimore: Williams & Wilkins, 1971:111–120.
97. Adams HR, Teske RH, Mercer HD. Anesthetic-antibiotic relationships. J Am Vet Med Assoc 169:409–412, 1976.
98. Lumb WV, Jones EW. In: Veterinary anesthesia, 2nd ed. Philadelphia: Lea & Febiger, 1984.
99. Muir WW, Bednarski RM. Equine cardiopulmonary resuscitation. Part II. Compend Cont Educ Pract Vet 5:S287–S295, 1983.
100. Short CE, Rebhun WC. Complications caused by the oculocardiac reflex during anesthesia in the foal. J Am Vet Med Assoc 176:630–631, 1980.
101. Heath RB. General anesthesia in ruminants. In: The practice of large animal surgery. Philadelphia: WB Saunders, 1984:202–204.
102. Brown SS, Lyons SM, Dundee JW. Intra-arterial barbiturates: a study of some factors leading to intravascular thrombosis. Br J Anesth 40:13–19, 1968.
103. Whitely RD, Moore CP. Ocular diagnostic and therapeutic techniques in food animals. Vet Clin North Am Large Anim Pract 6:553–575, 1984.
104. Ayres JW, Pearson EG, Riebold TW, Chang SF. Theophylline and dyphylline pharmacokinetics in the horse. Am J Vet Res 46:2500–2506, 1985.

chapter **20**D

SWINE

Introduction

SPECIAL CONSIDERATIONS

Swine (*Sus scrofa domestica*) present a special challenge to immobilization and anesthesia. A thorough understanding of their physiologic response to mechanical restraint, anesthesia, and surgery is essential for their safe handling.

Pigs come in all sizes. They range from piglets (0.5 to 3 kg) and miniatures (10 to 30 kg) to individuals that can weigh in excess of 400 kg. Most research is conducted in pigs weighing less than 50 kg, as is most field and hospital surgery. Exceptions include cesarean sections in mature sows and surgery in large boars.

The pig's anatomic structure is not conducive to manual restraint, especially when it has grown to large size. The pig's body is shaped such that, in the wild, it can scurry through underbrush and escape through small openings in an effort to elude its enemies. There is no part of its body that is easily grasped for restraint.

Pigs have only a few superficial veins (primarily on the dorsolateral surface of their ears) into which an injection can be made. As a result, drugs injected by the intramuscular route have become popular for immobilization and induction of anesthesia. Intramuscular injections must be made with needles in excess of 3 cm in length. Shorter needles may result in injection into fatty tissue, delaying drug absorption into the bloodstream and delivery to the CNS. Injection into fatty tissue is one of the most common reasons for alteration of the expected response to an intended intramuscular injection of an anesthetic.

Most discussions are directly related to the importance of swine as an agricultural entity because individual market pigs have limited economic value. Valuable breeding stock is an exception. The overall value of individuals and the species as a whole increases when we consider their selective breeding potential and contribution to human medicine, respectively. The pig is physiologically more closely related to people than are most other species. Because of this similarity, swine play an important role in human medical research. The cardiopulmonary system and other anatomic features including the skin and gastrointestinal tract are similar to those of people. Thus, pigs have become widely utilized as laboratory research animals.

Several recent publications have reviewed anesthetic and analgesic techniques in swine for research purposes.(1-4) Domestic or commercial species (i.e., food producing swine) have undergone genetic alterations that impact their reaction to stress and other responses to surgery and anesthesia. Veterinarians should be familiar with these variations. Otherwise, problems may arise that can only be dealt with on an emergency basis (e.g., malignant hyperthermia).

Sexual maturity occurs at approximately 6 months of age. Body weight among breeds is highly variable. Pigs are often unable to withstand the stress imposed by manual restraint. Studies comparing three miniature breeds of pigs at 4 months of age clearly revealed a significant difference in heart weight to body weight ratio. When measured under the same conditions, cardiovascular parameters were significantly different among these pigs.(5) This suggests that biologic measurements should not be extrapolated among breeds or from one age to another. This variability among swine implies a need for more basic studies designed to establish the norm for various ages, sizes, breeds, and sexes.

PREPARATION FOR ANESTHESIA

Elective surgery involving the abdominal organs is made easier when mature pigs are starved of food for 12 to 24 hours. It is less stressful for an isolated pig to be permitted to see and have nose contact with its fellow penmates while food is being withheld. Gastrointestinal gas will rapidly accumulate in improperly starved pigs. A full abdomen can produce enormous pressure upon the diaphragm, decreasing pulmonary functional residual capacity and decreasing alveolar ventilation as well as complicating intraabdominal organ manipulation. This is particularly true when surgery is 2 to 3 hours long. Bloat will often develop in unfasted pigs receiving an anticholinergic. The consequences of these alterations are complicated by deep general anesthesia and any position associated with a "head down" tilt. Pigs are often restrained by hoisting them by their rear legs. The head down position can interfere with breathing already depressed by the anesthetic. When surgery is completed, the pig should be placed in an independent stall until it has completely recovered from anesthesia. Otherwise, penmates may cannibalize the recovering pig.

Sows presented for cesarean surgery are often hypotensive. If labor has been prolonged, it is not uncommon for them to be suffering from shock. It is

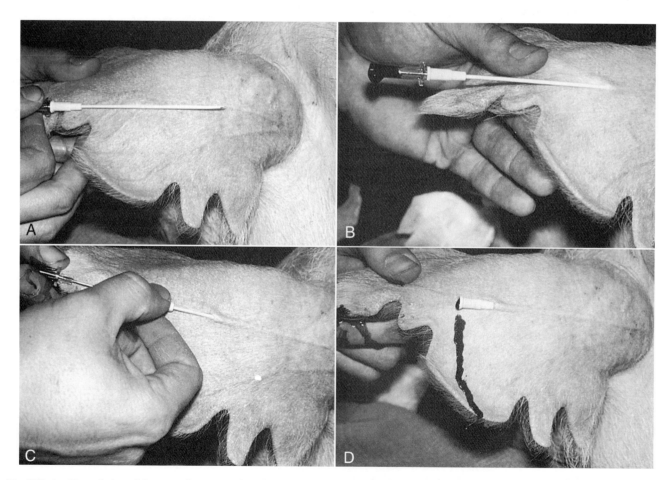

Fig. 20D–1.   Cannulation of the central ear vein of a landrace sow with a 16-gauge catheter. In photo A, a rubber band has been placed tightly around the base of the ear to engorge the veins so they are more easily identified. Photos B, C, and D sequentially illustrate the technique for inserting an over-the-needle catheter.

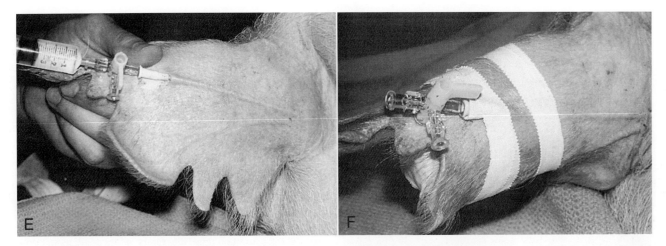

Fig. 20D–1 (continued). Photos E and F illustrate stopcock placement, flushing of the catheter following removal of the rubber band, and securing the catheter with a roll of gauze placed inside the ear and taped in place.

wise to administer large amounts of balanced electrolyte fluids and antibiotics prior to surgery. The mycin-derived antibiotics should be avoided because of their muscle-relaxing actions. Sows under these circumstances are not good candidates for extradural or subarachnoid analgesia (Chapter 16). Either may lead to hypotension, and heavy fluid loading combined with ephedrine or phenylephrine is recommended. Fluid loading is often found to be a difficult chore inasmuch as large peripheral veins are scarce in most breeds. An exception is found in mature landrace sows (Fig. 20D–1).

RESTRAINT

Baby pigs and small potbellied pigs are easily restrained by placing one hand over their back and the other under their sternum. Rough handling, particularly during hot weather, should be avoided. It can easily result in overheating and acute death. Mature swine may be restrained with a soft cotton rope looped around the maxilla just behind the upper canine teeth. A steel cable "hog catcher" snare is also used for this purpose but is painful, and pigs soon learn to avoid its placement. Head catches similar to those designed for cattle and small ruminants can be used, but because of the shape of the pig's head and neck, a considerable amount of pressure must be exerted on the squeeze to secure the head. This excessive pressure can result in airway occlusion. Once the pig is in the head squeeze, it must be observed closely in order to ensure that its airway remains functional.

A mobile device commonly used for restraint is a webbed-top stanchion (Fig. 20D–2). This apparatus is preferred over most commercial devices because it can be used to restrain pigs of all sizes. If the device is made of sufficient size, several pigs can be placed on it at one time for anesthetic induction or other minor procedures. Extradural injection is easily performed when the pig is restrained in the webbing. Furthermore, the stanchion can serve as an operating table for minor

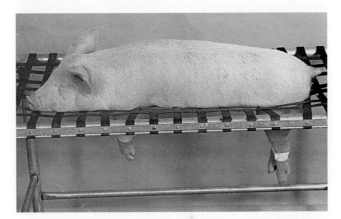

Fig. 20D–2. A homemade webbed stanchion used to restrain and transport swine. It may also be used as a surgical table for minor procedures following induction of anesthesia with injectable drugs or an inhalant administered by nose cone. Reprinted with permission from Thurmon JC, Tremquilli WJ. In: Stanton, Mersmann. Swine in Cardiovascular Research. Boca Raton, Fla: CRC Press, 1986.

elective procedures. When the webbing is made of nylon, it is easily sterilized by using a cold antiseptic solution or by steaming. The cart is mobile and can be used to weigh the patient and transport it into the surgery room for induction of anesthesia. Other devices are available but are expensive and designed to accommodate only one pig at a time. The size of the pig that can be restrained is also limited. The major disadvantage to this conveyance is the manual restraint that must be applied to get the pig into proper position atop the table so its legs can be secured. This problem can be easily overcome by constructing the four legs (cart corner posts) so they telescope. This will permit the table surface to be raised and lowered as required.

INJECTION SITES

Pigs have a proclivity to store body fat. Thus, any injection intended for intramuscular deposition must be

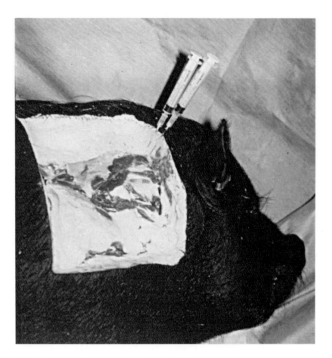

Fig. 20D–3. Injection into the neck region of an adult potbellied pig requires at least a 1½-inch needle to reach muscle tissue.

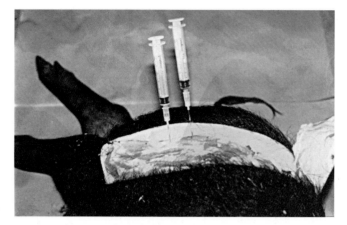

Fig. 20D–4. Injection into the rump of an adult potbellied pig requires at least a 1½-inch needle for intramuscular drug administration.

made with a needle that will reach muscular tissue. It is not desirable to inject into the "ham" muscles of pigs destined for human food. Although subcutaneous injections can be made, the pig's tight skin prevents injection of large volumes other than in the flank region and lateral side of the neck immediately posterior to the ear. The blood supply to fatty tissue is poor, and drug uptake and distribution from this tissue is very slow. Clinically, this often conveys a misconception about drug efficacy. The convenience of intramuscular injection is attractive, but if the drug is injected into fat, drug onset will be delayed and recovery will be prolonged. The possibility of injection into fatty tissue detracts from intramuscular injection technique in swine. This problem is frequently encountered in potbellied pigs when injections are made either in the neck or rump area (Figs. 20D–3 and 20D–4).

For induction of anesthesia, intravenous injection is preferred but the accessibility of veins is sparse in some breeds. In landrace swine, the auricular veins are usually large and easily cannulated. Most injections are made in the central or ventrolateral auricular veins. The major artery is located on the dorsolateral aspect of the ear. Injection of an anesthetic into the artery (e.g., barbiturates) can result in tissue slough of the distal end of the ear. Using a tourniquet, it is possible to raise the cephalic vein located on the dorsomedial aspect of the forelimb between the elbow and carpus. This is often difficult in a struggling pig. A single needle puncture is almost essential; otherwise a hematoma will form, resulting in venous constriction.

In the rear limb, the femoral vein is prominent. Patient restraint for injection is a problem that often

cannot be overcome unless a sedative is given. The medial and lateral saphenous veins are seldom used because of their size and the difficulty of patient restraint when attempting vena puncture. The jugular vein can be entered if appropriate restraint is applied, but only if the vein is well cannulated should an anesthetic be injected. Of concern is the close proximity of the carotid artery. An alternative to the jugular vein is the anterior vena cava. Entrance is made in the jugular furrow just lateral to the manubrium sterni, with the needle directed at the opposing shoulder. The right side is usually selected for vena puncture, even though the left side can be used. Injections should be given slowly. The anterior vena cava puncture is primarily used for blood sample collection.

TRACHEAL INTUBATION

The technique of inserting a tube into each individual nostril, connected by a Y piece (Carlen's adaptor) and attached to the anesthetic rebreathing system, should be discouraged. This method does nothing to protect the airway from aspiration of vomitus. Further, any attempt to ventilate an apneic pig with nasal intubation can result in gastric distension (meteorism) and displacement of the diaphragm anteriorly. Functional lung capacity is decreased, increasing the likelihood of hypoxemia. The importance of tracheal intubation cannot be overemphasized. It provides a means of alveolar ventilation and protects the airway and lungs from aspiration of foreign material.(6)

Two primary body positions, dorsal or sternal recumbency, are used for tracheal intubation. The technique that best serves the anesthetist should be chosen. Once proficiency has been gained, body position is of little or no importance. Sternal recumbency appears to be the best position for those individuals that have had little or no experience. Gauze strips or small cotton ropes are placed behind the upper and lower canine teeth to open the pigs mouth. A mouth wedge (Fig. 20D–5) designed specifically for swine may be used with or with out gauze strips. The head should be extended but excessive

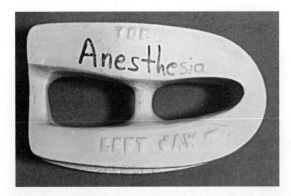

Fig. 20D–5. A mouth wedge that can be used in adult swine when intubating.

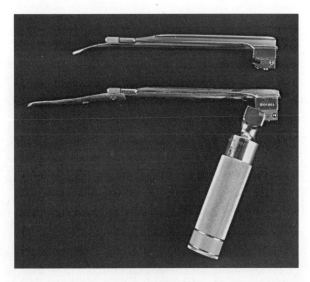

Fig. 20D–6. A human laryngoscope with a large "Miller" blade shown above. The blade attached to the laryngoscope handle has been modified with a 3½-inch metal extension for use in large adult swine.

extension will make the arytenoid cartilages (i.e., laryngeal opening) more difficult to identify and in some cases can actually occlude the airway. For pigs in excess of 50 kg, a laryngoscope with a 205-mm blade with an extension (4–8 cm in length) is desirable (Fig. 20D–6). Although some anesthetists use the blade tip to depress the epiglottis, it is more desirable to set the blade so that when the handle is raised the tip of the blade displaces the base of the epiglottis ventrally, providing maximal exposure of the laryngeal opening. A local anesthetic (e.g., 1–3 mL of a 2–4% solution of lidocaine sprayed directly into the laryngeal opening) will relieve laryngeal spasms and coughing when intubating a lightly anesthetized pig. Succinylcholine (1–2 mg/kg IV) may be given, but this drug may trigger malignant hyperthermia in susceptible swine. Furthermore, because the rimaglottidis is so small and because the mouth cannot be opened widely, a plastic "guide stylet" (three times the length of the endotracheal tube) placed a short distance into the trachea can be safely used to guide the endotracheal tube through the larynx. Only cuffed tubes should be used in mature swine. When using a guide tube, it must be held stationary as the endotracheal tube is being inserted over it. If the stiff stylet is advanced deeply into the respiratory passages, it can injure the bronchial and peribronchial tissues. Tension pneumothorax could be a sequela.

A quick review of the anatomy of the pig's larynx (Fig. 20D–7A and B) illustrates the tortuous course a tube must take in order to pass through the larynx and reach the trachea. When passing the tube without the aid of a stylet in a pig placed in a sternal position, the natural tube curvature is placed so that the tip is ventral. As the tube is advanced, it will meet resistance when the tip contacts the posterior floor of the larynx. At this point rotate the tube 180° and apply minimal pressure. If the correct size tube has been chosen, it will be felt to start its descent into the trachea, at which time it should again be rotated back to its original position (i.e., with the curvature dorsal and the tip ventral). In some individuals with extremely fat jowls (e.g., large potbellied pigs) intubation can often best be accomplished in lateral or dorsal recumbency (Fig. 20D–7B and C). These positions allow for a more direct route through the larynx and into the trachea. The size of the endotracheal tube is important. Practically, one should have three sizes at hand, the one thought to be correct, one size larger and one size smaller. Tube sizes will range from 3 to 4 mm for piglets up to 16 to 18 mm in large boars or sows (Table 20D–1).

Traumatic intubation resulting in injury to the delicate laryngeal mucosa can have a serious consequence. Formation of a hematoma or generalized laryngeal edema may go unnoticed, only to become evident when the tube is removed during recovery. Under all circumstances, the tube should not be removed until the pig is indicating laryngotracheal tube awareness as it awakens (e.g., coughing) or otherwise rejects the tube. A light spray of 2 to 4% lidocaine into the laryngeal opening just prior to or at the time of tube removal will often prevent laryngospasm after tube withdrawal.

Anesthetic Induction and Recovery

INDUCTION

The thiobarbiturates are the standard to which other injectable anesthetics are compared (Chapter 9). Two other major classes of anesthetics that are commonly used in swine are the dissociatives (e.g., ketamine) and the inhalants (Chapters 10 and 11). Induction drug popularity "ebbs and flows," but in large part is governed by proper preanesthetic medication. As in other species, so long as pigs are not overdosed, the chosen induction drug or drugs are of minimal importance.

The thiobarbiturates are considered monoanesthetics but are poor analgesics. The anesthetic dose is very close to the apneic dose. Repeated injection will result in tissue saturation and prolonged recovery. There is no specific antagonist for barbiturates. Some drug combi-

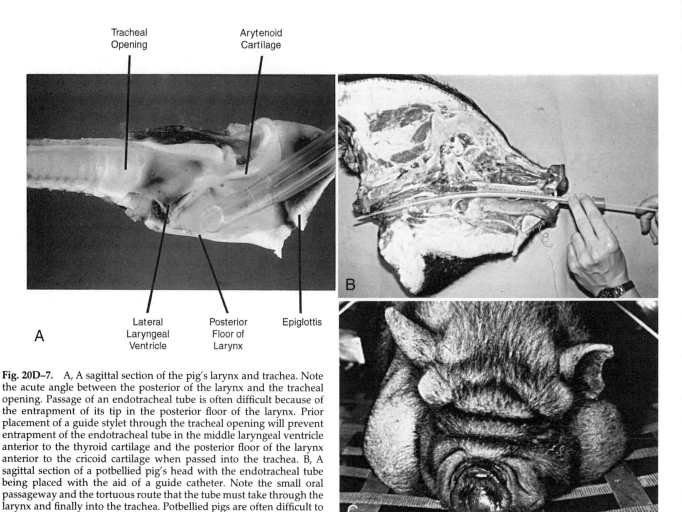

Fig. 20D–7. A, A sagittal section of the pig's larynx and trachea. Note the acute angle between the posterior of the larynx and the tracheal opening. Passage of an endotracheal tube is often difficult because of the entrapment of its tip in the posterior floor of the larynx. Prior placement of a guide stylet through the tracheal opening will prevent entrapment of the endotracheal tube in the middle laryngeal ventricle anterior to the thyroid cartilage and the posterior floor of the larynx anterior to the cricoid cartilage when passed into the trachea. B, A sagittal section of a potbellied pig's head with the endotracheal tube being placed with the aid of a guide catheter. Note the small oral passageway and the tortuous route that the tube must take through the larynx and finally into the trachea. Potbellied pigs are often difficult to intubate, especially when extremely brachycephalic (C).

Table 20D–1. Endotracheal Tube Sizes for Swine

Piglets	3–5mm
10–15 kg	5–7mm
20–50 kg	8–10mm
100–200 kg	10–14mm
larger	16–18mm

nations will provide better laryngeal relaxation than do barbiturates. A combination that provides good laryngeal relaxation consists of guaifenesin, ketamine, and xylazine ("Triple Drip").

When anesthesia is being induced with an inhalant in oxygen (e.g., isoflurane), there is a minimal amount of time to complete the intubation procedure once the nose cone is removed. Until regular breathing and signs of surgical anesthesia occur, the nose cone should be kept in place. Thus, the general procedure is to remove the nose cone, open the pig's mouth, and quickly spray the laryngeal opening with lidocaine, replace the nose cone, and continue with inhalant administration. For intubation, the laryngeal opening is exposed and identified with a laryngoscope, and the tube put in place

by one of two methods described earlier. After proper positioning of the tube the cuff is inflated so that when a pressure of 18 to 20 cm of H_2O is applied to the rebreathing circuit, a slight escapement of air can be heard from the pig's mouth (Chapter 17).

Apnea is simply dealt with by rhythmically squeezing the rebreathing bag four to eight times per minute or by the use of an Ambu resuscitator bag (Fig. 20D–8) when the patient is not connected to an anesthetic rebreathing system. With the latter either oxygen or ambient air can be used. Excessive ventilation will decrease blood carbon dioxide concentration and may prolong apnea. Experience gained in intubating pigs will increase the anesthetist's confidence and proficiency. Furthermore, an assistant who understands the anatomy of the pig's airway and appreciates the importance of keeping the head and neck properly positioned is essential for a clean, safe, tracheal intubation.

CARE DURING RECOVERY

Apnea resulting from laryngeal hematoma, edema, and/or spasms can occur and quickly result in death once the endotracheal tube is removed. Spraying the larynx with a modest amount of Neo-Synephrine prior

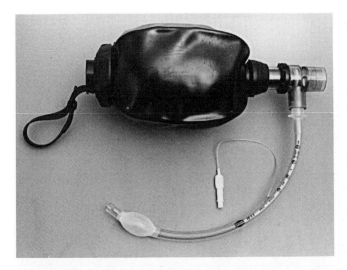

Fig. 20D–8. An Ambu resuscitator bag that may be used with either air or oxygen when connected to the endotracheal tube.

to tube removal may be helpful in decreasing vascular congestion and formation of edema in some cases. Thus, it is of the utmost importance to monitor respiration and other signs during recovery. Less vigilant monitoring is required once the pig has gained its righting reflex and is able to maintain sternal position. Difficulty in breathing and restlessness accompanied by hypoxemia are usually the first signs of a traumatic recovery that must be dealt with at once; time is crucial. Laryngeal edema can be treated by reintubation, but attempting to intubate a struggling pig is usually futile. If the intravenous catheter is still in place, the pig can be reanesthetized and an endotracheal tube quickly positioned to support ventilation. However, with the use of a local anesthetic, it may be more efficient and less time-consuming to quickly perform a tracheostomy.

It is important to keep piglets warm during recovery. If the chest or abdomen has been opened for any length of time in small pigs, it is essential to prevent further loss of body temperature and provide a source of external heat. This may be done by covering the pig with a blanket or by using a warm water circulating pad. Wrapping the extremities in bubble sheeting, the type used to pack fragile items for shipment, is helpful. Also, a sheet of this material between the patient and a cold surgical table top will help maintain body temperature.

Postoperative pain should be treated with appropriate analgesics. Alpha$_2$-adrenoceptor agonists, opioids, and local anesthetics can be administered alone or in combination to induce analgesia. These drugs have also been injected alone and in combination in the epidural space to provide postoperative analgesia (Chapter 16). Opioid agonist-antagonists that can be injected parenterally in pigs to relieve postoperative pain include Pentazocine (0.4 to 0.5 mg/kg IM), Butorphanol (0.1 to 0.5 mg/kg IM or IV), Nalbuphine (0.15 to 0.2 mg/kg IM) or Buprenorphine (0.004 to 0.008 mg/kg IM or IV) (Chapter 8).(1)

Injectable Drugs

PARASYMPATHOLYTIC DRUGS

The anticholinergic drugs atropine sulfate and glycopyrrolate are commonly used in swine. Because bradycardia is seldom a problem in anesthetized swine, their main use is to inhibit excessive salivation. Neither of these drugs is routinely required. Generally the pig has a heart rate greater than 80 beats a minute. Under clinical situations, a heart rate in excess of 120 beats a minute is not uncommon. Anticholinergics increase heart rate and thus myocardial work and oxygen consumption. Tachycardia can lead to a variety of other arrhythmias and, if not properly dealt with, can terminate in cardiac arrest. Preexisting bradycardia (i.e., heart rates below 50 beats per minute) should be treated with either atropine (0.02–0.04 mg/kg IM) or glycopyrrolate (0.005–0.01 mg/kg IM) prior to induction of anesthesia. Unlike cats and cattle, swine will respond to anticholinergics with a drier mouth. The airway will be drier and intubation easier. The major contraindication to this class of drugs is an existing tachycardia, as may be seen in patients with fever, extreme excitement, or hyperthyroidism.

Because swine occasionally vomit during the recovery period, glycopyrrolate would seem to be the anticholinergic of choice. This drug tends to decrease gastric fluid secretion and acid content, and unlike atropine, promotes gastric emptying. Further, glycopyrrolate is a large quaternary ammonia compound and does not readily cross the blood-brain barrier. In people, glycopyrrolate is considered to be about twice as potent an antisialagogue as atropine and to have a longer duration of action.(7)

ATARACTICS (TRANQUILIZERS)

Phenothiazine derivatives are not as effective in swine as in many other species. Although tranquilized swine are easier to approach, they will still resist mechanical restraint vigorously. It seems that the most effective tranquilizer in swine is azaperone (a butyrophenone derivative) (Chapter 8). Most tranquilizers offer little or no analgesia. Thus, their use in anesthetizing swine is limited unless they are combined with other drugs that induce analgesia and depress CNS activity. For example, Innovar-Vet will provide reasonable calming if administered in pigs experiencing pain. However, if aroused, pigs often sneeze and appear to become more excited after drug injection. When Innovar-Vet is combined with xylazine, sedation is more pronounced and pigs often lie quietly for some time. However, pigs will often respond vigorously to painful manipulation. Veterinary practitioners have reportedly given extremely large doses of phenothiazine tranquilizers along with local analgesics to induce intense quiescence in older sows undergoing cesarean section. These high doses can induce intense vascular alpha-receptor blockade, resulting in hypotensive shock, and should be discouraged. Many of these sows fail to recover, even though their piglets reportedly recover satisfactorily.

The use of high doses of a tranquilizer as a substitute for an anesthetic is improper in any species.

Butyrophenone tranquilizers include droperidol, flu-anisone, and azaperone. Only azaperone has been used extensively in swine. It is often used as a preanesthetic. However, its predominant use is to prevent fighting and anxiety among newly mixed pigs (2.5 mg/kg IM). Large doses will induce deep tranquilization and hypotension. The recommended intramuscular dose of azaperone for preanesthetic tranquilization ranges from 2 mg/kg in older, large swine to 8 mg/kg in young swine for purposes of immobilization.

The benzodiazepines (i.e., minor tranquilizers) are useful in swine but expensive. Although there are many benzodiazepine derivatives, diazepam and midazolam are most frequently used in North America. Reportedly, flurazepam (2 mg/kg IV) (8), lorazepam (0.1 mg/kg IV) (9), brotizolam (1–10 mg/kg PO) (10), and zolazepam (a component of Telazol) produce good effects in swine. Benzodiazepines induce hypnosis, sedation, and muscle relaxation, but little or no analgesia. Thus, they are generally combined with an anesthetic or strong analgesic to enhance anesthetic action. Diazepam (Valium, 1–10 mg/kg IM or 0.5–2 mg/kg IV) is usually combined with ketamine and xylazine or an inhalant for its additive muscle-relaxing and sedative effects. Diazepam, as is true of most benzodiazepine derivatives, will decrease anesthetic requirement even though it is not a strong analgesic. When given in large doses, benzodiazepines prolong recovery. This is particularly true in older sows and boars given large intramuscular doses. Midazolam, unlike diazepam, is water soluble and may be given by either the intravenous or intramuscular route without causing severe pain. The dose ranges from 0.1 to 0.5 mg/kg. Midazolam is approximately twice as potent as diazepam.

Flumazenil is a specific benzodiazepine antagonist. The minimal effective dose for reversal of diazepam or midazolam has not been established in swine. Clinical experience suggests that a dose of 1 part flumazenil to 13 parts of a benzodiazepine agonist will adequately antagonize lingering sedation and muscle relaxation (e.g., if 1.3 mg/kg of diazepam is given, 0.1 mg/kg of flumazenil is required). When using this ratio, flumazenil demonstrates good efficacy in antagonizing the residual actions of zolazepam (the benzodiazepine component of Telazol) in mature swine.

ALPHA-ADRENOCEPTOR AGONISTS

The alpha$_2$-adrenoceptor agonists available to the veterinarian in North America include xylazine and detomidine. Only xylazine has been used to any great extent in swine. Although xylazine is an extremely potent sedative in other animal species, it is not in swine. After injection of xylazine or detomidine some sedation is apparent. Pigs will usually lie down in 10 to 15 minutes, but when approached, they will rapidly rise and flee. Thus, in swine, xylazine is usually combined with other drugs. For example, xylazine and ketamine have be-

come a popular anesthetic drug combination for use in swine. The dose of xylazine ranges from 1 to 2 mg/kg IM or IV. The effects of xylazine when combined with ketamine or Telazol appear to be greater than additive (Chapter 10).

ALPHA$_2$-AGONIST EPIDURAL ANALGESIA

Xylazine has both alpha$_1$ and alpha$_2$ activity, while detomidine acts predominately at alpha$_2$-adrenoceptors. It has been demonstrated that both alpha subtype receptors are located in the dorsal horn of the spinal cord.(11-13) It has also been shown that analgesia can be induced by both alpha$_1$- and alpha$_2$-adrenergic agonists when injected intrathecally.(14) This finding supports the speculation that xylazine-induced analgesia is mediated in part by alpha-adrenoceptor stimulation. The ratio of alpha$_1$ to alpha$_2$ adrenoceptors in the spinal cord of domestic swine has not been determined. Xylazine induces more profound analgesia than does detomidine in this species.(13) In pigs receiving either intrathecal xylazine or detomidine, the response is different after a pure alpha$_2$-antagonist (i.e., atipamezole) is administered. In detomidine-treated pigs, sedation, analgesia, and immobilization are quickly abolished after intravenous injection of atipamezole. In xylazine-treated pigs, however, sedation is abolished but loss of motor and sensory responses posterior to the site of xylazine injection remains.(13) Seemingly, this indicates the presence of a xylazine-induced spinal local analgesic effect. This has also been reported in horses and cattle.(15, 16–18) In summary, epidural injection of xylazine or detomidine in swine induces sedation, analgesia, and immobilization. The intensity of analgesia is greater with xylazine than detomidine. Xylazine's superior analgesic action appears to be mediated by either its alpha$_1$-adrenoceptor activity located in the dorsal horn of the spinal cord and/or a local analgesic effect independent of alpha-adrenoceptor stimulation.(13)

With this knowledge, sows weighing from 150 to 225 kg scheduled for a cesarean section can be given an epidural injection of 10 mL of 2% lidocaine containing xylazine at a dose of 0.5 to 1.0 mg/kg. The onset of sedation analgesia and rear limb immobilization are rapid. Complete immobilization of the rear quarters remains for approximately 3 to 4 hours. Sows will lie quietly for over an hour, at which time some front limb movement may occur. Thus, even though there is some xylazine-induced sedation, the forelimbs should be tethered. Piglets are lively when delivered and experience no difficulty in breathing. Should sedation linger, it can be effectively antagonized with either yohimbine (0.15–0.2 mg/kg IV) or tolazoline (2–4 mg/kg IV). Although atipamezole is a very effective alpha-adrenoceptor antagonist, it is presently unavailable to the practicing veterinarian in North America. The local anesthetic effect of xylazine is not antagonized by administration of an alpha-adrenoceptor antagonist. Veterinarians skilled in the technique of epidural injection will find this a useful anesthetic regimen for use in swine when analgesia posterior to the umbilicus and mild sedation are both required.

BARBITURATES

Because barbiturates are given primarily by intravenous injection in the ear vein, dilute solutions are preferred (i.e., 5% concentration or less). Perivascular injection will often result in sloughing of the skin surrounding the vessel if not properly cared for. The thiobarbiturates (i.e., thiopental and thiamylal) and the oxybarbiturates have been given either by using a repeated bolus technique or by continuous infusion.(19, 20) If properly ventilated, pigs will survive extraordinary large doses over time, but recovery may be extremely long. In swine, the thiobarbiturates (e.g., thiopental) are preferred to the oxybarbiturates (e.g., pentobarbital) because of their rapid onset and shorter duration of action. The effect of a barbiturate may be enhanced with xylazine (1–2 mg/kg), ketamine (2–4 mg/kg), a benzodiazepine (diazepam 2–4 mg/kg), or another tranquilizer (e.g., azaperone 2–4 mg/kg). When a barbiturate is used alone for more than a brief period of surgical anesthesia, the patient's trachea should be intubated and there must be at hand a means of instituting positive pressure ventilation. An Ambu bag (Fig. 20D–8) will serve this purpose well because it may be used to ventilate with ambient air or oxygen. When pigs are properly ventilated they can tolerate three times the surgical dose of a barbiturate. Death of swine from barbiturates is usually a direct result of respiratory arrest.

Pentobarbital is vaguely classed as a short-acting barbiturate but when dosed repeatedly or administered as a constant infusion, recovery will be prolonged. The anesthetic dose of pentobarbital ranges from 20 to 40 mg/kg IV. When given as a continuous infusion, the recommended dose is 5 to 15 mg $\cdot$ kg^{-1} $\cdot$ h^{-1}.(19, 20) Xylazine will decrease the anesthetizing dose of pentobarbital measurably, as will diazepam or ketamine.(19)

Pentobarbital is an extremely effective anticonvulsant. Diazepam can be given for this purpose but has a shorter period of action and is much more expensive. In addition, dysphoria, often seen in swine recovering from ketamine administration, can be controlled with pentobarbital (6–10 mg/kg IV or IM). When possible, the smaller dose is given slowly intravenously. When intravenous injection is not possible, the larger dose (10 mg/kg) diluted to 3% or less with saline or water may be given intramuscularly. When administered intramuscularly as a dilute solution, pentobarbital should be injected deeply into a large muscle mass. In commercial swine the most appropriate site for intramuscular injection is in the neck muscle just rostral to the ear.

Commercially available thiobarbiturates are sold as desiccated powders and solubilized with either distilled water or saline. Concentrations of 2.5 to 5% are preferred. Until the recent removal of thiamylal from the market, it was the most widely used barbiturate in

veterinary patients, including swine. Thiobarbiturates are characterized as being ultra-short-acting. This is somewhat of a misnomer inasmuch as duration of action correlates directly with total dose. More correctly stated, these barbiturates have a more rapid onset of action than oxybarbiturates.

The thiobarbiturates are more soluble in blood and tissue than the oxybarbiturates (e.g., pentobarbital). Thus, the induction dose is less and recovery time is shorter after a single bolus injection of thiobarbiturate. As with the oxybarbiturates, thiobarbiturates may be used as monoanesthetics. Analgesia is minimal until deep planes of anesthesia occur. As previously stated, the dose for deep surgical anesthesia is very close to the apneic dose. The induction dose of either thiopental or thiamylal ranges from 10 to 20 mg/kg IV. The higher dose is given in unpremedicated young swine and the lower dose in sedate or tranquilized swine. To a large extent, the dose depends on the degree of analgesia and immobilization required. For example, procedures that are pain-free such as radiography will require a minimal dose. The dose will also depend on the physical condition of the patient and availability of respiratory support equipment. When thiamylal or thiopental is used as a continuous infusion to maintain anesthesia the recommended dose is 3 to 6 mg $\cdot$ kg^{-1} $\cdot$ h^{-1} IV. (19, 20)

Because the swallowing reflex remains intact after induction with a dissociative (e.g., ketamine, tiletamine), a small dose of thiopental (4–6 mg/kg IV) can be used to abolish laryngeal reflexes that interfere with endotracheal intubation. Specific antagonists for barbiturates are unavailable at this time. However, after ensuring a patent airway an analeptic such as doxapram (0.50–1.0 mg/kg IV) can be used to stimulate breathing. This effect can be short-lived in patients that have received large doses of a barbiturate. Under such circumstances, mechanical ventilation should be initiated and continued until the pig reinitiates spontaneous breathing (Chapter 17). In summary, the thiobarbiturates are useful drugs in swine, but they cannot be recommended as monoanesthetics for prolonged surgery without controlled ventilation and/or when rapid patient recovery is required.

Methohexital is a ultra-short-acting methylated oxybarbiturate, approximately three times as potent as thiopental. It is usually prepared in a 2.5% solution. In veterinary practice it has been used primarily in sight hounds because of its brief action. It has proven an effective induction anesthetic in many species when given by the intravenous route. It may also be given to maintain anesthesia by continuous infusion. However, it induces muscle fasciculations during induction, and recovery is often described as "rough" in swine not receiving preanesthetic medication (e.g., xylazine or azaperone). Methohexital is used most often to induce anesthesia, followed by maintenance with an inhalant. As with the thiobarbiturates, the dose varies considerably and depends on the type and amount of preanesthetic given. In healthy unpremedicated commercial swine, the dose ranges from 6 to 10 mg/kg IV. In potbellied pigs one half to two thirds the dose recommended for commercial swine appears to be appropriate.

Recovery from a single anesthetizing dose of methohexital is usually complete in 20 to 30 minutes. As with all barbiturates, respiratory depression and apnea are the most serious problems encountered when high doses are injected rapidly intravenously or when repeat doses are given. The necessity for repeat administration has been largely solved under field conditions by providing complete analgesia with local infiltration of the surgical site or epidural injection of a local anesthetic. Lidocaine (2%) is a reasonable choice and will often permit completion of minor surgery as the pig recovers from methohexital induced unconsciousness.

DISSOCIATIVES

Drugs disconnecting higher brain centers (thalamo-cortical) from lower centers (limbic systems) are referred to as *dissociative* anesthetics. The first dissociative used in veterinary anesthesia was phencyclidine hydrochloride. Although its use in swine and bears gained some popularity, illicit use as a "street drug" resulted in its removal from the medical market. Subsequently, tamer and perhaps less addictive derivatives were synthesized—namely, ketamine and tiletamine. These drugs have become popular for induction of anesthesia and short surgical procedures when combined with alpha$_2$-agonists, opioids, and/or benzodiazepines (Chapter 10).

Tiletamine, like ketamine, is available only in a proprietary compound. This drug combination consists of a 1:1 mixture of tiletamine and zolazepam. The latter is a benzodiazepine similar to diazepam but more potent. Anesthesia induced with dissociatives is characterized by incomplete muscle relaxation, often referred to as a *cataleptoid state*. Zolazepam tends to relieve this problem by providing muscle relaxation but does not seem to add measurably to analgesia.

Dissociative-induced analgesia appears to result from its action on N-methyl-D-aspartate (NMDA) and opioid receptors. However, attempts to antagonize ketamine's action with naloxone have not been effective.(21) With ketamine anesthesia, the patient's eyes remain open and the swallowing reflex usually remains intact. However, this does not prevent the patient from aspirating vomitus should vomiting occur during the course of anesthesia. Vomition can be a real threat when pigs are not properly fasted. In humans, ketamine-induced analgesia has been described as intense.(22) From clinical and laboratory observations, ketamine does not appear to induce analgesia in swine of the same magnitude as that described in people.(23)

Because ketamine induces excessive salivation in swine, it seems logical to administer an anticholinergic (atropine 0.04 mg/kg IM). However, atropine should be avoided in patients with tachycardia or fever. When given intramuscularly at a dose of 10 to 12 mg/kg,

ketamine will immobilize swine in approximately 5 minutes. Although xylazine does not provide good muscle relaxation or sedation when given alone, it will greatly enhance the anesthetic effects of ketamine. The xylazine dose range is 2–3 mg/kg IM or 1–2 mg/kg IV. When combined with ketamine, xylazine improves analgesia and muscle relaxation.(4) When necessary, anesthesia can be prolonged in the healthy patient with 2 to 4 mg/kg of ketamine and 0.5 to 1 mg/kg of xylazine mixed in the same syringe and injected slowly intravenously. When an auricular vein can be cannulated prior to induction, ketamine should be given by the intravenous route. A smaller dose will be required (4–6 mg/kg). Recovery will be quicker and excitement during recovery is less likely to occur with the lower intravenous dose. Excitement during recovery is most often seen in old mature sows and boars, but is less likely to occur when xylazine is a part of the anesthetic regimen.

Because physical restraint is frequently difficult in mature swine, the intramuscular route is often used to immobilize large patients. A drug combination that reportedly works well when administered intramuscularly is ketamine (4 mg/kg), oxymorphone (0.15 mg/kg), and xylazine (4 mg/kg). If an intravenous injection can be made, the dose of each drug is decreased by one half.(4, 24) This drug combination, although expensive, offers relatively good analgesia and muscle relaxation. Recovery is generally smooth and can be hastened with naloxone and yohimbine administration. It should be remembered that oxymorphone/xylazine reversal will antagonize postoperative analgesia and sedation. An excitatory response may ensue.

Ketamine (6–8 mg/kg) and xylazine (1–2 mg/kg) drawn into the same syringe may be safely used to anesthetize large boars for castration. One half of the drug combination is injected deep into the center of each testicle. Rapid castration will remove the remaining drug contained in the testicle, promoting a rapid recovery. Large doses of pentobarbital have also been administered intratesticularly for the same purpose, but recoveries are considerably longer.

Telazol is a proprietary drug combination. Five-milliliter vials contain 250 mg of tiletamine and 250 mg of zolazepam. Zolazepam is similar to diazepam, but it is water soluble and more potent than diazepam. As previously mentioned, zolazepam has a central muscle relaxant action that partially relieves the cataleptoid state induced by a dissociative. Excessive or repeat dosing of Telazol can cause prolonged recovery, particularly in older swine and other large species. Telazol is only approved for intramuscular use in dogs and cats but has been widely used in swine.

Telazol does not induce the intensity of analgesia required for most surgical procedures, but it is an effective anesthetic in swine when combined with the proper adjunct. Presently, xylazine is the most popular drug for this purpose. Alpha$_2$-agonists have been shown to decrease the requirement for inhalant anesthesia by as much as 90%. Telazol (6.6 mg/kg IM) combined with xylazine (2.2 mg/kg IM) immobilizes 20-

to 30-kg pigs in 1 to 2 minutes, and the anesthetic time extends up to approximately 1 hour. Tracheal intubation is easily performed.(25) These drugs can be mixed in the same syringe for easier administration. Prolonged recoveries have been experienced in old sows and boars when given the dosage reported for 20- to 30-kg pigs. Extended recoveries are more likely to occur when this drug regimen is given by the intramuscular route or after redosing to extend anesthesia. It appears that prolonged recovery is due in large part to zolazepam's lingering effects. Consequently, smaller intravenous doses are recommended for older swine (Telazol 2.2–4.4 mg/kg and xylazine 1.1 mg/kg). When using the IV route, anesthesia may be safely extended by giving one half the original dose as required.

Injectable Drug Combinations

TELAZOL-KETAMINE-XYLAZINE

Zolazepam appears to be responsible for the posterior weakness observed in recovering mature swine when Telazol is given intramuscularly in anesthetic doses. In order to minimize this problem, the dissociative content in the Telazol mixture can be increased by adding 2.5 mL of ketamine (100 mg/mL). Two and one-half mL (100 mg/mL) of xylazine can also be added to increase the sedative and analgesic effect of the mixture. This provides 100 mg of dissociative/mL (tiletamine plus ketamine) and 50 mg/mL each of xylazine and zolazepam. In this mixture zolazepam constitutes only 25% of the total drug dose rather than the 50% found in the proprietary mixture.

For commercial swine, the recommended dose of this drug combination is 1 mL/50–75 kg IM, depending on the depth of anesthesia required. For sedation and light anesthesia, potbellied pigs appear to require a smaller dose, approximately one half that given to commercial swine. Anesthesia may be extended by injecting one half the intramuscular dose slowly intravenously to avoid apnea or by administering either halothane or isoflurane in oxygen from a nose cone. The inhalation anesthetic requirement will be greatly decreased with this drug mixture.

Because of the recent popularity of potbellied pigs as companion animals, anesthesia in these small pigs deserves special consideration. Small animal practitioners are increasingly asked to perform selected surgical and diagnostic procedures (e.g., hoof trim, hernia repair, ovariohysterectomy, castration, cesarian section, ultrasound for pregnancy diagnosis, etc.). The potbellied pig's body appears to be sturdily built, but it is heavily covered with fatty tissue and drug injection can be problematic. Table 20D–2 lists a variety of drugs and combinations used in this breed.

GUAIFENESIN-KETAMINE-XYLAZINE ("TRIPLE DRIP")

This drug combination is prepared by adding 2 mg of ketamine and 1 mg of xylazine to each mL of 5% guaifenesin prepared in 5% dextrose in water. The drug combination must be given by the intravenous route. This can be a major problem because of the absence of accessible auricular veins in some individuals. The induction dose ranges from 2/3 to 1 mL of the mixture per kg. The average anesthetic maintenance dose is 2.2 $mL \cdot kg^{-1} \cdot h^{-1}$. Using a standard intravenous delivery set (15 drops = 1 mL) the maintenance dose is calculated as follows: (body wt. kg) $\times$ (2.2 $mL \cdot kg^{-1} \cdot h^{-1}$) $\times$ 15 drops/mL divided by 60 = drops/minute and when divided again by 60 = drops/second. In a 150 kg sow, induction would require approximately 100 to 150 mL depending on the rate of injection. Maintenance would be calculated as follows: 150 $\times$ 2.2 $\times$ 15 = 4950 drops/hour divided by 60 = 83 drops/minute, divided by 60 again = approximately 1.4 drops/second. This dosage rate is sufficient for the average sow. Sows that have been in prolonged labor usually require a smaller dose. On the other hand, young vigorous sows, in labor for only a short time, may require an increased dose. Animal response will serve as a guide to dose requirement. As with any injectable mixture, it should be given to effect as measured by monitoring of vital signs.

Induction and recovery from this anesthetic mixture is rapid (recovery occurring in 30 to 45 min). Recovery time can be decreased by intravenous injection of a specific xylazine antagonist (e.g., yohimbine 0.06–0.1 mg/kg or tolazoline 2–4 mg/kg). When the alpha$_2$-antagonist is given, postoperative analgesia is diminished. Rapid arousal to the antagonist suggests that xylazine is most likely responsible for residual anesthetic effect during recovery following continuous infusion of Triple Drip.

When Triple Drip is used for cesarean section, it provides excellent relaxation and analgesia. Piglets are only minimally depressed. Clearly, neonatal depression is directly related to the total dose of Triple Drip prior to fetal delivery. Speed of surgery is of the essence. It is likely that xylazine is responsible for neonatal respiratory depression. This speculation is based on clinical observations that piglets will quickly commence breathing after administering a small dose of an alpha$_2$-antagonist. A minimal dose (i.e., 0.25–0.5 mg/kg) of doxapram can also be used to stimulate breathing once the airway is cleared.(4)

Inhalation Anesthetics

The inhalants are safe anesthetics in swine other than for those individuals susceptible to malignant hyperthermia. Because of the equipment required for administration, inhalants can only be used practically within the hospital. Halothane and isoflurane are the primary inhalants used in swine. Enflurane, an isomer of isoflurane, is of limited use without appropriate premedication. High inspired concentrations of enflurane can cause a seizurelike response.

Desflurane is an isomer of isoflurane. This inhalant is nonflammable and is more volatile than either halothane or isoflurane. Because of this physical characteristic, it requires a special vaporizer for its administration. These vaporizers are extremely expensive and

Table 20D–2. Doses of Preanesthetic and Anesthetic Induction Drugs Used in Potbellied Pigs (42)

Drug	Dose (mg/kg)	Route	Comments
Preanesthetic Drugs			
Acepromazine	0.03–0.1 2.0	IM	Slow onset of action, 20 to 30 minutes to peak effect; light sedation; no analgesia; maximum dose, 15 mg.
Xylazine	2.2 4.4	IM	Minimal sedation; may cause vomiting before surgery or during recovery; administer with atropine to block increased vagal tone; will offset hyperalgesic effect produced by thiobarbiturates.
Diazepam	0.5–1.0 5.5–8.5	IM	Effective central muscle relaxant; high doses produce ataxia and recumbency
Fentanyl citrate and droperidol	1.0 mL/10 kg	IM	Administer with atropine 20 to 30 minutes before induction; excitement and goose-stepping may occur.
Azaperone	0.23–1.0	IM	Light sedation produced
Induction drugs			
Ketamine	20	IM	Poor analgesia and muscle relaxation.
Tiletamine HCl–Zolazepam	4.4	IM	Inadequate for intubation; rough recovery, characterized by vocalization, excessive salivation, and paddling motions.
Thiobarbiturates Thiopental or Thiamylal	10–20 6–18	IV IV	Concentration should be 5% or less; administer ⅓ to ½ as rapid bolus to unpremedicated pig; supplemental doses will prolong recovery.
Injectable Drug Combinations			
Acepromazine plus	0.5	IM	Onset of recumbency within 5 minutes; unreliable; recovery 65 to 80 minutes.
Ketamine	15 (given 30 minutes after acepromazine injection)	IM	
Diazepam plus	1.0–2.0	IM	Analgesia not as profound as xylazine-ketamine; smooth recovery; mix together in one syringe.
Ketamine	10–18		
Xylazine plus	2.2	IM	Mix together in one syringe to administer; good induction combination; intubation easily performed; acceptable short-term anesthesia with smooth recovery.
Tiletamine HCl–Zolazepam	4.4		

will limit desflurane's use primarily to people and possibly to swine research. Its solubility in blood is much lower than that of the other halogenated drugs. Thus, induction of anesthesia and recovery are rapid and depth can be readily regulated. In swine, desflurane's MAC value is somewhere between 8 and 10% (Chapter 11).

In some circumstances nitrous oxide can be used to enhance effects of other inhalants (e.g., halothane and isoflurane). Normobaric extrapolation studies reveal that an inspired concentration of nearly 200% would be required for complete anesthesia in swine.(26) The requirement for high concentrations of nitrous oxide

(N_2O) to decrease the inhaled concentration of the major anesthetic can aggravate hypoxic conditions. Rapid movement of N_2O from the blood to the alveoli at the termination of anesthesia, when the pig is permitted to breathe ambient air, can also cause diffusion hypoxia. Thus, patients should be permitted to breathe a high concentration of oxygen for 5 to 10 minutes after discontinuing N_2O administration to avoid this potential complication.

Isoflurane has a broad safety margin. It is more insoluble in blood and tissue than halothane. This physical characteristic is highly desirable because it allows for a rapid induction and recovery. The depth of

Table 20D–2.   Doses of Preanesthetic and Anesthetic Induction Drugs Used in Potbellied Pigs (42)—cont'd

Drug	Dose (mg/kg)	Route	Comments
Injectable Drug Combinations–cont'd			
Atropine plus	0.044	IM	Similar to the xylazine/tiletamine HCl–zolazepam combination; smooth recovery in 2 hours
Xylazine plus	4.4	IM	
Tiletamine HCl– Zolazepam	6.0	IM	
Xylazine* Ketamine Tiletamine HCl– Zolazepam	1 mL/75 kg	IV	Anesthesia can be maintained with 0.5 mL/75 kg, IV; must be given slowly (over 60 seconds) to minimize respiratory depression
Xylazine* Ketamine Tiletamine HCl– Zolazepam	1 mL/25 kg	IM	Good induction combination; intubation possible; recovery smoother than tiletamine HCl–zolazepam alone; 80 minutes' duration.
Xylazine Ketamine Oxymorphone	2.20 2.0 0.075	IV	Mix together in one syringe; suitable for short-term anesthesia and minor surgery; rapid and shallow breathing; duration approximately 20 to 30 minutes; smooth, rapid recovery; all doses may be doubled for IM administration.
GKX for swine (triple drip)†	0.5–1.0 mL/kg (to induce unpremedicated pig); 2.0 mL/kg/h constant infusion to maintain anesthesia	IV	Decrease induction dose 50% if tranquilizer or sedative administered; administer atropine IM before induction; rapid recovery after discontinuing GKX infusion; recovery may be hastened by administration of yohimbine (0.125 mg/kg, IV).
Inhalation Agents			
Halothane	to effect	Inhalation (face mask)	Recommended for young or sick pigs; recovery rapid.
Isoflurane	to effect	Inhalation (face mask)	Recommended for young or sick pigs; recovery rapid.

*Make combination by reconstituting tiletamine HCl–zolazepam with 2.5 mL ketamine (100 mg/mL) and 2.5 mL xylazine (100 mg/mL). Each milliliter of the resultant combination will contain 50 mg tiletamine, 50 mg zolazepam, 50 mg ketamine, and 50 mg xylazine.

†Solution contains 50 mg/mL of glycerol guaiacolate, 2 mg/mL of ketamine, and 1 mg/mL of xylazine. The combination should be mixed in the desired quantity immediately before use because of the potential diminished potency of the mixture during storage. Concentration of drugs in this mixture varies among species.

IM, intramuscular; IV, intravenous.

anesthesia is easily regulated. Halothane also has many desirable characteristics. It is a potent inhalant that has stood the test of time. It has a rather low solubility and is economic and readily available to the veterinarian. Both inhalants quickly cross the placental barrier and depress the fetus. Of the two drugs, isoflurane is the more desirable when performing cesarean section surgery. After delivery and once breathing is initiated, piglets rapidly eliminate isoflurane from body tissues. Central nervous depression rapidly disappears. Although halothane is more economic, recovery time of the neonate will be longer. Because of their high vapor pressures, isoflurane and halothane should only be administered from equipment designed specifically for their use. Their high vapor pressures and relatively small safety margins prohibit use by the open drop method.

The physical characteristics of halothane and isoflurane are similar enough that they may be administered from the same precision vaporizer designed specifically for either drug. For example, isoflurane can be administered from a properly cleaned and calibrated halothane vaporizer (e.g., Fluotech). Regardless which anesthetic is chosen, for adult swine it should be administered in oxygen from a circle or a "to and fro" rebreathing system. Anesthetic machines and delivery systems designed for humans or small animals are adequate for most adult swine weighing up to 150 kg, provided the soda lime is fresh and actively absorbing carbon dioxide (Chapter 14).

In sedated sows, anesthesia may be safely induced with an inhalant and properly fitted nose cone. Generally the machine is set to deliver 4 to 8 liters of oxygen and 3 to 5% halothane or isoflurane. The higher percentage of isoflurane is usually chosen because isoflurane is less potent than halothane. When anesthesia has been induced, the trachea should be intubated. Oxygen flow and anesthetic concentration is gradually decreased. For maintenance, oxygen flow ranges from 1 to 3 L/min. Halothane maintenance concentration ranges from 1.5 to 2.5% (mean 2%), whereas 2 to 3% (mean 2.5%) isoflurane is usually required to maintain surgical anesthesia.

Nitrous oxide can be used to speed induction of anesthesia. When N_2O is part of the anesthetic induction regimen, the pig is permitted to breathe oxygen and either halothane or isoflurane via nose cone. When signs of sedation appear (i.e., usually 3 to 4 minutes), N_2O is quickly entrained with oxygen so that it contributes 60 to 70% of the fresh gas inflow (e.g., 2 liters of oxygen and 4 liters of N_2O) into the breathing system. Because of its high concentration gradient, it rapidly moves from the alveoli to the blood stream. This technique increases the alveolar concentrations of oxygen (i.e., initially, hyperoxic effect) and the primary anesthetic (e.g., halothane or isoflurane). This increase in concentration gradient of the inhalant increases the rapidity of movement from the alveoli to blood, and thus increases the speed of induction. This phenomenon is referred to as the *second gas effect*. When induction is complete, delivery of N_2O is either decreased to less than 70% of total fresh gas flow or discontinued altogether (Chapter 11).

Carbon Dioxide in Oxygen

Carbon dioxide in oxygen can be used to effectively induce anesthesia in piglets. However, induction and surgical time should be restricted to 10 minutes or less. Most veterinarians are concerned about humane treatment of all animals. For example, the processing of piglets (i.e., castration, tail docking, and ear notching) involves painful procedures. Because processed pigs are generally destined for human consumption, the use of most injectable anesthetics is not approved to relieve the pain associated with the processing procedures. Thus, when general anesthesia is used for this purpose it must of necessity be safe, simple, economic, effective, and leave no tissue residues. Further, the anesthetic must have a rapid onset and allow rapid recovery. An anesthetic technique utilizing carbon dioxide (a natural body byproduct of metabolism) and oxygen has been developed to meet these requirements. Fifty percent oxygen and 50% carbon dioxide (2 L/min O_2 and 2 L/min CO_2) administered by nose cone with a simple mechanical device is illustrated in Fig. 20D–9. When assessing this device in 34 piglets, the mean time to inducing unconsciousness was approximately 31 sec-

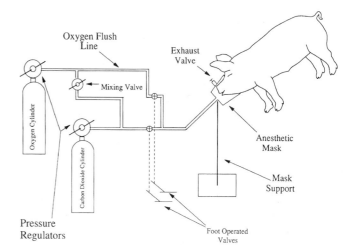

Fig. 20D–9. Schematic drawing of a device used to administer a 50:50 carbon dioxide–oxygen mixture to anesthetize piglets. This device utilizes a combination regulator-flowmeter to deliver gas flows to the anesthetic mask. Line pressures of 50 psi and flow rates of 2 L/min are adequate for rapidly anesthetizing piglets. (From Thurmon, J.C. and Benson, G.J. Anesthesia of Ruminants and Swine. In: Current Veterinary Therapy, 3rd ed. Food Animal Practice. Edited by J. Howard. Philadelphia: WB Saunders, 1993:58–76.)

onds whereas processing required 33 seconds. After CO_2 was discontinued, recovery was complete in 28 seconds. The time for induction processing and recovery was an average of 92 seconds.(27) The cost per piglet was less than 4 cents. This same technique is effective and safe in other neonatal species (e.g., lambs, kids, etc.).

Less Commonly Used Injectable Drugs

OPIOIDS

Opioids have been used in swine as adjuncts with other drugs to induce and maintain surgical anesthesia. They have also been used as constant infusions for maintenance. The first commercially available opioid drug combination was fentanyl and droperidol in a concentration of 0.4 and 20 mg/mL, respectively (Innovar-Vet). Pigs may become excited after Innovar-Vet injection. Salivation is often excessive unless atropine has been given. A major problem with this combination is the difference in drug half-life between the two drugs. That of fentanyl is quite short, whereas that of droperidol is rather long. Thus, the use of a specific opioid antagonist (e.g., naloxone) is ineffective in shortening a prolonged recovery because deep droperidol tranquilization often remains after the action of fentanyl has waned. In such situations pigs may respond violently if a high degree of postoperative pain persists. Innovar-Vet (1 mL/13–14 kg IM) combined with ketamine (11 mg/kg IM) will induce satisfactory anesthesia for 20 to 30 minutes in young swine.(1, 2, 28)

High-dose opioid infusion is most commonly used for anesthesia in cardiovascular research because of the drug's minimal effect on cardiovascular function.(29, 30) Fentanyl and sufentanil are the most commonly used drugs for this purpose. Sufentanil, a thienyl analog of fentanyl, is 5 to 10 times more potent than its parent compound (Chapter 8). In the atropinized pig 6–8 μg/kg IV of sufentanil followed by a constant infusion of 15–30 $\mu g \cdot kg^{-1} \cdot h^{-1}$ appears to be a reasonable rate of administration.(3) Fentanyl is given by the intravenous route in a wide range of doses (50–150 μg/kg) in people. Even with high doses there is excellent hemodynamic stability.(22) Anesthesia in swine can be maintained with fentanyl at a constant infusion of 45 to 90 $\mu g \cdot kg^{-1} \cdot h^{-1}$.

Mild tranquilization will generally prevent muscle rigidity after an intravenous opioid bolus and before infusion is commenced. In people, chest muscle rigidity following fentanyl administration is referred to as *woody chest syndrome*. Clinical experience suggests this may also occur in swine. When muscle rigidity is severe, it can be completely eliminated by a muscle relaxant.

Generally speaking, an opioid antagonist should only be given when an opioid severely depresses ventilation. In most instances an agonist-antagonist (e.g., butorphanol or nalbuphine) can be given to restore ventilation while retaining some degree of analgesia.(31) The half-life of nalbuphine in people ranges from 3 to 6 hours. However, fentanyl respiratory depression reversed by nalbuphine antagonism has been reported to recur in 2 to 3 hours.(22) A similar situation could be expected to occur in swine following butorphanol administration after long term fentanyl infusion. Naloxone (0.5–2 mg/kg IV or IM will antagonize the residual effects of fentanyl.

PROPOFOL

Propofol is an isopropylphenol derivative only administered by the intravenous route. This nonbarbiturate is supplied in an aqueous solution of 10% soybean oil, 2.5% glycerol, and 1.2% purified egg phosphatide in a concentration of 10 mg/mL (Chapter 9).(32) The drug is approximately twice as potent as thiopental and perhaps half as potent as methohexital. In people, consciousness returns more rapidly after a single injection or a constant infusion than with either thiamylal or thiopental. Residual CNS effect is less than that of the barbiturates. The clearance from plasma at a rate greater than the hepatic blood flow suggests that tissue sequestration plays an important role in its short duration of action.(22) Propofol is often described as a hypnotic offering only minimal analgesia. As a result it is generally used for induction of anesthesia or combined with a strong analgesic (e.g., an opioid or alpha$_2$-adrenoceptor agonist). Propofol has been used in combination with azaperone and thiopental in pigs. However, none of these are good analgesics. When propofol is used alone as an induction agent in dogs, the dose ranges from 6 to 8 mg/kg IV. Rapid injection may cause apnea. In swine deep sedation can be maintained with a constant infusion of 4 to 8 mg $\cdot kg^{-1} \cdot h^{-1}$. Propofol infused at a rate of 12 mg $\cdot kg^{-1} \cdot h^{-1}$ did not trigger malignant hyperthermia in susceptible swine.(33)

Medetomidine (20–40 μg/kg) and 2 to 4 mg/kg of propofol induces a light plane of anesthesia in 30- to 60-kg pigs. Xylazine (1–2 mg/kg) appears to be a reasonable substitute for medetomidine. Neither medetomidine nor xylazine is as effective in swine as in most other species, but when combined with propofol either provides a degree of analgesia commensurate with a light plane of anesthesia. Propofol is costly, and because it does not have a preservative, the possibility of bacterial contamination is a real threat if the entire vial is not used shortly after opening. A scrupulously sterile technique must be used after the heat-sealed vial has been opened. If the drug is to be stored for later use, complete sterility is essential.

ALPHAXALONE AND ALPHADALONE (SAFFAN)

Saffan has been used in swine for some time in Europe and Canada. Anesthetic response to this drug combination is short in duration, lasting only 10 to 15 min when a dose of 5 to 6 mg/kg is injected intravenously. The dose can be decreased by administering xylazine (1–2 mg/kg IM) or azaperone (4 mg/kg IM). The latter will prolong recovery time. Saffan anesthesia may be prolonged by intravenous injection of doses ranging from 2 to 4 mg/kg. Like propofol, this drug combination has been used without incident in swine susceptible to malignant hyperthermia.

ETOMIDATE

Etomidate is a carboxylated imidazole compound unrelated to other injectable anesthetics. It is a relatively poor analgesic and muscle relaxant, and is often classified as a sedative hypnotic when given in low doses (e.g., 2–4 mg/kg). Etomidate maintains cardiovascular stability but suppresses adrenocortical activity in people.(34) It does not trigger malignant hyperthermia in susceptible swine.(35) Etomidate in clinically recommended doses cause hemolysis in dogs. This has not been investigated in pigs. When pigs are treated with xylazine (1–2 mg/kg IM or IV) or azaperone (2–4 mg/kg IM), analgesia is increased, as is recovery time. Azaperone premedication prolongs recovery more than does xylazine. Furthermore, azaperone does not induce the degree of analgesia achieved with the coadministration of xylazine. Etomidate induction (0.6 mg/kg IV) followed by ketamine infusion at a rate of 10 mg $\cdot kg^{-1} \cdot h^{-1}$ has been used to maintain anesthesia in experimental swine.(19)

METOMIDATE

Metomidate (4 mg/kg IV) is a hypnotic similar to etomidate that provides rather stable cardiovascular function. In Europe, it is often used in combination with azaperone (2–4 mg/kg IM) to anesthetize swine. Azaperone is given as a preanesthetic, and metomidate is used to maintain anesthesia by repeat injection at 15- to 30-minute intervals.(36) The dose of metomidate can be doubled to prolong anesthesia. Under such circumstances it must be given slowly to prevent apnea.

Anesthesia with minimal analgesia has been maintained by continuous infusion of azaperone ($2\,mg \cdot kg^{-1} \cdot h^{-1}$) and metomidate ($8\,mg \cdot kg^{-1} \cdot h^{-1}$). Metomidate (15 mg/kg) has also been given by intraperitoneal injection.(1) However, because this route is often accompanied by peritonitis and intraabdominal adhesions, peritoneal injections are discouraged. Because metomidate provides poor analgesia, a local analgesic (e.g., lidocaine), an alpha$_2$-agonist, or an opioid is often administered concomitantly with metomidate and azaperone.

ALPHA-CHLORALOSE

This drug has been used in the research laboratory but probably has no place in swine practice. It is a poor analgesic and is usually accompanied by spontaneous leg movement. Blood pressure is unchanged or increased. Heart rate is usually increased, and respiratory depression does not occur until large doses are administered. Alpha-chloralose is relatively insoluble, and onset of peak effect is slow requiring approximately 15 to 20 minutes. Alpha-chloralose (55–86 mg/kg) can be combined with morphine (0.3–0.9 mg/kg) to provide anesthesia. However, continuous limb paddling is often experienced in pigs given this drug combination. Ketamine (5–10 mg/kg IV or IM) has also been combined with alpha-chloralose for research purposes where increased analgesia was required.(1)

Malignant Hyperthermia (MH)

This metabolic condition was first reported to occur in people in 1960. It wasn't until 1970 that E. W. Jones reported the occurrence of MH in swine. Prior to this report, healthy swine leaving the farm for market by truck and arriving dead were diagnosed as having *soft watery pork* syndrome. As people and swine with the disease were observed more closely, the condition later became known as *malignant hyperthermia*. The condition is characterized by striated muscle deterioration. Since that time, pigs possessing this genetic peculiarity have been identified in most swine breeds. Malignant hyperthermia has also been diagnosed in other species, including dogs, horses, cats, birds, deer and other wild animals (Chapter 11). In wild species the syndrome is often frequently referred to as *capture myopathy* (Chapter 22). However, of the mammalian species, MH is most commonly encountered in swine. Thus, swine have become the species of choice for studying the MH syndrome.

Early on, the predisposing factor appeared to be an autosomal dominant gene with complete penetrance.(37) Malignant hyperthermia seems to be most prevalent in individuals of breeds having a high ratio of muscle to total body mass and rapid growth.(38) Breeding for these market characteristics appears to have played a major role in increasing swine's predisposition to developing MH. The breeds most frequently carrying this genetic alteration are pietrain, landrace, spotted swine, large white, and Hampshire (not neces-

sarily in this order). Although others are not immune, the incidence of MH is encountered less frequently in the Duroc breed.(39) In highly susceptible individuals, MH may be triggered by the stress of restraint for blood sampling, castration, and other processing procedures in market swine. Malignant hyperthermia has been observed in young boars pursuing gilts that were unreceptive to breeding, particularly under hot summer conditions. Individuals arising from parentage with a strong inherent predisposition to MH were very common at one time, particularly in the landrace breed. Recognition of their predisposition in well-managed herds and elimination of individuals through death and marketing has in large part eliminated the problem in many of these herds, but individuals prone to MH are still occasionally encountered.

The incidence of MH in potbellied pigs is unknown. It can be expected to be small or nonexistent because this breed has a high fat to body mass ratio. Deaths in potbellied pigs attributed to MH may in fact be due to the stress of restraint. Anesthesia with halothane in hundreds of potbellied pigs has not uncovered the occurrence of a single death that could be attributed to MH. The most recent literature has not conclusively revealed the occurrence of MH in potbellied pigs. Presently, deaths attributed to MH appear to be speculative.

The occurrence of MH is associated with a sudden increase in muscle oxygen requirement and thus, lactate production. Body temperature increases as does respiration rate. Metabolic acidosis is accompanied by muscular contraction, sympathetic activation, and increased muscle cellular permeability. Initially, serum magnesium, calcium, phosphorus, and potassium ion concentrations are increased. These changes are followed by a decrease in serum potassium and calcium ion concentration. Myoglobinuria often appears shortly thereafter if the affected animal does not succumb. The syndrome appears to result from the individual's inability to regulate calcium ion concentrations in muscle tissue as a result of alteration in cellular membrane permeability. Individual susceptibility is diagnosed by muscle tissue biopsy reaction when exposed to caffeine, halothane, potassium, and succinylcholine in vitro. In addition, herd history and increased serum CPK concentrations are strong indicators of the MH trait.

Clinically, the MH syndrome in swine is characterized by rapid onset of tachycardia, hyperthermia, muscle rigidity (i.e., activation of limb extensor muscles), tachypnea progressing to dyspnea, and finally apnea. Rapidly increasing end-tidal carbon dioxide concentration is the most revealing clinical sign of impending MH.(40) In the later stages of the syndrome, tachycardia is accompanied by dysrhythmias that lead to bradycardia and finally cardiac arrest. Current findings indicate that metabolic status during MH is characterized by a demand ischemia of the heart and skeletal muscle. Insufficient coronary blood flow and increased metabolism as a result of tachycardia and increased concentrations of catecholamines are dominant factors contributing to the dramatic alteration in cardiac performance during porcine MH.(41) When tachycardia is accompanied by malignant dysrhythmias, treatment success is unlikely. Most patients will die regardless of treatment.

In susceptible swine, signs of MH appear shortly after exposure to halothane. An exception to this occurs when swine have been given a phenothiazine tranquilizer (e.g., acetylpromazine) and anesthesia is induced with a thiobarbiturate (e.g., thiopental). Under such circumstances, the onset of MH is delayed when anesthesia is continued with a halogenated hydrocarbon (i.e., halothane) or a halogenated ether (e.g., isoflurane). However, MH may occur in susceptible swine when the effects of the tranquilizer and/or the barbiturate have waned. Thus, it is important to understand that time of onset of MH is influenced by drugs used in various anesthetic regimens and is not always an acute response to halothane or succinylcholine administration. Succinylcholine injected into susceptible swine can easily trigger the MH syndrome, whereas nondepolarizing muscle relaxants (e.g., pancuronium) are less likely to do so (Chapter 13).

PREVENTION AND TREATMENT

The drug used most commonly to prevent and treat MH in swine is dantrolene (Dantrium, 2–5 mg/kg IV). This muscle relaxant is also an antipyretic. It suppresses calcium ion release but does not appear to inhibit uptake of calcium by muscle tissue cells. Even though it acts directly within muscle cells, its depressant effect upon respiratory muscle function is minimal. Dantrolene has proven to be a valuable prophylactic treatment for MH in susceptible swine and people.

Dantrolene is dosed per os (5 mg/kg) 8 to 10 hours prior to surgery. There is evidence that it should be repeated (3–5 mg/kg IV) preoperatively and postoperatively should surgery be prolonged. When a known triggering drug has been used to maintain anesthesia (e.g., halothane, isoflurane), the patient should be closely monitored for 24 hours postoperatively.

Symptomatic treatment includes rapid termination of the inhalant, changing of the anesthetic machine "rubber goods" (i.e., hoses and rebreathing bag), or switching to a clean machine, for administering 100% oxygen, procaine (1–2 mg/kg IV), intravenous corticosteroids, sodium bicarbonate (2–4 mEq/kg IV), and body cooling. Whole body cooling may be achieved with an ice water–alcohol mixture and cold fluids intravenously, orally, or by infusion per rectum.

Anesthetic drugs least likely to trigger MH in susceptible swine include thiopental, propofol, etomidate, metomidate and epidural anesthesia.(40) In highly susceptible swine, restraint for intravenous or epidural drug injection can precipitate the MH syndrome. In MH-susceptible swine, preanesthetic medications (e.g.,

acetylpromazine) known to inhibit the MH syndrome should be given intramuscularly prior to induction of anesthesia.

References

1. Thurmon JC, Tranquilli WJ. Anesthesia for cardiovascular research. In: Stanton HC, Mersmann HJ, eds. Swine in cardiovascular research, vol. 1. Boca Raton, FL: CRC Press, 1986:39–59.
2. Riebold TW, Thurmon JC. Anesthesia in swine. In: Tumbleson ME, ed. Swine in biomedical research, vol. 1. New York: Plenum Press, 1986:243–254.
3. Swindell MM. Anesthetic and perioperative techniques in swine. Wilmington, MA: Charles River Laboratories, CRL Tech. Bull. (winter) 1991.
4. Thurmon JC, Benson GJ. Anesthesia in ruminants and swine. In: Howard J, ed. Current veterinary therapy 3, food animal practice. Philadelphia: WB Saunders, 1993:58–76.
5. Smith AC, Spinale FG, Swindle MM. Cardiac function and morphology of Hanford miniature swine and Yucatan miniature and micro swine. Lab Anim Sci 40(1):47–50, 1990.
6. Thurmon JC, Benson GJ. Special anesthesia considerations of swine. In: Short CE, ed. Principles and practice of veterinary anesthesia. Baltimore: Williams & Wilkins, 1987:308–322.
7. Cohn MS, Lichtiger, M. Premedications. In: Lichtiger M, Moya F, eds. Introduction to the practice of anesthesia, 2nd ed. Hagerstown, MD: Harper & Row, 1978:13
8. Ochs HR, Greenblatt DJ, Eichelkraut W, Bakker C, Gobel R, Hahn N. Hepatic vs. gastrointestinal presystemic extraction of oral midazolam and flurazepam. J Pharmacol Exp Ther 243(3):852–856, 1987.
9. Pender KS, Pollack CV, Woodall BN, Parks BR. Intraosseous administration of lorazepam: same-dose comparison with intravenous administration in the weanling pig. J Miss State Med Assoc 1991:365–368.
10. Danneberg P, Bauer, R, Boke-Kuhn K, et al. General pharmacology of brotizolam in animals. Department of Pharmacology, Boehringer-Ingelheim, Ingelheim-Rhein (Germany), 1986.
11. Unnerstall JR, Kopajtic TA, Kuhar MJ. Distribution of alpha-^{2} agonist binding sites in the rat and human central nervous system: analysis of some functional, anatomic correlations of the pharmacologic effects of clonidine and related adrenergic agonists. Brain Res Rev 1:69–101, 1984.
12. Giron LT, McCann SA, Crist-Orlando SG. Pharmacological characterization and regional distribution of alpha-noradrenergic binding sites of rat spinal cord. Eur J Pharmacol 115:285–290, 1985.
13. Ko JCH, Thurmon JC, Benson. GJ, Tranquilli WJ , Olson WA. Evaluation of analgesia induced by epidural injection of detomidine or xylazine in swine. J Vet Anaesth 19:56–60, 1992.
14. Yaksh TL. Pharmacology of the spinal adrenergic system which modulate spinal nociceptive processing. Pharmacol Biochem Behav 22:845–856, 1985.
15. LeBlanc PH, Caron JP, Patterson JS, Brown M, Matta. MA. Epidural injection of xylazine for perineal analgesia in horses. J Am Vet Med Assoc 193:1405–1408, 1988.
16. Fikes LW, Lin HC, Thurmon JC. A preliminary comparison of lidocaine and xylazine as epidural analgesics in ponies. Vet Surg Anesth 18:5–86, 1989.
17. Ko JCH, Althouse GC, Hopkins SM, Jackson LL, Evans LE, Smith RP. Effects of epidural administration of xylazine or lidocaine on bovine uterine motility and perineal analgesia. Theriogenology. 32:786–797, 1989.
18. Skarda RT, Muir WW, Bednarski LS. A preliminary study of caudal epidural and subarachnoid analgesia after detomidine administration in horses [Abstract]. Proceedings, Sixth Annual Meeting, Midwest Anesthesia Conference, University of Illinois, Champaign-Urbana, 1990.
19. Worek FS, Blumel G, Zaravik, J, Zimmerman GJ, Pfeiffer UJ. Comparison of ketamine and pentobarbital anesthesia with the conscious state in a porcine model of pseudomonas aeriginosa septicemia. Acta Anesth Scand 32:509–515, 1988.

20. Swindell MM, Smith AC, Hepburn BJS. Swine as models in experimental surgery. J Invest Surg 1:65–79, 1988.
21. Reich DL, Silvay, G. Ketamine: an update on the first twenty-five years of clinical experience. Can J Anesth 36:186–197, 1989.
22. Stoelting RK. Pharmacology and physiology in anesthetic practice, 2nd ed. Philadelphia: JB Lippincott 1991:134–147.
23. Thurmon JC, Nelson DR, Christie GJ. Ketamine anesthesia in swine. J Am Vet Med Assoc 160:1325–1330, 1972.
24. Breese CE, Dodman NH. Xylazine-Ketamine-Oxymorphone: an injectable anesthetic combination in swine. J Am Vet Med Assoc 184:182–183, 1984.
25. Thurmon JC, Benson GJ, Tranquilli WJ, Olson WA, Tracy CH. The anesthetic effects of telazol and xylazine in pigs: evaluating clinical trials. Vet Med August:841–845, 1988.
26. Tranquilli WA, Thurmon JC, Benson GJ. Anesthetic potency of nitrous oxide in young swine (Sus scrofa). Am J Vet Res 46:58–60, 1985.
27. Thurmon JC, Lin HC, Curtis SE. Carbon dioxide and oxygen anesthesia for castration of baby pigs [Abstract]. 71st Conference of Research Workers in Animal Disease, Chicago, Illinois, November 5–6, 1990:34.
28. Benson GJ, Thurmon JC. Anesthesia of swine under field conditions. J Am Vet Assoc 174:594–596, 1979.
29. Merin RG, Verdouw PD, Jong JW. Myocardial functional and metabolic responses to ischemia in swine during halothane and fentanyl anesthesia. Anesthesiology 56:84–92, 1982.
30. Schuman RE, Swindle MM, Knick BJ, Case CL, Gelette PC. High dose narcotic anesthesia using sufentanil in swine for cardiac catheterization and electrophysiologic studies. J Invest Surg 5(13):283, 1992.
31. Baily PL, Clark NJ, Pace NL, et al. Antagonism with post operative opioid-induced respiratory depression: nalbuphine versus naloxone. Anesth Analg 70:8–15, 1990.
32. Sebel PS, Lowdon JD. Propofol: a new intravenous anesthetic. Anesthesiology. 67:260–277, 1989.
33. Raff M, Harrison GG. The screening of propofol in MH swine. Can J Anaesth 36:186–197, 1989.
34. Fragen RJ, Shanks CJ, Molteni A, Abram MJ. Effects of etomidate on hormonal responses to surgical stress. Anesthesiology 61:652–656, 1984.
35. Suresh MS, Nelson TE. Malignant hyperthermia: is etomidate safe? Anesth Analg 64:420–424, 1985.
36. Svendsen P, Carter AM. Blood gas tensions, acid-base status and cardiovascular function in miniature swine anesthetized with halothane and methoxyflurane or intravenous metomidate hydrochloride. Pharmacol Toxicol 64:88–93, 1989.
37. Gronert GA, Milde GH, Theye RA. Dantrolene in porcine malignant hyperthermia. Anesthesiology 44:488–495, 1976.
38. Gronert GA. Malignant hyperthermia. Anesthesiology 53:395–423, 1980.
39. Wagner AJ. The porcine stress syndrome. Vet Med Rev 1:68–77, 1972.
40. Kaplan RF. Malignant hyperthermia. Am Soc Anesth Annual Refresher Course Lectures, no. 231, San Francisco, California, 1991:1–7.
41. Roewer N, Dziadzka A, Greim C, et al. Cardiovascular and metabolic responses to anesthetic-induced malignant hyperthermia in swine. Anesthesiology 83:141–159, 1995.
42. Wertz EM, Wagnert AE. Anesthesia in potbellied pigs. Compend Cont Educ 17(3):369–382, 1995.

chapter 20 E

BIRDS

John W. Ludders, Nora Matthews

Introduction

The principles and practices of avian anesthesia depend on an understanding of anatomy, physiology, and pharmacology. A primary focus of this chapter is on the pulmonary and cardiovascular systems, both of which are important in the anesthetic management of birds, but where appropriate, other organ systems will be discussed. Although drugs will be discussed in general terms, this chapter is not a compendium of drugs and doses useful for anesthetic management of birds; the reader is referred to Dr. R. M. Fedde's article, which discusses this information in considerable detail.(1)

Data derived from mammalian studies are not applied to birds except for general physiologic, pharmacologic, and anesthetic principles that are applicable to avian species.

Form and Function

PULMONARY SYSTEM

The avian pulmonary system is very different from that of the mammalian system. A brief description of avian pulmonary anatomy and physiology will help to explain earlier misconceptions and current realities concerning the effects of anesthetics on birds, especially inhalant anesthetics. The avian respiratory system consists of two separate and distinct functional components: a component for ventilation (conducting airways, air sacs, thoracic skeleton, muscles of respiration), and a component for gas exchange (parabronchial lung).

Ventilation component. **Larynx and trachea.** The avian larynx protrudes into the pharynx as a somewhat heart-shaped mound and consists of four laryngeal cartilages: the cricoid, procricoid, and the right and left arytenoid cartilages.(2) Unlike in mammals, the thyroid and epiglottic cartilages are absent in birds.(2) In birds the larynx functions as a barrier to foreign material entering the airway, opens the glottis during inspiration, assists in swallowing, and may modulate sound production.(2)

In all avian species the trachea consists of four layers: mucous membrane, submucosa, cartilage, and adventitia. The tracheal cartilages form complete rings.(2) The internal lining of the larynx and trachea consists of simple and pseudostratified, ciliated columnar epithelium within which are large numbers of simple alveolar mucous glands composed of typical mucus-secreting cells.(2, 3) The mucous glands give way to mucous goblet cells in the caudal portion of the trachea and within the lining of the syrinx.(2, 3)

There are significant species-related variations in tracheal anatomy. For example, the emu and ruddy duck have an inflatable saclike diverticulum (tracheal sac) that opens from the trachea.(2) In the emu the sac arises from the ventral surface of the trachea approximately three quarters of the way down the neck where there is a slitlike opening where the tracheal rings are incomplete ventrally (Fig. 20E–1).(2) The caudal end of the sac may extend almost to the level of the sternum. This sac is present in both sexes and is responsible for the characteristic booming call of the emu.

In the ruddy duck the sac opens in a depression on the dorsal wall of the trachea immediately caudal to the larynx, thus lying between the trachea and esophagus.(2) In this bird the sac is found only in the male, in which it may act as a sounding board for the bill-drumming display of the male.(2)

The male of many anseriform species (waterfowl such as ducks and mergansers) have a unique anatomic feature of the trachea, the tracheal bulbous expansion. It is a bulblike structure in the trachea, and its exact function is not clear.

A double trachea, found in some penguins and petrels, consists of a median septum dividing part of the trachea into right and left channels.(2) In both groups of birds the septum extends cranially from the bronchial bifurcation, but the length of the septum is quite variable. For example, in the jackass penguin the septum extends to within a few centimeters of the larynx, whereas in the rockhopper penguin the septum is only 5 mm in length.(2)

Some species of birds have complex tracheal loops or coils that, depending on the species, may be located in

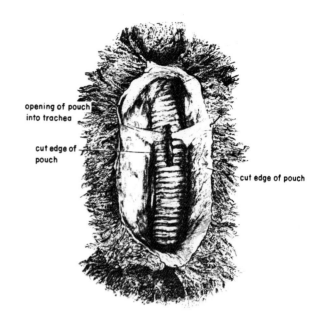

Fig. 20E–1. Opened tracheal sac exposing the tracheal slit of the emu (*Dromaius novaehollandiae*). (From McLelland, J. Larynx and trachea. In: Form and Function in Birds, vol. 4. Edited by A.S. King and J. McLelland. London, Academic Press, 1989:69–103; with permission.)

the caudal neck, within the keel, or within the thorax and the keel (Fig. 20E–2). Studies in cranes have demonstrated that tracheal coiling enables these birds to produce extremely loud calls using very low driving pressures.(4)

The fact that birds generally have relatively long necks, not to mention tracheal loops and coils, has important implications for the functional morphology of the trachea, especially tracheal dead space. Studies indicate that the typical bird trachea is 2.7 times longer than that of comparably sized mammals, but because the bird trachea is 1.29 times wider, the tracheal resistance in birds and mammals is comparable.(2) Tracheal dead space volume is increased in birds to about 4.5 times that of comparably sized mammals, but the relatively low respiratory frequency of birds, approximately one third that of mammals, ensures that the effect of the larger tracheal dead space volume is decreased.(2) As a result the minute tracheal ventilation rate is only about 1.5 to 1.9 times that of mammals.(2)

Syrinx. The syrinx, the sound-producing organ in birds, is located at the junction of the trachea and mainstem bronchi. Its shape, size, and location are extremely variable among avian species. For a thorough review of this anatomic structure the reader is referred to the work by A. S. King.(5) The location and structure of the syrinx explains why gas flowing through the trachea, especially during positive pressure ventilation, can produce sound in an intubated bird.

Bronchi. The bronchial system of birds consists of three orders of branching including a primary bronchus (extrapulmonary and intrapulmonary), secondary bronchi, and tertiary bronchi (parabronchi), which,

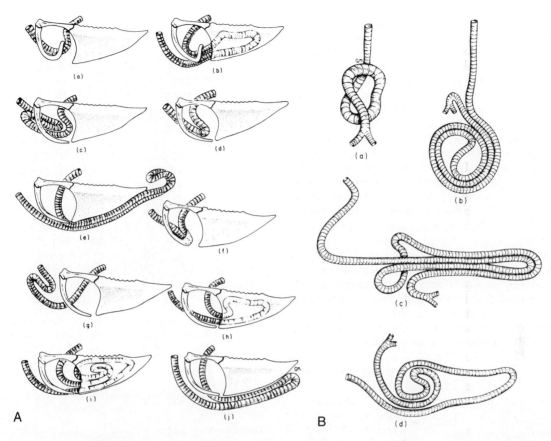

Fig. 20E-2. Tracheal loops found in birds. (From McLelland, J. Larynx and trachea. In: Form and Function in Birds, vol. 4. Edited by A.S. King and J. McLelland. London, Academic Press, 1989:69–103; with permission.) A, Different forms of tracheal loops: (a) black swan (*Cygnus atratus*); (b) whooper swan (*Cygnus cygnus*); (c) white spoonbill (*Platalea leucorodia*); (d) black curassow (*Crax alector*); (e) helmeted curassow (*Crax pauxi*); (f) crested guineafowl (*Guttera edouardi*); (g) capercaillie (*Tetrao urogallus*); (h) crane (*Grus grus*); (i) whooping crane (*Grus americana*); (j) a bird of paradise (*Manucodia sp.*). B, Extreme forms of tracheal loops: (a) *Platalea sp.*; (b) trumpet bird (*Phonygammus keraudrenii*); (c) magpie goose (*Anseranas semipalmata*); (d) whooping crane (*Grus americana*).

along with the paraperibronchial mantle of tissue, form the gas exchange tissues of the lung.(6)

The primary bronchus enters the lung ventrally and obliquely at the junction of the cranial and middle thirds of the lung, then passes dorsolaterally to the lung surface, where it turns caudally in a dorsally curved course until at the caudal lung margin it opens into the abdominal air sac.(7) The primary bronchi, both extrapulmonary and intrapulmonary, are lined with low columnar, pseudostratified epithelium containing goblet cells, intraepithelial mucous alveoli and projecting ridges carrying cilia.(3, 8) Below the mucosa there is a well-developed layer of smooth muscle. There are a series of C-shaped cartilaginous rings at the junction of each primary bronchus and lung. These C-shaped rings are lost just before the primary bronchus bends caudally within the lung. After losing the cartilaginous rings, the intrapulmonary primary bronchus possesses a well-developed, internal circular smooth muscle layer and longitudinally oriented smooth muscles.(9) Studies have shown that the smooth muscles, in response to a variety of stimuli, can change the internal diameter of the primary bronchus. Acetylcholine, pilocarpine, and

histamine induce strong contraction of the bronchial smooth muscle, while atropine blocks their effects but has no effect when given alone.(10)

Secondary bronchi. Any bronchus arising from a primary bronchus is a secondary bronchus, and in most birds the secondary bronchi are arranged into four groups: medioventral, mediodorsal, lateroventral, and laterodorsal secondary bronchi.(6) The medioventral secondary bronchi arise from the primary intrapulmonary bronchus close to where it enters the lung, and these secondary bronchi occupy the ventral surface of the lung.(11) The mediodorsal, lateroventral, and laterodorsal secondary bronchi arise from the caudal curved portion of the primary intrapulmonary bronchus. Between the medioventral group of secondary bronchi and the three remaining groups of secondary bronchi, depending on the species, there is a section of primary bronchus devoid of secondary bronchi.(6)

For a short distance the secondary bronchi have the same histologic structure as the primary bronchus, but subsequently they develop simple squamous epithelium.(3, 8) There are single small circular bands of smooth muscle over which there is ciliated epithelium.(9) Many of the medioventral and lateroventral secondary bronchi open into the cervical, clavicular, cranial thoracic, or abdominal air sacs.

Air sacs. Birds have nine air sacs including the two cervical, an unpaired clavicular, two cranial and two caudal thoracic, and two abdominal air sacs. Histologically, the air sacs are thin-walled structures composed of simple squamous epithelium covering a thin layer of connective tissue, although close to the secondary bronchial openings into the air sacs there are groups of ciliated cuboidal and columnar cells.(6) The air sacs are poorly vascularized and do not significantly contribute to gas exchange in birds.(12) To a varying extent, depending upon the species, diverticula from the air sacs aerate the cervical vertebrae, some of the thoracic vertebrae, vertebral ribs, sternum, humerus, pelvis, and head and body of the femur.(6)

In terms of function the air sacs serve as bellows to the lungs in that they provide tidal air flow to the relatively rigid avian lung.(13) Based on their bronchial connec-

tions, air sacs are grouped into a cranial group consisting of the cervical, clavicular, and cranial thoracic air sacs, and a caudal group consisting of the caudal thoracic and abdominal air sacs.(14) The volume is distributed approximately equally between the cranial and caudal groups of air sacs.(15) During ventilation, all air sacs are effectively ventilated, with the possible exception of the cervical air sacs, and the ratio of ventilation to volume is similar for each air sac.(15)

Muscles of respiration and the thoracic skeleton. In birds, unlike in mammals, both inspiration and expiration are active processes requiring muscular activity (Table 20E–1). With contraction of the inspiratory muscles the internal volume of the thoracoabdominal cavity increases (Fig. 20E–3), and since the air sacs are the only significant volume-compliant structures within the body cavity, volume changes occur mainly in the air sacs.(15) Pressure within the air sacs becomes negative relative to ambient atmospheric pressure, and air flows from the atmosphere into the pulmonary system,

Table 20E–1. Muscles of Respiration in Birds

Inspiratory Muscles	*Expiratory Muscles*
Principal	Principal
M. scalenus	Mm. intercostales interni (in 3rd and 6th spaces)
Mm. intercostales interni (in 2nd space)	Mm. intercostales externi (in 5th and 6th spaces)
Mm. intercostales externi (except in 5th and 6th spaces)	M. costosternalis par minor
M. Costosternalis pars major	M. obliquus externus abdominis
M. levatores costarum	M. obliquus internus abdominis
Accessory	M. rectus abdominis
M. serratus profundus	M. transversus abdominis
	Mm. costoseptales
	Accessory
	M. serratus superficialis pars cranialis et caudalis
	M. rhomboideus superficialis
	M. rhomboideus profundus
	M. latissimus doris
	Mm. iliocostalis et longissimus dorsi

Adapted from Fedde, M.R. Respiratory Muscles. In: Bird Respiration, vol. I. Edited by T.J. Seller. Boca Raton, FL: CRC Press, 1987.

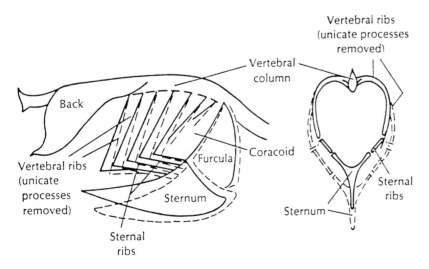

Fig. 20E–3. Changes in the position of the thoracic skeleton during breathing in a bird. The solid lines represent thoracic position at the end of expiration while the dotted lines show the thoracic position at the end of inspiration. (Reprinted with permission from Fedde, M.R. Respiration. In: Avian Physiology, 4th ed. Edited by P.D. Sturkie. New York: Springer-Verlag, 1986:191–220.)

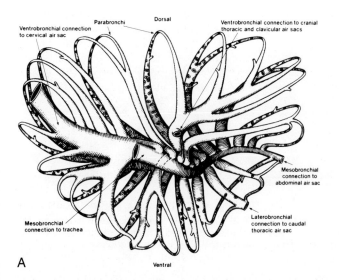

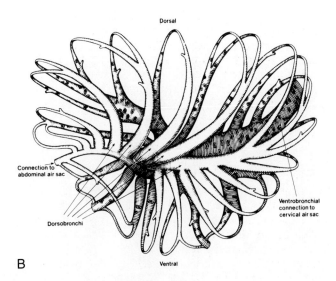

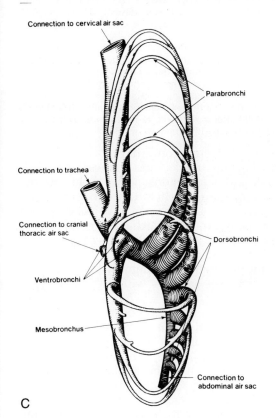

Fig. 20E–4. Three views of secondary bronchi and parabronchi (A, B, and C) in the right lung of a goose. (From Brackenbury, J.H. Ventilation of the lung-air sac system. In: Bird Respiration, vol I. Edited by T.J. Seller. Boca Raton, FL: CRC Press, 1987; with permission.) A, Medial view of the lung. B, Lateral view of the lung. C, Dorsal view of the lung.

specifically into the air sacs and across the gas exchange surfaces of the lungs.

Gas exchange component. The basic unit for gas exchange is the tertiary bronchus or parabronchus and its mantle of surrounding tissue. The parabronchi, which connect the two main sets of secondary bronchi, are long, narrow tubes that display only a mild degree of anastomosing (Fig. 20E–4).(11) There is a network of smooth muscle surrounding the entrances to the parabronchi, and this smooth muscle, upon electric

stimulation of the vagus nerve, can contract and cause narrowing of the openings to the parabronchi.(16) The inner surfaces of the tubular parabronchi are pierced by numerous openings into chambers called atria that are separated from each other by interatrial septa (Fig. 20E–5). The atrial openings also are surrounded by bundles of smooth muscle.(6) Since the avian lung is richly innervated with vagal and sympathetic nerves, it is possible that efferent and afferent pathways exist for controlling pulmonary smooth muscle, and with it the

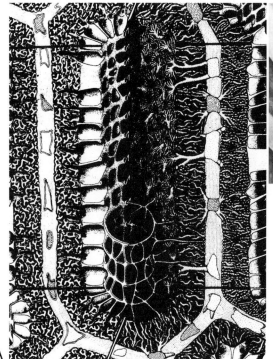

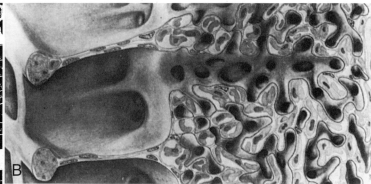

Fig. 20E–5. Three-dimensional drawings of a parabronchus. A, Drawing at left. On the left side are atria with infundibula departing from them and the three-dimensional air capillary meshwork arising from the infundibula. On the right side within the interparabronchial septa are the arterioles (dense stippling) from which the capillaries originate and run radially to the lumen. The infundibula lie between the capillaries, which are surrounded by a well-developed three-dimensional air capillary network. (From Duncker, H-R. Structure of the Avian Respiratory Tract. Respir Physiol 22:1, 1974; with permission.) B, Drawing above. At the left, two of the circular smooth muscle bundles surrounding the lumen of the parabronchus are shown in cross section. The atria are separated by this septa running horizontally and vertically. Originating from each atrium a few infundibula pass perpendicularly into the parabronchial mantle. At the right an infundibulum is shown in longitudinal section with air capillaries arising from it at all levels. The air capillaries cross-link and interlace, making up a three-dimensional meshwork around the blood capillaries. The very thin epithelium of the air capillaries and its surfactant film are shown as a single dark line. (From Duncker, H-R. Structure of the Avian Respiratory Tract. Respir Physiol 22:1, 1974; with permission.)

flow of air through the parabronchial lung, in response to a variety of stimuli.(14) Arising from the floor or abluminal surface of the atria are funnel-shaped ducts, the infundibula, that lead to air capillaries. The air capillaries measure 3 to 10 microns in diameter and form an anastomosing three-dimensional network intimately interlaced with a similarly structured network of blood capillaries.(6, 7) It is within this mantle of interlaced air and blood capillaries, this periparabronchial tissue, that gas exchange occurs.

A feature of the small radius of curvature of air capillaries is the very high surface tensions, which work against the anatomic integrity and gas exchange function of these air capillaries. The high surface tensions may explain why avian lungs consist of rigid tubes.(7) However, the avian lung is somewhat distensible, and surfactant, which is present in the avian lung, may decrease surface tensions, thus maintaining the structural integrity of the air capillaries and preventing transudation and filling of the air capillaries with fluid.(6)

There are two types of parabronchial tissue in the avian lung. The paleopulmonic parabronchial tissue, consisting of essentially parallel, minimally anastomosing parabronchi, is found in all birds (Fig. 20E–6A). By comparison, neopulmonic parabronchial tissue is a meshwork of anastomosing parabronchi located in the caudolateral portion of the lung, and its degree of development is species dependent (Fig. 20E–6B and

C).(6) Penguins and emus only have paleopulmonic parabronchi. Pigeons, ducks, and cranes have both paleopulmonic and neopulmonic parabronchi with the neopulmonic accounting for 10 to 12% of the total lung volume in these species, whereas in fowl-like birds and song birds the neopulmonic, which is more developed, may account for 20 to 25% of the total lung volume.(14) Although the paleopulmonic and neopulmonic parabronchi are histologically indistinguishable from each other, the direction of gas flow within the two types differs.

During inspiration and expiration the direction of gas flow in the paleopulmonic parabronchi is unidirectional, whereas that in the neopulmonic parabronchi is bidirectional (Fig. 20E–7).(14, 15) The unidirectional flow of gas through the intrapulmonary primary bronchus, the secondary bronchi, and the paleopulmonic parabronchi is governed by processes of aerodynamic valving and not by mechanical valving mechanisms.(17-21) Aerodynamic valving occurs as a consequence of the orientation of secondary bronchial and air sac orifices to the direction of gas flow, elastic pressure differences between the cranial and caudal group of air sacs, and gas convective inertial forces. The potential advantage of unidirectional gas flow to birds is discussed later.

A cross-current model of gas exchange describes the relationship between gas and blood flows within the avian lung. In birds there is no equivalent of alveolar gas

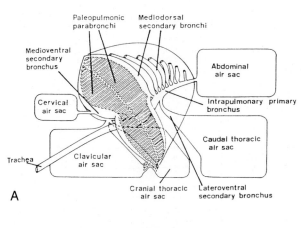

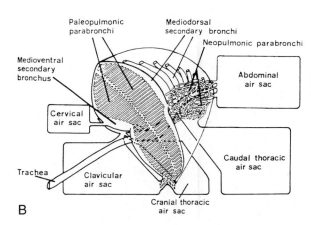

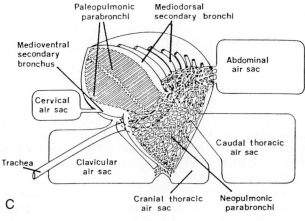

Fig. 20E–6. Drawings of paleopulmonic and neopulmonic lungs. (From Fedde, M.R. Structure and Gas-Flow Pattern in the Avian Respiratory System. Poultry Sci 59:2642, 1980; with permission.) A, The paleopulmonic lung found in penguins and emus. B, The paleopulmonic and neopulmonic lung found in storks, ducks and geese. C, The paleopulmonic and more highly developed neopulmonic lung found in chickens, sparrows and other song birds.

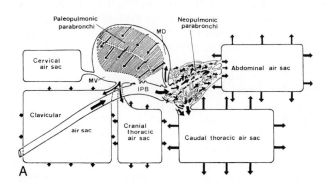

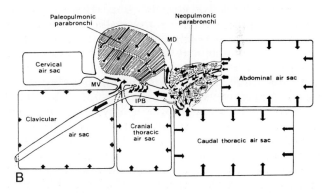

Fig. 20E–7. Schematic representation of the pathway of gas flow through the avian lung during inspiration and expiration; MV, medioventral secondary bronchus; MD, mediodorsal secondary bronchus; IPB, intrapulmonary primary bronchus. (Reprinted with permission from Fedde, M.R. Structure and Gas-Flow Pattern in the Avian Respiratory System. Poultry Sci 59:2642, 1980.) A, Inspiration. B, Expiration.

because parabronchial gas continuously changes in composition as it flows along the length of the parabronchus.(22) The degree to which capillary blood is oxygenated and carbon dioxide is eliminated depends on where along the length of the parabronchus the blood contacts the blood/gas interface. As a result arterial blood is formed by the mixing of streams of end-capillary blood of widely varying gas composi-

tion.(23) In addition, blood perfusing the inspiratory end of the parabronchus can equilibrate with gas entering the parabronchus that has a high partial pressure of oxygen. Thus, the partial pressure of oxygen in end-parabronchial gas can be lower than in arterial blood, while the partial pressure of carbon dioxide in end-parabronchial gas may exceed the partial pressure of CO_2 in arterial blood. This potential overlap of

Table 20E–2. Gas Exchange Variables in Awake Resting Birds

Variable	Pigeon	Domestic Fowl (♀)	Pekin Duck	Muscovy Duck (Cairina moschata)	Common Starling (Sturnus vulgaris)	Black Duck (Anas rubripes)
Weight (kg)	0.38	1.6	2.38	2.16	0.08	1.30
M_{O_2} (mmol · min^{-1})	0.35	1.09	1.67	—	0.13	0.84
f_{resp} (min^{-1})	27	23	8 to 15	10	92	27
V_T (mL)	7.5	33	16 to 98	69	0.67	30
V_E (L · min^{-1})	0.204	0.760	0.807 to 0.910	0.700	0.061	0.79
Q (L · min^{-1})	0.127	0.430	0.423 to 0.973	0.844	—	—
P_aO_2 (torr)	95	87	93 to 100	96	—	—
P_aCO_2 (torr)	34	29	34 to 36	36	—	—

M_{O_2}, oxygen consumption; f_{resp}, respiratory frequency; V_T, tidal volume; V_E, minute ventilation; Q, cardiac output.
(Adapted from Powell F.L. and Scheid P. Physiology of Gas Exchange in the Avian Respiratory System. In: McLelland Form and Function in Birds, vol. 4. Edited by A.S. King and J. McLelland. London: Academic Press, 1989:393–437.)

blood-gas partial pressures, which cannot occur in mammalian lungs, demonstrates the high gas exchange efficiency of the avian lung.(24, 25)

A number of factors limit gas exchange efficiency in the avian lung, including mismatching of ventilation and perfusion, diffusion barriers, and inhomogeneities within the lung.(25) It is generally assumed that diffusion is the primary gas transport mechanism in the air capillaries.(26) The gas exchange efficiency of the avian lung usually is not apparent under resting conditions (Table 20E–2), but becomes readily apparent under conditions of exercise or stress such as during flight at altitude or hypoxia.(27-30)

Despite its relative efficiency the avian lung does have some limitations. By using casting methods and gas washout techniques the specific volume (respiratory gas volume per unit body mass) of the avian respiratory system is estimated at between 100 and 200 mL/kg (by comparison the specific volume for the dog is 45 mL/kg).(15) However, in birds the volume of gas in the parabronchi and air capillaries is only 10% of the total specific volume, whereas that in the mammalian lung is 96% of the total specific volume. Because the ratio of residual gas volume to tidal volume is so much smaller in birds than in mammals, it has been suggested that cyclic changes in parabronchial gas flow, such as reversal of gas flow, could produce significant and intolerable cyclic changes in parabronchial gas exchange somewhat analogous to breath holding.(13) The unidirectional flow of gas within the avian lung solves this problem. In addition, it appears that the volume of parabronchial gas available for gas exchange may be larger than the anatomic studies would indicate and may be due to factors such as cardiogenic mixing or pulsations of blood flow within the pulmonary capillaries.(13)

Control of ventilation. Birds have many of the same physiologic components for respiratory control as mammals, such as a central respiratory pattern generator, central chemoreceptors that are sensitive to PCO_2, and

many similar peripheral chemoreceptors.(31) Birds have a unique group of peripheral receptors located in the lung called *intrapulmonary chemoreceptors* (IPCs) that are not mechanoreceptors, are acutely sensitive to CO_2, and are insensitive to hypoxia.(32, 33) The IPCs affect the rate and depth of breathing on a breath-to-breath basis by acting as the afferent limb of an inspiratory-inhibitory reflex that uses as the afferent signal the timing, rate, and extent of CO_2 washout from the lung during inspiration.(31)

There may be species differences in CO_2 responsiveness depending upon the ecologic niche that a given species occupies. The CO_2 responsiveness of IPC in chickens, ducks, emus, and pigeons is greater than the IPC of burrowing owls, a species of bird that lives underground, where the concentration of CO_2 is higher than that of above ground-dwelling birds.(34, 35)

CARDIOVASCULAR SYSTEM

The avian heart is a four-chambered muscular pump that separates venous blood (low in oxygen content and high in carbon dioxide content) from arterial blood (high in oxygen and low in carbon dioxide). Birds have larger hearts, larger stroke volumes, lower heart rates, and higher cardiac output than mammals of comparable body mass.(36) Birds also have higher blood pressures than do mammals.(36, 37) The atria and ventricles are innervated by sympathetic and parasympathetic nerves.(37) Norepinephrine and epinephrine are the principal sympathetic neurotransmitters in birds, and acetylcholine is the principal parasympathetic neurotransmitter. Excitement and handling can increase the concentration of norepinephrine and epinephrine, especially epinephrine, in the heart and blood.(37) This has significant implications for the anesthetic management of birds because inhalant anesthetics, especially halothane, sensitize the myocardium to catecholamine-induced cardiac arrhythmias. Hypoxia, hypercapnia, and anesthetics, the last depending on the type and dose, depress cardiovascular function.

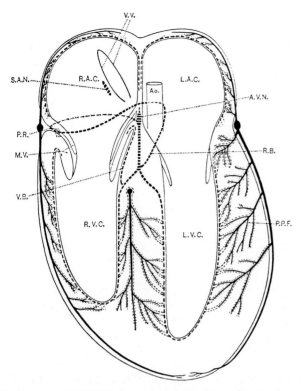

Fig. 20E–8. Diagram of the conducting system of the pigeon heart. The unbroken lines represent branches of the coronary arteries while the broken lines represent the various parts of the conducting system. Ao., Aorta; A.V.N., atrioventricular node; L.A.C., left atrial cavity; M.V., muscular right atrioventricular valve; P.P.F., periarterial Purkinje fibers; P.R., ring of Purkinje fibers around right atrioventricular orifice; R.A.C., right atrial cavity; R.V.C., right ventricular cavity; R.B., left recurrent branch of atrioventricular bundle; S.A.N., sinoatrial node; V.B., branch of right limb of atrioventricular bundle to muscular valve; V.V., right and left venous valves. (From Hodges, R.D. The Histology of the Fowl. London: Academic Press, 1974:200; with permission.)

The conduction system of the avian heart consists of the sinoatrial node, the atrioventricular node and its branches, and Purkinje fibers.(38) Two groups of animals can be identified by the depth and degree to which Purkinje fibers ramify within the ventricular myocardium, and the pattern of ramification is classified as type 1 or 2.(39) The pattern of Purkinje fiber distribution within the ventricular myocardium is responsible for QRS morphology. In birds, Purkinje fibers completely penetrate the ventricular myocardium from endocardium to epicardium (Fig. 20E–8), and the pattern of ventricular activation is described as type 2b, a pattern that may facilitate synchronous beating at high heart rates.(40) Electrocardiograms have been described for a number of avian species (38, 40-44), and the salient features of the avian electrocardiogram are summarized in Table 20E–3.

RENAL PORTAL SYSTEM

The avian kidney receives venous blood from the legs through the renal portal circulation as well as arterial blood through the arterial circulation (Fig. 20E–9).(45, 46) The flow of afferent venous blood, unlike in other nonmammalian vertebrates, is not obligatory, since blood can either perfuse the renal parenchyma or bypass it and enter the central circulation (Fig. 20E–10). A unique valvelike structure, the shape of which ranges from a thin membrane to a thickened funnel with one or many openings, depending on the species, is located within the external iliac vein at the point where the efferent renal vein joins the external iliac vein.(45) The valve contains smooth muscle innervated by cholinergic and adrenergic nerves. Epinephrine causes the valve to relax, whereas acetylcholine causes it to contract. When the valve contracts (closes), venous blood from the legs perfuses the kidney, but when the valve is relaxed (open), the venous blood is directed to the central circulation. The control of renal valve activity is complex, and its function is not fully understood.

Form and Function: Implications For Anesthetic Management

Air sacs. As previously noted, the air sacs of birds, because they are vessel poor, do not significantly participate in the process of gas exchange. For this same reason they do not play a major role in the uptake of inhalant anesthetics, nor, as has been suggested, do they accumulate or concentrate anesthetic gases.(47) Indeed, in a study of anesthetized spontaneously breathing pigeons it was found that the concentration of isoflurane in the abdominal air sacs was always lower than the concentration measured at the end of the endotracheal tube.(48)

Fluidic valving and mechanical positive pressure ventilation. During positive pressure ventilation it is possible that the direction of gas flow within the avian lung may be reversed, but such a reversal does not affect gas exchange, since the efficiency of the cross-current model is not dependent on the direction of flow.(15) Studies in which blood gases were collected from mechanically, bidirectionally ventilated birds, did not show an adverse effect of mechanical ventilation on gas exchange.(49, 50)

Effects of anesthesia and body position on ventilation. As mentioned earlier, the avian lung is very efficient at gas exchange, but this efficiency is compromised by anesthesia, and there probably are a number of causative factors responsible. In mammalian species it has been amply demonstrated that injectable and inhalant anesthetics, through their effects on the central nervous system and peripheral chemoreceptors, significantly depress ventilatory responses to hypoxia and hypercapnia.(51-53) Since birds have many of the same mechanisms for controlling ventilation as mammals it seems reasonable to assume that anesthetics will similarly depress avian ventilatory control mechanisms. A number of studies have shown that inhalants depress the responsiveness of a number of peripheral control mechanisms that directly or indirectly affect ventilation.(54-56)

Table 20E–3. Some Avian Electrocardiogram Configurations and Characteristics

Bird	Parakeet[42,43]						Parrot[42,43]					
Leads	I	II	III	aVR	aVL	aVF	I	II	III	aVR	aVL	aVF
P wave	+	+	+	−	±	+	+	+	+	− (80%) ± (20%)	+ (20%) ± (80%)	+
V E N T R I C U L A R D E P O L A R I Z A T I O N	QS or rS	QS or rS	RS or QS or rS	qR or R or QR	QR or R or qR	rS or QS or Rs	R (50%) or QS (30%) or RS (20%)	QS or rS	QS or rS	R or qR	R or qR	QS or rS
T wave	UI	+	+	−	−	+	Var.	+	+	−	−	+
MEA	−118° (−90° to −162°)						−86° (−83° to −108°)					

Barbiturates depress ventilation in birds but they retain the ability to respond to inspired CO_2.(57, 58) Furthermore, electromyograms from cocks lightly anesthetized with pentobarbital demonstrated that inspiratory and expiratory muscles of ventilation were equally depressed by the anesthetic.(59) Muscle relaxation is a feature of general anesthesia, and the degree of relaxation depends on the anesthetic. Because inspiratory and expiratory muscle activity is essential for ventilation in birds, any depression of muscle activity will affect ventilatory efficiency.

The position of the bird during anesthesia can significantly affect ventilation. As early as 1896 it was recognized that ventilation was much reduced in birds placed on their backs.(60) There are a number of factors that contribute to this phenomenon, not the least of which is the weight of the abdominal viscera compressing the abdominal air sacs and thus reducing their effective volume. Thus a number of factors regulating ventilation are affected by anesthetics.

By understanding how anesthetics affect these control mechanisms it is possible to make appropriate adjustments in anesthetic management, thus minimizing or eliminating anesthetic-induced deleterious effects on pulmonary function in anesthetized birds.

Lung gas volume, anesthesia, and the dive response. During anesthesia the lack of a significant functional residual volume in birds limits the period of time that a bird can remain apneic. During induction of anesthesia in birds, especially waterfowl, apnea and bradycardia can occur and last for 3 to 5 minutes. Anesthetic gases are not required to elicit this response, as it can occur by placing a mask snugly over a bird's beak and face. This response has been referred to as a *dive response,* but it is actually a stress response that appears to be mediated by stimulation of trigeminal receptors in the beak and nares of diving ducks.(61–63) During the stress response blood flow is preferentially distributed to the kidneys, heart, and brain.(64) This stress response makes safe induction of anesthesia in these birds a challenge. This response may be ameliorated by the use of premedicants such as diazepam or midazolam.

Unidirectional ventilation: Implications for anesthesia and artificial respiration. Because of the flow through nature of the avian respiratory system, it is possible to ventilate birds by flowing a continuous stream of gas through the trachea and lungs, and out through a ruptured or cannulated air sac.(65, 66) This same technique can be used to induce and maintain anesthesia in birds.(65, 67, 68) This technique also offers an effective means by which to ventilate and resuscitate an apneic bird or a bird with an obstructed airway.(69, 70) In one study in which arterial blood gases were compared before and after cannulation of the clavicular air sac in ducks, the arterial blood gases (PaO_2 and $PaCO_2$) remained unchanged by air sac cannulation.(71) Despite the lack of change in blood gases, tidal volume increased significantly and coupled with a slight but insignificant increase in respiratory frequency, there was a doubling of minute ventilation.

Intramuscular injections and the renal portal system. For walking birds, intramuscular injections are most commonly administered in the pectoral muscles and in the leg muscles for flying birds. Because birds possess a renal portal system there has been some concern that injections in the leg muscles might result in excessive

Table 20E-3. Some Avian Electrogardiogram Configurations and Characteristics (continued)

Bird	Pigeon[44]						Owl[42]					
Leads	I	II	III	aVR	aVL	aVF	I	II	III	aVR	aVL	aVF
P wave	+ (88%) ± (12%)	+	+ (43%) ± (57%)	−	±	+	+	+	+	−	−	+
VENTRICULAR DEPOLARIZATION	rS or qs	rS or QS	rS or QS	R or qR	R or qR	rS or QS	−	−	−	+	+	−
T wave	±	+	+	−	−	+	AB	+ or AB	+ or AB	− or AB	− or AB	+ or AB
MEA	−92° (−83° to −99°)						−102° (−81° to −127°)					

Definitions: +, positive wave; −, negative wave; ±, biphasic wave; UI, unidentifiable; Var., variable; ABS, absent; MEA, mean electric axis.

drug loss through the kidneys.(72) The renal portal system may play an important role in those situations in which drug efficacy depends on a constant blood level, as is the case for antimicrobial drugs. In a study of pigeons that were injected with flumequine in the pectoral and leg muscles, significant differences in bioavailability were found between the two injection sites, but whether this was caused by the renal portal system or of differences in blood flow was undetermined.(73) Although the renal portal system may be an important variable in antimicrobial therapy, its effect on anesthetic drugs injected into the leg muscles is probably unimportant. Injectable anesthetics are given to effect, and if a first dose does not produce the desired result, an additional smaller dose can be given to achieve the desired effect.

General Considerations for Anesthesia

PHYSICAL EXAMINATION

Every bird should be given a thorough physical examination prior to anesthesia. A number of excellent texts describe in detail the techniques for physical examination and what to look for in specific avian species.(69, 74, 75) In general, quiet observation of a bird in its cage will provide a great deal of information. Awareness of and attention to its surrounding environment, body form and posture, feather condition, and respiratory rate all provide clues to a bird's physical condition. Birds should be removed from their cage and examined, with particular attention given to the nares and mouth. A stethoscope with a pediatric head for small species should be used to examine the heart and lungs. At the same time the sharpness of the keel should be determined, as this is a good indicator of muscle mass and body fat.

ACCLIMATION

When possible a bird should be allowed to acclimate to the clinic or hospital environment prior to anesthesia. A bird brought into a new environment will be stressed. Time allows the bird to calm down after the initial physical examination and also gives the veterinarian time to evaluate the results of blood work. It is not unusual that once a bird has acclimated to the new environment, other signs of disease may become apparent that were masked at first presentation.

FASTING

There is some controversy about fasting birds prior to anesthesia and surgery. In general it has been recommended that birds either not be fasted or be fasted for no more than 2 to 3 hours prior to anesthesia because of their high metabolic rate and poor hepatic glycogen storage.(76, 77) However, because of the hazards associated with regurgitation in minimally fasted birds, some practitioners recommend that avian species, regardless of size, be fasted overnight.(78) Our experience with waterfowl, cranes, and ratites also suggests that an overnight fast is not deleterious to the bird and reduces the incidence of regurgitation-associated problems.

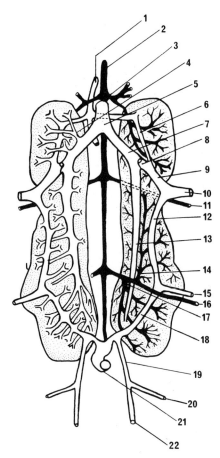

Fig. 20E–9. Ventral view of the kidneys of *Gallus* drawn as though transparent to reveal blood vessels within. The left side of the diagram shows renal portal and efferent veins; the right side shows arteries. 1, internal vertebral venous sinus; 2, aorta; 3, cranial renal artery; 4, one of several cranial renal veins; 5, caudal vena cava; 6, cranial renal portal vein; 7, common iliac vein; 8, portal valve; 9, common iliac vein; 10, external iliac vein; 11, external iliac artery; 12, caudal renal portal vein; 13, caudal renal vein; 14, middle renal artery; 15, ischiadic vein; 16, ischiadic artery; 17, caudal renal artery; 18, caudal renal portal vein; 19, internal iliac vein; 20, lateral caudal vein; 21, caudal mesenteric vein; 22, pudendal vein. (From Johnson, O.W. Urinary organs. In: Form and Function in Birds, vol. 1. Edited by A.S. King and J. McLelland. London: Academic Press, 1979:212; with permission.)

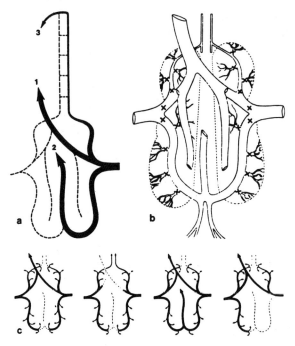

Fig. 20E–10. Ventral views of renal portal shunts, portal sphincters and variations in portal blood flow. (From Johnson, O.W. Urinary organs. In: Form and Function in Birds, vol. 1. Edited by A.S. King and J. McLelland. London: Academic Press, 1979:215; with permission.) A, The three renal portal shunts as marked on the left kidney: 1, through the portal valve to the caudal vena cava; 2, caudal renal portal vein to the caudal mesenteric vein; 3, cranial renal portal vein to the internal vertebral venous sinuses. Shunts 1 and 2 can function individually, or all three collectively, to provide a complete bypass of the kidney. B, Numerous combinations of vasoconstriction (marked by crosses) result in highly varied patterns of blood flow. C, Selected examples of routes of blood flow through the avian kidney.

PHYSICAL RESTRAINT

Proper physical restraint is an important part in the handling and anesthetic management of any bird. Improper capture or restraint can cause physical trauma, including wing or leg fractures. Because birds cannot dissipate heat through the skin, they can become stressed and easily overheated with prolonged restraint. Psittacine owners often judge the expertise of a veterinarian by his or her ability to restrain their bird without bruising it around the face. In general, a bird must be restrained so that the wings and legs are controlled and not allowed to flap or kick about. For long-necked birds such as herons and cranes, the neck must also be controlled so that head, eye, and neck trauma is avoided.

Proper restraint is also necessary to protect personnel working around birds. Each avian species has its own unique and effective mechanisms for defense. Birds of prey will use their talons and inflict severe physical trauma on a handler or assistant, and the risk of infection from such wounds is quite real. Although most birds of prey do not bite, some, such as great horned owls, will use their talons and beak to great effect. Psittacines have very strong beaks that can cause severe soft tissue injury. Cranes and herons will use their long, pointed beaks in a spearing manner, and they seem to focus on handlers' eyes. Understanding the physical characteristics and defensive means of birds is crucial to provide restraint that is safe both for the bird and for the people working with the bird.

INJECTABLE ANESTHETICS

Injectable anesthetics are used frequently to produce anesthesia in birds. There are many advantages associated with their use including their low cost, ease of use, and the rapidity with which anesthesia can be induced. In addition, expensive equipment is not required for delivery or maintenance of anesthesia, and pollution of the work environment is not an issue (Chapter 2).

However, there are inherent disadvantages associated with the use of injectables, including great individual and species variation among birds in terms of dose and response, difficulty in delivering a safe volume to small birds, ease in overdosing by any route, difficulty in maintaining surgical anesthesia without severe cardiopulmonary depression, and the potential for prolonged and violent recoveries.(76)

Pharmacologic considerations. Pharmacologic principles that apply to mammals apply to birds as well. Pharmacokinetics describes the bioavailability, absorption, distribution, biotransformation, and excretion of a drug (Chapter 2). Pharmacokinetics also is used to determine dosage and route of administration. The fate of a drug in the body, including protein binding, volume of distribution, biotransformation, and excretion, differs from species to species because the relationship between biotransformation and excretion is determined by metabolic factors and heredity.(73) A frequent assumption is that all birds are similar and pharmacologically belong to one group. This assumption can lead either to limited efficacy or to intoxication even among closely related species.(73) The veterinarian does have alternative methods available to determine safe yet effective doses for drugs used in birds. Allometric scaling and the concepts of physiologic time are recognized and accepted alternatives for determining drug doses in lieu of pharmacokinetic data.(79–81) More important, the general principles underlying allometric scaling serve as a rational basis for understanding how drug doses are affected by body mass or metabolic rate. A simple but specific example puts these principles and concepts into a clinically relevant perspective. Dosage guidelines for the use of ketamine in birds reflect the allometric concept that drug doses are inversely related to body mass. For example, a recommended dose for ketamine in a small psittacine weighing under 100 grams is 0.07 – 0.10 mg/g IM, while a bird weighing over 500 grams would receive 0.03 – 0.06 mg/g IM.(82)

There is very little information about the pharmacodynamics of drugs commonly used in birds. It is known that there can be significant differences in response among avian species given the same drug.(73, 83) For example, the commercially available form of ketamine consists of a racemic mixture of the L^- and D^+ forms of ketamine (Chapter 10). In great horned and snowy owls this racemic mixture characteristically induces chemical restraint and anesthesia of poor quality.(83) When great horned owls receive only the D^+ form of ketamine, anesthesia induction is smoother and there are fewer cardiac arrhythmias, whereas the L^- form of ketamine is associated with inadequate muscle relaxation, cardiac arrhythmias, and excited behavior during recovery.(83) Whether these differences are due to differing pathways for drug metabolism among birds, production of pharmacologically active metabolites, or differences in types of receptors or receptor sensitivity is not known.

Injection sites. Subcutaneous injection sites include the area over the back between the wings, the wing web,

and the skin fold in the inguinal region. The pectoral and thigh muscles can be used for intramuscular injections. The ulnaris vein, dorsal metatarsal vein, and jugular vein can be used for intravenous injections as well as for catheterization. In general the right jugular vein is larger and easier to visualize than the left jugular vein, and it is an easy vessel to draw blood from or to catheterize.

Drugs. Ketamine, diazepam, and xylazine have been used to induce anesthesia of relatively short duration (Chapter 10). Ketamine, a cyclohexamine, produces a state of catalepsy and can be given by any parenteral route. Doses range from 10 to 200 mg/kg depending on species and route of administration. Drugs such as diazepam or xylazine have been combined with ketamine in order to prolong or improve the quality of anesthesia, to provide muscle relaxation, or provide additional analgesia. When used alone, ketamine is suitable for chemical restraint for minor surgical and diagnostic procedures, but it is not a suitable general anesthetic for major surgical manipulations.(84, 85) Higher doses of ketamine only serve to prolong its duration of action while decreasing its margin of safety.(85)

Diazepam is a tranquilizer with excellent muscle relaxant properties. As with all tranquilizers it lacks analgesic properties and should not be viewed as providing additional analgesia when combined with primary anesthetics such as ketamine. Diazepam can be used to tranquilize a bird prior to mask induction with an inhalant anesthetic, thus reducing the stress and struggling associated with anesthetic induction. An important feature of diazepam is that its duration of action is short and recovery is not prolonged.

Midazolam is a more potent, longer-acting benzodiazepine that has been used in birds. In Canada geese, midazolam (2 mg/kg IM) induced adequate sedation for purposes of radiography, and the effective sedation lasted up to 20 minutes after injection.(86) Mean arterial blood pressure remained stable, and arterial blood gases, which were measured in a select number of birds, were unchanged from baseline values.(86) As with diazepam, midazolam can be given to facilitate induction of anesthesia. The effects of midazolam given to raptors and pigeons last for several hours after the termination of anesthesia. Although there have not been complications associated with prolonged recovery, it can be considered an undesirable feature.

Xylazine, an alpha$_2$–adrenergic agonist with sedative and analgesic properties, has been used for minor surgical and diagnostic procedures. It has profound cardiopulmonary effects, including second-degree heart block, bradyarrhythmias, and increased sensitivity to catecholamine–induced cardiac arrhythmias (Chapter 8). To enhance sedative and analgesic properties, xylazine is frequently combined with other anesthetic drugs such as ketamine. When used alone in high doses, xylazine is associated with respiratory depression, excitement, and convulsions in some species.(87) Hypoxemia and hypercapnia were observed in Pekin ducks given xylazine and a combination of xylazine and ketamine.(88)

To hasten recovery or to treat an overdose following the use of an alpha-adrenergic agonist such as xylazine, an alpha-adrenergic antagonist such as tolazoline or yohimbine can be used. Turkey vultures anesthetized with a combination of xylazine and ketamine regained consciousness approximately 4 minutes after tolazoline (15 mg/kg) was given intravenously.(89) Red-tailed hawks anesthetized with a combination of xylazine and ketamine recovered from anesthesia significantly faster after receiving yohimbine than birds not receiving the antagonist.(90) The results of the study indicated that a yohimbine dose of 0.1 mg/kg would be effective while not causing profound cardiopulmonary changes.(90)

Propofol is a substituted phenol derivative (2,6-diisopropylphenol) developed for the intravenous induction and maintenance of general anesthesia (Chapter 9). Its actions are characterized by a rapid onset and recovery. In pigeons, propofol produced respiratory depression and apnea, and was considered to have a narrow margin of safety.(91)

Surgical anesthesia can be maintained for relatively long periods of time (1 to 12 hours) by using intermediate to long-acting barbiturates or combinations of drugs with intermediate durations of effect. Pentobarbital can be used to produce anesthesia of several hours' duration using a dose of 25 to 30 mg/kg given intravenously.(1) Since it requires 10 to 15 minutes for full onset of action, the drug should be administered initially as a bolus consisting of half the total dose and the remainder titrated over several minutes until the desired plane of anesthesia is achieved.

Phenobarbital is a long-acting barbiturate and produces anesthesia lasting for as long as 24 hours when administered at 130 mg/kg (Chapter 9).(1) Its onset of action is very slow, requiring as much as 30 minutes before surgical anesthesia is achieved. As is true for pentobarbital, additional doses of phenobarbital can be administered as needed to deepen the plane of anesthesia, but there is a narrow margin between anesthesia and severe cardiac depression and death.

Equithesin is a combination of pentobarbital, chloral hydrate, and magnesium sulfate. It does not produce a surgical plane of anesthesia when used alone, but does produce surgical anesthesia lasting for as long as 90 minutes when combined with diazepam.(47)

Local anesthetics. Local anesthetics have been used in birds with unfortunate consequences including seizures and cardiac arrest.(1) The problem is related to the small size of some avian species and inappropriate doses (Chapter 12).(76) For example, 0.1 mL of 2% lidocaine administered intramuscularly or subcutaneously to a 30-gram parakeet is equivalent to 67 mg/kg, a gross and toxic overdose for any animal. Lidocaine can be used in birds for local anesthesia if the dose does not exceed 4 mg/kg, a dose that is difficult to achieve in very small birds. Although local anesthetics provide suffi-

cient local analgesia, they do nothing for stress induced by physical restraint and handling of an awake bird.

Opioids. In birds the lack of an anthropocentric type of response to pain does not necessarily mean that they do not perceive pain or that pain does not cause them distress. It may be that the behavior or physiologic variables associated with pain in birds have not been adequately characterized, and there are a number of reasons for this. The problem of recognizing pain in birds has been confused by research into the analgesic efficacy of opioids in birds. In contrast to studies of the analgesic effects of opioids in mammals, the objective of opioid studies in birds has been to evaluate the effect on learned behavior, not analgesia.(92–96) The few studies that have evaluated the analgesic effects of opioids in birds are conflicting. In one study morphine produced hyperalgesia (97), while in another it produced analgesia.(98) The results of a recent study in chickens indicate that motor deficits associated with the administration of morphine may mask the analgesic effects of the drug.(99) Studies have shown that kappa opioid receptors account for 76% of the radiolabeling of pigeon forebrain tissues.(100) Thus butorphanol, a kappa-agonist, may be a better analgesic for birds than mu opioid agonists. Butorphanol appears to reduce the concentration of isoflurane necessary to maintain anesthesia in cockatoos.

INHALANT ANESTHETICS

Early investigators stated that inhalant anesthetics would be lethal in birds because of their unique pulmonary system and that only injectable anesthetics could be used.(101) This proved not to be the case (102, 103), and inhalants, especially isoflurane, are considered the anesthetics of choice for use in birds.

Inhalant anesthetics offer several advantages for patient management not provided by injectable drugs. Their advantages include rapid induction and recovery, especially when inhalant anesthetics of low blood gas solubility are used (halothane and isoflurane), easier control of anesthetic depth, the concurrent use of oxygen with inhalants thus providing respiratory support, and fast recovery that does not depend on metabolic or excretory pathways (Chapter 11). A disadvantage is that the delivery of the potent inhalants requires special equipment such as a source of oxygen, a vaporizer, a breathing circuit, and a mechanism for scavenging waste anesthetic gases (Chapter 14).

Breathing circuits and fresh gas flows. Nonrebreathing circuits, such as the Bain circuit or Norman elbow, are ideal for use in birds because they offer minimal resistance to patient ventilation. An additional advantage to the plastic Bain circuit is that it is light in weight, an advantage when used in very small birds. When a nonrebreathing circuit is used, oxygen flows should be two to three times minute ventilation, or 150 to 200 mL · kg^{-1} · min^{-1} (Chapters 14 and 17).

Induction methods. The number and variety of techniques for inducing gas anesthesia in birds are only limited by the anesthetist's imagination. Birds can be induced with commercially available small animal masks, or with homemade masks fabricated from plastic bottles, syringe cases, syringes, or breathing hose connectors. Mask induction techniques can be used in a wide variety and sizes of birds, from the very small up to and including the emu. Mask inductions are unsatisfactory in adult ostriches.

Other techniques include the use of plastic bags or chambers. Birds can be induced by inserting their heads into plastic bags (preferably clear plastic) into which oxygen and anesthetic vapor are introduced via a nonrebreathing circuit. Plastic bags have been used to completely enclose a bird cage in order to induce anesthesia in a bird that is difficult to manage.(104)

An anesthetic chamber can be used to induce anesthesia. A disadvantage to this technique is that the anesthetist is not in physical contact with the bird and is unable to get a feel for how the bird is responding to the anesthetic. In addition, birds can injure themselves as they pass through stage II (involuntary excitement) anesthesia (Chapter 2).

Whatever technique is used, the anesthetist must take precautions to control and eliminate anesthetic gas pollution in the work environment. If a mask is used it should fit snugly over the bird's beak and face, or over its entire head. If a plastic bag or chamber is used, it should be free of leaks. Once induction is completed, the bag or chamber must be removed from the area without "dumping" the contents into the workplace environment.

Intubation. Any bird larger than a cockatiel or larger than 100 grams can be intubated.(105) However, unique anatomic features that can interfere with intubation, such as the median tracheal septum found in some penguins or the large bills of toucans and flamingos, must be kept in mind as one plans an intubation strategy. In most birds the glottis is easy to visualize and, depending on the size of the bird, the larynx and trachea are easily intubated. Some birds are difficult to intubate either because of their unique oropharyngeal anatomy or because of their size. Psittacine species, especially the smaller birds such as parakeets, can be difficult to intubate because of the awkward location of the glottis at the base of the humped, fleshy tongue.(106)

Intubation in small birds is not without risk. Tubes with very small internal diameters can impose significant resistance to ventilation, a feature that becomes an even greater hazard when an endotracheal tube develops a partial or complete obstruction caused by a mucus plug. During anesthesia, especially when an anticholinergic is not used, mucus production can be copious, and because of the drying effects of the inspired cold and dry gases, the mucus becomes thick and tenacious. Obstruction of an endotracheal tube can be detected by observing the bird's pattern of ventilation. As the airway becomes occluded, the duration of the expiratory phase is observed to become prolonged. An artificial sigh usually confirms the presence of an obstruction because the air sacs can be observed to fill in

a seemingly normal manner, but they empty slowly or not at all. This problem can be quickly corrected by extubating the bird and cleaning the tube or replacing it altogether. Airway noises may be heard as the tube becomes more obstructed with mucus. An anticholinergic, such as atropine (0.04 mg/kg) or glycopyrrolate (0.01 mg/kg), reduces mucus production and minimizes the formation of mucus plugs.

During intubation care must be exercised not to traumatize the trachea. The tube should not fit tightly, and if the endotracheal tube has a cuff, it either should not be inflated or must be inflated with extreme care. Since the trachea is composed of complete rings of cartilage an overly inflated cuff can traumatize and even rupture the tracheal mucosa and rings. Damage to the trachea may not become evident until 5 to 7 days after intubation, when the processes of healing and fibrotic narrowing of the trachea cause signs of dyspnea. When an endotracheal tube cuff is overinflated, the tracheal rings may rupture longitudinally rather than circumferentially.

MAC. The minimum alveolar concentration (MAC) that produces anesthesia in mammals exposed to noxious stimuli is referred to as *MAC* (Chapters 2 and 11). It is a measure that provides a description of concentration and effect, it can be used to quantify factors that influence anesthetic requirements, and it is a term equally applicable to all inhalation anesthetics.(107) As defined, the term *MAC* is not appropriate for discussions concerning inhalation anesthesia in birds because it presupposes the presence of an alveolar lung. In birds MAC has been defined as the minimal anesthetic concentration required to keep a bird from responding by gross purposeful movement to a painful stimulus.(50)

Although the avian pulmonary system anatomically and physiologically differs from the mammalian pulmonary system, MAC values for halothane and isoflurane in birds (Table 20E–4).(108–110) are similar to MAC values reported for mammals.(111) This lends support to the observation that different species or classes of animals do not show large variations in effective concentrations for inhalant anesthetics.(112)

Halothane and isoflurane. A number of inhalant anesthetics, including chloroform, cyclopropane, ether, methoxyflurane, and halothane, have been used in birds

Table 20E–4. Minimum Anesthetic Concentrations for Halothane and Isoflurane in Cockatoos, Chickens, Ducks, and Sandhill Cranes

	Halothane	Isoflurane
Birds		
Cockatoo	—	1.44*
Chicken	0.85%[108]	—
Ducks	1.05%[110]	1.32%[109]
Sandhill cranes	—	1.35%[50]

*Personal communication from Thomas G. Curro, DVM, Department of Surgical Sciences, School of Veterinary Medicine, University of Wisconsin, Madison, WI.

References superscripted.

to induce general anesthesia.(113–116) Although these drugs are historically interesting, this review focuses on halothane and isoflurane, the two most commonly used inhalant anesthetics at this time. Of these two inhalants, isoflurane is preferred for anesthesia in birds. Its introduction has revolutionized avian medicine and surgery because it is so well tolerated by birds of all sizes.(117)

Halothane and isoflurane, at all end-tidal anesthetic concentrations and in a dose-dependent manner, depress ventilation.(50, 108-110) More specifically, as the concentration of anesthetic increases the partial pressure of carbon dioxide increases. The anesthetic index (AI), a measure of the tendency for an inhalant anesthetic to cause respiratory depression and apnea, is derived by dividing the end-tidal concentration of an anesthetic at apnea by the MAC for the anesthetic (Chapter 11).(119) The lower the AI for an anesthetic, the greater is its depressant effect on ventilation. In ducks anesthetized with halothane the AI was found to be 1.51 or lower (110), while the AI for ducks anesthetized with isoflurane was 1.65.(109) These AI values are considerably lower than those reported for dogs (120, 121), cats (120), or horses.(122) Thus, halothane and isoflurane appear to depress ventilation more in birds than in mammals.

The effect of halothane on blood pressure can be variable. In chickens and ducks, increasing concentrations of halothane can cause a decrease in mean arterial blood pressure (108, 118, 123), or no change.(110) In contrast, isoflurane appears to consistently cause a dose-dependent decrease in mean arterial blood pressure.(50, 109, 118, 123) This may be because isoflurane causes peripheral vasodilation.

In mammals, positive pressure ventilation depresses mean arterial blood pressure by creating positive intrathoracic pressures that compress the great vessels, thus impeding the venous return of blood to the heart. In sandhill cranes anesthetized with isoflurane, mean arterial blood pressure was actually higher in the birds during positive pressure ventilation than it was during spontaneous ventilation.(50)

Cardiac arrhythmias frequently occur in animals, including birds, anesthetized with halothane. Cardiac stability is one of the perceived advantages of isoflurane and is one of the reasons why it has so readily gained wide acceptance in clinical avian practice. However, in a study in which an electric fibrillation model was used to investigate the myocardial irritant effects of isoflurane and halothane, isoflurane was found to lower the threshold for electric fibrillation more than halothane.(123) The reasons for the discrepancy between clinical experience and the result of this study are not clear.

Hypoventilation makes it difficult to control the plane of anesthesia. Furthermore, the hypercapnia associated with anesthetic-induced ventilatory depression can have a variety of adverse effects on cardiopulmonary function through direct or indirect mechanisms. For these reasons, ventilation in birds should be assisted or controlled during general inhalant anesthesia.

Nitrous oxide. Nitrous oxide can be used as an adjunct to general anesthesia in birds. However, it is not suitable for use as the sole anesthetic in birds.(113) As with other anesthetic gases and vapors, nitrous oxide is not uniquely sequestered or concentrated in the air sacs. The considerations for using nitrous oxide are the same as for its use in mammals: Pulmonary function should be adequate, and sufficient oxygen should be provided to meet the patient's metabolic demands. Thirty percent oxygen is generally accepted as the minimum inspired oxygen that should be provided (Chapter 11). Nitrous oxide may pose problems in some avian species. Diving birds such as pelicans have subcutaneous pockets of air that do not communicate with the respiratory system, and the use of N_2O in these birds can result in subcutaneous emphysema.(124)

ADJUNCTS TO GENERAL ANESTHESIA

Muscle paralytics may prove to be very useful in the anesthetic management of birds, especially during long surgical procedures requiring adequate muscle relaxation and immobility. All too often a bird may appear to be adequately anesthetized, lying still on the surgical table with complete muscular relaxation, slow respiration, closed eyelids, and relaxed feathers. The bird may accept a surgical scrub and draping, and a skin incision may be completed, when suddenly the patient displays unequivocal signs of being unsuitably anesthetized for surgery by throwing itself about on the table with flopping wings and neck.(106)

Atracurium is a nondepolarizing muscle relaxant with short duration of effect and minimal cardiovascular effects (Chapter 13). The neuromuscular and cardiovascular effects of atracurium given to 24 anesthetized chickens has been reported.(125) The effective dose associated with 95% twitch depression in 50% of the birds ($ED_{95/50}$) was calculated to be 0.25 mg/kg and $ED_{95/95}$ was calculated to be 0.46 mg/kg. The duration of action for the 0.25 mg/kg dosage was 34.5 ± 5.8 minutes, and 47.8 ± 10.3 minutes at the highest dose of 0.45 mg/kg. Edrophonium (0.5 mg/kg IV) reversed the effects of atracurium. There were small but statistically significant changes in cardiovascular variables in that heart rate decreased and blood pressure increased after administration of atracurium, but these changes were considered to be clinically unimportant.(125)

MONITORING THE AVIAN PATIENT

Birds must be monitored during anesthesia. Physiologic variables to monitor include respiratory rate and volume, heart rate and rhythm, body temperature, and muscle relaxation. Both respiratory rate and tidal volume should be monitored during anesthesia in order to assess the adequacy of ventilation and the depth of anesthesia. Respiratory frequency can be misleading as a single indicator of the adequacy of ventilation and anesthetic depth. High respiratory frequencies in an anesthetized bird do not necessarily indicate that the bird is light and hyperventilating. High respiratory rates can be associated with small tidal volumes, resulting in more dead space ventilation than effective ventilation.(50)

Ventilation should be monitored by watching the frequency and degree of motion of the sternum or movements of the reservoir bag on the breathing circuit. Respiratory pauses longer than 10 to 15 seconds should be treated by lightening the plane of anesthesia and ventilating the bird by periodically squeezing the reservoir bag or by using a positive pressure mechanical ventilator. During positive pressure ventilation, airway pressure should not exceed 15 to 20 cm H_2O pressure to prevent volotrauma to the air sacs. Ventilation also can be assessed by noting the color and capillary refill time of mucous membranes. The color of the cere, beak, or bill, as well as coloration on the head can give an indication of the adequacy of cardiopulmonary function.

The heart is an electromechanical pump, and the blood vessels are the conduits for its output. The adequacy of pump function can be assessed by monitoring mucous membrane color and refill time as noted earlier, as well as monitoring the ECG and blood pressure, and by palpating peripheral pulses. An electrocardiogram (ECG) is used to monitor the electric activity of the heart. Standard bipolar and augmented limb leads can be used to monitor and record the avian ECG. To assure adequate skin contact for an interference-free signal, ECG clips can be attached to hypodermic needles inserted through the skin at the base of each wing and through the skin at the level of each stifle. An alternative technique is to attach the ECG clips to stainless steel wires that have been inserted through the prepatagium of each wing and the skin at the lateral side of each stifle. The wire size selected depends on the size of the bird. Twenty- or 22-gauge wire can be used in birds larger than 500 grams. Appropriately sized hypodermic needles are used to insert the wires through the skin.

Pump function can be assessed by monitoring the pulsations of blood through a peripheral artery or by monitoring blood pressure. It is possible to directly monitor arterial blood pressure in birds larger than 4 kg, but this technique is not feasible in smaller birds. The Doppler flow probe (Parks Electronics, Aloha, Oregon) is an effective device for monitoring blood flow or blood pressure in either small or large birds. With the Doppler probe secured in position over a peripheral artery, pulse rate and rhythm can be determined. The probe can be placed over a digital artery, and a sphygmomanometer attached to a cuff placed around the leg can be used to measure arterial blood pressure indirectly.

Body temperature should be monitored for a number of reasons. The stress associated with anesthesia and surgery is minimized when birds are maintained at or near their normal body temperature. During anesthesia it is not unusual to see major fluctuations in body temperature. Hypothermia is the most common problem, and it decreases the requirement for anesthetic, causes cardiac instability, and prolongs recovery. In well–insulated birds (feathers, drapes, heating pads) hyperthermia can occur and also cause cardiac instability and an increased oxygen demand. Body temperature can be reliably monitored with an electronic thermometer and a long flexible thermistor probe inserted into the esophagus to the level of the heart. Temperature monitored from the cloaca can vary significantly over time owing to movements of the cloaca that affect the position of the thermometer or a thermistor probe. Body temperature can be adjusted by inserting or removing pads or blankets between the bird and cold surfaces, using circulating warm water blankets (not electric heating pads), maintaining a light plane of surgical anesthesia, raising or lowering the environmental temperature, or wetting the bird's legs with alcohol.

RECOVERY

Precautions should be taken to protect birds while they recover from anesthesia. Birds must be kept from flopping around, as this can lead to serious neck, wing, or leg injuries. Struggling and flopping behavior can be prevented by lightly wrapping a bird with a towel, but wrapping poses its own hazards. If a bird is wrapped too tightly, sternal movements will be impeded and breathing will be difficult if not impossible. Wrapping can lead to excessive retention of body heat and cause hyperthermia. If a bird has not been fasted prior to anesthesia, regurgitation can occur during recovery. Keeping a bird intubated during the recovery phase helps to maintain an open airway.

Ratites

In other countries, ratites have been raised for commercial purposes for almost 100 years, and there is an extensive base of knowledge concerning the commercial management of these birds. Only recently have they been imported into the United States. Little information is available about anesthesia because in their native countries where the value of individual birds is low, they are not presented for extensive veterinary care. However, in the United States, because of their high value, they are likely to be presented for treatment of conditions that require sedation or anesthesia. In general, young ratites (ostriches under 30 kg, emus under 18 kg) may be treated with the same considerations as given to other birds because the same problems of hypoglycemia, hypothermia, hypotension, and hypoventilation tend to occur. Hypoglycemia and hypothermia do not appear to be common in adult birds, but restraint and handling are more difficult.

RESTRAINT

Restraint of adult ratites is challenging. For this reason it is important to work with personnel, such as the owner, who are experienced in handling adult birds. An

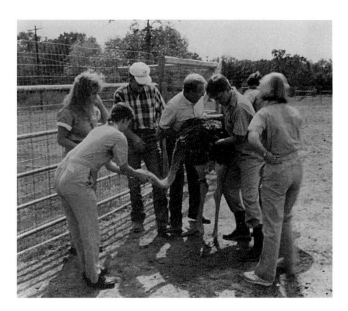

Fig. 20E–11. Manual restraint of an ostrich, including hooding.

adult ostrich may average 114 kg and stand 6 feet tall. They can move very quickly, peck accurately at objects, and have large-toed feet with which they can strike forward. Most farm-raised birds have been handled, and information about the bird's individual temperament can be obtained from the owner or handler. As in other birds, they can be hooded to facilitate handling. Hoods can be made from surgical stockinette, and the head can be manually restrained (Fig. 20E–11). Distracting the bird by allowing it to peck at a shiny object, which is held firmly to prevent ingestion, may be sufficient for completing minor procedures. The ostrich can be "herded" into a corner or chute by using a solid object such as a sheet of plywood or a large pad, or by holding one wing at the base of the humerus and pushing the bird in front of the handler. It is important always to work from behind or beside the bird to remain out of forward striking range of the feet. If the bird is recumbent, as can occur after sedation, it is best to transport the bird in sternal recumbency with it sitting on its hocks. This position allows control of the feet. In smaller birds, the handler may be able to safely restrain the bird by stepping over its back, grasping the hocks from behind and folding the legs up to the body.

INJECTIONS AND CATHETER PLACEMENT

Intramuscular injections are best given into the large muscle mass of the thigh. Although ratites are reported to have a renal portal system (126), drugs are effective when given in this location. Intravenous injections can be given into the jugular vein. As is generally true for all birds, the right jugular is more prominent than is the left jugular. Routinely placing a catheter (14 gauge, 10 cm) in the jugular vein is recommended in order to prevent hematoma formation from repeated needle sticks. In ostriches, the branchial vein (127) may also be used for

injections and catheterization (18 gauge, 3-4.5 cm). In emus, because of their vestigial wings, the brachial vein is very difficult to use, but the metatarsal vein can be used. The thick, cornified skin on the lower limbs of the ostrich makes it difficult to use the metatarsal vein.

PREOPERATIVE ASSESSMENT

Performing a good physical examination and preoperative assessment in an adult ostrich can be challenging and is often impossible. It is an unfortunate fact that it is not possible to reliably judge a bird's state of health by its behavior. Ill adult ostriches may appear to be quite normal and active. Some blood work is needed, preferably a complete blood count and chemistry profile. Acid-base imbalances and dehydration should be corrected before any bird is anesthetized. Normal hematologic and chemistry values have been reported.(128-131) It is important to get an accurate weight. Visual estimation of body weight is difficult because the feathers may conceal a very thin bird. Other preparations for anesthesia will depend on a bird's temperament and the facilities and personnel available. Adult ostriches and emus are routinely fasted overnight, but water is not withheld.

PREANESTHETICS

Although a wide variety of tranquilizers and sedatives have been used as preanesthetics in ratites (Tables 20E–5 and 20E–6) (131–137), a caveat is necessary before discussing the effects of preanesthetics in ratites. Almost all of the information relating drug and effect has been generated from clinical cases. In our opinion much of the variability in response to anesthetics is owing to variations in drug requirements imposed by disease conditions, as well as a lack of controlled studies. In point of fact, only one study reports dose effects for anesthetics in ratites (Chapter 10).(136) In addition, the practical problems of restraint impose restrictions on the acquisition of clinical data. For these reasons, the following guidelines should be taken as guidelines derived from clinical experience and studies.

For healthy, large ratites, premedication with xylazine (1-2 mg/kg IM) appears to facilitate handling, placement of catheters, and induction of anesthesia. This dose of xylazine would produce excessive cardiovascular depression in a sick bird, which emphasizes the importance of an accurate preoperative assessment. Diazepam (0.4-1.0 mg/kg IM) is especially effective in sick or debilitated ratites, or may be combined with xylazine in healthy ratites. Midazolam (0.4 mg/kg IM) also appears to be an effective preanesthetic, but it is expensive to use in a 100-kg ostrich.

INDUCTION OF ANESTHESIA

Ketamine appears to induce the most reliable and smoothest inductions in ratites.(138), especially when combined with diazepam, or following xylazine or midazolam premedication (Tables 20E–5 and 20E–6). Intravenous injection rapidly induces anesthesia and

Table 20E–5. Induction Drugs, Procedure, Body Weight, ASA Class, Heart and Respiratory Rates, Blood Pressure (Systolic/Diastolic, Mean) and Complications in Nine Ostriches Anesthetized at the College of Veterinary Medicine, Texas A&M University, 1992

| | | | | HR (bpm) | | | | BP (mm HG) Systolic/Diastolic/Mean | | | | RR (bpm) | | | | |
| | | | | | | | | *Minutes of Anesthesia* | | | | | | | | |
Induction	Procedure	Wt (kg)	ASA Class	15	30	45	60	15	30	45	60	15	30	45	60	Complications
Diaz 0.35 mg/kg IM & IV Ket 6.3 mg/kg IV	Entertomy	79	4E	45	45	45	40	100/75 85	85/76 78	90/65 75	80/55 65	10	10	10	10	Cardiac arrest hypovolemia anemia
Diaz 0.5 mg/kg IM Ket 6.6 mg/kg IV	Skin graft	91	2	45	45	45	60	N/A	165/125 145	150/100 130	165/120 145	10	10	10	10	None reported
Iso mask	Proventriculotomy	30	3	68	60	68	60	70/20 30	60/20 30	90/27 45	115/30 45	8	8	8	8	Anemia blood transfusion
Xyl 3.6 mg/kg IM Ket 16.5 mg/kg IM	Tendon repair	112	2	60	60	58	80	N/A	230/215 225	225/205 215	250/230 240	15	6	8	8	None reported
Diaz 0.2 mg/kg IV Ket 16.4 mg/kg IV	Proventriculotomy	95	4E	35	35	38	35	N/A	N/A	205/175 185	210/190 200	8	8	8	8	Bradycardia
Xyl 3.2 mg/kg IM Ket 16.4 mg/kg IM	Phacofragmentation	87	1	40	45	75	65	N/A	N/A	130/70 88	130/60 82	6	6	6	6	None reported
Xyl 1.9 mg/kg IM Diaz 0.1 mg/kg IV Ket 7.1 mg/kg IV	Proventriculotomy	106	3	60	95	90	85	N/A	N/A	N/A	110/95 105	10	10	10	10	Bradycardia in recovery
Xyl 3.5 mg/kg IM Ket 17.7 mg/kg IM Diaz 0.1 mg/kg IV Ket 2.6 mg/kg IV	Proventriculotomy	85	2	70	70	68	68	65/45 50	105/85 95	115/95 105	N/A	16	16	16	16	None reported
Mid 0.57 mg/kg IM Ket 6.8 mg/kg IV	Cast application	88	2	65	48	48	50	N/A	90/50 65	120/72 95	145/195 120	10	10	10	10	None reported

N/A, Data not available.

Table 20E–6. Induction Drugs, Procedures, Body Weight, ASA Class, Heart and Respiratory Rates, Blood Pressure (Systolic/Diastolic, Mean) and Complications in 10 Emus Anesthetized at the College of Veterinary Medicine, Texas A&M University, 1992

Induction	Procedure	Wt (kg)	ASA Class	HR (bpm)				BP (mm HG) Systolic/Diastolic Mean — Minutes of Anesthesia				RR (bpm)				Complications
				15	30	45	60	15	30	45	60	15	30	45	60	
Diaz 0.37 mg/kg IM Ket 7.3 mg/kg IV	Egg bound	41	2	155	150	145	125	N/A	50/40 45	75/45 62	110/60 95	12	12	12	12	Hypotension
Diaz 0.56 mg/kg IM Ket 14.8 mg/kg IV	Proventric-ulotomy	27	3E	58	60	72	58	135/60 88	125/95 108	115/90 105	100/80 90	15	15	15	15	None reported
Mid 0.4 mg/kg IM Ket 1 mg/kg IV	Egg bound	40	2	135	125	90	122	N/A	N/A	88/40 52	100/55 75	14	14	14	14	None reported
Azaperone 2.7 mg/kg IM Ket 3.8 mg/kg IV	Skin graft	26	2	50	30	30	40	N/A	N/A	N/A	N/A	8	8	8	8	Bradycardia
Diaz 1.0 mg/kg IM Ket 10 mg/kg IV	Wound debridement	31	2	85	65	70	65	N/A	N/A	N/A	N/A	10	10	10	10	None reported
Diaz 1.0 mg/kg IV Ket 19 mg/kg IV	Tracheal endoscopy	21	4	105	110	140	142	175/105	182/125	200/130	170/130	15	17	17	15	None reported
Diaz 0.7 mg/kg IM Ket 6.7 mg/kg IV	Endoscopy	45	2	92	92	80	70	N/A	N/A	N/A	N/A	6	6	10	8	Regurgitation at recovery
Xyl 4.5 mg/kg IM Ket 21 mg/kg IM	Papilloma removal	35	2	20	30	40	40	N/A	128/100 115	150/125 135	140/130 135	10	10	10	10	Bradycardia
Diaz 0.5 mg/kg IV Ket 7.0 mg/kg IV	Endoscopy		2	100	130	90	125	120/155 175	195/140 160	170/115 135	155/100 120	25	25	32	32	None reported
Xyl 4.7 mg/kg IM Ket 25 mg/kg IM	Osteotomy	17	2	40	35	35	32	128/70 95	100/50 65	100/40 48	80/40 50	12	12	12	12	None reported

N/A, Data not available.

allows the anesthetist to titrate the drug to achieve a desired effect. However, this may not be possible in fractious birds or where there is little assistance for restraint. Doses for intramuscular injection may be metabolically scaled (139) using an intermediate value between passerine and nonpasserine birds. Induction with tiletamine-zolazepam (140), either intramuscularly or intravenously, produces satisfactory inductions, but recoveries are rough and prolonged. Carfentanyl has been used for induction, but induction and recovery are reported to be rough.(134) In smaller ratites and debilitated birds, mask induction with isoflurane is effective and fairly smooth. In contrast, mask inductions in adult ostriches, even if they are debilitated, is not recommended because induction can take as long as 30 to 45 minutes.

INTUBATION

Intubation of ratites is similar to that for many other avian species. The larynx is readily accessible, the beak opens widely, and there is no epiglottis. Although the tracheal rings are complete, portions of the trachea are collapsible, so some caution must be used when advancing the endotracheal tube. In a recent report of an ostrich with a collapsed trachea, intubation was successfully performed following induction with diazepam (0.3 mg/kg IV) and ketamine (7 mg/kg IV).(141) Depending on their size, ostriches can be intubated with endotracheal tubes with internal diameters of 10 to 18 mm, while emus generally require endotracheal tubes measuring 9 to 14 mm. Careful inflation of the cuff is usually necessary to allow good ventilation of adult ratites. The tracheal cleft in emus (Fig. 20E–1), which is more highly developed in females but present in both sexes, does not complicate intubation. The cleft does make effective positive pressure ventilation difficult, but this problem can be overcome by placing a tight wrap (Vetrap) around the distal third of the neck.

MAINTENANCE AND MONITORING

Maintenance of anesthesia with isoflurane in oxygen and delivered from a precision vaporizer is recommended. The breathing circuit should be appropriate for the size of the ratite. Emus and ostriches under 130 kg can be maintained on a small animal breathing circuit. Larger ostriches can be maintained on a large animal breathing circuit. Ventilation of the larger ratites is recommended for two reasons. First, ventilation, as judged by respiratory rate and analysis of arterial blood for carbon dioxide, appears to be markedly depressed by anesthetic induction drugs. Second, ventilation appears to facilitate the uptake of inhalant anesthetics. Despite high vaporizer settings (3-5%), it may take 30 to 60 minutes to stabilize the plane of anesthesia. The reasons for this are not completely clear. A large respiratory volume (approximately 15 liters in a 70- to 100-kg bird) certainly contributes, but the ostrich may have a functional shunting system, which affects uptake of anesthetic gas.(142) Unlike flighted birds, in which

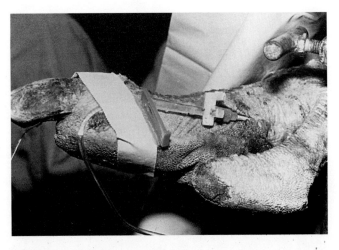

Fig. 20E–12.   Catheter in the digital artery of an ostrich for measuring arterial blood pressure and collecting arterial blood samples for analysis of pH, PaCO$_2$, and PaO$_2$.

increased ventilation tends to be linked to the increased muscular activity of flight, the ostrich pants to cool itself. Apparently this mechanism allows ostriches to cool themselves without effectively hyperventilating.(143)

Because of their larger size, ratites are generally easier to monitor than other avian species. An ECG should be utilized. The leads can be positioned by attaching one electrode to the neck, one to a wing fold, and the third electrode near the keel or on the opposite wing. Standardizing the placement of leads can be difficult because of the large size, tight skin, and surgical incision sites.

Blood pressure can be measured directly or indirectly. Indirect measurement with an oscillometric technique or a Doppler flow probe, can be accomplished in the emu or ostrich. The cuff is placed on the leg above the tarsus over the tibial artery. In the ostrich, direct arterial blood pressure can be monitored with a catheter placed in the brachialis or ulnaris artery of the wing, or in the metatarsal artery of a pelvic limb (Fig. 20E–12). In the emu, since the wing is vestigial, the brachial artery is very small and difficult to catheterize, so the pedal artery must be used. The transducer is zeroed at the level of the keel. Normal blood pressure values for awake or anesthetized ratites have not been reported. Ostriches have been observed to have high blood pressures (Tables 20E–5 and 20E–6) that increase over time with anesthesia, and are not the result of hypoxia, hypercarbia, or a light plane of anesthesia. In fact, if the pressures are not higher than those expected in anesthetized normal small animals, hypovolemia or anesthetic depression of cardiovascular function should be suspected. In emus, blood pressures appear to be somewhat lower than in ostriches. Tourniquet-induced hypertension has been reported in an ostrich undergoing surgery for removal of a bone sequestrum on the tarsometatarsal bone. Immediately after tourniquet release blood pressure

Table 20E–7. Arterial Blood Gas Values from Nine Ostriches Anesthetized with Isoflurane and Mechanically Ventilated. Values were corrected for body temperature using a Ciba Corning blood gas analysis machine. Arterial blood samples taken approximately 30 minutes after the induction of anesthesia. Values shown are mean ± SD shown in parenthesis

pH	CO₂	O₂	HCO₃⁻	BE	TV	BPM
7.53	24.1	471	20	0.6	13 mL/kg	11
(0.06)	(3.9)	(97)	(2.4)	(2.4)	(1)	(3)

Table 20E–8. Arterial Blood Gas Values from 10 Emus Anesthetized with Isoflurane and Breathing Spontaneously. Values were corrected for body temperature using a Ciba Corning blood gas analysis machine. Arterial blood samples taken approximately 30 minutes after the induction of anesthesia. Values shown are mean ± SD shown in parenthesis

pH	CO₂	O₂	HCO₃⁻	BE
7.20	56.7	355	20.1	−7.0
(0.08)	(2.9)	(24)	(0)	(4)

decreased from approximately 240 mm Hg to 175 mm Hg.(144)

Oxygen saturation of hemoglobin can be monitored with a pulse oximeter probe placed on the upper or lower beak. Oxygen-hemoglobin dissociation differs among species. The oxygen-hemoglobin dissociation curve for birds is qualitatively similar to that for mammals, but there are quantitative differences.(13) For this reason, the accuracy of pulse oximetry in birds is unknown. Clinical experience indicates that SpO_2 and PaO_2 are generally high.

Rate and depth of ventilation can be monitored as a measure of anesthetic depth, in the same manner as for other avian species. During controlled ventilation, tidal volumes of 10 to 13 mL/kg, respiratory rates of 8 to 16 breaths per minute (bpm), and inspiratory pressures of 10 to 15 cm H_2O have been used for controlled positive pressure ventilation. These settings effectively ventilate or slightly hyperventilate ostriches, as judged by analysis of arterial blood for oxygen and carbon dioxide (Tables 20E–7 and 20E–8). Similar settings are used for emus, but because of the greater difficulty in collecting arterial blood gas samples, correlation with mechanical ventilation has not been reported.

Muscle relaxants appear to be effective in ratites. Both atracurium (0.3 mg/kg IV) and vecuronium (0.08 mg/kg IV) have been used during general anesthesia (Chapter 13). Duration of effect appears to be similar to that in mammalian species. A peripheral nerve stimulator, with its electrodes placed on the proximal and distal ends of the wing, can be used to assess the block.

RECOVERY

Recoveries from inhalant anesthesia are generally prolonged, even when every attempt has been made to maintain a light anesthetic plane or decrease the anesthetic plane in the later stages of surgery. Weaning from the ventilator is also slow, and ventilation is often maintained with an Ambu bag after disconnection and while moving to the recovery area. Ratites are recovered in a darkened, padded area or a well-bedded stall. In the ideal setting, a ratite recovery box would be small and narrow, yet tall enough to allow the bird to stand, and would be padded to protect the head. Manual restraint as a means of controlling recovery of adult ratites is dangerous and is not recommended.

COMPLICATIONS

Many of the complications, such as bradycardia associated with visceral manipulation, do not require treatment or are manageable. It is not clear if the high incidence of complications is typical of ratites or is due to health-related factors, since many of the birds are debilitated. Cardiac problems are particularly common, and include bradycardia (heart rate under 30 bpm), atrial and ventricular premature beats (145), cardiac fibrillation, and arrest. Bradycardia usually responds to glycopyrrolate (0.01 mg/kg) or reversal with yohimbine when xylazine has been used. This high incidence of complications points out the need for good preoperative assessment, stabilization of the patient prior to anesthesia, and adequate intraanesthetic monitoring.

Summary

Anesthetic management of birds is an art and a science. There is a pressing need for pharmacokinetic and dose-response studies of drugs commonly used in avian anesthesia. Without this scientific information, anesthesia will be limited to anecdotal information and clinical judgment.

References

1. Fedde MR. Drugs used for avian anesthesia: a review. Poultry Sci 57:1376, 1978.
2. McLelland J. Larynx and trachea. In: King AS, McLelland J, eds. Form and function in birds, vol. 4. London: Academic Press, 1989:69–103.
3. Hodges RD. The histology of the fowl. London: Academic Press, 1974.

4. Gaunt AS, Gaunt SLL, Prange HD, Wasser JS. The effects of tracheal coiling on the vocalizations of cranes (Aves; Gruidae). J Comp Physiol 161:43, 1987.

5. King AS. Functional anatomy of the syrinx. In: King AS, McLelland J, eds. Form and function in birds, vol. 4. London: Academic Press, 1989:105–192.

6. McLelland, J. Anatomy of the lungs and air sacs. In: King AS, McLelland J, eds. Form and function in birds, vol. 4. London: Academic Press, 1989:221–279.

7. Duncker, Hans-Rainer. Structure of avian lungs. Respir Physiol 14:44, 1972.

8. King AS, McLelland J, eds. Birds—their structure and function, 2nd ed. London: Balliere Tindall, 1984.

9. Duncker, Hans-Rainer. Structure of the avian respiratory tract. Respir Physiol 22:1, 1974.

10. King AS, Cowie AF. The functional anatomy of the bronchial muscle of the bird. J Anat 105:323, 1969.

11. Scheid P, Piiper J. Gas exchange and transport. In: Seller TJ, ed. Bird respiration, vol 1. Boca Raton, FL: CRC Press, 1987.

12. Magnussen H, Willmer H, Scheid, P. Gas exchange in air sacs: contribution to respiratory gas exchange in ducks. Respir Physiol 26:129, 1976.

13. Scheid, P. Mechanisms of gas exchange in bird lungs. Rev Physiol Biochem Pharmacol 86:138, 1979.

14. Fedde MR. Structure and gas-flow pattern in the avian respiratory system. Poultry Sci 59:2642, 1980.

15. Scheid P, Piiper J. Respiratory mechanics and air flow in birds. In: King AS, McLelland J, eds. Form and function in birds, vol. 4. London: Academic Press, 1989:369–391.

16. Barnas GM, Mather FB, Fedde MR. Response of avian intrapulmonary smooth muscle to changes in carbon dioxide concentration. Poultry Sci 57:1400, 1978.

17. Jones JH, Effmann EL, Schmidt-Nielsen, K. Control of air flow in bird lungs: radiographic studies. Respir Physiol 45:121, 1981.

18. Kuethe DO. Fluid mechanical valving of air flow in bird lungs. J Exp Biol 136:1, 1988.

19. Butler JP, Banzett RB, Fredberg JJ. Inspiratory valving in avian bronchi: aerodynamic considerations. Respir Physiol 72:241, 1988.

20. Wang, N, Banzett RB, Butler JP, Fredberg JJ. Bird lung models show that convective inertia effects inspiratory aerodynamic valving. Respir Physiol 73:111, 1988.

21. Scheid P, Piiper J. Aerodynamic valving in the avian lung. Acta Anaesth Scand 33(suppl 90):28–31, 1989.

22. Scheid P, Piiper J. Analysis of gas exchange in the avian lung: theory and experiments in the domestic fowl. Respir Physiol 9:246, 1970.

23. Piiper J, Scheid P. Comparative physiology of respiration: Functional analysis of gas exchange organs in vertebrates. In: Widdicombe JG, ed. International review of physiology—respiratory physiology, vol 2. Baltimore: University Park Press, 1977.

24. Powell FL, Scheid, P. Physiology of gas exchange in the avian respiratory system. In: King AS, McLelland J, eds. Form and function in birds, vol. 4. London; Academic Press, 1989:393–437.

25. Piiper J, Scheid P. Gas exchange in avian lungs: models and experimental evidence. In: Bolis L, Schmidt-Nielsen K, Maddrell SHP, eds. Comparative physiology. Amsterdam, North-Holland, 1973.

26. Powell FL. Diffusion in avian lungs. Fed Proc 41:2131–2133, 1982.

27. Faraci FM, Kilgore DL, Fedde MR. Oxygen delivery to the heart and brain during hypoxia: Pekin duck vs bar-headed goose. Am J Physiol 247:R69–R75, 1984.

28. Faraci FM, Kilgore DL, Fedde MR. Blood flow distribution during hypocapnic hypoxia in Pekin ducks and bar-headed geese. Respir Physiol 61:21–30, 1985.

29. Black CP, Tenney SM. Oxygen transport during progressive hypoxia in high-altitude and sea-level waterfowl. Respir Physiol 39:217–239, 1980.

30. Shams H, Scheid P. Efficiency of parabronchial gas exchange in deep hypoxia: measurements on the resting duck. Respir Physiol 77:135–146, 1989.

31. Gleeson M, Molony, V. Control of breathing. In: King AS, McLelland J, eds. Form and function in birds, vol. 4. London: Academic Press, 1989:439–484.

32. Barnas GM, Mather FB, Fedde MR. Are avian intrapulmonary CO_2 receptors chemically modulated mechanoreceptors or chemoreceptors? Respir Physiol 35:237, 1978.

33. Hempleman SC, Burger RE. Receptive fields of intrapulmonary chemoreceptors in the Pekin duck. Respir Physiol 57:317, 1984.

34. Hempleman SC, Burger RE. Comparison of intrapulmonary chemoreceptor response to PCO_2 in the duck and chicken. Respir Physiol 61:179, 1985.

35. Kilgore DL, Faraci FM, Fedde MR. Static response characteristics of intrapulmonary chemoreceptors in the pigeon and burrowing owl, a species with a blunted ventilatory sensitivity to carbon dioxide. Fed Proc 43:638, 1984.

36. Grubb BR. Allometric relations of cardiovascular function in birds. Am J Physiol 245:H567, 1983.

37. Sturkie PD. Heart and circulation: anatomy, hemodynamics, blood pressure, blood flow. In: Sturkie PD, ed. Avian physiology, 4th ed. New York: Springer-Verlag, 1986.

38. Sturkie PD. Heart: contraction, conduction, and electrocardiography. In: Sturkie PD, ed. Avian physiology, 4th ed. New York: Springer-Verlag, 1986.

39. O'Callaghan MW. Regulation of heart beat. In: Phillipson AT, Hall LW, Pritchard WR, eds. Scientific foundations of veterinary medicine. London: William Heinemann Medical Books, 1980.

40. Keene BW, Flammer, K. ECG of the month. J Am Vet Med Assoc 198:408, 1991.

41. Kisch, B. The electrocardiogram of birds (chicken, duck, pigeon). Exp Med Surg 9:103, 1951.

42. Zenoble RD, Graham DL. Electrocardiography of the parakeet, parrot and owl. Proceedings of the Annual Meeting of the American Association of Zoo Veterinarians, Denver, Colorado, 1979:42.

43. Zenoble RD. Electrocardiography in the parakeet and parrot. Compend Cont Educ 3:711, 1981.

44. Lumeij JT, Stokhof AA. Electrocardiogram of the racing pigeon (Columba livia domestica). Res Vet Sci 38:275, 1985.

45. Burrows ME, et al. Avian renal portal valve: a reexamination of its innervation. Am J Physiol 245:H628–H634, 1983.

46. Palmore WP, Ackerman N. Blood flow in the renal portal circulation of the turkey: effect of epinephrine. Am J Vet Res 46:1589, 1985.

47. Christensen J, et al. Comparison of various anesthetic regimens in the domestic fowl. Am J Vet Res 48:1649, 1987.

48. Hellebrekers LJ, Sap R, van Wandelen RM. Spontaneous ventilation versus intermittent positive pressure ventilation in birds. Proceedings of the 4th International Congress of Veterinary Anaesthesia, Utrecht, The Netherlands, August 1991:81.

49. Piiper, J, Drees F, Scheid, P. Gas exchange in the domestic fowl during spontaneous breathing and artificial ventilation. Respir Physiol 9:234, 1970.

50. Ludders JW, Rode J, Mitchell GS. Isoflurane anesthesia in sandhill cranes (Grus canadensis): minimal anesthetic concentration and cardiopulmonary dose-response during spontaneous and controlled breathing. Anesth Analg (Cleve) 68:511, 1989.

51. Hirshman CA, et al. Hypoxic ventilatory drive in dogs during thiopental, ketamine or pentobarbital anesthesia. Anesthesiology 43:628, 1975.

52. Hirshman CA, et al. Depression of hypoxic ventilatory response by halothane, enflurane and isoflurane in dogs. Br J Anaesth 49:957, 1977.

53. Pavlin EG, Hornbein TF. Anesthesia and the control of ventilation. In: Cherniak NS, Widdicombe JG, eds. Handbook of physiology, sec. 3. The respiratory system, vol. 2. Bethesda, MD: American Physiological Society, 1986.

54. Molony, V. Classification of vagal afferents firing in phase with breathing in Gallus domesticus. Respir Physiol 22:57, 1974.

55. Pizarro J, et al. Halothane effects on ventilatory responses to changes in intrapulmonary CO_2 in geese. Respir Physiol 82:337, 1990.

56. Bagshaw RJ, Cox RH. Baroreceptor control of heart rate in chickens (*Gallus domesticus*). Am J Vet Res 47:293, 1986.

57. Osborne JL, Mitchell GS. Regulation of arterial PCO_2 during inhalation of CO_2 in chickens. Respir Physiol 31:357, 1977.

58. Osborne JL, Mitchell GS. Ventilatory responses during arterial homeostasis of PCO2 at low levels of inspired carbon dioxide. In: Piiper J, ed. Respiratory function in birds, adult and embryonic. Berlin: Springer-Verlag, 1978.

59. Fedde MR, Burger RE, Kitchell RL. Electromyographic studies of the effects of bodily position and anesthesia on the activity of the respiratory muscles of the domestic cock. Poultry Sci 43:839–846, 1964.

60. King AS, Payne DC. Normal breathing and the effects of posture in *Gallus domesticus*. J Physiol (Lond) 174:340–347, 1964.

61. Butler PJ. The exercise response and the "classical" diving response during natural submersion in birds and mammals. Can J Zoo 66:29–39, 1988.

62. Jones DR, et al. Forced and voluntary diving in ducks: cardiovascular adjustments and their control. Can J Zoo 66:75, 1988.

63. Woakes AJ. Metabolism in diving birds: studies in the laboratory and the field. Can J Zoo 66:138, 1988.

64. Jones DR, et al. Regional distribution of blood flow during diving in the duck (*Anas platyrhynchos*). Can J Zoo 57:995, 1979.

65. Burger RE, Lorenz FW. Artificial respiration in birds by unidirectional air flow. Poultry Sci 39:236–237, 1960.

66. Burger RE, et al. Gas exchange in the parabronchila lung of birds: experiments in unidirectionally ventilated ducks. Respir Physiol 36:19, 1979.

67. Whittow GC, Ossorio N. A new technique for anesthetizing birds. Lab Anim Care 20:651–656, 1970.

68. Wijnberg ID, Lagerweij E, Zwart, P. Inhalation anaesthesia in birds through the abdominal air sac, using a unidirectional, continuous flow. Proceedings of the Fourth International Congress of Veterinary Anaesthesia, Utrecht, The Netherlands, August 25–30, 1991.

69. Harrison GJ. Selected surgical procedures. In: Harrison GJ, Harrison LR. Clinical avian medicine and surgery. Philadelphia: WB Saunders, 1986.

70. Rosskopf WJ Jr. Surgery of the avian respiratory system. Proc Am Coll Vet Sur 16(1):373–382, 1988.

71. Rode JA, Bartholow S, Ludders JW. Ventilation through an air sac cannula during tracheal obstruction in ducks. J Assoc Avian Vet 4:98, 1990.

72. Clark CH, et al. Plasma concentrations of chloramphenicol in birds. Am J Vet Res 43:1249, 1982.

73. Dorrestein GM, Van Miert ASJPAM. Pharmacotherapeutic aspects of medication of birds. J Vet Pharmacol Ther 11:33, 1988.

74. Cooper JE. Veterinary aspects of captive birds of prey, 2nd ed. Gloucestershire, England: The Standfast Press, 1985.

75. Fowler ME, ed. Zoo and wild animal medicine, 2nd ed. Philadelphia: WB Saunders, 1986.

76. Franchetti DR, Klide AM, Restraint and anesthesia. In: Fowler ME, ed. Zoo and wild animal medicine. Philadelphia: WB Saunders, 1978:359–364.

77. Altman RB. Avian anesthesia. Compend Cont Educ 2:38, 1980.

78. Harrison GJ. Pre-anesthetic fasting recommended. J Assoc Avian Vet 5:126, 1991.

79. Sedgwick CJ, Pokras MA. Extrapolating rational drug doses and treatment periods by allometric scaling. Proc 55th Annu Mtg Am Anim Hosp Assoc, Washington, DC, 1988:156.

80. Boxenbaum, H. Interspecies scaling, allometry, physiological time, and the ground plan of pharmacokinetics. J Pharmacokinet Biopharm 10:201, 1982.

81. Schmidt-Nielsen, K. Scaling—why is animal size so important? New York: Cambridge University Press, 1991.

82. McDonald, S. Common anesthetic dosages for use in psittacine birds. J Assoc Avian Vet 3:186, 1989.

83. Redig PT, Larson AA, Duke GE. Response of great horned owls given the optical isomers of ketamine. Am J Vet Res 45:125, 1984.

84. Salerno A, Van Tienhoven A. The effect of ketamine on heart rate, respiration rate and EEG of white leghorn hens. Comp Biochem Physiol 55C:69, 1976.

85. McGrath CJ, Lee JC, Campbell VL. Dose-response anesthetic effects of ketamine in the chicken. Am J Vet Res 45:531, 1984.

86. Valverde A, et al. Determination of a sedative dose and influence of midazolam on cardiopulmonary function in Canada geese. Am J Vet Res 51:1071, 1990.

87. Samour JH, et al. Comparative studies of the use of some injectable anaesthetic agents in birds. Vet Rec 115:6, 1984.

88. Ludders JW, Rode JA, Mitchell GS. Pulmonary effects of ketamine, xylazine, and a combination of ketamine and xylazine in Pekin ducks. Am J Vet Res, 50:245, 1989.

89. Allen JL, Oosterhuis JE. Effect of tolazoline on xylazine-ketamine-induced anesthesia in turkey vultures. J Am Vet Med Assoc 189:1011, 1986.

90. Degernes LA, et al. Ketamine-xylazine anesthesia in red-tailed hawks with antagonism by yohimbine. J Wildl Dis 24:322, 1988.

91. Fitzgerald G, Cooper JE. Preliminary studies in the use of propofol in the domestic pigeon (*Columba livia*). Res Vet Sci 49:334–338, 1990.

92. France CP, Woods JH. Morphine, saline and naltrexone discrimination in morphine-treated pigeons. J Pharmacol Exp Ther 242:195–242, 1987.

93. Ruskoaho H, Karppanen H. Xylazine-induced sedation in chicks is inhibited by opiate receptor antagonists. Eur J Pharmacol 100:91–966, 1984.

94. Leander JD. Opioid agonist and antagonist behavioural effects of buprenorphine. Br J Pharmac 78:607–615, 1983.

95. Herling S, et al. Narcotic discrimination in pigeons. J Pharmacol Exp Ther 214:139–146, 1980.

96. Leander JD, McMillan DE. Meperidine effects on schedule controlled responding. J Pharmacol Exp Ther 201:434–443, 1977.

97. Hughes RA. Codeine analgesic and morphine hyperalgesic effects on thermal nociception in domestic fowl. Pharmacol Biochem Behav 35:567–570, 1990.

98. Bardo MT, Hughes RA. Shock-elicited flight response in chickens as an index of morphine analgesia. Pharmacol Biochem Behav 9:147–149, 1978.

99. Rager DR, Gallup GG. Apparent analgesic effects of morphine in chickens may be confounded by motor deficits. Physiol Behav 37:269–272, 1986.

100. Mansour A, Khachaturian LME, Akil H, Watson SJ. Anatomy of CNS opioid receptors. Trend Neurosci 11:308–314, 1988.

101. Biester HE, Schwarte LH. Diseases of poultry, 3rd ed. Ames, IA: Iowa State College Press, 1952.

102. Marley E, Payne JP. Anaesthesia for young animals. J Physiol (Lond) 162:35, 1962.

103. Jones RS. Halothane anaesthesia in turkeys. Br J Anaesth 38:656–658, 1966.

104. Bednarski RM, et al. Isoflurane-nitrous oxide-oxygen anesthesia in an Andean condor. J Am Vet Med Assoc 187:1209, 1985.

105. Klide AM. Avian anesthesia. Vet Clin North Am 3:175, 1973.

106. Sedgwick CJ. Anesthesia of caged birds. In: Kirk R, ed. Current veterinary therapy, 7th ed. Philadelphia: WB Saunders, 1980.

107. Eger E III. Anesthetic uptake and action. Baltimore: Williams & Wilkins, 1974.

108. Ludders JW, Mitchell GS, Schaefer SL. Minimum anesthetic dose and cardiopulmonary response for halothane in chickens. Am J Vet Res 49:929, 1988.

109. Ludders JW, Mitchell GS, Rode J. Minimal anesthetic concentration and cardiopulmonary dose response of isoflurane in ducks. Vet Surg 19:304, 1990.

110. Ludders JW. Minimal anesthetic concentration and cardiopulmonary dose-response of halothane in ducks. Vet Surg 21:319, 1992.

111. Eger E III. Isoflurane: a compendium and reference, 2nd ed. Madison, WI: Anaquest, 1985.

112. Quasha AL, Eger EI, Tinker JH. Determination and application of MAC. Anesthesia 53:315–334, 1980.

113. Arnall L. Anaesthesia and surgery in cage and aviary birds. I. Vet Rec 73:139, 1961.

114. Dolphin RE, Olsen DE. Anesthesia in the companion bird. Vet Med Small Anim Clinic 56:1961, 1977.

115. Gandal CP. Avian anesthesia. Fed Proc 28:1533, 1969.

116. Myers RE, Stettner LJ. Safe and reliable general anesthesia in birds. Physiol Behav 4:277, 1969.

117. McDonald Scott E. Avian anesthetics. J Assoc Avian Vet 3:181, 1989.

118. Goelz MF, Hahn AW, Kelley ST. Effects of halothane and isoflurane on mean arterial blood pressure, heart rate, and respiratory rate in adult Pekin ducks. Am J Vet Res 51:458, 1990.

119. Regan MJ, Eger EI. Effect of hypothermia in dogs on anesthetizing and apneic doses of inhalation agents: determination of the anesthetic index (apnea/MAC). Anesthesiology 28:689, 1967.

120. Steffey EP, et al. Isoflurane potency in the dog and cat. Am J Vet Res 38:1833, 1977.

121. Steffey EP, Howland, D. Potency of enflurane in dogs: comparisons with halothane and isoflurane. Am J Vet Res 39:573, 1978.

122. Steffey EP, et al. Enflurane, halothane, and isoflurane potency in horses. Am J Vet Res 38:1037, 1977.

123. Greenlees KJ, et al. Effect of halothane, isoflurane, and pentobarbital anesthesia on myocardial irritability in chickens. Am J Vet Res 51:757, 1990.

124. Reynold WT. Unusual anesthetic complication in a pelican. Vet Rec 113:204, 1983.

125. Nicholson A, Ilkiw JE. Neuromuscular and cardiovascular effects of atracurium in anesthetized chickens. Am J Vet Res 53:2337–2342, 1992.

126. Fowler ME. Comparative clinical anatomy of ratites. J Zoo Wildl Med 22:204, 1991.

127. Bezuidenhout AJ, Coetzer DJ. The major blood vessels of the wing of the ostrich (Struthio camelus). Onderstepoort J Vet Res 53:201, 1986.

128. Levy A, et al. Reference blood chemical values in ostriches (Struthio camelus). Am J Vet Res 50:1548, 1989.

129. Palomeque J, Pinto D, Viscor, G. Hematologic and blood chemistry values of the masai ostrich (Struthio camelus). J Wildl Dis 27:34, 1991.

130. Levi A, et al. Haematological parameters of the ostrich (Struthio camelus). Avian Pathol 18:321, 1989.

131. Stoskopf MJ, et al. Immobilization of large ratites: blue necked ostrich and double wattled cassowary with hematologic and serum chemistry data. J Zoo Anim Med 13:160, 1982.

132. Jacobson ER, et al. Ventriculostomy for removal of multiple foreign bodies in an ostrich. J Am Vet Med Assoc 198:1117, 1986.

133. Fowler JD, et al. Surgical correction of tibiotarsal rotation in an emu. Compend Anim Pract 1:26, 1987.

134. Cornick JL, Jensen J. Anesthetic management of ostriches. J Am Vet Med Assoc 220:1661, 1992.

135. Honnas CM, et al. Proventriculotomy to relieve foreign body impaction in ostriches. J Am Vet Med Assoc 199:461, 1991.

136. Van Heerden J, Keffen RH. A preliminary investigation into the immobilizing potential of tiletamine/zolazepam mixture, metomidate, a metomidate and azaperone combination and medetomidine in ostriches (Struthio camelus). J S Afr Vet Assoc 62:114, 1991.

137. Ensley DK, Launer DP, Blasingame JP. General anesthesia and surgical removal of a tumor-like growth from the foot of a double-wattled cassowary. Zoo Anim Med 15:35, 1984.

138. Grubb, B. Use of ketamine to restrain and anesthetize emus. Vet Med Small Anim Clin 78:247, 1983.

139. Sedgwick C, Pokras M, Kaufman, G. Metabolic scaling: using estimated energy costs to extrapolate drug doses between different species and different individuals of diverse body sizes. Proceedings of the Am Assoc Zoo Vet, South Padre Island, Tex, 1990:249–254.

140. Schobert, E. Telazol use in wild and exotic animals. Vet Med 82:1080, 1987.

141. McClure SR, Taylor TS, Johnson JH, Heisterkamp KB, Sanders EA. Surgical repair of traumatically induced collapsing trachea in an ostrich. J Am Vet Med Assoc 207:479–480, 1995.

142. Jones JH. Pulmonary blood flow distribution in panting ostriches. J Appl Physiol 53:1411, 1982.

143. Schmidt-Nielsen K, et al. Temperature regulation and respiration in the ostrich. Condor 71:341, 1969.

144. Cornick-Seahorn JL, Martin GS, Tulley TN, Morris JM. Tourniquet-induced hypertension in an ostrich. J Am Vet Med Assoc 207(3):344–346, 1995.

145. Matthews NS, Burba DJ, Cornick JL. Premature ventricular contractions and apparent hypertension during anesthesia in an ostrich. J Am Vet Med Assoc 198:1959, 1991.

REPTILES AND AMPHIBIANS

Juergen Schumacher

Reptiles

INTRODUCTION

In general, reptiles present a unique challenge to veterinarians, since there are over 6400 known species. The order squamata with over 5400 species represents the largest order, while the orders *rhynchocephalia, chelonia,* and *crocodilia* consist of approximately 241 species. Although it is impossible to have detailed knowledge about the specific requirements of each species, a thorough knowledge and understanding of reptilian anatomy and physiology is essential for proper medical treatment and anesthesia.

Reptile medicine is growing, reference data is becoming available, and knowledge about infectious and noninfectious diseases, their diagnosis and treatment, is increasing. A variety of advanced diagnostic and sur-

gical procedures are now routinely performed. The use of specialized diagnostic equipment such as fiber-optic instruments for diagnosis and surgery is common. There is a need for improved techniques for restraint and anesthesia of the reptilian patient. A variety of anesthetic drugs, doses, and anesthetic techniques have been described with variable success. There is general agreement that successful anesthesia of any reptile depends on the veterinarian's experience, skills, and knowledge of the species. This includes critical evaluation of the patient's overall health, the veterinarian's experience with the surgical procedure being performed, and knowledge of anesthetic drugs and techniques.

The need for adequate immobilization and anesthesia is obvious in the case of large and dangerous reptiles such as *crocodilia* and large or poisonous snakes.

Harmless tortoises may also represent a challenge for the clinician when performing a physical examination or attempting to collect diagnostic samples. Because of their protective behavior they may first require chemical immobilization for a complete examination or specimen collection. Chemical restraint in these cases will protect the animal from stress as well as possible injury caused by handling.

Reptilian morphology and physiology is very unique and differs in many ways from mammalian anatomy and physiology. Reptiles are ectothermic animals, and their response to anesthetic drugs depends on their environmental temperature. Since many body functions are temperature dependent, a variable response of reptiles to anesthetic drugs will be seen if the patient is kept above or below the preferred temperature range. Drugs and dosages successfully used in one animal may prove to be inadequate in another. The clinician's choice of drug depends on personal experience but even more on the purpose for which sedation or anesthesia is required.

It is not the purpose of this chapter to review all of the anesthetic techniques that have been used in reptiles, for example, electroanesthesia.(1) Several commonly used drugs and anesthetic regimens that have proven to be of clinical value are reviewed. There are several excellent reviews on reptile restraint and anesthesia to which the reader is referred.(2–12)

ANATOMY AND PHYSIOLOGY

Of particular interest for the anesthesiologist is the unique reptilian respiratory system. The total lung volume is greater in reptiles than in mammals, but the gas exchange surface is smaller when compared to a mammal of equal body mass.(13, 14) Among reptiles, crocodilians have the most developed lungs. In snakes, the left lung is either absent or vestigial, except in snakes of the family *Boidae,* where the left lung is developed.(13, 15–17) Depending on the species of snake, the right lung continues into an air sac, which is best developed in arboreal and terrestrial snakes. Aquatic snakes have a more developed vascular lung, and their gas exchange surface is larger than in terrestrial species.(17, 18) Although the trachea of chelonians and crocodilians consists of complete rings, the trachea of a snake contains incomplete rings.(13) Snakes have a very long trachea, while chelonian tracheas are relatively short and care should be taken not to intubate one of the primary bronchi. The position of the glottis is different among different species of reptiles. Although it is positioned rostrally and easily visible in snakes, in chelonians the glottis is positioned at the base of the tongue and may be difficult to visualize.(17) In marine turtles the presence of papillae on the tongue and their ability for breath holding makes tracheal intubation more challenging. Reptiles do not have a functioning diaphragm, and thus the thoracic and abdominal cavity are not separated.(13, 17, 19) In crocodilians a well-developed structure resembling a diaphragm has been described.(13)

Because of the absence of a functioning diaphragm, the force to move air into the lungs and air sacs comes from the movement of respiratory muscles.(14) In snakes, intercostal muscles will expand the volume of the lung and the air sac, thus creating a negative pressure. Because of the pressure difference with the atmosphere, gas will enter the lungs. Upon expiration the volume of the lung and the air sacs is reduced by contracture of the intercostal musculature, creating a positive pressure and forcing gas back to the atmosphere. In chelonians, the ability to change intrapulmonary volume and pressure comes from the movement of the front and hind limbs. With deep anesthesia, these muscles may become paralyzed and artificial ventilation may be needed. Induction of inhalation anesthesia may be complicated by some turtles' ability to metabolize anaerobically (*Pseudemys* spp.).(4, 20)

PHYSICAL RESTRAINT

Physical restraint, collection of samples, and route of drug administration require knowledge of the size, anatomic specificities, and potential danger of certain reptile species. Although the safety of the veterinarian and the personnel involved in the procedure is the highest priority, every effort should be made to avoid potential injury to the animal and minimize stress. It is essential to prepare all equipment prior to handling.

Chelonia. Prior to physical restraint and handling the animal should be observed undisturbed in its tank or cage. Level of activity, respiratory efforts, normal signs, and signs of illness should be noted. Careful examination of the shell to identify injuries and identifying nutritional disorders or infectious processes are helpful in assessing the health status of the animal. The legs should be examined as well as the cloacal region. The head should be examined, with particular focus on the eyes, tympanic membranes, and nares. The oral cavity should be inspected and evaluated for oral abscesses or traumatic lesions, which might interfere with endotracheal intubation and maintenance of anesthesia.

Examining tortoises and turtles requires patience and knowledge of how to manipulate these animals. Aquatic turtles are often very agile and can inflict a painful bite. Members of larger species are potentially dangerous, and great care should be taken when manipulating them. Snapping turtles and adult marine turtles are capable of crushing the examiner's hand, and in some cases it is advisable to perform physical examination and collection of diagnostic samples after the animal has been sedated or anesthetized. Often it is a major challenge to secure the head for examination. Pressure on the hind limbs may encourage tortoises to protrude the head from the shell so that it can be grasped quickly. Care should be taken to avoid injury to the animal, and excessive force should not be applied in order to pull out legs or the head. Legs have been broken when too much force was employed. In manipulating giant tortoises, care must be taken to prevent crushing injuries to the examiner's hands. Hands have been caught between legs or legs and the shell of the animal. In some cases, placement of the tortoise in dorsal recumbency will encourage it to protrude legs and head.

Crocodilia. Members of this reptilian group are dangerous. Self-inflicted injuries and damage to the handler can occur if precautions are disregarded. In general, alligators are more docile and easier to work with than crocodiles. Members of both species up to 3 feet in length may be manually restrained by an experienced person. The greatest potential for injury are from teeth and the tail, which will be violently thrashed around for defense and attack purposes. The first step should be to secure the mouth. The strength to open the jaws is relatively small in alligators and crocodiles, and one person may be able to hold the mouth closed while another tapes it shut with a strong tape (duct tape). When transporting the animal, it should be supported along the whole body axis and the head and tail should be secured. For ease of capturing, a pole with a sling at the end (snare) is very suitable, especially for animals beyond 3 feet in length. As soon as the snare is around the neck, the head and tail have to be restrained to prevent the animal from twirling. Large crocodilians require the efforts of several experienced people. The animal can be restrained with ropes around the head and the tail, the mouth can be taped when the animal is secured, and an examination or treatment can be performed. If necessary, large animals should be sedated prior to handling.

Squamata. **Sauria.** Restraint of this group of reptiles is relatively easy to accomplish. The only exception are larger species such as Komodo dragons (up to 100 kg in body weight) and some large monitors, which are potentially dangerous. They should be handled similarly to crocodiles. Most smaller species, although capable of inflicting serious and painful bites (adult green iguanas or some lizards) can be manually restrained if gloves are worn for protection from bites and scratches. In all cases a secure and firm grip should be placed around the head. Thumb and index finger should be placed around the neck, and one front leg should be placed between the other fingers to prevent the animal from spinning. The other hand can then, depending on the animal's size, be used either for manipulation of the animal or to support the rest of the body. Under no circumstances should iguanas and lizards be restrained by holding the tail alone. To support the body, the hand should be placed under the abdomen at the base of the tail to prevent it from hitting. Pet iguanas used to handling are relatively easy patients to work with. As a rule, when visually examining the iguana let it sit on your hand and arm, supporting the whole body, but with no restraint. This is a stress-free situation for the animal, and visual examinations can be made this way. Gentle, manipulative examinations can be made by palpating the abdomen and the limbs, as well as examining the head.

In poisonous species such as the gila monster and the beaded lizard, the head should be secured before examination begins.

Serpentes. Physical restraint of nonpoisonous snakes is, with the exception of large boid snakes, easy to accomplish. First, the head should be secured by placing the thumb and middle fingers on either side of the head and the index finger on the top of the head. With the other hand the body should be supported. Plexiglas tubes, which are available in different sizes, are very useful. The snake can be manipulated to crawl into the tube. This device allows for easy access for injections or other manipulations. They are especially useful when handling poisonous snakes. The most useful tool when working with poisonous or aggressive nonpoisonous snakes is a snake hook. It can be used for lifting the animal from its container, for manipulating it to crawl in a certain direction, or for pinning the head prior to manual restraint. Large boas and pythons should always be restrained by several people. If possible, remove the snake from its cage or box. This way there is more room to work in and the snake may be less territorial. For examination of the head, the body of the snake can be left in a large pillow case, with only the head exposed. As a rule, one person is responsible for the head and one person for each 3 feet of body length of a large snake. The head should be secured first. A plastic shield can be held in front of the snake to prevent it from striking.

Poisonous snakes can be handled with a snake hook or long forceps. They should be manipulated to crawl into a plexiglas tube for further evaluation. For procedures in the oral cavity, such as abscess debridement, chemical restraint of the snake is advisable in most cases. Experience is necessary when handling poisonous snakes to prevent potentially fatal injuries. When working with poisonous snakes on a regular basis, one should contact local breeders, zoos, or research facilities that store antivenom of the most commonly kept species. A snake hook and plastic tubes are essential tools when working with poisonous snakes. The tube can be held with a Pilstrom snake tong while the hook is used to manipulate the snake. Care should be taken to select a tube of proper diameter so that the snake cannot turn around within the tube. Pinning the snake with a hook and holding the head between the fingers should only be done by experienced people. If inexperienced, one should practice restraint on calm, nonpoisonous snakes first.

Blood sampling techniques. Depending on the species of reptile, blood can be collected from various sites. Hematologic and plasma biochemical determinations will help in identifying the health status and underlying diseases. Unfortunately, only limited reference data are presently available. The method of collecting a blood sample and the volume of blood depend on the size and the species of reptile. Minimally, packed cell volume and total protein should be determined prior to anesthesia. In most species of reptiles the total blood volume accounts for approximately 10% of the body weight. In a healthy reptile 10% of the total blood volume can be withdrawn safely.

In tortoises and turtles, blood can be collected from several sites. Although small volumes can be obtained by clipping a toenail, larger volumes require access to a peripheral vessel. The most common site for collecting a blood sample in chelonians is from the front legs. The brachial vein and artery, however, are surrounded by lymphatic structures. Therefore, hemodilution may occur when collecting blood from this site. Vessels cannot be visualized, and the sampling will be blind. In some larger tortoises, the vessels can be palpated. If pure lymph is obtained, it is advisable to discard the syringe and needle and retry. In larger species, samples can be obtained from the ventral coccygeal vein. The best site for collecting a pure blood sample in many turtles and tortoises is the jugular vein, which is beneath the skin at the lateral side of the neck. The major problem is restraint and fixation of the head while attempting to collect the sample. In some cases sedation may be necessary to avoid injury and excessive stress to the animal. A sample can also be obtained from the occipital sinus. For collecting blood from the heart, a hole must be drilled into the plastron with a 1½-inch bit. Sterile techniques must be employed to avoid contamination. Success in utilizing these techniques depends on the skills of the clinician.

In crocodiles and alligators blood can easily be obtained from a vertebral sinus located caudal to the occipita and dorsal to the spinal cord. Other sites include the heart, which is located in the ventral midline, and the ventral coccygeal vein. Most lizards can easily be bled from the ventral tail vein, and small amounts of blood can be collected by clipping a toenail.

The most common sites for collection of blood in snakes are the ventral tail vein, the heart, and in larger specimens, the palatine veins. Cardiac puncture is safe as long as the clinician employs the proper technique and does not traumatize the heart with multiple needle punctures. The heart can be either visualized by its beating and movement of the scales or examined by palpation. In most snake species the heart is located after the first third to first quarter of the body length. Once the heart is identified, it has to be stabilized by holding it between two fingers. Depending on the size of the snake, a 23- to 25-gauge needle is inserted between two ventral scales caudal to the heart at a 45° angle, with the tip of the needle aimed cranially and toward the apex of the heart. Only gentle suction should be employed when withdrawing the sample. If done properly with a sterile technique, there is only minimal risk involved for the snake. When collecting a sample from the ventral tail vein, care should be taken not to injure the hemipenis in male snakes. The needle is inserted in the ventral midline at either a 45 or 90° angle until it hits bone. Under gentle aspiration the needle is then withdrawn until blood flows into the syringe (Fig. 20F–1).

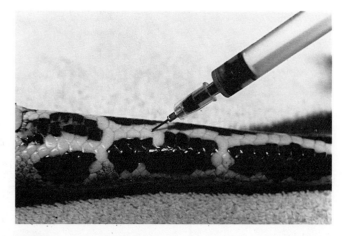

Fig. 20F–1. Blood sampling from the ventral tail vein in a Burmese python (*Python molurus bivittatus*). A 25-gauge needle is inserted at a 45° angle.

Routes of drug administration. In most cases injectable anesthetic agents are administered by intramuscular injection. Oral administration is less reliable and clinically not practical owing to variances in uptake and distribution of the drug. Subcutaneous administration will also result in prolonged induction times. A renal portal system has been described in reptiles; therefore, drugs that are eliminated by the kidneys, such as ketamine, should be given in the forelimbs or the rostral half of the body. In snakes, intramuscular injections are given in the front half of the body into the paravertebral muscles (Fig. 20F–2A). In chelonians and lizards intramuscular injections are given into the muscles of the forelegs (Figs. 20F–2B and 20F–2C) or the gluteal muscles of the hind leg. Intravenous injection is more difficult and often reserved for research purposes. With practice, intravenous injections of fluids and drugs can be given into the jugular vein in chelonians. An intravenous catheter can be inserted relatively easily and sutured or taped to the skin (Fig. 20F–3). In snakes, the right jugular vein is accessible for venous access. A cut-down and dissection of the vein will allow placement of a catheter and intravenous administration of drugs and fluids. The catheter can be secured to the skin by sutures and/or an adhesive. The catheter should then be protected with bandage material. In lizards (especially in green iguanas) the presence of a large abdominal vein allows for easy collection of blood, intravenous injection or placement of an intravenous catheter (Fig. 20F–4). A 1-cm-long cut-down through the ventral scales after a subcutaneous injection of 2% lidocaine is performed. The vein can be easily visualized within the connective tissue underneath the skin. Depending on the size of the iguana, a 20- to 24-gauge catheter may be inserted into the vein and secured to the skin by sutures and adhesives. A bandage will protect the catheter while the animal is moving.

In tortoises, crocodilians, and lizards an intraosseous catheter may be placed in the ulna or tibia for ad-

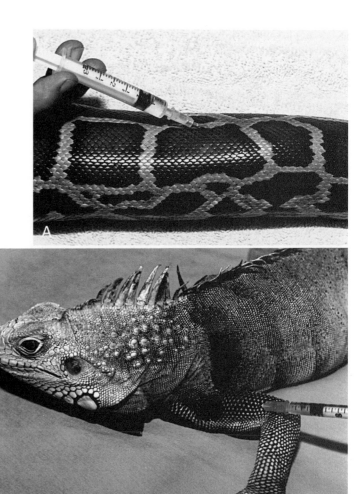

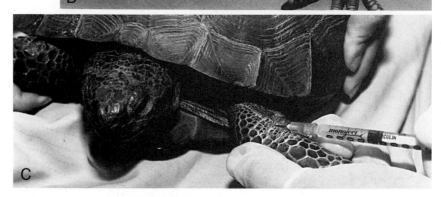

Fig. 20F–2. Intramuscular injection of ketamine HCl in the paravertebral muscle group of a Burmese python (*Python molurus bivittatus*) (A), the front leg of a green iguana (*Iguana iguana*) (B), and a gopher tortoise (*Gopherus polyphemus*) (C).

ministration of fluids. Depending on the size of the patient a spinal or hypodermic needle is suitable. Following aseptic preparation, the lateral notch on the distal ulna is identified and the needle advanced into the marrow cavity. Once the needle is secured in place, it should be flushed with heparinized saline.

PREANESTHETIC EVALUATION

Careful and critical assessment of the patient's health status is as important in reptilian as in avian and mammalian anesthesia.(21) Prior to anesthesia, an ac-

curate body weight is required to calculate the dose of the anesthetic agent. Ideally, the reptilian patient should be maintained at and acclimated to its optimum body temperature for several days prior to anesthesia. A complete physical examination including radiographs, hematology, plasma biochemistries, and fecal examinations should be performed, and samples for microbiologic determinations should be obtained to assess the patient's health status. Many infectious and noninfectious diseases in reptiles can effect renal and hepatic function. Supportive care, initiated prior to anesthesia, including administration of a balanced electrolyte solution (5–10 mL · kg^{-1} · h^{-1}), heat, nutritional support, and antimicrobial therapy will decrease anesthetic and surgical risk. Fluids, such as lactated Ringer's solution may be given intravenously, subcutaneously, or intracelomically. Guidelines for reptile fluid requirements have not been reported but may be calculated on the basis of those known for mammals. To reduce stress, handling of the reptile should be kept to a minimum.

PREMEDICATION

There is some controversy concerning the routine use of preanesthetic medications. Some authors recommend the use of parasympatholytics such as atropine sulfate at a dose of 0.04 mg/kg intramuscularly or intraperi-

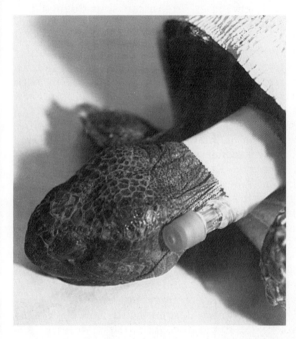

Fig. 20F–3. Intravenous catheter placed in the jugular vein of a gopher tortoise (*Gopherus polyphemus*).

toneally to prevent excessive secretions and to minimize the risk of bradycardia after induction of anesthesia. Routine use of parasympatholytic agents is not recommended, since excessive respiratory and salivary secretions are not commonly seen in anesthetized reptiles. If profound or prolonged bradycardia does occur, atropine can be given at the dose just mentioned. Glycopyrrolate is an excellent alternative to atropine, since it is more potent, longer acting, and more selective in its antisecretory properties. A decrease in heart rate during anesthesia is commonly seen but has not been associated with any complications in anesthetized reptiles. Although knowledge of cardiopulmonary responses and adaptations in snakes is extensive (18, 22, 23), little is known about the effects of anesthetics even on simple cardiopulmonary variables such as heart rate and blood pressure.

Administration of sedatives prior to induction of anesthesia will reduce the dose of ketamine HCl or an inhalational agent for maintenance of anesthesia. In many mammals, benzodiazepines produce a dose-dependent state of hypnosis and muscle relaxation.(24) However, they do not produce analgesia. Diazepam can be used in American alligators (*Alligator mississippiensis*) at a dose of 0.22–0.62 mg/kg IM, 20 minutes prior to injection of succinylcholine. This reduces the dose of succinylcholine necessary to produce immobilization.(25) The pronounced sedative effects would appear to be caused by diazepam. Midazolam (2 mg/kg), although more expensive than diazepam, has been used in combination with ketamine (20 or 40 mg/kg) to produce sedation and muscle relaxation in turtles.(26)

LOCAL ANESTHESIA

The skin of reptiles is very sensitive to painful stimuli.(10) The use of local anesthetics such as 2% lidocaine for abscess removal, repair of skin lacerations, and other minor procedures is recommended.(3, 6, 27) In venomous snakes or large crocodilians, local anesthesia alone is not safe and additional drugs are

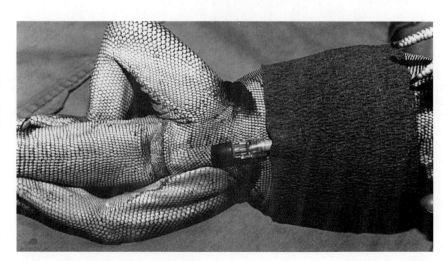

Fig. 20F–4. Intravenous catheter placed in the ventral abdominal vein in a green iguana (*Iguana iguana*).

Table 20F–1. Summary of Anesthetic Parameters for Drugs used to Anesthetize Green Sea Turtles

No. of Turtles	Drug	Dosage (mg/kg)	Route	Induction Time (min)	Duration of Anesthesia (min)	Recovery Time (hr)
8	Sodium pentobarbital	10.0–25.0	IV	14–120	40–240	4–24
11	Ketamine hydrochloride	38.0–71.0	IP	2–10	2–10	<4
26	Sodium thiopental	18.8–31.4	IV	5–10	5–120	<6

(From Wood, F.E., Critchley, K.H., and Wood, J.R. Anesthesia in the Green Sea Turtle, *Chelonia mydas.* Am J Vet Res 43:1882, 1982.)

recommended to immobilize the patient. In most other reptiles the combination of manual restraint or chemical immobilization with the use of local anesthetics is a practical way to perform minor surgical procedures.

PARENTERAL ANESTHESIA

Reptiles arc most commonly anesthetized with injectable anesthetics. Injectables offer the advantages of ease of administration and a relatively low cost. A major disadvantage of parenteral agents is that once they are administered, the depth of anesthesia cannot be controlled and untoward anesthetic effects are not readily reversible. Except for smaller species, an accurate weight is sometimes impossible to obtain prior to anesthesia, increasing the chance of overdosing. A major disadvantage following injectable anesthesia is prolonged recovery, which may take several days. Recovery depends on the drug and the species anesthetized. Injectable drugs are more commonly given by the intramuscular route, often requiring higher doses than needed with intravenous administration. Venous access is often difficult to achieve.(16, 28, 29) Most frequently, dissociative anesthetics in combination with benzodiazepines are the drugs of choice.(30)

Chelonia. Ketamine HCl alone or in combination with diazepam or midazolam has been used to produce sedation and anesthesia in tortoises and turtles. Ketamine (22–44 mg/kg IM or SQ) induces good sedation. A dose of 55 to 88 mg/kg is recommended for a surgical plane of anesthesia.(31-33) Induction time is between 10 and 30 minutes, but recovery may be prolonged, ranging up to 96 hours.(31-33) As a rule to induce anesthesia, smaller tortoises and turtles require more ketamine per unit body weight than larger species. It is recommended that ketamine be used in combination with diazepam (0.2–1 mg/kg IM) or midazolam (up to 2 mg/kg IM) to enhance muscle relaxation. Ketamine (10–30 mg/kg IM) is routinely administered in combination with butorphanol (0.5–1.5 mg/kg IM) for minor surgical procedures such as shell repairs or limb trauma. Because of prolonged recoveries following high doses of ketamine, it has been recommended that it be used only as a preanesthetic prior to inhalational anesthesia.

In Galapagos tortoises a dose of 0.22 mg/kg etorphine HCl produces adequate sedation for minor surgical procedures.(34) Large tortoises may be given tiletamine/zolazepam at a dose of 5–10 mg/kg IM or IV to facilitate tracheal intubation. If sedation of the animal is too light for tracheal intubation after Telazol has been given, mask induction with isoflurane is preferred instead of repetitive dosing with Telazol. This will significantly shorten recovery times. In African spur-thighed tortoises, high-dose Telazol anesthesia resulted in a recovery time of up to 3 days. Although mask induction might be a time-consuming challenge in marine turtles and many aquatic species that are capable of breath-holding for long periods of time, minimal dosing with the injectable drug will usually shorten the induction period.

Green sea turtles (*Chelonia mydas*) have been anesthetized with pentobarbital, thiopental, or ketamine (Table 20F–1). Pentobarbital is satisfactory but causes prolonged recovery. Recovery from thiopental is more rapid, but anesthesia is erratic. Ketamine is satisfactory when given intraperitoneally.

Alphaxalone/alphadolone (Althesin) has been recommended as a preanesthetic prior to inhalation anesthesia in reptiles.(35) If administered intravenously, induction time is between 2 and 4 minutes, allowing for rapid tracheal intubation and administration of an inhalant anesthetic. In contrast, after intramuscular administration, induction may take up to 30 minutes.(27) The optimum dose in lizards and chelonians is 15 mg/kg IM to produce 15 to 30 minutes of anesthesia. Its action in snakes is more variable. Since relatively large volumes are required, multiple intramuscular injection sites may be necessary. Complete recovery after alphaxalone/alphadolone may require 2 to 4 hours.

Propofol is an ultra-short-acting hypnotic commonly used in human anesthesia. Its use is followed by a rapid induction time, minimal accumulation after repeated administrations, and rapid, excitement-free recoveries. Disadvantages include depression of the cardiovascular system and respiratory depression. Furthermore, its high cost may make prolonged anesthesia very expensive. In reptiles its major disadvantage is its requirement for intravenous administration. Since catheter placement is often difficult or even impossible in some species of reptiles, the use of propofol is limited to patients where venous access has been established. In these cases, propofol is certainly the induction agent of choice in chelonians.(7) A propofol dosage of 5–10 mg/kg IV will induce anesthesia in most chelonians. Further doses (1 mg/kg^{-1} · min^{-1}) of propofol may be given for short procedures where it is used as a maintenance agent.

Crocodilia. Although smaller crocodiles, up to 3 feet in length, may be handled and restrained manually with subsequent administration of an injectable agent, larger animals require experienced personnel and potent and reliable anesthetic drugs. Both alligators and crocodiles detoxify drugs slowly, predisposing them to prolonged recovery when anesthetized with injectable drugs. Pentobarbital has been given both orally and intraperitoneally to alligators and crocodiles. Alligators given tricaine methanesulfonate (MS-222) intramuscularly at the rate of 80.0 to 90.0 mg/kg are completely relaxed in 10 minutes, with recovery in 9 to 10 hours (Chapter 9).

Neuromuscular blocking agents have been used in American alligators and crocodiles to produce various degrees of immobilization.(25) Succinylcholine has been recommended for use in large tortoises and crocodilians either prior to inhalation anesthesia or in combination with other drugs to facilitate physical examination and sample collection. The use of succinylcholine alone has been recommended for transporting crocodilians.(19, 36) Following administration of neuromuscular blocking agents, one has to be prepared for paralysis of the respiratory musculature. Equipment for tracheal intubation and positive pressure ventilation should be available, especially when higher dosages are administered. When using neuromuscular blocking agents, it must be understood that the animal is only paralyzed and analgesia is absent. Therefore, painful procedures should not be performed.

Succinylcholine (3–5 mg/kg IM) produces immobilization in less than 4 minutes when given to alligators.(37) American crocodiles reportedly require 9.5 mg/kg IM for immobilization.(36) Diazepam (0.37 mg/kg IM) given prior to succinylcholine has been shown to greatly decrease the succinylcholine (0.24 mg/kg IM) dose requirement. Spontaneous respiration is maintained, but recovery may take up to 3 hours.(25) Gallamine can be given to crocodiles at a dose of 0.4–1.25 mg/kg IM to induce immobilization.(38–40) In large crocodilians either ketamine (12–15 mg/kg IM) or tiletamine/zolazepam (2–10 mg/kg IM) can be given, followed by tracheal intubation and maintenance of anesthesia with isoflurane. This regimen provides safe inductions and recoveries. Tracheal in tubation in the adequately sedated animal is achieved by using a mouth gag and manual placement of the endotracheal tube. Smaller specimens can be given Telazol or ketamine alone or with diazepam to achieve sedation prior to tracheal intubation (Chapter 11).

Etorphine HCl is a highly potent synthetic opioid that has been used extensively for capture and restraint of domestic and wild mammals (Chapters 9, 21, 22). Etorphine has also been used in reptiles with variable success. Most often it has been used for capture and restraint of large crocodilians.(41) Major disadvantages for its use include potential danger for the veterinarian and relatively high cost. It may not be possible to achieve a surgical plane of anesthesia with the use of etorphine alone, and the dose is much higher when compared to a mammal of similar body mass. The route of administration largely determines the dose necessary to achieve immobilization. Intraperitoneal administration results in shorter induction times than intramuscular injection, although the duration of anesthesia is similar. It appears that smaller crocodilians require a larger dose on a per weight basis of etorphine. Although American alligators receiving 0.5 to 1.5 mg/kg etorphine IM developed short-term analgesia; in caimans little or no analgesia was reported following a dose of 0.5 mg/kg IM.(42) In another study, a dose of 4.4 mg/kg was required to anesthetize a caiman. Induction time was 11 minutes, and the animal recovered after 45 minutes.(34)

Sauria. With the exception of larger monitors or poisonous species such as the Gila monster (*Heloderma suspectum*), it is relatively safe for an experienced handler to manually restrain most lizards. At present the green iguana is probably one of the most popular pet reptiles, and many can be manually restrained for diagnostic procedures such as blood sampling or radiographs. For the majority of animals, anesthetic agents have to be used to facilitate diagnostic and surgical procedures. Like the green iguana, many species are capable of holding their breath for long periods of time, making a mask induction without premedication a time-consuming experience. Consequently a low dose of ketamine followed by tracheal intubation and maintenance with isoflurane is preferred. The administration of a low dose of ketamine (5–10 mg/kg IM) will decrease the incidence of breath holding significantly. Also, placement of the animal in an induction chamber will more likely decrease the incidence of breath holding. Clinical experience indicates that butorphanol (1–1.5 mg/kg IM) administered 30 minutes prior to induction with isoflurane will provide smoother and shorter inductions and analgesia during surgery.

Serpentes. Although many injectables have been used in snakes, ketamine HCl, either alone or in combination with diazepam, is preferred for sedation. Although the use of these drugs may provide satisfactory sedation for diagnostic procedures, it is recommended that an inhalant be used for prolonged procedures or if a surgical plane of anesthesia is required. An injectable anesthetic regimen is less reliable, is less safe for the patient, and may result in a prolonged recovery. Inhalational anesthesia administered via an endotracheal tube secures the airway, provides the means for

Table 20F–2. **Recommended Doses of Ketamine HCl for Tranquilizing and Anesthetizing Snakes**

Doses (mg/kg)	Remarks
(A) 22 to 44	Dose usually effective for tranquilizing effect; used mainly in small (<2 kg) snakes and as the initial injection to test response to anesthesia; slight mobility is retained.
(B) 55 to 88	Dose required for most surgical procedures; effects last 1 to 3 days.
(C) 99 to 132	Total accumulative dose (mg/kg) recommended for snakes that do not reach depth of anesthesia required from doses (A) or (B). Effects last 2 to 6 days; at 132-mg/kg dose levels, respiratory-support measures may be required.

(From Glenn, J.L., Straight, R., and Snyder, C.C. Clinical Use of Ketamine Hydrochloride as an Anesthetic Agent for Snakes. Am J Vet Res 33:1901, 1972.)

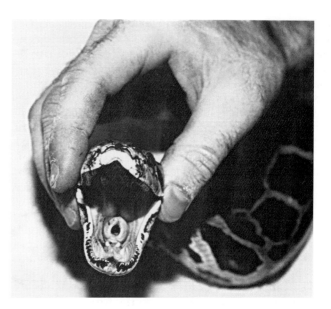

Fig. 20F–5. Glottis in a Burmese python (*Python molurus bivittatus*).

positive pressure ventilation, and will give more control over the depth and duration of anesthesia.

For a surgical plane of anesthesia a dose of 55 to 88 mg/kg ketamine HCl given intramuscularly has been recommended in snakes (Table 20F–2). For sedation, a dose of 22 to 44 mg/kg has been reported.(31-33) It is recommended that diazepam (0.2–0.8 mg/kg IM) or butorphanol (up to 1.5 mg/kg IM) be given to improve muscle relaxation. Induction times after ketamine administration may be up to 30 minutes. Complete recovery after administration of ketamine may take up to 4 days.

Several agents have been injected into the pleuroperitoneal cavity of snakes in the posterior third of the body on the ventral midline. Etorphine hydrochloride, thiopental sodium, and pentobarbital sodium have all been used. Thiopental and thiamylal administered intraperitoneally at doses of 2 to 6 mg/kg of body weight results in a very slow recovery (often requiring 48 to 72 hours) and a high mortality rate.

Metomidate is a nonbarbiturate that has been used for anesthesia in birds of prey as well as in domestic and nondomestic mammals. It reportedly is useful as a sedative in snakes to facilitate noninvasive diagnostic procedures.(8) It has a rapid onset of action even after intramuscular injection and results in profound sedation within 10 to 20 minutes. Metomidate has no analgesic properties and should only be used for sedation or as a preanesthetic prior to inhalation anesthesia.(3)

INHALATIONAL ANESTHESIA

The advantages of using inhalants include better controllability of anesthetic depth and a more rapid induction and recovery than are possible with injectable agents. Establishment of an airway allows for positive

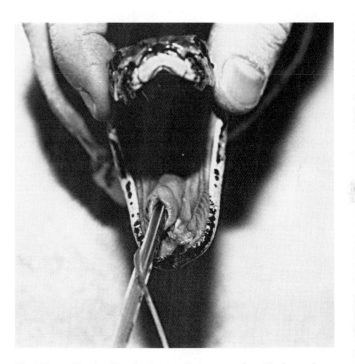

Fig. 20F–6. Tracheal intubation in a Burmese python (*Python molurus bivittatus*).

pressure ventilation and administration of oxygen. In most reptiles endotracheal intubation is easily achieved and can be performed either after a sedative dose of an injectable agent or after mask induction (Fig. 20F–5). In chelonians and crocodilians the tracheal rings are complete, and care should be taken not to overinflate the cuff, which may cause damage to the tracheal mucosa. A tight-fitting uncuffed tube may be more beneficial and safer. When intubating chelonians, care should be taken not to intubate one bronchus, since they have relatively short tracheas. Depending on the patient's size, commercially available endotracheal tubes (or in very small patients, an intravenous catheter) may be used (Fig. 20F–6). If endotracheal intubation is not performed and anesthesia is maintained via face mask, a clear plastic mask available for dogs and cats or syringe cases are recommended (Figs. 20F–7 and 20F–8).

When using inhalant anesthetics, the use of a precision vaporizer is recommended.(24) This will allow maintenance of long-term anesthesia more safely. In reptiles weighing less than 10 kg the use of a non-rebreathing system has the advantage of little resistance and minimal dead space.(2, 16) In small patients an oxygen flow rate of 300 to 500 $mL \cdot kg^{-1} \cdot min^{-1}$ is recommended. Since the normal respiratory rate of anesthetized reptiles is 2 to 4 breaths/minute, it is recommended that positive pressure ventilation also be set at a rate of 2 to 4 breaths/minute.(2) Breath holding is a common problem in reptiles, especially in

turtles and crocodiles. Increasing the anesthetic concentration in increments will tend to decrease breath holding, and the addition of nitrous oxide to the volatile anesthetic will often decrease induction times.(2, 16) Generally, when using a glass aquarium or induction chamber for inducing anesthesia in small or poisonous reptiles, the animal can be carefully removed from the chamber and intubated when it no longer is capable of righting itself when tipped onto its back.

Although in experienced hands, methoxyflurane and halothane are relatively safe for reptile anesthesia (43–45), isoflurane is the inhalant of choice. Methoxyflurane is a halogenated ether that is approximately twice as potent as halothane. Nevertheless, because of its high tissue solubility, it has the disadvantage of requiring longer induction and recovery times. Its use has been associated with the death of cobras.(46)

Halothane, a fluorinated hydrocarbon, is more insoluble and thus more rapid acting than methoxyflu-

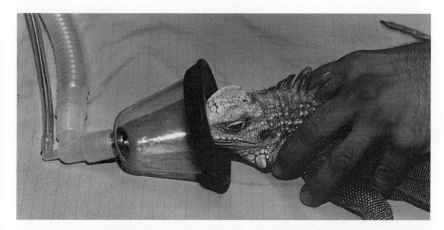

Fig. 20F–7. Mask induction of a green iguana (*Iguana iguana*). A suitable face mask may also be constructed from an empty syringe case.

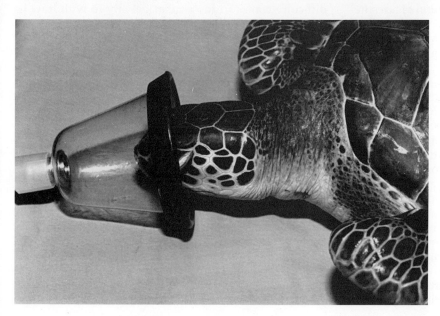

Fig. 20F–8. Mask induction of a green sea turtle (*Chelonia mydas*).

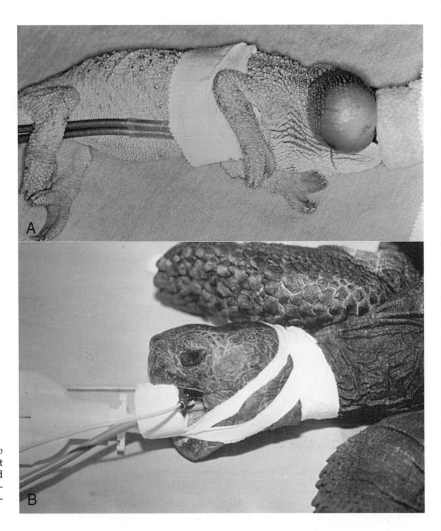

Fig. 20F–9. Jackson's chameleon (*Chameleo jacksoni*) with Doppler flow probe positioned at the level of the heart to monitor cardiac rate and rhythm (A). Galapagos tortoise (*Geochelone elephantopus*) after tracheal intubation and placement of an esophageal ECG (B).

rane.(24) Like methoxyflurane and isoflurane, it produces moderate muscle relaxation and dose-dependent cardiopulmonary depression. For induction of anesthesia of most reptiles a concentration of 3 to 5% in O_2 is used and may require 20 to 30 minutes. Maintenance of anesthesia is usually accomplished with a concentration of 1.5 to 2.5%.(2)

Isoflurane has anesthetic properties similar to halothane but has fewer depressant effects on cardiac output than other inhalational agents. In debilitated metabolically compromised reptiles, isoflurane is the anesthetic agent of choice. Because induction and recovery are more rapid than with other inhalation agents, it is often used alone. For induction in a chamber or by mask, concentrations between 3 and 5% are required. It is interesting that, in one report, snapping turtles administered 5% isoflurane over a period of 90 minutes were not satisfactorily anesthetized (likely due to breath holding).(26) In contrast, a rhino iguana induced with 4 to 5% isoflurane became anesthetized in 6 minutes, and recovery was considered complete after 1 hour.(47) Anesthesia was safely maintained with an isoflurane concentration of 1 to 2.5% in O_2.(47) It is

possible to anesthetize the turtle or tortoise using the face mask as the sole means of administration. The difficulty comes in the animal's ability to withdraw its head into the safety of its shell. Box turtles and several other varieties are capable of enclosing the soft portions of their bodies within the carapace and plastron, making the mask method unusable. Another alternative is to open the mouth manually and spray the larynx with topical anesthetic, after which a wooden dowel with a hole through it is positioned crosswise in the mouth and an endotracheal tube is inserted.

HYPOTHERMIA

Deliberate cooling below a reptile's optimum minimal external temperature has been mentioned as a useful means of reptilian restraint.(7, 16) However, rapid cooling will not provide analgesia and may be painful and stressful. Since reptiles are poikilothermic animals, cooling reduces the patient's metabolism.(3, 17, 48) Lower temperatures have been associated with necrotic changes in the brain of snakes and tortoises.(2) The use of body cooling as a substitute for anesthesia in reptiles is inappropriate. At present, safer and more humane anesthetic methods are available for diagnostic and surgical procedures. Placing an animal on a heating blanket set at the reptile's optimal external temperature is helpful in preventing rapid body cooling during and following anesthesia.

MONITORING

Monitoring the anesthetized reptile is critical to the successful outcome of anesthesia. Familiar reflexes are of limited value, and invasive means of monitoring, such as placement of an arterial catheter for direct blood pressure measurements, are limited to experimental conditions. Heart rate and rhythm, as well as respiratory rate should be monitored. An esophageal stethoscope or placement of a doppler flow probe at the level of the heart will facilitate cardiac monitoring (Figs. 20F–9A and B). Monitoring respiratory rate may be difficult in some reptiles, especially in snakes.(15) In most lizards, movement of the intercostal musculature is easier to observe.(15) In turtles, the tonus of the head, neck, and limbs can be used to judge the depth of anesthesia. Respiratory movements can be observed as alternating concavity and convexity of the skin adjacent to the limbs and tail. With such rudimentary methods to determine depth of anesthesia, close and frequent examination of the subject is necessary. ECG leads may be placed in reptiles in the conventional fashion (Fig. 20F–10).(49) Leads can be connected to hypodermic needles or alligator clips to improve lead contact. The heart is usually located after the first third to quarter of the body length in snakes.

The presence or absence of reflexes has been described as a useful way to monitor anesthetic depth in reptiles. The righting reflex, or the ability to turn over when placed in dorsal recumbency, is lost in relatively light planes of anesthesia.(16, 31, 50) Its presence or absence is most useful during the recovery period. In snakes not fully anesthetized, touching the muscles firmly along the vertebral column produces a spastic reaction. In snakes and some lizards the tongue withdrawal reflex should still be present in a surgical plane of anesthesia.(50) The patient is too deep if this reflex is absent. There is an obvious dilation of the pupils in deep surgical anesthesia. In chelonians the head withdrawal reflex is helpful.(16, 20)

Several definitions have been used to describe the anesthetic period of reptiles. Most useful are those given by R.A. Bennett. *Induction time* is the time between administration of the anesthetic agent and loss of the righting reflex.(51) *Total anesthesia time* is the time between the loss and the return of the righting reflex. A *surgical plane of anesthesia* is defined by the loss of the tail and foot withdrawal reflex, and *recovery time* is the time between the return of the righting reflex to the return of the preanesthetic state.(51)

ANALGESIA

At present, information about the uses and effects of analgesic agents in reptilian medicine is scant. Every animal is capable of feeling pain. Although it is sometimes difficult to assess and evaluate pain in the reptilian patient, there is no reason to believe that the lack of more familiar responses to pain such as vocalization and so forth is equivalent with no pain sensation. Routine administration of analgesics to any reptile that undergoes invasive or painful surgery is recommended. Although no information is available on drugs and doses, the higher end of the dose range recommended for mammalian species is commonly used. Sedation as well as pain-free behavior has been observed after administration of butorphanol to tortoises, turtles, and iguanas. A dose of 0.4 mg/kg to 1 mg/kg given intramuscularly appears beneficial. In addition, analgesic agents given pre- or intraoperatively will

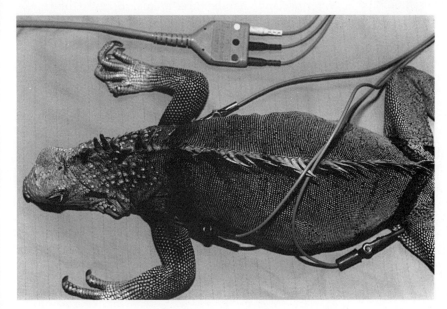

Fig. 20F–10. Green iguana with ECG leads placed in a conventional configuration.

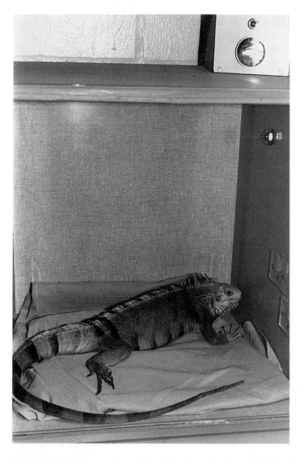

Fig. 20F–11. Recovery of a green iguana in an incubator after isoflurane anesthesia.

reduce the amount of anesthetic required to maintain surgical anesthesia.

RECOVERY

During the postoperative period, ectotherms should be placed in an incubator at a temperature and relative humidity within the optimal range for the species (Fig. 20F–11).(19) Recovery times in reptiles tend to be longer than those of birds and mammals.(3) Because drug metabolism and elimination is temperature dependent, some authors recommend placing the reptile at temperatures higher than 30° C to shorten recovery. This is not generally recommended, however. Most reptiles will be in a state of respiratory depression during the recovery period.(15, 50) Respiration should be carefully monitored especially after administration of ketamine or tiletamine/zolazepam. If necessary, ventilation should be assisted until the animal is capable of breathing spontaneously. When using inhalants in snakes, recovery may be hastened by gentle evacuation of the lungs. This is accomplished by a milking action of the hand drawn from the cloacal end of the snake toward the head. Prior to extubation, spontaneous ventilation should be observed. The administration of doxapram (0.2–0.6 mL/kg IV or IM) will stimulate breathing in most reptiles. Return of the righting reflex is the most useful indicator of recovery. To prevent drowning, aquatic species such as marine turtles should only be placed in deep water once recovery is complete.(37, 52)

Amphibians

INTRODUCTION

Only a limited number of anesthetic agents have been used in amphibians. Information about pharmacologic data of anesthetic agents and their effect on cardiopulmonary function is scant. For more detailed information on amphibian medicine and husbandry, the interested reader is referred to several excellent publications.(53-55)

ANATOMY AND PHYSIOLOGY

The class *amphibia* consists of three orders, representing over 4000 species. The order *gymnophiona* represents over 160 species, which are wormlike burrowers and rarely found in captivity. The order *caudata* includes about 350 species of salamanders, and the order *anura* is represented by over 3000 species of frogs and toads. The majority of amphibians found in captivity are in this order. Amphibians may range in weight from only a few grams to over 2 kg.

Amphibians are aquatic animals that will spend at least the reproductive phase of their lives in an aquatic environment. They have adapted to a wide diversity of habitat and can be found in aquatic, tropical, or desertlike climates. One adaptation to their lives in the water is the development of skin glands for protection of the skin. The secretions from these glands prevent the animal from desiccation and protect it from microorganisms. They also function to discourage predators. Especially in the case of toads, secretions from the parotid glands have repulsive effects on potential predators. Skin secretions make it difficult for the veterinarian to handle these animals because they make the body slippery. The secretions may act as an irritant to the handler's skin and damage to the film of secretions on the amphibian's skin may predispose the animal to infections. Additionally, the skin of some amphibians serves as a supplemental respiratory organ. Amphibians are highly sensitive to changes in humidity and may rapidly dehydrate.

PHYSICAL EXAMINATION

In order to appreciate changes from normal appearance, body condition, and behavior, knowledge of "normal" is a prerequisite. The animal's reflexes, such as the righting reflex, and postural changes should be assessed. A sick amphibian often has changes in skin color and may appear congested. Ascites, indicating infectious disease processes, and osmotic imbalances are commonly seen. The general body condition should be critically assessed based on abdominal contents, visibility of the skeleton, and musculature. Fecal examination is recommended to assess parasite infestation. The use of antiparasitic agents may be beneficial prior to anesthesia. In general, every effort should be made to improve the health status of the animal prior to anesthesia.

PHYSICAL RESTRAINT

Most amphibians can be handled manually for transfer and physical examination. In order to protect their sensitive skin, it is recommended that hands be moistened when handling aquatic species. A wet paper towel also serves well. The restraint period should be kept as brief as possible. Almost all frogs and toads secrete a venom from their glands. Gloves should be worn and contact with the eyes avoided. A few species secrete a poison, which in the case of the arrow-poison frog is highly toxic. Although smaller species rarely bite, larger individuals, especially large toads, are capable of inflicting a painful bite. In general toads are less slippery than frogs and may be restrained by supporting the body and holding on to the hind limbs.

ANESTHESIA

Although radiographs can be taken with the animal awake and placed in a box to prevent it from moving, procedures such as biopsies or removal of foreign bodies require sedation or general anesthesia. Anesthetic variables are evaluated by the loss of the righting reflex, loss of reflexes to pain (toe pinch), and respiratory rate and pattern. Although at a surgical plane of anesthesia the ventilation rate will often be greatly depressed, cutaneous respiration will provide sufficient oxygenation. One can take advantage of the amphibian's ability of cutaneous fluid absorption by immersion of the animal in a solution of anesthetic agent. Although information about pain sensation of amphibians is scant, it should be assumed that they are sensitive to pain. Like reptiles, amphibians require an optimum temperature for proper metabolism and function of various organ systems. Before anesthetizing the amphibian patient, it should be kept in its optimum temperature range to reduce stress and metabolic compromise.

Local anesthesia. Although not commonly reported in the literature, local anesthesia is a safe and effective method for certain procedures. Two percent lidocaine in combination with ketamine HCl for minor surgical procedures such as removal of subcutaneous abscesses or amputation of digits is effective. A combination of local anesthetic with a parenteral anesthetic offers the advantage of reduced dosage requirements for each drug. As an analgesic, butorphanol at a dosage of 0.2 to 0.4 mg/kg given intramuscularly has been used with good success.

Parenteral anesthesia. The use of parasympatholytic agents such as atropine or glycopyrrolate to reduce secretions has not been reported and is not routinely used in amphibians. One of the more commonly used amphibian anesthetics is tricaine methanesulfonate (MS-222) (Chapter 21). This drug may be administered to frogs, salamanders, newts, and mudpuppies by bath or through injection. In frogs and toads, injections can be given in the dorsal lymph sac. The dorsal lymph sacs are paired organs located on either side of the last vertebra. Location of these paired lymph hearts can be determined by observation of their rhythmic beating. In an adult leopard frog, 2 to 3 mL of anesthetic can be injected at one time into these sacs. Anesthesia can be maintained by keeping the animal partially submerged in the bath and taking advantage of its capability of cutaneous uptake of the drug. When using a bath, a 0.1 to 0.3% solution should be prepared. Induction time may take up to 30 minutes and recovery up to 24 hours. Benzocaine has also been used in a bath by some investigators and may be superior to MS-222.

In leopard frogs, pentobarbital has been used at a dose of 40 to 50 mg/kg administered into the dorsal lymph sac or intraperitoneally. Induction is prolonged (approximately 30 minutes), anesthesia may last 9 hours, and recovery may require up to 24 hours. The combination of ketamine (20–40 mg/kg IM) and diazepam (0.2–0.4 mg/kg IM) has been used with variable success. Although in some animals adequate anesthesia to perform surgical procedures was achieved, others required additional inhalant anesthetic. Tiletamine/zolazepam (10 to 20 mg/kg) given intramuscularly produces variable states of tranquilization or anesthesia in leopard frogs and bullfrogs. A dose of 50 mg/kg induces anesthesia consistently in bullfrogs but results in some mortalities. This same dose is uniformly fatal in leopard frogs.(56) Sites for intramuscular injection of drugs are the muscles of the front and hind limbs. In

Table 20F–3. Data for Methoxyflurane Anesthesia in *Rana pipiens* (Acclimatized to 21° C)*

Number Frogs (and Sex)	Body Weight (g)	Induction Time (min) for Deep Anesthesia (mean ± SD)	Duration (min) of Deep Anesthesia (mean ± SD)	Time (h) for Full Recovery† (mean ± SD)
15 (male)	48–98	2.0 ± 0.1	37.9 ± 21.1	7 ± 0.5
15 (female)	69–101	2.0 ± 0.2	38.7 ± 20.5	7 ± 0.4

*All data are bound to the ambient temperature, in frogs as in other ectotherms.

†Recovery time is the time from the end of the period of deep anesthesia to the time that such processes as righting reflexes, sensation, and locomotion are reestablished.

(From Wass, J.A., and Kaplan, H.M. Methoxyflurane Anesthesia for *Rana pipiens.* Lab Anim Sci 24:669, 1974.)

frogs and toads injections can be given into the dorsal lymph sac.

Inhalational anesthesia. In the laboratory setting, methoxyflurane-soaked cotton in a semiclosed jar has been used to produce anesthesia in frogs (Table 20F–3). Following a brief period of excitement, deep anesthesia occurs in approximately 2 minutes. This technique, although inexpensive, is fraught with danger of overdose and is discouraged. Presently, the inhalant of choice for amphibians is isoflurane because it provides a more rapid induction and recovery. Induction of anesthesia is usually achieved with an induction chamber. With concentrations of 3 to 5%, loss of the righting reflex may take up to 30 minutes. Anesthesia is maintained with 1 to 2% isoflurane. Tracheal intubation is easily accomplished by the use of a 2-mm uncuffed endotracheal tube or in smaller species by the use of plastic catheters connected to the anesthetic circuit. In frogs and toads, the tracheal opening is positioned at the base of the tongue. During recovery, amphibians should be kept moist over their entire body and in a warm environment. As with aquatic species of reptiles, in order to prevent drowning, care must be taken that terrestrial species of amphibians do not become completely immersed until recovery is complete.

References

1. Northway RB. Electroanesthesia of green iguanas (*Iguana iguana*). J Am Vet Med Assoc 155:1034, 1969.
2. Bennett RA. A review of anesthesia and chemical restraint in reptiles. J Zoo Wildl Med 22(3):282–303, 1991.
3. Burke TJ. Reptile anesthesia. In: Fowler ME, ed. Zoo and wild animal medicine. Philadelphia: WB Saunders, 1986:153–155.
4. Fowler ME. Reptiles. In: Fowler ME, ed. Restraint and handling of wild and domestic animals. Ames, IA: Iowa State University Press, 1978:286–310.
5. Frank W. Lokalanaesthesie, Sedation, Narkose, Euthanasie. In: Isenbuegel E, Frank W, eds. Heimtierkrankheiten. Stuttgart: Verlag Eugen Ulmer, 1985:187–194.
6. Jackson OF, Cooper JE. Anesthesia and surgery. In: Cooper JE, Jackson OF, eds. Diseases of the reptilia, vol. 2. New York: Academic Press, 1981:535–549.
7. Kaplan HM. Anesthesia in amphibians and reptiles. Fed Proc 28:1541–1546, 1969.
8. Lawton MPC. Anaesthesia. In: Beynon PH, ed. Manual of reptiles. Gloucestershire, England: Br Small Anim Vet Assoc, 1992:170–183.
9. Schildger BJR, Baumgartner W, Haefeli A, Ruebel E. Isenbuegel Narkose und Immobilisation bei Reptilien. Tierarztl Prax :361–376, 1993.
10. Sedgewick CJ. Anesthesia of reptiles. In: Kirk RW, ed. Current veterinary therapy, 7th ed. Philadelphia: WB Saunders, 1980: 618–620.
11. Sedgewick CJ. Anesthesia for reptiles. In: Paddleford RR, ed. Manual of small animal anesthesia. New York: Churchill Livingstone, 1988:309–321.
12. Wallach JD. Anesthesia of reptiles. In: Kirk RW, ed. Current veterinary therapy, 6th ed. Philadelphia: WB Saunders, 1977: 807–808.
13. Davies PMC. Anatomy and physiology. In: Cooper JE, Jackson OF, eds. Diseases of the reptilia, vol. 1. New York: Academic Press, 1981:9–73.
14. Wood SC, Lenfant CJM. Respiration: mechanics, control and gas exchange. In: Gans C, Dawson WR, eds. Biology of the reptilia. New York: Academic Press, 1976:223–274.
15. Brazenor CW, Kaye G. Anesthesia for reptiles. Copeia 3:165, 1953.
16. Calderwood HW. Anesthesia for reptiles. J Am Vet Med Assoc 159:1618–1625, 1971.
17. Millichamp NJ. Surgical techniques in reptiles. In: Jacobson ER, Kollias GV, eds. Exotic animals. New York: Churchill Livingstone, 1988:49–59.
18. Lillywhite HB. Behavioral control of arterial pressure in snakes. Physiol Zoo 58:159–165, 1985.
19. Messel H, Stephens R. Drug immobilization of crocodiles. J Wildl Managm 44:295–296, 1980.
20. Brannian RE, Kirk C, Williams D. Anesthetic induction of kinosternid turtles with halothane. J Zoo Anim Med 18:115–117, 1987.
21. Jacobson ER. The evaluation of the reptilian patient. In: Jacobson ER, Kollias GV, eds. Exotic animals. New York: Churchill Livingstone, 1988.
22. Lillywhite HB, Pough FH. Control of arterial pressure in aquatic sea snakes. Am J Physiol 244:R66–73, 1983.
23. Lillywhite HB. Circulatory adaptations of snakes to gravity. Am Zoo 27:81–95, 1987.
24. Hall LW, Clarke KW. Veterinary anesthesia. London: Balliere Tindall, 1991.
25. Spiegel RA, Lane TJ, Larsen RE, Cardeilhac PT. Diazepam and succinylcholine chloride for restraint of the American alligator. J Am Vet Med Assoc 185:1335–1336, 1984.
26. Bienzle D, Boyd CJ. Sedative effects of ketamine and midazolam in Snapping turtles. J Zoo Anim Med 23(2):201–204, 1992.
27. Lawrence K, Jackson OF. Alphaxalone/alphadolone acetate anesthesia in reptiles. Vet Rec 8:26–28, 1983.
28. Bush M, Smeller JM. Blood collection and injection techniques in snakes. Vet Med Small Anim Clin 73:211–214, 1978.
29. Harper RC. Anesthetizing reptiles. Vet Rec 115:475–476, 1984.
30. Boever WJ, Caputo F. Telazol (Cl 744) as an anesthetic agent in reptiles. J Zoo Anim Med 13(2):59–61, 1982.
31. Cooper JE. Ketamine hydrochloride as an anesthetic for East African reptiles. Vet Rec 95:37–41, 1974.
32. Glenn JR Straight R, Snyder CC. Clinical use of ketamine hydrochloride as an anesthetic agent for snakes. Am J Vet Res 33:1901–1903, 1972.
33. Jones DM. The sedation and anesthesia of birds and reptiles. Vet Rec 101:340–342, 1977.
34. Wallach JD, Hoessle C. M-99 as an immobilizing agent in poikilothermes. Vet Med Small Anim Clin 65:163–167, 1970.
35. Calderwood HW, Jacobson ER. Preliminary report on the use of saffan on reptiles. Proc Annu Mtg Am Assoc Zoo Vet, Denver, Colorado, 1979:23–26.
36. Klide AM, Klein LV. Chemical restraint of three reptilian species. J Zoo Anim Med 4(1):8–11, 1973.
37. Brisbin IL. Reactions of the American alligator to several immobilizing drugs. Copeia 1:129–130, 1966.
38. Loveridge JP. The immobilization and anesthesia of crocodilians. Int Zoo Yearbook 19:103–112, 1979.
39. Loveridge JP, Black DK. Techniques in the immobilization and handling of the Nile crocodile, *Crocodylus niloticus*. Amoldia (Rhod.) 5:1–14, 1972.
40. Morgan-Davies AM. Immobilization of the Nile crocodile (*Crocodylus niloticus*) with gallamine triethiodide. J Zoo Anim Med 11:85–87, 1980.
41. Jacobson ER. Immobilization, blood sampling, necropsy techniques and diseases of crocodilians: a review. J Zoo Anim Med 15:38–4527, 1984.
42. Hinsch H, Gandal CP. The effects of etorphine (M-99), oxymorphone hydrochloride and meperidine hydrochloride in reptiles. Copeia 2:404–405, 1969.
43. Bonath K. Halothane inhalation anesthesia in reptiles and its clinical control. Int Zoo Yearbook 19:112–115, 1979.
44. Gandal CP. A practical anesthetic technique in snakes utilizing methoxyflurane. J Am Anim Hosp Assoc 4:258–260, 1968.
45. Hackenbrock CR, Finster M. Fluothane: a rapid and safe inhalation anesthetic for poisonous snakes. Copeia 2:440–441, 1963.

46. Burke TJ, Wall BE. Anesthetic deaths in cobras (*Naja naja* and *Ophiophagus hannah*) with methoxyflurane. J Am Vet Med Assoc 157(5):620–621, 1970.

47. Faggella AM, Raffe MR. The use of isoflurane anesthesia in a water monitor lizard and a rhino iguana. Compend Anim Pract 1(2):52–53, 1987.

48. Terpin KM, Dodson P. Observations on ketamine hydrochloride as an anesthetic for alligators. Copeia 1:147–148, 1978.

49. Crane SW, Curtis M, Jacobson ER, Webb A. Neutralization bone-plating repair of a fractured humerus in an Aldabra tortoise. J Am Vet Med Assoc 177:945–948, 1980.

50. Betz TW. Surgical anesthesia in reptiles, with special reference to the water snake, *Natrix rhombifera*. Copeia 2:284–287, 1962.

51. Custer RS, Bush M. Physiologic and acid-base measures of gopher snakes during ketamine or halothane-nitrous oxide anesthesia. J Am Vet Med Assoc 177:870–874, 1980.

52. Wood FE, Critchley H, Wood JR. Anesthesia in the green sea turtle, *Chelonia mydas*. Am J Vet Res 43:1882–1883, 1982.

53. Crawshaw GJ. Amphibian medicine. In: Fowler ME, ed. Zoo and wild animal medicine. Philadelphia: WB Saunders, 1993:131–139.

54. Fowler ME. Amphibians and fish. In: Restraint and handling of wild and domestic animals. Ames, IA: Iowa State University Press, 1978:311–316.

55. Raphael BL. Amphibians. Vet Clin North Am Exotic Pet Med 23(6):1271–1286, 1993.

56. Letcher J, Durante R. Evaluation of use of tiletamine/zolazepam for anesthesia of bullfrogs and leopard frogs. J Am Vet Med Assoc 207:80–82, 1995.

chapter 21

ANESTHESIA OF WILD, EXOTIC, AND LABORATORY ANIMALS

Introduction

Veterinarians are frequently called upon to anesthetize a wide variety of mammals, birds, reptiles, and fish. Some species of mammals, such as rabbits, rats, and mice, have been used through the years to assess anesthetics, and a large amount of data is available concerning anesthesia in these species. Others have been anesthetized rarely if at all, and specific information on the effects of anesthetics and methods of achieving anesthesia is minimal. For additional information on anesthesia, restraint, and handling of wild and exotic animals, the reader is referred to additional texts.(1-4) Because restraint and control of wild and exotic species of ruminants, odd-toed hoofed mammals (Perissodactyla), procyonids, ursids, felids, canids, elephants, hippopotamus, sea mammals, and marsupials within modern zoologic parks and wildlife refuges require techniques similar to those used for capture and immobilization of free-ranging mammals, the reader is also referred to the text and tables in Chapters 10 and 22 for information on various drug combinations and capture techniques. In general, anesthesia for longer

Table 21–1. Recommended Concentrations and Actions of Drugs for Anesthetizing Fish

Anesthetic	Concentration*	Anesthetic Qualities		
		Induction Time, min	Maintenance	Recovery Time, min
Carbon dioxide	200 ppm	1–2	Good	5–10
Electricity		Immediate	Poor	5–30
Diethyl ether	10–50 mL	2–3	Fair	5–30
Secobarbital	35 mg	30–60	Good	60+
Amobarbital	7–10 mg	30–60	Good	60+
Urethan	5–40 mg	2–3	Good	10–15
Chloral hydrate	0.8–0.9 g	8–10	Poor	20–30
Tertiary amyl alcohol	0.5–1.25 mL	10–20	Fair	20–90
Tribromoethanol	4–6 mg	5–10	Fair	20–40
Chlorobutanol	8–10 mg	2–3	Good	30–60
2-Phenoxyethanol	0.1–0.5 mL	10–30	Fair	5–15
4-Styrylpyridine	20–50 mg	1–5	Good	20–30
Methyl pentynol	0.5–0.9 mL	2–3	Fair	5–20
Quinaldine	0.01–0.03 mL	1–3	Fair	5–20
Tricaine methanesul-fonate (MS-222)	25–100 mg	1–3	Excellent	3–15

*Expressed as milligrams or milliliters per liter of water unless otherwise noted.
(From McFarland, W.N., and Klontz, G.W. Anesthesia in Fishes. Fed Proc 28:1535, 1969.)

surgical procedures can be achieved with inhalant anesthetics delivered via modified large animal anesthetic machines and rebreathing systems (Chapter 14).

Crustaceans

The optimal effective concentration of tricaine methanesulfonate (MS-222) for two species of amphipods has been reported as 0.5 g/L.(5) Induction usually requires 25 minutes. Duration of anesthesia up to 2 hours does not prolong the recovery period. During anesthesia of gravid females, there may be premature release of eggs or young from the brood pouch. The effective dose of MS-222 in amphipods is quite high when compared with that for fish.

In aerated seawater at 10° C isobutyl alcohol is nontoxic to lobsters (*Homarus americanus*) at a concentration of 15 mL/L and can be effective at doses as small as 0.5 mL/L.(6) With lower concentrations induction is slowed. For routine use, concentrations between 1.5 and 7.0 mL/L are recommended. On immersion in the anesthetic solution, lobsters become agitated and gradually lose control of chelae and walking legs, which then become tangled and stiffened in an upright position. Once anesthetized, lobsters can be exposed to air and manipulated for at least 10 minutes before any response is noted. They can be out of water for periods of 1 hour after being anesthetized if then returned to seawater.

Fish

A large number of anesthetics have been used to anesthetize fish, a partial listing of which is shown in Table 21–1. Fish are affected by abrupt variations in

Table 21–2. Behavioral Changes in Fish at Various Levels of Anesthesia

	Stage	
Normal		Reactive to external stimuli; muscle tone normal
Light sedation	1	Slight loss of reactivity to external visual and tactile stimuli; equilibrium normal
Deep sedation	2	Total loss of reactivity to external stimuli except strong pressure; slight decrease in opercular rate; equilibrium normal
Partial loss of equilibrium	3	Partial loss of muscle tone; swimming erratic; increased opercular rate; reactive only to strong tactile and vibrational stimuli
Total loss of equilibrium	4	Total loss of muscle tone and equilibrium; rapid opercular rate (slow with some agents), reactivity only to deep pressure stimuli
Loss of reflex reactivity	5	Total loss of reactivity; opercular movements very shallow; heart rate very slow
Medullary collapse	6	Opercular movements cease immediately after gasping, followed by cardiac arrest

(From McFarland, W.N., and Klontz, G.W. Anesthesia in Fishes. Fed Proc 28:4, 1969.)

water temperature, pH, and mineral content. Therefore, water in which the fish is living is preferable for making anesthetic solutions. The degree of sedation and anesthesia is judged according to the criteria in Table 21–2. Squeezing the muscle at the base of the tail is a good test for anesthesia. The response should be diminished but not absent.

For handling fingerling trout for fin-clipping, ether anesthesia increases efficiency markedly. A 1% aqueous solution can be placed in a basin and additional ether added as required; thus, the eventual concentration that produces anesthesia can vary considerably.(7) Methyl pentynol is a liquid with an acrid odor and was once popular as a fish anesthetic. It is dissolved in water at the rate of 0.5 to 0.9 mL/L of water. Induction requires 2 to 3 minutes and recovery 5 to 20 minutes. Respiratory arrest tends to develop in deep anesthesia, making maintenance difficult.(8) Quinaldine is a water-insoluble, colorless, oily liquid that turns reddish brown when exposed to air. It can be dissolved in acetone for subsequent addition to water. The dose is 0.01 to 0.03 mL/L of water. Anesthetic induction requires 1 to 3 minutes, with recovery in 5 to 20 minutes. It may be used over a wide range of temperatures. Four-styrylpyridine is a fine white powder freely soluble in water. The dose for fish is 20 to 25 mg/L of water. This is one of the few fish anesthetics that is completely safe for handling by humans. Induction requires 1 to 5 minutes, with recovery in 20 to 30 minutes. Two-phenoxyethanol is an oily liquid with both anesthetic capability and chemotherapeutic properties against fish bacterial infections. The dose is 0.1 to 0.5 mL/L of water. Induction requires 10 to 30 minutes with recovery in 5 to 10 minutes.

Tricaine methanesulfonate has been approved by the Food and Drug Administration as a sedative-anesthetic for fish, providing they are not used as food for 21 days. The drug does not affect palatability. When anesthetizing most common fishes (teleosts), concentrations of 0.5 to 1.0 g/gal of fresh water are used while the water temperature is maintained between 40 to 60° F. Induction time varies depending on concentration and the period of exposure to the solution. The fish is immersed until it becomes immobilized, at which time it can be removed for examination, treatment, or surgery. While the fish is exposed to air, provision should be made to keep it wet. For longer anesthesia, the fish can be

reimmersed or the gills sprayed with solution. Repeated use tends to reduce the concentration of MS-222 in the solution. For best results a fresh solution should be used. Bluegill, bass, trout, and salmon have been anesthetized in concentrations of 1:3000 to 1:25,000 for weighing, tagging, and spawn collection, with anesthesia varying in duration from 3 minutes to several hours, depending again on concentration and immersion time. For large numbers of fish, a closed recirculating system may be advantageous.(9)

Tricaine methanesulfonate anesthesia has been used when transporting fish without water.(10) A dilution of 0.25 g/gal with water temperature of 5° C is used. When the fish turn over in the water, they are allowed to remain 8 minutes, at which time they are transferred to tanks containing layers of moss and chipped ice. Fish so anesthetized can be held for 4 to 4½ hours with a mortality of approximately 10%.

Treatment of fungal infections and other localized diseases in pet or ornamental fish can be performed following tricaine methanesulfonate anesthesia. For "tranquilization" of pet or ornamental fish for transportation, low concentrations are used. Depending upon the species of fish, size of container, and presence or absence of oxygen, doses ranging from 0.14 to 0.32 g/gal have been used (Table 21–3).(11) A recent report described pneumocystectomy in a fish (Midas cichlid) to correct a distended abdomen and inadequate buoyancy control. Anesthesia was induced by immersing the fish in an aqueous solution containing 100 mg of tricaine methanesulfonate/L for 6 minutes. An additional 50 mg of tricaine methanesulfonate/L of water was added to the aquarium, and after 2 minutes the fish had only mild opercular movements. While the opercula were moving, the movement was not sufficient to generate the water flow across the gills. After induction of anesthesia the fish was placed in dorsal recumbency in a V-shaped foam trough, and delivery tubes were placed in its mouth. Anesthesia was maintained with tricaine methanesulfonate (60 mg/L) at a constant flow rate of 2 L/min. Total duration of anesthesia was 71 minutes (Fig. 21–1).(12)

Large fish, such as sharks and rays, cannot be conveniently immersed in a solution. However, large fish have been anesthetized while hooked.(13) Tricaine in a concentration of 1:1000 (1 g/L of seawater) is used. The head of the fish is held above the water level by

Table 21–3. Dose of Tricaine Methanesulfonate for Ornamental Fish

Variety of Fish	Concentration	Anesthesia Time
Tropicals at 75 to 80° F:		
Live bearers	0.32 g per gal	to 12 h, uncrowded
Egglayers	0.24 g per gal	to 12 h, uncrowded
For uncrowded shipment of pugnacious species, without oxygen:		
Bettas, piranhas	0.25 g per gal	to 48 h
For goldfish, with oxygen:		
Goldfish variety	0.14 g per gal	to 48 h

(From Gossington, R.E. An Aid to Fish Handling—Tricaine. Aquarium J 28:318, 1957.)

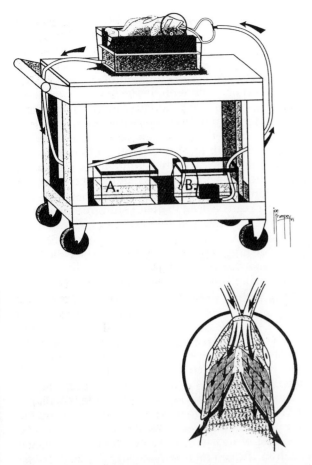

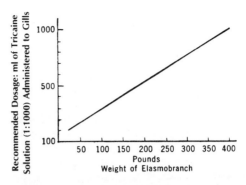

Fig. 21–2. Dose of tricaine solution (1 : 1000 concentration) recommended to anesthetize a shark or ray in 60 seconds or less. The solution should be sprayed over the gill exits of the pharynx while the head of the elasmobranch is held above the water level. If the head remains underwater, proportionally stronger concentration must be utilized. (From Gilbert, P.W., and Wood, F.G., Jr. Method of Anesthetizing Large Sharks and Rays Safely and Rapidly. Science 126:212, 1957.)

Fig. 21–1. (Top) Illustration of the anesthetic machine with submersible pump in tank B, which contains the anesthetic, and tank A, which is not in the recirculating system, but could be quickly used by removing the pump from tank B and placing it in tank A. Arrows indicate water flow, which is controlled by regulating the diameter of the outflow tube that drains the operating area. (Right) Illustration of how the water enters the mouth and is directed over the gills located deep to the opercula (gill plates). (From Lewbart, G.A., Stone, E.A., and Love, N. Pneumocystectomy in a Midas Cichlid. J Am Vet Med Assoc 207:319–321, 1995.)

means of a gaff or leader, whereas smaller fish may be temporarily removed from the water. By means of a water pistol, rubber bulb syringe, or small hand pump, the solution is introduced into the mouths of fish or the spiracles of rays and sprayed over the gill exits of the pharynx. Small species require approximately 100 mL and larger fish up to 1 L of solution. The action of the drug is quite rapid, 15 seconds being required for a visible effect to take place. A 400-pound shark may be anesthetized in 1 minute or less. The fish may then be manipulated either in or out of the water until recovery begins to take place. If additional anesthesia is required, more solution may be given. Recovery may be hastened by washing the gills with fresh seawater. This can be accomplished with large fish by "walking" the fish in a pool with its mouth open or by spraying a stream of fresh seawater into the mouth. Recovery usually begins to take place within 5 to 30 minutes after the fish is

returned to the water. The time elapsing before loss of muscular activity appears to be directly proportional to the concentration of drug used. Figure 21–2 shows the suggested dose for sharks. The effect of a given concentration varies inversely with the size of the fish. An increase in toxicity has been observed and correlated with a marked rise in temperature of the immersing solution.

Benzocaine (ethyl ester of paraaminobenzoic acid) is insoluble in water but can be dissolved in acetone (40 mg/mL) to be used as an anesthetic for fish. Sufficient immobilization for tagging, marking, and measuring is produced by 20 to 30 ppm (5 mL in 8 L of salt or fresh water), whereas 50 ppm induces surgical anesthesia.(3) Propoxate hydrochloride (R-7464) is one of several 1-substituted imidazole-5-carboxylic acid esters having hypnotic activity, and it is a safe anesthetic for cold-blooded vertebrates including fish.(3) Tranquilization for up to 16 hours results from 0.25 ppm in salt or fresh water, while light surgical anesthesia requires 4 ppm.

Metomidate in an aqueous solution has been used as an anesthetic in a variety of fish, including trout, salmon, and goldfish.(14) The optimal dose ranges from 7.5 (salmonids) to 15 ppm (goldfish). The onset of anesthesia requires 2 to 5 minutes, and recovery occurs in 6 to 12 minutes.

An inexpensive method for anesthetizing large fish in tank trucks or other large volumes of water is with the use of carbon dioxide.(15) Carbon dioxide is produced by addition of calculated amounts of technical-grade sodium bicarbonate and sulfuric acid to water with a temperature between 45 and 60° F. The carbon dioxide content of the water is determined by titration with N/44 sodium hydroxide. Some type of recirculating equipment must be available to disperse the reagents when added. Care must be taken in the storage and handling of sulfuric acid. Fish in carbon dioxide concentrations of 400 ppm for as long as 20 minutes appear to suffer no permanent ill effect.

The optimum carbon dioxide concentration for anesthetizing salmon and steelhead trout is 200 ppm. At this concentration, the fish gradually lose consciousness, turn over, and sink to the bottom of the tank within 90 seconds after the solution reaches full strength. The depth of respiration is used as a measure of the approaching lethal end point. When overdosed, respiratory movement gradually lessens and finally ceases, at which time the fish will not revive when placed in fresh water. After the period of exposure during which the fish are sorted or otherwise handled (which should not exceed 5 minutes), the carbon dioxide is neutralized by addition of a proper quantity of sodium carbonate. This quickly restores the original carbon dioxide concentration. Following neutralization with sodium carbonate, fish remain anesthetized for approximately 5 to 10 minutes.

Flying Mammals

BATS

Bats should be handled with thick leather gloves to prevent one from being bitten.(16) Fruit bats (*Eidolon helvum*) can be relaxed with chlorpromazine injected intramuscularly (2.5 mg/100 g). After the tranquilizer has taken effect, they can be mounted on a restraining board with wings extended and an inhalant anesthetic administered. Halothane or isoflurane alone delivered by mask or into an induction chamber can be used safely to anesthetize bats.(17)

Intraperitoneal pentobarbital injection at a dose of 0.05 mg/g of body weight has been used in a number of genera (*Rhinolophus, Hipposideros, Tadarida, Molussus, Eptesicus, Chilonycteris, Artibeus*) of bats to surgically implant electrodes on the round window of the cochlea or in the brain. Smaller doses (0.03 to 0.045 mg/g) have been used for *Myotis lucifugus* and *Pleocotus townsendii*.(18, 19)

Terrestrial Mammals

ARMADILLOS

There are ten living genera of armadillos. *Dasypus novemcinctus,* the most common, weighs 4 to 5 kg as an adult. Armadillos should be caught close to the base of the tail to avoid the hind claws. Because armadillos can incur a large oxygen debt, they may lie completely still without breathing for long periods. Armadillos also have the ability to recover spontaneously from repeated episodes of ventricular fibrillation.(20) Anesthetics may be given into the subcarpal tissues or the spinal muscles by inserting a needle between two bands slightly to one side of the midline. The site should be thoroughly cleansed to avoid danger of abscess formation.

Fentanyl-droperidol (0.20 to 0.25 mL/kg IM) produces sufficient depression and analgesia for surgery.(21) Long procedures have been performed with slow intravenous infusion of thiopental.(22) Five milliliters of 0.5% solution infused over a period of 1 hour are adequate and safe for most adults. The usual dosage is 5 to 6 mg $\cdot$ kg^{-1} $\cdot$ h^{-1}. Pentobarbital (25 mg/kg IV) can be administered via the superficial femoral vein.(23) Half the dose is given rapidly, followed by the remainder "to effect." Apnea and breath-holding is not reported to be a problem with this technique. Injections can be made into the two prominent superficial femoral veins. These are the only accessible superficial veins that can be easily catheterized. Midline cesarean section has been performed with local infiltration of lidocaine.

Inhalation anesthesia with halothane or isoflurane is easily achieved with a closed induction chamber. Premedication with intramuscular atropine sulfate (0.1 mg, total dose) can be used to diminish secretions. A soft polyethylene endotracheal tube 0.25 to 0.50 inches in external diameter is easily placed by exposing the laryngeal opening with a laryngoscope. Following intubation, anesthesia may be maintained with inhalant concentrations in the range of 1 to 3% delivered via a rebreathing system using a precision vaporizer.

WILD RODENTS

Chinchillas are easily removed from their cages by grasping them by the base of the tail and lifting them off their feet. Anesthesia can be achieved with 1.5 to 2.5% halothane or isoflurane. Alternatively, the intramuscular administration of 15 mg of meperidine approximately 30 minutes prior to surgery, followed by 1% lidocaine solution injected subcutaneously along the proposed line of incision, provides adequate analgesia and sedation for cesarean section surgery in chinchillas.(24) Recovery is rapid, and the young suckle within minutes after delivery. Intramuscular diazepam (5 mg/kg) plus ketamine (15 to 20 mg/kg) also produces relaxation and analgesia for up to 2 hours. Thiopental sodium in dilute solution can also be given intravenously "to effect" for minor surgical procedures. Epidural anesthesia can be used for cesarean section because the lumbosacral fossa is easily located and is comparatively large.(25)

Squirrels are best anesthetized with isoflurane or halothane administered into an induction chamber. Ketamine (10 to 20 mg/kg) is the most commonly used injectable anesthetic in grey and fox squirrels. It provides adequate immobilization for physical examination and diagnostic procedures. A combination of medetomidine and ketamine has also been used to immobilize squirrels (Table 21–4).

In prairie dogs intramuscularly administered ketamine (100 to 150 mg/kg) and xylazine (20 mg/kg) produce 1.5 to 2 hours of satisfactory surgical anesthesia.(26) Xylazine is administered 10 minutes prior to ketamine or may be given in the same syringe at the same time. For longer periods of anesthesia, inhalant anesthetics can also be administered via a mask or following endotracheal intubation.

Agoutis are large, excitable, agile rodents. They can injure themselves or handlers if not carefully restrained. Ketamine alone (25 to 35 mg/kg) has been used to immobilize agoutis.(27) Higher doses (63 to 83 mg/kg)

Table 21–4. Species and Medetomidine and Ketamine Dosages Used for Immobilization of Nondomestic Mammals

Species	Medetomidine (µg/kg)	Ketamine (mg/kg)	Plane*	Documentation†
Insectivora				
Hedgehog (*Erinaceus europaeus*)	100	5.0	2	+
Primate				
Baboon (*Papio hamadryas*)	100	5.0	1–2	+
Chimpanzee (*Pan troglodytes*)	50	5.0	3	+ +
Common marmoset (*Callithrix jacchus*)	100	5.0	1–2	+
Cotton-headed tamarin (*Saguinus oidipus*)	100	5.0	2–3	+ +
Emperor tamarin (*Saguinus imperator*)	100	5.0	2–3	+ +
Lar gibbon (*Hylobates lar*)	70	3.0	2	+
Lowland gorilla (*Gorilla gorilla*)	50	5.0	3	+
Red-bellied tamarin (*Saguinus labiatus*)	100	5.0	2	+
Rodentia				
Brown squirrel (*Sciurus vulgaris*)	100	5.0	1	+
Norwegian lemming (*Lemmus lemmus*)	200–300	—	2–3	+
Nutria (*Myocastor coypus*)	100	5.0	2–3	+ + +
Carnivora				
Amur leopard (*Panthera pardus orientalis*)	60–80	2.5–3.0	3	+ +
Blue fox (*Alopex lagopus*)	50	2.5	3	+ + +
Brown bear (*Ursus a. arctos*)	50	2.0	3	+
Ferret (*Mustela putorius*)	100	5.0	2	+
Golden cat (*Felis temmincki*)	80–100	3.0–4.0	3	+ +
Jaguar (*Panthera onca*)	60–80	2.5	3	+
Lion (*Panthera leo*)	60–80	2.0–3.0	3	+
Lynx (*Lynx lynx*)	80–100	2.5–3.5	3	+ +
Maned wolf (*Chrysocyon brachyurus*)	80	2.5	3	+
Mink (*Mustela vision*)	100	5.0	1–2	+
Pine marten (*Martes martes*)	100	5.0	2	+
Polar bear (*Thalarctos maritimus*)	30	2.5	3	+ +
Red panda (*Ailurus fulgens*)	80–100	2.5–4.0	2–3	+
Snow leopard (*Panthera uncia*)	60–80	2.5–3.0	3	+ + +
Ermine (*Mustela erminea*)	100	5.0	2–3	+ +
Sun bear (*Helarctos malayanus*)	60–80	2.0–3.0	2–3	+
Tiger (*Panthera tigris*)	60–80	2.5	3	+
Wolf (*Canis lupus*)	60–100	3.0–5.0	3	+ +
Wolverine (*Gulo gulo*)	100	5.0	3	+ +

*1, insufficient, animal sedated but able to struggle considerably or get up; 2, moderate, deep sedation but occasional muscle tension or mild struggling when handled; and 3, complete immobilization, good muscle relaxation and no arousal after handling or nociceptive stimuli.

†Subjective evaluation of how reliable the given recommendations are, ranging from + (least reliable) to + + + (most reliable). Modified from Jalanka H.J., and Koeken B.O. The Use of Medetomidine, Medetomidine-Ketamine Combinations, and Atipazmezole in Nondomestic Mammals: A Review. J Zoo Wild Med 21(3):259–282, 1990.)

are required for painful procedures. As might be expected, xylazine, phenothiazine tranquilizers, and fentanyl-droperidol alone are not as effective. Halothane and isoflurane delivered via a face mask or by endotracheal tube produce good surgical anesthesia following ketamine immobilization.

The coypu (Nutria) is difficult to restrain for intravenous injection. They have no readily accessible super-

Table 21–4.   **Species and Medetomidine and Ketamine Dosages Used for Immobilization of Nondomestic Mammals—cont'd**

Species	Medetomidine (μg/kg)	Ketamine (mg/kg)	Plane*	Documentation†
Perissodactyla				
Przewalski's wild horse (*Equus przewalski*)	60–80	1.5–2.0	2–3	+
Artiodactyla				
Alpine ibex (*Capra i. ibex*)	80–140	1.5	2–3	+ + +
Axis deer (*Axis axis*)	50	1.0–2.0	2	+ +
Bactrian camel (*Camelus bactrianus*)	40	–	1	+
Barbary sheep (*Ammotragus lervia*)	100–140	1.5	2–3	+ +
Blackbuck (*Antilope cervicapra*)	200–300	1.5–2.0	2–3	+
Chamois (*Rupicapra r. rupicapra*)	70–100	1.5–2.0	2–3	+ + +
Fallow deer (*Dama dama*)	100–150	2.0–2.5	2–3	+ +
Forest reindeer (*Rangifer tarandus fennicus*)	60–80	0.6–0.8	2–3	+ + +
Guanaco (*Lama guanicoe*)	60–100	1.5–2.0	2–3	+
Himalayan tahr (*Hemitragus jemlahicus*)	80–100	1.5	2–3	+ +
Llama (*Lama glama*)	50	1.0	2	+
Markhor (*Capra falconeri megaceros*)	60–100	1.5–2.0	2–3	+ + +
Moose (*Alces alces*)	60	1.5	2	+
Mouflon (*Ovis musimon*)	125	2.5	2	+
Pére David's deer (*Elaphurus davidianus*)	30	1.0	3	+
Red deer (*Cervus elaphus*)	50	1.5	3	+ +
Reindeer (*Rangifer tarandus tarandus*)	30	1.0	3	+ +
Rocky mountain goat (*Oreamnos americanus*)	60–80	1.5	2–3	+ + +
Roe deer (*Capreolus capreolus*)	50	1.0–2.0	2	+ +
Wapiti (*Cervus canadensis*)	60–80	1.5–2.0	2–3	+
White-tailed deer (*Odocoileus virginianus*)	60–80	1.5–2.0	2–3	+ +
Wisent (*Bison bonasus*)	50–80	1.5–2.5	2–3	+
Yak (*Bos mutus grunninens*)	70–100	2.0–3.0	2–3	+
Marsupiala				
Red-neck wallaby (*Macropus rufogriseus*)	100	5.0	2–3	+

ficial veins. Endotracheal intubation can be performed in anesthetized animals with a slightly flexible tube containing a curved stylet. Intubation can be performed without visualization of the laryngeal opening. Animals weighing 3 to 5 kg require a 5-mm internal diameter endotracheal tube. Upon insertion, apnea may occur. Following intubation either halothane or isoflurane can be used to maintain anesthesia. Chloralose (80 mg/kg) and pentobarbital (40 mg/kg) have been administered intraperitoneally for sedation but do not provide adequate surgical anesthesia at these dosages. Ketamine (10 to 20 mg/kg) plus 2 mg of xylazine have been used in 4- to 5-kg nutria for tail amputation. Twenty mg/kg of ketamine produces prolonged anesthesia, whereas 10 mg/kg is insufficient for surgery.(28) Medetomidine (0.1 mg/kg IM) and ketamine (5 mg/kg IM) induces rapid anesthesia in nutria (Table 21–4). Immobilization lasts

for approximately 40-60 minutes. Atipamezole (0.5–0.7 mg/kg IM) will awaken animals within 5 to 10 minutes of administration. The atipamezole dose should be 4 to 5 times the dose of medetomidine (Chapter 8). Atropine (0.1 mg/kg) is effective as a preanesthetic to decrease salivary secretions.

Intramuscular injections of pentobarbital, ketamine, or droperidol-fentanyl have been used to anesthetize wild marmots.(29) The proprietary combination of droperidol (20 mg/mL) and fentanyl (0.4 mg/mL) (Innovar) produced good anesthesia. Light anesthesia of 30 to 60 minutes' duration can be achieved with a dose of 0.3 to 0.4 mL/kg.

Voles have been anesthetized for nearly 3 hours with pentobarbital at a dose of 0.06 mg/g of body weight when given intraperitoneally. Surgical anesthesia of 15 to 20 minutes can be induced in meadow voles with a

0.06- to 0.09-mg/g dose of pentobarbital injected intramuscularly. Additional information on the dosing of dissociative combinations in wild rodents (e.g., beavers) can be found in Chapter 10.

MUSTELIDS

A metal or plexiglass tube is a convenient device for restraining mink. The dimensions of the tubes will vary according to the size of the mink being restrained.(30) One end is covered with hardware cloth, the other remaining open. The mink is inserted headfirst into the tube. Vaccinations or other injections can be given subcutaneously or intramuscularly on the inner surface of the hind leg while the animal is restrained. Anesthesia has been induced with $CO_2:O_2$ mixtures (1:1), but halothane and isoflurane are preferable for chamber inductions. Maintenance of anesthesia with halothane or isoflurane using rebreathing or nonrebreathing delivery systems is preferred.

Reserpine (0.036 to 0.05 mg) can be administered orally in feed to render mink less nervous and excitable.(31) Apparently, there is a wide margin of safety with little cumulative toxic effects. Adult mink have been safely anesthetized with a combination of propiopromazine (0.2 mL) followed by 0.2 mL (12 mg) of pentobarbital injected intraperitoneally. This combination can produce up to 5 to 6 hours of anesthesia.(32)

Ferrets are commonly induced with halothane or isoflurane in an anesthesia induction chamber. Atropine (0.04 mg/kg) is given either subcutaneously or intramuscularly prior to induction. To maintain anesthesia, inhalants are then delivered via a mask or through an endotracheal tube. Injectable mixtures for producing short periods of anesthesia in ferrets include ketamine (26 mg/kg IM) and acepromazine (0.22 mg/kg IM), ketamine alone (20 to 30 mg/kg IM) to produce light surgical anesthesia for 40 to 60 minutes, althesin (12 to 15 mg of total steroid/kg IM) to produce 15 to 30 minutes of light anesthesia, and Telazol (tiletamine/zolazepam) at a dose of 5 to 10 mg/kg IM. A mixture of Telazol (250 mg tiletamine and 250 mg zolazepam) solubilized in 4 mL of ketamine (400 mg) and 1 mL of 10% xylazine (100 mg/mL) commonly used in domestic cats can be used in ferrets and feral cats at a dose of 0.03–0.04 mL/kg IM. This mixture has been used for castrations, for declaws, and for intraabdominal surgery (Chapter 10).(33) Medetomidine (0.1 mg/kg IM) has also been combined with ketamine (5 mg/kg IM) to induce a short period of anesthesia (Table 21–4).

Veterinarians are occasionally asked to descent skunks. The operation is most often performed in young kittens. In general, rapid-acting volatile anesthetics such as halothane or isoflurane are preferred for producing anesthesia in this species. For small skunks, a transparent plastic disposable bag is an ideal container for induction with halothane or isoflurane. The skunk is induced in the bag, and the surgery is performed through a small opening cut in the bag. On conclusion, the skunk is removed and the bag discarded, eliminating the problem of an odoriferous container. This procedure should be done in a well-ventilated room to minimize human exposure to anesthetic gases. The best age for removal of the scent glands in skunks appears to be 5 to 6 weeks of age, when the skunk's weight is about 2 pounds.(34) Pentobarbital has been given intraperitoneally to induce anesthesia using a 2-mL syringe and 25-gauge needle; the usual dose ranges from 15 to 30 mg/kg in adult skunks.

An anesthetic technique for wild skunks caught in traps using a 9-foot pole syringe has been described.(35) The operator stands at a distance while making an injection and thus facilitates handling the skunk without exposure to musk or possibly being bitten. With this technique pentobarbital solution has been given at the rate of 20 mg/kg of body weight. Of over 50 striped skunks (*Mephitis mephitis*) given pentobarbital this way, only one died. With this technique, skunks are less likely to expel musk if the operator is slow and deliberate. Skunks that expel musk usually direct it at the pole syringe when the drug is injected. Additional anesthetic regimens are given in Chapter 10.

Stoat (*Mustela erminea*) and weasel (*Mustela nivalis*) are extremely fierce and difficult to handle. They will bite through thick leather gloves and if held tightly may be asphyxiated.(36) A satisfactory and nontraumatic method of inducing anesthesia is to place these animals in a plexiglass induction chamber (10″ × 4″ × 4″) attached to the end of the cage by means of a removable slide (Fig. 21–3). A 2½-inch-diameter hole connects the box to the cage. The animal is easily coaxed into this box. Isoflurane or halothane is then introduced into the box via the fresh gas line from the vaporizer. Safe induction concentrations range from 2.5 to 4.0%. Once the animal is unable to right itself it can be removed from the chamber and inhalant anesthesia maintained at lower concentrations by using a face mask or via delivery through an endotracheal tube. The intubation technique is similar to that used for ferrets. Light surgical anesthesia can be maintained with 1.5 to 2.0% concentrations of either isoflurane or halothane. Alternately, medetomidine (0.1 mg/kg IM) and ketamine (5 mg/kg IM) have been used to immobilize stoats with variable success (Table 21–4).

Badgers have a vicious disposition and are very difficult to handle. Historically, phencyclidine, acepromazine, chlorpromazine and succinylcholine had been successfully used for immobilizing badgers (*Taxidea taxus*) (Table 21–5). Ketamine has been found to be the most satisfactory drug for immobilizing the European badger (*Meles meles*).(37) The average effective dose is 20 mg/kg IM, and repeated smaller doses are sometimes administered. Complete recovery occurs in 90 to 180 minutes depending on the total dose of ketamine administered. Following immobilization with intramuscular administered ketamine (15–25 mg/kg) or a mixture of Telazol (8–12 mg/kg) and xylazine (0.5–1.0 mg/kg), anesthesia can be maintained with halothane or isoflurane delivered through a mask or endotracheal tube. For additional information on the use of injectable anesthetics in wild mustelids (e.g., otters) see Chapter 10.

WILD PROCYONIDS

Members of this family include the ring-tailed cat, raccoon, coatimundi, mountain coati, lesser panda, and giant panda. Anesthetic techniques used in these species are primarily based upon experience gained in the immobilization and anesthesia of the raccoon. These anesthetic techniques would appear applicable for most procyonids. Intravenous anesthesia is not practical because of difficulty in restraining these species. Ketamine and Telazol have been used extensively and are made more efficacious when supplemented with an alpha$_2$ agonist (e.g., xylazine or medetomidine). A phenothiazine (acepromazine) or benzodiazepine (diazepam) tranquilizer can also be combined with ketamine. Ketamine has been used alone at a dose of 20 to 30 mg/kg, given intramuscularly. Induction takes 3 to 7 minutes, and recovery can be expected in 45 to 90 minutes. A combination of ketamine (10 mg/kg IM) and xylazine (2 mg/kg IM) is often used to immobilize wild procyonids. Induction occurs in 3 to 5 minutes following IM injection. Anesthesia is excellent and lasts for 15 to 20 minutes, and can be prolonged by administering

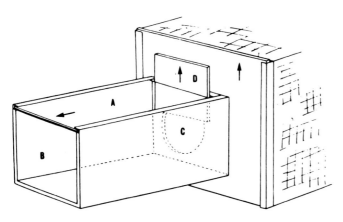

Fig. 21–3. Transfer box for anesthetizing small carnivores. Plexiglas sliding top (A) and end (B) allow visualization of animal. Access hole (C) can be blocked by sliding door (D) to prevent animal from returning to cage. (From Healey, P. A Simple Method for Anaesthetizing and Handling Small Carnivores. J Inst Anim Tech 18:37, 1967.)

one quarter to one half of the original dose intramuscularly or by the administration of halothane or isoflurane via a face mask or an endotracheal tube. Medetomidine (0.1 mg/kg IM) has also been combined with ketamine (4 mg/kg IM) to immobilize red pandas.

Innovar-Vet (1 mL/10 kg IM) can be used in raccoons, but auditory stimulation and bradycardia commonly occur. Bradycardia can be prevented with atropine or glycopyrrolate administration. Telazol has been used in a variety of procyonids for chemical restraint and short, minor surgical procedures. A dose of 10 mg/kg IM induces anesthesia lasting from 20 to 60 minutes. With this dose reflexes (including the palpebral, corneal, pinnal, pharyngeal and laryngeal) should persist.(38)

WILD AND FERAL CANIDS

Immobilization of these species has been achieved using dart guns with drugs such as nicotine, phencyclidine, etorphine, and succinylcholine. These drugs are rarely used today and have been replaced with various dose combinations of ketamine (e.g., 10 mg/kg IM) and xylazine (e.g., 2.0 mg/kg IM) or medetomidine (0.1 mg/kg IM; Table 21–4). With these dosages induction time averages 5 to 10 minutes. Anesthesia usually lasts 15 to 20 minutes, and recovery is complete in approximately 30 minutes. Medetomidine (0.025–0.1 mg/kg IM) can be used to produce dose-dependent sedation and immobilization of many wild canids. Nevertheless, for safety reasons ketamine is commonly given with medetomidine to ensure immobilization. The dose of ketamine should never be less than 2.5 mg/kg IM for immobilizing wild carnivores. Once captured, wild canids can be anesthetized with inhalants in the same manner as domesticated dogs. Induction of anesthesia is commonly performed in a squeeze cage. An injectable tranquilizer, narcotic, and/or ketamine or Telazol is administered, followed by administration of an inhalant such as halothane or isoflurane. Coyotes and other wild carnivores caught in steel traps often injure themselves struggling. A cloth-covered diazepam tablet has been described for attachment to the trap. The tablet may be

Table 21–5.   Dosages and Effects of Four Drugs Used on Captured Badgers

	Drug			
	Phencyclidine Hydrochloride	*Acepromazine Maleate*	*Chlorpromazine Hydrochloride*	*Succinylcholine Chloride*
Number	6	5	5	17
Average dose and range (mg/lb)	1.6(1.2–1.9)	1.2(1.0–1.4)	2.2(1.9–2.7)	0.16(0.12–0.26)*
Immobilization time (minutes after injection until animal was safe to handle)	6(3–9)	22.5(21–25)	14(9–20)	5.5(2–8)
Recovery time (minutes)	347(270–450)	252(220–270)†	312(280–340)†	47(20–68)

*Fifteen animals.
†Three animals.
(From Fitzgerald, J.P. Four Immobilizing Agents Used on Badgers Under Field Conditions. J Wildl Manag 37:418, 1973. Copyright The Wildlife Society.)

Table 21–6. Use of Ketamine in Nondomesticated Cats

Species	Sex	Age in Years M = Months)	Weight (kg)	Dose of Ketamine (mg/kg)	Onset Time (min)
Ocelot (Felis pardalis)	F	12	8	5.0	NM
Ocelot	F	12	8	6.0	NM
Ocelot	F	14	8	14.0	10
Serval (Felis serval)	M	8 M	11	9.0	10
Serval	F	4	9	15.0	NM
Leopard cat (Felis bengalensis)	M	10 M	3	14.0	NM
Leopard cat	M	10 M	3	8.0	U
Leopard cat	F	10 M	2	11.6	U
Leopard cat	F	10 M	1	15.0	10
Leopard cat	M	10 M	2	25.0	8
Clouded leopard (Neofelis nebulosa)	M	15	18	8.6	U
Chinese leopard (Panthera pardus Japonensis)	F	3.5	38	15.0	7 (C)
Black leopard (Panthera pardus)	F	13	54	15.0	19
Margay (Felis wiedii)	F	7	3	15.0	NM
Jaguar (Panthera onca)	F	14	60	13.0	10
Jaguar	M	5	83	18.0	U
Cheetah (Acinonyx jubatus)	M	7	34	8.0	U
Cheetah	M	7	33	11.0	NM
Cheetah	M	7	34	12.0	U
Cheetah	M	7	34	11.5	8 (C)
Cheetah	M	10	42	9.5	6
Cheetah	M	12	30.5	10.0	6
Puma (Felis concolor)	F	12	24	11.0	7
Puma	F	12	24	11.0	14
Puma	M	8 M	27	15.0	U
Puma	M	8 M	27	18.0	U
Puma	F	6	23	22.0	3
Puma	M	14	50	18.0	8
Puma	M	2	30	15.0	7
Puma	M	2	58	20.0	13
Puma	M	2.3	45	18.0	U
Puma	M	2.5	56	25.0	8
Lion (Panthera leo)	F	12	150	10.0	U
Lion	M	2	140	18.0	6
Lion	M	3	163	14.0	U (C)
Lion	F	2	95	20.0	5 (C)
Tiger (Panthera tigris)	M	15	130	7.0	7
Tiger	F	7	110	14.0	9

NM, not measured; U, never safe to handle; C, convulsions occured.
(From Hime, J.M. Use of Ketamine in Non-Domesticated Cats. Vet Rec 95:193, 1974.)

ingested by the coyote after capture, preventing additional self-inflicted harm to the animal.(39)

WILD FELIDS

Many species of nondomesticated cats have been immobilized with high doses of ketamine alone (Table 21–6).(40) However, salivation, muscle rigidity, and convulsions often occur with ketamine immobilization alone (Chapter 10). A combination of ketamine (10–20 mg/kg IM) and xylazine (2 mg/kg IM) can be used to induce short periods of anesthesia (i.e., 5–20 minutes) in wild felids. Additional doses can be given when necessary to prolong anesthesia. Xylazine can also be used to immobilize wild cats at a dose ranging from 1 to 3 mg/kg of body weight, but it should be understood that large felids immobilized with xylazine alone are

Table 21-7. Paralyzing Doses of Succinylcholine Chloride and Duration of Paralysis in Wild Animals

Animal	Scientific Name	Sex	No.	Age	Estimated Weight (lb)	Dose (mg)	Average Latent Period (min)	Maximum Latent Period (min)	Minimum Latent Period (min)	Duration Paralysis (min)
Deer, fallow	*Dama dama*	M	7	Adult	135	10	11½	17	7	13
Deer, axis	*Axis axis*	M	1	Adult	120	7	10	–	–	17
Deer, axis	*Axis axis*	F	1	Adult	120	7	8	–	–	19
Deer, sika	*Cervus nippon*	M	2	Adult	170	7	7	7	7	14
Deer, sika	*Cervus nippon*	F	4	Adult	130	7	7	7	7	14
Deer, barasingha	*Cervus dubauceli*	M	5	Adult	450	13	9½	11	7	15 7/10
Deer, barasingha	*Cervus dubauceli*	M	1	Adult	375	13	8½	–	–	20
Deer, barasingha	*Cervus dubauceli*	F	16	Adult	(170–360) Av. 227	6–10 7.2	8	12½	5	(10–30) 17½
Deer, barasingha	*Cervus dubauceli*	M	1	Adult	400	7	9½	–	–	20
Deer, barasingha	*Cervus dubaucelia*	M	1	Adult	325	6	9	–	–	30
Wapiti (elk)	*Cervus canadensis*	M	1	Adult	1,100	23	6	6	6	18
Wapiti (elk)	*Cervus canadensis*	F	4	Adult	550	15	5–3/10	7½	3½	2½
Wapiti (elk)	*Cervus canadensis*	M	1	Adult	450	15	5–3/10	7½	3½	21½
Deer, red	*Cervus elaphus*	M	5	Adult	260	15	7½	9½	6½	16
Bison	*Bison bison*	F	1	Adult	700	25	7	7	7	10
Antelope (eland)	*Taurotragus oryx*	F	1	Adult	250	6	9	–	–	14
Monkey, spider	*Ateles geoffroyi*	F	1	Adult	5	5	4½	–	–	20
Monkey, spider	*Ateles geoffroyi*	F	1	Adult	5	10	50 sec	–	–	30
Monkey, spider	*Ateles geoffroyi*	F	1	Adult	5	20	½	–	–	45
Lion, African	*Panthera leo*	F	1	Adult	275	60	6	–	–	11
Lion, African	*Panthera leo*	F	1	Adult	275	120	2½	–	–	60
Goat, domestic	*Capra prisca*	M	1	Adult	110	70	6½	–	–	60
Goat, domestic	*Capra prisca*	M	1	Adult	110	40	9	–	–	30
Goat, domestic	*Capra prisca*	M	1	Adult	110	20	14	–	–	15
Goat, domestic	*Capra prisca*	F	3	Adult	50–80	20	11	14	9	15
Goat, domestic	*Capra prisca*	F	3	Adult	60	15	11	11	11	17
Goat (Tahr), Himalayan	*Hemitragus jemiahious*	M	2	Adult	165	17½	6	–	–	21½
Goat (Tahr), Himalayan	*Hemitragus jemiahious*	F	2	Adult	115	15	6	–	–	20
Sheep, Barbary	*Ammotragus leroia*	M	2	Adult	200	20	15	17	12	7
Antelope, pronghorn	*Antelope Capra americana*	M	2	1 year	50	5	8	10	6	15

(From Thomas, W.D. Chemical Immobilization of Wild Animals. J Am Vet Med Assoc 138:264, 1961.)

easily aroused by auditory, visual, and physical stimuli. Medetomidine in combination with ketamine has also been used to immobilize a variety of wild felids (Table 21–4). For many years etorphine (M-99) has been used successfully to immobilize African lions and other wild cats.(41) For a 100-kg lion the suggested dose of M-99 is 0.5 mg/kg total dose. In adult lions tremors associated with M-99 injection can be controlled with acepromazine administration (25–30 mg; total dose). Appropriate doses of Telazol (1.5–5.0 mg/kg IM) will usually induce anesthesia in large felids in 2 to 5 minutes, providing 15 to 30 minutes of immobilization and analgesia (Chapter 10). The coadministration of atropine with dissociative anesthetics generally prevents excessive salivation. Tigers may be especially sensitive to Telazol.

Succinylcholine chloride has been used for immobilization of a large variety of wild species including large cats such as African and North American mountain lions (*Felis concolor*).(42) Paralyzing doses of succinylcholine used in a number of species are given in Table 21–7. However, with the availability of newer drugs and combinations for immobilization of wild and feral animals, succinylcholine alone is no longer considered an acceptable immobilizing drug.

Meperidine and promazine have been used as preanesthetics in some large cats such as the ocelot, leopard, and lion. In the lion, 11 mg/kg of meperidine and 4.4 to 9 mg/kg of promazine have been recommended.(43, 44) Subcutaneous and intramuscular injection is facilitated by use of a squeeze cage. After the preanesthetic takes effect, pentobarbital or thiopental can be given intravenously to effect. Once sedation is present, a tourniquet can be applied to the tail to help locate the caudal vein for intravenous injection of the barbiturate or dissociative.

When compared to smaller domestic cats, it appears that big cats require less anesthetic per kilogram to produce surgical anesthesia. For example, when combined with medetomidine (0.03 mg/kg IM), the required dose of ketamine is only 2.5 mg/kg IM for immobilization of tigers and lions (Table 21–4). Certain reflexes may persist, and the recovery period is usually longer in larger cats. The rate and character of ventilation are important criteria for assessing depth of anesthesia. Fewer than 10 breaths per minute should be cause for concern. It is suggested that local anesthetics be employed, whenever possible, to avoid large doses of general anesthetic in large undomesticated cats. Additional information on various injectable drug combinations used to immobilize wild felids can be found in Chapters 10 and 22.

Whenever possible halothane or isoflurane anesthesia is preferred for long periods of general anesthesia of large felids because they provide more control over depth and a more rapid emergence upon completion of the procedure. If the procedure is expected to be of considerable duration endotracheal intubation is preferable to mask delivery of the inhalant (Figs. 21–4A and

B). Tracheal intubation in large cats can be achieved with or without a laryngoscope. Large lions and tigers will require a medium Cole tapered tube (Figs. 21–5A and B) or an 18- to 24-mm-i.d. cuffed tube commonly used in small adult horses. Before the endotracheal tube is positioned in the trachea, the larynx should be sprayed with a local anesthetic to decrease the likelihood of laryngeal spasms.

WILD AND FERAL SWINE

Wild and feral hogs have been captured by placing alpha-chloralose on corn or in mixtures of flour, peanut butter, sardines, and syrup. The feeding site should be baited for several days prior to using the drugged bait. One teaspoonful of methocel per cup added to dampened shelled corn causes the relatively insoluble alpha chloralose to adhere to the corn. The maximum safe dosage for feral hogs is about 2.2 g/10 kg of body weight; the minimum effective dose is about 2.2 g/40 kg. Two grams of alpha-chloralose per cup of bait appear to be effective.(45) Bait should be removed after the trapping operation, since it is potentially dangerous to other wildlife. Once captured and restrained, wild swine and javelinas can be anesthetized with a dissociative or barbiturate such as thiopental (10 mg/kg IV). Following intubation, anesthesia is maintained with halothane or isoflurane. Once adequate restraint or immobilization

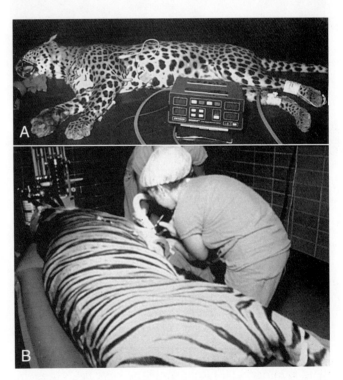

Fig. 21–4. Adult leopard (A) and tiger (B) anesthetized with isoflurane. In the leopard (A) indirect blood pressure was measured at 5-minute intervals using an oscillometric device and cuff placement around the metatarsal artery. Fluid administration is important during long procedures and will assure a ready venous access for drug administration.

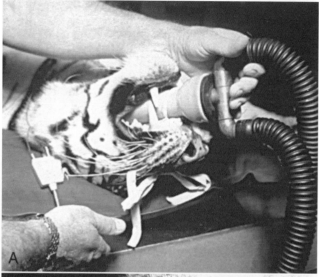

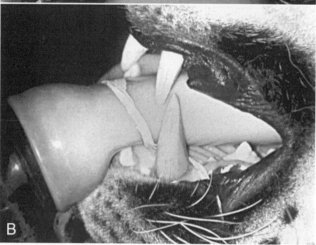

Fig. 21–5. Large animal Cole tube modified with rubber insert for attachment to adult rebreathing system for delivery of inhalation anesthetic to an adult tiger (A). Flow rates of 5 to 10 L/min are recommended. The tube should be secured in place to prevent movement and laryngeal trauma (B).

has been achieved, anesthetic techniques used in domestic breeds of pigs are effective in wild and feral swine (Chapter 20).

WILD RUMINANTS

Bovidae species. Prior to the availability of modern immobilizing drugs Beale and Smith reported on the immobilization of pronghorn antelope with 6–10 mg/45 kg of succinylcholine chloride.(46) Today, xylazine (1.0 to 3.0 mg/kg) or carfentanil are more commonly employed for sedation and capture of antelope and wild ruminants.(47) Roan antelope have been immobilized with 11 to 13 μg/kg of carfentanil combined with 0.75 mg/kg of azaperone.(48) Immobilizing doses of fentanyl, etorphine, and xylazine employed in African antelopes and other wild bovidae species are presented in Table 21–8. Xylazine alone and in combination with

ketamine has been used extensively for the immobilization of captive and free-ranging bovidae ruminants. Captive Dorcas gazelles have been immobilized for electroejaculation using xylazine (0.25 mg/kg IM) and ketamine (12 mg/kg IM).(49)

To capture bighorn sheep etorphine can be used at a dose of approximately 22 μg/kg IM.(50) The intramuscular injection of acepromazine (15 mg total dose in the adult animal) after capture prolongs the effect of etorphine and facilitates handling. Injection of cyprenorphine produces rapid recovery from the effects of etorphine. It is recommended that cyprenorphine or diprenorphine be given in a dose 2½ times the amount of etorphine and that half be given intravenously and half intramuscularly to smooth recovery and decrease the likelihood of renarcotization. To tranquilize bighorn sheep, diazepam can be mixed with feed at a dose of approximately 13 mg/kg of feed.

The domestic buffalo (*Bubalus bubalis*) is raised mainly in Asia as a producer of meat and milk. It has only distant relationship to the American bison (*Bison bison*). Most anesthetic techniques for the buffalo have been inferred from work with cattle. Recent studies have shown considerable species variation, however. The effects of xylazine on water buffalo calves at doses of 0.22 and 0.44 mg/kg IV and 0.44 mg/kg IM have been assessed.(51, 52) Recovery times were dose related and varied from 65 to 130 minutes for the intravenous doses, whereas the intramuscular dose produced an average of 150 minutes of recumbency. Administration of 0.04 mg/kg of atropine intramuscularly reduces salivary secretions and bradycardia observed with xylazine administration. Ketamine (2.0 mg/kg IV) can be combined with chlorpromazine (2.0 mg/kg IM) to anesthetize water buffalo calves. Pretreatment with chlorpromazine increases the duration of analgesia and recovery time beyond that achieved with ketamine alone. Short-term surgical procedures (5 to 10 minutes) have been performed in calves with this drug combination.(53)

The use of guaifenesin (165 mg/kg IV) alone in water buffalo calves to produce complete immobilization causes significant hypotension. Cardiovascular and respiratory effects produced by high doses of guaifenesin are generally undesirable.(54) A mixture of chloral hydrate (30 g), magnesium sulfate (15 g), and thiopental (2.5 g) in 1000 mL of distilled water has also been used to anesthetize water buffalo calves.(55) Thirty minutes following subcutaneous administration of atropine, the mixture is given intravenously at approximately 2.0 mL/kg. Anesthesia is adequate for 15 to 25 minutes following the initial injection and may be prolonged by additional injections. Halothane or isoflurane anesthesia have also proven satisfactory in water buffalo and are the preferred methods of achieving anesthesia when the appropriate delivery equipment is available.

Bison (*Bison bison*) are generally dangerous and difficult to handle, and mature animals require heavy equipment for restraint. Capture equipment is necessary to catch free-roaming animals (Chapters 2 and 22).

Table 21-8. Immobilizing Doses of Drugs in Several African Bovidae Species

Species	Age	Sex	Approx. Body Wt (kg)	Immobilized		Effective Doses of Drugs in Mg				Analgesic Antagonists	
				Total Times	No. of Animals	Fentanyl	Immobilon LA (Etorphine + Acepromazine)		Xylazine	Nalorphine	Diprenorphine
							Etorphine	Acepromazine			
Bongo	A	M	300	5	2	70	4.4–4.9	18–20	75	200	6.0
Boocercus eurycerus	A	F	220	12	5	40	2.45–2.94	10–20	50	120	3.6
	Imm.	M	50	2	1	10	—	—	10	30	—
			80	2		15	—	—	10	45	—
Zebra duiker	A	M/F	15	18	4	3.0	—	—	2.5–6.0	10	—
Cephalophus zebra	2 wks.	M	1.0	1	1	1.0	—	—	—	2.5	—
Red flanked duiker	A	M/F	9	9	4	2.0	—	—	2.0	6.0	—
Cephalophus rufilatus	Imm.	M	5	3	1	1.0	—	—	1.0	2.5	—
Jentink's duiker	A	M	80	5	1	15	—	—	10	50	—
Cephalophus jentinkii											
Maxwell's duiker	A	M/F	5.0	11	4	1.0–1.5	—	—	1.0–1.5	3–4	—
Cephalophus maxwellii											
Yellow-back duiker	A	M/F	65	11	4	15–20	—	—	10–20	50	—
Cephalophus sylviculator											
Black duiker	A	M	15	3	1	3	—	—	3	10	—
Cephalophus niger											
Eland	A	F	300	4	1	—	2.94	12	50	—	3.6
Taurotragus oryx	Imm.	M/F	150–200	14	6	—	1.96	8	40–50	—	2.4
	Imm.	M	120	4	2	15–20	1.46	6	20–40	50	2.0
	Imm.	F	60	1	1	12	—	—	12	30	—
Beisa oryx	Imm.	M/F	150	16	5	30	1.96–2.45	8–10	20–30	80	2.4–3.0
Oryx beisa											
Harnessed antelope	A	M/F	20		3	4.0	—	—	4	10	—
Tragelaphus scriptus											
Coke's hartebeeste	A	M/F	180	5	3	—	1.47	6	20–30	—	2.0
Alcelaphus buselaphus cokei											
Impala	A } Imm.	M/F	30–50	8	5	10	—	—	10	25	—
Aepyceros melampus											
Wildebeest	A	M/F	180–200	17	5	—	1.47–1.96	6–8	20–30	—	2.0–2.5
Connochaetes tourinus	Imm.	F	70	3	1	—	0.49	2	10	—	0.6
Defassa waterbuck	A	M	320	5	2	50	1.96–2.94	8–12	40–50	125	2.4–3.6
Kobus defassa											
Thomson's gazelle	A	M/F	18	5	3	5.0	—	—	5.0	12.5	—
Gazella thomsonii											
Buffalo	Near A	F	375	3	1	—	2.45	10	25	—	3.0
Syncerus caffer											

A = adult
(From Haigh, J.C. The Immobilisation of Bongo (Boocercus eurycus) and Other African Antelopes in Captivity. Vet Rec 98:237, 1976.)

Captured bison have been given chloral hydrate (250 mg/kg) to achieve deep surgical anesthesia.(56) Once bison have been restrained and/or immobilized by physical or chemical techniques, intravenous and inhalant techniques commonly used in large domestic cattle are quite effective (Chapters 20 and 22).

Cervidae species. The effects of intramuscular injections of 0.3 mg/kg up to 9 mg/kg of xylazine in red, fallow, and spotted deer have been reported.(57-59) With clinically effective doses the onset of sedation occurs within 3 to 10 minutes and usually lasts 1 to 2 hours. A degree of analgesia is produced, but supplementation with a local or regional anesthetic is required for surgery. During onset of sedation there is some salivation, but regurgitation of ruminal contents or ruminal tympany is rare. Alterations in respiratory rhythm, ranging from transient apnea to a Cheyne-Stokes respiration, is observed with higher doses of xylazine and is most frequently encountered in red deer, moose, sitatunga, and Barbary sheep. Xylazine has also been used to immobilize captive white-tailed deer.(60) Induction times are shorter in fawns and freshly trapped deer. Immobilization is prolonged with doses above 3 mg/kg, and higher doses than this should not be used. In general, xylazine produces good sedation and analgesia in wild cervidae species, but, with safe doses, immobilization and muscle relaxation are sometimes insufficient for handling.

When given alone the dose of ketamine for most deer species ranges from 10 to 20 mg/kg IM. Today, two of the more common drug mixtures for immobilizing wild deer are ketamine-xylazine and Telazol-xylazine (Chapters 10 and 22). Medetomidine has also been combined with ketamine at varying doses to immobilize several species of deer and other wild ruminants (Table 21-4). Atipamezole can be used to antagonize medetomidine-ketamine-induced immobilization at approximately five times the dose of medetomidine (Table 21-9).

Etorphine has been used extensively to immobilize many species of deer, and wild ruminants (Table 21-10).(41) For fallow and other species of deer intramuscularly administered mixtures of etorphine (2 mg/100 kg) and xylazine (30 mg/100 kg) or fentanyl (0.3 to 0.66 mg/kg) and xylazine (0.5 to 1.3 mg/kg) have also proven to be quite reliable and effective.(61, 62)

For tranquilization of deer prior to transportation, chlorpromazine can be given at a rate of 4.4 mg/kg intramuscularly.(63) Good results have also been obtained in elk with this dose. Full effect occurs in about an hour and lasts 16 to 24 hours. When used as preanesthetics prior to barbiturates, phenothiazine tranquilizers should be injected intramuscularly at least 1 hour in advance.

The reaction of deer to intravenous pentobarbital varies greatly. Deer must be watched closely during the recovery period. Salivation and bloating are common problems. If pentobarbital is to be used, it should be preceded by atropine and the animal should be deprived of feed and water for 24 hours prior to induction. In a series of approximately 50 deer anesthetized with pentobarbital, one death and several cases of postoperative pneumonia, caused by regurgitation of rumen contents, occurred.(64) As in other ruminants, endotracheal intubation is recommended during general anesthesia to eliminate such complications.

For short periods of anesthesia in deer, a 7% solution of chloral hydrate can be given intravenously "to effect." Combined chloral hydrate, halothane, and nitrous oxide anesthesia has also been used in mule deer.(64) The average dose of a 7% solution of chloral hydrate to induce anesthesia is 210 mL for a 200-lb deer. Atropine administration prevents excessive salivation.

As with bovidae species, diazepam alone has been used to produce sedation and muscle relaxation for capture of wild cervidae.(65) The dose ranges from 125 to 250 g/10 kg of feed. The effects vary depending upon the amount ingested but may persist for several days. Maximum effect occurs 4 to 8 hours after ingestion. Sedated individuals should be separated from untranquilized animals, since the latter may cause injury to less alert deer. As tranquilization deepens calm animals eat less, making the technique somewhat self-limiting.

Table 21-9. Total Atipamezole Doses and Atipamezole:Medetomidine Ratios (w/w) in Selected Ruminant Species to Reverse Medetomidine-Ketamine-Induced Immobilization

Species	n	Atipamezole (µg/kg)		Atipamezole:Medetomidine Ratio (w/w)	
		Median	Min–max	Median	Min–max
Alpine ibex	70	543	152–833	5.0	1.7–7.1
Barbary sheep	10	298	142–417	3.7	2.9–5.0
Chamois	41	328	197–653	5.0	3.0–7.1
Forest reindeer	41	309	185–522	5.0	3.0–7.0
Himalayan tahr	29	345	143–658	5.0	4.0–5.6
Markhor	62	409	194–698	5.0	4.0–5.6
Rocky Mountain goat	22	315	114–714	5.0	2.5–5.8
White-tailed deer	25	294	160–435	5.0	2.7–6.0

(From Jalanka H.J. and Koeken B.O. The Use of Medetomidine, Medetomidine-Ketamine Combinations and Atipamezole in Nondomestic Mammals: A Review. J Zoo Wildl Med 21(3)259–282, 1990.)

Table 21–10. Etorphine Immobilization of Wild Ruminants

Species	Sex	Est. Wt. (lb)	Etorphine (mg)	Ace (mg)	S (mg)	Imm. Time (min)	Nal (mg)	Lag Time (sec)	Remarks
Aoudad	M	275	1.0	5.0	5.0	13.0	100	15	Good state of immobility
Aoudad	M	200	1.0	5.0	5.0	8.0	200	I	Good state of immobility
Aoudad	F	150	1.0	5.0	5.0	3.0	100	I	Required additional 0.5 mg etorphine to trim
Aoudad	F	150	1.0	2.0	5.0	4.0	100	30	Required additional 0.4 mg etorphine to trim
Aoudad	F	150	2.0	2.0	5.0	3.5	100	I	Teeth grinding, twitching
Aoudad	F	150	2.0	2.0	5.0	6.0	100	I	Teeth grinding, twitching
Eland	F	650	2.0	10.0	25.0	11.0	250	60	Vomiting, pushing wall after nalorphine
Eland	F	650	2.0	10.0	25.0	9.0	250	120	Salivated, pushing wall after nalorphine
Reindeer	M	200	1.0	5.0	4.0	4.0	50	90	In rut, excellent results
Reindeer	M	200	1.0	5.0	4.0	6.0	100	45	Same animal as above, dehorned
Fallow deer	M	90	1.0	3.0	2.0	4.0	50	I	Good immobility, dehorned
Fallow deer	M	100	1.0	3.0	2.0	–	–	–	Dart bounced off, caught by hand 20 min
Fallow deer	M	100	0.5	2.0	2.0	4.0	100	30	Good state of immobility
Fallow deer	M	150	0.5	7.5	1.5	7.0	–	–	Up when approached; 120 min normal
Fallow deer	M	150	1.0	5.0	3.0	8.0	100	–	Free-ranging, died during manual restraint
Fallow deer	M	150	1.0	5.0	3.0	6.0	100	–	Free-ranging, died during manual restraint
Bison	M	250	1.0	5.0	2.0	7.0	100	–	Required minimal restraint
Bison	M	500	1.0	5.0	2.0	–	100	–	Required additional 0.5 mg etorphine, 2 mg Ap, 2 mg S
Bison	M	700	2.0	5.0	5.0	10.0	100	60	Required minimal restraint
Bison	M	1,200	2.5	5.0	25.0	9.0	125	240	Died in 2 hours— pulmonary emphysema
Lesser kudu	F	100	0.5	4.0	4.0	13.0	50	30	Required manual restraint
Greater kudu	M	450	2.5	5.0	5.0	15.0	100	60	Required manual restraint to cast leg
Black buck	M	60	0.5	10.0	10.0	–	50	–	Required additional 1 mg etorphine, 10 mg Ap, 10 mg S, deep analgesia
Giraffe	F	2,500	2.5	30.0	10.0	5.0	160	–	Five small doses of etorphine down 6 minutes after last injection; died following day from dystocia

Ace, acepromazine; S, scopolamine; Nal, nalorphine hydrochloride; Lag time, time elapsed from administration of nalorphine to animal standing; I, immediate recovery; –, drug not used; Imm. time, time elapsed from administration of drug to immobilization.

(From Wallach, J.D., Frueh, R., and Lentz, M. The Use of M.99 as an Immobilizing and Analgesic Agent in Captive Wild Animals. J Am Vet Med Assoc 151:870, 1967.)

A number of drugs have been used to immobilize and anesthetize caribou including fentanyl (0.3 to 0.6 mg/kg IM), xylazine (0.25 to 0.5 mg/kg IM), and azaperone (0.5 to 1.2 mg/kg IM).(66) Etorphine (0.02 to 0.1 mg/kg IM) has also proven effective in caribou when combined with acepromazine (0.02 to 0.1 mg/kg IM). North American elk (*Cervus canadensis*) have been immobilized with succinylcholine chloride or gallamine using capture equipment, but these drugs may result in bloating and severe respiratory depression. If other drugs (e.g., carfentanil) are not available, the following intramuscular doses of succinylcholine have been recommended for elk: 15 to 20 mg for calves 4 to 11 months of age; 20 to 25 mg for females 12 months and older; and 25 to 35 mg for males 12 months and older.(67) Xylazine alone produces long-lasting immobility in moose. Sedate animals require constant supervision. A mixture of xylazine (0.15 to 0.5 mg/kg) and fentanyl (0.15 to 0.5 mg/kg) delivered by dart syringe has proven effective in helicopter-assisted capture of moose (62.) Hyaluronidase (150 to 300 N.F. units) added to the mixture decreases the induction times 36 to 45%.

Camelids. Large camelidae can be sedated with xylazine (Chapter 20). Intramuscular doses ranging from 0.4 to 0.9 mg/kg have been used in Arabian and Bactrian camels. In most instances there is no resistance to positioning and manipulation of feet once sedation is evident. Onset of sedation usually occurs within 10 minutes and can vary in duration from 45 minutes to 5 hours. Larger doses produce sedation for up to 24 hours. Regurgitation of rumen contents and ruminal tympany are not common and recovery is unaccompanied by struggling and excitement.(68) Sedation in Bactrian camels achieved with xylazine doses of 0.25 to 0.50 mg/kg IM can be antagonized with doxapram administration (0.05 to 0.13 mg/kg IV).(69) Premedication with intramuscular chlorpromazine (1 mg/kg) decreases the dose of chloral hydrate or pentobarbital sodium necessary to induce anesthesia while prolonging its duration. Satisfactory intravenous anesthesia has been achieved in adult camels with a combination of chlorpromazine (0.5 mg/kg), pentobarbital (2.0 g total dose), and 2.5 g/50 kg of body weight of chloral hydrate. Anesthesia can be prolonged with supplemental doses of pentobarbital.

For laparotomy and rumenotomy procedures, regional analgesia can be used in camels by infiltration of 2% lidocaine in a reverse seven pattern along the caudal edge of the last rib and the distal tips of the lumbar transverse processes (Chapter 16). Epidural anesthesia can also be used in camels with the animal fastened in the sitting position. Injection is made with a 5-cm needle at the sacrococcygeal or first coccygeal space, slanting the needle forward about 45° from vertical. Twelve to 16 mL of 2% lidocaine produces analgesia of the anus, udder, vagina, scrotum, and hind limbs. Fifty mL produces anesthesia of the hindquarters posterior to the umbilicus.

A mixture of guaifenesin (110 mg/kg) and thiopental (4.4 mg/kg) can be given intravenously for induction of anesthesia in camels. For maintenance of general anesthesia, 5% guaifenesin in 5% dextrose plus thiopental (2 mg/mL) are given "to effect." As with other large ruminants, once intubated, inhalant anesthetics such as halothane or isoflurane can be used to maintain longer periods of anesthesia (Chapter 20).

Giraffe. Some investigators feel that xylazine alone is unsuitable for restraint of giraffes.(71) When combined with etorphine, however, results are more satisfactory. Intramuscular doses for Masai and reticulated giraffes range from 0.3 to 0.4 mg/kg of xylazine along with a 1.5- to 2.0-mg total dose of etorphine.(38) The sedative/anesthetic effects of this drug combination can be antagonized with diprenorphine (2–4 mg total dose IV) and an alpha$_2$-antagonist such as yohimbine (0.1–0.15 mg/kg IV) or tolazoline (1–2 mg/kg IV). Etorphine alone has been used for surgical analgesia and restraint of adult reticulated giraffes (*Giraffa camelopardalis reticulata*) (71) but is usually given intramuscularly (total dose of 2.5 mg) along with xylazine (0.3 mg/kg IM) or acepromazine (30 mg IM total dose). This combination produces recumbency and when supplemented with an additional 1 mg of etorphine produces surgical analgesia. Carfentanil can also be combined with xylazine to safely immobilize free-ranging giraffes.(72)

PERISSODACTYLS

Wild and feral equids. Etorphine (0.017 mg/kg IM) alone or in combination with acepromazine (0.04 mg/kg IM) has been used to restrain captive onagers and kiang for electroejaculation procedures.(49, 73) Using similar doses of 0.015 to 0.033 mg/kg IM, carfentanil has been used to immobilize zebras (*E. burchelli*) and Mongolian wild (Przewalski's) horses.(74–76) Immobilization usually occurs within 10 minutes following injection. Xylazine (0.6 mg/kg IM) is often used as a synergist to decrease the dose of carfentanil (0.02 mg/kg IM) and reduces narcotic induced muscle rigidity. Following injection mild tachycardia, hypertonia, and hyperthermia have been observed in some wild horses. In a recent study, when xylazine (1 mg/kg IM) and carfentanil (0.015 mg/kg IM) were administered to three domestic horses, severe physiologic disturbances were observed in each animal.(74) These changes were characterized by a hypermetabolic state including tachycardia, vigorous muscle activity, tachypnea, and increased rectal temperature. One horse was euthanatized because of the onset of severe pulmonary edema that was unresponsive to treatment.(74) The authors speculate that these untoward responses may have been the result of insufficient dosage. Medetomidine (0.06–0.08 mg/kg IM) combined with ketamine (1.5–2.0 mg/kg IM) has been used to effectively immobilize wild horses (Table 21–4). This combination produces good muscle relaxation, and recovery is rapid and complete following intravenous or subcutaneous atipamezole administration. Generally speaking, once sedated, wild equidae may be given injectable and inhalant general anesthetics in the same manner as domesticated horses (Chapter 20).

Rhinoceros. White rhinoceros (*Dicerus simus simus*) can be immobilized with an intramuscularly administered mixture of morphine and chlorpromazine.(77) The doses used are approximately 1.5 g morphine, 175 mg scopolamine, and 725 mg chlorpromazine. Complete immobilization requires 30 to 45 minutes in a 1600-kg animal. A variation of this mixture is made by substituting diethylthiambutene for morphine. For a 1400-kg animal, the dose of diethylthiambutene is approximately 3.0 g. These mixtures have also been used successfully in black rhinoceros. Black rhinoceros have been immobilized with combinations of etorphine and acepromazine, etorphine, acepromazine and azaperone, or etorphine and azaperone (Table 21–11).(78) Carfentanil alone can also be used to immobilize rhinos. The total intramuscular dose ranges from 1.0 to 1.5 mg in juveniles to 2.5 to 3.0 mg in adults. At these doses, deep sedation is achieved. The effects of carfentanil are readily antagonized with diprenorphine.(48, 79) Recommended carfentanil dosages for immobilizing rhinoceros and a variety of other wild African species are given in Table 21–12.

ELEPHANTS

Several drugs have been used to immobilize and anesthetize elephants. Over 40 years ago meperidine hydrochloride was successfully administered intravenously to an elephant at the dose of 2.2 mg/kg of body weight to allow manipulation of a painful fracture.(80) Over 25 years ago Indian elephants were anesthetized with pentobarbital administered in the middle auricular vein.(81) Today, elephants are more commonly immobilized with etorphine. It is interesting to note that for Ceylon elephants, the dose of etorphine (2.2 mg/1000 kg) is approximately twice that for the African elephant.(82) The intramuscular dose of etorphine for the African elephant varies from 4 to 8 mg total dose, or approximately 1.5 mg/1000 kg. A commercial mixture of etorphine-acepromazine (2.45 mg/mL of etorphine and 10 mg/mL of acepromazine; Immobilon LA) has been used to sedate and control adult Asian elephants. The dose is based on an unusual measurement: 1 mL/4 ft of shoulder height. Immobilon appears to induce more predictable actions than does etorphine alone.(83) Etorphine administration (total doses ranging from 4 to 6 mg) in African elephants (*Loxodanta africana*) ranging in weight from 2700 to 6000 kg usually results in the animals becoming either sternal or laterally recumbent.(84) The latter is preferred because sternal recumbency places great pressure on the diaphragm. Large elephants may become immobilized in the standing position when using the lower dose (4 mg total dose). If this occurs, elephants may be given acepromazine to improve sedation and immobilization. In summary, etorphine alone immobilizes adult African elephants satisfactorily (total dose of 6 mg) but the addition of acepromazine (25 to 50 mg total dose) enhances and prolongs the tranquil state. The inclusion of scopolamine along with etorphine and acepromazine appears to be of little value in deepening the anesthetic effect. However, a more prolonged state of depression occurs. Adult Asian elephants have been successfully sedated for air transport with xylazine alone (100 to 175 mg total dose). Animals remain standing in cages and are

somnolent. Injections of xylazine can be repeated at the same dose rate at approximately 3-hour intervals to maintain standing sedation.(85)

A report on repeated inhalation anesthesia of an African elephant has recently been published.(86) Food was withheld for 24 hours and water for 12 hours prior to induction. Chemical restraint and sternal recumbency were induced with 0.0017 mg/kg etorphine administered intramuscularly. Atropine (0.04 mg/kg IM) was administered prior to an additional 0.0006 mg/kg etorphine intravenously. Following the second dose of etorphine, the elephant was placed in lateral recumbency. A stomach tube was placed into the larynx by digital palpation, as is done in adult cattle. A 40-mm-i.d. cuffed endotracheal tube was passed into the trachea using the stomach tube as a guide, the cuff was inflated, and the endotracheal tube was connected to two large animal breathing circuits joined in parallel at the Y-piece. Initially, each machine was set to deliver 5% isoflurane in 15 L/min of oxygen. After 45 minutes, the two vaporizers were reset to deliver 2 to 3% isoflurane in 5 liters of oxygen per minute. Anesthesia was maintained for 155 minutes, at which time end-tidal isoflurane concentration ranged from 1.05 to 1.15 vol %. At the completion of surgery, isoflurane administration was discontinued. Twenty-five to 40 minutes later, diprenorphine was administered intravenously and the elephant stood unaided in 3 to 4 minutes.(86)

In a recent report of an Asian elephant anesthetized for cesarean section for removal of a dead fetus, excitement was induced following the intravenous injection of atropine.(87) In this elephant azaperone (0.035 mg/kg IM) administration was followed 90 minutes later by a 0.05 mg/kg intravenous dose of atropine. Within 1 minute of atropine injection, the elephant began swaying, kicking, and moving in an agitated manner around the stall. Normally responsive to commands, the elephant refused to obey verbal direction. When this behavior had not abated after 30 minutes, an additional dose of azaperone (0.018 mg/kg IM) was administered. Within 15 minutes, the elephant became calm and responsive to commands, and anesthesia was induced with etorphine (0.002 mg/kg IV). Following intubation, anesthesia was maintained with two large animal anesthetic machines arranged in parallel delivering 100% oxygen and was supplemented with additional doses of etorphine when necessary. The authors speculated that the excitement observed following atropine administration was due primarily to atropine rather than a drug interaction with azaperone. Atropine has often been used in elephants, and suggested dosages vary from 0.11 mg/kg IM to 0.01 mg/kg IV. As with domestic animals, differences in sensitivity to the toxic effects of atropine may exist in elephants, especially when preexisting pathology or abnormal physiologic conditions are present.(87) Additional data on the use of injectable drugs and drug combinations for immobilization of free-ranging and captive elephants can be found in Tables 21–12, 21–13, and 21–14.

Table 21-11. Drug Immobilization Data on 11 Black Rhinoceros in East Africa

Intramuscular Doses of Drugs in mg (and μg/kg)

Sex	Weight (kg) A-actual E-estimated	Analgesic		Neuroleptic		Antidote		Elapsed Time (Min) from Injection to:				
		Etorphine	Fentanyl	Ace-promazine	Azaperone	Nalorphine	Route	Ataxia	Immob.	Down	Antidote	Up
Female	818 E	2.0 (2.44)		25.0 (30.5)		200.0 (244.5)	IM	7	10	15	118	126
Male	1185 A	2.0 (1.69)		20.0 (16.8)	250.0 (210.9)	200.0 (168.7)	IM	5	21	25	258	270
Male	1085 A	2.0† (1.84)	20.0* (18.43)	10.0 (9.2)	300.0 (276.5)	300.0 (276.5)	IM	7	5	7	63	81
Male	1196 A	2.0 (1.76)		20.0 (18.4)		300.0 (250.8)	IM	5	20	25	170	177
Male	955 E	2.0 (2.09)		25.0 (21.7)	200.0 (209.5)			8	13	18	Drowned in lake	
Male	1033 A	2.0 (1.93)		25.0 (26.1)	200.0 (193.6)	300.0 (290.4)	IM	7	–	42	74	77
Male	700 E	2.0 (2.86)		25.0 (24.2)	200.0 (285.7)	250.0 (357.1)	IM	5	–	12	66	79
Female	400 E	1.0 (2.50)		25.0 (35.7)	200.0 (250.0)	200.0 (250.0)	IM	7	10	12	46	55
Male	600 E	2.0 (3.33)		20.0 (25.0)	350.0 (583.3)	200.0 (333.3)	IM	7	–	13	60	65
Male	750 E	2.5 (3.33)			400.0 (533.3)	250.0 (333.3)	IM	4	7	9	51	63
Female	820 E	2.25 (2.74)			400.0 (487.8)	180.0 (219.5)	IM	5	6	10	65	77

*First syringe, little effect other than slight ataxia after 28 minutes.
†Second syringe.

(From Denney, R.N. Black Rhinoceros Immobilization Utilizing a New Tranquilizing Agent. East Afr Wildl J 7:159, 1969.)

Table 21–12. Recommended Optimal Intramuscular Dosage of Carfentanil (Wildnil) and Additives for the Immobilization of 19 Free-Ranging Wild Animal Species

	Adult Body Weight (kg)	Analgesic (Narcotic) Carfentanil		Additive Xylazine		Azaperone		Analgesic Antagonist Naloxone		Cyprenorphine	
		Dosage Rate (µg per kg)	Total Dose* (mg)	Dosage Rate (µg per kg)	Total Dose* (mg)	Dosage Rate (µg per kg)	Total Dose* (mg)	Multi-plication Factor	Total Dose† (mg)	Multi-plication Factor	Total Dose† (mg)
African elephant	5000	1	5	—	—	—	—	6–10	40	10–12	50
Square-lipped rhinoceros	2000	1	2	—	—	100	200	6–10	16	10–12	20
Black rhinoceros	1000	1.5	1.5	—	—	150	150	8–10	10	10–12	12
Giraffe	1000	3(1.5)§	3(1.5)§	40	40	100	100	3–4	12	4–5	15
African buffalo	700	5	3.5	50	35	150	105	2–3	10	3–4	12.5
Eland	800	8	6.4	200	160	300	240	2–3	15	3–4	20
Roan antelope	250	10	2.5	100	25	300	75	2–3	7	3–4	10
Blue wildebeest	220	8	1.75	80	17.5	240	52.5	2–3	5	3–4	6
Black wildebeest	150	8	1.2	80	12	240	36	2–3	3.5	3–4	5
Red hartebeest	140	10	1.4	100	14	300	42	2–3	4	3–4	5
Tsessebe	140	10	1.4	100	14	300	42	2–3	4	3–4	5
Blesbok	90	10	0.9	100	9	300	27	2–3	2.5	3–4	3.5
Common waterbuck	240	10	2.4	100	24	300	72	2–3	7	3–4	8
Greater kudu	260	10	2.6	100	26	300	78	2–3	7	3–4	8
Gemsbok	180	10	1.8	100	18	300	54	2–3	5	3–4	7
Impala	50	7	0.35	100	5	300	15	3–4	1.4	4–5	1.7
Springbok	35	10	0.35	100	3.5	300	10.5	3–4	1.4	4–5	1.7
Steenbok	12	10	0.12	100	1.2	300	3.6	3–4	0.4	4–5	0.5
Warthog	80	12.5	1	100	8	300	24	3–4	4	4–5	5
Burchell's zebra‡											

*Analgesic or additive total dose = Analgesic rate × body weight.
†Analgesic antagonist total dose = Analgesic total dose × multiplication factor.
‡Carfentanil is not recommended for the zebra. Etorphine is recommended as the principal immobilizing agent.
§Figures in parentheses denote noncasting dosage levels for giraffe.
The dosages listed are for free-ranging wild animals. Wild animals adapted to captive conditions usually require lower dosages.
When a short induction period is required, the (carfentanil) dosage rate can be drastically increased.
Carfentanil can be used without an additive. In cases of excitable species and warthog, a mixture or "cocktail" is preferred.
Although diprenorphine is not listed as an antagonist, it can be used with equal success in dosages slightly less than cited for cyprenorphine.
Nalorphine hydrobromide can also be used as an antagonist.
(From DeVos, V. Immobilisation of Free-Ranging Wild Animals Using a New Drug. Vet Rec 103:64, 1978.)

Table 21–13. Dosage Rates of Drugs Used for Neuroleptic Narcosis in Species of Hoofed Wild Animals in South African National Parks

Species	No. of Successful Cases	Mortality	Sex	Range Adult Body Weight (lb)	Dissociative Phencyclidine (mg)	(Major Tranquilizer Fluanisone† (mg)
Elephant (*Loxodonia africana africana*)	34	2	M M F	12,000–15,000 7000–12,000 7000–12,000		
Square-lipped Rhinoceros (*Dicerus simus simus*)	3	1	M M & F	3000–5000 2500–4000		
Hippopotamus (*Hippopotamus amphibius capensis*) (on land)	2	1	M F	3500–4500 3000–3800		
Giraffe (*Giraffa camelopardalis giraffa*)	73	8	M & F M & F	2000–3000 Young 600–1200		
Warthog (*Phacochoerus aethiopicus sundevalli*)	2	—	M & F	140–220		10
Zebra (*Equus burchelli antiquorum*)	106	7	M & F M & F	550–750 Young 250–350		20 10
Impala (*Aepyceros melampus melampus*)	47	2	M & F	100–165		
Blue wildebeest (*Connochaetes (Gorgon) taurinus taurinus*)	124	8	M & F M & F	450–650 Young 200–450		20 (or 10 + 10 Ace prom.§) 10
Red hartebeest (*Acelaphus buselaphus caama*)	5	—	M F	350–450 280–380		10 10
Tsessebe (*Damaliscus lunatus lunatus*)	1	—	M & F	250–350		10 (or 5 + 5 Ace prom.)
Buffalo (*Syncerus caffer caffer*)	19	—	M F	1300–2000 1000–1500		40 (or 30 + 20 Ace prom.) 30 (or 20 + 15 Ace prom.)
Waterbuck (*Kobus ellipsiprymnus ellipsiprymnus*)	5	—	M F	475–600 350–500		Preferable to Ace prom. alone. *20 + 10 Ace prom. *20 + 10 Ace prom.
Kudu (*Trogelaphus strepsiceros strepsiceros*)	13	1	M F	550–650 280–400	75–100 50	Alternative to Sernylan‖ *50 *40
Eland (*Taurotragus oryx oryx*)	2	—	M F	1200–2000 500–850	100–150 75–100	Alternative to Sernylan. 50–60 *50
Sable antelope (*Hippotragus niger niger*)	2	1	M & F	450–550		*20 (or 10 + 20 Trifluopromazine)
Roan antelope (*Hippotragus equinus equinus*)	1	—	M & F	450–600 +		*20–30 (or 15 + 20 Trifluopromazine)

*The dosages marked with an * are subject to further confirmation.
†Fluanisone (R2028) is a neuroleptic of the butyrophenone series.
‡M-183 is the acetyl ether of etorphine (M-99) and is not commercially available.
§Ace prom, acepromazine.
‖Sernylan (phencyclidine) is not available commercially.
(From Pienaar, U.D., Van Niekerk, J.W., Young, E., and Van Wyk, P. Neuroleptic Narcosis of Large Wild Herbivores in South African National Parks with the New Potent Morphine Analogues M-99 and M-183. J S Afr Vet Med 37:277, 1966.)

Dosages (Total Average Dose for Adult Animals)

Ataractic (Tranquilizer)			Narcotic		Parasympatholytic	Morphine Antagonist	
Acepromazine (mg)	Trifluopromazine (mg)	Chlorpromazine (mg)	Etorphine (mg)	M-183‡ (mg)	Hyoscine (mg)	Cyprenorphine (mg)	Nalorphine (mg)
50–60			7–8			60	1500–4000
40–60			5–6			40	(Not recommended)
40–50			5–6			40	
40 (optional)			2–3		100 (optional)		250–500
40 (optional)			1.5–2.5		75 (optional)		250–500
40 (optional)			5		100 (optional)		250–500
40 (optional)			4		100 (optional)		250–500
40				4–5	100		250–500
20				2	50		100–200
20			1.0–1.5		5–10		50–100
Alternative to Fluanisone			2	Alternative 2	20	5	100
20			1	1	20		50–100
10							
5			0.25–0.5	Alternative 0.25–0.5	5		10 (immediately) +40
20			2		20 (optional)		100
			1		10 (optional)		50–100
15			1.0		10 (optional)		100
10			0.75		10 (optional)		75–100
10			0.75–1.0		10 (optional)		100
20			4–6		75–100 (optional)		200–400
20			3–4		50–100 (optional)		200
20			*3.0–3.5		20–30 (optional)		200
20			*2.0–2.5		20–30 (optional)		100–200
Not recommended							
Not recommended	50	Alternative to trifluopromazine. 1.5–2.0 mg/lb body weight	4		50 (optional)		200
	50		2.5–3		30 (optional)		100–200
Not recommended	50–100		5–6		100 (optional)		200–400
	50		4		50 (optional)		200
Not recommended	20–30		2	Alternative 2	20 (optional)		200
Not recommended	20–30		2–3	Alternative 2–3	20 (optional)		200–300

HIPPOPOTAMUS

Relatively little information is available on restraint and anesthesia of the hippopotamus. These large artiodactyls live in and around rivers and shallow lakes and have raised eyes and nostrils that allow them to float partially submerged while viewing and breathing. Their nostrils have valves, and a hippopotamus can remain completely submerged for up to 4 minutes. Large males may weigh up to 2800 kg. Etorphine can be administered intramuscularly at a total dose of 4 to 8 mg alone or in combination with xylazine (0.1 mg/kg IM) (Table 21–12). Animals will often seek the safety of their water pools once injected and should be kept away from water when immobilization procedures are attempted. Phencyclidine (0.6–1.1 mg/kg IM) has also been combined with xylazine or acepromazine to immobilize free-ranging animals in large African parks. Many animals have been injected while in the water or near it. It is reported that animals that remain in water will float to the surface once sedated. These animals can be safely roped and hauled to the shore. Animals have remained immobilized for approximately 40 minutes following injection with these drug mixtures.(38)

URSIDS

Several anesthetic techniques have been used for capturing, immobilizing, and anesthetizing bears. Alpha-chloralose has been mixed with honey to capture black bears (*Ursus americanus*) in the field. The effective dose for wild bears is 2 grams per 3 to 8 kg of feed. Recovery usually occurs between 8 to 10 hours from the time of ingestion.(88)

Ketamine and xylazine combined in a ratio of approximately 2:1 on a per mg basis produces good anesthesia in captive and wild black bears (*Ursus americanus*). The optimum dose range is 4.5 to 9.0 mg/kg of ketamine and 2.0 to 4.5 mg/kg of xylazine when injected intramuscularly. Smaller bears appear to be induced more quickly. Supplemental injections have been used to maintain tractability for as long as 31

Table 21–14.   Etorphine (M991) Restraint of Large, Feral Animals Kept in Captivity

Family Groups	Suggested Drugs and Dosage	Comments on Other Drugs	Other Comments
Kangaroos and wallabies	Etorphine—0.1 mg per 20 lb body wt	Phenothiazine-derivative tranquilizers are not effective for restraint.	
	Etorphine—1 mg per 200 lb	Succinylcholine is effective, but hazardous.	
Elephants	Etorphine—1 mg per 2000 lb body wt given intramuscularly		If this dosage is ineffective, further attempts for restraint should not be made for 24 hours; then the dosage can be increased by half the original dosage.
Zebras and other wild equines	Etorphine—1 mg per 200 lb body wt. Can be mixed with acepromazine—2 mg per 100 lb body wt	Phenothiazine tranquilizers are ineffective as sole restraint agents.	Care must be exercised not to cause severe exertion and excitement in these animals. A tie-up syndrome has been seen in sedentary individuals that were exerted.
Camels and llamas	Etorphine—2 mg per 500 lb body wt		Emprosthotonic reflexes have occurred.
Tapir	Etorphine—1 mg per 100 lb body wt		
Elk and large deer	Etorphine—1 mg per 100 lb body wt		This drug is not very effective in small deer.
Giraffes	Etorphine—3 mg per 400 lb body wt		Etorphine has variable effect on giraffes. A relatively high dose is suggested because of the effectiveness of the antagonist, cyprenorphine.
American bison	Etorphine—1 mg per 200 lb body wt		Great care must be taken with herds because of their tendency to charge a single downed animal and human handlers.

(From Sedgtwick, C.J., and Acosta, A.L. Capture Drugs. Mod Vet Pract 50:32, 1969.)

Table 21–15. Intramuscular Etorphine Immobilization in Bears

Species	Sex	Est. Wt (lb)	Etorphine (mg)	Ace (mg)	S (mg)	Imm. Time (min)	Nal (mg)	Lag Time (sec)	Remarks
Spectacled	M	300	1.0	5.0	4.0	3.0	250	300	Good immobility, deep analgesia
Black	F	110	0.5	5.0	5.0	12.0	100	200	Good immobility, deep analgesia
Black	F	110	0.5	5.0	2.0	10.0	50	..	Same animal as above
Black	M	125	0.1	1.0	1.0	..	..	..	Tranquil, required additional 0.5 mg etorphine to immobilize
Black	M	125	0.5	2.0	2.0	15.0	50	30	Excellent stage of immobility, deep analgesia
Black	M	140	0.5	5.0	5.0	..	..	..	Tranquil, dart bounced off, hand caught
Black	M	140	0.5	5.0	5.0	..	..	..	Tranquil, dart bounced off, additional 0.25 mg etorphine, good immobility

Ace, acepromazine; S, scopolamine; Nal, nalorphine hydrochloride; Lag time, time elapsed from administration of nalorphine to animal standing; .., drug not used; Imm. time, time elapsed from administration of drug to immobilization.

(From Wallach, J.D., Frueh, R., and Lentz, M. The Use of M.99 as an Immobilizing and Analgesic Agent in Captive Wild Animals, J Am Vet Med Assoc, 151:870, 1967.)

hours.(89) Free-ranging polar bears (*Ursus maritimus*) can be immobilized with a concentrated solution of ketamine and xylazine containing 200 mg of ketamine and 200 mg of xylazine/mL. Cubs require approximately 3 mg/kg of each drug, whereas adults require 7 mg/kg.(90) Relatively low doses of medetomidine (0.03–0.06 mg/kg IM) and ketamine (2.5–4.0 mg/kg IM) have also been used to immobilize brown and polar bears (Table 21–4). Etorphine, acepromazine, and scopolamine have been used in combination to immobilize bears with relatively good success (Table 21–15).(41)

Small bears can be anesthetized with intravenous thiopental, thiamylal, or pentobarbital sodium given in the cephalic or saphenous vein. A squeeze cage facilitates the procedure. If this is not available, the caged animal is offered a favorite food; when it reaches for it, the paw is grasped by an assistant wearing gloves. A rope is tied around the limb to act as a tourniquet and to distend the vein. With this technique, 715 mg of pentobarbital produced surgical anesthesia in a 35-kg Malayan sun bear for 2 hours.(91) It has been reported that an average dose of 13.5 mg/kg of pentobarbital intravenously permits safe handling and minor surgery of American and Himalayan black bears.(92) Following induction with an intravenous thiobarbiturate, bears can be maintained with halothane or isoflurane via a muzzle mask or endotracheal tube. Inhalants are the preferred drugs to maintain anesthesia for long procedures because they provide good reliable muscle relaxation and more rapid emergence. As with most large carnivorous animals, endotracheal intubation can be easily accomplished. Additional information on the various drugs and techniques used for restraint and anesthesia of bears may be found in Chapters 10 and 22.

Sea Mammals

SEALS AND SEA LIONS

It has been reported that some phenothiazine-derived tranquilizers are ineffective in seals and sea lions.(93) For example, chlordiazepoxide produces a true ataractic effect in the California sea lion but has no effect on harbor seals, whereas diazepam produces an ataractic effect on harbor seals but apparently has no effect on California sea lions. Northern fur seals have been successfully anesthetized with propriopromazine (4 mg/kg IM) followed in 30 minutes by ketamine (11 mg/kg IM) for ovariohysterectomy surgery.(94) Ketamine alone (4.5 to 11.0 mg/kg IM) has been used to immobilize ringed seals and sea lions.(95) Atropine (0.3 to 0.6 mg total dose) can be given concurrently to prevent excessive salivation. Animals with respiratory problems should not be given high doses of ketamine alone. Phocid seals have been repeatedly anesthetized with a combination of ketamine (1.5 mg/kg) and diazepam (0.05 mg/kg) intramuscularly or intravenously.(96) The investigators preferred this combination over ketamine alone because induction and recovery were smoother. Weddell seals have also been safely immobilized with intramuscular ketamine (2 mg/kg) prior to administration of halothane.(97)

A 2.5-mg/kg dose of succinylcholine has proven effective in immobilizing adult Southern elephant seals (*Mirounga leonina*).(98) These seals are generally so lethargic that they can be injected at close range with a pole syringe. Sixteen- to eighteen-gauge needles up to 4 inches long are necessary to penetrate the skin and underlying blubber. The use of succinylcholine is not recommended without concomitant analgesic or anesthetic drug administration and ventilatory support equipment readily at hand.

For intravenous injections, sea lions are best restrained in a squeeze cage to allow access to a protruding flipper. A vein on the ventral aspect of the flipper, approximately 3 cm anterior to its posterior edge, can be used for intravenous administration. Thiopental or thiamylal can be given at the rate of 2.2 to 4.4 mg/kg to produce anesthesia.(99) Barbiturates should be given rapidly to minimize struggling and to produce relaxation. Alternatively, isoflurane or halothane can be administered by means of a face mask to induce anesthesia. Sea lions can hold their breath for as long as 5 minutes. When they do breathe, their air intake is enormous and rapid. For this reason, the respiratory pattern during anesthetic induction is not an accurate gauge of CNS depression. Once the animal is induced, the trachea is easily intubated for further inhalant administration. Concentrations of 0.75 to 1.5% are usually sufficient to maintain anesthesia.

Numerous combinations of injectable drugs have been assessed in sea otters, including Telazol, butorphanol-diazepam, oxymorphone-acepromazine-diazepam, azaperone-fentanyl-diazepam, and fentanyl-diazepam. Of these, the most effective combination appears to be the combinations of fentanyl (0.1 mg/kg) with either acepromazine or diazepam (0.22 mg/kg) administered intramuscularly.(100)

PORPOISES

Porpoises breathe through a modified nasal orifice, called the *blowhole,* located on the dorsum of the head just anterior to the cranial vault. It appears on the surface as a single, transversely crescentic opening with a forward-facing concavity. It is closed by a muscular nasal plug and opens through the action of forehead muscles. Normally it remains closed. Ventral to the blowhole are vestibular and tubular air sacs connected to the paired nares, which begin a few centimeters down the respiratory passage. A septum divides the nares for 10 to 12 cm, after which the respiratory passage becomes single again just above the glottis. The larynx forms an arytenoepiglottal tube giving a direct opening from the internal nares to the lungs, thus allowing the animal to breathe only through the blowhole (Fig. 21–6).

Approximately 10 cm from the base of the larynx the trachea gives off a separate right bronchus, and at about 15 cm it bifurcates into two main bronchi. It is important, when the porpoise is intubated, that the endotracheal tube extend only about 20 cm past the proximal tip of the glottis so that all of the lungs will be ventilated. Porpoises can take one full respiration in 0.3 seconds. With a tidal volume of 5 to 10 L, the flow rates through the air passages range from 30 to 70 L/s during expiration and inspiration. Porpoises breathe 2 or 3 times each minute. Each breath is deep (approximately 80% tidal air). After inspiration, the animal holds an apneustic plateau for 20 to 30 seconds followed by rapid exhalation.

To produce a calming effect, paraldehyde-impregnated fish have been fed to porpoises.(101) Thiopental-halothane anesthesia in the porpoise has been described.(102) Porpoises can be intubated while awake, but intubation is more easily accomplished after injection of 10 mg/kg of thiopental into one of the tail fluke veins. A 24- to 30-mm modified equine endotracheal tube with an inflatable cuff is used. The mouth is held open with towels by assistants. The hand inserted into the pharynx grasps the larynx, pulls it from its

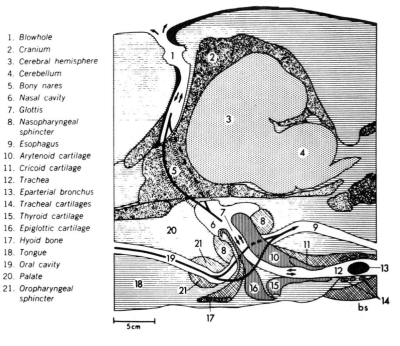

1. Blowhole
2. Cranium
3. Cerebral hemisphere
4. Cerebellum
5. Bony nares
6. Nasal cavity
7. Glottis
8. Nasopharyngeal sphincter
9. Esophagus
10. Arytenoid cartilage
11. Cricoid cartilage
12. Trachea
13. Eparterial bronchus
14. Tracheal cartilages
15. Thyroid cartilage
16. Epiglottic cartilage
17. Hyoid bone
18. Tongue
19. Oral cavity
20. Palate
21. Oropharyngeal sphincter

Fig. 21–6. Sagittal view of the head and neck of the bottlenose dolphin. (From Nagel, E.L., Morgane, P.J., and McFarland, W.L. Anesthesia for the Bottlenose Dolphin. Vet Med Small Anim Clin 61:230, 1966.)

intranarial position and, with two fingers inserted into the glottis, guides the tube in along the palm of the hand. In *Delphinus delphis* and *Stenella styx* a method of introducing the tube through the blowhole has been described.(103) For induction without thiopental, 3.5% isoflurane or halothane is administered for 5 to 15 minutes via a mask or endotracheal tube, after which 1.0 to 1.25% is used to maintain surgical anesthesia. If thiopental is used to induce anesthesia before intubation, 1.5 to 2.0% isoflurane or halothane is sufficient for maintenance.

Loss of swimming movements of the tail flukes indicates surgical anesthesia and occurs after loss of strong corneal and eyelid reflexes. The swimming reflex is considered the best criterion for assessing the depth of anesthesia. During the recovery period the endotracheal catheter is kept in position until the blowhole reflex returns. This requires 15 to 45 minutes following cessation of inhalant administration. Anesthesia with halothane has been maintained for periods up to 21 hours. The heart rate under anesthesia is generally 100 to 120 a minute. Arterial pH averages 7.35, PaO_2 is maintained at 100 to 200 mm Hg, and $PaCO_2$ is 35 to 50 mm Hg. In awake animals breathing ambient air, arterial PaO_2 reportedly ranges from 65 to 98 mm of Hg, and $PaCO_2$ from 40 to 60 mm of Hg.

Injection of thiopental alone (10 mg/kg IV) produces 10 to 15 minutes of light anesthesia and 45 minutes of respiratory depression during which the animal may require artificial ventilation. A dose of 15 to 25 mg/kg IV produces surgical anesthesia for 10 to 25 minutes, with respiratory depression lasting 1 to 2½ hours. Sensitivity to barbiturates has been further demonstrated following high doses of intraperitoneal pentobarbital (10 to 30 mg/kg), which has resulted in respiratory failure and death.(104) An apneustic plateau control unit for use with the Bird Mark 9 respirator has been developed to imitate the natural respiration of the porpoise. It inflates the lungs rapidly, holds an apneustic plateau for a variable period, and then deflates the lungs.(105) Because plasma cholinesterase is not present in *Tursiops truncatus,* the use of succinylcholine during anesthesia to produce muscle relaxation is contraindicated.

Reflexes that may be observed for depth of anesthesia in the porpoise include (a) contraction of the eyelid on tapping the inner canthus of the eye, (b) contraction of the eye muscles when the cornea is touched, (c) contraction of the throat muscles when the hand is inserted into the pharynx, (d) retraction of the tongue on being pulled, (e) reflex movements of the body when the anus is distended, (f) tail movements, (g) movements of the pectoral flippers in response to scratch or pinprick of the chest or axillary region, (i) movement of the blowhole on insertion of the finger into the nares or vestibular sacs, and (j) vaginal or penile movements when the vagina or prepuce is distended by insertion of the fingers or instruments.

Timing of removal of the endotracheal tube is critical. The correct time is when the animal is completely capable of breathing on its own, as manifested by movements of the blowhole and thorax, and by struggling and "bucking." When the endotracheal tube is removed, the larynx must be placed into its normal intranarial position. If the animal does not blow within 3 minutes or if the heart rate falls below 60, the tube must be reinserted and the animal ventilated for a few more minutes. In water porpoises are near neutral in buoyancy. Out of water it is more difficult for them to breathe and maintain circulation. For this reason, the animal should be returned to water as soon as possible.

Marsupials

Care should be used when catching and restraining kangaroos, since the claws on the hind limbs are well developed and may cause severe lacerations. Occasionally, a kangaroo will bite or claw with its forepaws. For capture of macropods, ketamine (3.0 mg/kg) has been combined with etorphine (0.005 mg/kg) and administered intramuscularly for successful immobilization.(106) Immobilization occurs in 3 to 4 minutes. Ketamine has also be combined with xylazine (8 mg/kg IM of each) to induce satisfactory anesthesia.(107) Althesin at the rate of 15 mg of total steroid per kg administered intramuscularly produces anesthesia and good muscle relaxation. Generally phenothiazine tranquilizers have a slow onset of action in marsupials, and effects may last for 2 to 3 days. For this reason diazepam has been considered a better drug for tranquilization.(106)

Red and gray kangaroos can be anesthetized by intravenous administration of thiopental in the recurrent tarsal vein. Small kangaroos (tammar wallabies and quokkas) have been anesthetized with thiopental (28 mg/kg IV), intubated, and maintained with halothane-oxygen.(108) The rat kangaroo (*Potorous tridactylus Kerr*) or potoroo, is a small species that can be picked up by the tail. It will bite, kick, and scratch if not handled carefully. A large plastic tube has been devised (6" diameter by 13" long) with a slot in the end gate to allow access to the tail for venipuncture. The vein, located at the lateral aspect of the base of the tail, can be distended with a tourniquet. Rat kangaroos appear to have a low tolerance to thiopental and pentobarbital.(109) Several anesthetics and dosages commonly used for inducing anesthesia in marsupials are given in Table 21–16.

Opossums can be carried by the tail, with precaution being taken to prevent the animal from crawling up its tail and attacking the handler. When removing an animal from a cage, it is wise to distract or immobilize the head while grasping the tail.(110) Ketamine (20 to 25 mg/kg IM) or fentanyl-droperidol (0.75 to 1.0 mL/kg IM) provides satisfactory immobilization for handling.(111) Inhalants and pentobarbital sodium have been commonly used to anesthetize opossums. Inhalants can be administered via a closed system and mask once the opossum is sedate.(112) For prolonged procedures, thiopental can be given for induction of anesthesia and intubation, followed by administration of halothane or

Table 21–16. Anesthesia in Marsupials

Agent	Dose and Route	Species and Comments
Azaperone 40 mg/mL	2–4 mg/kg by IM injection	Tranquilization in large macropods
Diazepam 5 mg/mL	2–4 mg/kg IM or IV	All marsupials; tranquilization or anti-convulsant
Diazepam	Oral (in feed) 2 mg/kg	Tranquilization in all marsupials
Acepromazine	0.1 mg/kg IJM	Indications of some delayed effect (lasts some days); needs quiet and dark for some hours to have maximum effect
Ketamine HCl	20 mg/kg IM	Monotremes for light surgical anesthesia
	25 mg/kg IM	Anesthesia (light) in dasyurids macropods, wombat, koala
	30–50 mg/kg IM	Phalangers for light anesthesia; variable; give 30 mg/kg first, then if insufficient give additional 20 mg/kg
Thiopental	20 mg/kg as 5 or 2.5% sol. (exactly as small animals) by IV injection	All marsupials (tail veins usually easy to use)
Alphaxolone 9 mg/mL Alphadolone 3 mg/mL	0.25–0.5 mL/kg IV to effect	Macropods and phalangers; short duration, can top up; recover fast
Halothane	Inhalation to effect	Bell jar for tiny dasyurids; anesthetic machine and mask or tube in larger species
Etorphine and combinations	0.5 ml of "large animal immobilon" per large kangaroo by IM projectile	Only for capture; restricted availability; can cause excitement and self-injury
Ketamine and xylazine	5 mg/kg ketamine; 2 mg/kg xylazine in same projectile	Capture of macropods

(Adapted from Reddacliff, G. Therapeutic Index—Marsupials. Proc Postgrad Committee Vet Sci Univ of Sidney, 39:1037, 1978.)

isoflurane. Pentobarbital at a dose of 36 mg/kg produces satisfactory anesthesia when given intravenously. Intraperitoneal injection is less reliable and provides a narrower margin of safety. Alpha-chloralose has been safely used in opossums to produce long periods of anesthesia. Induction is achieved with thiopental given intravenously followed by alpha-chloralose administered at a dose of approximately 12 mg intravenously every 2 hours.

Laboratory Animals

RODENTS

Prior to anesthesia, rodents should be weighed and given a physical exam, and their history should be reviewed. Because of their small size and high metabolic rate, preanesthetic fasting should be limited to 1 or 2 hours to avoid hypoglycemia. Water should not be withheld. In addition, owing to their high body surface to body volume ratio, care should be taken to avoid excessive hypothermia in the perioperative period.

If injectable anesthetics are to be used, consideration should be given to their volume, the site(s) of administration, their irritant properties, and the method of administration (i.e., single or repeated IV bolus, IV infusion). Irritant or highly concentrated agents can be diluted to reduce irritation at the site of injection and to aid in accurate delivery of the proper dose. If irritating drugs are used, multiple sites of injection can be used to further decrease tissue damage.

Intraperitoneal injection has been commonly used in laboratory rodents because it requires minimal skill and does not result in lesions or signs of pain when irritating drugs are administered, and because of the scarcity of readily accessible peripheral veins, especially in hamsters and guinea pigs. Intraperitoneal injections should be made into the lower left quadrant of the abdomen while the animal is restrained in a head down position. Adult hamsters and guinea pigs may be fasted for 4 to 6 hours to reduce the abdominal contents and thereby decrease the likelihood of injecting into the bowel. Care should be taken to assure that injection is indeed into the peritoneum and not into the abdominal wall or fat.

Intramuscular injections should be made into the caudal thigh or epaxial muscles. Tissue damage occurs following injection of irritating drugs such as ketamine or Innovar-Vet. The severity ranges from subclinical inflammation to ulceration, necrosis, and self-mutilation. Irritation can be minimized by use of small needles, deep injections, multiple injection sites, and dilution of the drug(s). Intravenous injections can be made into the lateral tail vein of mice, rats, and gerbils. Vasodilation of the vein induced by a heated restrainer or heat lamp will facilitate injection. Other, less accessible veins, such as the dorsal metatarsal or sublingual veins, could also be used in anesthetized subjects for intraoperative drug administration. Intravenous drug delivery is seldom attempted in hamsters or guinea pigs, although the lateral saphenous vein can be cannulated for drug or fluid administration in the anesthetized guinea pig.(113)

Injectable anesthetics, although easy and inexpensive to use, have several disadvantages in that they may not always induce adequate anesthesia at recommended doses and may induce a prolonged duration of action and delayed recovery. Nevertheless, they can be quite useful. Tables 21–17 to 21–21 give doses, routes, and duration of anesthesia for injectable anesthetic drugs and drug combinations used in laboratory rodents. Table 21–22 gives doses of analgesics for use in various laboratory rodents.

Inhalation agents can be safely administered to small rodents and have the advantage of greater control of anesthetic depth and duration. Induction can be readily induced in a chamber and maintenance of anesthesia achieved with a face mask or head chamber. Face or head masks can be made from a disposable syringe. Because of the animals' size and anatomy, endotracheal intubation is not often attempted. Nevertheless, endotracheal intubation allows control of the airway and provides a means to administer inhalation agents efficiently either as the sole anesthetic or to supplement and extend anesthesia induced with injectables. Intubation is most readily done via direct visualization. Pediatric laryngoscopes can be modified to a width sufficient to allow their use in rats, hamsters, and guinea pigs. Alternatively, an otoscope cone can be used as an oral speculum and the pharynx transilluminated with an external light source such as a penlight to allow visualization of the larynx. Fourteen- to 20-gauge over-the-needle catheters can be used as an endotracheal tube and adapted to connect to the breathing circuit. Guinea pigs are particularly difficult to intubate because their large tongue and upwardly projecting epiglottis makes visualization of the larynx difficult. All of the available inhalation anesthetics provide safe predictable anesthesia in laboratory rodents.

Mice. Mice may be lifted by the tail for handling but should be supported lest they climb their tail and bite the handler. Methods for restraining and holding mice are illustrated in Figure 21–7. It is possible to inject mice in the lateral vein of the tail, though extensive practice is necessary for proficiency.(114) The dorsal metatarsal vein may also be used after the hair has been clipped. A 27- or 28-gauge needle is used for injection (Fig. 21–8). Intraperitoneal or intramuscular injections of ketamine may be used in mice. Smoother anesthesia can be achieved by adding xylazine (Table 21–17).

Isoflurane and halothane are commonly used to anesthetize mice. The animal is usually placed in a chamber or other container and is removed when anesthetized. Anesthesia may be maintained by means of a small nose cone. Anesthetic chambers have been developed for mice and other small laboratory animals that enable anesthetization of several animals simultaneously. These chambers produce better control of anesthetic concentrations and carbon dioxide levels. For brief periods of anesthesia (1 minute or less), high concentrations of carbon dioxide may be used (see "Guinea Pigs"). Intravenous or intraperitoneal pentobarbital or thiopental can be used in mice. Anesthetized mice are particularly susceptible to cold and therefore should be kept in a warm, draft-free location until fully conscious.

Rats. Rats that are not tame can be difficult to handle. Although gloves may be worn, it is preferable to avoid their use, since they impede the fingers and there is a tendency to crush the animals rather than to grasp them securely. Using the thumb and forefingers of the left hand, the anesthetist grasps the tail near its base, lifts the animal out of the cage quickly, and places it head down on the upper surface of the right thigh. Degloving can occur if the rat is picked up by the distal portion of the tail. With the thumb and forefinger of the right hand, the anesthetist then quickly grasps the animal by the scruff of the neck and, without the left hand releasing its hold on the tail, turns it on its back. The rat, when placed on the thigh, will strain to pull away from the hand grasping the tail. However, if the animal is not caught immediately in the right hand, it cannot be carried by the tail for any length of time, as it will turn and climb its own tail far enough to bite the hand restraining it. A second method is to grasp the animal with the palm of the hand over the back and, with the thumb and forefinger, to fold the forelegs across each other under the animal's chin. When the legs are held correctly, the animal cannot depress its chin to bite.

A Turkish towel may be used for restraint while making intravenous injections into the tail veins or obtaining blood samples from them. The towel is folded over the rat, rolled, and pinned with safety pins, making sure the legs are secure. Rats may be left so restrained for hours without harm. Rats and mice readily enter and accept tunnel restrainers. A commercial rat restraining cage is shown in Figure 21–9.

The dorsal metatarsal vein is suitable for intravenous injection of rats and mice after the hair has been clipped. A 27- or 28-gauge needle is optimal. For intravenous injection of anesthetized rats, the lingual vein can be used. Once the rat is anesthetized, a small suture can be passed through the tip of the tongue for traction, which aids in exposure.

There are age and sex differences in the response of rats to ketamine.(115) Sleeping time decreases as young rats mature from 1 to 3 weeks. After 3 weeks, females sleep longer than males. Ketamine potentiates the production of restraint-induced stress ulcers in the stomachs of rats. This effect is presumably due to splanchnic vasoconstriction. Ketamine does not produce ulcers in unstressed rats.(116) Neither ketamine nor xylazine given alone will produce satisfactory

Table 21–17. Anesthetics and Tranquilizers for Use in Mice

Drug	Dosage	Route of Injection	Duration of Anesthesia	Reference
Barbiturates				
Thiopental	25–50 mg/kg	IV	10 min	148
	50 mg/kg	IP		149, 150
EMTU (Inactin)	80 mg/kg	IP		151
Methohexitone	8–16 mg/kg	IV	2 min	148
Pentobarbital	30–40 mg/kg (sedation)	IP	10–300 min	—
	50–90 mg/kg (anesthesia) dilute in saline to give a volume of 0.1 mL/10 gm body weight	IP		152
	50–60 mg/kg	IV		149
Dissociatives				
Ketamine	80–100 mg/kg	IM		153
	100 mg/kg	IP		150
	50 mg/kg	IV		150
Ketamine +	100 mg/kg	IM		154
Acetylpromazine	2.5 mg/kg	IM		155
Xylazine	2.5 mg/kg	IM		
Ketamine +	200 mg/kg	IM		
Diazepam	5 mg/kg	IP		
Ketamine +	100–200 mg/kg	IM		156
Xylazine	5–16 mg/kg or 0.1 mL/30 g of a solution containing 1 mL ketamine + 1 mL xylazine (100 mg/mL conc.) + 4.6 mL sterile water, yielding 50 mg/kg of each component per 0.1 mL	IP	60–100 min (Anesthetic depth varies from sedation to anesthesia)	157 154
Tiletamine + Zolazepam (Telazol)	80–100 mg/kg (restraint)	IP		158
Neuroleptanalgesics				
Fentanyl + Droperidol (Innovar-Vet)	0.001–0.01 mL/g (using a 10% solution of the commercial Innovar-Vet solution)	IM		159 160
Fentanyl + Droperidol (Innovar-Vet) + Diazepam	using a 1/10 saline dilution of Innovar-Vet, 0.1 mL/30 g after injecting 5 mg/kg diazepam	IP		
Fentanyl + Fluanisone (Hypnorm)	0.01 mL/30 g	IP		155
Fentanyl + Fluanisone (Hypnorm) + Diazepam	0.1–0.2 mL/30 g of 1/10 dilution of Hypnorm 5 mg/kg	IP, SQ IP, SQ	60–90 min	155 161
Fentanyl + Fluanisone (Hypnorm) + Midazolam	10–13.3 mL/kg	IP		155
Carfentanyl + Etomidate	0.003 mg/kg 15 mg/kg	IM IM		156

surgical anesthesia in rats. When combined, however, they are satisfactory.

For prolonged anesthesia, pentobarbital sodium may be used. The animal's weight in grams is determined.

For convenience, pentobarbital solution should be diluted so that each mL contains 30 mg (3% solution). A 0.25-mL syringe with a scale of 0.01 mL should be used. The dose on the scale is then the same as the animal's

Table 21–17. Anesthetics and Tranquilizers for Use in Mice—cont'd

Drug	Dosage	Route of Injection	Duration of Anesthesia	Reference
Other				
Alpha Chloralose (5% conc.)	114 mg/kg	IP		150
Alphaxalone-Alphadolone	7–25 mg/kg	IV bolus	7–8 min (14 mg/kg dosage)	162
(Saffan)	(14 mg/kg is optimal dose) maintain with 4–6 mg/kg every 15 minutes	IV bolus	10 min (25 mg/kg dosage)	148, 149
Chloral Hydrate	60–90 mg/kg 370–400 mg/kg	IP IP		162 150
Etomidate (Hypnomidate)	23.7–33.0 mg/kg 11.2 mg/kg	IP IV	20 min 20 min	163 163
Propofol	12–26 mg/kg	IV	5.6–6.9 min	148
Tribromoethanol (1.2% solution)	125–250 mg/kg	IP		164 165
Inhalants				
Carbon Dioxide	50–70% mixed with oxygen; vaporized dry ice	Inhalant		166 164

weight in grams divided by 10. For light anesthesia, 3 mg/100 g are sufficient; 4 to 5 mg/100 g will produce deep surgical anesthesia. The solution is given intraperitoneally just lateral to the umbilicus. Complete anesthesia will develop in 5 to 15 minutes and will be effective for approximately 45 minutes. Injection can be made subcutaneously, but the effect develops more slowly and is of longer duration. If anesthesia lightens before the desired time has elapsed, a second dose approximately one quarter of the first can be given after 45 minutes. In rats, intraperitoneal injection of 3.5% chloral hydrate solution at the rate of 1 mL/100 g of body weight produces adynamic ileus, and its use by this route is contraindicated.(117, 118)

There is a difference in the ability of various rat strains to respond to the nephrotoxic effects of inorganic fluoride, a metabolic end product of methoxyflurane and enflurane. Fischer 344 rats are particularly susceptible, whereas Long-Evans and Sprague-Dawley strains are not.(119) However, there is no difference in the ability of hepatic microsomes of these three strains of rats to enzymatically release inorganic fluoride from methoxyflurane.(120)

Carbon dioxide anesthesia is effective for short procedures in rats. It may be administered into a chamber from a cylinder mixed with oxygen (1:1 or 3:2), or by evaporation of dry ice (see "Guinea Pigs"). Little effect on hematologic parameters, except blood glucose, were found when this technique was used for orbital blood collection.(121)

Over 60 years ago, hypothermia was first reported for castration of 12-hour-old rats.(122) Rats were wrapped in filter paper, placed in a test tube, and immersed in a thermos bottle filled with ice. The test tube must be dry or the rat will freeze to it. The rat is cooled until its body temperature falls to about 2° C, at which temperature it is immobile and shows no reaction to stimuli. Anesthesia lasts for 3 to 10 minutes after the rat is removed from the thermos, and the operation is performed during this period. Gradual rewarming is then allowed by placing the animal in a cool place for 10 to 30 minutes followed by warming in the palm of the hand for 20 minutes. When the animal has recovered, it is cleaned and returned to its mother. At least one young should be left in the nest with the mother during the procedure, and the operated animal should be returned in front of the nest rather than placed in it. The mother then retrieves it. A cold room at 7° C has been used to induce hypothermia in neonatal rats for short periods (5 to 7 min) of surgery.(123)

Gerbils. The Mongolian gerbil is grasped by the base of the tail during handling because it is agile and may easily wriggle free and escape. The gerbil can be lifted by the tail (with caution, because it readily degloves). For intraperitoneal injection it can be restrained similarly to mice. Table 21–19 lists several anesthetic drugs and drug combinations that can be safely used in gerbils.

Guinea pigs. Guinea pigs are best restrained by grasping them around their pectoral and pelvic girdles. Methoxyflurane, halothane, and isoflurane are commonly employed for inhalation anesthesia of guinea pigs. Nitrous oxide–oxygen (1:1 or 2:1) may be employed as carrier gases for these volatile agents. Because guinea pigs produce copious secretions in the respiratory tract when exposed to inhalant agents, atropine

Table 21–18. Anesthetics and Tranquilizers for Use in Rats

Drug	Dosage	Route of Injection	Duration of Anesthesia	Reference
Sedatives/Tranquilizers				
Droperidol	0.5–2.0 mg/kg (sedation)	SQ		167
Diazepam	5.0–15.0 mg/kg (sedation)	SQ		167
Barbiturates				
Thiopental (1.25% solution)	20–40 mg/kg 40 mg/kg	IV IP	5–10 min	150 150
EMTU (Inactin)	80–100 mg/kg	IP		150, 151
Methohexital (1% solution)	10–15 mg/kg 40 mg/kg	IV IP	5–10 min 15–20 min	168
Methohexital + Pentobarbital	40 mg/kg (induction) 20 mg/kg (maintenance)	IP IP	2 hours	169
Pentobarbital	40–60 mg/kg	IP	80–95 min	170, 171
	60–100 mg/kg induce with 50 mg/kg then 500 µg/kg/min	IM IP Continuous IV infusion		172
Dissociatives				
Ketamine	50–100 mg/kg (sedation)	IM		153
Ketamine + Acetylpromazine	75–80 mg/kg 2.5 mg/kg	IM IM		155
Ketamine + Diazepam	45–60 mg/kg 5–10 mg/kg or 2.5 mg/kg	IP IP IM		170
Ketamine + Medetomidine	60–75 mg/kg 0.25–0.5 mg/kg	IP SQ		173 174
Ketamine + Xylazine	40–87 mg/kg 5–13 mg/kg	IP, IM IP, IM		153, 170, 174, 175, 176
Tiletamine + Zolazepam (Telazol)	20–40 mg/kg 20 mg/kg	IP IM		158, 177
Tiletamine + Zolazepam (Telazol) + Xylazine	20–40 mg/kg 5–10 mg/kg	IP IP		178
Tiletamine + Zolazepam + Butorphanol	20–40 mg/kg 1.25–5 mg/kg	IP IP		178
Neuroleptanalgesics				
Fentanyl + Droperidol (Innover-Vet)	0.02–0.06 mL/100 g or 0.3 mL/kg	IP IM		170
Fentanyl + Droperidol (Innover-Vet) +	0.1 mL/30 g of a 1/10 dilution of the commercial preparation	IP		
Diazepam	5 mg/kg (inject diazepam 5 min prior to Innovar-Vet)	IP		

Table 21–18. Anesthetics and Tranquilizers for Use in Rats—cont'd

Drug	Dosage	Route of Injection	Duration of Anesthesia	Reference
Neuroleptanalgesics—cont'd				
Fentanyl + Fluanisone (Hypnorm)	0.4–0.5 mL/kg	IM or IP	20–90 min	161, 179
Fentanyl + Fluanisone + Midazolam (2 parts water for injection, 1 part Hypnorm and 1 part Midazolam, the latter at 5 mg/mL conc.)	0.20–0.22 mL/kg	IP		179, 180
Other				
Alpha-Chloralose (5% conc.)	31–65 mg/kg	IP		150
Alpha-Chloralose + Urethane	50–60 mg/kg 500–800 mg/kg (administer urethane 20–30 min prior to alpha chloralose)	IP IP	500 min	172, 181
Alphaxalone + Alphadolone (Saffan)	10–12 mg/kg (supplement with 3–4 mg every 15–20 min or 0.25–0.45 mg/kg/min	IV bolus Continuous IV infusion	5–12 min Up to 8 hours	162 162
Chloral Hydrate (5% conc.)	300–450 mg/kg	IP	60–136 min	182, 183
Propofol	7.5–10.0 mg/kg (induction) 44–45 mg/kg/h	IV Continuous IV infusion	8–11 min	148
Tribromoethanol (0.25% conc.)	300 mg/kg	IP		

administration and periodic endotracheal aspiration are indicated.

When pentobarbital sodium is given by intraperitoneal injection, anesthesia requires approximately 15 minutes to develop and lasts 1 to 2 hours. The recommended dose is 28 mg/kg; the fatal dose is 56 mg/kg.(114) Complete recovery may require 12 hours, and supplementary heat should be provided during this period. Intravenous injection is difficult to accomplish and is seldom used in guinea pigs. When necessary, the marginal vein of the ear, the lingual vein, or the pudic vein in the male are possible sites. The caudal auricular vein has been used for intravenous injections following ketamine (44 mg/kg) immobilization. For short periods of anesthesia, such as those needed for inoculation, carbon dioxide can be used effectively. Approximately 2 pounds of dry ice are broken into pieces 1 to 2 inches square and placed in the bottom of an open metal container, measuring 18 × 12 × 14 inches deep. The guinea pig is placed on a removable wire platform 5 inches above the bottom of the container. Carbon dioxide liberated from the dry ice produces general anesthesia in 10 to 15 seconds, following which the animal should be removed promptly. Anesthesia lasts approximately 45 seconds, and recovery occurs in about 1 minute. In a group of 1460 guinea pigs anesthetized by this method, 1 death occurred.(124) There is no excitement during induction, and no adverse side effects are seen. The respiration is increased temporarily. Chinchillas, rabbits, rats, mice, neonatal pigs (Chapter 20) and other small species also respond in a similar fashion to this method of anesthesia.

Fentanyl-droperidol (0.88 mL/kg IM) produces excellent anesthesia in guinea pigs. However, injected animals often develop swelling and lameness in the injected limb, which may eventually result in self-mutilation.(125, 126) Therefore, this mixture can only be recommended for acute studies.

A method for epidural anesthesia in the guinea pig has been developed for use in bilateral removal of the adrenal glands.(127) Following sedation, the guinea pig is held on its side with the back flexed to facilitate introduction of the needle into the lumbosacral space. A 23-gauge, 1-inch needle is directed at a 30° angle anteriorly through the skin and into the space until it strikes the floor of the vertebral canal. If no blood or cerebrospinal fluid can be withdrawn, 0.2 to 0.25 mL of warm 1% lidocaine is slowly injected into the epidural

Table 21–19. Anesthetics and Tranquilizers for Use in Guinea Pigs

Drug	Dosage	Route of Injection	Duration of Anesthesia	Reference
Sedatives/Tranquilizers				
Diazepam	2.5–5.0 mg/kg	IP	Sedation	161
Xylazine	5–40 mg/kg	IP	Mild sedation	161
Barbiturates				
Pentobarbital	15–40 mg/kg	IP	60 min	184
	30 mg/kg	IV	60 min	150, 154
Pentobarbital + Diazepam	20–25 mg/kg 1–8 mg/kg	IM IM		185
Dissociatives				
Ketamine	40–200 mg/kg (40 mg/kg is optimal dose)	IM		153, 184
*Ketamine + Acetylpromazine	33–44 mg/kg 0.1–1.6 mg/kg or 125 mg/kg ketamine 5 mg/kg acepromazine	IM IM	Sedation Anesthesia	
Ketamine + Diazepam	60–100 mg/kg 5–8 mg/kg	IM IM		186
Ketamine + Droperidol	125–150 mg/kg 1 mg/kg	IM	35 min	187
Ketamine + Medetomidine	40 mg/kg 0.5 mg/kg	IM or IP SQ		173
Ketamine + Xylazine	30–44 mg/kg	IM	77 min	188
	0.1–5.0 mg/kg or 40–100 mg/kg ketamine 4–5 mg/kg xylazine (Optimal dose is 87 mg/kg ketamine + 13 mg/kg xylazine)	IM IM SQ or IM	(sedation) 60 min (general anesthesia)	
Tiletamine + Zolazepam (Telazol)	10–80 mg/kg (sedation)	IM or IP		189
Neuroleptanalgesics				
Fentanyl + Fluanisone (Hypnorm)	0.5–1.5 mL/kg	IM	25–30 min (sedation)	161
Fentanyl + Fluanisone (Hypnorm) + Diazepam	0.2–1.5 mL/kg	IM	60–70 min	161, 185
	2.5–5 mg/kg prolong with Hypnorm, 0.05 ml/kg	IP, IM IM	Up to 3.5 h (with supplementation)	190 185
Fentanyl + Fluanisone (Hypnorm) + Midazolam	8.0 mL/kg of a mixture of 1 part Hypnorm, 2 parts water + 1 part Midazolam (5 mg/mL conc.) supplement with 0.1–0.3 mL/kg	IP IP		191, 192
*Fentanyl + Droperidol (Innovar-Vet)	0.44–0.88 mL/kg	IM		159
Fentanyl + Droperidol (Innovar-Vet) + Diazepam	1 mg/kg 2.5 mg/kg	IM IP		192

*IM injection of ketamine + acepromazine or fentanyl-droperidol may lead to self-mutilation in guinea pigs.

Table 21–19. Anesthetics and Tranquilizers for Use in Guinea Pigs—cont'd

Drug	Dosage	Route of Injection	Duration of Anesthesia	Reference
Neuroleptanalgesics—cont'd				
Fentanyl + Droperidol (Innovar-Vet) +	0.4 mg/kg	IM	60 min	188
Pentobarbital	15 mg/kg (pentobarbital is given 20 min prior to Innovar-Vet)	IP		
Fentanyl Diazepam	0.32 mg/kg 5 mg/kg (diazepam given 20 min prior to fentanyl)	IM IP	60–90 min	188
Other				
†Alphaxalone/ Alphadolone	40–45 mg/kg or 16–20 mg/kg	IP or IM IV bolus	40–90 min (sedation) 10–20 min (anesthesia)	161, 188 162
Alphaxalone/ Alphadolone + Diazepam	45 mg/kg 5 mg/kg (diazepam is injected 20 min prior to alphaxalone-alphadolone)	IM IP	60 min	188
Alpha Chloralose (1%) + Urethane (40%), in a 7:1 mixture	0.8 mL/100 g	IP	greater than 120 min	188
Chloral Hydrate	400 mg/kg	IP		150

†Attempts to prolong the duration of alphaxalone-alphadolone anesthesia in guinea pigs by repetitive bolus administration may lead to pulmonary edema.

space. Successful injection is indicated by a twitching of the hind limbs followed by relaxation of the posterior half of the guinea pig. Guinea pigs under 500 g are given 0.2 mL of lidocaine; those over 550 g are given 0.25 to 0.3 mL. Anesthesia lasts for 45 minutes. This technique has been modified for continuous epidural administration (Chapter 16).(128) Following sedation, the guinea pig is restrained in lateral recumbency with the vertebral column flexed to enlarge the intervertebral space at the lumbosacral junction. After skin preparation, the lumbosacral joint is palpated one vertebral space caudal to the iliac crests. A 19-gauge needle with an intravenous catheter attached is inserted, with the needle slanted forward at a 30° angle. The site of insertion is approximately 1.5 cm caudal to the lumbosacral fossa and just lateral to the spinous processes of the sacral vertebrae. As the needle point is felt piercing the intervertebral ligament, it is slipped forward into the vertebral canal for approximately 1 cm. The catheter is then introduced through the needle into the epidural space for about 1 cm. No resistance should be felt. Fibrillation of the muscles of the hind limbs may occur, indicating the catheter is positioned properly. A 1% lidocaine solution with 1:100,000 epinephrine is warmed to body temperature and injected slowly over a period of 1 to 2 minutes. Guinea pigs weighing less than 500 grams may be given up to 0.2 mL, and those weighing more, 0.25 mL.

The effect is prompt and lasts 40 to 50 minutes. Repeated injections may be made, subsequent doses usually being smaller than the initial dose and varying between 0.15 and 0.20 mL. Anesthetic and tranquilizing drugs commonly used in guinea pigs are given in Table 21–19.

Hamsters. Hamsters are nocturnal and greatly resent being disturbed during the day, which results in a definite tendency to bite. They should not be surprised, but warned of your presence. They are best picked up by being trapped against the side of their cage and gently encircled by the hand. Hamsters can be scruffed, but their scruff is quite voluminous and must be grasped accordingly. Hamsters will attempt to bite when scruffed, so it must be done aggressively. If they are scruffed, they should be cupped in the hands and stroked prior to release. Tunnel restrainers work well for hamsters and gerbils as well as rats and mice (Fig. 21–9).

Methoxyflurane, halothane, isoflurane, and pentobarbital sodium are anesthetics commonly employed in hamsters. The procedures for induction and administration of anesthesia are similar to those for the guinea pig, though fasting and atropine administration are not essential.

Pentobarbital is given intraperitoneally approximately ¼-inch lateral to the umbilicus. Intravenous injection is extremely difficult. Methohexital (7.5 mg/

Table 21–20. Anesthetics and Tranquilizers for Use in Hamsters

Drug	Dosage	Route of Injection	Duration of Anesthesia	Reference
Barbiturates				
Pentobarbital	70–80	IP	60–75 min	150
Methohexital + Diazepam (combined in a mixture containing 7.5 mg/mL methohexital + 1.25 mg/mL diazepam)	2–4 mL/kg of mixture	IP	15–30	129, 150
EMTU	200 mg/kg	IP		150
Dissociatives				
Ketamine	40–80 mg/kg	IP	Sedation	153
	200 mg/kg	IP	Anesthesia	150
	100 mg/kg	IM	Sedation	150
Ketamine + Acetylpromazine	150mg/kg 5 mg/kg	IM IM		
***Ketamine + Xylazine	80–100 mg/kg 7–10 mg/kg	IP IP		153
Tiletamine + Zolazepam (Telazol)	20–40 mg/kg (sedation) 50–80 mg/kg (anesthesia)	IP or IM IP		158
Tiletamine + Zolazepam (Telazol) + Xylazine	20–30 mg/kg 10 mg/kg	IP	10–30 min	193
Neuroleptanalgesics				
†Fentanyl + Droperidol (Innovar-Vet)	0.15 mL/100 g	IP		194
Fentanyl + Droperidol (Innovar-Vet) + Diazepam	1 mL/kg 5 mg/kg	IP IP		194
Fentanyl + Fluanisone (Hypnorm)	1 mL/kg (of a 1/10 dilution of Hypnorm)	IM or IP	Sedation	155, 161
Fentanyl + Fluanisone (Hypnorm) + Diazepam	1.0 mL/kg (of a 1/10 dilution of Hypnorm) 5 mg/kg	IP IP	55–60 min	155, 161
Other				
Alpha-Chloralose (1% w/v)	8–10 mg/100 g	IP	Hypnosis only	195
Alphaxalone/Alphadolone (Saffan)	120–160 mg/kg or 14 mg/kg, induction, maintain with 4–6 mg/kg every 15 min	IP IV bolus IV bolus	40–60 min 6–9 min	162 162
Urethane (50% w/v)	150 mg/100 g	IP	6 hours	195
Urethane (50%) + Alpha-Chloralose (10%) + Pentobarbital	38 mg/100 g 3.8 mg/100 g 2.6 mg/100 g supplement with 13.5 mg/100 g urethane and 1.4 mg/100 g chloralose	IP IP IP	1.5–2 hours Up to 6 hours	195 195

***Intramuscular ketamine + xylazine may cause irritation, lameness and self-mutilation in hamsters.
†Innovar-Vet may be contraindicated in hamsters because it induces CNS abnormalities.

Table 21–21. Anesthetics and Tranquilizers for Use in Gerbils

Drug	Dosage	Route of Injection	Duration of Anesthesia	Reference
Barbiturates				
Pentobarbital	36–100 mg/kg	IP	50–60 min	196
Dissociatives				
Ketamine	44–100 mg/kg	IM, IP	30 min (mild sedation)	196
	150–200 mg/kg	IP	15 min (anesthesia)	197
Ketamine +	75 mg/kg	IM	74 min (sedation)	196
Acetylpromazine	3 mg/kg	IM		
Ketamine +	50 mg/kg	IM	51 min (sedation)	196
Diazepam	5 mg/kg	IP		
Ketamine +	50 mg/kg	IM	41 min (sedation)	196
Xylazine	2 mg/kg	IM		
Tiletamine + Zolazepam	20–40 mg/kg (sedation)	IM		158
(Telazol)	60 mg/kg (anesthesia)	IM		
Neuroleptanalgesics				
Fentanyl + Fluanisone	0.5–1 mL/kg	IM or IP		155
(Hypnorm)				
Fentanyl + Fluanisone	1 mL/kg	IM or IP	21 min	196
(Hypnorm) +				
Diazepam	5 mg/kg	IP		
Fentanyl + Fluanisone	0.6 mL/kg	IM	Sedation	196
(Hypnorm) +				
Xylazine	5 mg/kg	IP		
Fentanyl +	0.05 mg/kg	SQ	72 min	196
Metomidate	50 mg/kg	SQ		
Other				
Alphaxalone + Alphadolone	80–120 mg/kg	IP	75 min	196
(Saffan)				
Tribromoethanol	225–325 mg/kg	IP	10–35 min (anesthesia)	198
	225–450 mg/kg	SQ	20–63 min (sedation)	198

mL) and diazepam (1.25 mg/mL) can be mixed in the same syringe in a ratio of 3:1 and administered intraperitoneally at the rate of 2.0 to 4.0 mL/kg.(129) Onset of anesthesia is rapid, and it lasts approximately 20 to 25 minutes. The mixture turns white but does not precipitate. Althesin (150 mg/kg IP) produces deep sedation with analgesia for 20 to 60 minutes. Tranquilizers and anesthetics commonly used in hamsters are listed in Table 21–20.

RABBITS

Rabbits should be handled with care to avoid self-injury. Forceful thrusting of the unrestrained hind limbs can result in fracture or subluxation of the lumbar spine. Immediate paralysis will occur if the spinal cord is severed. Paralysis usually accompanies the development of edema and hematomyelia. Rabbits should be caught by firmly grasping the scruff of the neck and can be initially restrained with downward pressure against the floor of their cage until they relax. Rabbits can be picked up by the scruff of the neck and

withers while supporting the hindquarters. If the rabbit is to be carried for more than a short distance, it can be carried in the forearms with its head tucked into the crook of the elbow like a football. When placing the rabbit on a table it should be held down until it relaxes to avoid kicking. It is also helpful to use a mat or towel to provide the rabbit with some traction and thereby avoid the scrambling that occurs in response to a smooth surface.(130)

Restraint of rabbits can be done manually or with the use of a restraint device. Manual restraint is greatly facilitated by wrapping the rabbit in a towel with one or both forelimbs incorporated into the wrap such that they cannot be extended. Rabbits can be calmed and assured by scratching the forehead and area behind the ears or by petting or stroking the back.(130) It is important to remember that rabbits display akinesis when alarmed or threatened and should be handled gently. In addition, during periods of stress, rabbits may increase their respiratory rate from 35 to 50 breaths per minute up to 200 breaths per minute. This

Table 21–22. Analgesics for Use in Laboratory Rodents

Drug	Rats and Mice	Guinea Pig	Duration of Effect	Reference(s)
Acetaminophen	110–305 mg/kg PO, IP	?	?	179
Alfentanil	0.05–1.5 mg/kg IP (mouse)	?	15 min	199
Aspirin	20 mg/kg SQ, 100–120 mg/kg PO	20 mg/kg SQ	?	179, 199
Buprenorphine	2.5 mg/kg SQ, IP (mouse) 0.5–1.0 mg/kg SQ 0.25–1.6 mg/kg IP (rat)	0.5–0.8 mg/kg SQ	6–12 h	155, 169, 179
Butorphanol	5.6 mg/kg PO (mouse) 0.05–5.4 mg/kg SQ (mouse) 0.04–23.3 mg/kg SQ 2.1 mg/kg PO (rat)	?	2–4 h	169, 179
Codeine	6.4–20 mg/kg SQ 12.5–25 mg/kg IP (mouse) 60–90 mg/kg PO (mouse) 60 mg/kg SQ (rat) 30–50 mg/kg IP (rat)	25–40 mg/kg SQ	4 h	179, 200, 201, 202
Diclofenac	14–100 mg/kg PO (mouse)	?	?	199
Fentanyl	0.032 mg/kg SQ (mouse ED_{50})* 0.0125–1.0 mg/kg IP (mouse)	? ?	? 15 min	200
Ibuprofen	7.5 mg/kg PO (mouse)	?	?	179, 199
Indomethacin	1.5–10 mg/kg PO (mouse)	?	?	199
Ketorolac	0.7–10 mg/kg PO (mouse)	?	?	199
Meperidine	12.5–25 mg/kg IP 20 mg/kg SQ or IM (rat) 3–12 mg/kg IP, SQ (mouse)	20 mg/kg SQ or IM 25–45 mg/kg IP	2–3 h	179, 200, 201, 202, 203
Methadone	1.6–2.0 mg/kg SQ (mouse) 1.0 mg/kg IP, 3.75 mg/kg SQ (rat)	3.6 mg/kg SQ	?	179, 203, 204
Morphine	1–4 mg/kg IV (rat) 2–10 mg/kg SQ 5–24 mg/kg IP (rat) 2–4 mg/kg IP (mouse ED_{50})*	5–12 mg/kg SQ or IM	2–4 h	169, 179, 201, 204, 205, 206
Naproxen	57–350 mg/kg PO (mouse)	?	?	199
Nalbuphine	40 µg/kg bolus followed by 100 µg/kg/min continuous IV infusion, 1 mg/kg SQ	? ?	? 4–6 h	206
Oxymorphone	0.22–0.33 mg/kg SQ (rat) 0.051 mg/kg SQ (mouse ED_{50})*	?	4 h	169, 200
Piroxicam	3.4–20 mg/kg PO (mouse)	?	?	199
Pentazocine	1–21 mg/kg SQ (mouse) 59–60 mg/kg PO (mouse ED_{50})* 8–10 mg/kg SQ 25–75 mg/kg IP (rat)	?	3–4 h	169, 179, 200, 203, 205
Phenylbutazone	31–250 mg/kg IP (mouse)	?	?	201
Sufentanil	0.0023 mg/kg SQ (mouse ED_{50})*	?	?	200
Xylazine	5–12 mg/kg SQ (rat)	?	2 h	169

*ED_{50}, effective analgesic dose in 50% of experimental animals.

high-frequency ventilation does not result in hyperventilation because minute volume does not increase.(131),

Respiratory disease, usually caused by pasteurellosis, is a common problem in rabbits. Many older rabbits may appear to be healthy but have significantly reduced functional lung tissue due to multilobular consolidation. Three- to 5-year-old unspayed females frequently develop uteroadenocarcinoma with pulmonary metastasis. Identification of pulmonary disease by auscultation is difficult in the rabbit. Therefore, thoracic radiography to assess the lungs may be prudent in older rabbits prior to anesthesia.

Rabbits produce atropinase, which rapidly inactivates atropine. As a result, the recommended doses are high (1–2 mg/kg) and the redosing interval is short (10–15 minutes).(131, 132) Alternatively, glycopyrrolate (0.01–0.02 mg/kg) may be used when an anticholinergic is desired.(132)

Drugs may be administered intramuscularly, subcutaneously, or intravenously. The muscles of the thigh and the lumbar muscles are the most common site of injection. The lateral ear vein can be used for intravenous administration of anesthetic drugs (Fig. 21–10).

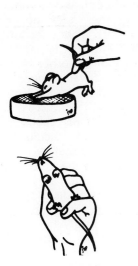

Fig. 21–7. Handling mice for injections. The upper figure illustrates the proper positioning of the animal. The lower figure shows its proper restraint. (From Taber, R., and Irwin, S. Anesthesia in the Mouse. Fed Proc 28:1528, 1969.)

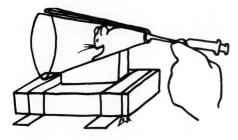

Fig. 21–8. Device for intravenous injection in mice. (From Taber, R., and Irwin, S. Anesthesia in the Mouse. Fed Proc 28:1528, 1969.)

The cephalic and lateral metatarsal veins can be catheterized for fluid administration. The central auricular artery can be catheterized for obtaining arterial blood for blood gas analysis or direct determination of arterial blood pressure, or to obtain large volumes of blood. Lidocaine-prilocaine (a eutectic mixture) patches can be used to desensitize the skin prior to catheterization. Plucking the hair over the vessel and use of a heat lamp to induce vasodilation are helpful. Table 21–23 gives anesthetic doses and various injectable anesthetic combinations for use in the rabbit. Table 21–24 provides suggested dose rates of analgesics for clinical use in rabbits.

Intubation in rabbits is relatively difficult compared to the more commonly encountered domestic species. The oropharynx is long and narrow, and the long incisors limit access to the mouth directly from the front. The tongue is fleshy, thick, friable, and easily torn. It is best to avoid traction on the tongue to avoid injury. The soft palate is long, and the epiglottis is large. The diameter of the larynx is less than that of the trachea, limiting the size of endotracheal tube that can be passed. Nevertheless, endotracheal intubation can be accomplished by direct visualization or by blind passage of the tube. Following induction of anesthesia, the mouth is opened and a straight premature infant laryngoscope blade is passed into the oropharynx at the diastema between the incisors and premolars and advanced over the base of the tongue until the larynx can be seen. The head and neck should be held in atlantooccipital extension to displace the epiglottis and provide a straight line of passage for the endotracheal tube. The larynx may be sprayed or swabbed with local anesthetic to prevent laryngospasm. A semirigid stylet can then be used as a guide to aid in passage of the tube into the larynx.

Blind passage of the endotracheal tube is possible even in small rabbits (<1.5 kg). Following induction, the rabbit's head is held in extension as previously described. An endotracheal tube is placed into the mouth at the diastema and advanced over the base of the tongue (Fig. 21–11). The tube is advanced into the larynx during inspiration by listening for breath sounds through the tube. Rotation of the tube facilitates placement and proper placement is verified by sounds and air flow through the tube. Cole or straight infant endotracheal tubes of 2.5 to 4.0 mm i.d. work well in rabbits.

Ketamine alone (44 mg/kg IM) does not produce adequate analgesia or muscle relaxation in rabbits. When it is combined with acepromazine or xylazine, analgesia and relaxation are of longer duration and recovery is smoother.(133) The optimum dose of fentanyl-droperidol for rabbits appears to be 0.22 mL/kg (1 mL/10 lb).(134) At this rate, it can be used as the sole anesthetic agent or supplemented with inhalants. Naloxone and doxapram can be used to partially antagonize the CNS effects of this combination.(135)

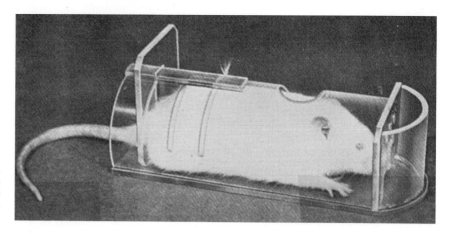

Fig. 21–9. A plastic restrainer for rats. Methoxyflurane-soaked cotton can be placed in the well at right to anesthetize the animal. (Courtesy of Fisher Scientific Company, Pittsburgh, Pennsylvania.)

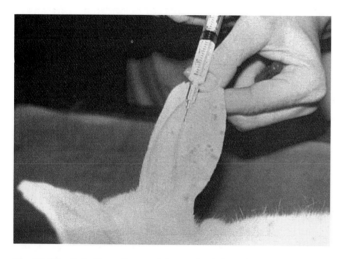

Fig. 21–10. Injection of propofol anesthetic into the lateral ear vein of a rabbit. Rabbits will often react vigorously to the injection and are best sedated with xylazine or ketamine prior to induction with a barbiturate or propofol.

The intravenous dose of pentobarbital usually recommended for rabbits is 30 mg/kg, but there is wide variation in response. A dose of 15 mg/kg may be sufficient for one, whereas another may require 50 mg/kg. Generally speaking, intravenous injection of 30 to 50 mg/kg of pentobarbital sodium satisfactorily anesthetizes cottontail rabbits (*Sylvilagus floridanus*).(136) Arousal time also varies widely, ranging from 1 to 10 hours. The depth of respiration is the best sign of anesthesia; it should be regular, deep, and slower than in the unanesthetized animal. Thiopental can also be used in rabbits. The average dose is about 50 mg/kg. Recovery from thiopental anesthesia is rapid.

When barbiturates are administered to rabbits, they are usually given intravenously in the marginal vein of the ear. The animal is weighed and prepared by clipping the hair over the vein. If rabbits are anesthetized only occasionally, it is recommended that the animal be wrapped in a towel with the forelegs securely included. With practice, use of a towel becomes un-

necessary. An assistant stands behind the animal and puts both hands over its eyes, directing the ear toward the anesthesiologist with the thumbs. The animal's rear is placed against the chest of the assistant, who leans forward with the forearms lightly restraining the animal on either side. The assistant can compress the marginal ear vein at the base of the ear. The veterinarian grasps the ear between thumb and second finger at its distal end, holding the index finger extended under the ear for support. The injection should be made toward the distal end of the ear so that if the first attempt is unsuccessful another may be made more proximally. A 24- or 25-gauge needle is inserted with the bevel upward and is threaded up the vein for 4 or 5 mm.

In laboratories where anesthetization of rabbits is carried out frequently, a restraining box facilitates handling and allows injections to be done by one person (Fig. 21–12). Thiopental should be injected slowly. During injection, respirations should be carefully observed. After the rabbit gives a deep sigh, injection of anesthetic should pause. Leaving the syringe and needle in place gripped firmly between the thumb and forefinger of the left hand, the animal's reflexes should be tested. While the veterinarian holds the rabbit's head with the right hand, the assistant lightly pinches the Achilles tendon at the heel. If anesthesia is not deep, the animal may give a forcible jerk; for this reason, the head should be held firmly. Further injection of thiopental is made until the Achilles tendon reflex produces only a moderate withdrawal response or tensing of the leg muscles. At this stage the animal is in surgical anesthesia, but the corneal reflex is still present and the pupil moderately dilated. In the rabbit, loss of the corneal reflex is a sign of dangerously deep anesthesia. With surgical anesthesia, respirations are regular. When the needle is withdrawn, a cotton pledget can be held over the insertion site with slight compression between the thumb and forefinger for a minute or two. Should the need arise for supplementary anesthesia, the assistant should hold the head firmly

Table 21–23. **Suggested Doses of Anticholinergics, Sedatives, Tranquilizers, and Anesthetics for Clinical Use in the Rabbit***

Drug	Dosage	Route of Administration	Reference
Anticholinergics			
Atropine	0.04–2.0 mg/kg (0.5 mg/kg commonly recommended)	IM, SQ	132
Glycopyrrolate	0.01–0.02 mg/kg	IM, SQ	132
Sedatives/Tranquilizers			
Diazepam	5–10 mg/kg 1–2 mg/kg	IM IM, IV	131, 153, 207
Midazolam	2 mg/kg	IP, IV	191
Acetylpromazine	0.75–10.0 mg/kg (0.75–1.0 mg/kg is most frequently used)	IM	208
Xylazine	3–9 mg/kg	IM, IV	161, 209
Medetomidine	0.25 mg/kg	IM	210
Barbiturates			
Thiopental	15–30 mg/kg	IV (1% sol) GTE†	131, 154
Thiamylal	15 mg/kg 29 mg/kg	IV (1% sol) GTE IV (2% sol) GTE	131, 154
EMTU	47.5 mg/kg	IV to effect	212
Methohexital	5–10 mg/kg	IV (1% sol) GTE†	161
Pentobarbital	20–60 mg/kg	IV	161, 207, 213
Pentobarbital + Chlorpromazine	20–30 mg/kg 2 mg/kg	IV IM prior to pentobarbital	161
Pentobarbital + Xylazine	11.8–28.4 mg/kg 5 mg/kg	IV SQ follow in 10 min by pentobarbital	212
Dissociatives			
Ketamine	20–60 mg/kg	IM	131, 154, 161, 211
Ketamine + Xylazine	10 mg/kg 3 mg/kg	IV IV	192
Ketamine + Xylazine (reverse with Yohimbine)	22–50 mg/kg 2.5–10 mg/kg 0.2 mg/kg	IM IM IV	131, 154, 214, 215 216
Acetylpromazine + Ketamine + Xylazine (preop with atropine, 0.04 mg/kg IM)	0.75–1.0 mg/kg 35–40 mg/kg 3–5 mg/kg	SQ IM IM	212 214
Ketamine + Acetylpromazine	75 mg/kg 5 mg/kg	IM IM (given 30 min prior to ketamine)	154
Ketamine + Diazepam	60–80 mg/kg 5–10 mg/kg	IM IM (given 30 min prior to ketamine)	131
Ketamine + Medetomidine	25 mg/kg 0.5 mg/kg	IM SQ	173
Tiletamine† + Zolazepam	32–64 mg/kg	IM	217
Tiletamine† + Zolazepam + Xylazine	15 mg/kg 5 mg/kg	IM (inject all simultaneously but use separate syringes)	215

*Modified from Wilson SK, Hobbs BA, Karchner LE, et al. Determination of appropriate analyesics for relief of pain in laboratory rats. J Invest Surg 4:359, 1991.
†GTE, given to effect.

Table 21–23.   Suggested Doses of Anticholinergics, Sedatives, Tranquilizers, and Anesthetics for Clinical Use in the Rabbit*—cont'd

Drug	Dosage	Route of Administration	Reference
Neuroleptanalgesics			
Fentanyl-droperidol	0.125 mL/kg 0.15–0.44 mL/kg (0.22 mL/kg is optimal dose)	SQ IM	134, 159, 218
Fentanyl-fluanisone	0.2–0.6 mL/kg	IM, SQ	155, 161, 191
Diazepam + Fentanyl-fluanisone	1.5–5 mg/kg 0.2–0.5 mL/kg (administer diazepam 5 min prior to fentanyl-fluanisone)	IM, IV, IP IM, SQ	155, 161, 207
Midazolam + Fentanyl-fluanisone	2 mg/kg 0.3 mL/kg (administer midazolam 5 min prior to fentanyl-fluanisone)	IP, IV IM	155, 191
Etorphine + Methotrimeprazine	0.025–0.05 mL/kg	IM	155, 207
Diazepam + Etorphine + Methotrimeprazine	1.0 mg/kg 0.25 mL/kg	IV, IP IM	155, 207
Other			
Alphaxalone + Alphadolone	6–20 mg/kg (optimal dose, 12 mg/kg)	IV	162
Propofol	7.5–15 mg/kg	IV	219
Medetomidine + Propofol	0.25 mg/kg followed in 5 min by 4 mg/kg	IM IV	210
Medetomidine + Midazolam + Propofol	0.25 mg/kg 0.5 mg/kg 2 mg/kg	IM IM IV	210
Intermittent Bolus or Continuous IV Infusion Regimens			
Sedate with Fentanyl + Droperidol	0.05 mg/kg 2.5 mg/kg	IM	220
Dilute Hypnorm 1:10	Infuse 1–3 mL/kg/h	IV	155
Midazolam + Xylazine + Alfentanil	1 mg/kg 1 mg/kg 0.1 mg/kg	IV	213
Sedate with Ketamine + Xylazine	35 mg/kg 5 mg/kg	IM IM	221
Maintain with Ketamine Xylazine	1 mg/min 0.1 mg/min	Continuous IV infusion	221
Ketamine + Xylazine	25 mg/kg 5 mg/kg	IV ⅓ bolus over 1 min, remainder over 4 min	213
Pentobarbital	40 mg/kg	IV ⅓ bolus dose initially over 1 min, remainder over 4 min	213
Propofol	Sedate with 1.5 mg/kg Maintain with 0.2–0.6 mg/kg/min "Utilization rate" of 1.55 mg/kg/min	IV bolus Continuous IV infusion IV	222 148
Alphaxalone + Alphadolone	Sedate with 1 mg/kg Maintain with 0.1 mg/kg/min	IV bolus continuous IV infusion	222

when the ear is punctured, since the rabbit may otherwise jerk violently at this time.

When respiratory arrest does occur, it is usually caused by too rapid administration of barbiturate. If one holds the rabbit's chest in the hand to compress it

Table 21–24. Suggested Dose Rates of Analgesics for Clinical Use in the Rabbit

Analgesic	Dose Rate	Reference(s)
Buprenorphine	0.01–0.05 mg/kg SQ, IV each 6–12 h	223
Butorphanol	0.1–0.5 mg/kg IV, each 4 h	223
Flunixin	1.1 mg/kg IM, each 12 h	224
Meperidine	5–10 mg/kg SQ, each 2–3 h	—
Methadone	1 mg/kg IV	225
Morphine	2.5 mg/kg SQ, each 2–4 h	—
Nalbuphine	1–2 mg/kg IV, each 4–5 h	223
Pentazocine	5 mg/kg IV, each 2–4 h	223
Piroxicam	0.2 mg/kg per os, 8 h	224

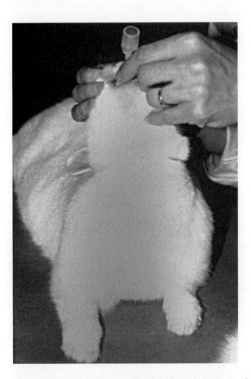

Fig. 21–11. Positioning the head and neck in full extension will facilitate blind passage of an endotracheal tube in rabbits. Small Cole or 2.5- to 4.0-mm-i.d. endotracheal tubes work well in rabbits using this technique.

lightly, the animal will resume respiration. Because this continues only as long as the chest is squeezed and stops when pressure is removed, it is only a temporary measure. Artificial respiration can be performed by rocking the animal alternately head down and head up. When done gently this technique is usually effective. Oxygen administration and other resuscitative measures should also be undertaken if necessary. Rabbits should be placed on a heating pad while on the operating table. Following surgery they can be placed in a baby incubator at 95° F until completely recovered from the anesthetic.

PRIMATES

In anesthetizing primates, the chief problem lies in restraint of the animals during induction because of their agility, strength, and defensive nature. Gauntlets and a net are essential pieces of equipment. Larger species, such as chimpanzees weighing over 30 lb, have tremendous strength coupled with a nasty disposition and are often extremely dangerous. For this reason, they should never be handled by persons working alone. If large numbers are to be anesthetized, a squeeze cage is effective and time-saving. In baboons and other large primates, the route of injection for anesthetics is usually intramuscular or into the posterior "pad." Several drugs and combinations commonly used for immobilizing and anesthetizing primates are given in Table 21–25.

The use of dissociatives for restraint, as preanesthetics, and as anesthetics revolutionized the handling of primates. By using squeeze cages, which allow easy intramuscular injection, one individual can immobilize many animals in a short time. As a guideline, ketamine at doses of 10 to 15 mg/kg intramuscularly in most primates results in immobilization that is adequate for performing examination, urethral and cardiac catheterization, blood collection, treatment of wounds, tattooing, and tuberculosis testing. Fifteen to thirty mg/kg IM will usually provide surgical anesthesia. Larger doses (20–30 mg/kg) of ketamine are usually necessary to produce surgical anesthesia for smaller primates and prosimians, but smaller doses (6–10 mg/kg) are sufficient for the great apes. Tolerance to repeated ketamine administration does not appear to be a problem in primates.(137)

The proprietary mixture of tiletamine and zolazepam (Telazol) has been used extensively for immobilizing and anesthetizing a large number of primate species. Reported doses range from 1.5 mg/kg IM in large primates to 10 mg/kg IM in smaller species. A combination that is effective for inducing anesthesia and allowing easy intubation of smaller monkeys such as the *Rhesus macaque* consists of 0.15 mg/kg of oxymorphone, 3 mg/kg of Telazol, and 0.04 mg/kg of atropine IM (Table 21–25). To prolong anesthesia and/or improve muscular relaxation, ketamine or Telazol injection can be followed by halothane or isoflurane administration. Inhalant administration produces surgical anesthesia and

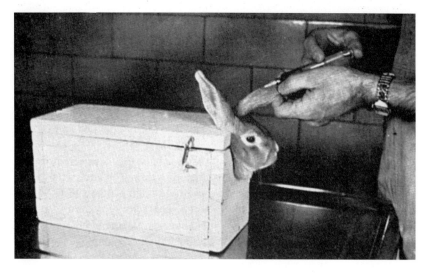

Fig. 21–12. Injection of the marginal ear vein of a rabbit using a restraining box.

prevents the involuntary movement observed with ketamine alone. A laryngoscope is helpful in intubating smaller monkeys such as the rhesus. Endotracheal tubes ranging from 4 to 6 mm i.d. are adequate for adult rhesus monkeys. Following induction, succinylcholine (1.5–2.0 mg/kg) can be given to produce laryngeal paralysis of short duration (1–1½ min) in order to facilitate intubation.

The anesthetic effects of various ketamine:xylazine dose ratios in monkeys (*Macaca mulatta*) have been studied.(138) Intramuscular ketamine alone at a dose of 2.5 mg/kg does not produce anesthesia. Xylazine alone at less than 2 mg/kg IM induces sedation, whereas the addition of xylazine to ketamine produces anesthesia whose duration is a logarithmic function of the xylazine dose (Fig. 21–13). The effect of a 5-mg/kg intramuscular dose of ketamine on cardiovascular function in baboons (*Papio cynocephalus*) has been assessed.(139) Cardiac output, peak aortic flow velocity, and peak aortic flow acceleration were all depressed; heart rate and stroke volume were slightly decreased. Primates immobilized with ketamine have near-normal acid-base balance.(140)

Neuroleptanalgesia with droperidol and fentanyl has been accomplished in a wide variety of primates ranging from squirrel monkeys to a gorilla.(141) The mixture may be given intramuscularly or orally in milk or fruit juice. Sufficient analgesia for 30 to 60 minutes of surgery is produced with either technique.
Intramuscular Technique:
  Droperidol 1 mg/kg
  Fentanyl 0.020 mg/kg (anthropoids)
  0.040 mg/kg (monkeys)
Oral Technique:
  Droperidol 1 mg/kg
  Fentanyl 0.040 mg/kg
Administration of etorphine to several species of primates is summarized in Table 21–26.(41) Intramuscularly administered meperidine at the rate of 11 mg/kg will produce a calming effect in most primates. Intra-

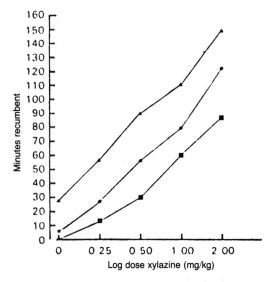

Fig. 21–13. Time recumbent as a function of increasing xylazine dose superimposed on ketamine dose. Ketamine: 2.5 mg/kg ■; 5 mg/kg ●; 10 mg/kg ▲. Each point represents a mean of 5 or 6 trials (1 trial per animal). (From Naccarato, E.F., and Hunter, W.S., Anaesthetic Effects of Various Ratios of Ketamine and Xylazine in Rhesus Monkeys (*Macaca mulatta*). Lab Anim 13:317, 1979.)

muscular injection of these agents can be accomplished by grasping the hand or forearm. Caged monkeys that are hard to manage can sometimes be enticed to reach for fruit held close to the cage bars. Tranquilizers can be administered to chimpanzees by dissolving the drug in canned pineapple juice. Other tantalizing vehicles for drug administration include maple syrup and peanut butter. After preanesthetics have taken effect, thiopental can be administered intravenously using veins of either the forearm or hind limb. Restraint for this procedure is necessary in most instances despite preanesthetic medication. The assistant can best hold small primates by grasping their arms and holding them behind the animal's back.

A wide variety of sedatives and anesthetics have been assessed in baboons including morphine, methadone, chloral hydrate, chloralose, pentobarbital, hexobarbital, amobarbital, paraldehyde, chlorpromazine, ether, chloroform, and nitrous oxide.(142) Morphine administered orally or by injection in doses up to 1000 mg caused severe skin irritation of the palms and soles with loss of appetite. Sedation was not produced. Pentobarbital sodium given by intramuscular injection was unpredictable, with animals reacting differently to equal doses on different days. After several hundred injections, pentobarbital was considered unpredictable. Chlorpromazine proved the most valuable sedative, but the response still varied widely. Doses of up to 3.5 mg/kg IV made the animals apathetic and slow, but they could not be easily handled. When doses were given intramuscularly, the action was slow, maximum effect occurring at 2½ to 6 hours after injection.

The use of halothane in various species of primates has been assessed.(143-146) For example, during spontaneous and controlled ventilation in stump-tailed macaques (Macaca actoides) a dose-dependent depression of cardiovascular function produced by halothane was greater than that observed in dogs, suggesting that there was a smaller margin of safety in this species.(146) Similarly, both halothane and enflurane produce dose-related decreases in heart rate, mean arterial pressure, and peak left ventricular dp/dt in rhesus monkeys.(147) Central venous pressure was increased with both inhalants. At equal MAC levels, no significant differ-

Table 21–25. Drugs and Combinations Used to Immobilize and Anesthetize Primates

Drug	Route of Administration	Doses (mg/kg)	Induction (min)	Duration (min)	Recovery (min)	Comments on Effects
Ketamine	IM	8–10	4–8	20–40	60–180	Immobilization good, quick induction, sedation, restraint, fair muscle relaxation, good for short procedures such as translocation, T.B. testing, blood collection, radiography, etc. Slight salivation.
Ketamine	IM	15–30	3–6	30–50	60–180	Immobilization excellent, quick induction, analgesia and anesthesia excellent, good muscle relaxation. Good for all procedures including major surgery. Slight salivation. Available in 100 mg/mL only—difficult to get enough volume into larger primate.
Ketamine	Oral	20–30	Variable	Variable	Variable	Variable
Telazol	IM	2–6	2–5	15–40	60–120	Immobilization excellent, quick induction, excellent analgesia and anesthesia. Good muscle relaxation.
M-99	IM	0.005–0.008	15–20	30–120	Reverse with naloxone	Immobilization fair, poor muscle relaxation, advantage of reversal with opioid antagonists.
M-99	Oral	0.1	Variable	Variable	Variable	Variable
Pentobarbital	IV	25–30	1–2	15–30	60–180	Immobilization good, excellent anesthesia and analgesia, good muscle relaxation. Drug must be administered intravenously.
Drug Combinations						
Ketamine + Thiopental	IM IV	5–10 10–15	1–2	20–30	60–120	Good muscle relaxation and analgesia for short period of surgery.
Xylazine + Ketamine	IM IV	2 to effect	1–2	60–120	120–180	Duration of anesthesia is dependent upon ketamine dose (see Fig. 21–13).
Oxymorphone + Telazol	IM IM	0.15 3.0	2–5	30	—	Used primarily for induction to be followed by intubation and inhalation anesthesia.

ences in anesthetic effects were noted between these anesthetics.

Administration of volatile inhalants can be accompanied by 50 to 70% N$_2$O to speed induction. This usually requires premedication and heavy sedation. Following administration of 0.2 to 0.5 mg of scopolamine and 10 mg/kg of meperidine, anesthesia may be induced with thiopental (8 to 10 mg/kg). An alternative for larger primates is induction with ketamine. Either method produces heavy sedation or light anesthesia so that the animal will readily accept a face mask. Human face masks are suitable for use with most small primates. Once relaxation is accomplished, an endotracheal tube is passed.

During prolonged surgery, small primates should be positioned on a heating pad to maintain body heat. Following removal from the operating table, they can be recovered in an infant incubator maintained at 95° F. Supplemental oxygen should be supplied by flowing it through a nebulizer to maintain the humidity within the incubator. These support procedures will help in shortening recovery time. The importance of postoperative analgesia cannot be overemphasized following major surgery in primates. Analgesic drugs, doses,

routes, and their duration of action that have been used in primates include morphine (1–2 mg/kg IM or SQ; 4 h), meperidine (2–4 mg/kg IM; 3–4 h), butorphanol (0.2–0.4 mg/kg IM; 3–4 h), buprenorphine (0.01 mg/kg IV or IM; 8–12 h), and aspirin (10–20 mg/kg, PO; 4–6 h). Spinal anesthesia is very difficult to perform safely in primates without heavy sedation or prior anesthesia.

Insectivora

HEDGEHOG

The African pygmy hedgehog (*Atelerix albiventris*) is rapidly becoming a popular household pet within the United States. These small insectivorous and carnivorous animals weigh from 11 to 16 oz. Their diet consists primarily of insects and larvae, but hedgehogs will thrive on canned dog or cat food. These pets are generally allowed to roam freely within the home but should be provided a large cage for sleeping and feeding. Although timid by nature, they will become accustomed to handling and placid as adults. If they should lick your hand, beware, they may subsequently bite this spot.

Hedgehogs and other insectivores such as tenrecs, shrews, and moles are easily anesthetized with isoflu-

Table 21–26. Etorphine Immobilization of Primates (Total Dose Values)

Species	Sex	Est. Wt (lb)	Etorphine (mg)	Ace (mg)	S (mg)	Imm. Time (min)	Nal mg	Lag Time (sec)	Remarks
Woolly monkey	F	15	0.03	..	..	4.0	..	..	Recovered in 1 hour, without nalorphine; dilated pupils
Woolly monkey	M	15	0.06	..	..	4.0	50	60	Salivated, muscle tremors
Woolly monkey	F	15	0.03	..	..	5.0	..	..	Recovered in 45 minutes without nalorphine; tractable, not dilated
Woolly monkey	M	18	0.1	..	..	5.0	..	..	Reduced effect 3-day-old solution
Spider monkey	F	4	0.03	..	..	4.0	..	..	Recovered in 3 hours without nalorphine; analgesia in 5 minutes
Spider monkey	F	6	0.03	..	1.0	4.0	..	..	Recovered in 3 hours without nalorphine; analgesia in 5 minutes
Spider monkey	M	5	0.03	1.0	1.0	4.0	..	..	Required additional 0.01 mg etorphine
Chimpanzee	F	35	0.06	..	..	10.0	..	..	Additional 0.04 mg etorphine; good immobility; recovered in 1 hour without nalorphine
Chimpanzee	M	55	0.05	1.0	1.0	5.0	50	300	Sternal recumbency, visual reflex
Chimpanzee	M	65	0.1	1.0	1.0	4.0	75	15	Good immobility, deep analgesia
Orangutan	M	50	0.25	..	..	7.0	125	..	Cardiac arrest, cardiac massage effected recovery

Ace, acepromazine; S, scopolamine; Nal, nalorphine hydrochloride; Lag time, time elapsed from administration of nalorphine to animal standing; .., drug not used; Imm. time, time elapsed from administration of drug to immobilization.

(From Wallach, J.D., Frueh, R., and Lentz, M. The Use of M.99 as an Immobilizing and Analgesic Agent in Captive Wild Animals. J Am Vet Assoc 151:870, 1967.)

rane in oxygen in an induction chamber or box. Maintenance of anesthesia can be achieved with isoflurane delivered via a face mask or endotracheal tube at a concentration ranging from 0.5 to 1.5%. The most commonly used injectable anesthetic is ketamine (5–20 mg/kg IM), alone or in combination with diazepam (0.5–2 mg/kg IM), xylazine (0.5–1.0 mg/kg IM) or medetormidine (Table 21–4). Telazol can also be used at a dose of 1–5 mg/kg IM. Hypothermia is a real threat because of the hedgehog's small body size. Fluids can be given intravenously or subcutaneously in the loose tissue beneath the spines. Subcutaneous fat may account for up to 50% of the hedgehog's body weight and can cause delayed absorption of fluids and injectable anesthetics when injected. Intramuscular injections require a needle length sufficient to extend through fatty subcutaneous tissues (Smith, A personal communication).

References

1. Fowler ME. Restraint and Handling of Wild and Domestic Animals. Ames, IA: Iowa State Univ. Press, 1978.
2. Fowler ME. Zoo and Wild Animal Medicine. Philadelphia: WB Saunders, 1978.
3. Green CJ. Animal Anaesthesia. London: Laboratory Animals Ltd., 1979.
4. Nielson L, Haigh JC, Fowler ME. Chemical Immobilization of North American Wildlife. New York: IR Publications Ltd., 1983.
5. Gamble JC. An Anaesthetic for *Corophium volutater* (Pallas) and *Marinogammarus obtusatus* (Dahl), Crustacea, Amphipoda. Experientia 25:539, 1969.
6. Foley DM, Stewart JE, Holley RA. Isobutyl Alcohol and Methyl Pentynol as General Anesthetics for the Lobster, *Homarus americanus* Milne–Edwards. Can J Zoo 44:141, 1966.
7. Eschmeyer PH. The Effect of Ether Anesthesia on Fin-Clipping Rate. Progressive Fish Culturist 15:80, 1953.
8. McFarland WN, Klontz GW. Anesthesia in Fishes. Fed Proc 28:1535, 1969.
9. Hublou WF. A Method of Using an Anesthetic in Marking Fins. Progressive Fish Culturist 19:40, 1957.
10. Martin NV, Scott DC. Use of Tricaine Methanesulfonate (MS222) in the Transport of Live Fish Without Water. Progressive Fish Culturist 27:183, 1959.
11. Gossington RE. An Aid to Fish Handling Tricaine. Aquarium J 28:318, 1957.
12. Lewbart GA, Stone EA, Love N. Pneumocystectomy in a Midas cichlid. J Am Vet Med Assoc 207:319–321, 1995.
13. Gilbert PW, Wood FG Jr. Method of Anesthetizing Large Sharks and Rays Safely and Rapidly. Science 126:212, 1957.
14. Scordelis P. Internal Communication. Redmond, WA: Tavolek, 1977.
15. Fish FF. The Anaesthesia of Fish by High Carbon Dioxide Concentrations. Trans Am Fisheries Soc 72:25, 1942.
16. Church JCT, Noronha RFX. The Use of the Fruit Bat in Surgical Research. East Afr Med J 42:348, 1965.
17. Ladhani FW, Thies RE. Fiber Lengths and End-Plate Locations in Fruit Bat Web Muscles. Proc Soc Exp Biol Med 127:787, 1968.
18. Grinnell AD. The Neurophysiology of Audition in Bats: Intensity and Frequency Parameters. J Physiol 167:38, 1963.
19. Suga N: Single Unit Activity in Cochlear Nucleus and Inferior Colliculus of Echolocating Bats. J Physiol 172:449, 1964.
20. Hoff HE, Coles SK, Szabuniewicz M, McCrady JD. The Respiratory Heart Rate Relationship in the Armadillo. Cardiovasc Res Cent Bull 21:37, 1982.
21. Szabuniewicz M, McCrady JD. Some Aspects of the Anatomy and Physiology of the Armadillo. Lab Anim Care 19:843, 1969.
22. Anderson JM, Benirschke K. The Armadillo in Experimental Biology. Lab Anim Care 16:202, 1966.
23. Wampler SN. Husbandry and Health Problems of Armadillos, *Dasypus novemcinctus*. Lab Anim Care 19:391, 1969.
24. Hayes FA. Modifications for Cesarian Section in Chinchillas. Vet Med 50:367, 1955.
25. Riddell WK. Caudal Anesthesia in Canine Surgery. J Small Anim Med 1:159, 1952.
26. Roslyn J, Thompson JE Jr, DenBesten, L. Anesthesia in Prairie Dogs. Lab Anim Sci 29:542, 1979.
27. Bacher JD, Potkay S, Baas JE. An Evaluation of Sedatives and Anesthetics in the Agouti (*Dasyprocta* spp.) Lab Anim Sci 26:195, 1976.
28. Van Foreest, A. Use of Ketamine/Xylazine Combination for Tail Amputation in Nutria. J Zoo Anim Med 11:19, 1980.
29. Noyes DH, Siekierski DM. Anesthesia of Marmots with Sodium Pentobarbital, Ketamine Hydrochloride, and a Combination of Droperidol and Fentanyl. Lab Anim Sci 25:557, 1975.
30. Hummon OJ. A Device for the Restraint of Mink During Certain Experimental Procedures. J Am Vet Med Assoc 106:104, 1945.
31. Lafortune JG, Rheault JPE. Essai d'Evaluation Clinique de la Reserpine (Serpasil) Chex le Vison. Can J Comp Med Vet Sci 24:243, 1960.
32. Padgett GA. Personal Communication. Washington State University, Pullman, Washington, 1964.
33. Ko JCH, Thurmon JC, Benson GJ. An Alternative Drug Combination for Use in Declawing and Castrating Cats. Vet Med 1061–1065, 1993.
34. Barry JA. Removal of Scent Glands in Skunks. MSU Vet 19:77, 1958.
35. Verts BJ. A Device for Anesthetizing Skunks. J Wildl Man 24:344, 1960.
36. Healey P. A Simple Method for Anaesthetizing and Handling Small Carnivores. J Inst Anim Tech 18:37, 1967.
37. Mackintosh CG, MacArthur JA, Little TWA, Stuart P. The Immobilization of the Badger. Br Vet J 132:609, 1976.
38. Wallach JD, Boever WJ. Diseases of Exotic Animals, Medical and Surgical Management. Philadelphia: WB Saunders, 1983: 469–470.
39. Balser DS. Tranquilizer Tabs for Capturing Wild Carnivores. J Wildl Man 29:438, 1965.
40. Hime JM. Use of Ketamine Hydrochloride in Non–Domesticated Cats. Vet Rec 95:193, 1974.
41. Wallach JD, Frueh R, Lentz, M. The Use of M.99 as an Immobilizing and Analgesic Agent in Captive Wild Animals. J Am Vet Med Assoc 151:870, 1967.
42. Hornocker MG, Craighead JJ, Pfeiffer EW. Immobilizing Mountain Lions with Succinylcholine Chloride and Pentobarbital Sodium. J Wildl Man 29:880, 1966.
43. Clifford DH. Observations on Effect of Preanesthetic Medication with Meperidine and Promazine on Barbiturate Anesthesia in an Ocelot and a Leopard. J Am Vet Med Assoc 133:459, 1958.
44. Clifford DH, Stowe CM Jr, Good AL. Pentobarbital Anesthesia in Lions with Special Reference to Preanesthetic Medication. J Am Vet Med Assoc 139:111, 1961.
45. Austin DH, Peoples JH. Capturing Hogs with Alpha Chloralose. Proc 21st Annu Conf Southeast Assoc Game and Fish Comm, New Orleans, Louisiana, 1967.
46. Beale DM, Smith AD. Immobilization of Pronghorn Antelopes with Succinylcholine Chloride. J Wildl Man 31:840, 1967.
47. Gaukler, VA, Kraus, M. Zur Immobilisierung von Wild-wiederkauern mit Xylazin (Bay Va 1470). Der Zoologische Garten 38:1, 1970.
48. Hofmyer JM. Immobilization of Black Rhinos, Eland and Roan Antelope with R33799. Report, Etosha Ecological Institute, South–West Africa, October, 1978.
49. Howard JG, Pursel, VG, Wildt DE, Bush, M. Comparison of Various Extenders for Freeze–Preservation of Semen from Selective Captive Wild Ungulates. J Am Vet Med Assoc 179:1157, 1981.
50. Logsdon HS. Use of Drugs as a Capture Technique for Desert Bighorn Sheep [Dissertation]. Colorado State University, Fort Collins, 1969.

51. Peshin PK, Kumar A, Singh, H. Xylazine in Buffaloes I: Cardiovascular, Respiratory and Sedative Effects. Pantnagar J Res 3:245, 1978.

52. Peshin PK, Kumar A. Physiologic and Sedative Effects of Xylazine in Buffaloes. Indian Vet J 56:864, 1979.

53. Pathak SC, Nigam JM, Peshin PK, Singh AP. Anesthetic and Hemodynamic Effects of Ketamine Hydrochloride in Buffalo Calves (*Bubalis bubalis*). Am J Vet Res 43:875, 1982.

54. Singh J, Sobti VK, Kohli RN , Kumar VR, Khanna AK. Evaluation of Glyceryl Guaiacolate as a Muscle Relaxant in Buffalo Calves. Zentralbl Veterinarmed [A] 28:60, 1981.

55. Johari MP, Sharma SP. General Anaesthesia in Buffaloes by Intravenous Use of Chloral–Thiopentone Sodium Mixture. Indian J Vet Sci 32:235, 1962.

56. Lasater GM, Stowe CM, Good AL, Short EC, Pacheco–Perez, D. Some Effects of Autonomic and Curariform Drugs in Bison. Cornell Vet 55:309, 1965.

57. Kloppel, G. Zur Immobilisation von Zoo– und Wiltieren. Kleintier–Praxis 14:203, 1969.

58. Hime JM, Jones DM. The Use of Xylazine in Captive Wild Animals. Zoological Society of London; Sonderdruck aus Verhandlungsbericht des XI Internationalen Symposiums uber die Erkrankugen der Zootiere, Budapest, 1970.

59. Honich, M. Untersuchungen uber wirtung van BAY Va 1470 biem wild. From the Laboratory for Game Diseases, Ministry of Agriculture, Budakeszi, Hungary. Presented at the 12th International Symposium on Diseases of Zoo Animals, Budapest, 1970.

60. Roughton RD. Xylazine as an Immobilizing Agent for Captive White–Tailed Deer. J Am Vet Med Assoc 167:574, 1975.

61. Harrington R. Immobilon–Rompun in Deer. Vet Rec 94:362, 1974.

62. Haigh JC, Stewart RR, Frokjer R, Hauge, T. Capture of Moose with Fentanyl and Xylazine. J Zoo Anim Med 8:22, 1977.

63. Davis RW. Personal Communication. Colorado State University, Fort Collins, 1963.

64. Wolff WA, Davis RW, Lumb WV. Chloral Hydrate–Halothane–Nitrous Oxide Anesthesia in Deer. J Am Vet Med Assoc 147:1099, 1965.

65. Thomas WD. Chemical Immobilization of Wild Animals. J Am Vet Med Assoc 138:263, 1961.

66. Haigh JC. Capture of Woodland Caribou in Canada. Proc Am Assoc Zoo Vet, Knoxville, Tennessee, 1978:110.

67. Flook DR, Robertson JR, Hermanrude OR, Buechner HK. Succinylcholine Chloride for Immobilization of North American Elk. J Wildl Man 26:334, 1962.

68. Custer R, Kramer L, Kennedy S, Bush, M. Hematologic Effects of Xylazine When Used for Restraint of Bactrian Camels. J Am Vet Med Assoc 171:899, 1977.

69. Said AH. Some Aspects of Anaesthesia in the Camel. Vet Rec 76:550, 1964.

70. Bush M, Ensley PK, Mehren K, Rapley, W. Immobilization of Giraffes with Xylazine and Etorphine Hydrochloride. J Am Vet Med Assoc 169:884, 1976.

71. Williamson WM, Wallach JD. M99–Induced Recumbency and Analgesia in a Giraffe. J Am Vet Med Assoc 153:816, 1968.

72. Bush M, deVos V. Observations on field immobilization of free-ranging giraffe (*Giraffa camelopardalis*) using carfentanyl and xylazine. J Zoo Wild Anim Med 18:135–140, 1987.

73. Seidel VB, Straub G, Carlo WR, Effert, W. Anasthesie, Hamatologie und Biochemie beim Kiang (Equus hemionus kiang, Moorcroft, 1981). Sonderdruck aus Verhandlungsbericht des XXIVInternationalen Symposiums uber die Erkrankungen der Zootiere, Veszprem, 1982.

74. Shaw ML, Carpenter JW, Leith DE. Complications with the use of carfentanil citrate and xylazine hydrochloride to immobilize domestic horses. J Am Vet Med Assoc 206:833–836, 1995

75. Allen, JL. Renarcotization following carfentanil immobilization of nondomestic ungulates J Zoo Wildl Med 20:423–426, 1989.

76. Allen JL. Immobilization of Mongolian wild horses (*Equus przewalski przewalski*) with carfentanil and antagonism with naltrexone. J Zoo Wildl Med 23:422–425, 1992.

77. Harthoorn AM, Player IC. The Narcosis of the White Rhinoceros: A Series of Eighteen Case Histories. Tijdschr Diergeneeskd 89:225, 1964.

78. Denney RN. Black Rhinoceros Immobilization Utilizing a New Tranquillizing Agent. East Afr Wildl J 7:159, 1969.

79. DeVos, V. Immobilization of Free–Ranging Wild Animals Using a New Drug. Vet Rec 103:64, 1978.

80. Counsilman JW. Demerol Hydrochloride as an Anaesthetic for an Elephant. N Am Vet 35:835, 1954.

81. Anderson IL. Tutu Poisoning in Two Circus Elephants. N Z Vet J 16:146, 1968.

82. Gray CW. Personal Communication. National Zoological Park, Washington DC, 1969.

83. Bongso TA, Perera BMAO. Observations on the Use of Etorphine Alone and in Combination with Acepromazine Maleate for Immobilization of Aggressive Asian Elephants (*Elephas maximus*). Vet Rec 102:339, 1978.

84. Wallach JD, Anderson JL. Oripavine M99 Combinations and Solvents for Immobilization of the African Elephant. J Am Vet Med Assoc 153:793, 1968.

85. Bongso TA. Use of Xylazine for the Transport of Elephants by Air. Vet Rec 107:492, 1980.

86. Dunlop CI, Hodgson DS, Cambre RC, Kenny DE, Martin HD. Cardiopulmonary Effects of Three Prolonged Periods of Isoflurane Anesthesia in an Adult Elephant. J Am Vet Med Assoc 205:1439, 1994.

87. Gross ME, Clifford CA, Hardy DA. Excitement in an Elephant After Intravenous Administration of Atropine. J Am Vet Med Assoc 205(10):1437–1438, 1994.

88. Stafford SK, Williams LE, Jr. Data on Capturing Black Bears with Alpha–Chloralose. Proc 22nd Annual Conference Southeastern Assoc of Game and Fish Commissioners, Baltimore: Maryland, 1968.

89. Addison EM, Kolenosky GB. Use of Ketamine Hydrochloride and Xylazine Hydrochloride to Immobilize Black Bears (*Ursus americanus*) J Wildl Dis 15:253, 1979.

90. Lee J, Schweinsburg R, Kernan F, Haigh J. Immobilization of Polar Bears (*Ursus maritimus, Phipps*) with Ketamine Hydrochloride and Xylazine Hydrochloride. J Wildl Dis 17:331, 1981.

91. Fowler ME. Extracting Canine Teeth of a Bear. J Am Vet Med Assoc 137:60, 1960.

92. Clarke NP, Huheey MJ, Martin WM. Pentobarbital Anesthesia in Bears. J Am Vet Med Assoc 143:47, 1963.

93. Hubbard RC, Poulter TC. Seals and Sea Lions as Models for Studies in Comparative Biology. Lab Anim Care 18:249, 1968.

94. Keyes MC. Personal Communication. National Marine Fisheries Service, St. Paul Island, Alaska, 1971.

95. Geraci JR : An Appraisal of Ketamine as an Immobilizing Agent in Wild and Captive Pinnipeds. J Am Vet Med Assoc 163:574, 1973.

96. Geraci JR, Skirnisson K, St. Aubin DJ. A Safe Method for Repeatedly Immobilizing Seals. J Am Vet Med Assoc 179:1192, 1981.

97. Hochachka PW, Liggins GC, Quist J, Schneider R, Snider MY, Wonders TR, Zapol WM. Pulmonary Metabolism During Diving: Conditioning Blood for the Brain. Science 198:831, 1977.

98. Ling JK, Nicholls DG, Thomas CDB. Immobilization of Southern Elephant Seals with Succinylcholine Chloride. J Wildl Man 37:468, 1967.

99. Ridgway SH, Simpson JG. Anesthesia and Restraint for the California Sea Lion, *Zalophus californianus*. J Am Vet Med Assoc 155:1059, 1969.

100. Sawyer DC. Chemical Restraint and Anesthesia of Sea Otters Affected by the Oil Spill in Prince William Sound, Alaska. ACVA Scientific Proceedings. New Orleans, LA, 1989:30.

101. McBride AF, Kritzler, H. Observations on Pregnancy, Parturition, and Postnatal Behavior in the Bottlenose Dolphin. J Mamml 32:251, 1951.

102. Ridgway SH, McCormick JG. Anesthetization of Porpoises for Major Surgery. Science 158:510, 1967.

103. Rieu M, Gautheron, B. Preliminary Observations Concerning a Method for Introduction of a Tube for Anesthesia in Small Delphinids. Laboratorie d' Acoustique Animals. Jouy–en–Josas, France, 78, 1968.

104. Lilly JC. Man and Dolphin. New York: Doubleday, 1961.
105. Bird FM. Personal communication. Palm Springs, California, 1964.
106. Keep JM. Marsupial Anaesthesia. Proc Postgrad Committee Vet Sci Univ of Sidney, 36:123, 1978.
107. Wilson GR. Intramuscular Anaesthesia in the Red Kangaroo. Aust Vet Pract 6:51, 1976.
108. Richardson KC, Cullen LK. Anesthesia of Small Kangaroos. J Am Vet Med Assoc 179:1162, 1981.
109. Cisar CF. The Rat Kangaroo (*Potorous tridactylus*). Handling and Husbandry Practices in a Research Facility. Lab Anim Care 19:55, 1969.
110. Krupp JH, Quillin R. A Review of the Use of the Opossum for Research: Husbandry, Experimental Techniques and Routine Health Measures. Lab Anim Care 14:189, 1964.
111. Feldman DB, Self JL. Sedation and Anesthesia of the Virginia Opossum. Lab Anim Sci 21:717, 1971.
112. Luschei ES, Mehaffey JJ. Small Animal Anesthesia with Halothane. J Appl Physiol 22:595, 1967.
113. Nau R, Schunck O. Cannulation of the Lateral Saphenous Vein–A Rapid Method to Gain Access to the Venous Circulation in Anaesthetized Guinea Pigs. Lab Anim 27:23–25, 1993.
114. Croft PG. An Introduction to the Anaesthesia of Laboratory Animals. The Universities Federation for Animal Welfare, London, 1960.
115. Waterman AE, Livingston A. Effects of Age and Sex on Ketamine Anesthesia in the Rat. Br J Anesth 50:885, 1978.
116. Cheney DH, Slogoff S, Allen GW. Ketamine–Induced Stress Ulcers in the Rat. Anesthesiology 40:531, 1974.
117. Leary SL, Manning PJ. Adynamic Ileus in Rats after Intraperitoneal Chloral Hydrate Anesthesia. Abstract 83, Publication 81–3, Am Assoc Lab Anim Sci 1981.
118. Leary SL, Manning PJ. Fat Rats. Lab Anim 11:17, 1981.
119. Cousins MJ, Mazze RI, Barr GA, Kosek JC. A Comparison of the Renal Effects of Isoflurane and Methoxyflurane in Fischer 344 Rats. Anesthesiology 38:55, 1973.
120. Van Dyke RA, Wood CL. Metabolism of Methoxyflurane: Release of Inorganic Fluoride in Human and Rat Hepatic Microsomes. Anesthesiology 39:613, 1973.
121. Fowler SL, Brown JS, Flower EW. Comparison between Ether and Carbon Dioxide Anaesthesia for Removal of Blood Samples from Rats. Lab Anim 14:275, 1980.
122. Weisner BP. The Post–Natal Development of the Genital Organs of the Albino Rat. J Obstet Gynecol 41:867, 1934.
123. Libbin RM, Person, P. Neonatal Rat Surgery: Avoiding Maternal Cannibalism. Science 206:66, 1979.
124. Hyde JL. The Use of Solid Carbon Dioxide for Producing Short Periods of Anesthesia in Guinea Pigs. Am J Vet Res 23:684, 1962.
125. Leash AM, Beye RD, Wilber RG. Self–Mutilation Following Innovar–Vet Injection in the Guinea Pig. Lab Anim Sci 23:720, 1973.
126. Newton WM, Cusick PK, Raffe MR. Innovar-Vet–Induced Pathologic Changes in the Guinea Pig. Lab Anim Sci 25:597, 1975.
127. Hopcroft SC. A Technique for the Simultaneous Bilateral Removal of the Adrenal Glands in Guinea Pigs, Using a New Type of Safe Anesthetic. Exp Med Surg 24:12, 1966.
128. Tan E, Snow HD. Continuous Epidural Anesthesia in the Guinea Pig. Am J Vet Res 29:487, 1968.
129. Ferguson JW. Anaesthesia in the Hamster Using a Combination of Methohexitone and Diazepam. Lab Anim 13:305, 1979.
130. Kesel ML. Handling, Restraint and Common Sampling and Administration Techniques in Laboratory Species. In: The Experimental Animal in Biomedical Research, vol. 1. Edited by BE Rollin and ML Kesel. Boca Raton, FL: CRC Press, 1990:333.
131. Sedgwick CJ. Anesthesia for Rabbits. Vet Clin North Am Food Anim Pract 2:731, 1986.
132. Hall LW, Clarke KW. Veterinary Anaesthesia, 9th ed. London: Balliere Tindall, 1991.
133. White GL, Holmes DD. A Comparison of Ketamine and the Combination Ketamine–Xylazine for Effective Surgical Anesthesia in the Rabbit. Lab Anim Sci 26:804, 1976.
134. Strack LE, Kaplan HM. Fentanyl and Droperidol for Surgical Anesthesia of Rabbits. J Am Vet Med Assoc 153:822, 1968.
135. Khanna VK, Pleuvry BJ. A Study of Naloxone and Doxapram as Agents for the Reversal of Neuroleptanalgesic Respiratory Depression in the Conscious Rabbit. Br J Anaesth 50:905, 1978.
136. Casteel DA, Edwards WR. Surgical Anesthesia for Cottontails. J Wildl Man 29:196, 1965.
137. Kuhn USG III, Arko RJ. Repeated Ketamine Anesthesia in the Chimpanzee. J Am Vet Med Assoc 165:838, 1974.
138. Naccarato EF, Hunter WS. Anaesthetic Effects of Various Ratios of Ketamine and Xylazine in Rhesus Monkeys (*Macaca mulatta*). Lab Anim 13:317, 1979.
139. Chimoskey JE, Huntsman LL, Gams E, Flanagan WJ. Effect of Ketamine on Ventricular Dynamics of Unanesthetized Baboons. Cardiovasc Res Cent Bull 14:53, 1975.
140. Bush M, Custer R, Smeller J, Bush LM. Physiologic Measures of Nonhuman Primates During Physical Restraint and Chemical Immobilization. J Am Vet Med Assoc 171:866, 1977.
141. Marsboom R, Mortelmans J, Vercruysse J. Neuroleptanalgesia in Monkeys. Vet Rec 75:132, 1963.
142. Newsome J, Robinson DLH. Sedatives and Anaesthetics for Baboons. Br Vet J 113:163, 1957.
143. Clark GC, Kesterson JW, Coombs DW, et al. Comparative effects of repeated and prolonged inhalation exposure of beagle dogs and Cynomolgus monkeys to anesthetic and subanesthetic concentrations of enflurane and halothane. Anaesth Scand 71:1, 1979.
144. Day PW. Anesthetic Techniques for the Chimpanzee. In: Experimental Animal Anesthesiology. Edited by DC Sawyer. USAF School of Aerospace Medicine, Brooks Air Force Base, Texas, 1965.
145. Aronson HB, Robin GC, Weinberg H, Nathan H. Some Observations on General Anesthesia in the Baboon. Anesth Analg 44:289, 1965.
146. Steffey EP, Gillespie JR, Berry JD, Eger EI, Rhode RA. The Cardiovascular Effects of Halothane in the Stumptail Monkey During Spontaneous and Controlled Ventilation. Am J Vet Res 35:1315, 1974.
147. Ritzman JR, Erickson HH, Miller ED. Cardiovascular Effects of Enflurane and Halothane on the Rhesus Monkey. Anesth Analg 55:85, 1976.
148. Glen JB. Animal Studies of the Anaesthetic Activity of ICI 35 868. Br J Anaesth 52:731, 1980.
149. Rank J, Jensen AG. The Value of Anaesthetic Steroids alphaxalone-alphadalone in pregnant mice. Scand J Lab Anim Sci 16:115, 1989.
150. White WJ, Field KJ. Anesthesia and Surgery of Laboratory Animals. Vet Clin North Am Small Anim Pract 17(5):989, 1987.
151. Buelke-Sam J, Holson JF, Bazare JJ, Young JF. Comparative Stability of Physiological Parameters During Sustained Anesthesia in Rats. Lab Anim Sci 28:157, 1978.
152. Lovell DP. Variation in Pentobarbitone Sleeping Time in Mice. Lab Anim 20:85, 1986.
153. Green CJ, Knight J, Precious S, Simpkin, S. Ketamine Alone and Combined with Diazepam or Xylazine in Laboratory Animals: A 10 Year Experience. Lab Anim 15:163, 1981.
154. Clifford DH. Preanesthesia, Anesthesia, Analgesia, and Euthanasia in Laboratory Animal Medicine. Edited by JG Fox, BJ Cohen, and FM Loew. New York: Academic Press, 1984:527.
155. Flecknell PA. Laboratory Animal Anaesthesia. London: Academic Press Ltd., 1987.
156. Erhardt W, Hebestedt A, Aschenbrenner GA. Comparative Study with Various Anesthetics in Mice (Pentobarbitone, Ketamine-Xylazine, Carfentanyl-Etomidare). Res Exp Med 184:159, 1984.
157. Mulder KJ, Mulder JB. Ketamine and Xylazine Anesthesia in the Mouse. Vet Med Small Anim Clin 74:569, 1979.
158. Silverman J, Huhndorf M, Balk M, et al. Evaluation of a Combination of Tiletamine and Zolazepam as an Anesthetic for Laboratory Rodents. Lab Anim Sci 33:457, 1983.
159. Walden NB. Effective Sedation of Rabbits, Guinea Pigs, Rats and Mice with a Mixture of Fentanyl and Droperidol. Aust Vet J 54:538, 1978.

160. Lewis GE, Jennings PB. Effective Sedation of Laboratory Animals using Innovar-Vet. Lab Anim Sci 22:430, 1972.

161. Green CJ. Neuroleptanalgesic Drug Combinations in the Anesthetic Management of Small Laboratory Animals. Lab Anim 9:161, 1975.

162. Green CJ, Halsey MJ, Precious S, et al. Alphaxalone-Alphadolone Anaesthesia in Laboratory Animals. Lab Anim 12:85, 1978.

163. Gomwalk NE, Healing TD. Etomidate: A Valuable Anesthetic for Mice. Lab Anim 15:151, 1981.

164. Taber R, Irwin S. Anesthesia in the Mouse. Fed Proc 28:1528, 1969.

165. Papaioannou VE, Fox JG. Use and Efficacy of Tribromoethanol Anesthesia in the Mouse. Lab Anim Sci 43:189, 1993.

166. Urbanski HF, Kelley ST. Sedation by Exposure to Gaseous Carbon Dioxide-Oxygen Mixture: Application to Studies Involving Small Laboratory Animal Species. Lab Anim Sci 41:80, 1991.

167. Quinn RH, Dannemen PJ, Dysko RC. Efficacy of Sedating Rats with Diazepam or Droperidol Prior to Noninvasive Manipulation. Contemp Top Lab Anim Sci 32:25, 1993.

168. Wixson SK. Anesthesia and Analgesia for Rabbits. In: Biology and Diseases of the Rabbit, 2nd ed. Orlando, FL: Academic Press, 1994:87–109.

169. Wixson SK, Hobbs BA, Karchner LE, Lawrence W. Determination of Appropriate Analgesics for Relief of Pain in Laboratory Rats. J Invest Surg 4:359, 1991.

170. Wixson SK, White WJ, Hughes HC, et al. A Comparison of Pentobarbital, Fentanyl-Droperidol, Ketamine-Xylazine, and Ketamine-Diazepam Anesthesia in Adult Male Rats. Lab Anim Sci 37:726, 1987.

171. Field KJ, White WJ, Lang CM. Anaesthetic Effects of Chloral Hydrate, Pentobarbitone and Urethane in Adult Male Rats. Lab Anim 27:258, 1993.

172. Seyde WC, McGowan L, Land N, et al. Effects of Anesthetics on Regional Hemodynamics in Normovolemic and Hemorrhaged Rats. Am J Physiol 249:H164, 1985.

173. Nevalainen T, Pyhala L, Hanna-Maija V, et al. Evaluation of Anaesthetic Potency of Medetomidine-Ketamine Combination in Rats, Guinea Pigs, and Rabbits. Acta Vet Scand 85:139, 1989.

174. Smiler KL, Stein S, Hrapkiewicz KL, et al. Tissue Response to Intramuscular and Intraperitoneal Injections of Ketamine and Xylazine in Rats. Lab Anim Sci 40:60, 1990.

175. Hsu WH, Bellin SI, Dellmon HD, et al. Xylazine-Ketamine Induced Anesthesia in Rats and its Antagonism by Yohimbine. J Am Vet Med Assoc 189:1040, 1986.

176. Van Pelt LF. Ketamine and Xylazine for Surgical Anesthesia in Rats. J Am Vet Med Assoc 171:842, 1977.

177. Ward GS, Johnson DO, Roberts CR. The Use of CI 744 as an Anesthetic for Laboratory Animals. Lab Anim Sci 24:737, 1974.

178. Wilson RP, Zagon IS, Larach DR, et al. Antinociceptive Properties of Tiletamine-Zolazepam Improved by Addition of Xylazine or Butorphanol. Pharmacol Biochem Behav 43:1129, 1992.

179. Flecknell, PA. The Relief of Pain in Laboratory Animals. Lab Anim 18:147, 1984.

180. Royer CT, Wixson SK. A Comparison of Fentanyl-Fluanisone (Hypnorm) with Fentanyl-Droperidol (Innovar-Vet) for Anesthesia and Analgesia in Laboratory Rats. J Invest Surg 5:282, 1992.

181. Hughes EW, Martin-Brody RL, Sarelius IH, Sinclair JD. Effects of Urethane-Chloralose Anesthesia on Respiration in the Rat. Clin Exp Pharmacol Physiol 9:119, 1982.

182. Silverman J, Muir WW. A Review of Laboratory Animal Anesthesia with Chloral Hydrate and Chloralose. Lab Anim Sci 43(3):210–216, 1993.

183. Field KJ, White WJ, Lang CM. Anaesthetic Effects of Chloral Hydrate, Pentobarbitone and Urethane in Adult Male Rats. Lab Anim 27:258–269, 1993.

184. Frisk CS, Hermann MD, Senta KE. Guinea Pig Anesthesia Using Various Combinations and Concentrations of Ketamine, Xylazine, and/or Acepromazine. Lab Anim Sci 32:434, 1982.

185. Carter AM. Acid-Base Status of Pregnant Guinea Pigs During Neuroleptanalgesia with Diazepam and Fentanyl-Fluanisone. Lab Anim 17:114, 1983.

186. Gilroy BA, Varga JS. Ketamine-Diazepam and Ketamine-Xylazine Combinations in Guinea Pigs. Vet Med Small Anim Clin 75:508, 1980.

187. Tena E, Ramirez C, Caldreon J. Anesthesia in Suckling Guinea Pigs Using a Combination of Ketamine Hydrochloride and Droperidol. Lab Anim Sci 32:434, 1982.

188. Brown JN, Thorne PR, Nutall AL. Blood Pressure and Other Physiologic Responses in Awake and Anesthetized Guinea Pigs. Lab Anim Sci 39:142, 1989.

189. Ward GS, Johnson DO, Roberts CR. The Use of CI 744 as an Anesthetic for Laboratory Animals. Lab Anim Sci 24(5):737–742, 1974.

190. Mulvey, S. Anaesthesia of Guinea Pigs. Vet Rec 120:309, 1987.

191. Flecknell PA, Mitchell, M. Midazolam and Fentanyl-Fluanisone: Assessment of Anaesthetic Effects in Laboratory Rodents and Rabbits. Lab Anim 18:143, 1984.

192. Flecknell PA. Anaesthesia of Guinea Pigs. Vet Rec 120:167, 1987.

193. Forsythe DB, Payton AG, Dixon D, et al. Evaluation of Telazol-Xylazine as an Anesthetic Combination for Use in Syrian Hamsters. Lab Anim Sci 42:497, 1992.

194. Thayer CB, Lowe S, Rubright EC. Clinical Evaluation of a Combination of Droperidol and Fentanyl as an Anesthetic for the Rat and Hampster. J Am Vet Med Assoc 161:665, 1972.

195. Reid WD, Davies C, Pare PD, Pardy RL. An Effective Combination of Anaesthetics for 6-Hour Experimentation in the Golden Syrian Hamster. Lab Anim 23:156, 1989.

196. Flecknell PA, John M, Mitchell M, Shurey C. Injectable Anaesthetic Techniques in 2 Species of Gerbil (Meriones libycus and Meriones unguiculatus). Lab Anim 17:118, 1983.

197. Marcoux FW, Goodrich JE, Dominick MA. Ketamine Prevents Ischemic Neuronal Injury. Brain Research 452:329, 1988.

198. Norris ML, Turner WD. An Evaluation of Tribromoethanol (TBE) as an Anesthetic Agent in the Mongolian Gerbil (Meriones unguiculatus). Lab Anim 17:324, 1983.

199. Walter T, Chau TT, Weichman BM. Effects of Analgesics on Bradykinin-induced Writhing in Mice Presensitized with PGE2. Agents and Actions 27:375, 1989.

200. Schmidt WK, Tam SW, Schotzberger GS, et al. Nalbuphine. Drug Alchohol Depend 14:339, 1985.

201. Nilsen PL. Studies on Algesimetry by Electrical Stimulation of the Mouse Tail. Acta Pharmacol Toxicol 18:10, 1961.

202. Lightowler JE, Wilder-Smith AE. B-(N-pyrolidyl)-butyroanilid (WS10), Its Subacute Toxicity, Influence on Morphine Analgesia in the Rat and Morphine Analgesia and Respiratory Depression in the Rabbit. Arch Int Pharmacodyn 144:97, 1963.

203. Collier HOJ, Warner BT, Skerry R. Multiple Toe-Pinch Method for Testing Analgesic Drugs. Br J Pharmacol 17:28, 1961.

204. Paazlow, L. An Electrical Method for Estimation of Analgesic Activity in Mice. Acta Pharm Suecica 6:207, 1969.

205. Cowan A, Doxey JC, Harry EJR. The Animal Pharmacology of Buprenorphine, an Oripavine Analgesic Agent. Br J Pharmacol 60:547, 1977.

206. DiFazio CA, Moscicki JC, Magruder MR. Anesthetic Potency of Nalbuphine and Interaction with Morphine in Rats. Anesth Analg 60:629, 1981.

207. Flecknell PA, John M, Mitchell M, Shurey C, Simpkin S. Neuroleptanalgesia in the Rabbit. Lab Anim 17:104, 1983.

208. McCormick MJ, Ashworth MA. Acepromazine and Methoxyflurane Anesthesia of Immature New Zealand White Rabbits. Lab Anim Sci 21:220–223, 1971.

209. Sanford TD, Colby ED. Effect of Xylazine and Ketamine on Blood Pressure, Heart Rate, and Respiratory Rate in Rabbits. Lab Anim Sci 30:519, 1980.

210. Ko JCH, Thurmon JC, Tranquilli WJ, Benson GJ, Olson WA. Comparison of Medetomidine-Propofol and Medetomidine-Midazolam-Propofol Anesthesia in Rabbits. Lab Anim Sci 42:503, 1992.

211. Green CJ. Orders Lagomorpha, Rodentia, Insectivora and Chiroptera. In: Animal Anesthesia, Laboratory Animal Handbook, Vol 8, 1982:131.

212. Hobbs BA, Rolhall TG, Sprenkel TL, Anthony KL. Comparisons of Several Combinations for Anesthesia in Rabbits. Am J Vet Res 52:669, 1991.
213. Borkowski GL, Danneman PJ, Russell GB, Lang CM. Evaluation of Three Intravenous Anesthetic Regimens in New Zealand Rabbits. Lab Anim Sci 40:270, 1990.
214. Lipman NS, Marini RP, Erdman SE. Comparison of Ketamine/Xylazine and Ketamine/Xylazine/Acepromazine Anesthesia in the Rabbit. Lab Anim Sci 40:395, 1990.
215. Popilskis SJ, Oz MC, Gorman P, Florestal A, Kohn DF. Comparison of Xylazine with Tiletamine-Zolazepam (Telazol) and Xylazine-Ketamine Anesthesia in Rabbits. Lab Anim Sci 41:51, 1991.
216. Lipman NS, Phillips PA, Newcomer CE. Reversal of Ketamine/Xylazine Anesthesia in the Rabbit with Yohimbine. Lab Anim Sci 37:474, 1987.
217. Brammer DW, Doerning BJ, Chrisp CE, Rush HG. Anesthetic and Nephrotoxic Effects of Telazol in New Zealand White Rabbits. Lab Anim Sci 41:432, 1991.
218. Tillman P, Norman C. Droperidol-Fentanyl as an Aid to Blood Collection in Rabbits. Lab Anim Sci 33:181, 1983.
219. Adam HK, Glen JB, Hoyle PA. Pharmacodynamics in Laboratory Animals of ICI 35 868, a New IV Anaesthetic Agent. Br J Anaesth 52:743, 1980.
220. Guierreiro D, Page CP. Effect of Neuroleptanalgesia on Some Respiratory Variables in the Rabbit. Lab Anim 21:205, 1987.
221. Wyatt JD, Scott RAW, Richardson ME. Effects of Prolonged Ketamine-Xylazine Intravenous Infusion on Arterial Blood Pressure, Heart and Respiratory Rates, Rectal Temperature and Reflexes in the Rabbit. Lab Anim Sci 39:411, 1989.
222. Blake DW, Jover B, Mc Grath BP. Hemodynamic and Heart Rate Reflex Responses to Propofol in the Rabbit. Br J Anaesth 61:194, 1988.
223. Flecknell PA, Liles JH. Assessment of Analgesic Action of Opioid Agonist-Antagonists in the Rabbit. J Assoc Vet Anaesth 17:24, 1990.
224. More RC, Kody MH, Kabo JM, Dorey FJ, Meals RA. The Effects of Two Non-Steroidal Anti–Inflammatory Drugs on Limb Swelling, Joint Stiffness, Bone Torsional Strength Following Fracture in a Rabbit Model. Clin Orthop. 247:306, 1989.
225. Piercey MF, Schroeder LA. A Quantitative Analgesic Assay in the Rabbit Based on the Response to Tooth Pulp Stimulation. Arch Int Pharmacodyn Ther 248:294, 1980.

chapter 22

CHEMICAL IMMOBILIZATION OF FREE-RANGING TERRESTRIAL MAMMALS

Leon Nielsen

Introduction

The capture of free-ranging, wild mammals by remote delivery of a dart loaded with an immobilizing drug is a relatively new technique, which has developed independent of the evolution of other forms of veteri-nary anesthesia. The need to capture large terrestrial mammals unharmed for marking, sampling, translocation, medical treatment, and research has brought this technique from a limited, embryonic stage to a highly sophisticated and widely used animal management procedure in the short span of 35 to 40 years.(1–6)

The concept is not new. Hunting people of South America, Asia, and Africa have used arrows and spears prepared with plant or animal poisons for combat and hunting for thousands of years. Because they are simple to make, silent, and effective, such weapons are still used in some areas of the world. *Curare* (or woorare), a term used by South American Indians to describe a group of related plant poisons, was used sporadically after 1835 in the treatment of equine tetanus and some human nervous disorders. The results were not encouraging. Curare causes paralysis by blocking the peripheral neuromuscular junctions, but has no effect on the central nervous system (Chapter 13). Overdosing usually results in paralysis of the diaphragm and death through respiratory failure.

In the 1940s and early 1950s, curare had been rediscovered and was being synthetically manufactured in several forms as a muscle relaxant for use in human surgical procedures. At that time wildlife researchers began to experiment with these drugs as a means of capturing animals. At first, drug delivery equipment was improvised and crude. Air guns and CO_2 rifles were modified and used to deliver darts with the drug attached to the tips.(7, 8) Some researchers used long bows (9); others preferred the crossbow.(10)

The most commonly used drugs were gallamine triethiodide, nicotine alkaloid, succinylcholine chloride, and tubocurarine chloride. Their major disadvantage was a narrow safety margin, and many animals died from respiratory muscle paralysis. Regurgitation was also a problem in ruminants, and since the drugs did not affect the central nervous system, stress levels were high and predictably detrimental to the health of the animals (Chapter 4). The objective, however, was to capture the animal, not to render it senseless through anesthesia. That would come later, with a better understanding of the process and the introduction of new drugs.

In the late 1950s, the first complete remote delivery system became available.(11) One of the most important features of the system was a drug dart, which injected the animal on impact. The injection mechanism was an effervescent tablet released into acid. The pressure caused by the mixture forced the plunger forward. Because the mechanism was unreliable, it was later replaced by a small explosive charge in the tail of the dart.

At the same time, some centrally acting drugs were being tested in South Africa. Phencyclidine HCl was used for primates and felidae (12, 13) but was not safe or effective for capturing ungulates.(14) Combinations of morphine, sedatives, and scopolamine were used successfully on white rhinoceros.(15) Buffalo, young elephants, rhinoceroses, hippopotamuses, and antelope were captured with thiambutene HCl (Chapter 21).(16)

With the availability of the oripavine derivative etorphine HCl (M99) in 1963, a new chapter in the evolution of animal capture by chemical immobilization began. Etorphine, a potent opioid derived from the opium alkaloid thebaine, soon proved to be the drug of choice for many species.(17, 18) Relatively fast acting and concentrated to facilitate high doses in small volumes, etorphine acts at specific opioid receptors in the central nervous system.

Depending on the dose given and the species, etorphine's effects range from extreme agitation to deep depression. Etorphine has been particularly useful in ungulates, elephants, and rhinoceroses.(19–22) An important advantage of the opioid drugs was that their effect could be antagonized by a specific antagonist (Chapter 8). The greatest disadvantage was their toxicity to humans, which made them hazardous to handle.

Just as important as the evolution of safe and effective drugs for animal immobilization has been the development of a technology that could reliably and safely deliver the drugs.(23, 24) The primitive, but ingenious, darting devices of the past have been replaced by more sophisticated drug delivery systems. At the leading edge of this technology are dart velocity controls, trackable transmitter darts, silencers, night vision scopes, and laser sights.

General Considerations

Field immobilization (anesthesia) of wild animals is a sequence of connective events each of which contains elements of risk to personnel and to the animals. Mortalities among immobilized animals and injuries to personnel are still too common and are often the inevitable result of lack of experience and appreciation of the complexity of the technique.

To minimize the risks and maximize the chances for success, it is important that personnel not only understand the functioning, potential, and limitations of the delivery equipment and immobilizing drugs, but also have a sound knowledge of animal behavior, physiology, and anesthesiology. In addition, the personnel must be cognizant of any species-specific condition or risk unique to a particular species or individual animal.

In preparation for field immobilization, the following guidelines are suggested:

The first consideration of any capture or restraint technique should be its suitability, safeness, and potential risk (to both personnel and animals). The objective should be to capture the animal while inflicting the least amount of injury, pain, or stress, and taking every possible precaution to safeguard its health and welfare throughout the process. The responsibility for the life of an immobilized or captured wild animal must be accepted by the person who captures it. If that person is not prepared or qualified to do so, he or she should not be capturing animals.

Chemical immobilization is not universally applicable to every situation, and some species are better or more safely captured in traps or by other physical methods. The decision to use chemical immobilization in preference to physical capture should be based on the need to capture the animal, the species, the animal's condition, the environment, the technology available, and the experience of the personnel. In some cases, physical capture in snares, traps, nets, or bomas with subsequent administration of immobilizing drugs or sedatives to facilitate nontraumatic, safe handling may be the optimum method. Darting should be limited to the larger animals. As a rule, animals under 12 to 15 kg should not be captured by means of remote drug delivery. Regardless of the species, smaller animals are easily injured or killed by the impact of the dart. An exception is the use of lightweight darts propelled from a blowgun. Only the muscle masses of the shoulder, upper hind leg, and rump should be used as injection sites for remote drug delivery. In larger animals, the neck may also present a suitable site (Fig. 22–1). The risk of impact injury will greatly increase if the animal is darted in any other area. Also, since these muscle masses are rich in blood vessels, the drug will be absorbed more quickly and this will result in faster immobilization of the animal.

Field immobilization is animal anesthesia administered under the most difficult circumstances and imposed without the benefit of any preanesthetic evaluation and preparation. Except for a brief visual inspection before darting, little is known about the animal's health and physical condition. Factors such as nutrition, disease, parasite load, infection, estrus, pregnancy, and lactation are major anesthetic considerations, but usually cannot be determined or assessed with certainty at a distance. Bearing this in mind, one must proceed with caution. There should be a real and justifiable purpose for capturing any wild animal. If that is not the case and capture is neither justified or necessary, the life and welfare of the animal should not be jeopardized.

Instrumentation

The development of safe, reliable, and efficient drug delivery equipment is an ongoing process, and potential buyers should keep informed on new systems as they become available. During the past 30 years, existing systems have been field-tested exhaustively, and equipment that was less suitable has come and gone with some frequency. There is a vast body of literature and information on the technology, use, advantages, and disadvantages of the older and commercially established systems.(2, 23–26) Resource agencies or individuals who have little experience with chemical immobilization but want to purchase darting equipment should seek the advice and guidance of other agencies or individuals with experience before deciding on equipment purchase.

The choice of drug delivery equipment should be made on the basis of practical considerations including present and projected needs, species to be captured, choice of immobilizing drugs, environmental conditions, and delivery techniques, as well as the ability and experience of the personnel using the equipment in the

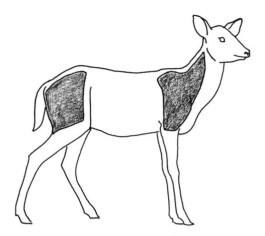

Fig. 22–1. Only the muscle masses of shoulder, upper hind leg and neck (in larger animals) should be used as injection sites for remote drug delivery.

field. Cost should not be a major factor in the choice of purchase. Good equipment will last for many years with proper maintenance. The short-term savings that may be gained by purchasing less suitable equipment are usually not worth the loss in performance, versatility, and safety on a long-term basis.

As a guideline, the drug delivery equipment should
- Be safe, uncomplicated to operate and easy to clean, service and repair.
- Be practical and relatively fast to use in the field and not noticeably affected by temperature, humidity or altitude changes.
- Provide trouble-free, reliable performance.
- Deliver consistent dart accuracy at desired maximum range.
- Cause minimum impact trauma, tissue damage, and animal anxiety.
- Be versatile for use on different species and under varying environmental conditions.
- Be sturdily constructed, with darts, charges, accessories, and other parts that are readily available.

The instructions supplied with the equipment should be learned and the manufacturer's recommendations followed. Components from different systems are usually not interchangeable, although some .50 caliber darts may be used in other systems. Before actual field use, personnel should familiarize themselves with the equipment through target practice and preparation of the drug delivery darts.

The *hypodermic syringe* is the simplest type of drug delivery equipment. The syringe is used to hand-inject a liquid drug into a suitable site of the animal. Use of the syringe requires that the animal be inactive or sufficiently restrained. Hypodermic syringes are usually disposable and are available in different sizes. The needles, also disposable, are available in different lengths and gauges.

The *pole syringe* is a hypodermic syringe contained at the end of an extension pole. This device makes it possible to inject an animal that may not be restrained but contained in a trap, snare, cage or similar small enclosure or may be walking through a narrow passage. Pole syringes are commercially available. Some models are spring activated; others require manual pressure against the animal in order to inject. A pole syringe can be easily and inexpensively manufactured from a disposable syringe with a 16-gauge needle and a wooden dowel (Fig. 22–2A).

The *blow gun* is the most basic of all remote drug delivery systems. By blowing into a 1- to 2-meter pipe, a trained operator can accurately propel a lightweight (3 mL) drug dart a distance of up to 10 or 15 meters. Blow guns are effective. They have been used by hunting people of South America and southeast Asia for thousands of years against birds and small mammals. Made from wood or cane and using palm wood splinters for darts, the blow gun is about 3 meters long and has an effective range of up to 40 meters in the hands of an experienced hunter.

In recent years the modern blow gun has become very popular as a short-range, limited-volume drug delivery system. It is commonly used in zoo work, wildlife rescue, and urban animal control work. The blow gun is silent, uncomplicated to use and maintain, and well suited for immobilization of smaller animals. Because of their light weight, limited mass, and low velocity, blow-gun darts cause minimal impact damage and tissue trauma. The discharge mechanism in most blow-gun darts is compressed air or butane gas (Fig. 22–2B and C).

Practice with the blow gun is required before range and accuracy can be attained. Leaky darts can be hazardous to the operator, and pressurized darts should be carefully inspected before loading. Several excellent blow gun systems are commercially available, but they can also be home manufactured inexpensively from disposable syringes and plastic or conduit pipes. (24, 27–29)

Power projection systems are commercially available in the form of rifles and pistols. Dart propulsion is either a blank .22 caliber powder charge, carbon dioxide (CO_2) gas, or compressed air.

Powder-charged projectors utilize the gas expansion from a fired .22 caliber charge to propel the drug dart. There are two basic types of this projector. The first uses different .22 caliber charges to compensate for various distances. It is very important that the correct charge be used for the dart size and distance, and that the manufacturer's recommendations be followed. The use of long-range charges at short distances will result in serious impact damage and dart penetration. Dart velocity may also be regulated by pushing the dart farther down the barrel of the projector. The farther the dart is moved toward the muzzle, the lower will be its velocity. A rod with markings for different settings and distances is useful for consistency in positioning the dart in the barrel. This method is particularly useful when darting at short distances (as from a helicopter) with this type of projector.

The second type of powder projector vents the gas from a single blank .22 caliber charge through a ported velocity control. By opening or closing the control, velocity and range of the drug dart can be regulated in accordance with dart size and distance. This system affords greater versatility and faster operation in cases where the distance to the animal may change frequently or suddenly. It is also more difficult to learn to use, and the velocity control must be kept clean to maintain consistency and accuracy.

Carbon dioxide–powered projectors utilize gas from a CO_2 cartridge to propel the drug dart. The range potential of a CO_2-powered projector is affected by the ambient temperature. Warm weather will increase CO_2 pressure and extend the range of the projector; cold temperatures will decrease CO_2 pressure and reduce range and dart velocity. This makes these projectors less suitable for darting in colder climates or during winter. When stored, CO_2 projectors should be kept charged and cocked to preserve internal seals. When put into use, all CO_2 cartridges should be replaced with fresh cartridges. The carbon dioxide–powered projectors are short- to medium-range systems; they do not have the range potential of the powder-charged projectors.

Compressed air–powered projectors utilize compressed air from a tank or pump to propel the dart. A control valve and/or gauge on the projector, pump, or tank provides a means for regulating the air pressure for dart size and distance. Air propulsion systems are often used in connection with blow-gun components and to propel lightweight drug darts for short to medium distances. The system is almost silent, which is an advantage when darting timid or easily disturbed animals.

Sights. Unless otherwise specified, all power projectors are delivered with open sights. Depending on the distance and light conditions under which the projector will be used, this may or may not be adequate. Telescopic sights in 2× to 4× magnification can be

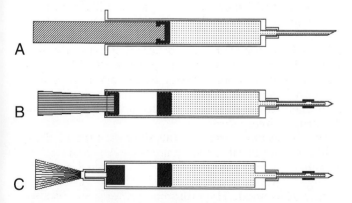

Fig. 22–2. A, Pole syringe manufactured from a disposable syringe, a 16-gauge needle, and a wooden dowel. B, Blow gun dart manufactured from a disposable syringe. Discharge mechanism is butane introduced through the tail. C, Commercial blow gun dart. Discharge mechanism is compressed air introduced through a tail valve.

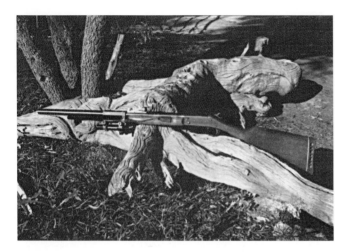

Fig. 22–3. Laser sight mounted on a dart projector (rifle). Laser sights can increase accuracy when darting during twilight and in moonlight.

mounted on most rifle- and pistol-type projectors. When mounted and sighted correctly, telescopic sights will provide a consistent sight picture and will enhance available light when darting during poor visibility. A good telescopic sight is a necessity when darting at maximum range. Night vision rifle scopes and laser sights (although expensive) are commercially available and can greatly improve darting success in darkness, during twilight and in moonlight (Fig. 22–3).

Three major types of drug delivery darts are used with the power projectors:

The *dart with explosive discharge mechanism* consists of an aluminum or plastic body into which a small explosive cap is placed between the plunger and the tail. Upon impact, a firing pin inside the cap is forced forward, against the resistance of a spring, detonating the charge. The expanding gas pushes the plunger forward and the drug is expelled through the needle. The speed of injection, 0.001 second, may cause tissue damage. The explosive caps are very sensitive to moisture and must be kept dry. When placed in the dart, the cap must have its open end against the tail. If it is turned around, detonation and expulsion of the drug will occur at the moment the projector is fired (Fig. 22–4A).

Before loading the prepared dart into the breech of the projector, test it by inserting the dart in the muzzle. If it slides in and out with ease, the dart is not deformed and can be loaded. If the dart jams in the muzzle, the dart barrel is deformed and should not be loaded. With repeated use, the dart barrel may expand where the aluminum is weakened by the threads cut into it. This is a result of the high-pressure created in the dart when gases from the explosive charge pushes the plunger forward at great speed. The deformation may also cause fine cracks in the dart barrel through which gas pressure and atomized drug will escape during impact.

All the darts with explosive discharge mechanisms inject frontally through the tip of the needle. In order to retain the needle in the animal during injection, it should be barbed. If there is no barb or if the barb is removed, the force of the frontal expulsion of the drug may be sufficiently powerful to drive the dart out of the animal with only part of the drug injected.

The *dart with an air-activated mechanism* consists of an aluminum or plastic body into which air is introduced through a one-way valve in the tail piece and compressed behind the plunger. At impact a silicone seal is displaced, exposing a port in the side of the needle. The plunger is pushed forward by air pressure, and the drug is expelled through the port (Fig. 22–4B). Most of these darts are made of plastic, which facilitates visual inspection. When the dart is filled, a small air bubble should be left in the drug. As air is introduced and pushes the plunger forward, the air bubble will be compressed, so it provides a quick reference of the status of the dart. If pressure is lost, the air bubble will increase in size. Depending on the type and usage, plastic darts can be used repeatedly but will eventually begin to leak or lose air pressure. At temperatures below freezing, plastic darts may become brittle and the drug may freeze. Either condition will cause the dart to shatter on impact. The darts should be kept warm in an inside pocket, motor vehicle, or aircraft until used.

The *dart with a spring-activated discharge mechanism* consists of an aluminum or plastic body that contains a coil spring behind the plunger. After the drug is loaded into the front of the dart, a rubber seal is placed over the needle tip. The tail piece with the coil spring is then screwed into the dart, compressing the spring behind the plunger. Upon impact, the needle tip penetrates the rubber seal and the coil spring pushes the plunger forward, expelling the drug (Fig. 22–4C).

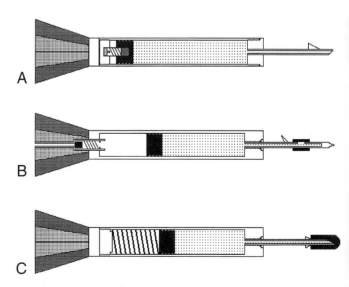

Fig. 22–4. A, Dart with explosive drug discharge mechanism. B, Dart with air-activated drug discharge mechanism. C, Dart with coil spring–activated drug discharge mechanism.

Pharmacology

The drugs used for animal immobilization have histori-cally been classified in two categories: (a) paralyzing compounds, and (b) centrally acting compounds.(2) This classification may still be valid, although the drugs in the former category were mostly used in the past. With the introduction of new, superior drugs, the use of these compounds has experienced a precipitous decline.

PARALYZING COMPOUNDS

This category of drugs includes three classes of neuro-muscular blockers (Chapter 13):
1. *Competitive neuromuscular blockers.* These are curari-form drugs that act on the neuromuscular junction of skeletal muscles or motor end plates, causing paralysis (Chapter 7). Drugs in this class are d-tubocurarine chloride and gallamine triethiodide.
2. *Depolarizing neuromuscular blockers.* These drugs act on the motor end plates, causing depolarization and consequent paralysis. Succinylcholine chlo-ride is in this class.
3. *Ganglionic neuromuscular blockers.* These drugs stimulate autonomic ganglia, causing paralysis. Drugs included in this group are nicotine salicylate and other nicotine alkaloids.

The drugs in this category produce immobilization through paralysis of voluntary muscles. They have no effect on the central nervous system. An animal immo-bilized with any of these drugs may be unable to move, but is conscious and sensitive to stress and pain. The margin between an effective dose and a lethal dose is narrow. Death may occur during immobilization as a result of overdosing, which causes paralysis of the muscles of respiration and respiratory failure. Other undesirable side effects are associated with the use of neuromuscular blockers, and some of them are also highly toxic to humans. The availability of safer and more suitable immobilizing drugs has largely made the paralyzing compounds obsolete. There is no justifi-able use for these drugs in mammalian species unless they are combined with drugs that produce uncon-sciousness.

CENTRALLY ACTING COMPOUNDS

This category includes five classes of drugs that act on the central nervous system. Immobilization is produced by an action in the central nervous system and may range from light sedation to deep anesthesia, depend-ing on the drug, its mode of action, the dose given, and the sensitivity of the animal.(30, 31) The five drug classes are
1. *Opioids.* These are potent synthetic opiates, primar-ily oripavine derivatives or 4-amino-piperidine compounds. They are commonly used for immo-bilization of ungulates (Chapters 8 and 21).
2. *Cyclohexamines.* Drugs in this class are rapid-acting, dissociative anesthetics. They are used in many species, but have been particularly effective in carnivores, bears, primates, and birds (Chapters 10, 20, and 21).
3. *Central alpha$_2$-adrenergic agonists.* Used alone or with the opioids or cyclohexamines, these drugs are powerful depressants. Drug response in treated animals may range from mild sedation to immobilization, depending on the dose given and species. They have been used in a variety of species (Chapters 8, 20, and 21).
4. *Neuroleptics.* These drugs are short-acting sedatives or tranquilizers. They are seldom used alone for immobilization, but are included with other drugs to potentiate their effect and mitigate side effects (Chapters 8, 20, and 21).
5. *Long-acting neuroleptics (LANs).* A new category, which includes certain drugs with a longer-lasting CNS depressant effect. They are most commonly used for calming newly caught wild animals while in captivity and while transporting. Table 22–1 provides dosage recommendations for immobilization of selected species when using the potent opioids carfentanil and etor-phine, the cyclohexamines ketamine and Telazol (tiletamine and zolazepam), and the alpha$_2$-agonist xylazine.

Opioids

The opioids used for animal immobilization are pri-marily oripavine derivatives or 4-amino-piperidine compounds. They are considerably more potent than morphine and act through central nervous system depression. The opioids have good analgesic but only limited muscle relaxant properties. They have a wide margin of safety, are predictable in action, and can be reversed with the administration of a suitable an-tagonist. The opioids have been used in a wide range of species, but have been particularly effective in ungulates. They have been used alone or with the addition of a neuroleptic synergist. This inclusion will potentiate the opioid, produce a smoother induction by counteracting the excitatory state often associated with opioid induction, and prevent some undesirable side effects. The opioids are relatively fast acting. Underdosing may result in a prolonged induction time and lead to hyperthermia, exhaustion, loss, and/or death of the animal. If not reversed, the duration of immobilization is lengthy, often several hours, during which the animal is at risk from opioid-induced respiratory depression and environmental hazards. The side effects of opioid immobilization include (a) excitation following administration, resulting in aim-less running, pacing, or walking, which may lead to hyperthermia or capture myopathy; (b) regurgitation of ruminal content or vomiting; (c) critical depression of respiration; (d) muscular tremors, (e) hyper- or hypotension; (f) tachycardia; and (g) recycling. Opi-oids require hepatic metabolism before renal excretion. They are highly toxic and must be handled with the

Table 22–1. Drug and Dosage (mg/kg) Recommendations for Immobilization of Selected Terrestrial Mammals

Species	Carfentanil	Etorphine	Ketamine	Telazol	Xylazine	Reference
Aardwolf			10.0–20.0 + 0.15–0.40 acetylpromazine			65
(Proteles cristatus)			10–15			66
Addax	1.8–2.4 mg*	+			10 mg	67
(A. nasomaculatus)		5.0–8.0 mg				68
				7.0–9.0		68
Aoudad		2.0–4.0 mg				68
(Ammotragus lervia)				3.5–8.6		25
Baboon				2.0–4.0		69
(Papio hamadryas)			2.5–5.0			70
Bandicoot, short-nosed				10.0		71
(Isoodon macrourus)			20–30			68
Bear, black				7.0		72
(Ursus americanus)			5.0–9.0	+	2.0–4.5	73
				4.0–4.2		74
Bear, grizzly				7.0–9.0		75
(Ursus a. horribilis)			11.1	+	11.1	76
Bear, polar				8.0–9.0		77
(Ursus maritimus)	0.02					33
Bear, sun			10.0			78
(Thalarctos malayanus)			10–12			68
Bighorn sheep		4.5 mg	+		7.0–10.0 mg	25
(Ovis canadensis)	0.044					79
Bison		0.011–0.013		+	0.6–1.0	80
(Bison bison)	0.0024	+			0.07	81
Blackbuck	1.2–1.5 mg					67
(Antilope cervicapra)		2.0–3.0 mg + 5.0 mg acepromazine				82
				4.5–10		68
Blesbok	1.2 mg					67
(Damaliscus dorcas)		2.0 mg		+	5.0–10 mg	83
Bobcat			15.2			84
(Felis rufus)			2.5–5.0			25
Bongo	1.5–2.0 mg					67
(Tragelaphus eurycerus)		2.5–3.2 mg	+		50–75 mg	66
Bontebok		2.0 mg	+		5–10 mg	83
(Damaliscus d. dorcas)		1.0–2.0 mg + 25–50 mg azaperone				85
Brush-tailed rock wallaby				11.2		71
(Petrogale penicillata)			15–30			68
Buffalo, African	6.0 mg					67
(Syncerus caffer)		6.0–8.0 mg	+		50 mg	83
		2.5–4.5 mg	+		20–30 mg	66
Bushbuck		1.0–2.0 mg	+		10 mg	83
(Tragelaphus scriptus)		1.0 mg	+		100 mg	86
		1.0–1.5 mg	+		8.0–12 mg	66
Bush dog			20.0 + 2.0 promazine			87
(Speothos venaticus)				10.0		87
Bushpig		0.03	+		0.2	66
(Potamochoerus porcus)				5.0–20		88
Caribou		2.45–6.12 mg + 10–25 mg acepromazine				89
(Rangifer tarandus)		4.0–5.0	+		30–80 mg	25
Cat, domestic			5.0	+	1.0	u/p
(Felis catus)			11–44			88

Dosages are in mg/kg unless otherwise noted. When dose is followed by (mg) this indicates total dose.

*Where a dosage range is listed, the low value is for adult females and the high value is for adult males. Dosages used for immature animals should be appropriately adjusted.

u/p, unpublished data, personal experience.

Before using the above listed drug and dosage recommendations in the field, it is suggested that the literature referenced be consulted.

Table 22–1. Drug and Dosage (mg/kg) Recommendations for Immobilization of Selected Terrestrial Mammals—cont'd

Species	Carfentanil	Etorphine	Ketamine	Telazol	Xylazine	Reference
Cheetah				2.0–6.0		88
(*Acinonyx jubatus*)			10.0	+	1.0	66
Chimpanzee			6.0–8.0			90
(*Pan troglodytes*)					2.0–10.0	88
Coyote			10.0 + 1.0 promazine			87
(*Canis latrans*)				10.0		87
Deer, axis		2.0–3.5 mg + 10–15 mg acepromazine				82
(*Axis axis*)				2.6		69
Deer, Barasingha	2.1 mg					67
(*Cervus duvauceli*)		2.0–2.5 mg		+	45–60 mg	82
Deer, fallow	1.2 mg					67
(*Dama dama*)		1.2–2.0 mg		+	35–70 mg	82
Deer, hog	0.30–0.45 mg					67
(*Axis porcinus*)		1.0–1.5 mg + 5.0–7.0 mg acepromazine				82
Deer, marsh		0.02				88
(*Blastocerus dichotomus*)		2.8–4.5 mg	+	20–50 mg		25
Deer, mule	0.03		+		0.70	25
(*Odocoileus hemionus*)			9.2	+	0.73	91
Deer, pampas		0.02				88
(*Ozotoceros bezoarticus*)		2.8–4.5 mg	+		20–50 mg	25
Deer, red		2.0–4.5 mg + 9.0–20 mg acepromazine				82
(*Cervus elaphus*)		0.02–0.04				3
Deer, roe	0.6 mg					67
(*Cervus capreolus*)		1.0–1.2 mg		+	15–20 mg	82
Deer, rusa	0.6 mg		+		15 mg	67
(*Cervus timorensis*)		1.5–2.0 mg + 7.0–10 mg acepromazine				82
Deer, sambar	1.2–2.1 mg		+		15–30 mg	67
(*Cervus unicolor*)		2.5–4.0 mg + 10–15 mg acepromazine				82
Deer, sika	1.5 mg					67
(*Cervus nippon*)		2.0–3.5 mg + 9.0–15 mg acepromazine				82
Deer, white-tailed		2.7 mg	+		40 mg	92
(*Odocoileus virginianus*)			6.6	+	5.6	93
Dingo			10.0 + 1.0 promazine			87
(*Canis dingo*)				10.0		87
Dog, domestic			5.0		1.0	51
(*Canis familiaris*)				5.0–10.0		88
Eland, common	6.0 mg		+		50 mg	67
(*Taurotragus oryx*)		10–14 mg		+	150–200 mg	83
Elephant, African	2.1 μg/kg					94
(*Loxodonta africana*)		14–18 mg				83
		14–20 mg				95
Elephant, Asian		0.0025 + 0.01 acepromazine				96
(*Elephas maximus*)		14–20 mg				95
		0.0022				88
		6.75 mg				97
Elk	1.2–12.0 μg/kg					98
(*Cervus elaphus*)	0.55 μg/kg					37
	0.019				0.23	25
		4.7–6.0 mg		+	30–50 mg	25
Fox, bat-eared			20.0 + 2.0 promazine			87
(*Otocyon megalotis*)				10.0		87
Fox, gray			20.0 + 2.0 promazine			87
(*Urocyon cinereoargenteus*)				8.8		87
Fox, red			20.0 + 2.0 promazine			87
(*Vulpes vulpes*)				10.0		87

Table 22–1.   Drug and Dosage (mg/kg) Recommendations for Immobilization of Selected Terrestrial Mammals — cont'd

Species	Carfentanil	Etorphine	Ketamine	Telazol	Xylazine	Reference
Gaur	5.0–7.0 mg		+		50–100 mg	99
(Bos gaurus)	5.0–6.0 mg		+		75 mg	67
		6.0–8.0 mg				u/p
Gazelle, Addra	1.0 mg					67
(Gazella d. ruficollis)		2.0–3.0 mg				68
Gazelle, Grant's		0.6–0.7 mg	+		30 mg	66
(Gazella granti)				2.5–15		68
Gazelle, Mohrr	1.5–1.8 mg					67
(Gazella d. mhorr)		2.0–3.0 mg				68
Gazelle, Persian	1.2–1.5 mg					67
(Gazella s. subgutturosa)				2.5–15		68
Gazelle, Roosevelti	1.2–1.5 mg					67
(Gazella roosevelti)		2.0–3.0 mg				68
Gazelle, sand	0.60–0.75 mg					67
(Gazella s. marica)				2.5–15		68
Gazelle, sl.-horned	0.9–1.0 mg					67
(Gazella leptoceros)		2.0–3.0 mg				68
Gazelle, Thompson	1.0–1.2 mg					67
(Gazella t. thomsoni)		0.4–0.5 mg				66
Gemsbok	2.7–3.0 mg					67
(Oryx g. gazella)		3.0–5.0 mg	+		20–40 mg	85
Giant forest hog		0.03	+		0.2	66
(Hylochoerus meinertzhageni)				5.0		66
Giraffe	8.0 mg + 10 mg atropine		+		100 mg	100
(Giraffa camelopardalis)		8.0–10 mg (Antidote immediately)				83
		3.0–5.0 mg + 30 mg acepromazine				85
		5.0–6.0 mg	+		20 mg	66
Gorilla			6.0–8.0			90
(Gorilla gorilla)				2.0–4.0		69
Gnu, white-tailed	1.2–1.5 mg					67
(Connochaetes gnou)		2.0–3.0 mg	+		10–15 mg	83
Gnu, white-bearded	1.5 mg					67
(C. taurinus)		3.0–4.0 mg	+		15 mg	83
		2.0–3.0 mg + 50 mg azaperone				85
Grey duiker		0.2–0.3	+		4 mg	66
(Sylvicapra grimmia)		0.03	+		0.4–0.8	83
Guanaco		0.007				88
(Lama guanicoe)			7.5–15.0			101
Hartebeest, red		2.0–3.0 mg + 100 mg azaperone				86
(Alcelaphus buselaphus)		3.0–4.0 mg	+		20 mg	83
Hippopotamus		3.0–5.0 mg				102
(Hippopotamus amphibius)		2.0 mg + 200 mg azaperone				83
Horse, Przewalski's	0.02					103
(Equus p. przewalskii)		0.02 + 0.08 acepromazine		+	0.2	104
Hyena, spotted			13.2	+	6.3	105
(Crocuta crocuta)			10–15	+	1.0	66
Hyena, striped			10–15	+	1.0	66
(Hyaena hyaena)			10.0	+	0.5	68
Hunting dog			10.0 + 1.0 promazine			87
(Lycaon pictus)				10.0		87
Ibex	1.5 mg					67
(Capra ibex)		1.0–3.0 mg				68
Impala	1.2–1.5 mg					67
(Aepyceros melampus)		0.6–0.7 mg	+		30 mg	66
Jackal, black-backed			20.0 + 2.0 promazine			87
(Canis mesomelas)					10.0	87

Table 22–1.   Drug and Dosage (mg/kg) Recommendations for Immobilization of Selected Terrestrial Mammals—cont'd

Species	Carfentanil	Etorphine	Ketamine	Telazol	Xylazine	Reference
Jackal, golden			20.0 + 2.0 promazine			87
(Canis aureus)				10.0		87
Jackal, side-striped			20.0 + 2.0 promazine			87
(Canis adustus)				10.0		87
Jaguar			15–20		1.0–1.5	106
(Panthera onca)				3.5–4.4		69
Jaguarundi			10–15 + tranquilizer and atropine			106
(Felis yagouaroundi)				6.6		69
Koala				2.9–4.3		71
(Phascolarctos cinereus)			15–30			68
Kob, Uganda	2.1 mg		+		5 mg	67
(Kobus k. thomasi)		1.2–2.0 mg		+	10 mg	u/p
Kudu, greater	2.7–3.0 mg		+		25–35 mg	67
(Tragelaphus strepsiceros)		3.0–4.0 mg		+	200–300 mg	86
		5.0–8.0 mg		+	30–50 mg	83
Lechwe, Kafue	1.2–1.5 mg		+		5 mg	67
(Kobus l. kafuensis)		1.2–1.9 mg				66
Lechwe, Nile	1.5–2.1 mg					67
(Kobus megaceros)						
Leopard				3.5–6.0		69
(Panthera pardus)				2.2		66
Leopard, snow				3.5–6.0		69
(Panthera uncia)			10.9	+	2.2	107
Lion, African			7.6	+	3.5	108
(Panthera leo)				2.13		108
				2.2		66
Lion, mountain				2.2–3.3		69
(Felis concolor)			7.5–8.0	+	1.5–1.6	25
Llama		3.0 mg + 0.1 mg/kg acepromazine				109
(Llama glama)					1.0–2.0	68
Lynx			11.0			84
(Felis lynx)			2.5			25
Markhor	0.9–1.2 mg					67
(Capra falconeri)		1.0–3.0 mg				68
Moose	5.5–12.0 µg/kg					98
(Alces alces)	4.5 mg					37
	0.010					25
		7.0 mg		+	300 mg	110
Mouflon	1.2–1.5 mg					67
(Ovis orientalis)		1.0–2.0 mg				68
Mountain goat	2.75 mg					25
(Oreamnos americanus)		4.0 mg		+	30 mg	25
Muskox		0.022–0.030				111
(Ovibos moschatus)		7.0–8.0 mg				112
Nilgai	3.0–3.9 mg					67
(Boselaphus tragocamelus)		4.0–6.0 mg				68
Nyala		2.0–3.5 mg		+	15–25 mg	83
(Tragelaphus angasi)		1.0–3.0 mg		+	15–30 mg	85
Ocelot			22.0–33.0			25
(Felis pardalis)				4.0–5.0		69
Orangutan			6.0–8.0			90
(Pongo pygmaeus)					2.0–5.0	69
Oryx, fringe-eared	2.7–3.0 mg		+		5–10 mg	67
(Oryx g. callotis)		4.0 mg		+	50 mg	66
Oryx, sci.-horned	2.5–3.0 mg		+		10 mg	67
(Oryx g. dammah)						

Table 22–1. Drug and Dosage (mg/kg) Recommendations for Immobilization of Selected Terrestrial Mammals — cont'd

Species	Carfentanil	Etorphine	Ketamine	Telazol	Xylazine	Reference
Otter, river			22.0			84
(*Lutra lutra*)				2.0–6.0		25
Otter, sea		0.022 + 0.22 diazepam				84
(*Enhydra lutris*)					1.0–2.0	113
Peccary, collared		1.0–2.0 mg				68
(*Tayassu tajacu*)			20.0			114
Pronghorn		2.5–3.0 mg + 10 mg acepromazine				80
(*Antilocapra americana*)		4.0–5.0 mg	+		40–50 mg	80
Pudu		0.4–0.6 mg	+		3.0–5.0 mg	82
(*Pudu puda*)						
Raccoon			3.0–4.0			25
(*Procyon lotor*)			5.0	+	1.0	u/p
Red-necked wallaby				5.6–11.1		71
(*Macropus rufogriseus*)						
Reedbuck		1.0–2.0 mg	+		10 mg	83
(*Redunca arundinum*)		1.0–2.0 mg	+		20 mg	85
Rhinoceros, black		4.0–5.5 mg + 225–250 mg azaperone				115
(*Diceros bicornis*)		3.0 mg	+		100 mg	116
Rhinoceros, Indian		2.0–2.5 mg				117
(*Rhinoceros unicornis*)						
Rhinoceros, white	1.2 mg					67
(*Ceratotherium simum*)		2.0 mg + 50 mg hyoscine hydrobromide				118
		3.0–4.0 mg				83
Roan antelope		3.0–5.0 mg	+		25–30 mg	85
(*Hippotragus equinus*)		5.0–7.0 mg	+		40 mg	83
Sable antelope		2.0–4.0 mg	+		25–30 mg	85
(*Hippotragus niger*)		4.0–6.0 mg	+		15 mg	83
Saiga, Russian	2.1 mg					67
(*Saiga t. tatarica*)						
Sitatunga	0.9 mg					67
(*Tragelaphus spekii*)		1.1–1.7 mg	+		30–40 mg	66
Skunk, striped			6.0–6.5			25
(*Mephitis mephitis*)			5.0	+	1.0	u/p
Springbok	0.9 mg					67
(*A. m. angolensis*)		1.0 mg	+		10 mg	83
Tahr	1.2 mg		+		5 mg	67
(*Hemitragus jemlahicus*)		2.0–4.0 mg				68
Tapir		0.007				119
(*Tapirus terrestris*)					6.0	120
Tasmanian devil					7.5–10.0	71
(*Sarcophilus harrisii*)			15–30			68
Tiger				4.0–5.0		69
(*Panthera tigris*)				3.3–7.9		121
Tsessebe		3.0–4.0 mg	+		20 mg	83
(*Damaliscus l. lunatus*)		2.0–4.0 mg	+		20–30 mg	85
Tur	1.5 mg					67
(*Capra caucasia*)						
Urial	1.0–1.2 mg					67
(*Ovis cycloceros*)						
Vervet monkey			12–20 + 0.1 diazepam			66
(*Cercopithecus aethiops*)			5.0	+	1.0	u/p
Wart hog		4.0–5.0 mg	+		20 mg	83
(*Phacochoerus aethiopicus*)				2.0–8.8		69
Waterbuck	3.0 mg		+		25 mg	67
(*Kobus ellipsiprymnus*)		3.0–6.0 mg	+		30–50 mg	85
		5.0–7.0 mg	+		50 mg	83

Table 22–1. Drug and Dosage (mg/kg) Recommendations for Immobilization of Selected Terrestrial Mammals — cont'd

Species	Carfentanil	Etorphine	Ketamine	Telazol	Xylazine	Reference
Wild boar		1.0–3.0 mg + 5–15 mg acepromazine				25
(Sus scrofa)				2.0–8.8		69
Wolf, gray			10.0 + 1.0 promazine			87
(Canis lupus)				10.4		122
Wolf, maned			10.0 + 1.0 promazine			87
(Chrysocyon brachturus)				10.0		87
Wolf, red			10.0–1.0 promazine			87
(Canis rufus)				10.0		87
Wolverine	0.02–0.13		+		2.7–4.8	25
(Gulo gulo)			17.2–25.5			123
Wombat, common				4.0–20.0		71
(Vombatus ursinus)						
Zebra, common		2.0–4.0 mg + 200 mg azaperone				85
(Equus burchelli)		4.5–7.0 mg	+	80–150 mg		83
		4.5 mg	+		40 mg	66
Zebra, Grevy's		6.0–8.5 mg	+	40–60 mg		66
(Equus grevyi)		0.01 + 0.05 acepromazine		+	0.1	104
Zebra, mountain		4.0–7.0 mg	+	80–150 mg		83
(Equus zebra)		2.0–3.0 mg + 200 mg azaperone				85

greatest care to avoid accidental exposure in humans.(32)

Opioids used for immobilization include etorphine HCl (M99. Lemmon Co., Sellersville, Pennsylvania), fentanyl citrate (Janssen Lab., Beerse, Belgium), carfentanil citrate (Wildnil; Wildlife Lab., Ft. Collins, Colorado), and A-3080 (Anaquest Div., British Oxygen Co., Montvale, New Jersey).

ETORPHINE HCl

Etorphine hydrochloride is the most commonly used opioid for wild animal immobilization. It is a potent analgesic and at optimum doses produces relatively fast central nervous system depression. Etorphine was until, recently, available in the United States in a 1-mg/mL aqueous solution. Although it is no longer on the market in the United States, many wildlife agencies,
zoos, and veterinarians still have stores of the drug on hand. In other parts of the world it is available in two formulations: 2.45 mg/mL etorphine with 10 mg/mL acepromazine (Large Animal Immobilon) and 0.07 mg/mL etorphine with 18 mg/mL methotrimeprazine (Small Animal Immobilon) (Chapter 8). Another formulation of 9.8 mg/mL etorphine is available in Europe and Africa (Game Immobilization Div., R&C Pharmaceuticals [Pty] Ltd., Merebank, South Africa). Etorphine has been used successfully in many species, but has been particularly effective in ungulates, rhinoceroses (Fig. 22–5), and elephants (Chapter 21). It can be used alone or in combination with a suitable neuroleptic synergist. Course of induction, induction time, and duration of immobilization are dose dependent. Underdosing can cause excitation with associated problems. At optimum dose, the first effects

may be observed 10 to 15 minutes following intramuscular injection. The full effect may be reached in 20 to 30 minutes. Recovery is slow, at times up to 7 or 8 hours, if no antagonist is given. When antagonized, the animal will recover in 1 to 3 minutes after intravenous injection and in 5 to 10 minutes following intramuscular injection. The most serious side effect is respiratory depression. For that reason, an animal should not be kept immobilized longer than necessary, but reversed as soon as possible. Other side effects are often dose or species dependent and may include excitement, muscle tremors, convulsions, regurgitation, bloat, bradycardia, tachycardia, hypertension, hyperthermia, and enterohepatic recycling.

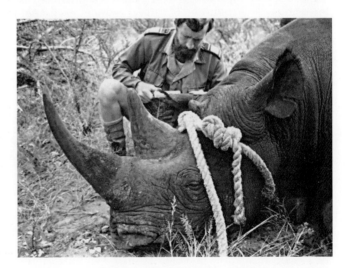

Fig. 22–5. Free-ranging black rhinoceros immobilized with etorphine HCl and azaperone. Notice third horn between ears.

FENTANYL CITRATE

Fentanyl, a 4-amino-piperidine derivative, is not commonly used in North America for immobilization of wild animals. It has been used extensively in Africa, Europe, and New Zealand. Fentanyl is available in the United States in a 0.4-mg/mL solution with 20 mg/mL droperidol (Innovar-Vet; Pitman-Moore Co., Washington's Crossing, New Jersey) and as a 0.05 mg/mL solution (Janssen Lab., Beerse, Belgium). These solutions are too dilute to be useful in larger species. Fentanyl may also be obtained in powder form (Sigma Chemicals, St. Louis, Missouri). Until recently, fentanyl was available in New Zealand and Australia in a solution of 10 mg/mL with 80 mg/mL azaperone (Fentaz; Smith Kline and French NZ, Ltd., Auckland, New Zealand). Not as potent as etorphine, fentanyl has nevertheless been effective in a variety of species. It has been used with xylazine for immobilization of a wide range of deer. Animals immobilized with fentanyl may remain standing, but approachable and handleable, which can be an advantage when such animals must be crated for transport.(32) It is not effective in equids and is not reliable in mature elephants. Fentanyl is fast acting, with onset of effect in 3 to 5 minutes and maximum effect reached in 15 to 20 minutes. When compared to etorphine, it is short acting, with effects beginning to abate in 60 to 80 minutes. The effect of fentanyl may be reversed with a suitable antagonist.

CARFENTANIL CITRATE

Carfentanil is a relatively new derivative of fentanyl and is one of the most potent opioids (Chapter 8). It is available in a 3-mg/mL solution. Carfentanil has been used successfully for immobilization of a variety of species. The first published report on the use of carfentanil in North American wildlife was in the polar bear (*Ursus maritimus*) in 1983.(33) Carfentanil is fast acting, with onset of effects 2 to 10 minutes following intramuscular injection. It can be used alone, but the inclusion of a neuroleptic may reduce excitement during induction and improve the quality of immobilization. When it is not reversed, the recovery is prolonged. When it is reversed, the animal is up and moving within minutes following antagonist administration. Side effects may include excitement, tachycardia, tachypnea, muscle tremors, excessive salivation, and regurgitation. Depending on the dose, species, and choice of antagonist, enterohepatic recycling may be a serious consideration following immobilization with carfentanil.(32, 34)

A-3080

A-3080 is a new, experimental, short-acting opioid analgesic that produces rapid and reversible immobilization. It is also a 4-amino-piperidine derivative and appears to be 63% as potent as carfentanil.(35) A-3080 produced induction times of 1.6 to 2.3 minutes in elk (*Cervus elaphus*). Respiratory depression was not excessive, and heart rate and temperature remained unal-

tered. Recovery time was dose dependent, but considerably shorter than experienced with carfentanil. Diprenorphine HCl and naltrexone were effective antagonists. Renarcotization was not observed.

A-3080 has also been used for immobilization of elk (*Cervus elaphus*), moose (*Alces a. shirasi*), African buffalo (*Syncerus caffer*), eland (*Taurotragus oryx*), greater kudu (*Tragelaphus strepsiceros*), and common waterbuck (*Kobus e. ellipsiprymnus*).(36, 37)

Opioid Antagonists

The ability to remobilize animals within minutes to a normal state with their natural functions and reflexes intact has given wildlife managers a degree of control that was not possible before the event of the opioids and their antagonists. At present several opioid antagonists are available.

DIPRENORPHINE HCl

Diprenorphine hydrochloride (M50-50;. Lemmon Co., Sellersville, Pennsylvania) is the antagonist used to reverse the effects of etorphine. It has agonistic properties of its own. Reversal is rapid following intravenous injection, with the animal ambulatory in 1 to 3 minutes (Fig. 22–6). If the antagonist is injected intramuscularly, reversal takes longer, up to 15 to 20 minutes. Side effects are rare. Overdosing with the antagonist may cause continued immobilization. Following human accidental exposure to etorphine, diprenorphine HCl should not be used as an antagonist because of its agonist effects. Naloxone is the preferred human antagonist.

NALOXONE HCl

Naloxone hydrochloride is a pure narcotic antagonist. It has no known agonistic properties (Chapter 8). Naloxone may be used to reverse the effects of all the opioids described. Presently, it is also the opioid antagonist of

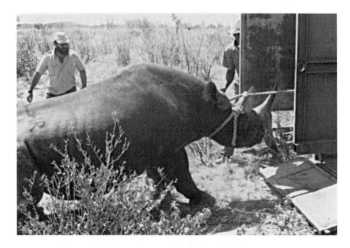

Fig. 22–6. Black rhinoceros immobilized with etorphine HCl and reversed with diprenorphine HCl. At the moment of recovery the rhino is pulled into a steel crate for transport.

choice after accidental human exposure.(38) Reversal occurs within 1 to 3 minutes following intravenous injection. Naloxone has a relatively short half-life. Some animals may revert to a state of immobilization within a few hours and require repeated treatment with naloxone.

NALORPHINE HCl

Nalorphine hydrochloride is one of the earliest commercially available opioid antagonists. As with diprenorphine, it has its own agonistic properties (Chapter 8). Overdosing may prolong immobilization. Nalorphine has been used to reverse the effects of fentanyl and etorphine in a variety of species. After intravenous injection, reversal takes place within 1 to 3 minutes.

Naltrexone (Sigma Chemicals, St. Louis, Missouri) and nalmefene HCl (Nalmefene HCl; Key Pharmaceuticals, Miami, Florida) are two new pure narcotic antagonists. They are similar in action to naloxone, but longer lasting.

Cyclohexamines

The drugs in this category are cyclohexanone derivatives, which produce rapid immobilization and analgesia by selective actions within the central nervous system (Chapter 10). During the state of unconsciousness known as *cataleptoid-dissociative anesthesia,* the treated animal retains normal pharyngeal and laryngeal reflexes while being unresponsive to stimulation. The cyclohexamines do not produce muscle relaxation but may cause muscle rigidity or twitching. Other side effects are excessive salivation, hyper- or hypotension, vocalization, or convulsions. The cyclohexamines are fast acting, have a relatively wide margin of safety, and cause only moderate depression of respiration and circulation at optimum doses. Under normal circumstances, recovery is quick because of rapid metabolism of the drug. The cyclohexamines may be used alone or in combination with neuroleptics for animal immobilization. The addition of a neuroleptic synergist will potentiate the cyclohexamine, produce a smoother induction and recovery, and alleviate the undesirable side effects common to dissociative anesthesia. The cyclohexamines have been used in a wide variety of species, but are particularly known for their effectiveness in carnivores (Fig. 22–7), bears, primates, and birds (Chapters 10 and 20). There are no known antagonists for this class of drugs. The drugs in this category include ketamine HCl (Ketamine; Bristol Lab., Syracuse, New York), and the tiletamine HCl–zolazepam HCl combination (Telazol; Fort Dodge Laboratory, Fort Dodge, Iowa).

KETAMINE HCl

Ketamine hydrochloride is a nonbarbiturate, dissociative anesthetic related to phencyclidine hydrochloride. It is available in a 100-mg/mL aqueous solution. Since this solution may be too dilute for efficient delivery to larger species, it may be lyophilized and reconsti-

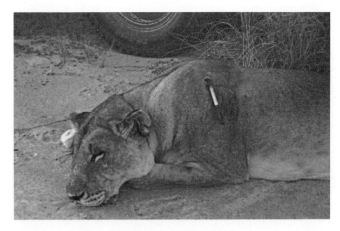

Fig. 22–7. Adult female African lion immobilized with ketamine HCl and xylazine HCl in a 5:1 mixture.

tuted at 200 mg/mL. Ketamine has been used successfully in many species, and doses vary widely from one species to another (Chapters 20, 21, 23). Induction time and duration of immobilization are dose and species dependent. At optimum doses, the first effects are observed in 2 to 5 minutes following intramuscular injection, with the full effects reached in 5 to 10 minutes. Immobilization usually lasts from 45 to 120 minutes, but in some cases may last considerably longer. Recovery is usually uneventful in carnivores but can be stormy in ungulates. This may be remedied by the inclusion of a neuroleptic in the drug regimen. In most species ketamine is metabolized in the liver and the metabolites are excreted through the kidneys. The principal metabolite has some anesthetic activity, and in domestic cats metabolism does not proceed further. Cats with renal dysfunction tend to stay anesthetized for longer than normal following ketamine induction.

Side effects of ketamine immobilization may include convulsions, catatonia, apnea, excessive salivation, and hyperthermia as a consequence of catatonia. Many of these side effects can be negated by adding a suitable neuroleptic or by treating the animal specifically after immobilization. There is no known antagonist for ketamine.

TILETAMINE HCl–ZOLAZEPAM HCl COMBINATION

The tiletamine hydrochloride–zolazepam hydrochloride combination, available as Telazol, is a cyclohexanone dissociative anesthetic agent (tiletamine HCl) combined with a benzodiazepine (zolazepam HCl) (Chapter 10). Tiletamine is a congener of phencyclidine HCl and ketamine HCl. The combination is available as a freeze-dried powder 250 mg/250 mg, which is reconstituted with a diluent. When dissolved the zolazepam becomes unstable and will only last 4 days at room temperature and 14 days if refrigerated at 4° C. Telazol is effective in a variety of species. Induction time and duration of effect is dose dependent and is comparable to ketamine. At optimum doses, first effects may be noticeable at 1 or 2 minutes following intramuscular injection, with full effects reached in 15 to 30 minutes. The induction is usually smooth, with good muscle relaxation and somatic analgesia. The duration varies with species but may persist for several hours. Because tiletamine and zolazepam are metabolized at different rates in some species, the quality of emergence and duration of recovery may be affected. Recovery occurs is 3 to 5 hours in most cases, but may be prolonged in some species. Telazol is metabolized and excreted through the kidneys.

The tiletamine-zolazepam combination may cause hypertension and increase heart rate and cardiac output. Other side effects are excessive salivation, with rare reactions of muscle rigidity, vomiting, vocalization, apnea, and cyanosis. During high ambient temperatures or in heavy-coated animals, hyperthermia may also be observed. There is evidence of behavioral problems associated with the use of this combination in tigers. Work done with midazolam (another benzodiazepine) in domestic cats has shown some behavioral effects, excitement, aggression, and disorientation. Telazol's effects in tigers appear similar, implicating the zolazepam fraction, and for that reason some workers have stopped using it in this species. There is no known antagonist for the tiletamine-zolazepam combination, although zolazepam can be effectively antagonized with flumazenil (Chapter 8).

Alpha$_2$-Adrenergic Agonists

The alpha$_2$-adrenergic agonists are potent central nervous system depressants with sedative, muscle relaxant, and some analgesic properties (Chapter 8). They block neural transmission in the brain and spinal cord by stimulating the synaptic alpha$_2$ adrenoreceptors in the noradrenergic neurons, inhibiting the release of norepinephrine and causing a decrease in central nervous system activity (Chapters 4 and 7). They may be used singly for immobilization or as synergists with opioids or cyclohexamines. Their effect is dose dependent and ranges from mild sedation to deep sleep. At high doses, the central alpha$_2$-adrenergic agonists may cause critical depression of respiration and circulation (Chapters 5 and 6). In very excited animals, they do not produce a satisfactory level of immobilization. They may also disrupt the thermoregulatory mechanisms, leading to hyper- or hypothermia. Unreversed recovery from high dosages is usually prolonged and difficult. The development of specific antagonists has increased the usefulness of the alpha$_2$-adrenergic agonists for animal immobilization.(39)

Alpha$_2$-agonists presently available include xylazine HCl (Rompun; Haver-Mobay Corp., Shawnee, Kansas), detomidine HCl (Dormosedan; Pfizer Inc., Westchester, Pennsylvania) and medetomidine HCl (Domitor; Pfizer Inc., Westchester, Pennsylvania)

XYLAZINE HCl

Xylazine hydrochloride is available in 20- and 100-mg/mL aqueous solutions, or in powder form. The 20-mg/mL solution is too dilute to be useful for field work. The 100-mg/mL solution may be lyophilized and reconstituted to >300 mg/mL. Induction, response, and length of recovery is dose dependent. Given alone, xylazine does not produce reliable immobilization. Its effectiveness is decreased in excited or stressed animals. Xylazine may induce a recumbent sleeplike or anesthetic state; however, stimulation may cause rapid arousal with defense responses intact. In calm animals, the initial effect may be seen in 4 to 5 minutes following IM injection, with full effect reached in 15 to 20 minutes. If left alone, the animal may "sleep" for several hours depending on the dose given. The side effects of xylazine are few at low doses. At higher doses, side effects may include respiratory and circulatory depression, bradycardia, hypotension and shock (Chapter 8).

Xylazine has been used effectively as a synergist with opioids and cyclohexamines (Chapters 20, 21, 23). The inclusion of xylazine has decreased dose requirements of the primary immobilizing drugs, produced a faster and smoother induction, and countered some of the undesirable side effects of these drugs. The response to high doses of xylazine may conceal a recovery from the primary immobilizing drug and place the workers at risk if the animal is suddenly aroused by noises, touch, or other stimulation. The effects of xylazine may be reversed with the administration of an alpha$_2$-adrenergic antagonist. If xylazine is used in combination with a cyclohexamine, its effects should not be reversed before the animal has metabolized the latter drug. In case of early reversal, an emergence of the cyclohexamine side effects can be expected.

DETOMIDINE HCl

Detomidine hydrochloride is an alpha$_2$-adrenergic agonist, developed for use in horses. It is about 50 times as potent as xylazine in horses and is available in a 10-mg/mL solution. The effects of detomidine have been studied in other species (40), but information on its use for immobilization of captive and free-ranging wild animals is presently somewhat limited. The action of detomidine is much like that of xylazine. Its effects may be reversed by an appropriate alpha$_2$-adrenergic antagonist.

MEDETOMIDINE HCl

Medetomidine hydrochloride is a new alpha$_2$-adrenergic agonist, developed primarily for use in dogs and cats. It is about 30 to 40 times as potent as xylazine in dogs and cats. Medetomidine has been studied in other animals (41-43) and appears to be useful for immobilization of wild animals (Chapter 21). The action of medetomidine is comparable to xylazine. Its effect may be reversed by giving an appropriate alpha$_2$-adrenergic antagonist. The drug is currently manufactured in Finland and is awaiting approval in the United States.

Alpha₂-Adrenergic Antagonists

The alpha₂-adrenergic antagonists block the effect of the alpha₂-adrenergic agonist at the synapse and permit resumption of neural transmission (Chapter 8). The appropriate dose may cause complete reversal in 2 to 5 minutes. There are several alpha₂-adrenergic antagonists.

YOHIMBINE HCl

Yohimbine hydrochloride (Antagonil; Wildlife Lab., Fort Collins, Colorado) is an effective alpha₂-antagonist for reversal of xylazine in a variety of species. Its effectiveness appears to be species related. Some species may respond reliably, whereas others may show no or only partial recovery. Yohimbine may cause tachycardia and hypertension in treated animals. It is not the most effective antagonist for medetomidine (Chapter 8).

ATIPAMEZOLE

Atipamezole (Antisedan; Pfizer Inc., Westchester, Pennsylvania) is a very selective alpha₂-antagonist for medetomidine and is effective in reversing the actions of medetomidine, detomidine, and xylazine. This is the most specific and potent alpha₂-antagonist currently available.

IDAZOXAN

Idazoxan (RX781094; Reckitt and Coleman, Hull, UK) is an alpha₂-antagonist currently under investigation. It has proven to be an effective antagonist for xylazine in some species.

RX821002

RX821002 (Reckitt and Coleman, Hull, UK) is an alpha₂-antagonist currently under investigation.

TOLAZOLINE HCl

Tolazoline hydrochloride (Priscoline; Ciba Pharmaceutical, Summit, New Jersey) is a peripheral vasodilator with moderate competitive alpha-adrenergic properties. It is used in human medicine for treatment of pulmonary hypertension in newborn. Tolazoline has proven to be an effective alpha₂-antagonist in some wild and domestic species. Because of its alpha-antagonist properties, tolazoline may produce systemic hypotension, although there are no controlled studies showing tolazoline-induced hypotension to be of major concern when appropriately dosed in healthy animals.

Neuroleptics

Although the neuroleptics are placed in several classes, they all exert similar effects in treated animals. Through depression of the central nervous system, the neuroleptics produce a calming or tranquilizing effect with little or no analgesia (Chapter 8). They do not produce

immobilization and are primarily used as synergists with opioids or cyclohexamines. In that capacity they have proven effective in potentiating the immobilizing drug, decreasing the total dose, causing a smoother and more speedy induction, and negating undesirable side effects of the immobilizing drug. Some opioids and cyclohexamines are only available with a neuroleptic included in the product. Because of their tranquilizing properties, these drugs are also used to calm wild animals for captivity and transport. The drugs in this group include the phenothiazine derivatives, the butyrophenones, and the benzodiazepines.

PHENOTHIAZINES

This class includes acepromazine, chlorpromazine, and promazine. The phenothiazines may cause hypotension and disturbance of the thermoregulatory mechanism in treated animals. For this reason they are not ideal drugs for use during high ambient temperatures or for transport when the animals are overheated or ventilation may be compromised.

BUTYROPHENONES

This class includes azaperone, droperidol, and haloperidol. The butyrophenones have a wide safety margin with no significant effect on the cardiovascular system. Azaperone has been used with good results as an adjunct to opioids for immobilization and for tranquilization in many species. It has also been shown to counteract fentanyl induced respiratory depression. Haloperidol has been used for calming captive wild animals.

BENZODIAZEPINES

This class includes diazepam, midazolam, and zolazepam. The benzodiazepines have a wide margin of safety and produce sedation and muscle relaxation in treated animals (Chapter 8). They have dose-related anxiolytic and anticonvulsant properties and may be used for induction of general anesthesia. The benzodiazepines have little effect on the cardiopulmonary system or on heart rate and blood pressure. When mixed with ketamine, diazepam may cause pain on intramuscular injection. It is not well absorbed by this route, but midazolam as an aqueous suspension is. Zolazepam is only available in combination with tiletamine HCl. Midazolam is about twice as potent as diazepam. Flumazenil is an effective antagonist for benzodiazepine-induced sedation and muscle relaxation. The drug has been released for use in humans in Europe and North America.[39] Flumazenil is marketed as Romizacon in the United States (Hoffman-LaRoche, Nutley, New Jersey).

Long-Acting Neuroleptics

The use of long-acting neuroleptics (LANs) in newly caught wild animals to facilitate adaptation or transportation is a relatively new concept.[44] Activities such as capture, confinement, and transportation are traumatic events for any wild animal. Some are particularly susceptible to stress and are unable to calm down in captivity. This may lead to high anxiety levels, which in turn can result in refusal of food and water, self-injury, injury by other animals, and exhaustion with fatal consequences. Stress induced by confinement may exacerbate aggression and lead to territorial or dominance conflicts causing injury or death. There is clearly a need for neuroleptics with a more prolonged duration of effect. One answer has been the long-acting neuroleptics used to relieve anxiety, aggressiveness, and dysphoria in humans.

The currently used long-acting (depot) neuroleptics are derived from the phenothiazines or thioxanthenes. Through the process of esterification the drug is dissolved in an oil, which permits a slow release into the tissue and hydrolyzation in the blood. Depending on the product and dose given (IM), effects can be maintained up to 30 days. Some effects observed in wild antelopes treated with long-acting neuroleptics were modification/alteration of mood, indifference to surroundings, and loss of fear of humans.(44) Little research has been published on the use of long-acting neuroleptics. Most of the work has taken place in South Africa.(45, 46)

Some of the currently available long-acting neuroleptics are perphenazine enanthate, pipothiazine palmitate, fluphenazine decanoate, zuclopenthixol decanoate, flupenthixol decanoate, and zuclopenthixol acetate. Of these only fluphenazine decanoate is available in the United States at this time.

In summary, it should be remembered that phenothiazine derivatives may cause disturbance of thermoregulation and fetal depression. Their tranquilizing effects may suppress normal functions of the treated animal. The approach to the use of these drugs should be conservative and reflect a regimen based on the lowest effective dose.

Drug Combinations

Field experiences have demonstration that a combination of compatible and complementary drugs may constitute the safest and most effective method for immobilization for selected species.(47-50) Such combinations, or cocktails, are widely used by wildlife workers. The most common mixture of drugs for animal immobilization consists of a primary drug, usually an opioid or cyclohexamine, with a neuroleptic (tranquilizer) or alpha$_2$-agonist (sedative) added (Chapters 10 and 21). The drugs of these two classes will potentiate the primary drug and alleviate its side effects. This will result in a smoother, more rapid induction and safer immobilization. To speed absorption of the drug and reduce the induction time, an enzyme (to speed drug absorption) may be added to the dose.

An example of a widely used immobilization drug combination is the five-to-one mixture of ketamine HCl and xylazine HCl. Ketamine, as the primary drug, will cause a rapid onset of drug action, and the inclusion of

xylazine will result in a smoother induction and also counteract the adverse side effects of ketamine. This drug combination has been used effectively in carnivores such as bears, cats, coyotes, dogs, foxes, raccoons, skunks, and wolves. The suggested dose is 5.0 mg/kg ketamine and 1.0 mg/kg xylazine (IM) for all species. This combination and dosage produces recumbency (immobilization) in dogs in 2 to 4 minutes, with recovery times of 110 to 130 minutes.(51)

Field Immobilization Techniques

Most commonly, the drug dart is loaded after the target animal has been located and observed. How an animal responds to a drug and the level of immobilization achieved are influenced by several factors. In addition to weight, age, sex, physical condition and mental state at time of darting, individual animals have varying degrees of sensitivity to a given drug. This may produce different and unexpected results from one animal to another even within the same species. Excited animals will usually require a higher dose than calm animals. Old, debilitated, ill, or exhausted individuals may require a lesser dose than young, healthy animals, and, in some cases, females may need a higher dose than males to achieve satisfactory immobilization. On these considerations the immobilizing drug is chosen, the dose is calculated, and the dart is loaded. This is the safest method and provides the best control for dosing, induction time, and depth of immobilization.

There may be times when it is more practical to load the darts before the target animal has been located. In that case, drug doses are calculated for specific sizes or age groups, and the darts are preloaded and marked accordingly. Metal darts, however, should not be kept loaded for more than a 12-hour period due to the possibility of internal corrosive action by the drug, which may impair the injection mechanism and damage the dart. Plastic darts can be kept loaded for several weeks, but since the drug contained in the darts may corrode or crystallize in the needle, clearance of the needle or replacement before use is recommended. Preloaded darts with air-activated discharge mechanisms should not be pressurized, and spring-activated darts should not be fully assembled (i.e, compression of spring) before they are to be used. Both of these dart types have a tendency to leak, or lose pressure, if maintained armed for an extended period of time.

As a safety precaution, the immobilizing drugs may be colored with a biologically inert coloring agent. With few exceptions, most of the drugs used are colorless, which makes them difficult to identify once extracted from the vial. This is particularly important when working with opiates, which can be extremely dangerous if the person handling the drug is accidently self-injected.

To facilitate range and accuracy, the smallest darts should be used with the highest available drug concentration. The smaller darts have the best ballistic properties, are least affected by the wind, and have less total mass, which will reduce impact damage to the animal. If the dart is equipped with an explosive discharge mechanism, which does not permit adjustment of the drug compartment volume, saline or sterile water must be added when the drug volume is less than required to fill the dart. This is necessary to ensure stability in flight and complete injection.

The length of the dart needle should be chosen to suit the species being immobilized. A barbed needle of 25 to 35 mm is sufficient for most species. In cases where the needle must penetrate a layer of subcutaneous fat or heavy fur, a needle of greater length should be used. This is particularly relevant in bears and other species which gain a considerable amount of seasonal body fat. Large, thick-skinned animals such as the elephant, giraffe, and rhinoceros will require special needles of 35 to 60 mm in length. The barb should not be removed from darts that inject frontally. As previously stated, without the barb to secure the dart in place, it may be expelled by the force of discharge, resulting in incomplete injection. As an aid for later excision of the barbed needle, the position of the barb should be indicated on the dart barrel with a marker.

DARTING TECHNIQUES

Because of the relatively limited range of drug delivery equipment, a free-ranging animal must be approached by the worker or must move toward the worker in order to be within a practical darting distance. For most types of darting equipment, this distance is 30 to 60 meters, although some projectors using smaller darts may be accurate at a greater distance.

The most common method of bringing the animal within range of the drug delivery equipment is by stalking. The approach is made slowly, quietly, and into the wind. Most mammals have acute senses of smell and hearing. Any concealment offered by the terrain must be used. If the terrain is open and does not facilitate a hidden approach, carefully crawling toward the animal with frequent stops and maintaining as small a physical presence as possible is often successful. Depending on the species, this can be dangerous, since the decreased human size may encourage the animal to attack. The secret of stalking lies in knowing where to find the animal, how to track it, and how to approach it. Successful stalking of free-ranging, wild mammals requires patience and skill.

As an alternative, the animal may be carefully guided, driven, or maneuvered toward a shooting blind by natural or constructed barriers, or by other workers. The blind should be placed downwind and be well concealed. If the animal is known to frequent specific areas or moves along identified paths, it may be darted from a blind when it passes. In both cases, absolute silence must be observed in the blind and attention should be given to the wind direction.

When natural food or water is scarce, animals may be attracted to a suitable area and darted from a blind. Deer are often darted at feeding stations in winter. African lions may be baited with a carcass left at a location suitable for darting. Tigers and leopards may be attracted by staking out live bait animals such as goats or sheep. In arid and semiarid areas, water holes provide an opportunity for darting animals from permanent blinds. Night darting at water holes is also possible with the right equipment. Laser sights are particularly useful in moonlight, and night vision scopes may be used on darker nights. The projector should preferably be silenced, and only red light should be used for working purposes. The most serious problem with night darting, especially when there is no moon, is the possibility of losing the darted animal in the dark. If that happens, any number of circumstances including predation, injury, and malposition may cause the death of the animal.

Some animals are more productively and economically caught in traps, snares, or nets before they are physically restrained and chemically immobilized to facilitate handling. African and North American ungulates have been successfully captured in drive nets or large corrals; bighorn sheep and other species have been baited and caught under drop nets or caught individually with net guns; deer have been captured in different types of traps; and bears are commonly caught in foot snares or culvert traps and subsequently immobilized.[52] Animals caught in snares or traps should be attended to quickly to reduce stress, trauma, and self-inflicted injury. Traps or snares can be monitored electronically by the use of radio transmitters.[53]

Animals that are accustomed to motor vehicles (traffic or tourists) and animals that are fed from vehicles or associate their arrival with food may be more successfully darted from a vehicle than on foot. Under other circumstances, it may be possible to approach the target animal closer or more safely on horseback or from the back of elephants.

Free-ranging, wild animals may also be captured by pursuit and darting from vehicles or from aircraft. It is vitally important that the actual chase time be kept as short as possible. Wild animals are usually not in condition to run hard for more than a short distance. Capture myopathy has been associated with high mortalities in animals which had been pursued extensively.[54] *To prevent capture myopathy and related conditions, it is recommended that animals should not be chased for more than 2 minutes, prior to darting. If an animal cannot be darted within this time, the chase should be discontinued. Helicopter pursuit is particularly traumatic to wild animals.*

When darting is done from a helicopter, it is important that the pilot have experience with animal pursuit. Otherwise, most of the time allotted will be used teaching the pilot. Pursuing and darting animals from a helicopter can be very risky if the pilot is not experienced in low-level flight. The usual darting distance is short, and the pilot must not only be aware of the position of the animal but also mindful of anything in the flight path that might cause the helicopter to crash (Fig. 22–8). A good pilot with "animal sense" will often make the difference between a successful operation and failure.(55, 56)

The sequence of pursuit and darting from a helicopter will vary from one scenario to another but usually consists of (a) spotting the animal from a higher altitude and preparing the drug delivery equipment; (b) dropping and starting the pursuit, placing the helicopter slightly behind and above the running animal on the shooter's side of the craft (a darting distance of 8 to 10 meters is optimum); and (c) darting the running animal keeping the trajectory of the dart as vertical as possible to negate the effect of the rotor downwash. When the animal is darted (d), the helicopter is immediately taken to a higher altitude, which permits the animal to calm down while still being observed. It may be necessary to use the helicopter to keep it from entering water, dense growth, or hazardous terrain during the induction time. When the animal is recumbent (e), the helicopter lands and postcapture monitoring and treatment is begun without delay.

In addition to the immobilization process itself, the physical act of approaching and darting free-ranging, wild animals is inherently dangerous. The risks may be mitigated by caution and a thorough knowledge of the behavior and social organization of the animals pursued. Depending on the species, it may be advisable to have a conventional firearms "backup" escort to protect the worker with the darting equipment. Knowledge is important. Even timid animals may attack in defense of young and during mating season. When in rut, male deer of all species can become aggressive. It would be unwise to dart an elephant in a cow-calf group. Most likely, the other cows in the group will protect the immobilized animal and drive off the workers. On the other hand, a group of bulls will usually scatter with seemingly little concern for the welfare of an immobilized member of the group. African lions are opportu-

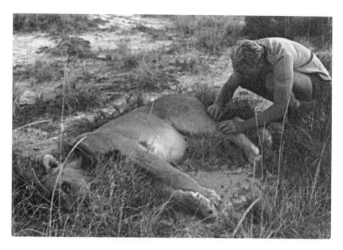

Fig. 22–9. When darting African lions, one should be watchful of the approach of other lions in the area, particularly at night. They are opportunistic predators and can be dangerous to humans.

nistic predators and can be dangerous if only some of the members of a pride are immobilized (Fig. 22–9), leaving others to menace the workers. This is particularly dangerous at night and in parks, where the lions have lost much of their natural fear of humans. Aquatic mammals such as polar bears and hippopotamuses will usually seek water when darted and, if they are not prevented from entering it, may drown (Chapter 21). Mothers and young may become separated during the capture process, causing death of the young for lack of parental care. It is well to remember that each species has its own peculiarities, which should be known and understood to facilitate successful capture.

INDUCTION

In order to have any effect, the immobilizing drug must be absorbed from the injection site and conveyed in sufficient volume through the circulatory system to the brain. The time from injection to a satisfactory immobilization is known as the *induction time*. The induction time is influenced by several factors.

Malfunction of the drug delivery equipment is a common cause for lack of response to the drug or prolonged induction. Failure of the discharge mechanism in the dart may result in only partial or no injection. Dirt, corrosion, crystallized drugs, or bone and skin cores might occlude the needle and prevent expulsion of the drug. If the animal is hit at an oblique angle or if bone is struck, the needle may bend or break. Hitting with excessive force can cause the needle to bounce out, and in cases of severe bleeding from the dart wound, the drug might bleed out of the injection site.

In order to facilitate quick absorption of the drug, the injection must take place in the muscle masses of the neck, shoulder, or hindquarter, which are rich in blood vessels. Darting in other areas, such as the thorax, abdomen, head, or extremities, may not only cause

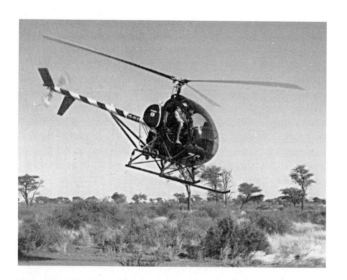

Fig. 22–8. Helicopters are excellent for spotting, pursuing, and darting free-ranging, wild animals, but they can also be dangerous in the hands of an unskilled pilot.

injury but will also result in prolonged induction, since blood circulation is more limited in these areas.

In addition to mechanical problems or misplacement of the dart, other factors may influence induction. These include the drug dose received, the animal's physical and mental condition, its age and sex, and its sensitivity to the immobilizing drug. If, for example, the animal has been chased or stressed, the induction time might be considerably longer than in calm animals. Wild animals that have gained their "winter fat" for the year may present yet another problem. Drugs injected into the fat layer are not readily absorbed, which may result in unsuccessful immobilization. The needle should be sufficiently long to penetrate the fat layer and reach the muscle.

After the animal is darted, the worker should make a note of the time and keep the animal within sight. Chasing it or following too closely will cause it to flee, which may result in a lost animal. It may also increase the induction time and make it more difficult to find the immobilized animal. If the worker is skillful at tracking, the darted animal may be carefully tracked while giving time for the drug to take effect. This method is useful in the winter after a snowfall. If, following a reasonable time, the animal does not appear to respond to the drug, it may be darted again. It is recommended that at least 30 minutes elapse between repeat injections.

POSTCAPTURE HANDLING

When the animal is recumbent, it should be approached cautiously to ascertain that it is satisfactorily immobilized (Fig. 22–10). Be careful with large mammals. The approach of a human may be enough stimulation to trigger an aggressive response. Avoid loud noises or talking. If the animal is not sufficiently immobilized, it may be necessary to give an additional half-dose by hand injection. In case the animal has gone down in difficult terrain from which recovery will be difficult,

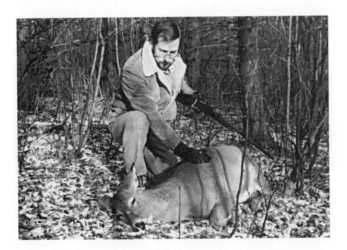

Fig. 22–10. Approach immobilized animals carefully and quietly. They may not be satisfactorily immobilized, and the approach of a human may be sufficient stimulation to trigger a defensive response.

immobilization should be reversed and the animal permitted to leave on its own.

With the animal secured, open airways are established by pulling the tongue forward and clearing the mouth. Respiration is observed to ensure that the animal is breathing regularly. Doxapram HCl (Dopram V; Fort Dodge Laboratories, Fort Dodge, Iowa) may be given in case of respiratory depression after a patent airway is established. Respiratory distress should be countered immediately by reversal of the immobilizing drug and appropriate emergency procedures. The animal's vital signs (respiration, heart rate, temperature, color of mucous membranes, and capillary refill time) should be recorded immediately following capture, after 5 minutes, and then at 10- to 15-minute intervals throughout the time of immobilization. Any deviation from acceptable parameters could be an indication that the animal's condition requires supportive treatment. Field workers should have sufficient knowledge and experience to identify unacceptable deviations from normal vital signs for the species.

After a bland eye ointment is applied to prevent drying, the animal's eyes are covered with a blindfold or soft bandage for protection against light, dirt, damage, and visual stimulation. It may be beneficial to decrease noise stimulation by plugging the ears of the animal. The next step is to protect it against the effects of inclement weather and extreme temperatures. On cold, rainy, or snowy days, the animal must be kept warm and dry. Conversely, on warm, sunny days, it should be kept shaded and cool. Some of the drugs used may affect the animal's ability to regulate its body temperature. Heating or cooling then depends on muscle activity or inactivity, ambient temperatures, and precipitation.

During immobilization and until recovery, all ruminants must be maintained in sternal recumbency, which is a natural position for these animals (Chapters 2 and 20). The legs should be flexed and the head lifted. This position is necessary to prevent inhalation of regurgitated ruminal content and reduce the possibility of bloat (Fig. 22–11). Other species may be kept in lateral recumbency but must be turned ventrally every 30 minutes until recovery is evident. It is essential to keep the airways open.

Very large, heavy animals are sensitive to damage of the muscles and tendons in the legs if the weight of the recumbent animal is on the legs for a prolonged period of time. Such animals should have their weight shifted every half hour to prevent damage. Large species of wild cattle and rhinoceroses are particularly prone to this problem. Elephants should not be kept in sternal recumbency for more than 15 minutes, but pulled over in lateral recumbency. Otherwise, massive pressure may be exerted on the lungs, heart, and diaphragm, resulting in impairment of respiration and cardiovascular function often causing death (Chapter 21).

The immobilized animal should not be manipulated or transported in any position that would not be natural for the species. Small antelopes, gazelles, deer, sheep, or

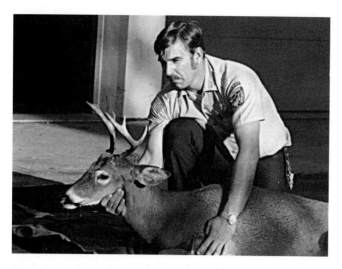

Fig. 22–11. All immobilized ruminants should be kept in sternal recumbency. This position will prevent inhalation of regurgitated ruminal content and reduce the possibility for bloat.

goats, for example, should not be carried upside down by the legs. Injury to the head, spine, or extremities is often the result of incorrect handling. Care must be taken to protect the head, neck, and legs from injury during handling and transport. Physical restraint with rope or wire is not recommended. Tying the limbs or head may result in impairment of circulation or strangulation. If restraint becomes necessary, and depending on the size of the animal, it can be wrapped in a large canvas or hobbled (front to hind legs on each side, not cross-tied) with broad, padded leather straps. Small mammals, up to the size of coyote and lynx, are best kept in dark, ventilated cages or crates.

Barbed darts are excised surgically rather than being pulled out. After disinfecting the wound with an antiseptic solution, a small incision is made with a scalpel to free the barb and guide the needle out. The wound is flushed with a disinfectant and filled with antibiotic ointment. Simple dart wounds are treated as puncture wounds and are not sutured, but permitted to drain. More complicated wounds or tears should be cleaned or sutured, with a drain inserted. Otherwise the wound may become infected and abscess. The dart wound should be protected against insects and birds by applying a suitable repellant compound. After removing the dart, prophylactic injection of a broad spectrum penicillin is recommended. If the animal is to be transported, a tranquilizer or long-acting neuroleptic may be given at this time.

Transportation

In smaller operations, a few animals can be transported either crated or bedded in straw in the darkened back of small trucks. Drugged or immobilized animals must be maintained in the proper position, and all animals should ride with their posterior toward the front of the vehicle. In this way, head and neck injuries are prevented if the vehicle suddenly stops. It is important to monitor the animals during transport, to provide adequate ventilation, and to protect against extreme temperatures, precipitation, or windchill.

Individual animals may also be airlifted by helicopter. Animals can be carried by the helicopter in a sling, cargo net, or cloth bag, or on a tubular steel–framed, net platform.(56-58) It is critical that the animal be secured and carried in such manner that the possibility of injury or strangulation is minimized. Special care must be taken with the positioning of ruminants to prevent bloat and aspiration of regurgitated ruminal content. A helicopter airlift has a cooling effect on the animal. This may be beneficial to overheated animals in the summer, but it can result in hypothermia during winter operations, especially if the animal has become wet previous to the airlift.

Large numbers of animals may be transported in individual crates or in groups. The use of well-designed and sturdy individual crates has been advocated as the best method of transporting wild animals, but there may be cases in which crating of certain species may induce undue stress in isolated animals.(59, 60) As a guideline, all larger and potentially dangerous animals should be individually crated, as should the carnivores, the bears, and the larger, more aggressive primates. Communal crates that can contain several animals may be used for species that are better transported as a group. This method also permits segregation of age and sex groups.

It may be necessary for the safety of the animals and the workers to immobilize or sedate individuals or groups of animals during transport. Because of their effect on the thermoregulatory mechanisms, the phenothiazine derivatives should be used with caution. Benzodiazepine derivatives are safer and more useful drugs for this purpose. On long journeys, it is particularly important that the transport be accompanied by experienced and knowledgeable workers. In case of an emergency, their presence and attentiveness to the problem is invaluable.

For transportation of animals by road, night is often the best time. In addition to the advantage of darkness, which will calm the animals, there is less traffic on the road and less noise to stimulate the animals, and the transport will move faster, making the actual time on the road shorter than by day. In warm climates or during the warm season, when temperatures are highest at midday, the night and early morning would also be the preferable time for transport. In cold climates or during the cold season, it may be better to transport by day to avoid extremely low temperatures. Off-the-road transport usually takes place during the day to ensure visibility and safe driving.

The route should be as direct as possible. The speed should be kept constant while avoiding sharp turns, rapid acceleration, and sudden stops. Most animals will settle down if a steady pace is maintained. It is recommended that brief stops be made to check on the animals and give them an opportunity to change position and stimulate circulation. Some species will not urinate or defecate while moving, which may cause health problems associated with waste retention.

Release

Depending on species and circumstances, there are different methods by which the animals may be released. Upon arrival at the release site, the animals may be released directly and immediately. This phase can be very traumatic and potentially dangerous to both animals and personnel. Ungulates transported in groups are prone to accidents and injuries at this time. Animals that are not sedated or immobilized will come tumbling off the transport disoriented and panicked. They should not be made to jump or fall off the back of the transport. A ramp of sufficient height and width constructed to form a gentle slope from the vehicle to the ground should be prepared in advance. The release site should be carefully chosen and away from watercourses, precipitous terrain, and other hazards. The transport should be turned so that the first visual impression is of relatively open, nonthreatening terrain, free of obstacles, vehicles, and humans. As soon as the doors of the transport are opened, the workers should step aside quietly and let the animals exit at their own pace. Carnivores, primates, or other species transported in individual crates should be permitted to come out at their own volition.

Individual animals that are chemically immobilized with a reversible drug are placed on the ground away from the transport before the antagonist is given. All personnel should move back and allow the animal to recover and leave at its own will. This is very important with the larger or aggressive species, which may be dangerous to humans.

Heavily sedated animals or animals immobilized with a nonreversible drug should be positioned correctly and monitored until recovery. Animals that are ambulant, but still depressed, should be guided away from any obstacle that might be injurious to them. To prevent poaching, predation, or other interference, drugged animals should be monitored by at least one experienced person until they have recovered sufficiently to respond naturally.

Under different circumstances, it may be beneficial to release the animals into a temporary enclosure from which they are released over a period of time. This gives them time to calm down and recover from the trauma of capture and transport. It also provides an opportunity to feed and water the animals before release and to identify any individuals that may need veterinary care. Another method consists of releasing the animals into permanent enclosures where they may be kept for an extended period of time before being released.

Field Emergencies

Various medical emergencies may occur in association with chemical immobilization and capture.(54, 61–63) They may happen at any time during the process, and workers should be prepared to provide supportive field treatment as required. Immobilization-related emergencies may be caused by a number of factors, including stress, accidents, trauma, infections, illness, parasite load, poor condition, unusual drug reaction, inclement weather, extreme ambient temperatures, and malposition while immobilized. The most commonly encountered field emergencies are summarized next.

Physical Trauma

During the process of immobilization and capture, physical injuries such as contusions, lacerations, abrasions, punctures, and fractures may be inflicted on the animal accidentally or as a result of mishandling. Minor injuries can be treated successfully in the field, but fractures and other serious conditions are difficult to treat effectively and will often require that the animal be euthanatized for humane reasons. Standard first aid procedures consist of the following steps: (a) maintain patent airway; (b) stop bleeding; (c) prevent infection, protect the wound; (d) prevent shock, decrease stress; (e) immobilize fractures.

Minor lacerations (<35 mm) should be cleaned, treated with a topical antibiotic ointment, and protected with an insect repellant. An appropriate antibiotic may be given intramuscularly to help prevent infection. Larger lacerations (>35 mm) should be closed with a long-lasting absorbable suture material. Antibiotics should be given as indicated.

Physical trauma may be prevented by taking notice of any hazard in the environment that may cause injury to the animal during capture and by careful handling. If traps, snares, nets, or other forms of manual capture or restraint are used, they should be appropriate for the species. It is important that release procedures be planned to cause the least amount of trauma.

Hyperthermia

Hyperthermia (overheating) is one of the most often encountered capture-related emergencies. It is a major cause of mortality in animals immobilized during high ambient temperatures. The most immediate symptom is a critical rise in body temperature to above 41° C. At this temperature oxygen needs exceed cardiovascular capability, leading to cellular damage of the brain, liver and kidney. Excessive vasodilation as a mechanism of heat dissipation leads to hypotension, depression, cardiovascular dysfunction, shock and death. Other symptoms are rapid, shallow breathing, panting, and weak, rapid, or irregular heart rate.

Causative factors of hyperthermia are (a) external heat absorption (high ambient temperatures, exposure to sun); (b) internal heat production (muscular exertion during pursuit, physical restraint, stress); and (c) interference with thermoregulatory mechanism (drug response, ventilatory depression, poor ventilation, crating). Supportive procedures consist of an immediate attempt to lower body temperature. Move the animal into shade, or immerse it in or spray it with cold water.

Pack ice or snow around the animal, fan the abdomen and inside the hind legs, or place it in an air-conditioned environment. Give cold water enemas. Cold saline given intravenously will cool the animal and counteract metabolic acidosis. Flunixin meglumine administered intravenously may help to decrease body temperature. Treat for shock and monitor closely.

Hyperthermia may be prevented by avoiding immobilization or capture on very warm days or limiting activities to the coolest part of the day. Avoid prolonged pursuit, keep stress to a minimum, and use the least severe method of physical restraint. Protect the animal from high ambient temperatures and direct exposure to the sun. Transport only in well-ventilated crates or vehicles.

Hypothermia

Hypothermia (excessive cooling) is a concern when animals are immobilized during low ambient temperatures. This condition is characterized by a precipitous decrease in body temperature, below 35° C. Other symptoms are unresponsiveness, respiratory and circulatory depression, and shock. Low body temperature generates an attempt to minimize heat loss through peripheral vasoconstriction. If prolonged, decreased circulation and compromised oxygen flow may lead to anoxia, vasodilation, hypotension, shock and death.

Causative factors of hypothermia are (a) external heat loss (low ambient temperature); (b) evaporative cooling (windchill, wetness, precipitation); and (c) prolonged inactivity (drug response, trauma). Supportive procedures consist of an immediate attempt to increase body temperature by immersing the animal in or spraying it with warm water and drying thoroughly. In addition, the animal can be wrapped in a blanket with hot water bottles and/or warmed with a heat lamp. Small animals can be placed in an incubator.

Hypothermia may be prevented by avoiding immobilization or capture on very cold days or limiting activities to the warmest part of the day. Protect the immobilized animal from low ambient temperatures and exposure to wind and precipitation. Keep it warm and dry. Do not keep the animal immobilized (inactive) longer than is necessary for the job. Minimize conductive heat loss by maintaining the animal insulated from direct ground contract. An electric heating pad may be used for prolonged procedures on smaller animals.

Bloat

Bloat is a potentially life-threatening condition that can affect all animals, although ruminants are particularly susceptible. The condition is caused by excessive gas retention in the rumen and stomach associated with blockage of or external pressure on the esophagus. As the volume of unrelieved gases increases, pressure is exerted on the diaphragm and vena cava, compromising respiration and decreasing venous return to the right heart. This may result in asphyxia, shock, and death. Symptoms are abnormal distension of the abdomen and rapid and shallow breathing.

Bloat is commonly caused by malposition with consequent blockage of the esophagus. This results in the inability to relieve gases from the rumen or stomach through eructation (belching). Other causes of bloat are external pressure (restraint) on the esophagus, drug-induced ruminal atony, excessive exposure to sun, and esophagal blockage by regurgitated ruminal content. Supportive procedures consist of placing the immobilized animal in sternal recumbency with the neck extended and the head forward, permitting saliva to drain. Clear the mouth of regurgitated material. Move the animal from side to side over the brisket and elevate the front quarters of small animals. If positioning does not relieve the bloat, insert a lubricated and properly sized tube via the esophagus into the rumen to relieve pressure. The last resort is trocharization of the rumen. A 14- to 16-gauge needle of sufficient length may be used instead of a trochar. This often works well and is usually not associated with any major leakage from the rumen into the abdominal cavity. Bloat may be prevented by keeping immobilized animals in sternal recumbency and protecting them from exposure to the sun. If possible, withhold food and water for 12 hours prior to immobilization.

Shock

Shock is a life-threatening condition characterized by failure of the cardiovascular system and its consequent inability to deliver oxygen to the tissues, leading to cellular hypoxia and death (Chapters 5, 23, 24). Symptoms are rapid and weak heart rate, shallow and rapid breathing, depression, pale mucous membranes, and slow capillary refill time.

Shock may be caused by loss of blood volume (hypovolemic shock), heart failure (cardiogenic shock), infection, bloat, hyperthermia, hypothermia (vascular shock), and stress (neurogenic shock). Treatment of shock in the field is difficult. Treatment consists of controlling loss of blood, eliminating stress, maintaining a patent airway and supporting respiration. The animal should be kept warm and quiet while administering a balanced electrolyte solution intravenously. Prednisolone sodium succinate (50 mg/kg IV) or dexamethasone (4–8 mg/kg IV) can be administered along with a broad spectrum antibiotic. Prevention of shock is usually much easier than treatment. Minimize stress and trauma inflicted on the animal during capture. Avoid excessive handling and stimulation of the immobilized animal. Use the least severe method of restraint.

Capture Myopathy

Most free-ranging, wild animals are exerting themselves only infrequently to escape danger. Their time is primarily occupied with foraging or resting. As a result, they are not conditioned for running hard over long distances. Chasing wild animals with helicopter or motor vehicle for capture or trapping imposes a tremendous amount of fear, which in turn causes intensive muscular activity. The effects of sympathetic exhaustion from sustained stress, combined with intense muscular exertion are the causative factors of various life-threatening syndromes known as *capture myopathy*.(54, 62)

Intense sustained muscular exertion associated with capture pursuit or resisting physical restraint, leads to the production and buildup of lactic acid in muscle cells and nonrespiratory acidosis (Chapter 18). High levels of lactic acid leads to destruction of muscle fibers. Heart muscle destruction (myocardial necrosis) compromises cardiac function and leads to heart failure. Lactic acid may also cause the death of skeletal muscle fibers, causing them to release cellular potassium (K^+), calcium (Ca^{++}), and the red muscle pigment myoglobin into the blood. The toxicity of myoglobin causes kidney failure, and K^+ and Ca^{++} alter electric conduction within the heart. In association with high levels of K^+ or Ca^{++}, epinephrine causes disorganization of the heart rhythm. Cardiac arrest may occur as a result of these random, unproductive contractions (ventricular fibrillation). Intracellular enzymes LDH, CPK, and SGOT are also released, and the likelihood of capture myopathy is easily confirmed by their presence at increased concentrations in the blood.

In addition to the destruction of muscle fibers by high concentrations of lactic acid, the imposition of stress and intense fear on the animal causes the release of epinephrine. Normally, this assists in the short-term flight response by mobilizing glycogen and through selective vasodilation increases oxygen delivery to the brain and muscles. Prolonged epinephrine release, as may occur during sustained pursuit or resisting restraint, will result in lack of oxygen in vasoconstricted tissues and loss of responsiveness to epinephrine and dilation. Blood may stagnate and pool in this tissue. Blood pressure will drop, leading to shock and death. Four common clinical syndromes of capture myopathy have been identified.

Acute death syndrome (signs and/or death within 3-4 hours). The animal appears depressed, it is weak and remains recumbent after reversal, breathing is rapid and shallow, heart rate is rapid and weak, and hypotension persists, progressing to shock. Causative factors are exhaustion, lactic acidemia, hypoglycemia, hyperthermia, and the multiple organ dysfunction syndrome (MODS) (Chapter 24).

Supportive procedures consist of fluid replacement therapy to increase blood volume and pressure, restoration of electrolytes to normal concentrations, correcting acidosis, increasing renal perfusion, and the rehydration of tissues.

Delayed peracute death syndrome (death after 24 hours). In this syndrome the animal appears to be in reasonably good condition. When stressed again, it dies from ventricular fibrillation and cardiac arrest. The pathogenesis of this syndrome is muscle destruction,

with potassium release sensitizing the heart to catecholamines.

Ataxic-myoglobinuric syndrome (death in hours or days after capture). This condition is characterized by ataxia and brownish stained urine. Increased SGOT, CPK, LDH, and BUN is associated with lesions in skeletal muscles and kidneys. Death may occur acutely or in 4 to 5 days from kidney failure associated with myoglobin toxicity. There are survivors.

Muscle rupture syndrome (death in 3 or 4 weeks). The first signs of this syndrome are observed 24 to 48 hours following capture. The animal seems unable to support weight on the hind legs. Hocks are hyperflexed. CPK, LDH, and SGOT are increased, but BUN is normal. The animal will usually die within 3 or 4 weeks. There are extensive, light-colored areas in the large muscles used for flight.

Capture myopathy may be prevented by reducing capture stress, fear and exertion. Limit chase time to 2 minutes and abort the procedure for 24 hours. Keep visual and auditory stimulation, handling, and restraint of the captured animal to a minimum. Provide a stress-free postcapture environment. Captured wild animals should not be handled or stressed for at least 6 weeks following capture. Dietary vitamin E and selenium may be of value in the prevention of capture myopathy.(59)

Respiratory Distress

Respiratory distress is a serious emergency that may be caused in immobilized animals by several factors. Airway obstruction as a result of malposition, physical restraint, regurgitated stomach contents, the tongue falling back, pressure on the chest or diaphragm from malposition, excessive restraint, or bloat. Respiratory depression can also be caused by drug action causing an excessive buildup of carbon dioxide that alters respiratory patterns. Any departure from regular, effortless, and noiseless breathing may be a sign of respiratory distress.

Supportive procedures consist of clearing the airway by placing the animal in sternal recumbency with neck extended, pull the tongue forward, clear the mouth of vomit, and check for bloat and for any physical restraint which may inhibit respiration. If the animal is still not breathing, assist respiration with mouth-to-nose resuscitation at the rate of 15 inhalations/exhalations per minute. Mechanical resuscitation is more efficient using a self-inflating bag with an appropriately sized nose cone or, better, with a cuffed endotracheal tube. It is important that the proper size of tube be used. Transtracheal ventilation is a last resort.

Animals that have been immobilized with opioids should be given the antagonist immediately if respiratory arrest occurs and let go as they recover. Doxapram HCl may be used to alleviate respiratory depression by stimulation of the respiratory center of the brain, but it is not effective in case of serious airway obstruction or irreversible respiratory center tissue damage.

Respiratory distress may be prevented by using no higher a drug dose than is necessary for immobilization, by avoiding severe physical restraint, and by keeping the immobilized animals in the proper position while maintaining a patent airway. Also, guard against bloat and transport only in well-ventilated crates or vehicles.

Circulatory Failure

Circulatory failure (cardiac arrest) is the most serious of all emergencies and is usually preceded by respiratory arrest. Unless respiration and circulation can be restored, irreversible brain damage will occur in 2 to 4 minutes and the animal will expire.

Supportive procedures consist of immediately reversing opioid immobilizing drugs. Place the animal on its side and establish a patent airway. Begin mouth-to-nose or mechanical resuscitation at the rate of 15 breaths per minute. Simultaneously apply cardiac stimulation by compressing the lower chest behind the shoulders by 3 to 5 cm. The rate of compression should be 60 per minute, or 4 compressions for each breath. The resuscitation attempt is continued until respiration and circulation have been restored or until death of the animal has been ascertained.

Immune Resistance

It has been found that mitogen response in captured deer goes to zero 2 days postcapture and slowly returns to normal over a 40-day period.(64) This suggests that there is a rather defined period of time following capture when animals are particularly susceptible to stress, infection, and disease. Accordingly, handling, testing, or translocation should be avoided within 6 weeks of capture. If animals must be transported after capture, it should be done either immediately or wait for 6 weeks.

Field Emergency Kit

Recommendations for a field immobilization emergency kit are listed in Table 22–2.

Personnel Safety

Whenever drugs are used for capturing animals, personnel safety should be given a high priority.(38) All the drugs employed for this purpose are potentially hazardous to humans. In addition to the toxicity of specific drugs, the doses administered for animal immobilization usually exceed by far the safe levels in humans.

Throughout the immobilization process, the human worker is subject to a number of risk factors that may expose him or her to the toxic effects of the drugs used. Accidental exposure may include the absorption of drugs through broken skin or mucous membranes, by inhalation of powdered drug, or by injection. This is most likely to occur when preparing solutions of high-potency drugs and when loading and unloading drug darts. It is also important to recognize the hazards caused by incorrect use or malfunction of the delivery equipment, leaky darts, or untimely discharge. Caution

Table 22–2.　Recommended Field Immobilization Emergency Kit

1. **Equipment**
   Self-inflating resuscitation bag w/nose cone(s)
   Human face mask for self-inflating bag
   Endotracheal tubes in various sizes
   Laryngoscope
   Speculum
   Oxygen tank
   Transtracheal auger
   Stomach tubing in various sizes
   Trochar
   Syringes/hypodermic needles in various sizes/gauges
   Perfusion equipment
   Small sterile surgery pack w/needles/suture material
   Small stainless steel trays
   Cold sterilant
   Thermometer
   Stethoscope
   Stopwatch
2. **Wound treatment and sampling supplies**
   Disinfectant
   Eye ointment
   Topical antibiotic ointment and/or spray
   Insect/fly repellent
   Drains for puncture wounds, abscesses, etc.
   Antiseptic swabs
   Bandaging material
   Adhesive tape
   Scissors
   Containers for blood, bacteria, tissue samples
3. **Drugs**
   Antagonist(s) for immobilizing drug(s) used
   Atropine sulfate
   Calcium chloride (10%)
   Dexamethasone
   Dextrose (50%)
   Doxapram HCl
   Epinephrine
   Flunixin meglumine
   Furosemide
   Physiologic saline
   Physostigmine salicylate
   Prednisolone sodium succinate
   Ringer's solution
   Sodium bicarbonate

should be observed when handling immobilizing drugs. Because of their high toxicity, exposure to even minute amounts may cause fatality in humans.

As a rule, no one should work alone or be permitted to work alone with these drugs. Work in pairs and be aware of what the other person is doing. The use of disposable surgical gloves or splash boxes can greatly reduce the risk of accidental exposure when mixing drugs and loading darts. Direct contact with the drugs should be avoided and care taken not to inhale or ingest spilt, powdered, or atomized drugs. Firearms safety rules should be observed, and all projectors should be handled as carefully as conventional firearms. An accidentally discharged drug dart, propelled at more than 700 feet per second (fps), can cause serious injury. Loaded darts should be stored, handled, and carried so they do not present a safety hazard.

The opioids etorphine, fentanyl, and carfentanil, often potentiated with neuroleptics, are the most commonly used immobilization drugs for free-ranging, wild animals. These high-potency opioids are extremely toxic to humans. Depending on the dose, accidental exposure may cause sudden and precipitous depression of the central nervous system, loss of consciousness, respiratory failure, and death. The cyclohexamines and neuroleptics may not be as toxic as the opioids, but they can still cause serious complications, which in some cases may result in human fatality. Accidental exposure to ketamine and tiletamine, for example, may cause disorientation, excitation, and behavior modification. Death may occur as a result of events caused by personality or behavior change. Large doses of xylazine, if untreated, may produce respiratory and circulatory depression, coma, and death. The neuroleptics are less hazardous, but through their potentiation of the opioids and cyclohexamines contribute to the overall toxicity.

Emergency first aid treatment for accidental opioid exposure, consists of the immediate administration of an appropriate antagonist and respiratory support. Naloxone HCl (Narcan) is the currently recommended human opioid antagonist. An initial dose of 1 mg (IV) followed by 0.4 to 0.8 mg (IV) every 2 to 4 minutes until the central nervous system depression is reversed, is recommended.(38) To maintain stability and prevent recycling, an intramuscular dose of twice the successful intravenous dose should be given. Injections should be given slowly to prevent hypertension and tachycardia. This regimen is repeated as indicated until the patient is under medical care. Simultaneous respiratory support is given by maintaining a patent airway and resuscitating by mouth-to-mouth or with a self-inflating bag. In case of cardiac arrest, cardiopulmonary resuscitation (CPR) must be started at once. All field personnel should be trained and proficient in first aid and CPR. Recommendations for an emergency kit for human drug exposure are listed in Table 22–3.

There are no antagonists for the cyclohexamines. Emergency treatment consists of keeping the patient in a nonstimulating environment and careful monitoring for behavioral changes. Cranberry juice may help in metabolizing the drug. Exposure to large doses may require respiratory support and medical care. Xylazine exposure requires monitoring and if necessary respiratory support and antagonist administration. Large doses may cause fatal depression of respiration and circulation and require immediate hospitalization and life support.

In addition to the risk of accidental exposure to immobilizing drugs, there is also a possibility for physical injuries. Bites, cuts, bruises, lacerations, and fractures are not uncommon, and field personnel should be equipped and trained to provide treatment as necessary. First aid supplies should be readily available for this purpose.

Safety is an important consideration when helicopters are used in animal capture operations. Operational helicopters should only be approached from the front or side and with visual contact to the pilot. Wait for the pilot's sign to approach. Do not approach the tail rotor or walk under the tail boom. In uneven terrain, only approach and leave the helicopter on the downhill side. Crouch when walking under moving rotor blades. Secure hats and other loose items. Load and secure equipment as instructed by the pilot. Wear a seat belt in the helicopter and a safety harness when darting from it. Smoking is not permitted, and firearms should not be carried loaded in the helicopter. There should be a radio link between the pilot and the worker darting the animals. Again, the importance of an experienced pilot with "animal sense" cannot be overemphasized.(25, 55, 56)

When animals are immobilized in public access areas, such as national and state parks, game ranches, wildlife preserves, and zoos, there is an additional risk to public safety. Missed darts not recovered might be found by the public and through careless handling cause accidental drug poisoning. A dart missing its intended target might hit a bystander. Animal immobilization in areas utilized by the public should be conducted with great caution. All expended darts, drug vials, syringes, and needles must be recovered. Equipment and drugs should not be left unattended, but kept under lock in a secure container, compartment, or room. Care should be taken to protect the drugs and equipment from theft or

Table 22–3. Recommended Emergency Kit for Human Drug Exposure

1. Equipment
  Self-inflating resuscitation bag with face mask(s)
  Oropharyngeal airways
  Laryngoscope*
  Endotracheal tubes, size 8 and 9*
  Cuff inflating syringe*
  One liter bag crystalloid solution (e.g. Ringer's Lactate)
  Intravenous giving sets
  Sterile IV canulae
  Assorted disposable syringes/hypodermic needles
  Adhesive tape, scissors
  Antiseptic swabs
2. Drugs
  Naloxone HCl (at least 40 ampoules, preferably more)
  Physostigmine salicylate (10 ampoules)
  Hydrocortisone (250 mg vials)†
  Sodium bicarbonate (1 milliequivalent/ml)†
  Diazepam†

*For use by physician called to the scene or by properly trained personnel only.
†For use by physician called to the scene.
(From Parker, J.B.R., and Haigh, J.C. Human Exposure to Immobilizing Agents. In: Chemical Immobilization of North American Wildlife. Edited by L. Nielsen, J.C. Haigh, and M.E. Fowler. Milwaukee: Wisconsin Humane Society, 1982: 119–136.)

misuse. It should not be possible for unauthorized persons to gain access to the equipment or drugs.

In addition to all the aforementioned risks inherent to the use of drugs for immobilization of animals, the responsibility for public safety liabilities incurred as a direct or indirect result of the use of this technique in public access areas should be recognized.

References

1. Harthoorn AM. The capture and restraint of wild animals. In: LR Soma, ed. Textbook of Veterinary Anesthesia. Baltimore: Williams & Wilkins, 1971:404–437.
2. Harthoorn AM. The Chemical Capture of Animals. London: Balliere Tindall, 1976.
3. Hatlapa H-HM, Weisner H. Die Praxis der Wildtierimmobilisation. Hamburg: Paul Parey, 1982.
4. Nielsen L, JC Haigh, ME Fowler, eds. Chemical Immobilization of North American Wildlife. Milwaukee: Wisconsin Humane Society, 1982.
5. Nielsen L, RD Brown, cds. Translocation of Wild Animals. Milwaukee: Wisconsin Humane Society; Kingsville, TX: Caesar Kleberg Wildl Res Inst, 1988.
6. Young E, ed. The Capture and Care of Wild Animals. Cape Town, South Africa: Human & Rousseau, 1973.
7. Crockford JA, et al. Nicotine salicylate for capturing deer. J Wildl Man 21:213–220, 1957.
8. Hall TC, et al. A preliminary report on the use of flaxedil to produce paralysis in the white-tailed deer. J Wildl Man 17:516–520, 1953.
9. Anderson CF. Anesthetizing deer by arrow. J Wildl Man 25:202–203, 1961.
10. Short RV, JM King. The design of a crossbow and dart for the immobilization of animals. Vet Rec 76:707–708, 1964.
11. Green H. New techniques for using the CAP-CHUR gun. J Wildl Man 27:292–296, 1963.
12. Harthoorn AM. On the use of phencyclidine in narcosis in the larger animals. Vet Rec 74:410, 1962.
13. Spalding VT, Heyman CS. The value of phencyclidine in the anaesthesia of monkeys. Vet Rec 74:158, 1962.
14. Talbot LM. Field immobilization of large mammals. Serengeti-Mara Wildl Res Project, 1960.
15. Harthoorn AM. Capture of the white (square lipped) rhinoceros (Ceratoterium simum) (Burchell) with the use of drug immobilization technique. Can J Comp Med 26:203, 1962.
16. Royal Veterinary College of East Africa Expedition. The use of a thiambutene/phencyclidine/hyoscine mixture for the immobilization of the topi (Damaliscus korrigum) and the hippopotamus (Hippopotamus amphibius). Vet Rec 75:630, 1963.
17. Harthoorn AM. The tranquilization and handling of large animals. A field and laboratory study. Department of Physiology. University College, Nairobi, 1965.
18. Harthoorn AM. The use of a new orpavine derivative with potent morphine-like activity for the restraint of hoofed wild animals. Res Vet Sci 6:290, 1965.
19. Harthoorn AM. The drug immobilization of large wild herbivores other than the antelopes. In: E Young, ed. The Capture and Care of Wild Animals. Cape Town, South Africa: Human & Rousseau, 1973:51–61.
20. Harthoorn AM, Player IC. The narcosis of the white rhinoceros. A series of eighteen case histories. Proc 5th Int Symp Dis Zoo Anim, Amsterdam, 1963.
21. King JM, Carter BH. The use of the oripavine derivative M99 for the immobilization of black rhinoceros, and its antagonism with the related compound M285 or nalorphine. East Afr Wildl J 3:19, 1965.
22. Pienaar UDeV. Capture and immobilizing techniques currently employed in Kruger National Park and other South African national parks and provincial reserves. Kruger National Park. Report, 1966.

23. Bush M, V deVos. Remote drug delivery systems. J Zoo Wildl Med 23:159–180, 1992.
24. Fowler ME. Delivery systems for chemical immobilization. In: L Nielsen, JC Haigh, ME Fowler, eds. Chemical Immobilization of North American Wildlife. Milwaukee: Wisconsin Humane Society, 1982:18–45.
25. Jessup DA, et al. Wildlife Restraint Series. International Wildlife Veterinary Services. Salinas, California, 1990.
26. Pienaar UDeV. Darting and injection equipment and techniques. In: E Young, ed. The Capture and Care of Wild Animals. Cape Town, South Africa: Human & Rousseau, 1973:7–13.
27. Barnard SM, JS Dobbs. A handmade blowgun dart: its preparation and application in a zoological park. J Am Vet Med Assoc 177:951–954, 1980.
28. Bubenik AB, GA Bubenik. New, non-traumatic, disposable, automatic injection dart. CALAS/ACTAL Proc 1976:48–53.
29. Haigh JC, HC Hopf. The blowgun in veterinary practice: its uses and preparation. J Am Vet Med Assoc 169:881–883, 1976.
30. Haigh JC. Mammalian immobilizing drugs, their pharmacology and effects. In: L Nielsen, JC Haigh, ME Fowler, eds. Chemical Immobilization of North American Wildlife. Milwaukee: Wisconsin Humane Society, 1982:46–62.
31. Harthoorn AM. Review of wildlife capture drugs in common use. In: E Young, ed. The Capture and Care of Wild Animals. Cape Town, South Africa: Human & Rousseau, 1973:14–34.
32. Haigh JC. Opioids in zoological medicine. J Zoo Wildl Med 21:391–413, 1990.
33. Haigh JC, Lee LJ, Schweinsburg RE. Immobilization of polar bears with carfentanil. J Wildl Dis 19:140–144, 1983.
34. Allen JL. Renarcotization following immobilization of nondomestic ungulates. J Zoo Wildl Med 21:391–413, 1989.
35. Stanley TH, et al. Immobilization of elk with A-3080. J Wildl Man 52:577–581, 1988.
36. Janssen DL, et al. Field studies with the narcotic immobilizing agent A3080. Proc Am Assoc Zoo Vet, Calgary, Alberta, 1991.
37. Stanley TH, S McJames, J Kimball. Chemical immobilization for the capture and transportation of big game. Proc Am Assoc Zoo Vet, Greensboro, North Carolina, 1989.
38. Parker JBR, JC Haigh. Human exposure to immobilizing agents. In: L Nielsen, JC Haigh, ME Fowler, eds. Chemical Immobilization of North American Wildlife. Milwaukee: Wisconsin Humane Society, 1982:119–136.
39. Klein LV, AM Klide. Central alpha-2 adrenergic and benzodiazepine agonists and their antagonists. J Zoo Wildl Med 20:138–153, 1989.
40. Kock RA, Pearce PC, Taylor P. The use of detomidine and butorphanol in zoo equids. Proc Joint Annu Mtg Am Assoc Zoo Vet Am Assoc Wildl Vet, Toronto, 1988.
41. Barnett JEF, Lewis JCM. Medetomidine and ketamine anaesthesia in zoo animals and its reversal with atipamezole: a review and update with specific reference to work in British zoos. Proc Am Assoc Zoo Vet, South Padre Island, Texas, 1990:207–214.
42. Jalanka HH. Evaluation of medetomidine- and ketamine-induced immobilization in markhors (Capra falconeri megaceros) and its reversal by atipamezole. J Zoo Anim Med 19:95–105, 1988.
43. Jalanka HH. Medetomidine- and ketamine-induced immobilization of snow leopard (Panthera uncia): doses, evaluation, and reversal by atipamezole. J Zoo Anim Med 20:154–162, 1989.
44. Ebedes H. The translocation and adaptation of some southern African wild antelopes with long-acting neuroleptics (LAN) [Personal communication]. National Zoo Gardens of South Africa, Pretoria, 1989.
45. Hofmeyer JM. The use of haloperidol as a long-acting neuroleptics in game capture operations. J S Afr Vet Assoc 52:273–282, 1981.
46. Hofmeyr JM, HG Lucthenstein, PKN Mostert. Capture, handling and transport of springbok and the application of haloperidol as a long-acting neuroleptic. Madoqua 10:123–130, 1977.
47. Bush M, deVos V, Citino SB, Tell L. Telazol and Telazol/Rompun anesthesia in non-domestic cervids and bovids. Proc Am Assoc Zoo Vet and Am Assoc Wildl Vet, Oakland, California, 1992:251–252.

48. Fowler ME. Zoo and Wild Animal Medicine: Current Therapy, 3rd ed. Philadelphia: WB Saunders, 1993.
49. Kock MD, P Morkel. Capture and translocation of the free-ranging black rhinoceros: medical and management problems. In: ME Fowler, ed. Zoo and Wild Animal Medicine: Current Therapy, 3rd ed. Philadelphia: WB Saunders, 1993:466–475.
50. Snyder SB, MJ Richard, WR Foster. Etorphine, ketamine and xylazine in combination (M99KX) for immobilization of exotic ruminants: a significant additive effect. Proc Am Assoc Zoo Vet Am Assoc Wildl Vet, Oakland, California, 1992.
51. McWade DH. An evaluation of ketamine and xylazine in combination as agents for the remote chemical immobilization of feral and stray dogs. In: L Nielsen, JC Haigh, ME Fowler, eds. Chemical Immobilization of North American Wildlife. Milwaukee: Wisconsin Humane Society, 1982:175–187.
52. Nielsen L. Definitions, considerations, and guidelines for translocation of wild animals. In: L Nielsen and RD Brown, eds. Translocation of Wild Animals. Milwaukee: Wisconsin Humane Society; Kingsville, TX: Caesar Kleberg Wildl Res Inst, 1988: 12–51.
53. Tomkiewicz SM. Advances in capture technology. In: L Nielsen, JC Haigh, ME Fowler, eds. Chemical Immobilization of North American Wildlife. Milwaukee: Wisconsin Humane Society, 1982:1–17.
54. Spraker TR. An overview of the pathophysiology of capture myopathy and related conditions that occur at the time of capture of wild animals. In: L Nielsen, JC Haigh, ME Fowler, eds. Chemical Immobilization of North American Wildlife. Milwaukee: Wisconsin Humane Society, 1982:83–118.
55. Albers DF. Game Capture and Culling for the Helicopter Pilot. Fly-Safe Products. Weltevredenpark, South Africa, 1989.
56. Jessup DA. The use of the helicopter in the capture of free-roaming wildlife. In: L Nielsen, JC Haigh, ME Fowler, eds. Chemical Immobilization of North American Wildlife. Milwaukee: Wisconsin Humane Society, 1982:289–303.
57. Schmitt SM, RW Aho. Reintroduction of moose from Ontario to Michigan. In: L Nielsen and RD Brown, eds. Translocation of Wild Animals. Milwaukee: Wisconsin Humane Society; Kingsville, TX: Caesar Kleberg Wildl Res Inst, 1988:258–274.
58. Van Reenen, G. Field experiences in the capture of red deer by helicopter in New Zealand with reference to post-capture sequela and management. In: L Nielsen, JC Haigh, ME Fowler, eds. Chemical Immobilization of North American Wildlife. Milwaukee: Wisconsin Humane Society, 1982:408–421.
59. Harthoorn AM. Mechanical capture as a preliminary to chemical immobilization and the use of taming and training to prevent post capture stress. In: L Nielsen, JC Haigh, ME Fowler, eds. Chemical Immobilization of North American Wildlife. Milwaukee: Wisconsin Humane Society, 1982:150–164.
60. Hirst SM. Transportation of wild animals. In: E Young, ed. The Capture and Care of Wild Animals. Cape Town, South Africa: Human & Rousseau, 1973:119–125.
61. Basson PA, JM Hofmeyer. Mortalities associated with wildlife capture operations. In: E Young, ed. The Capture and Care of Wild Animals. Cape Town, South Africa: Human & Rousseau, 1973:151–160.
62. Harthoorn AM. Physical aspects of both mechanical and chemical capture. In: L Nielsen, JC Haigh, ME Fowler, eds. Chemical Immobilization of North American Wildlife. Milwaukee: Wisconsin Humane Society, 1982:63–71.
63. Silberman MS. Emergency medicine during immobilization. In: L Nielsen, JC Haigh, ME Fowler, eds. Chemical Immobilization of North American Wildlife. Milwaukee: Wisconsin Humane Society, 1982:72–82.
64. Griffin F. The impact of domestication on red deer immunity and disease resistance. In: The Biology of Deer. Proc Dept Wildl Fisheries. Mississippi State University, 1990:17.
65. Anderson MD, PRK Richardson. Remote immobilization of the aardwolf. S Afr J Wildl Res 22:26–28, 1992.
66. Sayer P, D Rottcher. Wildlife management and utilization in East Africa. In: ME Fowler, ed. Zoo and Wild Animal Medicine: Current Therapy, 3rd ed. Philadelphia: WB Saunders 1993:101–111.
67. Allen JL, et al. Immobilization of captive non-domestic hoofstock with carfentanil. Proc Am Assoc Zoo Vet, Calgary, Alberta, 1991.
68. Fowler ME, ed. Zoo and Wild Animal Medicine. Philadelphia: WB Saunders, 1978/1986.
69. Schobert E. Telazol use in wild and exotic animals. Vet Med 82:1080–1088, 1987.
70. Foster PA. Immobilization and anaesthesia of primates. In: E Young, ed. The Capture and Care of Wild Animals. Cape Town, South Africa: Human & Rousseau, 1973:69–76.
71. Holz P. Immobilization of marsupials with tiletamine and zolazepam. J Zoo Wild Med 23:426–428, 1992.
72. Gibeau ML, PC Paquet. Evaluation of Telazol for immobilization of black bears. Wildl Soc Bull 19:400–402, 1991.
73. Addison EM, GB Kolenosky. Use of ketamine hydrochloride and xylazine hydrochloride to immobilize black bear (Ursus americanus). J Wildl Dis 15:253–257, 1979.
74. Stewart GR, JM Siperek, VR Wheeler. Use of the cataleptoid anesthetic CI-744 for chemical restraint of black bears. Int Conf Bear Res and Man 3:57–62, 1980.
75. Taylor WP Jr, HV Reynolds III, WB Ballard. Immobilization of grizzly bears with tiletamine hydrochloride and zolazepam hydrochloride. J Wildl Man 53:978–981, 1989.
76. Lynch GM, W Hall, B Pelchat, JA Hanson. Chemical immobilization of black bear with special reference to the use of ketamine-xylazine. In: L Nielsen, JC Haigh, ME Fowler, eds. Chemical Immobilization of North American Wildlife. Milwaukee: Wisconsin Humane Society, 1982:245–266.
77. Stirling IC, C Spencer, D Andriashek. Immobilization of polar bears (Ursus maritimus) with Telazol in the Canadian arctic. J Wildl Dis 25:159–168, 1989.
78. Klos, H-G, EM Lang, eds. Zootierkrankheiten. Hamburg: Paul Parey, 1976.
79. Jessup DA, et al. Immobilization of free-ranging desert bighorn sheep, tule elk, and wild horses using carfentanil and xylazine: reversal with naloxone, diprenorphine and yohimbine. J Am Vet Med Assoc 187:1253–1254, 1985.
80. Thorne ET. Agents used in North American ruminant immobilization. In: L Nielsen, JC Haigh, ME Fowler, eds. Chemical Immobilization of North American Wildlife. Milwaukee: Wisconsin Humane Society, 1982:304–334.
81. Kock MD, J Berger. Chemical Immobilization of free-ranging North American bison (Bison bison) in Badlands National Park, South Dakota. J Wildl Dis 23:625–633, 1988.
82. Jones DM. Physical and chemical methods of capturing deer. Vet Rec 114(5):109–112, 1984.
83. Morkel P. Dosages for the chemical capture of African game. Namibian Game Capture Unit. Department report, 1990.
84. Jessup DA. Restraint and chemical immobilization of carnivores and furbearers. In: L Nielsen, JC Haigh, ME Fowler, eds. Chemical Immobilization of North American Wildlife. Milwaukee: Wisconsin Humane Society, 1982:227–244.
85. Young E. Wildboerdery & Natuurreservaatbestuur. Nylstroom, South Africa, 1984.
86. Pienaar UDeV. The drug immobilization of antelope species. In: E Young, ed. The Capture and Care of Wild Animals. Cape Town, South Africa: Human & Rousseau, 1973:35–50.
87. Kreeger TJ. A review of chemical immobilization of wild canids. Proc Am Assoc Zoo Vet Am Assoc Wildl Vet, Oakland, California, 1992.
88. Fowler ME. Restraint and Handling of Wild and Domestic Animals. Ames, IA: Iowa State Univ. Press, 1978.
89. Fong DW. Immobilization of caribou with etorphine plus acepromazine. J Wildl Man 46:560–562, 1982.
90. Robinson PT, D Lambert. A review of 226 chemical restraint procedures in great apes at the San Diego Zoo. Proc Annu Mtg Am Assoc Zoo Vet, Chicago, 1986.
91. Jessup DA, et al. Immobilization of mule deer with ketamine and xylazine, and reversal of immobilization with yohimbine. J Am Vet Med Assoc 183:1339–1340, 1983.
92. Nielsen L. Electronic ground tracking of white-tailed deer chemically immobilized with a combination of etorphine and

xylazine hydrochloride. In: L Nielsen, JC Haigh, ME Fowler, eds. Chemical Immobilization of North American Wildlife. Wisconsin Humane Society, 1982:355–362.

93. Nielsen L. Selective removal as an alternative in deer management. In: Deer Management in an Urbanized Region. Conf Proc Humane Soc US, Washington, DC, 1993:33–37.

94. Jacobson ER. Immobilization of African elephants with carfentanil and antagonism with nalmefene and diprenorphine. J Zoo Animal Med 19:1–7, 1987.

95. Kock RA, P Morkel, MD Kock. Current immobilization procedures used in elephants. In: ME Fowler, ed. Zoo and Wild Animal Medicine: Current Therapy, 3rd ed. Philadelphia: WB Saunders, 1993:436–441.

96. Franz W, B Seidel, A Jacob. Zur operativen behandlung einer pododermatitis purulenta beim Indischen elefanten (*Elephas maximus*). Verhandlungsbericht des 31. Internationalen Symposiums uber die Erkrankungen der Zoo- und Wildtiere. Dortmund, Germany, 1989.

97. Jainudeen MR, TA Bongso, BMOA Perera. Immobilization of aggressive working elephants (*Elephas maximus*). Vet Rec 89:686–688, 1971.

98. Meuleman T, et al. Immobilization of elk and moose with carfentanil. J Wildl Man 48:258–262, 1982.

99. Armstrong DL. An evaluation of carfentanil as an immobilizing agent for gaur (*Bos gaurus*). Proc Am Assoc Zoo Vet, Greensboro, North Carolina, 1989.

100. Bush M, V deVos. Observations on field immobilization of giraffa (*Giraffa camelopardalis*) using carfentanil and xylazine. J Zoo Animal Med 18:135–140, 1987.

101. Beck CC. Chemical restraint of exotic species. J Zoo Med 3:3–60, 1972.

102. Pienaar UDeV. The field-immobilization and capture of hippopotami in their aquatic element. Koedoe 10:149–157, 1967.

103. Allen JL. Immobilization of Mongolian wild horses (*Equus przewalskii przewalskii*) with carfentanil and antagonism with naltrexone. J Zoo Wildl Med 23:422–425, 1992.

104. Wiesner H. Chemical immobilization of wild equids. In: ME Fowler, ed. Zoo and Wild Animal Medicine: Current Therapy, 3rd ed. Philadelphia: WB Saunders, 1993:475–476.

105. Stander PE, WC Gasaway. Spotted hyaenas immobilized with ketamine/xylazine and antagonized with tolazoline. Afr J Ecol 29:168–169, 1991.

106. Seal US, Kreeger TJ. Chemical immobilization of furbearers. In: M Novak, JA Baker, ME Obbard, B Malloch, eds. Wild Furbearer Management and Conservation in North America. Toronto, Ontario: Ontario Ministry of Natural Resources, 1987: 191–215.

107. Jalanka HH. Evaluation and comparison of two ketamine-based immobilization techniques in snow leopard (*Panthera uncia*). J Zoo Anim Med 20:163–169, 1989.

108. Stander PE, PvdB Morkel. Field immobilization of lions using disassociative anaesthetics in combination with sedatives. Afr J Ecol 29:137–148, 1991.

109. Jessup DA, Lance WE. What every veterinarian should know about South American camelids. Calif Vet 36: 1982.

110. Franzmann AW. An assessment of chemical immobilization of North American Moose. In: L Nielsen, JC Haigh, ME Fowler, eds. Chemical Immobilization of North American Wildlife. Milwaukee: Wisconsin Humane Society, 1982:393–407.

111. Patenaude RP. Chemical immobilization of muskox. In: L Nielsen, JC Haigh, ME Fowler, eds. Chemical Immobilization of North American Wildlife. Milwaukee: Wisconsin Humane Society, 1982:439–44.

112. Hopf HC. Notes on muskoxen. Proc Am Assoc Zoo Vet Annu Mtg, Atlanta, Georgia,1974.

113. Williams TD, FH Kocher. Comparison of anesthetic agents in the sea otter. J Am Vet Med Assoc 173:1127–1130, 1978.

114. Hellgren EC, et al. Endocrine and metabolic response of the collared peccary (*Tajassu tajacu*) to immobilization with ketamine hydrochloride. J Wildl Dis 21:417–425, 1985.

115. Morkel P. Drugs and dosages for capture and treatment of black rhinoceros (*Diceros bicornis*) in Namibia. Koedoe 32(2):65–68, 1989.

116. Kock MD, M la Grange, R du Toit. Chemical immobilization of free-ranging black rhinoceros (*Diceros bicornis*) using combinations of etorphine (M99), fentanyl, and xylazine. J Zoo Anim Med 21:155–165, 1990.

117. Dinerstein E, S Shrestha, H Mishra. Capture, chemical immobilization, and radio-collar life for greater one-horned rhinoceros. Wildl Soc Bull 18:36–41, 1990.

118. Booth VR, AM Coetzee. The capture and relocation of black and white rhinoceros in Zimbabwe. In: L Nielsen and RD Brown, eds. Translocation of Wild Animals. Milwaukee: Wisconsin Humane Society; Kingsville, TX: Caesar Kleberg Wildl Res Inst, 1988:191–209.

119. Alford BTR, L Burkhart, WP Johnson. Etorphine and diprenorphine as immobilizing and reversing agents in captive and free-ranging mammals. J Am Vet Med Assoc 164:702–705, 1974.

120. Beck CC. Chemical restraint of exotic species. Proc Am Assoc Zoo Vet Annu Mtg, Honolulu, Hawaii, 1971.

121. Smith JLD, et al. A technique for capturing and immobilizing tigers. J Wildl Man 47:255–259, 1983.

122. Ballard WB, et al. Immobilization of gray wolves with a combination of tiletamine hydrochloride and zolazepam hydrochloride. J Wildl Man 55:71–74, 1991.

123. Hash SH, MG Hornocker. Immobilizing wolverines with ketamine hydrochloride. J Wildl Man 44:713–715, 1980.

section **VIII**

ANESTHESIA MANAGEMENT

ANESTHESIA FOR SELECTED DISEASES: CARDIOVASCULAR DYSFUNCTION

Robert R. Paddleford, Ralph C. Harvey

Introduction

The anesthetic management of a patient with cardiovascular dysfunction can be very challenging, since most preanesthetic and anesthetic agents capable of CNS depression are also capable of producing cardiovascular depression. Patients with cardiovascular dysfunction may be more prone to fluid overload and dysrhythmias. Extremes in heart rate may cause severe problems, including heart failure. Patients with cardiovascular dysfunction may lack sufficient cardiac reserve to compensate for anesthetic-induced depression.

Cardiovascular Physiology

The function of the myocardial cell is to rhythmically contract and relax with other myofibers so that the heart will act as a pump. The basic contractile unit of heart muscle is the sarcomere, which is composed of interdigitating protein filaments referred to as *actin* and *myosin*. Muscle shortening develops in the myocardial muscle when the actin and myosin filaments are activated. This activation is regulated by tropomyosin and troponin. Tropomyosin prevents the interaction of actin and myosin during diastole. When tropomyosin is no longer at its blocking position, systole is initiated. The availability of ionized calcium in the area of the troponin-tropomyosin protein unit acts as an immedi-

ate catalyst for the contraction-relaxation cycle. The contraction of the heart muscle is dependent on the amount of free calcium ions available around the myofibril. Part of the contractile-dependent calcium originates from superficial sites on cell membranes that are in equilibrium with extracellular calcium and therefore can be affected by drugs that do not penetrate the myocardial cell (Chapter 5).

Few clinically used drugs affect the actin-myosin proteins; however, many drugs can alter the availability of calcium for activation of the contractile process.(1) Digitalis increases calcium movement to the troponin-tropomyosin protein unit and thus increases contractile strength. Barbiturates and inhalant anesthetic agents seem to disrupt calcium movements and thus cause a reduced contractile strength. Myocardial intracellular acidosis also inhibits the binding of calcium to the troponin-tropomyosin unit, causing decreased myocardial contractile strength. Disease conditions or drugs that produce metabolic or respiratory acidosis may decrease contractility. Most anesthetics depress respiration and predispose the patient to respiratory acidosis.

Blood pressure is the product of peripheral vascular resistance and cardiac output. Cardiac output is the product of heart rate and stroke volume. Drugs that alter any or all of these parameters may greatly affect blood pressure and tissue blood flow. Preanesthetic and anesthetic agents can alter peripheral resistance (phenothiazine tranquilizers, alpha$_2$-agonists, barbiturates, inhalant agents), heart rate (narcotics, alpha$_2$-agonists, dissociative agents, inhalants) and stroke volume (inhalant anesthetics). Patients that suffer from diseases causing impaired cardiac output, patients with congenital heart disease, and those suffering from hypotension/hypovolemia, anemia, and/or heartworms are at a higher anesthetic risk.

Patients With Impaired Cardiac Output

Cardiomyopathies can be classified as hypertrophic or congestive. *Hypertrophic cardiomyopathy* is characterized by ventricular hypertrophy, decreased ventricular compliance, and impaired ventricular filling, which results in reduced cardiac output. Ventricular performance (pump function) is usually not impaired.(2) *Congestive cardiomyopathy* is characterized by marked ventricular dilation, increased ventricular diastolic volume, and poor ventricular performance. Often, congestive heart failure is present.(2) Commonly employed cardiovascular medications used for treatment of congestive heart failure are listed in Table 23A–1.

Pericardial tamponade and *constrictive pericarditis* are associated with impaired cardiac output secondary to reduced preload. There is limited expansion of the cardiac chambers, resulting in decreased ventricular filling, stroke volume, and cardiac output. Pump function is not impaired.(3)

Valvular heart disease is associated with impaired cardiac output, and when severe can cause congestive heart failure. *Mitral insufficiency* is probably the most common valvular disease. Characterized by ventricular hypertrophy and dilation and pulmonary vascular engorgement, it may eventually cause right heart failure.(4) Left ventricular pump function and systemic cardiac output are usually maintained until retrograde flow becomes severe.

The primary goals in the anesthetic management of patients with impaired cardiac output are to avoid tachycardia, decreased preload, and hypovolemia. These patients should be preoxygenated for 5 to 7 minutes prior to anesthetic induction. If pump function is adequate, the choice of anesthetic drugs is not specific for these patients; however, drugs that may produce tachycardia (anticholinergics, dissociative agents) are best avoided. The exception to this is congestive cardiomyopathy, in which an increased heart rate may help increase cardiac output.(5)

Narcotics are often used as preanesthetic medication because of their minimal effects on the myocardium, and they can be readily antagonized. They can be used in combination with acepromazine or a benzodiazepine tranquilizer for additional sedation. The fact that they slow the heart rate may be beneficial. However, if

Table 23A–1.   Chronic Therapy for Congestive Heart Failure (CHF) Enlists a Variety of Classes of Medications Including Digitalis, "Inodilators," Vasodilators, Angiotensin Converting Enzyme (ACE) Inhibitors, and Diuretics

| Classes | Trade Name | Mechanism of Action | Effects on | | Maintenance Dose[a] |
			Contractility	Afterload	
Inotropes					
Digitalis	Cardoxin; Lanoxin	Inactivates Na$^+$-K$^+$ exchange increasing Ca^{+2} intracellularly	↑	↑	*Dog:* 0.005 mg/kg PO, BID *Cat:* 0.007 mg/kg PO, q 48 hours
T3	Triostat	Increases Ca^{+2} adenosine ATPase activity; β receptor up regulation	↑	–	NA[c]
"Inodilators"					
Amrinone	Inocor	Class III phosphodiesterase inhibitors prevent breakdown of cAMP, which results from stimulation of β-adrenergic receptors. Enoximome is a more potent vasodilator than older "inodilators."	↑	↓	3 mg/kg IV slow to effect
Milrinone			↑	↓	0.5–1.0 mg/kg PO, BID
Enoximome			↑	↓	NA

[a] Patients will usually be stabilized on CHF medications prior to undergoing anesthesia. Medications should *not* be discontinued when contemplating anesthesia and surgery.

[b] EDRF, Endothelium-dependent relaxant factor, which is now known to be nitric oxide (NO). NO binds to a heme group in the enzyme guanylyl cyclase, activating the enzyme, resulting in the production of cyclic guanine monophosphate (cGMP). cGMP produces relaxation as a second messenger in vascular smooth muscle.

[c] NA, Dose is not available at this time for dog or cat.

[d] If one diuretic does not produce increased urine flow, another class may be effective. Some diuretics result in salt wasting, so serum K$^+$ should be monitored to avoid complicating arrhythmias in the congestive patient.

Table 23A–1. Chronic Therapy for Congestive Heart Failure (CHF) Enlists a Variety of Classes of Medications Including Digitalis, "Inodilators," Vasodilators, Angiotensin Converting Enzyme (ACE) Inhibitors, and Diuretics — cont'd

Classes	Trade Name	Mechanism of Action	Effects on Contractility	Effects on Afterload	Maintenance Dose[a]
Nitrovasodilators					
Na nitroprusside	Nitropress	Activation of EDRF[b] or nitric oxide (NO). These drugs act as substrates for the formation of NO. Nitroprusside is primarily an arterial dilator, whereas nitroglycerin is a venodilator.	—	↓	1–10 μg/kg/min IV (monitor pressure)
Nitroglycerin	Nitrostat; Nitrolpaste		—	↓	1–5 μg/kg/min IV; available in oral and transdermal paste formulations: *Dog:* ¼–½ in./20 kg QOD. *Cat:* ⅛ in. QOD.
Isosorbide dinitrate		Formation of NO.	—	↓	0.5–2.0 mg/kg PO, TID; also available as ointment
Hydralazine	Apresoline	Hydralazine interferes with Ca^{+2} transport in smooth muscle	—	↓	*Dog:* 1–3 mg/kg PO, BID. *Cat:* 2.5–5.0 mg/kg PO, BID
ACE Inhibitors					
Captopril	Capoten	Prevents conversion of Angiotensin I to Angiotensin II which decreases blood pressure and produces some venodilation. Produces balanced vasodilation and prevents renal fluid retention.	—	↓	*Dog:* 0.5–2.0 mg/kg PO, TID *Cat:* Same.
Enalapril	Enacard		—	↓	*Dog:* 0.5 mg/kg PO, SID-BID *Cat:* 0.25–0.5 mg/kg PO, SID-QOD
Benazepril	Lotensin		—	↓	*Dog:* 0.25–0.5 mg/kg PO, SID-BID *Cat:* 0.25–0.5 mg/kg PO, SID-QOD
Diuretics[d]					
Acetazolamide		Inhibits Na^+ from passing into proximal tubule osmotic effect at glomerulus.	—	↓	*Dog:* 10 mg/kg q 6 h
Mannitol			—	↓	*Dog and Cat:* 0.25–0.5 g/kg 5% solution IV
Aminophylline		Increases vascular perfusion of glomerulus.	↑	↓	*Dog:* 11 mg/kg PO, TID *Cat:* 5 mg/kg PO, BID-TID
Spironolactone	Aldactone	Inhibits aldosterone receptor in collecting tubule.	—	↓	*Dog:* 1–2 mg/kg PO, BID *Cat:* Same
Furosemide	Lasix	Inhibits Na^+, K^+, Cl^{-2} co-transporter in thick ascending loop of Henle.	—	↓	*Dog:* 1–4 mg/kg PO, SID, QOD *Cat:* 0.5–3.0 mg/kg PO, 8–48 h

significant bradycardia occurs, atropine or glycopyrrolate should be given to effect.

If only tranquilization is needed, a low dose of acepromazine (0.05 mg/kg IM to a maximum total dose of 1.5 mg) may be used. Acepromazine produces minimal direct myocardial depression. However, it can produce a decrease in peripheral vascular resistance, which can potentially lead to arterial hypotension. If acepromazine is utilized in these patients, they must be closely monitored for this effect. The alpha$_2$-agonists should be avoided in patients with impaired cardiac output (Chapter 8). These drugs can produce significant dysrhythmias including severe sinus bradycardia and SA and AV nodal blocks.

Induction of anesthesia can be accomplished by using thiopental, propofol, etomidate, or a neuroleptanalgesic (Chapter 9). Mask induction using one of the potent volatile inhalant anesthetics is also a very acceptable technique. Inhalant anesthetics are probably the preferred maintenance agent for these patients. Isoflurane is the preferred inhalant because of its preservation of a near normal cardiac index and its minimal dysrhythmic effects when compared to halothane (Chapter 11).

Patients With Congenital Heart Disease

When considering the anesthetic management of patients with congenital heart disease, the problems encountered are often similar to patients with congestive heart failure. The most common surgically correctable problems are patent ductus arteriosus (PDA) and persistent right aortic arch (PRAA).

Patent ductus arteriosus is usually recognized early in life before the patient deteriorates. If the patient is normal in other respects, the anesthetic protocol is designed for the pediatric patient undergoing a thoracotomy. There are no specific contraindications to any particular preanesthetic or anesthetic drug. Surgical manipulation around the heart may cause ventricular ectopic beats. These are usually transitory and do not require treatment. When the PDA is ligated, increased blood pressure may cause a reflex slowing of the heart rate. This is a normal physiologic response.(6) In some instances atropine may be needed to counteract sinus bradycardia. Because of their size, intraoperative hypothermia is often a problem with patients undergoing PDA surgery. Every effort should be made to minimize the loss of body heat.

Persistent right aortic arch is also usually recognized early in life and corrected at that time. If the patient is normal in other respects, the anesthetic protocol is designed for the pediatric patient undergoing a thoracotomy. It is important to remember that a patient with PRAA may be suffering from aspiration pneumonia. As with a PDA, surgical manipulation around the heart may cause ventricular ectopic beats and intraoperative hypothermia is of concern.

Patients With Hypotension/Hypovolemia — The Patient in Shock

Patients with hypotension/hypovolemia should be stabilized with fluids and/or whole blood prior to anesthesia. Many preanesthetic and anesthetic drugs are potentially hypotensive; therefore, these drugs can exacerbate preexisting hypotension.

Shock can be defined as an acute clinical syndrome characterized by progressive circulatory failure that leads to inadequate capillary perfusion and cellular hypoxia.(7) Shock is a complex, multisystem disorder that may be caused by a variety of insults. Shock may be classified as hypovolemic, cardiogenic, or vasculogenic. If one thinks of the cardiovascular system as a pump, fluid, and pipes to carry the fluid, then the three classifications reflect which component of the cardiovascular system is affected.

Hypovolemic shock occurs when there is an inadequate volume of fluid (blood) being pumped through the cardiovascular system. Hemorrhage (trauma, surgery), fluid loss (vomiting, diarrhea, burns, diuresis), and trauma (sequestered fluid) can all cause hypovolemic shock (Chapter 24).

Cardiogenic shock occurs when the heart is no longer an effective pump. It can be caused by a failure in ventricular filling (cardiac tamponade, tension pneumothorax, or collapse of the vena cava caused by inadvertent closure of the "pop-off" valve, resulting in airway pressure buildup) or by a failure of ventricular ejection (ruptured chordae tendineae, cardiac dysrhythmias, severe myocardial depression, or severe and prolonged increase in systemic vascular resistance).

Vasculogenic shock occurs when there are changes in venous capacitance or peripheral resistance. Numerous causes can lead to vasculogenic shock, including sepsis (vasodilation occurs due to release of vasoactive substances such as histamine, prostaglandins, and bradykinin), anaphylaxis (vasodilation occurs because of histamine release), neurogenic factors (loss of vasomotor tone caused by excessive general anesthesia, CNS trauma, spinal anesthesia), and a severe and prolonged increase in peripheral resistance (Chapter 5).

Regardless of the underlying cause, a common pathway of circulatory failure is present in shock. Reflex mechanisms may compensate for circulatory failure and result in recovery of the patient with mild or moderate shock. However, reflex compensating mechanisms may become deleterious to the patient if they are prolonged and may result in microcirculatory changes and further cellular hypoxia.

All forms of shock eventually result in decreased blood flow and hypoperfusion of the body tissues. Baroreceptors in the aorta and carotid artery and low-pressure receptors in the atria respond to the decreased cardiac output and blood pressure. This results in activation of the sympathoadrenal system. Hypothalamic sympathetic nerve centers increase release of norepinephrine from postganglionic sympathetic nerve endings and increase liberation of epinephrine and norepinephrine from the adrenal medulla into the blood (Chapters 5 and 7). This results in splenic contraction and a release of blood into the circulation. Epinephrine and norepinephrine stimulate alpha and beta receptors. Alpha stimulation results in vasoconstriction of both arteries and veins. Beta stimulation causes vasodilation in skeletal muscle and increased force and rate of cardiac contraction. This results in a redistribution of blood flow to the heart and brain. Blood flow to the splanchnic, renal, and cutaneous vessels is markedly decreased. The catecholamines produce tachycardia, increase myocardial contractility, and stimulate hepatic glycogenolysis. Venous constriction produces decreased vascular capacity. The decreased vascular capacity improves venous return and thus cardiac output.

An important compensatory mechanism in shock is the extravascular fluid shift. Owing to vasoconstriction, there is decreased capillary blood flow and thus capillary pressure. The decreased capillary pressure allows extravascular fluid to enter the blood vessels (Chapter 19). This is very important in expanding circulating fluid volume. Endocrine factors are also important in the compensatory mechanism of shock. Renin is released from the ischemic kidney to activate the renin-angiotensin-aldosterone system. This results in vascular constriction; renal absorption of sodium, chloride, and water; and renal excretion of potassium. Antidiuretic hormone is released because of hypovolemia, and this also promotes water retention. The overall effect is to increase extracellular fluid volume (Chapter 5).

These compensatory mechanisms cause a significant redistribution of blood flow to the heart, brain, and adrenals, and may aid patient recovery in mild to moderate shock. However, they may not be adequate in severe shock, and it may become irreversible. Irreversibility is characterized by inadequate tissue perfusion to vital organs, resulting in cardiac failure, disseminated intravascular coagulation, depression of the reticuloendothelial system, and peripheral vascular failure (Chapter 24). Hypotension and decreased capillary perfusion lead to cellular hypoxia, decreased delivery of energy substrates to the cell, and increased concentration of cellular metabolites.

Glucose is first used anaerobically by the cells as an energy source with production of pyruvate and limited amounts of ATP. Pyruvate is then aerobically utilized to produce large amounts of ATP, or it may be released into the circulation after being reduced to lactic acid. Large amounts of oxygen are needed by the cell to produce the ATP. In shock, cellular hypoxia occurs, and although ATP can be produced anaerobically, it may not be produced in adequate amounts.(7) The establishment of membrane ionic gradients depends on adequate ATP generation. Cellular edema may result if ionic gradients are not maintained. The lactic acidemia that occurs in shock results from the release of anaerobic energy in tissues unable to support adequate oxidative processes. Individual cells and then organs begin to die.

Increased cellular metabolites (lactic acid) in the capillary bed cause precapillary sphincters to relax, but postcapillary sphincters remain constricted. Blood flows into the capillary bed but is slow to leave, resulting in an increased hydrostatic pressure with net flow into the tissues and further volume deficits. Decreased perfusion of the splanchnic vasculature results in pancreatic ischemia and the release of myocardial depressant factor (MDF). MDF decreases myocardial contractility.(8) Splanchnic vasoconstriction and decreased capillary perfusion result in depression of the reticuloendothelial system (RES) in the spleen and liver. With an impaired RES, endotoxins, bacteria, and microemboli accumulate and produce further circulatory failure. Slow-moving (stagnant), acidic blood is hypercoagulable. Clot initiating factors are common in shock and include bacterial toxins and thromboplastin of red cells (released by hemolysis).(9) These factors result in disseminated intravascular coagulation (DIC). DIC results in a consumption of clotting factors, bleeding, and focal tissue infarcts due to microthrombi. Multiorgan failure (MODS) occurs, and the patient dies (Chapter 24).

Always stabilize the patient in shock prior to anesthesia. The treatment for shock is discussed elsewhere in this text (Chapter 19). Once a patient has been treated and stabilized, there are no particular contraindications to any of the preanesthetic or anesthetics.

Patients With Anemia/Hypoproteinemia

Anemic patients are of concern from an anesthetic standpoint because the oxygen carrying capacity is diminished. These patients should be preoxygenated prior to anesthetic induction. Whole blood transfusion should be considered if the dog or cat has a PCV of less than 25 to 30% prior to surgery or less than 20% following surgery (Chapter 19). Patients with chronic anemia seem to be able to better cope with the problem than those with acute anemia. Whole blood should be available for administration both intraoperatively and postoperatively. The rate and total amount of whole blood administered should be tailored to the requirements of the patient.

Many preanesthetic and anesthetic drugs are reversibly bound to plasma protein, making them inactive. If there is less plasma protein, more drug is pharmacologically active and therefore will have an increased effect in the patient (Chapters 2 and 3). Plasma protein is also required to maintain plasma oncotic pressure. Hypoproteinemic patients are less tolerant of fluid administration and more prone to fluid overload and pulmonary edema. Plasma proteins should be maintained above 3.5 grams percent. If the plasma proteins fall below this number, the administration of plasma proteins should be considered (Chapter 19).

Anemic and/or hypoproteinemic patients should have serial PCVs and total plasma protein values run during surgery and postoperatively. Supplemental oxygen may be very beneficial in the preanesthetic as well as the postoperative period in anemic patients. A high inspired oxygen tension will allow more oxygen to be dissolved into the plasma and thus help counteract the decreased oxygen carrying capacity due to low red blood cell numbers. A mask, nasal catheter, or oxygen cage can be used to deliver 40 to 100% oxygen to the patient (Chapter 17).

Patients With Heartworm Disease

Heartworm disease in itself does not contraindicate any particular anesthetic regimen or protocol. If the patient is not exhibiting clinical signs, any standard anesthetic protocol is probably satisfactory (Chapter 20). One should be aware that patients with heartworms may be more prone to spontaneous cardiac dysrhythmias while under anesthesia. If a significant number of heartworms are present, cardiac output may also be decreased. Heartworms may also lead to pulmonary dysfunction, which could compromise the patient's ability to ventilate.

References

1. Paddleford RR. Anesthetic considerations in patients with pre-existing problems or conditions. In: Paddleford RR, ed. Manual of small animal anesthesia. New York: Churchill Livingstone, 1988: 253–308.
2. Fox PR. Feline and canine myocardial disease. In: Fox PR, ed. Canine and feline cardiology. New York: Churchill Livingstone, 1988:435–493.
3. Olivier NB. Pathophysiology of cardiac failure. In: Slatter D, ed. Textbook of small animal surgery, 2nd ed. Philadelphia: WB Saunders, 1993:709–723.
4. Evans AT. Anesthesia for severe mitral and tricuspid regurgitation. Vet Clin North Am Small Anim Pract 22(2):465–466, 1992.
5. Bednarski RM. Anesthetic concerns for patients with cardiomyopathy. Vet Clin North Am Small Anim Pract 22(2):460–464, 1992.
6. Hellyer PW. Anesthesia in patients with cardiopulmonary disease. In: Kirk RW, Bonagura JD, eds. Current veterinary therapy xi. Philadelphia: WB Saunders, 1992:655–659.
7. Green EM, Adams HR. New perspectives in circulatory shock: pathophysiologic mediators of the mammalian response to endotoxemia and sepsis. J Am Vet Med Assoc 200(12):1834–1841, 1992.
8. Taboada J, Hoskins JD, Morgan RV. Shock. In: Emergency medicine and critical care: the compendium collection. Trenton, NJ: Veterinary Learning Systems, 1992:6–41.
9. Haskins SC. Management of septic shock. J Am Vet Med Assoc 200(12):1915–1924, 1992.

chapter **23** B

PULMONARY DYSFUNCTION

Robert R. Paddleford

INTRODUCTION
PHYSIOLOGY OF VENTILATION
EFFECTS OF PREANESTHETIC AND
  ANESTHETIC DRUGS ON VENTILATION

ANESTHETIC CONSIDERATIONS IN PATIENTS
  WITH RESPIRATORY DYSFUNCTION
CONTROLLED VENTILATION

Introduction

Patients with pulmonary dysfunction are often difficult to safely anesthetize. Most preanesthetic and anesthetic drugs depress respiratory function, further compromising patients with pulmonary dysfunction.

Physiology of Ventilation

The primary function of the lungs is to exhale carbon dioxide generated by body metabolism and oxygenate venous blood. Alveolar ventilation can be assessed by measuring arterial carbon dioxide tension ($PaCO_2$) or end-tidal carbon dioxide partial pressures. No conscious control is necessary to sustain ventilation. Many factors can alter ventilatory pattern: (a) arterial carbon dioxide tension, (b) arterial pH, (c) arterial oxygen tension, (d) pulmonary stretch and upper airway receptors, (e) heat regulation, (f) sensory input, and (g) emotional factors (Chapter 6).

The ventilatory control system is a series of complex feedback loops made up of sensors, controllers, and effectors. The principal ventilatory receptors or sensors are (a) the peripheral carotid-body chemoreceptors (located at the bifurcations of the carotid arteries), (b) the central chemoreceptors (located near the surface on the ventrolateral aspect of the medulla oblongata), and (c) receptors sensing stretch, irritation, and proprioception in the lungs, airways, and muscles of respiration. The carotid-body chemoreceptors are responsive to oxygen and stimulate respiration when hypoxemia is present (Chapter 7). The central chemoreceptors respond to carbon dioxide and stimulate ventilation when hypercarbia (respiratory acidosis) is present. Increased ventilation caused by metabolic acidosis may be mediated through either the central or peripheral chemoreceptors or the controllers of the ventilatory feedback loop located in the brain (Chapter 18).(1) Automatic breathing is governed by specialized regions in the brain stem. The cortex controls voluntary and behavioral modifications of ventilation, and respiratory rhythm is controlled by the medulla. Control functions are integrated both centrally (brain stem) and peripherally (spinal cord). The effectors of ventilation are the muscles of respiration and include the intercostal muscles, the diaphragm, and the muscles of the upper airways.

Many preanesthetic and anesthetic agents can alter a patient's ventilatory pattern. Most preanesthetic and anesthetic agents alter ventilation by altering the threshold of the respiratory centers to carbon dioxide, by altering the sensitivity of the respiratory centers to carbon dioxide, and/or by relaxing the muscles of ventilation.(2)

Effects of Preanesthetic and Anesthetic Drugs on Ventilation

Most preanesthetic and anesthetic drugs depress respiratory function, thereby further jeopardizing a patient with respiratory dysfunction (Chapter 8). Drugs depress or stimulate ventilation by acting directly or indirectly on one or more of the elements of the ventilatory control system.(3)

Atropine and glycopyrrolate decrease airway resistance by causing direct dilation of the airways. Atropine also increases respiratory dead space by dilating the larger bronchi. Both drugs will increase the viscosity of airway secretions.

Phenothiazine tranquilizers have minimal effects on ventilation at therapeutic doses, although large doses can depress ventilation. They produce a decrease in respiratory rate, but this is usually compensated for by an increase in tidal volume. Phenothiazines do not delay the central respiratory center response (threshold) to increases in arterial carbon dioxide, although the maximum ventilatory response (sensitivity) may be decreased.(2)

The alpha$_2$-agonists (xylazine, detomidine, medetomidine) vary in their pulmonary depressant effects and are somewhat unpredictable. Their depressant effects may range from mild to significant, depending on dose and individual patient response.(4) As with all general CNS depressants, this effect is more pronounced in patients already suffering from respiratory distress caused by pneumonia, hydrothorax, pneumothorax, and so on.

The benzodiazepine tranquilizers (diazepam, midazolam) usually produce minimal respiratory depression at therapeutic doses. However, both drugs have produced significant respiratory depression in isolated cases. This may be especially true when higher doses are administered intravenously.

Narcotics are potentially potent respiratory depressants. The depression is drug and dose dependent, and may occur at doses that do not produce marked CNS depression or analgesia. The narcotics directly depress the pontine and medullary centers, causing a decrease in respiratory rate and tidal volume. They also produce a delayed response (altered threshold) and a decreased response (altered sensitivity) to increases in arterial carbon dioxide.(2) The panting observed in some dogs following narcotic administration may be caused by an initial stimulation of the respiratory centers and/or alteration of the thermoregulation center.

The barbiturates are potent respiratory depressants (Chapter 9). At anesthetizing doses, the respiratory centers of the brain are depressed. The barbiturates can depress both the respiratory rate and tidal volume, and thus minute ventilation. The barbiturates also produce a delayed response (altered threshold) and a decreased response (altered sensitivity) to increases in arterial carbon dioxide and depress the carotid-aortic chemoreceptors.

The dissociative anesthetics (ketamine, tiletamine) may have a dual effect on ventilation (Chapter 10). They may effect ventilation at two or more anatomic sites, causing stimulation at one and depression at another. Both drugs can produce apneustic ventilation, that is, a ventilatory pattern characterized by a prolonged pause after inspiration. Although the respiratory rate may decrease, the tidal volume usually remains normal. In general, the respiratory alterations do not affect blood gases; however, in some patients the dissociative agents can produce marked hypoxia and hypercarbia, especially when additional CNS depressant drugs, such as tranquilizers, sedatives, or opioids, are used in combination with them. Dissociative agents do not depress the pharyngeal or laryngeal reflexes, although they may be activated with stimulation. Therefore, a patient may be more prone to laryngospasm, bronchospasm, and coughing. The dissociative agents increase salivation and respiratory secretions, sometimes resulting in aspiration and respiratory obstruction. For this reason, the use of an anticholinergic in combination with these drugs may be indicated.

Propofol (Diprivan) is a relatively new injectable anesthetic that produces respiratory depression in much the same manner as the barbiturates. The incidence of apnea with propofol is comparable to the barbiturates, but the duration of apneic episodes may be slightly longer. Etomidate (Amidate) is a carboxylated imidazole that can produce a mild to moderate dose-dependent respiratory depression (Chapter 9).

The inhalant anesthetics methoxyflurane, halothane, and isoflurane depress ventilation by decreasing tidal volume (Chapter 11). These anesthetics produce an increase in respiratory rate, but this is not adequate to compensate for the decrease in tidal volume. Potent inhalation anesthetics increase the level of arterial carbon dioxide at which spontaneous ventilation ceases (i.e., the "apneic threshold"). The degree of elevation in apneic threshold is directly related to the depth of anesthesia. Methoxyflurane, halothane, and isoflurane decrease the slope of the carbon dioxide response curve. There is a delayed response (altered threshold) and a decreased response (altered sensitivity) to increases in arterial carbon dioxide. Potent inhalation anesthetics depress the ventilatory response to hypoxemia. In addition, the interaction between hypoxemia and hypercarbia in stimulating ventilation is greatly attenuated or eliminated by moderate concentrations of these agents.

Nitrous oxide does possess some respiratory depressant properties, but they are minimal. However, nitrous oxide should be used with care in patients with pulmonary dysfunction to prevent hypoxemia.

Anesthetic Considerations in Patients with Respiratory Dysfunction

Patients with pulmonary dysfunction may lack the ability to properly expand the lungs (extrapulmonary dysfunction) and/or may have impairment of oxygen–carbon dioxide transfer across the alveolar membranes (intrapulmonary dysfunction). Examples of extrapulmonary dysfunction include diaphragmatic hernia, pneumothorax, hydrothorax, space-occupying lesions of the thorax, flail chest, and any condition that restricts chest wall expansion. Examples of intrapulmonary dysfunction include pneumonia, pulmonary edema, intrapulmonary hemorrhage (contusions), atelectasis, interstitial disease, and upper airway, tracheal, or bronchial obstruction.

Patients with respiratory dysfunction can be placed in one of four categories:

Category I: Dyspnea does not occur with exertion.
Category II: Dyspnea occurs with moderate exertion.
Category III: Dyspnea occurs with mild exertion.
Category IV: Dyspnea occurs at rest.

Patients in categories III and IV are definitely at higher anesthetic risk.

A thorough preanesthetic evaluation should be done on all patients with respiratory dysfunction. An extensive physical examination of the thorax should be performed, and thoracic radiographs should be taken.

An ECG should be done, and, if possible, arterial blood gases tension should be determined. A baseline CBC, serum electrolyte, and chemistry panel should be obtained.

If possible, surgery and anesthesia should be delayed in patients with pneumonia, pulmonary edema, lung contusions, atelectasis, pneumothorax, and/or hydrothorax to allow time for these problems to improve. A thoracocentesis should be done in patients with moderate to severe pneumo- or hydrothorax prior to anesthesia, and in some cases a chest tube may be needed.

Patients with respiratory dysfunction should be preoxygenated with oxygen for 5 to 7 minutes prior to anesthetic induction.(5) A mask, nasal catheter, or oxygen chamber may be used (Chapter 17). Supplemental oxygen should always be available both preoperatively and postoperatively.

Mild preanesthetic sedation may be necessary to allow the patient to be handled without causing stress and exacerbating the respiratory dysfunction. Preanesthetic drugs with minimal respiratory depression should be considered. Several preanesthetic drugs or combinations may be used, such as the combination of acepromazine and butorphanol. Acepromazine is a phenothiazine derivative tranquilizer that produces minimal respiratory depression, especially in low doses. Butorphanol (Torbugesic, Torbutrol) is a synthetic, noncontrolled opioid agonist-antagonist. Butorphanol can produce a dose-related respiratory depression similar to morphine; however, butorphanol seems to reach a "ceiling" beyond which higher doses do not cause significantly more respiratory depression. The dose of acepromazine is 0.05 mg/kg IM to a *maximum total* dose of 1 mg. It is not recommended that 1 mg of acepromazine be exceeded in any patient when combined with butorphanol. The recommended dose of butorphanol is 0.44 mg/kg IM to a *maximum total* dose of 20 mg. Because butorphanol can increase vagal tone, atropine at a dose of 0.044 mg/kg IM should be administered to the patient.

After the patient has been sedated, rapid induction of anesthesia may be needed to gain quick control of the airway to allow for positive pressure ventilation. Rapid anesthetic induction may be accomplished using thiopental, propofol, etomidate, or ketamine intravenously. A rapid mask induction using halothane or isoflurane may be used; however, because of the patient's inability to ventilate properly, this technique may result in delayed anesthetic induction and struggling. Whichever induction technique is utilized, rapid and accurate intubation must be accomplished.

Maintenance of anesthesia is best achieved with an inhalant anesthetic and controlled or positive pressure ventilation. Nitrous oxide should be used with care in patients with respiratory dysfunction. It can increase the severity of a pneumothorax, and it should be discontinued if cyanosis is evident. Even if a patient with respiratory dysfunction seems to have adequate spontaneous ventilation, assisted or controlled ventilation is desirable.

Controlled Ventilation

In spontaneous ventilation, the respiratory muscles increase the size of the thoracic cavity, the volume of air within it increases, and the pressure in the thorax falls. The intrapulmonary pressure falls. The difference between the intrapleural pressure and alveolar pressure overcomes the elasticity of the lungs, and the difference between the alveolar pressure and the pressure at the oral-pharyngeal area overcomes the airway resistance. There is a great difference between the intrapleural and alveolar pressures, and a small difference between the oral-pharyngeal pressure and airway resistance. The net effect is movement of air into the alveoli from the upper airway (Chapter 6).

Controlled ventilation is "positive pressure" ventilation. Air is forced into the alveoli. Intrapleural pressure and intrapulmonary pressure increase during controlled ventilation. Controlled ventilation may be provided manually ("squeezing" the rebreathing bag) or mechanically (using a ventilator) (Chapter 17).

One of three methods can be used to control a patient's ventilation and take over his or her ventilatory effort. The patient can be hyperventilated to decrease the arterial carbon dioxide levels and therefore decrease the stimulus for ventilation; the anesthetic level can be deepened in the patient; or the patient can be paralyzed using peripheral-acting muscle relaxants (Chapter 13). Of the three methods, hyperventilating the patient (i.e., manually or mechanically increasing the patient's respiratory rate and depth) is usually the easiest and is usually very effective.

Five components can be adjusted in the ventilatory cycle during controlled ventilation: (a) peak airway pressure, (b) mean airway pressure, (c) length of inspiratory phase, (d) length of expiratory phase, and (e) the inspiratory to expiratory ratio (Chapter 17).

Peak airway pressures are measured by a pressure manometer in the anesthesia circuit. Peak airway pressures of 15 to 20 cm H_2O are necessary to overcome lung resistance to expansion in dogs and larger species. In cats, slightly higher pressures may be needed. A decreased lung compliance will increase the peak airway pressures needed to expand the lungs. An increase in airway resistance will increase the peak airway pressure needed to expand the lungs.

The mean airway pressure is the average pressure generated during the inspiratory and expiratory phases of positive pressure ventilation. Mean airway pressure should be kept low. It is kept low by not maintaining the positive airway pressure for longer than is necessary. Mean airway pressure correlates most closely with decreases in cardiac output.

To produce minimal cardiovascular alteration, the inspiratory phase should be less than the expiratory phase. The inspiratory phase should last 1 to 1.5 seconds. Prolonged holding of the tidal volume at peak airway pressure will not increase tidal exchange but will increase mean airway pressure, and thereby decrease venous return and cardiac output. The expiratory phase should begin as soon as the inspiratory phase is complete. The increased pressure within the lung must be allowed to return to 0 cm H_2O pressure as soon as possible to prevent cardiovascular impairment.

The inspiratory to expiratory (I/E) ratio is very important during controlled or positive pressure ventilation. The inspiratory phase should be a third and no more than half of the total ventilatory cycle. An I/E ratio of 1:2 or 1:3 will help provide an adequate period for proper cardiac filling. A 1:2 ratio will provide for a ventilatory rate of approximately 20 cycles per minute. A 1:3 or 1:4 ratio provides for a rate of 15 or 12 breaths per minute respectively.

Although controlled or positive pressure ventilation is safe and effective, if it is done improperly, harmful side effects can occur. Interference with cardiac output can occur during controlled or positive pressure ventilation. During spontaneous ventilation, the intrapleural pressure at the height of inspiration is approximately a negative 8 to 10 cm H_2O. This augments the movement of blood in the great veins into the chest (thoracic pump). However, during controlled or positive pressure ventilation, the intrapulmonary pressure increases and may reach plus 3 to 5 cm H_2O pressure. Only during expiration is the intrapulmonary pressure the same in spontaneous ventilation and controlled ventilation. Increased alveolar pressure will also decrease pulmonary blood flow. This is why maintaining proper peak and mean airway pressures and a proper I/E ratio is so critical.

Lung damage or volotrauma during positive pressure ventilation is always a possibility. Volotrauma can range from mild trauma producing minimal alveolar hemorrhage to severe trauma producing airway rupture and a tension pneumothorax. Maintaining proper peak and mean airway pressures will help minimize pulmonary trauma.(6) If a major airway "blowout" occurs during positive pressure ventilation, it is due to excessive peak airway pressures and/or preexisting lung pathology.

Acid-base balance will be changed with any change in alveolar ventilation. Overventilation will cause a decreased arterial carbon dioxide level and an increased pH (alkalosis) (Chapter 18). Overventilation can also lead to cerebral vasoconstriction.(7) Underventilation will cause an increased arterial carbon dioxide and a decreased pH (acidosis). It is better to err on the side of overventilation. Overventilation is probably not harmful for short periods.

References

1. Tuker A. Pathophysiology of the respiratory system. In: Slatter D, ed. Textbook of small animal surgery, 2nd ed. Philadelphia: WB Saunders, 1993:709–723.
2. Paddleford RR. Anesthetic considerations in patients with preexisting problems and conditions. In: Paddleford RR, ed. Manual of small animal anesthesia. New York: Churchill Livingstone, 1988: 253–308.
3. Schatzmann URS. Clinical considerations of complications of the pulmonary system. In: Short CE, ed. Principles and practice of veterinary anesthesia. Baltimore: Williams & Wilkins, 1987:208–221.

4. Quandt JE, Raffe MR. Anesthesia for upper airway and thoracic surgery. In: Slatter D, ed. Textbook of small animal surgery, 2nd ed. Philadelphia: WB Saunders, 1993:2278–2283.
5. Dunlop CI. Anesthesia for patients with preexisting pneumonia and cyanosis. Vet Clin North Am Small Anim Pract 22(2):454–455, 1992.
6. Wilson DV. Anesthesia for patients with diaphragmatic hernia and severe dyspnea. Vet Clin North Am Small Anim Pract 22(2):456–459, 1992.
7. Nunn JF. Cyanosis. In: Applied respiratory physiology. London: Butterworths, 1987:276–278.

chapter **23**c

NEUROLOGIC DISEASE

Ralph C. Harvey, Michael H. Sims, Stephen A. Greene

Introduction

Veterinary patients frequently require anesthesia for diagnostic evaluation or surgical correction of neurologic disorders. Diagnostic procedures that require either general anesthesia or heavy sedation include electroencephalography (EEG), myelography, other imaging techniques, and electrodiagnostic testing. Veterinary neurosurgical anesthesia is more often required in patients with spinal cord rather than intracranial disorders. Intervertebral-disc disease is the most frequently performed neurosurgical procedure in veterinary medicine. However, the increased use of advanced imaging techniques, such as computed tomography and magnetic resonance imaging (MRI), has led to a greater frequency of intracranial operative procedures in small animal patients where these imaging modalities are available. In patients with neurologic disease, consideration of the dynamics of intracranial pressure (ICP), cerebral blood flow (CBF), and cerebrospinal fluid (CSF) production and flow is important in order to prevent neurologic morbidity or mortality.

Physiology

In normal awake animals, blood supply to the CNS is controlled by autoregulatory mechanisms. Alteration in CBF can result from a variety of changes in arterial oxygenation, carbon dioxide accumulation, mean arterial pressure, and venous outflow. The brain and spinal cord are protected by encasement within the bony skull and vertebral column. Increases in the flow of blood within the noncompliant cranial vault cause an increase in the intracranial volume and pressure.(1–3) Once increases in CBF cause the intracranial volume to exceed the limits of effective compliance, there is a sharp increase in intracranial pressure. When ICP is already increased by intracranial masses, trauma, or derangement of autoregulation, slight changes in intracranial volume greatly increase ICP.(2) Significant increases in ICP may lead to cerebral ischemia and eventually brain herniation.(1)

AUTOREGULATION OF CEREBRAL BLOOD FLOW

Autoregulation of brain blood flow is usually very effective in a pressure range of approximately 60 to 140 mm Hg. Within this range of blood pressures, many factors including intracranial tumors, hypercapnia, severe hypoxia, and many anesthetics interfere with autoregulation and cause changes in ICP (Fig. 23C–1).(1, 4, 5) Blood vessels in the brain supplying diseased tissue or neoplasms may be fully dilated and unaffected by normal autoregulation mechanisms.

The CNS depression of general anesthesia is usually accompanied by a decrease in cerebral metabolic rate (cerebral metabolic oxygen requirement, $CMRO_2$) (Chapter 7). This decrease in oxygen requirement is thought to be protective in the possible event of relative ischemia during anesthesia and neurosurgery. There are conflicting reports on the efficacy of various anesthetics in reducing $CMRO_2$, just as there are with regard to the relative effects of the anesthetics on CBF and ICP. Isoflurane, etomidate and the barbiturates are generally recognized as contributing substantially to reduction of $CMRO_2$, affording some cerebral protection.(5)

In patients with preexisting elevated ICP, further increases can result from gravitational or positional interference with drainage of venous blood from the head. Obstruction by occlusion of jugular veins through surgical positioning of the head or use of a neck leash,

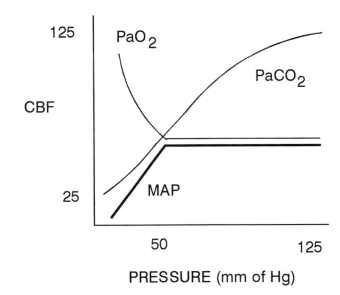

Fig. 23C–1. Alterations in cerebral blood flow (CBF), in mL per 100 grams of brain tissue per minute, caused by changes in arterial tension of oxygen (PaO_2), carbon dioxide ($PaCO_2$), and mean arterial blood pressure (MAP). (Redrawn after Shapiro, H.H. Neurosurgical anesthesia and intracranial hypertension. In: Anesthesia, 2nd ed. Edited by R.D. Miller. New York: Churchill Livingstone, 1986:1563–1620.)

or for purposes of obtaining blood samples or placement of jugular-vein catheters can rapidly result in dangerous increases in ICP.(6) For intracranial neurosurgery, a slight elevation of the head above the level of the heart (with the neck in a neutral position) will facilitate venous drainage, lowering ICP. Extreme elevation is avoided to minimize the risk of venous air embolization.(3)

Only at very low arterial oxygen tensions does the cerebral blood flow change. When arterial oxygen tension (PaO_2) decreases below a threshold of 50 mm Hg, CBF increases (Fig. 23C–1). The relationship between arterial carbon dioxide partial pressure ($PaCO_2$) and cerebral blood flow, on the other hand, is linear. Cerebral blood flow increases by about $2\,mL \cdot min^{-1} \cdot 100\,g^{-1}$ of brain tissue for every 1 mm Hg increase in arterial carbon dioxide over the range of arterial carbon dioxide partial pressures from 20 to 80 mm Hg.(7) Hyperventilation has been used extensively in neuroanesthesia to electively reduce cerebral blood flow as a result of cerebral vasoconstriction. This maneuver decreases tissue bulk, facilitating intracranial surgery. Although quite effective, this technique is somewhat controversial in some situations, since a potential exists for the diversion of remaining blood flow preferentially to diseased tissues lacking autoregulation at the expense of normal brain tissue.(8) Deliberate hyperventilation to decrease ICP may be risky when mean arterial blood pressures are reduced to below 50 mm Hg. The ensuing ischemia could be deleterious to normal brain tissues if a "steal" of CBF diverts remaining blood flow.(8, 9) The rapid and substantial reduction in CBF and ICP achieved by hyperventilation makes it a valuable tool for the immediate reduction in brain bulk to facilitate intracranial surgery and to reduce acute brain swelling.

Although controversial, restriction of intravenous fluids to only that volume necessary to maintain adequate circulating volume is usually recommended in neurosurgical patients with increased ICP.(10, 11) Excessive fluid volume has been associated with decreased venous outflow and increased risk of compounding cerebral edema. Diuretic therapy is frequently indicated in the medical management of patients with intracranial masses and elevated ICP or cerebral edema.(6) Dextrose administration is somewhat controversial and must be individualized to the situation. Hyperglycemia is associated with adverse outcome in animals with cerebral ischemia, and cerebral edema can be exacerbated by administration of isotonic dextrose. However, its use decreases the incidence of seizures in patients following metrizamide myelography and is indicated in hypoglycemic seizures or hypoglycemic coma.(1, 12, 13)

Glucocorticoids are effective in the treatment of some forms of cerebral edema.(14) Corticosteroids have been shown to be effective in reducing the increased ICP that is caused by brain tumors and hydrocephalus. Glucocorticoid therapy may be considered in the management of patients with cerebral edema associated with primary or metastatic brain neoplasia, trauma, some types of hemorrhage, and contusion. Since dexamethasone administration has been shown to reduce the rate of formation of CSF in dogs (14, 15), there may be some value to steroid administration in the preanesthetic management of hydrocephalic patients considered at risk of further increases in ICP. Corticosteroids would be contraindicated in cases of CNS diseases where an infectious etiology is considered possible. The value of steroids in treating cranial trauma is controversial. There are conflicting reports from well-controlled studies and clinical trials on the efficacy of steroid administration after head trauma. It is likely that steroid therapy is of relatively little value once cerebral ischemia has occurred. Administration of antiinflammatory doses of corticosteroids prior to a traumatic insult improves the compliance of the brain and ultimately reduces cerebral edema. The practicality of this observation is in preoperative steroid therapy (primarily with dexamethasone) as a means of reducing subsequent cerebral edema.(14) Glucocorticosteroid therapy should optimally begin the day before surgery. Dexamethasone is recommended at 0.25 mg/kg every 8 hours, with a dose of 0.25 to 1 mg/kg IV after the induction of anesthesia.(6)

Pharmacologic Considerations

SEDATIVES, TRANQUILIZERS, AND ANALGESICS

Increased seizure activity associated with administration of the phenothiazine (e.g., acepromazine) and butyrophenone (e.g., droperidol) tranquilizers contraindicates their use in seizure-prone patients and in patients for diagnostic electroencephalography (EEG).(16) Control of seizures with benzodiazepine tranquilizers (e.g., diazepam, midazolam) is desirable in the management of seizure-prone patients but can obscure characteristic patterns in diagnostic EEGs.

Use of xylazine in dogs and cats is controversial, yet clinical evidence for or against its use in the patient with neurologic disease is lacking. In healthy conscious horses, xylazine (1.1 mg/kg IV) decreased CSF pressure measured at the lumbosacral space.(17) Horses anesthetized with pentobarbital and subsequently given xylazine (1.1 mg/kg IV) had no change in either lateral ventricle or lumbosacral cerebrospinal fluid pressure.(18) Horses given detomidine (20 µg/kg IV) also have a reduction in CBF.(19) Dexmedetomidine, another alpha$_2$-agonist, decreases the CBF in both halothane and isoflurane anesthetized dogs (Chapter 7).(20, 21) Thus, although the effects of xylazine or detomidine on ICP may differ in horses with head trauma or neurologic disease, they appear to be rational choices to provide sedation for examination or as a preanesthetic medication in the horse. Venous congestion in the head, when positioned below the level of the heart, may be associated with an increase in ICP. Therefore, the dose of xylazine or detomidine should be titrated to prevent excessive head lowering and possible resultant increased ICP in the standing horse.

Opioids or neuroleptanalgesic combinations are sometimes used in anesthetic management of patients with increased ICP. The direct effects of opioids on CBF and ICP are minimal. However, opioids may indirectly increase CSF pressure and should be used cautiously in patients with cerebral trauma or space occupying tumors. Increases in pressure within the cranium may aggravate the underlying condition. The elevation in CSF pressure is caused by accumulation of CO_2, which in turn is due to opioid-induced hypoventilation. If the patient is ventilated to prevent hypercapnia, the increase in CSF pressure does not occur when opioids are administered.(22) When opioids are used in these cases, the respiratory status must be assessed, and when necessary the patient should be ventilated to prevent hypercapnia. The judicious use of opioids for pain management in the postoperative period often does not cause as much respiratory depression as does pain itself.(23) Thus, opioid analgesic medication is based upon the relative severity of pain in each animal.

INJECTABLE ANESTHETICS

Most injectable anesthetics cause significant reductions in $CMRO_2$, CBF, and ICP (Table 23C–1).(1–3, 5, 6, 12) Recognition of the barbiturate-induced reductions in $CMRO_2$, CBF, and ICP has contributed to the development of "barbiturate-coma" therapy for cerebral resuscitation following periods of cerebral ischemia as occurs in near-drowning and in cardiopulmonary resuscitation. The value of barbiturates as a therapy for cerebral ischemia/hypoxia is controversial at best. It is likely that barbiturates are protective if administered prior to the insult but of relatively little value if administered after clinical signs of brain ischemia have developed. As with glucocorticoids, barbiturates may be of value in

Table 23C–1. Effects of Anesthetics and Anesthetic Adjuncts on Cerebral Blood Flow (CBF), Intracranial Pressure (ICP), Blood Pressure (BP), and Cerebral Perfusion Pressure (CPP)

Agent	CBF	ICP	BP	CPP
Halothane	↑ ↑	↑ ↑	↓	↓
Isoflurane	↑	↑	↓	↓
Nitrous oxide	↔	↔	↔	↔
Thiobarbiturates	↓ ↓	↓ ↓	↓	↔
Fentanyl	↓	↓	↓	↔
Morphine	↓	↔	↔ or ↓	↔
Droperidol	↓	↓	↓	↔
Atracurium	↔	↔	↔	↔
Succinylcholine	↑	↑	↔	
Diazepam	↓	↓ or ↔	↓	↔
Midazolam	↓	↔	↔	↔
Ketamine	↑ ↑	↑ ↑	↑	↓
Halothane-thiopental	↔	↔	↓	↔ or ↓

voiding postoperative sequelae to surgical trauma. It must be recognized, however, that barbiturate anesthesia often prolongs anesthetic recovery. In neurosurgical patients, the CNS depression associated with residual barbiturates can seriously obscure postoperative evaluation and prevent meaningful neurologic evaluation.

The dissociative anesthetics represent a notable exception to the reduction in CBF, ICP, and $CMRO_2$ characteristic of most injectable anesthetics.(1–3, 6, 12) Electroencephalographic (EEG) activity also increases with dissociative anesthesia. Convulsant activity ranging from muscle twitching to seizures occurs as an infrequent adverse effect of the dissociatives. Patients with a history of seizure-related disorders and those with intracranial masses, closed-head traumatic injuries, and other conditions potentially increasing ICP should not receive dissociative anesthetics.

VOLATILE ANESTHETICS

Volatile anesthetics increase CBF and alter $CMRO_2$ to varying degrees (7, 10, 12, 24–27). Since increased CBF and ICP are also highly influenced by carbon dioxide retention, respiratory depression associated with volatile anesthesia can be responsible for increases in ICP that are clinically significant in neurosurgical patients. There is evidence that regional changes in the distribution of CBF result from administration of the volatile anesthetics such that our understanding of cerebrovascular effects may not be accurately based on global estimates of CBF in animals.(4)

Among the volatile anesthetics clinically used in veterinary medicine, halothane dramatically blocks autoregulation, increasing CBF and ICP.(25, 26) Methoxyflurane, enflurane, and isoflurane all interfere with autoregulation to a more limited extent than halothane.(3) At 1.1 MAC levels of anesthesia, cerebral blood flow increases almost 200% with halothane but by only about 40% with enflurane and is unchanged with

isoflurane.(2, 24) Higher concentrations of isoflurane cause increases in CBF. The loss of cerebral autoregulation with halothane is implicated in the greater degree of brain swelling noted during neurosurgery with this anesthetic. The increase in CBF occurs rapidly upon halothane administration and occurs independent of changes in arterial blood pressure, implicating halothane's direct cerebrovascular effects.

Fortunately, modest hyperventilation, reducing arterial carbon dioxide to about 30 mm Hg, eliminates the volatile anesthetic—induced increase in CBF.(25) Hyperventilation is rapidly effective in reducing CBF and ICP or in preventing their rise in patients at risk. It is easy, rather cost-free, and the safest method available. In light of the respiratory depression of general anesthesia and the potential rise in CBF and ICP, modest hyperventilation should be incorporated into the anesthetic technique for animals with intracranial masses or other disorders of autoregulation.

Nitrous oxide has substantial cerebrovascular effects. Although there are conflicting reports and a minority opposing opinion, adverse effects of nitrous oxide for neurosurgical patients have been well documented in animals.(5, 27) Nitrous oxide causes the most profound increase in both CBF and ICP of all the inhalant anesthetics (Chapter 11). Owing largely to the limited potency of nitrous oxide in veterinary patients, its use is primarily in combination with other general anesthetics. The combination of volatile anesthetic gases and nitrous oxide can produce greater increases in CBF and ICP. In rabbits, nitrous oxide administration produced a consistent increase in CBF and ICP regardless of whether it was combined with halothane, isoflurane or fentanyl/pentobarbital.(16) Furthermore, these potentially adverse effects were not blocked by hyperventilation.

In dogs, nitrous oxide increases $CMRO_2$ by 11 percent. In animal models of regional cerebral ischemia, the use of nitrous oxide worsens the neurologic outcome.(5) The disadvantages of nitrous oxide appear to be substantial for the neurosurgical patient.

Anesthetic Management of Specific Neurologic Problems

MYELOGRAPHY AND INTERVERTEBRAL DISC DISEASE

For the relatively common surgical procedures to decompress cervical or thoracolumbar intervertebral disc herniation, anesthetic management should address (a) protection from possible seizures and other potential complications associated with administration of myelographic contrast agents, (b) perioperative pain relief, (c) maintenance of adequate spontaneous ventilation, and (d) management of concurrent disorders such as urinary incontinence or other factors predisposing to adverse recovery.

Radiographic contrast myelography is frequently performed in the immediate preoperative period in order to localize the lesion(s) and to identify the proper site(s) for surgical decompression. As these procedures are often performed during the same anesthetic period, patient management is designed to optimize conditions for both the diagnostic (radiographic) and the therapeutic (surgical) procedures. Dural puncture for sampling of CSF and/or for administration of myelographic contrast agent requires a depth of anesthesia at less than a surgical plane but adequate to prevent patient movement with subsequent trauma. Considerations for an anesthetic protocol suitable for spinal cord surgery are listed in Table 23C–2.

Avoidance of potent respiratory depressants and a light surgical plane of anesthesia will optimally maintain spontaneous ventilation during myelography. Among the less frequent complications associated with myelography is respiratory depression or respiratory arrest and cardiac arrhythmias.(28) Respiratory depression is probably referable to effects of the contrast agent at the level of brain-stem and medullary respiratory centers. As such, respiratory effects are most likely to be associated with "high" myelograms, typically those showing contrast agent ascending to the brain and brain stem. The incidence of seizure activity and the other potential adverse side effects of myelography appears to be greatly reduced with use of the newer contrast agents iopamidol and iohexol rather than metrizamide.(29, 30) Hyperflexion of the cervical spine for cisternal CSF collection and for cervical administration of myelographic contrast can easily kink most endotracheal tubes, resulting in airway obstruction. Armored or spiral wire containing endotracheal tubes are quite resistant to kinking (Chapter 14). Metal or other radiopaque reinforcement in the armored tubes makes them unsuitable for use in cervical and cranial radiographic studies. Close attention to adequacy of the airway and spontaneous ventilation is of paramount importance.

In addition to the precautions and considerations appropriate for thoracolumbar disc disease, cervical disc disease can be associated with increased risk of cardiac arrhythmias.(3) Increased vagal stimulation during ventral approaches to the cervical spine may occur with retraction of the carotid sheath. Frequently there appears to be greater postoperative pain with cervical as opposed to thoracolumbar surgical repair. Patients having lost deep-pain perception are surgical emergencies. Rapid-sequence induction, using intravenous general anesthetics rather than inhalation-induction of anesthesia is indicated if the animal has or may have a full stomach. Additional management related to the emergent nature of their distress may be indicated. The fact that these animals do not feel painful stimuli to the rear limbs suggests that these areas preferentially can be used for placement of injections and intravenous catheters without contributing additional stress to an already highly stressed patient.

ANESTHESIA FOR HORSES WITH WOBBLER SYNDROME

The preanesthetic dose of xylazine administered to a horse with wobbler syndrome should be decreased to prevent the horse from becoming recumbent prior to induction of anesthesia. Xylazine should not be administered until the horse is moved to the induction area. Horses that are severely ataxic prior to drug administration may be anesthetized in the stall and returned there for recovery following the procedure.

Horses with wobbler syndrome are frequently anesthetized for myelography. For premedication, a low dose of xylazine (0.2-0.4 mg/kg IV) can be used. Induction of anesthesia may be accomplished using guaifenesin in combination with thiopental. Anesthesia can be maintained with halothane, isoflurane, or injectable agents such as guaifenesin/thiopental. Some clinicians prefer to administer guaifenesin alone until the horse becomes unsteady and then administer a bolus of thiopental (2-3 g/450 kg). Total dose of injectable anesthetics should be kept to a minimum so that recovery from anesthesia is optimized. As a rule of

Table 23C–2. Anesthetic Management for Myelography and Intervertebral Disc Disease

Myelography and Surgical Decompression:
  A. Benzodiazepine tranquilization (e.g., diazepam 0.4 mg/kg IM or IV)
  B. Low-dose opioid or partial-agonist opioid (analgesia without marked respiratory depression)
  C. Anticholinergics if indicated
  D. Intravenous induction with thiobarbiturate or inhalational induction with isoflurane or halothane by mask
  E. Avoid hyperextension of neck in cervical trauma, instability, and disc disease patients
  F. Maintenance of protected airway and spontaneous ventilation (for prevention of side effects of myelography and to minimize vertebral sinus blood flow during surgery)
  G. Fluid therapy with dextrose for metrizamide myelography
  H. Positioning to avoid venous occlusion
  I. Postoperative analgesics as needed

thumb, a total dose of 2 liters of the guaifenesin/ thiopental combination is not exceeded (5% guaifenesin with 0.3% thiopental). Most horses should have an acceptable recovery when anesthesia is maintained with this injectable combination for less than 1 hour. Controlled ventilation during the procedure is recommended.

Myelography or withdrawal of CSF may precipitate changes in cerebrospinal pressure, which can adversely affect function of the respiratory center in the brain stem.(31) Following administration of a contrast agent, the head should be elevated to minimize the agent's migration toward the brain. In one study, 32% of the horses with significant gait abnormalities that underwent myelography (using metrizamide as the contrast agent) had significant worsening of clinical signs after the procedure.(32) Iopamidol or iohexol used as the contrast agent for equine myelography may be associated with less toxicity and fewer side effects than metrizamide.(33, 34) Regardless of the contrast agent used, a sudden drop in arterial blood pressure may occur at the time of injection. Thus, monitoring of blood pressure is recommended during the procedure. At the end of the procedure, the horse is returned to spontaneous ventilation and allowed to recover after a minimum of 30 minutes since the last injection of contrast agent. Following prolonged lateral recumbency it is advised to allow the horse to recover with the same side down. Turning horses to the opposite side following procedures in lateral recumbency does not improve and may worsen arterial oxygenation.(35, 36) Recovery from anesthesia for myelography is often characterized by several hours of ataxia, which may be more severe than prior to anesthesia. Measures to observe and support the recovering horse should be available. Some horses benefit from being placed in a sling for a few hours after anesthesia. To promote a smooth recovery (and possibly to decrease the incidence of postmyelogram seizure or muscle tremor activity), a low dose of xylazine (25-100 mg IV) or diazepam (0.03 mg/kg IM) may be administered. Some clinicians use phenylbutazone to minimize postmyelogram muscle tremor activity. Phenylbutazone is a highly protein-bound drug. Therefore, it is recommended that phenylbutazone be administered before any anesthetic agents are given to minimize anesthetic displacement from protein binding sites. Phenylbutazone administration during anesthesia that is induced and/or maintained with injectable anesthetics may result in deepened anesthesia or prolonged recovery.

INTRACRANIAL MASSES AND ELEVATED ICP

Patients with intracranial masses, dysfunctional CBF autoregulation and/or increased ICP are at risk of rapid deterioration under anesthesia as described earlier. Anesthetic monitoring should address the physiologic

Table 23C–3. Anesthetic Management for Patients with Elevated CBF and/or ICP and for Intracranial Surgery

A. Preanesthetic critical care management and stabilization (including glucocorticosteroid and diuretic therapy as indicated)
B. Fluid therapy limited to minimize cerebral edema but adequate to support circulation
C. Avoid potent respiratory depression, jugular venous occlusion, and coughing at induction of anesthesia and during recovery
D. Avoid dissociatives, halothane, enflurane, and nitrous oxide
E. Intravenous barbiturate induction of anesthesia preferred
F. Minimal concentrations of isoflurane supplemented with opioids or barbiturates for maintenance of anesthesia
G. Modest hyperventilation to reduce CBF and/or ICP
H. Postoperative critical care with support of ventilation and circulation as indicated

variables associated with altered ICP. Venous and arterial pressures and airway or arterial sampling for CO_2 analysis should be included if possible. Optimal anesthetic management can substantially improve patient status and the outcome of intracranial surgical procedures. A recommended anesthetic technique is summarized in Table 23C–3.

MANAGEMENT OF SEIZURES IN THE PERIANESTHETIC PERIOD

Seizures are most commonly observed in animals with other signs of brain disease. Thus, horses anesthetized for diagnosis or treatment of CNS (especially brain) problems are likely to exhibit seizure activity during the perianesthetic period. The animal with seizure activity prior to anesthesia should be medically treated using the standard recommendations before anesthesia is attempted. In the horse, treatments for status epilepticus include use of anticonvulsants such as diazepam, pentobarbital, phenobarbital, phenytoin, primidone, xylazine, chloral hydrate, and the combination of guaifenesin with a thiobarbiturate.(37) Foals exhibiting seizure activity may be treated with diazepam (5-10 mg IV), phenytoin (5-10 mg/kg IV, IM, or PO), or phenobarbital (with plasma level monitoring).(38) A complication associated with treatment of seizures in neonatal foals is the altered disposition of drugs. Development of the hepatic microsomal enzymes and renal function in the neonate is immature in most species. Thus, concurrent medication with other drugs may cause unexpected interactions or changes in elimination, necessitating careful patient monitoring and alteration of the anticonvulsant dosage regime (Chapter 3).(39)

Phenothiazine tranquilizers have been shown to augment epileptiform activity on the electroencephalogram of dogs.(40) Intrathecal injection of radiographic contrast agents is frequently associated with seizures (Chapter 8).(41) Therefore, acepromazine and other phenothiazine tranquilizers are avoided in animals with preexisting seizures and in animals undergoing myelography (Table 23C–4).

Normal horses sedated with xylazine showed electroencephalographic slowing with irregular waveforms.(42) Xylazine (0.1 to 0.2 mg/kg IV) and diazepam (0.2 mg/kg IV) are both suggested as injectable treatments for seizures in horses recovering from anesthesia.(43) Seizures occurring after myelography that are not controlled by injections of xylazine or diazepam may be treated by reanesthetizing the horse using guaifenesin and a thiobarbiturate. Anesthesia with an inhalation anesthetic may be necessary for up to 1 or 2 hours.

In horses, accidental intracarotid injection of drugs such as xylazine may cause irritation of the brain resulting in violent behavior and seizures (Chapter 8). Management of this potentially dangerous situation should be directed toward manual and, preferably, chemical restraint to prevent injury. Intravenous injection of thiopental or guaifenesin combined with thiopental is recommended. Inspired oxygen should be supplemented, and intravenous fluids should be administered. In the case of intracarotid injection of xylazine, pharmacologic antagonism of xylazine with yohimbine is not suggested. Normal horses given intracarotid drug injections can be maintained for 30 minutes using the combination of guaifenesin and thiopental and often recover uneventfully. Some cases involving intracarotid injection of large doses of drug may have neurologic sequelae (presumably caused by brain edema) requiring symptomatic treatment.

ANESTHESIA FOR ELECTRODIAGNOSTIC TECHNIQUES

Electrodiagnostic procedures are those procedures that involve recording spontaneous or evoked electric activity from tissues or organs. Although consistent with the definition, electrocardiography is usually not considered under this rubric. In veterinary medicine, clinical electrodiagnostic techniques are used to record potentials that are recorded from muscle, peripheral nerves, spinal cord, brain stem, cortex, and retina in animals. In human beings, these procedures are performed without the use of general anesthetics, tranquilizers, or analgesics. With adequate instructions, most adults will tolerate some degree of discomfort or boredom in order to achieve good test results. Some procedures, such as nerve conduction studies or electromyography, cause some pain, whereas others, such as visual or auditory evoked potentials, may simply require human patients to concentrate or refrain from movement. A fundamental problem encountered in the use of electrodiagnostic techniques in veterinary medicine, however, is that of patient cooperation. Even during those procedures in which the stimulus is innocuous, artifacts caused by movement may render the technique ineffective. Therefore, many of the procedures are performed on anesthetized or tranquilized animals. This approach is usually less stressful to the animal, insures a minimum of recording artifacts, and often gives the examiner an opportunity to collect more useful data. The obvious trade-off is a nervous system that has been chemically altered to some degree.

The effects of anesthetics on the outcome of electrodiagnostic procedures range from insignificant to dramatic. In some instances, the use of anesthetic agents altogether precludes recording certain types of potentials. The order of increasing anesthetic effects on recordings is peripheral nerve and skeletal muscle, spinal cord and retina, brain stem, and cerebral cortex. Even so, as long as the effects are understood, the benefits of the recordings still outweigh the data alterations induced by anesthetics. Today, intraoperative monitoring has become standard practice in human beings when the physician desires direct and prompt feedback about neural function during surgical procedures. The use of intraoperative electrodiagnostic monitoring in veterinary medicine is not widespread, but many electrodiagnostic laboratories judiciously use anesthetics for their procedures. Certainly, the precautions will vary between animal species and the physical condition of the patient. An exhaustive review of anesthetic effects is not possible here, but some examples from the literature underscore the importance of this area.

ELECTROENCEPHALOGRAM AND ELECTROMYOGRAPHY

There are two procedures in which electric activity is recorded from spontaneously, reflexively, or volitionally active tissue. The first is the electroencephalogram

Table 23C–4. Anesthetic Management for Seizure-Prone Patients and for Diagnostic Electroencephalography

Control of Seizures:
A. Treatment or avoidance of hypoglycemia
B. Avoid phenothiazine (e.g., acepromazine) and butyrophenone (e.g., droperidol) tranquilizers
C. Benzodiazepine tranquilization (diazepam 0.4 mg/kg IM or IV) or barbiturate sedation (phenobarbital 2–5 mg/kg IM)
D. Intravenous induction with thiobarbiturate (thiamylal or thiopental) but not methohexital
E. Inhalational induction with isoflurane or halothane but not enflurane
F. Avoidance of increases in CBF and/or ICP

Diagnostic Electroencephalography:
A. Avoid preanesthetic tranquilizers and sedatives
B. Intravenous induction with thiobarbiturate
C. Maintain light plane of anesthesia with halothane or incremental thiobarbiturate if necessary to prolong duration
D. Infiltration of temporal muscles wth lidocaine as an alternative to general anesthesia

(EEG), activity produced by the cerebral cortex, and the second is the electromyogram (EMG), electric activity produced by skeletal muscle. Most other electrodiagnostic procedures require a stimulus to evoke activity from excitable tissue. The evoking stimulus may be electric, visual, auditory, or mechanical.

The effects upon the EEG depend on the anesthetic type and depth. Anesthesia initially causes an increase in the voltage and a decrease in the frequency of cortical potentials when compared to the record of an awake alert dog. Spikes and spindles may also riddle the EEG of lightly anesthetized dogs and cats.(44, 45) As anesthesia deepens, the overall voltage begins to diminish (Chapter 7). A dose-response decrease in cerebral oxygen consumption ($CMRO_2$) accompanies the use of isoflurane in dogs and causes the EEG to become isoelectric at an end-expired concentration of 3%.(46) The same type of cortical alteration of electric activity, sometimes referred to as "burst suppression," has been reported in swine.(47) Isoflurane anesthesia may thereby interfere with acquisition of diagnostic information. A recommended anesthetic technique for diagnostic EEG evaluation and for procedures other than EEGs in seizure-prone patients is summarized in Table 23C-4.

Dose-dependent CNS depression of electroencephalographic (EEG) activity by most anesthetics is characteristic and has led to the development of EEG-based anesthetic monitoring techniques.(48) Use of computer-analyzed "quantitative" EEG in isoflurane-anesthetized dogs has been reported.(49) Notable exceptions include the dissociatives (discussed earlier) and the volatile anesthetic enflurane. Enflurane anesthesia can be accompanied by increased EEG activity extending to seizures, particularly if the patient is hyperventilated and hypocarbic.(3, 12) Alterations in normal arterial carbon dioxide tension are associated with significant changes in the quantitative EEG of dogs during halothane anesthesia.(50) Methoxyflurane and halothane anesthetics cause a progression of cerebral depression in dogs, with the latter more likely to promote burst suppression than the former.(51) Similar results in dogs have been reported for sodium pentobarbital. In dogs, barbiturate anesthesia was accompanied by reduced EEG amplitude and burst suppression.(52)

With the exception of miniature end-plate potentials, skeletal muscle that is not volitionally or reflexively active does not produce electric potentials. Because general anesthesia prevents volitional movement, EMG activity is nonrecordable. However, light anesthesia will allow movement in response to judiciously applied painful stimuli, and the occurring EMG is recordable and useful. Potentials that occur in diseased muscle, such as fibrillation potentials and positive sharp waves, bizarre high-frequency discharges, and myotonic potentials, will continue to be produced in anesthetized animals. Compound muscle action potentials evoked by electric stimuli applied to peripheral nerves can be recorded in anesthetized animals and are essential

for determining motor and sensory nerve conduction velocity. Most clinically acceptable anesthetic protocols will not obtund these recordings.

NERVE CONDUCTION STUDIES

Nerve conduction velocity has been successfully recorded in dogs using a variety of anesthetic protocols. Because these procedures do cause pain in unanesthetized animals, the pure effects of anesthetics are largely unknown. Studies in dogs have been successful using thiamylal sodium and methoxyflurane for assessment of motor (53) and sensory (54) nerve function.

AUDITORY AND VISUAL EVOKED POTENTIALS

Auditory and visual evoked potentials may be altered by anesthetic agents depending upon the location of signal generators. Generally, cortical potentials are more likely to be affected than brain-stem potentials. In cats, pentobarbital (20 mg/kg IP) was shown to increase latency, increase area, and increase amplitude of auditory potentials.(55) In another study, brain-stem auditory evoked potentials recorded from cats were unaffected by sodium pentobarbital, ketamine, halothane, and chloralose.(56) Similar results were obtained from rats using ketamine and pentobarbital.(57) Ketamine in rats does, however, affect photic and field potentials recorded directly from various sensory relay nuclei using implanted microelectrodes.(58) The use of ketamine and xylazine in cats produces only minimal changes (latency increases) in the brain-stem auditory evoked responses (BAER) compared to xylazine alone.(59) Thiamylal sodium alters the BAER in dogs by increasing the latencies and decreasing the amplitudes of certain peaks.(60) The same dose of thiamylal sodium, however, completely obliterates middle latency components of the auditory evoked response in dogs.(61) Light pentobarbital anesthesia in cats produces an increase or no change in cortical auditory evoked responses, moderate levels cause some increases in amplitude, and deep anesthesia causes all waves to disappear.(62) Although paraldehyde, ether, and ethyl chloride produce effects similar to those of pentobarbital, chloralose and chloroform are associated with an earlier and more profound period of enhancement.

In rats, halothane (0.25-2.0%) affects auditory evoked responses in a dose-related fashion.(63) These potentials are more sensitive to halothane than are visual evoked responses, especially in the auditory cortex. Pentobarbital, given to rats in sufficiently high doses to cause coma, progressively depresses and then abolishes all peaks of the auditory brain-stem potential.(64) The use of atropine and xylazine in dogs in combination with ketamine or pentobarbital produces only slight changes in the latency of BAER wave VI when compared with xylazine and atropine alone.(65) When BAER waves in dogs anesthetized with methoxyflurane are compared to those in unanesthetized dogs, all waves have significantly longer latencies.(66) In gerbils, ketamine and xylazine induces only minor changes in the low- and high-frequency components of the auditory brain-stem response.(67)

Visual evoked potentials (VEPs) have been successfully recorded in dogs and cats with halothane (68, 69), and in cats with halothane and thiamylal sodium.(70) In dogs, a comparison of VEP from dogs anesthetized with chloralose with VEP from dogs anesthetized with halothane or halothane and thiopental did not reveal any differences in the waveform.(71)

ELECTRORETINOGRAM AND OSCILLATORY POTENTIALS

The electroretinogram and oscillatory potentials can be recorded from small animals under a variety of anesthetic agents.(72–74) The effects of clinical anesthetic protocols in animals is not well documented. Cone adaptation curves are retarded in monkeys as a result of methoxyflurane, halothane, enflurane, ether, and chloroform anesthesia.(75) Pentobarbital anesthesia in cats permits visual evoked responses to be recorded with only minor fluctuations over a period of 80 minutes.(76) Barbiturate anesthesia has no effect on the maturation of the visual evoked response during the first 2 weeks of life.(77) Beyond 2 weeks of age, anesthesia causes an increase in the amplitude of early components while eliminating later components altogether.

SOMATOSENSORY EVOKED POTENTIALS

Somatosensory evoked potentials (SEPs, SERs, or SSEPs) are also affected by anesthesia (Chapter 7). Isoflurane at 1% produces a sustained latency change in SSEP in newborn piglets.(78) Halothane does not affect peak latencies of lumbar spinal cord evoked potentials, but amplitudes are reduced.(79) In cats, increasing levels of pentobarbital can be used to achieve therapeutic coma levels.(80) The early brain-stem components are relatively unaffected, whereas late brain-stem and initial cortical responses show progressive latency increases. Late cortical waves are abolished at relatively low doses; central conduction is unaffected, and late waves of the visual evoked response are abolished even though a single potential survives massive doses. Components of sheep SEPs have been shown to be differentially sensitive to barbiturate anesthesia.(81)

MOTOR EVOKED POTENTIALS

The effects of isoflurane on motor evoked potentials in rats has been examined using concentrations ranging from 0.2–1.5%.(82) There is a progressive increase in onset latency of the compound muscle action potentials and a decrease in the peak-to-peak amplitude and duration. Spinal cord motor evoked potentials (MEPs) have been reported in dogs using a combination of fentanyl, droperidol, sufentanil, and nitrous oxide. It was observed that halogenated gas anesthetics raise the stimulus threshold for recording MEP as compared to narcotic/nitrous oxide anesthesia.(83) Peripheral nerve MEPs have been successfully recorded from dogs using thiopental sodium, isoflurane, and oxymorphone.(84)

References

1. Shapiro HH. Neurosurgical anesthesia and intracranial hypertension. In: Miller RD, ed. Anesthesia, 2nd ed. New York: Churchill Livingstone, 1986:1563–1620.
2. Stoelting RK. Pharmacology and physiology in anesthetic practice. Philadelphia: JB Lippincott, 1987.
3. vanPoznak A. Special consideration for veterinary neuroanesthesia. In: Short CE, ed. Principles and practice of veterinary anesthesia. Baltimore: Williams & Wilkins, 1987.
4. Hansen TD, Warner DS, Vust LH, Todd MM, Trawick DC. Regional distribution of cerebral blood flow with halothane and isoflurane. Anesthesiology 69:332–337, 1988.
5. Osborn I. Choice of neuroanesthetic technique. Anesthesiology Clin North Am 5:531–540, 1987.
6. Dayrell-Hart B, Klide AM. Intracranial dysfunctions: stupor and coma. Vet Clin North Am Small Anim Pract 19:1209–1222, 1989.
7. Grubb RL, Raichle ME, Eichling JO, Ter-Pogossian MM. The effects of changes in P_aCO_2 on cerebral blood volume, blood flow, and vascular mean transit time. Stroke 5:530–539, 1974.
8. Cottrell JE. Deliberate hypotension. Annual Refresher Course Lectures, Am Soc Anesthesiologists, Section 245, 1989:1–7.
9. Harp JR, Wollman H. Cerebral metabolic effects of hyperventilation and deliberate hypotension. Br J Anaesth 45:256, 1973.
10. Frost EAM. Central nervous system trauma. Anesthesiol Clin North Am 5:565–585, 1987.
11. Hirshfeld A. Fluid and electrolyte management in neurosurgical patients. Anesthesiol Clin North Am 5:491–505, 1987.
12. Gilroy BA. Neuroanesthesiology. In: Slatter D, ed. Textbook of small animal surgery. Philadelphia: WB Saunders, 1985.
13. Gray PR, Lowrie CT, Wetmore LA. Effect of intravenous administration of dextrose or lactated Ringer's solution on seizure development in dogs after cervical myelography with metrizamide. Am J Vet Res 48:1600–1602, 1987.
14. Franklin RT. The use of glucocorticoids in treating cerebral edema. Compen Cont Educ 6:442–448, 1984.
15. Sato O, Hara M, Asai T, et al. The effect of dexamethasone phosphate on the production rate of cerebrospinal fluid in the spinal subarachnoid space of dogs. J Neurosurg 39:480–484, 1973.
16. Gleed RD. Tranquilizers and sedative. In: Short CE, ed. Principles and practice of veterinary anesthesia. Baltimore: Williams & Wilkins, 1987.
17. Moore RM, Trim CM. Effect of xylazine on cerebrospinal fluid pressure in conscious horses. Am J Vet Res 53:1558, 1992.
18. Moore RM, Trim CM. Effect of hypercapnia or xylazine on lateral ventricle and lumbosacral cerebrospinal fluid pressures in pentobarbital-anesthetized horses. Vet Surg 22:151–158, 1993.
19. Short CE. Alpha$_2$ agents in animals—sedation, analgesia, and anaesthesia. Santa Barbara, CA: Veterinary Practice Publishing Co., 1992:13.
20. Karlsson B, Forsman M, Roald O, et al. Effect of dexmedetomidine, a selective and potent alpha$_2$-agonist, on cerebral blood flow and oxygen consumption during halothane anesthesia in dogs. Anesth Analg 71:125–129, 1990.
21. Zornow MH, Fleischer JE, Scheller MS, et al. Dexmedetomidine, an alpha-2 adrenergic agonist, decreases cerebral blood flow in the isoflurane-anesthetized dog. Anesth Analg 70:624–630, 1990.
22. Marsh ML, Marshall LF, Shapiro HM. Neurosurgical intensive care. Anesthesiology 47:149, 1977.
23. Bonica JJ. The management of pain, 2nd ed. Philadelphia: Lea & Febiger, 1990:471.
24. Eger EI. Isoflurane (forane). A compendium and reference. Madison, WI: Ohio Medical Products, 1984.
25. Drummond JC, Todd MM. The response of the feline cerebral circulation to P_aCO_2 during anesthesia with isoflurane and halothane and during sedation with nitrous oxide. Anesthesiology 62:268–273, 1985.
26. Drummond JC, Todd MM, Shapiro HH. CO_2 responsiveness of the cerebral circulation during isoflurane anesthesia and nitrous oxide sedation in cats. Anesthesiology 57:A333, 1982.
27. Kaieda R, Todd MM, Warner DS. The effects of anesthetics and P_aCO_2 on the cerebrovascular, metabolic, and electroencephalo-

graphic responses to nitrous oxide in the rabbit. Anesth Analg 68:135–143, 1989.
28. Riedesel DH. Diagnostic or experimental surgical procedures. In: Short CE, ed. Principles and practice of veterinary anesthesia. Baltimore: Williams & Wilkins, 1987.
29. Wheeler SJ, Davies JV. Iohexol myelography in the dog and cat: a series of one hundred cases and a comparison with metrizamide and iopamidol. J Small Anim Pract 26:247–256, 1985.
30. Cox FH. The use of iopamidol for myelography in dogs: a study of twenty-seven cases. J Small Anim Pract 27:159–165, 1986.
31. Kornegay JN, Oliver JE, Gorgacz EJ. Clinicopathologic features of brain herniation in animals. J Am Vet Med Assoc 182:1111, 1983.
32. Hubbell JAE, Reed SM, Myer CW, Muir WW. Sequelae of myelography in the horse. Equine Vet J 20:438–440, 1988.
33. May SA, Wyn-Jones G, Church S. Iopamidol myelography in the horse. Equine Vet J 18:199–202, 1986.
34. Burbridge HM, Kannegieter N, Dickson LR, et al. Iohexol myelography in the horse. Equine Vet J 21:347–350, 1989.
35. MacDonell WN, Hall LW. Radiographic evidence of impaired pulmonary function in laterally recumbent anaesthetized horses. Equine Vet J 11:24, 1979.
36. Mason DE, Muir WW, Wade A. Arterial blood gas tensions in the horse during recovery from anesthesia [Abstract]. Vet Surg 15:461, 1986.
37. Mayhew IG. Large animal neurology – a handbook for veterinary clinicians. Philadelphia: Lea & Febiger, 1989:116.
38. Adams R, Mayhew IG. Neurologic diseases. Vet Clin North Am Equine Pract 1:209–234, 1985.
39. Collatos C. Seizures in foals: pathophysiology, evaluation, and treatment. Comp Cont Educ Pract Vet 12:393–399, 1990.
40. Redman HC, Wilson GL, Hogan JE. Effect of chlorpromazine combined with intermittent light stimulation in the electro-encephalogram and clinical response of the beagle dog. Am J Vet Res 34:929, 1973.
41. Wright JA, Clayton-Jones DG. Metrizamide myelography in sixty-eight dogs. J Small Anim Pract 22:415, 1981.
42. Mysinger PW, Redding RW, Vaughan JT, et al. Electroencephalographic patterns of clinically normal, sedated, and tranquilized newborn foals and adult horses. Am J Vet Res 46:36, 1985.
43. Hodgson DS, Dunlop CI. General anesthesia for horses with specific problems. Vet Clin North Am 6:625–650, 1990.
44. Klemm WR. Subjective and quantitative analyses of the electroencephalogram of anesthetized normal dogs: control data for clinical diagnosis. Am J Vet Res 29:1267–1277, 1968.
45. Klemm WR, Mallo GL. Clinical electroencephalography in anesthetized small animals. J Am Vet Med Assoc 148:1038–1042, 1976.
46. Newberg LA Milde JH, Michenfelder JD. The cerebral metabolic effects of isoflurane at and above concentrations that suppress cortical electrical activity. Anesthesiology 39:23–28, 1983.
47. Rampil IJ, Weiskopf RB, Brown JG, Eger EI, Johnson BH, Holmes MA, Donegan JH. I-653 and isoflurane produce similar dose-related changes in the electroencephalogram of pigs. Anesthesiology 69:298–302, 1988.
48. Goodrich JT. Electrophysiologic measurements: intraoperative evoked potential monitoring. Anesthesiol Clin North Am 5:477–489, 1987.
49. Moore MP, Greene SA, Keegan RD, Gallagher LV, Gavin PR, Kraft SL, DeHaan C, Klappenbach KM. Quantitative electroencephalography in the dogs anesthetized with 2.0% end-tidal concentration of isoflurane. Am J Vet Res 52:551–560, 1991.
50. Smith LJ, Greene SA, Moore MP, Keegan RD. Effects of altered arterial carbon dioxide tension on quantitative EEG in halothane-anesthetized dogs. Am J Vet Res 55:467–471, 1994.
51. Prynn RB, Redding RW. Electroencephalographic continuum in dogs anesthetized with methoxyflurane and halothane. Am J Vet Res 29:1913–1928, 1968.
52. Tonuma E. Electroencephalography with barbiturate anesthesia in the dog. Can Vet J 8:181–185, 1967.
53. Sims MH, Redding RW. Maturation of nerve conduction velocity and the evoked muscle potential in the dog. Am J Vet Res 41:1247–1252, 1980.
54. Sims MH, Selcer RR. Occurrence and evaluation of a reflex-evoked

muscle potential (H reflex) in the normal dog. Am J Vet Res 42:975–983, 1981.
55. Guha D, Pradhan SN. Effects of mescaline, [D9]-tetrahydro-cannabinol and pentobarbital on the auditory evoked responses in the cat. Neuropharmacology 13:755–762, 1974.
56. Cohen MS, Britt RH. Effects of sodium pentobarbital, ketamine, halothane, and chloralose on brainstem auditory evoked responses. Anesth Analg 61:338–343, 1982.
57. Bobbin RP, May JG, Lemoine RL. Effect of pentobarbital and ketamine on brain stem auditory potentials. Arch Otolaryngol 105:467–470, 1983.
58. Dafney N, Rigor BM. Dose effects of ketamine on photic and acoustic field potentials. Neuropharmacology 17:851–862, 1978.
59. Sims MH, Horohow JE. Effects of xylazine and ketamine on the acoustic reflex and brain stem auditory-evoked response in the cat. Am J Vet Res 47:102–109, 1986.
60. Sims MH, Moore RE. Auditory-evoked response in the clinically normal dog: early latency components. Am J Vet Res 45:2019–2027, 1984.
61. Sims MH, Moore RE. Auditory-evoked response in the clinically normal dog: middle latency components. Am J Vet Res 45:2028–2033, 1984.
62. Pradhan SN, Galambos R. Some effects of anesthetics on the evoked responses in the auditory cortex of cats. J Am Vet Med Assoc 139:97–106, 1962.
63. Rabe LS, Moreno L, Rigor BM, Dafny N. Effects of halothane on evoked field potentials recorded from cortical and subcortical nuclei. Neuropharmacology 19:813–825, 1980.
64. Shapiro SM, Miller AR, Shiu GK. Brain-stem auditory evoked potentials in rats with high-dose pentobarbital. Electroencephalogr Clin Neurophysiol 58:266–276, 1984.
65. Toruriki M, Matsunami K Uzuka Y. Relative effects of xylazine-atropine, xylazine-atropine-ketamine, and xylazine-atropine-pentobarbital combinations and time-course effects of the latter two combinations on brain stem auditory-evoked potentials in dogs. Am J Vet Res 51:97–102, 1990.
66. Myers LJ, Redding RW, Wilson S. Reference values of the brainstem auditory evoked response of methoxyflurane anesthetized and unanesthetized dogs. Vet Res Commun 9:289–294, 1985.
67. Smith DI, Mills JH. Low-frequency component of the gerbil brainstem response: response characteristics and anesthetic effects. Hear Res 54:1–10, 1991.
68. Sims MH, Laratta LJ. Visual-evoked potentials in cats, using a light-emitting diode stimulator. Am J Vet Res 49:1876–1881, 1988.
69. Sims MH, Laratta LJ, Bubb WJ, Morgan RV. Waveform analysis and reproducibility of visual-evoked potentials in dogs. Am J Vet Res 50:1823–1828, 1989.
70. Pang XD, Bonds AB. Visual-evoked potential responses of the anesthetized cat to contrast modulation of grating patterns. Vision Res 31:1509–1516, 1991.
71. Bichsel P, Oliver JE, Coulter DB, Brown J. Recording of visual-evoked potentials in dogs with scalp electrodes. J Vet Intern Med 2:145–149, 1988.
72. Rubin LF. Clinical electroretinography in dogs. J Am Vet Med Assoc 151:1456–1469, 1967.
73. Gum GG, Gelatt KN, Samuelson DA. Maturation of the retina of the canine neonate as determined by electroretinography and histology. Am J Vet Res 45:1166–1171, 1984.
74. Sims MH, Brooks DE. Changes in oscillatory potentials in the canine electroretinogram during dark adaptation. Am J Vet Res 51:1580–1586, 1990.
75. van Norren DV, Padmos P. Influence of anesthetics, ethyl alcohol, and freon on dark adaptation of monkey cone ERG. Invest Ophthalmol Vis Sci 16:80–83, 1977.
76. Uzuka Y, Doi S, Tokuriki M, Matsumoto H. The establishment of a clinical diagnostic method of the visual evoked potentials (VEP's) in the cat: the effects of recording electrode positions, stimulus intensity and the level of anesthesia. Jpn J Vet Sci 51:547–553, 1989.
77. Rose GH, Gruenau SP, Spencer JW. Maturation of visual electro-cortical responses in unanesthetized kittens: effects of barbiturate

anesthesia. Electroencephalogr Clin Neurophysiol 33:141–158, 1972.

78. Boston JR, Davis PJ, Brandom BW, Roeber CM. Rate of change of somatosensory evoked potentials during isoflurane anesthesia in newborn piglets. Anesth Analg 70:275–283, 1990.

79. Hogan K, Gravenstein M, Sasse F. Effects of halothane dose and stimulus rate on canine spinal, far-field and near-field somatosensory evoked potentials. Electroencephalogr Clin Neurophysiol 69:277–286, 1988.

80. Sutton LN, Frewen T, Marsh R, Jaggi J, Bruce DA. The effects of deep barbiturate coma on multimodality evoked potentials. J Neurosurg 57:178–185.

81. Wilson RD, Beerwinkle KR. Somatosensory-evoked potential induced by stimulation of the caudal tibial nerve in awake and barbiturate-anesthetized sheep. Am J Vet Res 47:46–49, 1986.

82. Haghighi SS, Green KD, Oro JJ, Drake RK, Krache GR. Depressive effect of isoflurane anesthesia on motor evoked potentials. Neurosurgery 26:993–997, 1990.

83. Cook JR, Konrad PE, Tacker WA. Amplitude and latency characteristics of spinal cord motor-evoked potentials in dogs. Am J Vet Res 51:1340–1344, 1990.

84. Kraus KH, O'Brien D, Pope ER, Kraus BH. Evoked potentials induced by transcranial stimulation in dogs. Am J Vet Res 51:1732–1735, 1990.

chapter **23**D

RENAL DISEASE

Stephen A. Greene

RENAL BLOOD FLOW AND GLOMERULAR
  FILTRATION
ANESTHETIC EFFECTS ON RENAL FUNCTION
EFFECTS OF RENAL INSUFFICIENCY ON
  ANESTHESIA

TESTS OF RENAL FUNCTION
POSTOPERATIVE OLIGURIA
URETHRAL OBSTRUCTION
RUPTURED URINARY BLADDER

Renal Blood Flow and Glomerular Filtration

The kidneys have three primary functions: filtration, reabsorption, and secretion. To accomplish these functions they receive about 25% of the cardiac output. The renal tubules and collecting ducts reabsorb up to 99% of filtered solutes, indicating that the total filtration volume is much greater than daily urine production. Neurohumoral substances and physiologic factors that affect reabsorption of the filtered water and sodium include aldosterone, antidiuretic hormone (ADH), arterial blood pressure, atrial natriuretic factor, catecholamines, prostaglandins, renin-angiotensin, and stress.

Renal blood flow (RBF) is regulated by extrinsic nervous and hormonal control and by intrinsic autoregulation (Chapter 5). Renal vasculature is highly innervated by sympathetic constrictor fibers originating in the T4-L1 spinal cord segments. The kidneys lack sympathetic dilator fibers and parasympathetic innervation. Intrinsic autoregulation of RBF is defined by a constant flow when mean arterial blood pressure ranges from 80 to 180 mm Hg. When the mean arterial blood pressure is between 80 and 180 mm Hg, the kidney is able to control blood flow by altering resistance in the renal afferent arterioles. Although the exact mechanism of renal autoregulation is not known, the significance of this phenomenon relates to protection of glomerular capillaries during hypertension and preservation of renal function during hypotension. However, even within the range of blood pressure described for function of renal autoregulation extrinsic forces (e.g., neural, hormonal, pharmacologic) may cause alterations in RBF and the glomerular filtration rate (GFR). Catecholamines are the major hormonal regulators of RBF. Epinephrine and norepinephrine cause dose-dependent changes in RBF and the GFR. Low doses increase arterial blood pressure and decrease RBF with no net change in the GFR. Higher doses cause decreased RBF and GFR. The renal vascular anatomy is unique in its distribution to cortical and medullary zones. Because of this vascular dichotomy, local tissue ischemia and hypoxia may occur even though total organ blood flow is normal. Oxygen delivery to the kidney is complex, and selective regional hypoxia is a possible source of renal injury during renal hypoperfusion. Experimental evidence indicates that the medullary thick ascending limb of Henle's loop is selectively vulnerable to hypoxic injury.(1)

Anesthetic Effects on Renal Function

Effects of anesthetics on renal blood flow can be summarized with the following generalization: All anesthetics are likely to decrease the rate of glomerular filtration. Anesthetics may directly affect RBF, or they may indirectly alter renal function via changes in cardiovascular and/or neuroendocrine activity. Most anesthetics decrease the GFR as a consequence of decreased RBF (Table 23D–1). Anesthetics that cause catecholamine release (e.g., ketamine, tiletamine, and nitrous oxide) have variable effects on RBF. Inhalation anesthetics tend to decrease RBF and the GFR in a dose-dependent manner. Light planes of inhalation anesthesia preserve renal autoregulation of blood flow, whereas deep planes are associated with depression of autoregulation and decreases in RBF. Although isoflurane has little effect on RBF, it decreases the GFR and urine output.(2) Nitrous oxide in combination with halothane does not appear to alter autoregulation of RBF.(3) The new inhalation anesthetic, desflurane, has

Table 23D–1.   Effects of Anesthetics on Renal Blood Flow (RBF) and Glomerular Filtration Rate (GFR)

Drug	RBF	GFR
Diethyl ether	Decrease	Decrease
Desflurane	No change	?
Enflurane	Decrease	Decrease
Etomidate	No change	No change
Halothane	Slight decrease	Decrease
Isoflurane	Slight decrease	Decrease
Ketamine	Increase	Decrease or no change
Methoxyflurane	Decrease	Decrease
Thiopental	No change	No change or slight decrease

no effect on RBF at concentrations up to two times the minimal alveolar concentration (MAC).(4) The concentration of inhaled anesthetic that prevents purposeful movement in response to a noxious stimulus in 50% of a population is defined as MAC. Desflurane decreases renal vascular resistance at concentrations greater than 1.75 MAC.

Thiobarbiturates increase systemic vascular resistance but decrease renal vascular resistance with no net change in RBF. In contrast, ketamine increases RBF and renal vascular resistance.(5) Most anesthetics cause less disruption of renal autoregulation of blood flow at lower doses (lighter anesthetic planes). Different responses to anesthetics may occur in controlled studies of RBF compared to clinical use of anesthetics. Renal responses to anesthetics also depend on the preexisting hydration status and quantity of perioperative fluids administered.

Renal ischemia may occur during anesthesia due to systemic hypotension or renal vasoconstriction. Systemic hypotension may be caused by excessive depth of inhalation anesthesia, as all potent halogenated anesthetics cause peripheral vasodilation. Inhalant anesthetics also depress myocardial contractility and cardiac output in a dose-dependent manner. Hypotension may also be induced by phenothiazine or butyrophenone tranquilizers. Phenothiazine and butyrophenone tranquilizers block alpha adrenoceptors and dopamine receptors. Alpha-adrenergic blockade may induce peripheral vasodilation and hypotension. Dopamine receptor blockade by acepromazine premedication may prevent dopamine-induced increases in RBF during surgery.

Intraoperative administration of epinephrine for hemostasis may increase renal vascular resistance, resulting in up to 40% reduction in renal blood flow.(6) Renal failure likely occurs occasionally in animals that have been given epinephrine for hemostasis during otherwise uneventful anesthesia.(7) Following the initial ischemic insult, renal perfusion may remain altered because of other mechanisms. In experimental dogs injected intrarenally with norepinephrine, saline administration restored renal blood flow but did not correct oliguria.(8) Necropsy of animals following acute renal failure may not detect renal damage because histologic evidence may not be evident until 3 or 4 days postinjury.(9)

Anesthesia and the stress associated with surgery cause release of aldosterone, vasopressin, renin, and catecholamines. Thus, RBF and GFR (and therefore urine production) are generally decreased with surgery in any patient. For most patients, the effects of inhaled anesthetics on renal function are reversed at the termination of anesthesia. Some patients, however, may not regain the ability to regulate urine production for several days.(10) Postanesthetic oliguria should be evaluated (discussed later).

Some drugs used in the perianesthetic period have a significant effect on urine production. Xylazine can dramatically increase urinary output and reduce urinary osmolality.(11) Xylazine is believed to decrease antidiuretic hormone (ADH) concentration in the mare, accounting, in part, for increased urine production.(12) Detomidine-induced diuresis has also been reported in the horse.(13) Because they can induce diuresis, xylazine and detomidine should not be used in animals with urethral obstruction. Reports on the effects of opioids on ADH secretion are confusing. The antidiuresis following morphine administration in animals has been attributed to increased release of ADH.(14) Others suggest this is a response to stress associated with surgical stimulation.(15) Opioids may cause urine retention when administered systemically or as an epidural injection.

Nephrotoxic drugs administered during anesthesia may cause oliguria. Methoxyflurane is the only anesthetic known to cause nephrotoxicity as a consequence of biotransformation to oxalate and free fluoride ion. (16–18) Dogs appear to be more resistant to F-induced renal toxicosis than humans. Induction of hepatic enzymes with phenobarbital increases the risk of methoxyflurane-related renal failure. In addition, nephrotoxic activity of other drugs used during anesthesia may be enhanced by methoxyflurane (Table 23D–2). Methoxyflurane anesthesia combined with flunixin meglumine precipitates renal failure in dogs.(19) Ad-

Table 23D–2. Potential Nephrotoxins in the Perianesthetic Period

Aminoglycoside antibiotics
Amphotericin B
Bilirubin
Fluoride ion
Hemoglobin
Iodinated radiographic contrast agents
Methoxyflurane
Myoglobin
Nonsteroidal antiinflammatory agents
Oxalate

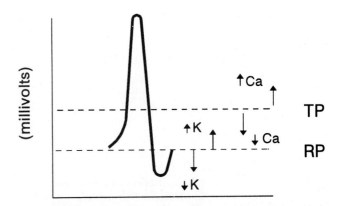

Fig. 23D–1. Relationships between extracellular concentrations of potassium (K^+) and calcium (Ca^{++}) and the resting (RP) and threshold potentials (TP). An action potential is generated when there is sufficient depolarization to reach the TP. Increased extracellular potassium will result in raised (less negative) RP, whereas increased extracellular calcium will result in raised TP.

ministration of aminoglycoside antibiotics also enhances renal toxicity of methoxyflurane.(20)

Effects of Renal Insufficiency on Anesthesia

Azotemia in the patient with renal insufficiency will alter the response to anesthetics. Azotemia may be associated with changes in the blood-brain barrier, leading to increased CNS drug sensitivity. Patients with renal insufficiency may be acidotic, which will increase the fraction of unbound barbiturate and other injectable drugs in the plasma. Increased unbound fraction of any injectable anesthetic will increase drug activity. Thus, lower doses of highly protein-bound injectable anesthetics are required in acidotic patients (Chapter 2).

Hyperkalemia may be present in animals with renal insufficiency, obstructed urethra, or rupture of the urinary bladder. Acidosis may be associated with a concurrent increase in serum potassium. Patients in renal failure with hypocalcemia are at even greater risk, since hypocalcemia potentiates the myocardial toxicity of hyperkalemia. Further, administration of succinylcholine will transiently increase serum potassium concentration.(21) Succinylcholine-induced increases in potassium are potentially life threatening in animals with hyperkalemia. In contrast, elevation in serum potassium is not observed following administration of nondepolarizing neuromuscular blocking agents (Chapter 13). Patients with hypermagnesemia associated with chronic renal failure may have prolonged recovery from nondepolarizing neuromuscular blocking agents.(22) As a rule, patients having a serum potassium concentration greater than 5.5 or 6.0 mEq/L should not be anesthetized. Electrocardiographic abnormalities are commonly associated with potassium concentrations exceeding 7 mEq/L (Chapters 15 and 19). The resting membrane potential of cardiac muscle is dependent on permeability and extracellular concentration of potassium (Fig. 23D–1). During hyperkalemia the membrane's resting potential is raised (partially depolarized) and fewer sodium channels are available to participate in the action potential. As the serum potassium concentration increases, repolarization occurs more rapidly and automaticity, conductivity, contractility, and excitability are decreased. These changes produce the classic electrocardiographic appearance of a peaked T wave with a prolonged PR interval progressing to wide QRS complexes and loss of P waves. Mild chronic hyperkalemia may not require treatment prior to anesthesia. If hyperkalemia is acute or electrocardiographic abnormalities are noted, treatment should be initiated prior to induction of anesthesia. The most rapid treatment for the cardiac effects associate with hyperkalemia is 10% calcium chloride (0.1 mg/kg IV). Calcium will increase the membrane's threshold potential, resulting in increased myocardial conduction and contractility. Because increased serum potassium concentration causes the resting potential to be less negative (partially depolarized), the calcium ion induced increase in threshold potential temporarily restores the normal gradient between resting and threshold potentials (Fig. 23D–1). It should be recognized that administration of calcium will not affect the serum potassium concentration, and its effects will therefore be short-lived. Regimens to decrease the serum potassium concentration by shifting potassium intracellularly include bicarbonate administration and combined infusion of glucose and insulin.

Patients in chronic renal failure are frequently anemic because of bone marrow suppression and decreased erythropoietin production. In response to anemia, the cardiovascular system may become hyperdynamic in an attempt to maintain oxygen delivery. Chronic renal disease may be associated with hypertension and increased cardiac output but reduced cardiac reserve. Patients undergoing anesthesia should have a red blood cell transfusion if the hematocrit is less than 18% (cat) or 20% (dog).

In dogs and cats with mild renal insufficiency, a rapid intravenous induction of anesthesia may be accomplished with thiobarbiturates, diazepam-ketamine, or diazepam-opioid combinations. Depressed patients can be mask-induced with isoflurane or halothane. Anesthesia may be maintained with isoflurane or halothane. Medications that are potentially nephrotoxic should be avoided.

Patients that are dehydrated or cachectic are more prone to pressure necrosis caused by poor positioning during anesthesia. Proper positioning with adequate padding should be provided. The urinary bladder should be catheterized and urine production monitored. Urine production is an indirect monitor of renal prefusion. Normal urine output for the dog is 0.5-1 $mL \cdot kg^{-1} \cdot h^{-1}$. In the normal horse, daily urine production has been estimated to be about 15 L; horses that are denied feed and water for 24 hours produce about 6 L.[23] Empty fluid bags can be saved for the purpose of collecting urine from catheterized patients. Intravenous fluids should be administered during anesthesia at the rate of 20 mL/kg for the first hour. A rate of 10 $mL \cdot kg^{-1} \cdot h^{-1}$ is used thereafter. The choice of intravenous fluid is based on the individual animal's particular electrolyte and acid-base status (Chapter 19). In general, animals with mild to moderate renal insufficiency that are well prepared for surgery or anesthesia are given lactated Ringer's solution. Measurement of arterial blood pressure is advised in order to detect systemic hypotension and prevent renal hypoperfusion. The mean arterial blood pressure should be maintained above 70 mm Hg. The central venous pressure (CVP) can be measured via a jugular catheter to evaluate the rate of intravenous fluid administration. Normal CVP should be between -3 and $+5$ cm H_2O. If the CVP rises more than 10 cm H_2O, the fluid administration should be slowed or stopped. If the CVP falls in response to stopping the fluids, they may be resumed at a slower rate. Maintenance of greater than 10 cm H_2O elevations in CVP after the fluids are discontinued indicates inadequate myocardial function. Myocardial function may be improved by infusion of dopamine (1-3 $\mu g \cdot kg^{-1} \cdot min^{-1}$) (Chapters 5 and 24). Low doses of dopamine will also improve RBF. Doses of dopamine above 10 $\mu g \cdot kg^{-1} \cdot min^{-1}$ may cause renal vasoconstriction and decreased RBF.

Tests of Renal Function

Measurements of the GFR and renal tubular function such as urine specific gravity and blood urea nitrogen (BUN) are not specific for renal disease. However, BUN concentrations greater than 50 mg/dL nearly always indicate renal insufficiency. Serum creatinine is a specific indicator of the GFR, but it may be eliminated via nonrenal routes. Thus, patients with mild renal insufficiency may not have elevated serum creatinine. In the absence of proteinuria or casts, normal BUN, creatinine, and urine concentrating ability may be present with up to 67% loss of renal parenchyma.

In addition to BUN and serum creatinine concentration, patients with renal insufficiency should be evaluated to determine acid-base balance, electrolyte concentrations (especially potassium), exercise intolerance, hematocrit, hydration, urine concentrating ability, and urine production.

Postoperative Oliguria

Postoperative oliguria (less than 0.5 $mL \cdot kg^{-1} \cdot h^{-1}$) should be investigated. If the animal does not have congestive heart failure or pulmonary edema, a fluid challenge of 5 mL/kg of isotonic saline may be given. If urine production resumes, the animal was hypovolemic and fluids should be continued. If not, dopamine may be initiated as an infusion at a rate of 1 to 3 $\mu g \cdot kg^{-1} \cdot min^{-1}$. Dopamine improves renal function when used at low doses by increasing the RBF, GFR, urine output, and sodium excretion, and by decreasing renal vascular resistance.[24] At moderate doses (5-10 $\mu g \cdot kg^{-1} \cdot min^{-1}$), dopamine activates beta adrenoceptors, which may dilate renal arterial beds and increase cardiac output. Doses above $10 \, \mu g \cdot kg^{-1} \cdot min^{-1}$ cause alpha-adrenoceptor stimulation, vasoconstriction, and decreased RBF. Dopamine may also be beneficial because it inhibits intrarenal norepinephrine release and has an antialdosterone effect.(1) Recall that in patients medicated with acepromazine, dopamine may be ineffective at increasing RBF because of dopaminergic receptor blockade.

The use of diuretics in the perioperative period is controversial. In a study of human patients, acute renal failure treated with diuretics such as mannitol and furosemide was not resolved.(25) In a dog model of uranyl nitrate-induced acute renal failure, a combination of furosemide and dopamine was effective in restoring renal blood flow and creatinine clearance, whereas either drug alone was not.(26) Furosemide is used to promote diuresis in patients with pulmonary edema but should not be used when the patient is known to be hypovolemic. In hypovolemia, furosemide will increase nephrotoxicity of other drugs by increasing their contact time in the renal tubules.(27) Mannitol can be given at 0.25 to 0.5 mg/kg to prevent pulmonary edema or hyponatremia if the patient does not respond to fluid administration.

Urethral Obstruction

Patients with urethral obstruction become hyperkalemic, azotemic, acidotic, and hyperphosphatemic. Selected species (e.g., cats) may also develop hyperglycemia, hypocalcemia, and hyponatremia. Hyponatremia is associated with leakage of urine into the periotoneal cavity.(28) Any metabolic abnormalities should be evaluated and corrected prior to anesthesia. Hyperkalemia is the primary concern in most cases of urethral obstruction. Treatment of hyperkalemia has been discussed in preceding paragraphs.

In small animals with urethral obstruction, centesis of the urinary bladder should be performed prior to anesthesia. Rupture of the urinary bladder during induction of anesthesia in a horse has been described.(29) Perineal urethrostomy may be performed in the stallion with urethral blockage using standing restraint and epidural anesthesia (Fig. 23D–2). If general anesthesia is required while the bladder is distended, every attempt should be made to gently place the animal into recumbency during induction.

Anesthesia may be induced using injectable or inhalation anesthetics. In many animals, distension of the urinary bladder is associated with increased heart rate. Cats that are chamber-induced with an arrhythmogenic inhalation anesthetic such as halothane should be preoxygenated and tranquilized prior to exposure to high concentrations of the anesthetic. Chamber induction with isoflurane is preferred over halothane for small animals with urethral obstruction. Ketamine has been used in obstructed cats even though active metabolites of the drug are excreted by the kidney. The rationale is that once the obstruction is relieved, excretion of the anesthetic will proceed normally.

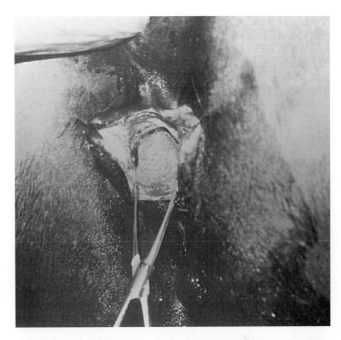

Fig. 23D–2. Photograph of a large urethral calculus being removed via perineal urethrostomy in a standing horse sedated with xylazine and butorphanol and given epidural analgesia using xylazine (0.17 mg/kg added to 8 mL of isotonic saline).

However, cats with a long duration of urethral obstruction may develop metabolic disturbances and renal insufficiency such that elimination of drugs is slowed even after removal of the obstruction. Thus, it is recommended that low doses of ketamine (2 mg/kg IV) in combination with acepromazine (0.05 mg/kg IV) be used in these circumstances. With low doses, termination of anesthetic action will occur following redistribution of the drug into body tissues and does not depend solely upon renal elimination.

Ruptured Urinary Bladder

Rupture of the urinary bladder is an emergency situation. Animals may become hyperkalemic, hyponatremic, hypochloremic, and acidotic following rupture of the urinary bladder.(30) Intravenous fluids, such as isotonic saline, should be given to aid in correcting electrolyte imbalances. Potassium enters the abdominal cavity from the ruptured bladder and is reabsorbed into the circulation, causing an increased serum potassium concentration. An electrocardiogram should be evaluated prior to induction of anesthesia to determine if cardiac arrhythmias or evidence of hyperkalemia are present. Hyperkalemia (serum $[K^+] > 5.5$ mEq/L) should be treated prior to anesthesia. Anesthesia may be induced by face mask administration of isoflurane or halothane. Young foals (weighing <200 kg) may be nasotracheally intubated while awake and then induced rapidly with halothane or isoflurane (Chapter 17). In larger foals, xylazine (1.1 mg/kg IV) and ketamine (2.2 mg/kg IV) can be used for induction.(31) Foals that are depressed may be induced with decreased doses of injectable drugs. Isoflurane is indicated in all species because of its minimal myocardial depressant action and its minimal potentiation of catecholamine-induced cardiac arrhythmias.(32)

References

1. Gelman S. Preserving renal function during surgery. International Anesthesia Research Society Review Course Lectures, 1992.
2. Gelman S, Fowler KC, Smith LR. Regional blood flow during isoflurane and halothane anesthesia. Anesth Analg 63:57, 1984.
3. Leighton KM, Macleod BA, Burce C. Renal blood flow: differences in autoregulation during anesthesia with halothane, methoxyflurane, or alphaprodine in the dog. Anesth Analg 57:389, 1978.
4. Merin RG, et al. Comparison of the effects of isoflurane and desflurane on cardiovascular dynamics and regional blood flow in the chronically instrumented dog. Anesthesiology 74:568, 1991.
5. Priano LL. Alteration of renal hemodynamics by thiopental, diazepam, and ketamine in conscious dogs. Anesth Analg 61:853, 1982.
6. Innes IR, Nickerson M. Nor-epinephrine, epinephrine, and the sympathomimetic amines. In: Goodman LS, Goodman A, eds. The pharmacologic basis of therapeutics, 5th ed. New York: Macmillan, 1977.
7. Trim C. Anesthesia and the kidney. Compend Cont Educ 1:843, 1979.
8. Levinsky NG. Pathophysiology of acute renal failure. N Engl J Med 296:1453, 1977.
9. Boba A, Landmesser CM. Renal complications after anesthesia and operation. Anesthesiology 22:782, 1961.
10. Hayes MA, Goldenberg IS. Renal effects of anesthesia and operation mediated by endocrines. Anesthesiology 24:487, 1963.
11. Thurmon JC, et al. Xylazine causes transient dose-related hyperglycemia and increased urine volumes in mares. Am J Vet Res 45:224, 1984.
12. Greene SA, Thurmon JC, Benson GJ, Tranquilli WJ. Antidiuretic hormone prevents xylazine induced diuresis in mares [Abstract]. Vet Surg 15:459, 1986.
13. Gasthuys F, Terpstra P, van den Hende C, DeMoor A. Hyperglycaemia and diuresis during sedation with detomidine in the horse. Zentralbl Veterinarmed 334:641, 1987.
14. Papper S, Papper EM. The effects of pre-anesthetic, anesthetic, and post-operative drugs on renal function. Clin Pharmacol Ther 5:205, 1964.
15. Philbin DM, Coggins CH. Plasma antidiuretic hormone levels in cardiac surgical patients during morphine and halothane anesthesia. Anesthesiology 49:95, 1978.
16. Crandell WB, Pappas SG, MacDonald A. Nephrotoxicity associated with methoxyflurane anesthesia. Anesthesiology 27:591, 1966.
17. Benson GJ, Brock KA. Halothane-associated hepatitis and methoxyflurane-related nephropathy: a review. J Vet Pharmacol Ther 3:187, 1980.
18. Brunson DB, Stowe CM, McGrath CJ. Serum and urine inorganic fluoride concentrations and urine oxalate concentrations following methoxyflurane anesthesia in the dog. Am J Vet Res 40:197, 1979.
19. Mathews K, Doherty T, Dyson D, Wilcock B. Renal failure in dogs associated with flunixin meglumine and methoxyflurane anesthesia [Abstract]. Vet Surg 16:323, 1987.
20. Kuzucu EY. Methoxyflurane, tetracycline, and renal failure. JAMA 211:1162, 1970.
21. Miller RD, Way WL, Hamilton WK, Layzer RB. Succinylcholine-induced hyperkalemia in patients with renal failure? Anesthesiology 36:138, 1972.
22. Ghonheim MM, Long JP. The interaction between magnesium and other neuromuscular blocking agents. Anesthesiology 32:23, 1970.
23. Rumbaugh GE, Carlson GP, Harrold D. Urinary production in the healthy horse and in horses deprived of feed and water. Am J Vet Res 43:735, 1982.
24. Schwartz LB, Bissell MG, Murphy M, Gewertz BL. Renal effects of dopamine in vascular surgical patients. J Vasc Surg 8:367, 1988.
25. Cantarovich F, et al. Furosemide in high doses in the treatment of acute renal failure. Postgrad Med J 47:13, 1978.
26. Lindner A, Cutler RE, Goodman WG. Synergism of dopamine plus furosemide in preventing acute renal failure in the dog. Kidney Int 16:158, 1979.
27. Stoelting RK. Pharmacology and physiology in anesthetic practice. Philadelphia: JB Lippincott, 1987.
28. Lees GE, Rogers KS, Wold AM. Diseases of the lower urinary tract. In: Sherding RG, ed. The cat-diseases and clinical management. New York: Churchill Livingstone, 1989.
29. Pankowski RL, Fubini SL. Urinary bladder rupture in a two-year-old horse: sequel to a surgically repaired neonatal injury. J Am Vet Med Assoc 191:560, 1987.
30. Finco DR. Kidney function. In Kaneko JJ, ed. Clinical biochemistry of domestic animals, 3rd ed. New York: Academic Press, 1980.
31. Tranquilli WJ, Thurmon JC. Management of anesthesia in the foal. Vet Clin North Am Equine Pract 6(3):651–663, 1990.
32. Eger EI III. Isoflurane: a review. Anesthesiology 55:559, 1981.

chapter 23E

HEPATIC DISEASE

Stephen A. Greene

HEPATIC BLOOD SUPPLY
DETERMINATION OF HEPATIC
  INSUFFICIENCY
PHARMACOLOGIC CONSIDERATIONS FOR
  PATIENTS WITH HEPATIC DISEASE
  Tranquilizers/Sedatives
  Opioids
  Thiobarbiturates

Propofol and Etomidate
Dissociative Anesthetics
Inhalation Anesthetics
Muscle Relaxants
GENERAL GUIDELINES FOR PATIENTS WITH
  HEPATIC DISEASE
PORTAL-CAVAL SHUNT

Hepatic Blood Supply

About 20% of cardiac output is delivered to the liver. The hepatic artery supplies 30% of the blood flow and 90% of the oxygen, and the remainder is supplied by blood flowing through the portal vein. Anesthetics may affect hepatic blood flow by altering vascular tone in the hepatic artery, the portal vein, or both (Table 23E–1). Methoxyflurane decreases both portal vein and hepatic arterial blood flow. Halothane decreases portal vein blood flow but has only a slight effect, if any, on hepatic arterial blood flow. Isoflurane decreases portal vein blood flow but increases hepatic artery blood flow and a net overall increase in flow. Nitrous oxide has no direct effect on liver perfusion. Desflurane maintains hepatic artery and portal vein resistance and is associated with decreased portal vein and total hepatic blood flow.(1) Decreased blood flow may occur in cirrhotic livers or patients with portocaval shunt syndrome. Detrimental effects of decreased blood flow are likely to be more significant when an animal is hypotensive. Significant decreases in blood flow may be associated with decreased hepatic extraction and, ultimately, elimination of drugs.(2)

Determination of Hepatic Insufficiency

Clinical signs of hepatic insufficiency include ascites, depression, seizures, jaundice, and petechial hemorrhage. Horses with colic have an increased incidence of concurrent hepatic disease.(3) Tests of substrate metabolism may give an indication of hepatic function. Low values for plasma proteins and albumin, urea nitrogen, and cholesterol are associated with poor hepatic function. Coagulation defects such as prolonged prothrombin time and increased fibrinogen values may also indicate decreased hepatic function. Bilirubin is formed by metabolism of degraded hemoglobin by macrophages and carried by albumin to the liver for conjugation to a diglucuronide. In the horse, fasting for more than 24 hours causes fatty acids to compete with bilirubin for hepatic metabolism. In this way, hyperbilirubinemia frequently causes icterus in the anorexic horse.

Blood ammonia concentration and retention of dyes such as sulfobromophthalein (BSP) or indocyanine green (ICG) indicate liver dysfunction as evidenced by the liver's inability to eliminate these substances in a normal manner. The dyes, like bile acids, are more

791

Table 23E–1. Effect of Inhaled Anesthetics on Hepatic Blood Flow

Agent	Portal Vein	Hepatic Artery
Desflurane	Decrease	No change
Halothane	Decrease	Decrease or no change
Isoflurane	Decrease	Increase
Methoxyflurane	Decrease	Decrease
Nitrous oxide	No direct effects	

sensitive indicators of liver dysfunction than is a change in bilirubin concentration.(4) Bile acids are produced by the liver and excreted in the bile. They undergo a process termed *enterohepatic circulation.* Following biliary excretion, bile acids are reabsorbed by the ileum and enter the portal circulation. Bile acids are then removed by the hepatocytes, leaving only a low concentration to enter the systemic circulation during normal circumstances. Fasting does not affect bile acid concentration. Normal fasting bile acid concentrations are below 5 μmol/L for the cat, below 10 μmol/L for the dog, and below 15 μmol/L for the horse.

Postprandial blood samples will demonstrate an elevation in bile acid concentration caused by gall bladder contraction. Within 2 hours the liver can remove most of the bile acids presented to it as a result of gall bladder emptying. Thus, marked increases in postprandial bile acid concentration indicates decreased hepatic function or the presence of a portal-caval vascular shunt. Normal 2-hour postprandial concentrations of bile acids are below 15 μmol/L in the cat and below 25 μmol/L in the dog. Because the horse lacks a gall bladder, postprandial elevations in bile acid concentrations are not expected. Use of bile acid concentrations to aid in assessment of hepatic disease in the horse is best when combined with other tests of hepatobiliary function.(5)

Tests of cell membrane integrity (i.e., alanine aminotransferase, gamma-glutamyltransferase, sorbitol dehydrogenase, lactate dehydrogenase, and serum alkaline phosphatase) indicate hepatocellular damage but may not reflect hepatic function.

Pharmacologic Considerations For Patients with Hepatic Disease

TRANQUILIZERS/SEDATIVES

Acepromazine, droperidol (a component of Innovar-Vet), and alpha$_2$-adrenergic agonists should be avoided in patients with moderate to severe liver disease. Hypotension may occur following administration of phenothiazine (acepromazine) or butyrophenone (droperidol) tranquilizers because of peripheral vasodilation mediated by alpha-adrenergic blockade. Dysrhythmias such as bradycardia or heart block and alterations of plasma glucose concentration may occur following

administration of xylazine or detomidine. Diazepam is generally considered safe when used in doses less than 0.2 mg/kg IV because it causes minimal changes in cardiovascular function. Diazepam may not consistently tranquilize the healthy young animal but frequently produces tranquilization in animals with liver disease. When diazepam is administered intravenously, it should be injected slowly to decrease irritation and prevent hypotension associated with the propylene glycol carrier (Chapter 8).

OPIOIDS

Opioids can be used in patients with liver disease. Morphine and meperidine can cause release of histamine, which may cause a decrease in total hepatic blood flow. Morphine also constricts the sphincter of Oddi, which could be of significance in obstructive biliary disease. Side effects of opioids should be treated if they appear to affect cardiac or respiratory function. Opioid-induced bradycardia will decrease cardiac output and should be prevented by administration of an anticholinergic agent. Respiratory depression from opioids may lead to decreased oxygen delivery to all body tissues including the liver. Titration of the opioid antagonist naloxone can relieve depression of respiration while maintaining some of the analgesic and sedative effects of the opioid agonist. Butorphanol is associated with less respiratory depression than other opioid agonists and is a reasonable choice for the patient with hepatic disease.

THIOBARBITURATES

Thiobarbiturates should be used in low doses or avoided altogether in patients with liver disease. A single, intubating dose of thiobarbiturate is not necessarily contraindicated because it will be redistributed from the brain to less well perfused tissues, terminating the anesthetic effect. However, liver disease may affect the duration and depth of thiobarbiturate induced-anesthesia because of increased sensitivity of the CNS or hypoalbuminemia and decreased protein binding of the anesthetic. Anesthesia should not be maintained by redosing thiobarbiturates in patients with liver disease.

Methohexital is a methylated oxybarbiturate, and although it is more rapidly metabolized than thiobarbiturates, it is associated with hyperexcitation and possible seizures during the recovery period. For this reason, methohexital should be avoided in patients with hepatic encephalopathy.

PROPOFOL AND ETOMIDATE

Propofol is an alkylphenolic compound used for induction of anesthesia that is supplied in a lecithin emulsion, giving it a milky white appearance. Redistribution and metabolism of propofol after a single injection are extremely rapid. The total body clearance of propofol exceeds hepatic blood flow, indicating sites other than the liver (lung?) may play a role in its elimination. Propofol is about 90% excreted by the kidneys as conjugated metabolites.(6) Indications for use of propofol are similar to those for the thiobarbiturates. The major advantage over a thiobarbiturate is the rapid rate of propofol elimination. In dogs, the incidence of apnea occurring immediately after injection seems to be greater than that associated with thiobarbiturates (Chapter 9).

Etomidate is an imidazole compound used for induction of anesthesia. It is supplied as a weak base in a propylene glycol vehicle. As with other drugs formulated with propylene glycol, it is irritating when injected intravenously.(7) Etomidate does not decrease hepatic perfusion. It has a short duration of action, primarily because of rapid redistribution from the brain to muscle tissue. Etomidate is metabolized by the hepatic microsomal enzyme system as well as by plasma esterases. The total body clearance rate for etomidate is five times as fast as for thiopental.(4) Etomidate has been shown to cause adrenocortical suppression with repeated administration.(8) The importance of etomidate's effect on steroidogenesis following single bolus administration in the patient with hepatic disease is unknown. In both humans (9) and dogs (10), etomidate infusion has been associated with hemolysis. Hemolysis appears to be caused by the propylene glycol vehicle in which etomidate is formulated. In dogs, blood cell counts during and 10 minutes after termination of a 60-minute infusion of etomidate were not significantly different from preinfusion values.(10) All dogs in the aforementioned study appeared normal after recovery from anesthesia maintained with etomidate. Thus, the clinical significance of etomidate–propylene glycol–induced hemolysis in dogs is not clear. Etomidate is a reasonable drug choice for induction of anesthesia in patients with cardiac and/or hepatic disease (Chapter 9).

DISSOCIATIVE ANESTHETICS

Dissociative anesthetics such as tiletamine (Telazol) or ketamine are generally acceptable for induction of anesthesia in patients with hepatic disease. Intravenous administration is preferred in order to minimize the dose required for tracheal intubation. In the dog, these drugs are largely metabolized by the liver, so maintenance of anesthesia should be with an inhalant. Dissociative anesthetics may induce seizures in dogs or cats. In the cat, ketamine is metabolized to a small extent by the liver to form norketamine, which has about 10% of the activity of ketamine.

Zolazepam, the benzodiazepine tranquilizer in Telazol, has been suspected of causing the prolonged recovery following intramuscular injection in the cat. Flumazenil (Romazecon) has been used intravenously (0.1 mg/kg) to antagonize midazolam in cats anesthetized with a combination of ketamine and midazolam.(11) Zolazepam's effect in the cat is similarly antagonized by flumazenil, providing an alternative to the apparently slow hepatic metabolism of the benzodiazepines in this species.

INHALATION ANESTHETICS

Inhalation anesthetics are the best choices for maintenance of anesthesia in patients with severe liver disease. Halothane decreases hepatic blood flow and is metabolized up to 20% by the liver.(12) Halothane anesthesia in ponies is associated with decreased bile acid excretion and increased conjugated bilirubin excretion.(13) It is recommended that halothane be avoided if possible in patients with liver disease. However, the presence of hepatic disease does not necessarily result in increased hepatotoxicity when the patient is subsequently exposed to an unpredictable hepatotoxin such as halothane.(14) Halothane has been implicated in causing liver disease in people and possibly in animals. This is a problem in about 1 of every 6000 to 10,000 people and is probably genetically related.(15, 16) Halothane is metabolized to trichloroacetic acid, which may undergo reductive metabolism to produce hepatotoxins during hypoxia. Recent studies indicate that the trifluoroacetate metabolite of halothane combines with an hepatic protein, resulting in the formation of a hapten.(17-19) The trifluoroacetate hapten is subsequently attacked by serum antibodies, causing hepatitis. A clinical test for this hapten is not yet available for animals. In a study of goats hyperimmunized for production of anti-human-lymphocyte serum that were subsequently exposed to 3, 6, or 9 hours of halothane anesthesia, 7 of 29 (24%) showed evidence of hepatic necrosis.(20) A rat model of halothane-induced hepatopathy showed that hepatic hypoxia was required to produce symptoms.(21) Precautions should be taken when using halothane (or any other anesthetic!) to ensure adequate blood pressure, flow, and oxygen delivery during anesthesia. Prevention of hepatic hypoxia during inhalation anesthesia is probably more important than choice of anesthetic in preventing the occurrence of postanesthetic hepatopathy.

Methoxyflurane decreases hepatic blood flow, and up to 50% of the inhaled dose is metabolized by the liver.(22) In addition, oxalate and fluoride ion metabolites of methoxyflurane are potential renal toxins. Of the volatile anesthetics, methoxyflurane is associated with the highest metabolite production of fluoride ion (Fig. 23E–1).

Isoflurane increases hepatic artery blood flow at both 1 and 2 MAC in man, whereas halothane preserves hepatic arterial flow at 1 MAC but decreases it at 2 MAC.(23) Less than 1% of inhaled isoflurane is metabolized. It has not been associated with hepatic or renal toxicity.(24) Cardiovascular function during isoflurane anesthesia is less depressed than with halothane or methoxyflurane. The higher cardiac output associated with isoflurane anesthesia is likely to maintain better hepatic perfusion and oxygen delivery than halothane. Thus, isoflurane appears to be the best choice for

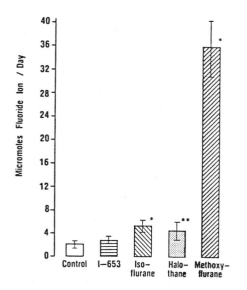

Fig. 23E–1. Twenty-four-hour excretion of fluoride ion in urine of rats pretreated with phenobarbital and anesthetized with 1.6 MAC desflurane (I-653), isoflurane, halothane, or methoxyflurane for 2 hours. (From Koblin, D.D., et al. I-653 Resists Degradation in Rats. Anesth Analg 67:534, 1988.)

maintenance of anesthesia in patients with hepatic disease.

The effects of desflurane on hepatic blood flow are similar to those of halothane (Table 23E–1). Desflurane differs from isoflurane structurally only by substitution of a fluorine atom for a chlorine atom. The substitution of a fluorine atom for other halogens generally makes a molecule more stable in terms of biotransformation. Indeed, desflurane metabolism to free fluoride ion is less than that of isoflurane (Fig. 23E–1).(25) Desflurane would appear to be a good anesthetic for the patient with hepatic disease due to its low metabolism, low blood solubility (allowing rapid induction and recovery from anesthesia) and cardiovascular stability (maintaining hepatic perfusion).

Nitrous oxide has been used in patients with hepatic disease in an effort to decrease the amount of volatile anesthetic required for anesthesia. There are no reports of direct hepatic injury caused by exposure to nitrous oxide as used in clinical practice. There is evidence of hepatic injury (centrilobular necrosis) caused by nitrous oxide in the hypoxic rat model.(26) It is unknown whether the mechanism of hepatic injury in hypoxic rats for nitrous oxide is the same as for halothane.

MUSCLE RELAXANTS

Nondepolarizing muscle relaxants such as pancuronium and vecuronium are metabolized by the liver (Chapter 13). Effects of these relaxants may be prolonged in patients with hepatic disease. Concurrent administration of aminoglycoside antibiotics with nondepolarizing muscle relaxants may also prolong neuromuscular blockade.(27) This is likely to be a problem in large animals such as the horse, for which prolonged recumbency may adversely affect recovery to standing. Atracurium is a nondepolarizing muscle relaxant whose metabolism is independent of hepatic function. Atracurium undergoes plasma degradation via a metabolic pathway termed *Hofmann elimination* that is primarily dependent on plasma pH and temperature.(28) For patients with hepatic disease requiring neuromuscular blockade, atracurium seems to be a good choice.

Succinylcholine is a depolarizing muscle relaxant that is degraded by plasma cholinesterase. Cholinesterases are produced by the liver. Organophosphate compounds have cholinesterase-inhibiting activity and may potentiate the action of succinylcholine.(29) The phenothiazine tranquilizers (e.g., acepromazine) may inhibit cholinesterase activity, so succinylcholine should be used cautiously in patients medicated with acepromazine. Both acepromazine and succinylcholine should be avoided in patients with hepatic disease.

Centrally acting muscle relaxants such as guaifenesin (glyceryl guaiacolate) or mephenesin are metabolized by the liver.(30, 31) Although the margin of safety for use of guaifenesin is wide, side effects following administration of large doses include moderate hypotension, decreased tidal volume, and concentration-dependent hemolysis. Toxic effects may be caused by the metabolite catechol, which causes seizures, opisthotonos, prolonged incoordination and respiratory paralysis (Chapter 13). Increased incidence in side effects or occurrence of toxic effects may be observed when guaifenesin is administered to animals with hepatic disease.

General Guidelines For Patients with Hepatic Disease

Most anesthetics are metabolized by the liver, so elimination may be significantly slowed in animals that are hypothermic. Use of heated circulating water blankets and administration of warm intravenous or irrigation fluids is advised.

Glucose metabolism is frequently affected by hepatic disease. Homeostasis of glucose can be maintained with loss of up to 80% of functional liver mass. Nevertheless, patients with severe hepatic disease that are stressed by anesthesia and surgery may become hypoglycemic. Hypoglycemia is present in 35% of dogs with portal-caval shunts.(32) For this reason blood glucose concentration is routinely determined and glucose (e.g, 5% dextrose in water) administered when indicated. If not corrected, hypoglycemia may delay recovery from anesthesia.

Excessive weight of ascitic fluid may impede lung expansion and pulmonary function. Ascitic fluid should be removed prior to anesthesia. Rapid removal of a large quantity of fluid may result in a fluid shift from the vascular space to the abdominal cavity as the formation of ascites continues. When removing massive amounts of ascitic fluid, intravenous fluids should be simultaneously administered to avoid cardiovascular collapse. Hypoalbuminemia is often present in patients with liver disease. When albumin concentration is less than 1.5 g/dL, the plasma oncotic pressure is decreased such that pulmonary edema may occur following intravenous fluid administration. Arterial blood pressure may be difficult to maintain when plasma oncotic pressure is significantly decreased. Replacement of albumin and plasma proteins is indicated in these cases. If matched plasma from a donor animal is not available, dextran 70 (up to 20 mL/kg) may be administered. Although dextran will aid in reestablishing plasma oncotic pressure, its duration of effect is not as great as that of plasma (Chapter 19).

Seizures resulting from hepatic encephalopathy may require treatment. Diazepam or phenobarbital are commonly used to control seizures. Avoid use of anesthetics that may induce seizure activity such as enflurane, ketamine, tiletamine (Telazol), or methohexital. There is increased cerebral sensitivity to gamma-aminobutyric acid (GABA) in some patients with hepatic disease. This increased sensitivity to GABAergic inhibition within the CNS may enhance the depressant effects of the barbiturates and benzodiazepine tranquilizers.

When there is concern about an animal's ability to metabolize anesthetics because of hepatic disease, use of local anesthesia should be considered. Although animals that are not depressed usually require tranquilization for effective use of local anesthesia, those with hepatic disease are likely to be depressed, and therefore may require less tranquilization or sedation. Local anesthetics of the ester class (e.g., procaine, tetracaine) are metabolized by plasma cholinesterases produced by the liver, whereas the amide class (lidocaine, mepivacaine, bupivacaine) is directly metabolized by the liver. For this reason, the generalized effects of local anesthetics may be prolonged in patients with severe hepatic disease long after local analgesia has waned. This is unlikely to be a major deterrent for their clinical use.

Because of the liver's role in production of coagulation factors, the coagulation profile should be evaluated before surgery in patients with hepatic disease. If coagulopathy exists, clotting factors or whole blood should be available and administered.

A major complication associated with major surgery in people is thromboembolic disease. Thromboembolic disease can be attenuated by anesthetic technique in selected surgical procedures. For example, there is less intraoperative activation of fibrinolysis and pulmonary thromboembolism in people undergoing total hip arthroplasty when using epidural or spinal anesthesia versus injectable or inhalation anesthesia.(33, 34) Women undergoing hysterectomy develop clinical signs of deep vein thrombosis with a frequency as high as 30%.(35) Higher Factor VIII Complex levels may account for the increased incidence of thromboembolic

disease following hysterectomy with general anesthesia compared to epidural anesthesia. Factor VIII Complex is increased to a lesser degree in women undergoing hysterectomy during epidural bupivacaine anesthesia compared to those anesthetized with enflurane.(36)

Epidural opioids are associated with similar benefits in terms of postoperative coagulation status and thromboembolic disease. In obese patients undergoing gastroplasty for weight reduction, those receiving epidural morphine postoperatively have fewer clinical signs of deep vein thrombosis and an earlier return to normal pulmonary function than patients given intramuscular morphine. It is unknown if epidurally injected local anesthetics and opioids alter neuroendocrine function in a similar fashion, resulting in altered postoperative coagulation.

Little is known about the influence of anesthetic technique on coagulation in animals. In dogs, platelet aggregation was significantly decreased following administration of acepromazine and atropine but returned to normal during subsequent halothane anesthesia and surgery.(37) Coagulation deficiencies such as thrombocytopenia, increased prothrombin time, increased activated partial thromboplastin time, hypofibrinogenemia, increased fibrin degradation products, and decreased antithrombin III are associated with gastric dilation/volvulus.(38) In dogs undergoing colonic anastomosis, there was less intraoperative bleeding and more advanced healing (detected histologically) 1 and 7 days after surgery following epidural bupivacaine and general anesthesia when compared to general anesthesia alone.(39) Much work remains to be done to identify anesthetic techniques having the least effect on normal coagulation and healing during the convalescent period.

Portal-Caval Shunt

Portal-caval shunt is most frequently encountered in the dog. Dogs with this congenital vascular anomaly are usually gaunt and small for their breed and age. Anesthetic management of the dog with portal-caval shunt should be based on presenting clinical signs and physical status (Table 23E–2). Signs of hepatic encephalopathy and hypokalemia may be present. Hypokale-

Table 23E–2. Problems Associated with Portal-Caval Shunt

Problem	Significance
Weight loss	May affect drug dose, disposition
Hypoalbuminemia	May affect drug dose, disposition, or plasma oncotic pressure
Hepatic shunt	Loss of hepatic metabolism of drugs
Low bile salts	Increase absorption of intestinal endotoxin
Portal hypertension	May require second surgery and central venous pressure monitoring

mia in animals with portal-caval shunt may be caused by gastrointestinal (vomiting and diarrhea) or urinary loss (diuresis). Hypokalemia ([K+] < 3.5 mEq/L) should be corrected prior to anesthesia. Intravenous potassium administration should not exceed the rate of $0.5 \text{ mEq} \cdot \text{kg}^{-1} \cdot \text{h}^{-1}$.

Chronic hepatic dysfunction may be associated with increased GABAergic sensitivity and permeability of the blood-brain barrier. The effect of anesthetics and anesthetic adjuncts may be greater than expected and unpredictable. Diazepam is frequently used as preanesthetic medication in dogs with portal-caval shunt. Antagonists of the benzodiazepine receptor such as flumazenil (Romazicon) have been reported to ameliorate signs of encephalopathy in a woman [40] and in animal models [41, 42] of portal-caval shunt. The value of flumazenil in the perioperative management of dogs with portal-caval shunt remains to be determined.

Animals with portal-caval shunt may have hepatic insufficiency. When termination of action is highly dependent upon drug hepatic metabolism (e.g., ketamine, acepromazine, xylazine) such drugs should be avoided. Drugs that are highly protein bound (e.g., barbiturates) will be more active in animals with hypoalbuminemia. Drugs such as methohexital and ketamine that may induce seizure activity are contraindicated in animals with hepatic encephalopathy. Of the inhaled anesthetics, methoxyflurane undergoes greatest metabolism by the liver. Thus, elimination of methoxyflurane may be prolonged in the animal with portal-caval shunt. Halothane may cause hepatopathy in animals with poor hepatic perfusion and oxygenation, and therefore should be used cautiously in patients with portal-caval shunt. Isoflurane is the preferred anesthetic in patients with this condition. Mask induction and maintenance with isoflurane is frequently used. Opioids may be used as analgesic supplements prior to or following anesthesia for surgical correction of the shunt.

Arterial blood pressure should be monitored during portal-caval shunt surgery. Hypoalbuminemia predisposes the patient to hypotension that may be revealed by isoflurane induced peripheral vasodilation. Judicious use of plasma or dextran 70 (10-20 mL/kg given over 1 h) to aid in maintenance of plasma oncotic pressure may be indicated. At high concentrations of isoflurane, myocardial contractility and cardiac output are also decreased. Hypotensive patients with portal-caval shunt may fail to respond to catecholamine infusions such as dobutamine or dopamine. Surgical retraction of the liver or compression of the caudal vena cava may further decrease venous return, cardiac output, and arterial blood pressure.

Intraoperative management of the patient for correction of portal-caval shunt is often uneventful until the shunt is ligated. In normal dogs, portal pressure is reported to be between 6 and 15 cm of H_2O, whereas portal pressure in dogs with portal-caval shunt is usually lower.[43] Following surgical correction of the shunt, portal venous pressure should not be more than 9 cm of H_2O above baseline measurement, or a maximum of 20 cm of H_2O.[44] Intraoperative measurement of central venous pressure is a useful method for estimating portal resistance and for predicting the development of postoperative portal hypertension.[45] A decrease in central venous pressure after ligation of a single portal-caval shunt indicates decreased transit of blood from the intestine to the vena cava. Central venous pressure should not decrease by more than 1 cm of H_2O from baseline measurement at 3 minutes after ligation to avoid postoperative portal hypertension.[46]

Animals with portal-caval shunts may have decreased production of bile salts. Lack of bile salts in the intestine allows absorption of endotoxin.[47] Intestinal ischemia associated with portal hypertension may enhance absorption of endotoxin. Flunixin meglumine (1 mg/kg IV) has been shown to improve cardiovascular function in dogs with experimental endotoxemia.[48] Consequently, use of flunixin meglumine in dogs with evidence of endotoxemia secondary to portal-caval shunt has been suggested.[49]

References

1. Merin RG, et al. Comparison of the effects of isoflurane and desflurane on cardiovascular dynamics and regional blood flow in the chronically instrumented dog. Anesthesiology 74:568, 1991.
2. Rowland M, Tozer TN. Clinical pharmacokinetics, 2nd ed. Philadelphia: Lea & Febiger, 1989.
3. Moore JN, Traver DS, Coffman JR. Large bowel obstruction and chronic active hepatitis in a horse. Vet Med Small Anim Clin 71:1457, 1976.
4. Meyer DJ, Embert HC, Rich LJ. Veterinary laboratory medicine: interpretation and diagnosis. Philadelphia: WB Saunders, 1992.
5. West HJ. Evaluation of total plasma bile acid concentrations for the diagnosis of hepatobiliary disease in horses. Res Vet Sci 46:264, 1989.
6. White PF. What's new in intravenous anesthetics? Anesthesiol Clin North Am 6:297, 1988.
7. Muir WW, Mason DE. Side effects of etomidate in dogs. J Am Vet Med Assoc 194:1430, 1989.
8. Kruse-Elliot KT, Swanson CR, Aucoin DP. Effects of etomidate on adrenocortical function in canine surgical patients. Am J Vet Res 48:1098, 1987.
9. Nebauer AE, Doenicke A, Hoernecke R, Angster R, Mayer M. Does etomidate cause haemolysis? Br J Anaesth 69:58–60, 1992.
10. Ko JCH, Thurmon JC, Benson GJ, Tranquilli WJ, Hoffmann WE. Acute haemolysis associated with etomidate-propylene glycol infusion in dogs. J Vet Anaesth 20:92–94, 1993.
11. Ilkiw JE. Other potentially useful new injectable anesthetic agents. Vet Clin North Am 22:281, 1992.
12. Cousins MJ, Sharp JH, Gourlay GK. Hepatotoxicity and halothane metabolism in an animal model with application for human toxicity. Anaesth Intensive Care 7:9, 1979.
13. Engelking LR, et al. Effects of halothane anesthesia on equine liver function. Am J Vet Res 44:607, 1984.
14. Dykes MHM. Anesthetic hepatotoxicity. In: Hershey SG, ed. Refresher courses in anesthesiology. Philadelphia: JB Lippincott, 1982.
15. Cahalan MK. Post-operative hepatic dysfunction. ASA Annual Refresher Course Lectures, Las Vegas, Nevada, 133:1, 1982.
16. Benson GJ, Brock KA. Halothane-associated hepatitis and methoxyflurane-related nephropathy: a review. J Vet Pharmacol Ther 3:187, 1980.
17. Bird GL, Williams R. Detection of antibodies to a halothane

metabolite hapten in sera from patients with halothane-associated hepatitis. J Hepatol 9:366, 1989.

18. Kenna JG, Satoh H, Christ DD, Pohl LR. Metabolic basis for a drug hypersensitivity: antibodies in sera from patients with halothane hepatitis recognize liver neoantigens that contain the trifluoroacetyl group derived from halothane. J Pharmacol Exp Ther 245:1103, 1988.

19. Pohl LR, et al. Hapten carrier conjugates associated with halothane hepatitis. Adv Exp Med Biol 283:111, 1991.

20. O'Brien TD, et al. Hepatic necrosis following halothane anesthesia in goats. J Am Vet Med Assoc 189:1591, 1986.

21. Cousins MK. Mechanisms and evaluation of hepatotoxicity. ASA Refresher Course Lectures, New Orleans, Louisiana, 204:1, 1984.

22. Halsey MJ, Sawyer DC, Eger EI. Hepatic metabolism of halothane, methoxyflurane, cyclopropane, ethrane, and forane in miniature swine. Anesthesiology 35:43, 1971.

23. Gelman S, Fowler KC, Smith LR. Regional blood flow during isoflurane and halothane anesthesia. Anesth Analg 63:557, 1984.

24. Eger EI. Isoflurane: a review. Anesthesiology 55:559, 1981.

25. Koblin DD. Characteristics and implications of desflurane metabolism and toxicity. Anesth Analg 75:S10, 1992.

26. Fassoulaki A, et al. Nitrous oxide, too, is hepatotoxic in rats. Anesth Analg 63:1076, 1984.

27. Forsyth SF, Ilkiw JE, Hildebrand SV. Effect of gentamicin administration on the neuromuscular blockade induced by atracurium in cats. Am J Vet Res 51:1675, 1990.

28. Hughes R, Chapple DJ. The pharmacology of atracurium: a new competitive neuromuscular blocking agent. Br J Anaesth 53:31, 1981.

29. Himes JA, Edds GT, Kirkham WW, Neal FC. Potentiation of succinylcholine by organophosphate compounds in horses. J Am Vet Med Assoc 151:54, 1967.

30. Funk KA. Glyceryl guaiacolate: a centrally acting muscle relaxant. Equine Vet J 2:173, 1970.

31. Davis LE, Wolff WA. Pharmacokinetics and metabolism of glyceryl guaiacolate in ponies. Am J Vet Res 31:469, 1970.

32. Armstrong PJ. Problem: Hypoglycemia. Proc Fourth Annual Vet Med Forum ACVIM, 1986:103.

33. Davis FM, et al. Influence of spinal and general anaesthesia on hemostasis during total hip arthroplasty. Br J Anaesth 59:561, 1987.

34. Modig J, et al. Thromboembolism after total hip replacement: role of epidural and general anesthesia. Anesth Analg 62:174, 1983.

35. Rakoczi I, Chamone D, Collen D, Verstraete M. Prediction of postoperative leg-vein thrombosis in gynaecological patients. Lancet 8:509, 1978.

36. Bredbacka S, et al. Pre- and postoperative changes in coagulation and fibrinolytic variables during abdominal hysterectomy under epidural or general anaesthesia. Acta Anaesthesiol Scand 30:204, 1986.

37. Barr SC, Ludders JW, Looney AL, Gleed RD. Platelet aggregation in dogs after sedation with acepromazine and atropine and during subsequent general anesthesia and surgery. Am J Vet Res 53:2067, 1992.

38. Millis DL, Hauptman JG. Coagulation abnormalities and gastric necrosis in canine gastric dilatation-volvulus [Abstract]. Vet Surg 20:342, 1991.

39. Blass CE, et al. The effect of epidural and general anesthesia on the healing of colonic anastomoses. Vet Surg 16:75, 1987.

40. Ferenci P, Grimm G, Meryn S, Gangl A. Successful loading-term treatment of portal-systemic encephalopathy by the benzodiazepine antagonist flumazenil. Gastroenterology 96:240, 1989.

41. Bassett ML, Mullen KD, Skolnik P, Jones EA. Amelioration of hepatic encephalopathy by pharmacologic antagonists of the $GABA_A$-benzodiazepine receptor complex in a rabbit model of fulminant hepatic failure. Gastroenterology 93:1069, 1987.

42. Baraldi M, et al. Supersensitivity of benzodiazepine receptors in hepatic encephalopathy due to fulminant hepatic failure in the rat: reversal by a benzodiazepine antagonist. Clin Sci 67:167, 1984.

43. Swalec KM. Portosystemic shunts. In: Bojrab MJ, ed. Disease mechanisms in small animal surgery, 2nd ed. Philadelphia: Lea & Febiger, 1993.

44. Breznock EM, Whiting PG. Portacaval shunts and anomalies. In: Slatter DH, ed. Textbook of small animal surgery. Philadelphia: WB Saunders, 1985.

45. Swalec KM, Smeak DD, Brown J. Effects of mechanical and pharmacologic manipulations on portal pressure, central venous pressure, and heart rate in dogs. Am J Vet Res 52:1327, 1991.

46. Swalec KM, Smeak DD. Partial versus complete attenuation of single portosystemic shunts. Vet Surg 19:406, 1990.

47. Bailey ME. Endotoxin, bile salts, and renal function in obstructive jaundice. Br J Surg 63:774, 1976.

48. Bottoms GD, Johnson MA, Roesel OF. Endotoxin-induced hemodynamic changes in dogs: role of thromboxane and prostaglandin I_2. Am J Vet Res 44:1497, 1983.

49. Trim CM. Anesthesia and the liver. In: Slatter DH, ed. Textbook of small animal surgery. Philadelphia: WB Saunders, 1985.

GASTROINTESTINAL DISEASE

Stephen A. Greene

CONDITIONS ASSOCIATED WITH THE ORAL
    CAVITY AND PHARYNX
REMOVAL OF ESOPHAGEAL FOREIGN
    BODIES
ANESTHESIA FOR DOGS WITH GASTRIC
    DILATION/VOLVULUS

ANESTHETIC MANAGEMENT OF HORSES
    WITH ACUTE ABDOMINAL DISTRESS
DISPLACED ABOMASUM
DISORDERS OF THE PANCREAS
OBESITY

Conditions Associated with the Oral Cavity and Pharynx

Animals with trauma or space-occupying masses of the head and neck frequently require general anesthesia. These patients are often difficult to intubate to secure and maintain a patent airway. Fractures of the mandible, maxilla, or temporomandibular joint may not permit examination to determine the range of jaw motion. Temporal myositis may prevent opening of the mouth even while the patient is anesthetized. General anesthesia without a secure airway may result in aspiration, which can be fatal (Chapter 17). Anesthetic management of these conditions should be initiated by preparing for placement of a tracheostomy tube. In the dog, a combination of acepromazine (0.05 mg/kg IM) and oxymorphone (0.2 mg/kg IV) will induce neuroleptanalgesia, permitting the mouth and jaw to be examined without inducing apnea or severe respiratory depression. Owing to oxymorphone-induced vagal bradycardia, premedication with an anticholinergic is recommended. In dogs weighing over 40 lb, a maximum dose of 4 mg of oxymorphone is suggested to prevent excessive respiratory depression. In the cat, a low dose of ketamine (4 mg/kg IM) combined with acepromazine (0.05 mg/kg) usually permits examination of the oral cavity.

Intramuscular or subcutaneous administration of xylazine in the dog or cat may cause emesis (Table 23F-1). Dogs and cats with oral or pharyngeal masses are at high risk for aspiration pneumonia, so xylazine, morphine, and other drugs that induce emesis should be avoided. Xylazine administration in large animals is not associated with emesis and may be used to sedate horses (0.5 to 1 mg/kg IV) or cattle (0.1 mg/kg IM) for oral examination.

Removal of Esophageal Foreign Bodies

General anesthesia may be required for removal of esophageal foreign bodies in a variety of species. In the horse that has a foreign object lodged in the esophagus

Table 23F–1. Gastrointestinal Effects of Drugs Used During Anesthesia

Drug	Effect
Acepromazine	Antiemetic
Atropine	Decreased motility
Cholinesterase inhibitors	Increased motility
Detomidine	Decreased motility
Diazepam	Appetite stimulant
Halothane	Decreased mucosal blood flow
Morphine	Emetic, gastrointestinal stimulant
Xylazine	Decreased motility; emetic

("choke"), passage of a nasogastric tube or endoscope is facilitated by sedation with xylazine (0.5 mg/kg) or detomidine (10-20 µg/kg) (Dormoseden; Pfizer Inc., West Chester, Pennsylvania). If the foreign body cannot be retrieved or dislodged, the horse is anesthetized. Relaxation of the striated muscular coat of the esophagus may aid in removal of the obstruction. Skeletal muscle relaxation is enhanced at deeper planes of anesthesia. Muscle relaxation may also be improved by induction of anesthesia with guaifenesin (5% solution in 5% dextrose combined with 0.3% thiopental given to effect) or by administration of a neuromuscular blocker. In the horse and cat, the proximal two thirds of the esophagus has a striated muscle layer, whereas in the dog, the entire esophagus contains striated muscle.(1) In the anesthetized dog and horse, skeletal muscle relaxation of the esophagus may be improved with a short-acting muscle relaxant (e.g., atracurium; 0.2 mg/kg IV) (Chapter 19). Administration of atracurium must be accompanied by tracheal intubation and support of ventilation.

Anesthesia For Dogs with Gastric Dilation/Volvulus

It has been estimated that there are between 40 and 60 thousand cases of canine gastric dilation/volvulus per year in the United States.(2) The condition is associated with multiple system problems (Table 23F–2) resulting in a high mortality rate (40–60%).(2) The distended stomach severely restricts ventilation and decreases cardiac function. Metabolic alkalosis may develop from gastric sequestration of hydrogen ions. Later in the course of the disease, metabolic acidosis may occur from decreased cardiac output and poor ventilation resulting in tissue hypoxia and lactate production. Consequently, cardiac arrhythmias such as sinus tachycardia or ventricular premature contractions are frequently observed. Because the metabolic status is difficult to predict, it is suggested that serum electrolytes, blood pH, and plasma bicarbonate concentration be measured prior to anesthesia. In one study, hypokalemia was present in 33% of the dogs with gastric dilation/volvulus.(3) Electrolyte abnormalities, acid-base imbalance, and gastric distension should be corrected as soon as possible. The derangements in acid-base balance frequently lead to shock if untreated. Restoration of circulating plasma volume should be initiated using high doses of isotonic saline (90 mL/kg IV) or hypertonic saline solution (7%, 4 mL/kg IV) (Chapter 19). In dogs with experimentally induced gastric dilation/volvulus and shock a combination of 7% hypertonic saline in 6% dextran 70 (5 mL/kg IV) was superior to isotonic saline (60 ml/kg IV) for resuscitation.(4)

Cardiac arrhythmias should be identified and treated prior to induction of anesthesia. Lidocaine (4 mg/kg IV, then 20–80 $\mu g \cdot kg^{-1} \cdot min^{-1}$) and procainamide (0.5–2 mg/kg IV, then 20–40 $\mu g \cdot kg^{-1} \cdot min^{-1}$) separately or in combination have been used for treating premature ventricular contractions or ventricular tachycardia. Quinidine (6–8 mg/kg IM every 6 hours) has also been

Table 23F–2. Problems Associated with Gastric Dilation/Volvulus

Problem	Significance
Acidosis/alkalosis	pH should be measured.
Cardiac arrhythmias	Attempt correction prior to anesthesia.
Gastric necrosis	May cause arrhythmias
Hypokalemia/hyperkalemia	K^+ should be measured
Impaired venous return	Correct by decompressing stomach; treat shock.
Respiratory impairment	Correct by decompressing stomach; ventilate.
Peritonitis	Begin antibiotics; poor prognosis.
Shock	Correct underlying problems.

recommended for treatment of arrhythmias in dogs with gastric dilation/volvulus. Postoperative treatment of cardiac arrhythmias may also be necessary. A continuous lidocaine infusion may be prepared by adding 25 mL of 2% lidocaine to each 500 mL of fluid given at a daily maintenance rate of 66 mL $\cdot$ kg^{-1} $\cdot$ day^{-1}.

Administration of oxygen via face mask should be begun before induction of anesthesia. Large doses of arrhythmogenic agents such as thiobarbiturates or halothane should be avoided. Xylazine should be avoided as a sedative because it may cause aerophagia.(5) In addition, xylazine causes decreased gastrointestinal sphincter pressure and may allow increased gastric reflux.(6) Xylazine decreases intestinal motility in the dog and may prolong recovery of normal gastrointestinal function following correction of the gastric distension.(7) Neuroleptanalgesic combinations such as Innovar-Vet (0.5 mL/20 kg IV) or the combination of diazepam (0.2 mg/kg IV) and oxymorphone (0.1 mg/kg IV) are good choices for induction of anesthesia in dogs with unstable cardiovascular function. Opioids may decrease intestinal motility, but this effect is usually of minor clinical significance.(8) Diazepam-ketamine has also been suggested as a good choice for induction of anesthesia. For maintenance of anesthesia, isoflurane appears to be superior to other inhalants. Nitrous oxide is contraindicated prior to gastric decompression because it will equilibrate with gas in the stomach, increasing the intragastric volume and pressure.

Succinylcholine initially causes contraction of skeletal muscle. The distended stomach is predisposed to rupture if succinylcholine is administered prior to relief of excessive gastric pressure. If a neuromuscular blocking agent is used in the anesthetic management of gastric dilation/volvulus, it should be a nondepolarizing drug such as pancuronium or atracurium.

Of the dogs that die from gastric dilation/volvulus, 50% die on the day of surgery.(9) Death is usually associated with septic shock or peritonitis secondary to gastric necrosis or perforation.(10) Reperfusion injury has also been implicated as a factor associated with the high mortality from this condition.(11) Iron chelating drugs such as deferoxamine (Desferal) are currently being evaluated for their ability to decrease injury in anoxic tissues that are subsequently reperfused.

Anesthetic Management of Horses with Acute Abdominal Distress

Acute abdominal distress in horses is often characterized by severe pain. Pain elicits a variety of responses that include release of catecholamines and corticosteroids.(12) The stress response and sympathetic stimulation resulting from pain are detrimental to the animal's well-being. It is often difficult to perform diagnostic procedures or examine a horse in severe pain. Judicious use of analgesics in horses with acute abdominal distress is essential.

The alpha$_2$-agonists xylazine and detomidine are used extensively in horses with acute abdominal pain because of their strong analgesic and sedative effects (Chapter 8). Depending upon the amount of xylazine or detomidine administered in the preoperative period, the induction dose of anesthetic may need to be decreased. Cardiovascular depression associated with alpha$_2$-agonists will persist longer than either sedation or analgesia. Even though the sedative effects of these drugs may have waned, the anesthetic requirement will be decreased. At a comparable dose, detomidine is more potent than xylazine and has a longer analgesic and sedative action.(13–15) High doses of detomidine (i.e., 0.02 mg/kg IV) decrease cardiac output by 50%.(16) The increased potency and duration of side effects may limit the use of detomidine as a premedicant for horses undergoing surgery to correct intestinal problems.

Xylazine is a suitable alternative to detomidine in the compromised horse. However, the 1.1-mg/kg intravenous dose of xylazine should be decreased (or avoided altogether) to prevent excessive cardiovascular depression. Xylazine prolongs gastrointestinal transit time in a variety of species.(17) In the horse, xylazine (0.55 mg/kg IV) has been shown to decrease the motility index of circular and longitudinal muscle layers for 30 minutes.(18) In ponies, xylazine (1.1 mg/kg IV) induces increased intestinal vascular resistance, motility, and oxygen consumption.(19) In a study of cecal and right ventral colon myoelectric activity in ponies, xylazine (0.5 mg/kg IV) and/or butorphanol (0.04 mg/kg IV) resulted in decreased coordinated spike bursts for 20 minutes or longer.(20) It should be appreciated that the results of these studies were derived from horses or ponies with healthy gastrointestinal function. Clinically, it appears that these effects are rarely a disadvantage to using xylazine for preanesthetic medication in horses with colic. Furthermore, a study comparing myoelectric activity in equine intestine following three anesthetic regimens found no prolonged effect associated with (a) xylazine and ketamine, (b) thiopental and halothane, or (c) thiopental in guaifenesin and halothane.(21) The conclusion from that study was that the particular regimen of general anesthesia is relatively unimportant in the development of motility disturbances in horses after anesthesia.

Excessive cardiovascular depression is avoided in the compromised patient by decreasing the preanesthetic dose of xylazine (0.1–0.5 mg/kg IV) and the subsequent administration of diazepam (0.02–0.04 mg/kg IV) or guaifenesin (55–80 mg/kg IV) when inducing anesthesia with ketamine (1.5–2 mg/kg IV). Induction may be accomplished with ketamine as a bolus or in combination with guaifenesin (1 to 2 grams ketamine per liter of 5% guaifenesin). An alternative induction regime is to combine thiopental (2–4 mg/kg) with guaifenesin, given to effect. Induction of anesthesia when using thiopental and guaifenesin does not depend on heavy sedation to prevent rigidity or excitement as does induction with ketamine.

Anesthesia may be maintained with either halothane or isoflurane (1.5–2.5%) in oxygen. Halothane has been associated with a 62% decrease in intestinal blood flow in ponies anesthetized at one minimal alveolar concentration (MAC).(22) However, clinically significant deleterious effects of halothane on recovery from colic surgery have not been demonstrated. Horses anesthetized with isoflurane have higher cardiac outputs than horses anesthetized with a similar MAC of halothane.(23) Isoflurane anesthesia in the horse undergoing surgery for colic was associated with a higher heart rate and lower arterial CO_2 concentration as compared with halothane.(24) Horses anesthetized with isoflurane recover more rapidly than those anesthetized with halothane.(24, 25) Thus, there are advantages to using isoflurane for the horse undergoing surgery for colic that may outweigh the added expense of isoflurane.

Damaged intestinal tissue may release toxins into the systemic circulation, which can lead to cardiovascular dysfunction and decreased tissue perfusion. Release of eicosanoids (leukotrienes, prostacyclins, prostaglandins, and thromboxanes) has been associated with colonic volvulus in ponies.(26) Administration of flunixin meglumine (1 mg/kg IV) may counteract deleterious effects of toxins released during abdominal surgery. In addition, generation of free radicals in the equine intestine following anoxia and subsequent reoxygenation has been demonstrated in vitro.(27) Such studies may be the basis for the empiric intraoperative treatment of certain cases of equine colic with free radical quenchers such as dimethylsulfoxide (DMSO).

Opioid agonists such as oxymorphone, morphine, and meperidine can be safely used in horses experiencing pain.(28) These drugs frequently induce undesirable excitement in horses that are pain free, unless preceded with a suitable sedative or tranquilizer (e.g, xylazine or acepromazine). Use of an opioid agonist-antagonist such as butorphanol may be advantageous because this drug provides analgesia but has a "ceiling" on respiratory depression.(29)

In addition to pain control, support of the respiratory and cardiovascular systems is paramount in managing anesthesia for colic surgery. The bulk and weight of the gastrointestinal tract filled with ingesta and/or gas impair venous return to the heart and consequently decrease cardiac output. Diaphragmatic excursion and pulmonary function are impaired by a full stomach during anesthesia. These effects decrease tissue perfusion and oxygenation creating metabolic acidosis and complicating the anesthetic management of the horse. Evaluation of acid-base status will aid in determining adequacy of ventilation. Respiratory acidosis (pH < 7.2) can be avoided by use of controlled ventilation (Chapter 18). Aggressive fluid therapy with lactated Ringer's solution will aid in correcting mild to moderate metabolic acidosis if normovolemia is reestablished (Chapter 19).(30) It is not uncommon for a horse to require 30 or more liters of isotonic intravenous fluids during colic surgery.

Monitoring arterial blood pressure is recommended in all species in order to provide some indirect information concerning cardiac output and tissue perfusion (Chapter 15). Low tissue perfusion has been implicated in the occurrence of postanesthetic myositis (Chapter 2).(31) Maintenance of a mean arterial blood pressure above 70 mm Hg may be achieved by fluid administration, by adjusting anesthetic depth, and by careful infusion of dobutamine (3–5 $\mu g \cdot kg^{-1} \cdot min^{-1}$ IV) or another sympathomimetic drug. Improved cardiac output will result when intravenous fluids are administered to the hemoconcentrated patient. A decreased packed cell volume will decrease blood viscosity and improve cardiac output. Hypertonic saline (7% at 4 mL/kg IV) has been recommended for use in the hypovolemic horse to rapidly expand plasma volume.(32) One advantage of hypertonic saline administration over isotonic crystalloid solutions is that a small volume is required. Correction of an extracellular volume deficit via administration of a small volume of hypertonic saline is accomplished more rapidly than with the administration of a large volume of isotonic fluids. However, the beneficial effects of hypertonic saline administration are short-lived and should be preserved during anesthesia with subsequent isotonic crystalloid therapy (Chapters 18 and 19).

Cardiac arrhythmias may occur during anesthesia for surgical correction of an intestinal disorder. Bradycardia caused by increased vagal tone elicited from intestinal manipulation has been observed. Anticholinergic agents are occasionally used in horses for treatment of vagal-induced bradycardia. However, high doses of these drugs may decrease gastrointestinal motility for up to 12 hours in horses.(33) Horses treated with anticholinergics are more likely to develop postanesthetic colic if they have been fed within 4 to 6 hours of anesthesia.(34) Perhaps a more important concern during anesthesia is the effect of atropine administration on cardiac arrhythmogenicity. Administration of atropine to halothane-anesthetized horses was associated with an increased incidence of tachycardia after administration of epinephrine (35) or dobutamine (36). Thus, treatment of hypotension with a catecholamine may induce a life-threatening cardiac arrhythmia in the halothane-anesthetized horse that has been medicated with atropine.

Displaced Abomasum

Displaced abomasum is frequently a problem in adult dairy cattle and occasionally in other ruminants such as the llama. In adult cattle a standing laparotomy is the standard surgical approach. Regional anesthesia for standing laparotomy may be accomplished by a number of techniques including the distal paravertebral block, the proximal paravertebral block, and the line block (Chapter 16). For small ruminants such as the goat, sheep, or llama, general anesthesia will provide a more immobilized patient on which to perform surgery. General anesthesia in small ruminants is discussed elsewhere (Chapter 20).

Particular anesthetic concerns for animals with displaced abomasum include disturbances in acid-base balance and electrolyte abnormalities. Similar to the pathogenesis of gastric dilation/volvulus in the dog, displaced abomasum in the ruminant may initially present with metabolic alkalosis caused by abomasal sequestration of hydrogen chloride. Hypokalemia is a common concurrent finding as potassium is excreted by the kidneys in an attempt to retain hydrogen ions in response to metabolic alkalosis. As the disease progresses, metabolic acidosis occurs because of poor tissue perfusion and lactate accumulation. Shock, followed by death, is expected in untreated animals. Correction of dehydration, poor circulatory volume, and electrolyte abnormalities are required. Serum chloride less than 79 mEq/L and heart rate greater than 100 are associated with a poor prognosis.(37)

Disorders of the Pancreas

Acute pancreatitis in dogs and cats is frequently associated with vomiting, anorexia, and abdominal pain. However, the diagnosis of acute pancreatitis is often difficult to make antemortem. Classic laboratory findings associated with pancreatitis (increased amylase and lipase activity) may not be observed. Conversely, increased pancreatic enzyme activity is not specific for pancreatitis. Intestinal foreign bodies are frequently associated with increased lipase activity. Exploratory laparotomy in healthy dogs (without signs of pancreatitis) in which abdominal tissues were examined but not surgically altered was associated with a threefold increase in serum lipase activity.(38) Morphine administration may cause elevation of amylase and lipase activity caused by increased smooth muscle contraction in the pancreatic duct.(39) In addition, most dogs with pancreatitis have a concurrent disease such as diabetes mellitus, hyperadrenocorticism, renal failure, neoplasia, congestive heart failure, or autoimmune disorders.(40) Acute pancreatitis has been induced by drugs, including corticosteroids, nonsteroidal antiinflammatory agents, organophosphates, thiazide diuretics, sulfonamides, tetracycline, valproic acid, furosemide, and estrogen.(41) Thus, it is likely that animals with acute pancreatitis are anesthetized for reasons unrelated to diagnosis or treatment of pancreatitis. Iatrogenic pancreatitis may also occur following abdominal surgery. Human beings occasionally develop acute pancreatitis following renal transplantation, gastrectomy, and biliary tract surgery.(42) The "incidental" finding of acute pancreatitis at necropsy of many patients with an unknown cause of death is not uncommon.

Medical management of acute pancreatitis basically consists of maintaining adequate fluid therapy and nothing per os. Establishing normal pancreatic circulation is paramount for tissue healing. Preanesthetic preparation of the patient with pancreatitis is accomplished by withholding oral intake of food and water and administering intravenous fluids to correct hydration and/or electrolyte imbalances.

The choice of anesthetics for use in the patient with pancreatitis is often based on other complicating factors identified for the patient. Intravenously administered alpha$_2$-adrenergic agents have a hyperglycemic effect owing to inhibition of insulin release by the beta cells in the islets of Langerhans of the pancreas. This effect has been observed with epinephrine and with the potent sedative-analgesics such as detomidine and xylazine.(43-48) Alpha$_2$-adrenergic agonist-induced hyperglycemia is prevented by pretreatment with yohimbine.(43, 49, 50) It is unknown whether the alpha$_2$-adrenergic effects on the pancreas are of clinical significance in patients with pancreatitis. However, a conservative approach to anesthetic management of these patients generally avoids use of these drugs. Opioid analgesics (oxymorphone, buprenorphine, or butorphanol) are a suitable alternative to provide sedation and analgesia prior to induction of anesthesia. Morphine causes spasm of the sphincter of Oddi in the gall bladder duct in 1 to 3% of the human population and may be associated with complications in patients with pancreatitis.(39) Other opioids cause less spasm of the sphincter and are useful when indicated for treatment of pain associated with pancreatitis. In human beings, epidural administration of morphine is preferred for treatment of pain associated with pancreatitis because of better pain relief with fewer side effects.(51)

There is no clear "best choice" for induction of anesthesia for the patient with pancreatitis. Halothane would not be the anesthetic of choice in patients with concurrent liver disease or in patients with cardiac dysrhythmias. Maintenance of anesthesia with isoflurane is preferred in such cases. During surgery, the anesthetist should attempt to provide vigilant monitoring of anesthetic depth, prevention of hypotension, and maintenance of adequate vascular volume.

Obesity

Obese patients often have underlying physiologic problems in addition to the condition for which anesthesia is required. Evaluation of obese animals for presence of pancreatitis, diabetes mellitus, hepatic insufficiency, or cardiac disease should be included in the diagnostic workup. The obese animal's veins may be more difficult to locate and catheterize. Drug dose should be adjusted to the patient's lean weight in order to avoid overdosing with anesthetic drugs. Obese animals anesthetized with halothane or methoxyflurane will also have a longer recovery time than other patients because of sequestration of anesthetic in fat. Isoflurane is the most desirable inhalation anesthetic for an obese animal because of its minimal biotransformation and low tissue solubility (Chapter 11).

Preoperative hypoxemia (Pickwickian syndrome) is a common feature of obesity in man and is markedly worsened by anesthesia. Obesity decreases the ventilatory capacity of a patient during anesthesia owing to decreased chest wall compliance. Hypoventilation may occur because of limited diaphragmatic excursion from the increased weight of the abdominal contents. The increased mass of the pharyngeal tissues and tongue may lead to upper airway obstruction after premedication with tranquilizers or during induction of anesthesia. Obese patients given sedatives or tranquilizers prior to anesthesia should be continuously observed for airway obstruction. Rapid control of the airway at induction and positive pressure ventilation during anesthesia is recommended. During recovery from anesthesia, obese patients should be kept intubated until they will no longer tolerate the endotracheal tube. Obese animals must regain normal muscle function in order to maintain an adequate tidal volume and a patent airway after extubation.

References

1. Nickel R, Schummer A, Seiferle E, Sack WO. The viscera of the domestic animals. New York: Springer-Verlag, 1973.
2. Canine bloat panel offers research and treatment recommendations. Friskies Res Dig 24:1, 1985.
3. Muir WW. Acid-base and electrolyte disturbances in dogs with gastric dilatation-volvulus. J Am Vet Med Assoc 181:2, 1982.
4. Allen DA, et al. Hypertonic saline/dextran resuscitation of dogs with experimentally induced gastric dilatation-volvulus shock. Am J Vet Res 52:92, 1991.
5. Booth NH. Non-narcotic analgesics. In: Booth NH, McDonald LE, eds. Veterinary pharmacology and therapeutics, 5th ed. Ames, IA: Iowa State University Press, 1982.
6. Strombeck DR, Harrold D. Effects of atropine, acepromazine, meperidine, and xylazine on gastroesophageal sphincter pressure in the dog. Am J Vet Res 46:963, 1985.
7. Hsu WH, McNeel SV. Effect of yohimbine on xylazine-induced prolongation of gastrointestinal transit in dogs. J Am Vet Med Assoc 183:297, 1983.
8. McDonell WN. General anesthesia for equine gastrointestinal and obstetric procedures. Vet Clin North Am Large Anim Pract 3:163, 1981.
9. Betts CW, et al. A retrospective study of gastric dilatation-torsion in the dog. J Small Anim Pract 15:727, 1974.
10. Matthiesen DT. The gastric dilatation-volvulus complex: medical and surgical considerations. J Am Anim Hosp Assoc 19:925, 1983.
11. Lantz GC, Badylak SF, Hiles MC, Arkin TE. Treatment of reperfusion injury in dogs with experimentally induced gastric dilatation-volvulus. Am J Vet Res 53:1594, 1992.
12. Yeager MP. Outcome of pain management. Anesthesiol Clin North Am 7:241, 1989.
13. Short CE, Matthews N, Harvey R, Tyner CL. Cardiovascular and pulmonary function studies of a new sedative/analgetic

(Detomidine/Domosedan) for use alone in horses or as a preanesthetic. Farmos Report 2:139, 1986.

14. Saarinen H. Preanesthetic use of detomidine in horses–some clinical observations. Acta Vet Scand 82:157, 1986.
15. Clarke KW, Taylor PM. Detomidine: a new sedative for horses. Equine Vet J 18:366, 1986.
16. Wagner AE, Muir WW, Hinchcliff KW. Cardiovascular effects of xylazine and detomidine in horses. Am J Vet Res 52:651, 1991.
17. Greene SA, Thurmon JC. Xylazine – a review of its pharmacology and use in veterinary medicine. J Vet Pharmacol Ther 11:295, 1988.
18. Clark SE, Thompson SA, Becht JL, Moore JN. Effects of xylazine on cecal mechanical activity and cecal blood flow in healthy horses. Am J Vet Res 49:720, 1989.
19. Stick JA, Chou CC, Derksen FJ, Arden WA. Effects of xylazine on equine intestinal vascular resistance, motility, compliance, and oxygen consumption. Am J Vet Res 48:198, 1987.
20. Rutkowski JA, Ross MW, Cullen K. Effects of xylazine and/or butorphanol or neostigmine on myoelectric activity of the cecum and right ventral colon in female ponies. Am J Vet Res 50:1096, 1989.
21. Lester GD, Bolton JR, Cullen LK, Thurgate SM. Effects of general anesthesia on myoelectric activity of the intestine in horses. Am J Vet Res 53:1553, 1992.
22. Manohar M, Goetz TE. Cerebral, renal, adrenal, intestinal, and pancreatic circulation in conscious ponies and during 1.0, 1.5, and 2.0 minimal alveolar concentrations of halothane-O_2 anesthesia. Am J Vet Res 46:2492, 1985.
23. Steffey EP, Howland D. Comparison of circulatory and respiratory effects of isoflurane and halothane anesthesia in horses. Am J Vet Res 40:821, 1980.
24. Harvey RC, et al. Isoflurane anesthesia for equine colic surgery. Vet Surg 16:184, 1987.
25. Matthews NS, Miller SM, Hartsfield SM, Slater MP. Comparison of recoveries from halothane vs isoflurane anesthesia in horses. J Am Vet Med Assoc 201:559, 1992.
26. Stick JA, et al. Thromboxane and prostacyclin production in ponies with colonic volvulus. Am J Vet Res 53:563, 1992.
27. Johnston JK, Freeman DE, Gillette D, Soma LR. Effects of superoxide dismutase on injury induced by anoxia and reoxygenation in equine small intestine in vitro. Am J Vet Res 52:2050, 1991.
28. Muir WW. Drugs used to produce standing chemical restraint in horses. Vet Clin North Am Large Anim Pract 3:17, 1981.
29. Nagashima H, et al. Respiratory and circulatory effects of intravenous butorphanol and morphine. Clin Pharmacol Ther 19:738, 1976.
30. Hartsfield SM, et al. Effects of sodium acetate, bicarbonate and lactate on acid-base status in anaesthetized dogs. J Vet Pharmacol Ther 4:51, 1981.
31. Lindsay WA, Robinson GM, Brunson DB, Majors LJ. Induction of equine postanesthetic myositis after halothane-induced hypotension. Am J Vet Res 50:404, 1989.
32. Schmall LM, Muir WW, Robertson JT. Hypertonic saline resuscitation in experimentally induced hemorrhagic shock in the horse [Abstract]. Proc SALT II Forum, Monterey, California, 1987:21.
33. Ducharme NG, Fubini SL. Gastrointestinal complications associated with the use of atropine in horses. J Am Vet Med Assoc 182:229, 1983.
34. Short CE. Special considerations for equine anesthesia. In: Short CE, ed. Principles and practice of veterinary anesthesia. Baltimore: Williams & Wilkins, 1987.
35. Lees P, Travernor WD. Influence of halothane and catecholamines on heart rate and rhythm in the horse. Br J Pharmacol 39:149, 1970.
36. Light GW, Hellyer PW, Swanson CR. Parasympathetic influence on the arrhythmogenicity of graded dobutamine infusions in halothane-anesthetized horses. Am J Vet Res 53:1154, 1992.
37. Benson GJ. Anesthetic management of ruminants and swine with selected pathophysiologic alterations. Vet Clin North Am Food Anim Pract 2:677, 1986.
38. Bellah JR, Bell G. Serum amylase and lipase activities after exploratory laparotomy in dogs. Am J Vet Res 50:1638–1641, 1989.
39. Stoelting RK. Opioid agonists and antagonists. In: Pharmacology and physiology in anesthetic practice. Philadelphia: JB Lippincott, 1987:79.
40. Cook AK, Breitschwerdt EB, Levine JF, Bunch SE, Linn LO. Risk factors associated with acute pancreatitis in dogs: 101 cases (1985–1990). J Am Vet Med Assoc 203:673–679, 1993.
41. Soergel KH. Acute pancreatitis. In: Sleisinger MH, Fordtran JS, eds. Gastrointestinal disease, 4th ed. Philadelphia: WB Saunders, 1989.
42. Estabrook SG, Levine EG, Bernstein LH. Gastrointestinal crises in intensive care. Anesthesiol Clin N Am 9:367–391, 1991.
43. Thurmon JC, et al. Xylazine hydrochloride-induced hyperglycemia and hypoinsulinemia in thoroughbred horses. J Vet Pharmacol Ther 5:241, 1982.
44. Thurmon JC, Nelson DR, Hartsfield SM, Rumore CA. Effects of xylazine hydrochloride on urine in cattle. Aust Vet J 54:178, 1978.
45. Trim CM, Hanson RR. Effects of xylazine on renal function and plasma glucose in ponies. Vet Rec 118:65, 1986.
46. Benson GJ, et al. Effect of xylazine hydrochloride upon plasma glucose and serum insulin concentrations in adult pointer dogs. J Am Anim Hosp Assoc 20:791, 1984.
47. Gasthuys F, Terpstra P, van den Hende C, DeMoor A. Hyperglycaemia and diuresis during sedation with detomidine in the horse. Zentralbl Veterinarmed 34:641, 1987.
48. Mengozzi G, et al. Adrenergic regulation of blood glucose levels and insulin release in horses: role of alpha-2 agonists and antagonists. Acta Vet Scand Suppl 87:336, 1991.
49. Greene SA, Thurmon JC, Tranquilli WJ, Benson GJ. Yohimbine prevents xylazine-induced hypoinsulinemia and hyperglycemia in mares. Am J Vet Res 48:676, 1987.
50. Hsu WH. Yohimbine increases plasma insulin concentrations and reverses xylazine-induced hypoinsulinemia in dogs. Am J Vet Res 49:242, 1988.
51. Mulholland MW, Debas HT, Bonica JJ. Diseases of the liver, biliary system, and pancreas. In: Bonica JJ, ed. The management of pain, 2nd ed. Philadelphia: Lea & Febiger, 1990:1225.

ENDOCRINE DISEASE

Robert R. Paddleford, Ralph C. Harvey

| DIABETES MELLITUS | HYPOTHYROIDISM |
| HYPOADRENOCORTICISM (ADDISON'S DISEASE) | HYPERTHYROIDISM |

Diabetes Mellitus

Insulin is essential for normal cellular function. The effects of insulin on normal cellular function include (a) inhibition of glycogenolysis, (b) inhibition of gluconeogenesis, (c) inhibition of lipolysis, (d) stimulation of glucose uptake into cells, (e) stimulation of potassium transport into cells, and (f) suppression of ketogenesis.(1)

Carbohydrate, protein, and fat metabolism are all affected with an insulin deficiency. There is a decreased uptake of glucose, especially in fat and muscle. There is loss of control of hepatic gluconeogenesis, with the resultant hyperglycemia leading to osmotic diuresis. There is catabolism of muscle for energy, and protein synthesis is inhibited resulting in muscle wasting. There is production of acetylcoenzyme A and ketone bodies for energy. There is inhibition of lipolysis regulation and a resultant accumulation of ketone bodies with osmotic diuresis and metabolic acidosis. Prolonged hyperglycemia and ketonemia can lead to (a) metabolic acidosis, (b) dehydration, (c) circulatory collapse, (d) renal failure, and/or (e) coma and death.(1)

Diabetes mellitus should be suspected in any patient with the following clinical signs: (a) a recent history of polyuria, polydipsia, weight loss, or rapid onset of cataracts; (b) dehydration, weakness, collapse, mental dullness, hepatomegaly and/or muscle wasting; and/or (c) increased rate and depth of respiration and a sweet acetone odor to the breath. Diabetes mellitus occurs more frequently in female dogs and male cats. These clinical signs should alert the clinician to the possibility of diabetes mellitus in a patient. The presence of glucose and ketones in the urine is diagnostic. A resting blood glucose of greater than 250 mg/dL with ketonemia is a common finding. Electrolyte and renal function tests may be altered and serum alkaline phosphatase may be increased due to hepatic fatty infiltration.

The patient with diabetes mellitus should be stabilized and regulated prior to anesthesia. The anesthetic protocol is probably not as critical as the adjunct support during and after anesthesia and surgery. The key to the anesthetic management of a diabetic is to use preanesthetic and anesthetic agents that will result in the shortest anesthetic recovery time with the least amount of drug hangover. Drugs that can be antagonized (narcotics, alpha$_2$-agonists, benzodiazepine tranquilizers) or are readily eliminated from the patient (propofol, etomidate, inhalant anesthetics) should be considered. The goal is to get the patient awake as soon as possible so that the patient can resume its normal feeding schedule.

The procedure should be scheduled early in the morning following the administration of the patient's normal dose of insulin.(2) Preoperative and serial intraoperative and postoperative blood glucose levels should be determined. Ideally the blood glucose should be maintained between 150 to 250 mg/dL. During the procedure, 5% dextrose in a balanced electrolyte solution should be administered to prevent hypoglycemia.(3) Depending on the blood glucose values, the dextrose drip may need to be continued following the procedure. A rate of 11 to 15 mL $\cdot$ kg^{-1} $\cdot$ h^{-1} is usually adequate. As soon as the patient starts eating, it is probably not necessary to maintain the dextrose drip.

Close monitoring of the patient should be continued after the procedure, since the stress of anesthesia and surgery may cause a diabetic to decompensate. The use of corticosteroids may also cause decompensation and should not be used unless absolutely necessary.

Hypoadrenocorticism (Addison's Disease)

Hypoadrenocorticism is a deficiency of aldosterone and/or glucocorticoids resulting from adrenal cortex dysfunction. As with the diabetic, the patient with hypoadrenocorticism should be stabilized and regulated prior to anesthesia and surgery.

Hypoadrenocorticism can be caused either by diseases or destruction of the adrenal glands or by decreased corticotropin secretion. Primary idiopathic hypoadrenocorticism is the most common cause of hypoadrenocorticism in dogs and may be immune mediated. It is characterized by an acute necrosis of the adrenal cortex. Other diseases that may cause destruction of the adrenal glands include systemic mycosis, metastatic tumors, hemorrhagic infarction, amyloidosis of the cortices, and canine distemper, and therapy for hyperadrenocorticism that may inadvertently produce a selective deficiency of glucocorticoids caused by destruction of the zona fasciculata.(4)

Decreased corticotropin secretion may also lead to hypoadrenocorticism. Adrenocorticotropic hormone (ACTH) directly controls glucocorticoid secretion and is secreted by the pituitary gland. Decreased ACTH secretion may develop with diseases or tumors of the pituitary gland or with decreased secretion of corticotropin releasing factor (CRF) owing to hypothalamic lesions. Prolonged negative feedback from exogenous corticosteroid therapy also results in decreased ACTH secretion and atrophy of the adrenal cortex. Decreased ACTH secretion usually produces glucocorticoid insufficiency, although mineral corticoid secretion often remains normal.

The clinical signs of hypoadrenocorticism will depend on the particular adrenal hormone (aldosterone, glucocorticoids) most affected by the disease. Aldosterone's primary function is to stimulate absorption of sodium in the distal renal tubules and promote the excretion of potassium. Aldosterone deficiency produces hyponatremia and hyperkalemia. Hyponatremia with concurrent water loss can produce lethargy, nausea, impaired cardiac output, hypovolemia, hypotension, and/or impaired renal perfusion. Hyperkalemia will produce muscle weakness, decreased cardiac conduction and excitability and bradycardia.

Glucocorticoid deficiency can result in significant problems. Cortisol stimulates gluconeogenesis, increases blood glucose, enhances extravascular fluid movement to the intravascular compartment, stabilizes lysosomal membranes, and counteracts the effects of stress. Cortisol depletion impairs renal excretion of water and energy metabolism, decreases stress tolerance, and can cause anorexia, vomiting and/or diarrhea. Cortisol depletion rarely produces electrolyte imbalances.(4)

Hypoadrenocorticism should be suspected in any dog with a history of anorexia, vomiting, diarrhea, and lethargy when there are clinical findings of muscle weakness, dehydration, and bradycardia. Electrolyte imbalance may be suggestive of hypoadrenocorticism. Serum sodium levels are often less than 135 mEq/L, and serum potassium levels may be greater than 5.5 mEq/L. The Na:K ratio may be less than 25:1 (normal is 33:1).

Confirmation of hypoadrenocorticism is made by measuring serum cortisol. Resting plasma cortisol is often less than 10 ng/mL and won't respond to exogenous ACTH stimulation in a hypoadrenocorticism patient. Plasma cortisol levels are the most accurate method of diagnosing hypoadrenocorticism. Glucocorticoid replacement therapy must be withheld for 2 hours before testing.(4)

Other diagnostic aids that may be helpful include the CBC, BUN, and ECG. The CBC reflects dehydration and decreased cortisol will cause eosinophilia and lymphocytosis. The BUN may be elevated due to prerenal uremia or renal failure. The ECG may show evidence of hyperkalemia.

The anesthetic protocol used in the patient with hypoadrenocorticism is not as critical as the medical management prior to anesthesia. A patient with hypoadrenocorticism must be stabilized. The treatment objectives are to (a) correct the dehydration and treat the hypovolemic shock, (b) return renal function to normal, (c) correct electrolyte imbalances, and (d) supply glucocorticoids.(5)

Addisonian patients have decreased stress tolerance. The key is to provide adequate intravenous fluid volume replacement during and following surgery and to provide exogenous glucocorticoids. A balanced electrolyte solution should be administered intraoperatively at a rate of 15 to 22 mL $\cdot$ kg^{-1} $\cdot$ h^{-1}. The rate may be adjusted depending on the patient's physiologic status. The fluid rate may be decreased postoperatively to approximately 90 mL $\cdot$ kg^{-1} $\cdot$ day^{-1}. Again, this rate can be adjusted depending on the patient's physiologic status.

Glucocorticoids should be given concomitantly with initiation of the anesthetic regimen. Preoperatively 2 to 4 mg/kg of dexamethasone should be given intravenously or subcutaneously. Intraoperatively, a rapid-acting glucocorticoid such as prednisolone sodium succinate (Solu-Delta-Cortef) at a dose of 11 to 22 mg/kg IV or prednisolone calcium phosphate (Cortisate-20; 11 mg/kg IV) should be given and repeated as necessary. Postoperatively, additional glucocorticoids are given as needed. The patient with hypoadrenocorticism should be closely monitored for signs of hypotension and shock.

Hypothyroidism

A hypothyroid patient often has a decreased metabolic rate. This can prolong the effects of many preanesthetic and anesthetic drugs. Any anesthetic drug should be used in low doses and ideally should require minimal or no metabolism or can be readily antagonized. Narcotics, low doses of tranquilizers, propofol, and inhalants are the preferred preanesthetic and anesthetic drugs.

A hypothyroid patient is often obese and may suffer from anemia. This may cause ventilatory problems under anesthesia caused by the excess amounts of abdominal and intrathoracic fat. Assisted or controlled ventilation may be necessary in these patients to keep them adequately ventilated. Anemia may range from subclinical to severe. If the anemia is severe, whole blood transfusion should be considered prior to anesthesia and surgery.(6)

Hyperthyroidism

Patients with thyroid adenomas or adenocarcinomas may exhibit evidence of hyperthyroidism. Several factors may place these patients at higher anesthetic risk. A thyroid tumor may place mechanical pressure on the trachea, causing a partial obstruction and interfering with respiration. The surgical area may be highly vascular, and this can lead to excessive bleeding.

Hyperthyroid patients may develop "thyroid storm" during the procedure as a result of excessive thyroid hormone production. This is precipitated by catecholamine release and is characterized by an increased heart rate, increased blood pressure, cardiac dysrhythmias, elevated body temperature, and shock. Hyperthyroid patients often have increased metabolic rates, making them more prone to developing hypoxemia. There is increased oxygen and glucose demand, and increased carbon dioxide production. Hyperthyroid patients may be more prone to heart failure. They have an increased heart rate and myocardial oxygen consumption, and are more prone to cardiac dysrhythmias during anesthesia.

Because of their increased metabolic rate, hyperthyroid patients may rapidly metabolize anesthetic drugs. Adequate oxygenation must be provided because of the increased oxygen consumption and demands of the patient. Intubation may be difficult if the tumor is compressing the trachea. Preanesthetic and anesthetic agents that decrease catecholamine response and myocardial irritability are preferred. Low doses of acepromazine or an alpha$_2$-agonist can be used as a preanesthetic in hyperthyroid patients. Acepromazine decreases myocardial irritability, and it blocks alpha-adrenergic receptors and thus may help counteract hypertension. An opioid can be combined with acepromazine because opioids generally slow heart rate and decrease myocardial oxygen consumption similar to alpha$_2$-agonists.

Anesthesia may be induced with low-dose thiopental, propofol, etomidate, or an inhalant by mask. Isoflurane is the inhalant of choice because cardiac output is better maintained and the drug has minimal dysrhythmic properties. Cardiovascular and respiratory parameters should be monitored closely and ventilation controlled when necessary. A 5% dextrose drip should be administered to counteract increased glucose demands.

References

1. Nelson RW. Disorders of the endocrine pancreas. In: Ettinger SJ, ed. Textbook of veterinary internal medicine. Philadelphia: WB Saunders, 1989:1676–1720.
2. Trim CM. Anesthesia and the endocrine system. In: Slatter D, ed. Textbook of small animal surgery, 2nd ed. Philadelphia: WB Saunders, 1993:2290–2294.
3. Paddleford RR. Anesthetic considerations in patients with preexisting problems or conditions. In: Manual of small animal anesthesia. New York: Churchill Livingstone, 1988:253–308.
4. Feldman EC. Adrenal gland disease. In: Ettinger SJ, ed. Textbook of veterinary internal medicine. Philadelphia: WB Saunders, 1989:1721–1776.
5. Peterson ME. Pathophysiological changes in the endocrine system. In: Short CE, ed. Principles and practice of veterinary anesthesia. Baltimore: Williams & Wilkins, 1987:251–260.
6. Peterson ME, Ferguson DC. Thyroid disease. In: Ettinger SJ, ed. Textbook of veterinary internal medicine. Philadelphia: WB Saunders, 1989:1632–1675.

AIRWAY DISEASE

Stephen A. Greene, Ralph C. Harvey

INTRODUCTION
RESPIRATORY DEPRESSION IN THE
   PERIANESTHETIC PERIOD
AIRWAY TRAUMA

BRACHYCEPHALIC AIRWAY SYNDROME
LARYNGOSPASM
MISHAPS INVOLVING THE AIRWAY

Introduction

Airway obstruction may be associated with trauma, congenital anatomic abnormalities, aspiration of foreign material, or laryngospasm. Management of airway obstruction in the perianesthetic period is based on the severity of the obstruction and the underlying factors associated with its cause.

Respiratory Depression in the Perianesthetic Period

When possible, potent respiratory depressant medications should be avoided in patients with respiratory disease during the perianesthetic period. When sedative/analgesics with respiratory depressant effects (e.g., opioids) are used for premedication, respiration of the patient should be closely monitored. Mixed agonist-antagonist opioids such as butorphanol minimize respiratory depression. Butorphanol's effects are characterized by a "ceiling effect" on respiratory depression and analgesia (Chapter 8).(1) Naloxone can be used to antagonize respiratory depression associated with opioid analgesics but will also antagonize analgesia.(2) Analgesia may be preserved to some extent by titrating naloxone "to effect" when reversing opioid-induced respiratory depression. Rapid intravenous administration of naloxone has been associated with development of cardiac dysrhythmias and sudden death.(3, 4) Administration of a mixed-agonist/antagonist opioid such as butorphanol may effectively antagonize severe respiratory depression while maintaining some analgesic action via kappa opioid receptors.(5) Incremental dos-

ing of butorphanol (0.05 mg/kg at a time) for antagonism of full agonist opioids is advised to prevent sudden arousal and dysphoria.

Regional analgesia is gaining in popularity for postoperative analgesia. This technique causes less respiratory depression than parenteral opioids. Following thoracotomy, analgesia may be achieved by intrapleural injection of bupivacaine (1.5 mg/kg).(6) For control of pain associated with procedures involving the hind limbs (and possibly procedures more rostral), epidural analgesia is a useful adjunct to general anesthesia. Epidural analgesia prior to surgery will decrease the requirement for the general anesthetic.(7) Inhalation anesthetics are associated with dose-dependent respiratory depression. Therefore, use of epidural analgesia as an adjunct to inhalation anesthesia may decrease respiratory and cardiovascular depression. Epidural analgesia in the dog is often accomplished using morphine (0.1 mg/kg) in sterile water or isotonic saline solution q.s. to yield 1 mL per 4 kg of body weight (Chapter 16).(8)

Airway Trauma

Trauma to the head and neck can cause progressive respiratory distress (Chapter 24). Occlusion of the airways may result from collapse of the nasal or oral passages accompanied by tissue swelling, hemorrhage, and aspiration of tissues, blood, or foreign materials. Head trauma and secondary cerebral edema can decrease ventilation via neurologic mechanisms independent of physical obstructions. Additional respiratory depression must be avoided to prevent associated increases in intracranial pressure and neurologic morbidity (Chapter 23). In a retrospective study of 85 dogs undergoing cervical spinal decompressive surgery, respiratory arrest was a significant factor in 3 of 7 (42%) dogs that died from complications arising during surgery.(9)

Surgical procedures of the nasal airway, pharynx, larynx, or trachea can be followed by obstructive postoperative swelling. Delicate surgical technique combined with perioperative antiinflammatory doses of corticosteroids minimize this potential. Administration of pediatric strength phenylephrine nose drops in each nostril will counteract nasal passage hyperemia, improving ventilation and often stimulating increased swallowing.

Animals with thick or copious secretions in the respiratory tract have increased risk for airway obstruc-

tion. Endotracheal intubation restricts the diameter of the trachea and increases the likelihood of airway obstruction from viscid secretions. Particular attention should be given to patients with small (e.g., < 5 mm i.d.) endotracheal tubes. Difficult positive pressure ventilation (by squeezing the rebreathing bag) in a patient with abnormal respiratory tract secretions should prompt the anesthetist to inspect the airway. Suction of secretions from the endotracheal tube may be required periodically during anesthesia. In some cases, the best solution may be to reintubate the trachea with a different endotracheal tube. Pharyngeal suction prior to anesthetic recovery from nasal, pharyngeal, or oral surgery decreases risk of aspiration of blood and debris. When regurgitated material or blood has accumulated in the pharynx, the risk of aspiration can be reduced further

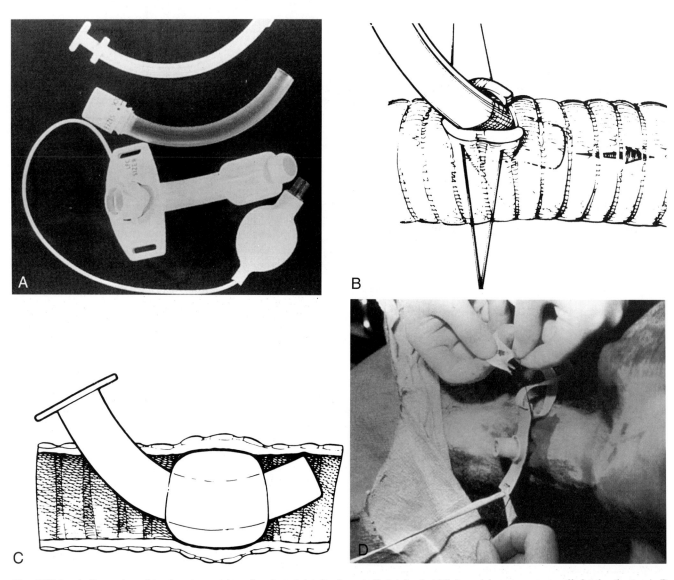

Fig. 23H–1. A, Examples of tracheostomy tubes showing stylet (top), uncuffed tube (middle), and low-pressure, cuffed tube (bottom). B, Schematic of surgical approach and insertion of the tracheostomy tube. C, Schematic illustrating final position of cuffed tracheostomy tube. D, Photograph of tracheostomy tube being secured to the neck using umbilical tape. (Figure courtesy of Dr. Karen Tobias.)

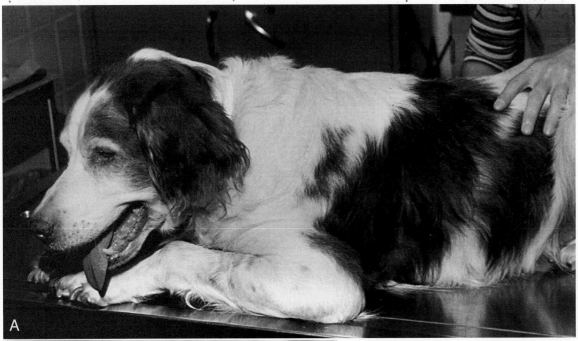

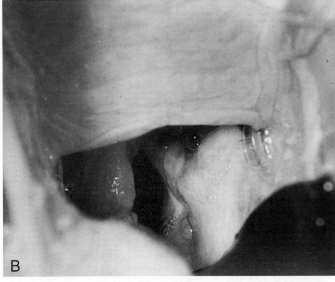

Fig. 23H–2. A, Photograph illustrating typical appearance of a dog with upper airway obstruction caused by collapse of the arytenoid cartilages. Note the facial expression. B, Photograph of glottis from dog in A. The soft palate is at the top, and the laryngoscope blade is at lower right. Note the edema and asymmetrical appearance of the arytenoid cartilages. (Photographs courtesy of Dr. Joseph Harari.)

by gently withdrawing the endotracheal tube with the cuff partially inflated. After delivery to the pharynx, matter can be removed by suction.

Administration of oxygen should continue throughout recovery from anesthesia when there is risk of postoperative airway obstruction. If obstruction develops, supplementary oxygenation increases the time available for institution of airway control. Rapid-sequence induction of anesthesia with an injectable anesthetic may be necessary to regain control of the upper airway via an endotracheal tube. After reestablishment of a secure airway, it may be possible to resolve the underlying problems and then successfully recover the patient from anesthesia. In brachycephalic animals, resection of an elongated soft palate may be necessary in order to prevent airway obstruction associated with tissue swell-

ing that has developed during anesthesia for other procedures. In severe cases of obstruction, an emergency tracheostomy may be necessary (Fig. 23H–1).

Brachycephalic Airway Syndrome

Anatomic abnormalities of the upper airway syndrome in brachycephalic dogs can severely compromise their ability to adequately ventilate. The primary defects of stenotic nares, elongated soft palate, and hypoplastic trachea are exacerbated in extreme cases with eversion of laryngeal saccules and redundant pharyngeal tissues. Dogs with arytenoid cartilage or tracheal collapse present similar anesthetic challenges (Fig. 23H–2). Reduction of the cross-sectional area of the trachea greatly increases resistance to air flow and the work of breathing. In addition, vagal tone is frequently high in brachycephalic dogs. Vagal stimulation associated with pharyngeal manipulation (difficult intubation) or vagotonic drugs can contribute to significant bradycardia. Preanesthetic administration of anticholinergic agents is indicated in these cases. The anesthetist's goals are to avoid deep sedation, especially in animals that are not continuously monitored; intubate the trachea using a rapid intravenous induction technique when practical; and maintain tracheal intubation until the dog demonstrates adequate recovery from anesthesia. Induction of anesthesia should be preceded by having the dog breathe oxygen using a face mask. Respiratory support during anesthesia may be required, especially in overweight animals. Obesity further impairs ventilatory function by decreasing tidal volume and functional residual capacity of the lung.

Recovery from anesthesia is judged to be adequate when the dog strongly objects to the presence of the endotracheal tube. At the time of extubation, reversal of opioids by naloxone administration may aid in rapid return of the dog's ability to maintain its airway. Because of the presence of redundant tissue in the pharynx, most brachycephalic breeds (e.g., bulldog, shar pei) benefit from having the anesthetist hold the tongue and/or extend the neck immediately following extubation of the trachea. A source of 100% oxygen should be available. Ventilatory function of brachycephalic dogs should be closely monitored for at least an hour following recovery from anesthesia.

Laryngospasm

Laryngospasm during the perianesthetic period occurs most frequently in cats, swine, rabbits, and primates, but has also been observed in dogs and horses. Laryngospasm may occur following irritation of laryngeal tissues by secretions or blood. It has been estimated that laryngospasm occurs postsurgically in 22% of children undergoing tonsillectomy.(10) Spasm of the larynx may be caused by touching the larynx during a light plane of anesthesia. Topical application of a local anesthetic such as lidocaine is recommended prior to tracheal intubation in these species in order to minimize tactile stimulation-induced laryngospasm. Neuromuscular blocking agents such as atracurium may be useful for preventing laryngospasm at the time of tracheal

Table 23H–1. Factors Associated with Development of Pulmonary Edema Following Acute Airway Obstruction

Severe negative intrathoracic pressure
Decreased interstitial hydrostatic pressure
Catecholamine release
Vasoconstriction
Increased vascular hydrostatic pressure
Hypoxia
Increased permeability of pulmonary vasculature
Net accumulation of interstitial fluid
Inadequate lymphatic removal of interstitial fluid

intubation. Extubation of the trachea can also trigger laryngospasm in susceptible animals. In one case a Vietnamese potbellied pig apparently developed laryngospasm 4 hours after tracheal extubation in spite of an uneventful recovery from inhalation anesthesia. Treatment of laryngospasm that occurs at the time of tracheal extubation (or later) includes reintubation using anesthetics and neuromuscular blocking agents if necessary. Nasotracheal intubation is an effective means of reestablishing a patent airway in some species such as the horse. Oxygen should be administered and the patient should be evaluated for subsequent development of pulmonary edema over the next 1 to 4 hours.

Acute pulmonary edema following laryngospasm has been reported in human beings.(11, 12) Pulmonary edema may occur with delayed onset after laryngospasm with clinical signs of dyspnea, tachypnea, and production of pink frothy material in the airway becoming apparent during recovery from anesthesia.(13) Dogs with upper airway obstruction can acutely develop life-threatening pulmonary edema.(14) Factors associated with generation of pulmonary edema following airway obstruction are listed in Table 23H–1. The extreme negative pressure produced by an animal with airway obstruction when attempting to inspire causes decreased interstitial hydrostatic pressure in the lung. Simultaneous release of catecholamines causing increased vascular hydrostatic pressure may result in a net accumulation of interstitial fluid. Hypoxia associated with an acutely obstructed airway may promote fluid movement into the interstitial spaces by increasing permeability of pulmonary vasculature. It is likely that pulmonary edema formation after airway obstruction is multifactorial, so treatment is symptomatic. Oxygen (40%) supplementation, diuretics, and corticosteroids have been used to treat pulmonary edema. Emergency tracheostomy may be required to rapidly establish a patent airway. Tracheal intubation and positive pressure ventilation are routinely used for human patients with pulmonary edema in whom the syndrome is rarely fatal.

Large animals are more difficult to maintain on mechanical ventilators for a prolonged period and have higher mortality associated with laryngospasm-induced pulmonary edema. Horses may develop airway obstruction at the time of tracheal extubation after anesthesia. Potential causes include laryngospasm, paralysis of the arytenoid cartilages, and mechanical obstruction. Laryngospasm is associated with cessation of airflow, whereas paralysis of the arytenoid cartilages is characterized by stridor and decreased airflow. Laryngospasm may result from laryngeal irritation at the time of extubation. Paralysis of the arytenoid cartilages has been associated with poor function of the recurrent laryngeal nerve. In the horse, the recurrent laryngeal nerve may be susceptible to damage by hyperextension of the neck for a prolonged period during anesthesia.(15) Postanesthetic paralysis of the arytenoid cartilages has also been observed following 2- to 4-hour procedures in which the horse's trachea was intubated with an excessively large (in retrospect) endotracheal tube. Mechanical obstruction of the airway may occur during recovery from anesthesia if the horse becomes cast or positioned such that the neck is improperly flexed. Pulmonary edema following transient mechanical airway obstruction in a horse has been reported.(16) Horses anesthetized with the head lower than the body may be at risk for accumulation of fluid in laryngeal tissues. These horses develop mechanical airway obstruction by edema of the glottis following tracheal extubation. Many anesthetists prefer to recover horses at risk for upper airway obstruction with a nasotracheal tube in place until the horse is standing (Chapter 17). Treatment of the horse with postanesthetic airway obstruction is initiated by placement of a nasal or oral endotracheal tube. If one of these techniques is not successful, an emergency tracheostomy is indicated. Supportive treatment includes administration of oxygen, diuretics, corticosteroids, antibiotics, and analgesics.

Mishaps Involving the Airway

Unfortunately, mishaps or accidents involving management of the airway during anesthesia increase morbidity and mortality among animal patients. It is imperative that the anesthetist become familiar with the anesthetic machine, ventilator, and intubating equipment available to prevent such mishaps. Vigilance in preventing excessive pressure buildup within an anesthetic circuit is required. The function of the "pop-off" valve should be continuously monitored. Sudden or unexplained increases in circuit or airway pressure should be immediately investigated. Equipment failure should be ruled out while anesthesia is maintained using a different delivery system (Chapter 14). An unusual cause of increased inspiratory plateau pressure has been attributed to a leak in the bellows of a mechanical ventilator that allowed the driving gas of the bellows to enter the breathing circuit.(17) Increased airway pressure may also occur from development of tension pneumothorax.

Venipuncture may be associated with iatrogenic trauma to vital structures in the neck that results in airway obstruction. Injury of the recurrent laryngeal nerve may cause temporary paralysis of the arytenoid cartilage in the horse. Aspiration pneumonia secondary to choke caused by a periesophageal hematoma following venipuncture has been reported in a llama.(18)

Airway obstruction may occur in intubated patients following administration of nitrous oxide. Nitrous oxide may diffuse into the air-filled endotracheal tube cuff causing increased cuff pressure and endotracheal tube collapse.(19) Overexpansion of the endotracheal tube cuff when administering nitrous oxide may be prevented by filling the cuff with an appropriate nitrous oxide/oxygen mixture (i.e., gas aspirated from the breathing circuit) rather than with air. Nitrous oxide may also diffuse into small bubbles of air found in some endotracheal tubes as a manufacturing defect. Expansion of these air bubbles with nitrous oxide has caused airway obstruction in guarded endotracheal tubes (endotracheal tubes with a spiral wire used to prevent kinking of the tube).(20) Prior to use, endotracheal tubes

should be examined for material defects such as presence of air bubbles that contraindicate administration of nitrous oxide.

Inadvertent displacement of the endotracheal tube may cause airway obstruction. Subtle changes in position of the endotracheal tube may occur during radiography or surgical positioning. Flexion of the neck of the anesthetized dog may result in caudal displacement, endobronchial placement, or total occlusion of the endotracheal tube.(21)

References

1. Nagashima H, Karamanian A, Malovany R, et al. Respiratory and circulatory effects of intravenous butorphanol and morphine. Clin Pharmacol Ther 19:738–745, 1976.
2. Copland, VS, Haskins SC, Patz J. Naloxone reversal of oxymorphone effects in dogs. Am J Vet Res 50:1854–1858, 1989.
3. Michealis LL, Hickey PR, Clark TA, et al. Ventricular irritability associated with the use of naloxone hydrochloride. Ann Thor Surg 18:608–614, 1974.
4. Andree RA. Sudden death following naloxone administration. Anesth Analg 59:782–784, 1980.
5. McCrackin MA, Harvey RC, Sackman JE, et al. Butorphanol tartrate for partial reversal of oxymorphone-induced postoperative respiratory depression in the dog. Vet Surg 23:67–74, 1994.
6. Thompson SE, Johnson JM. Analgesia in dogs after intercostal thoracotomy—A comparison of morphine, selective intercostal nerve block, and intrapleural regional analgesia with bupivacaine. Vet Surg 20:73–77, 1991.
7. Valverde A, Dyson DH, Cockshutt JR, et al. Comparison of the hemodynamic effects of halothane alone and halothane combined with epidurally administered morphine for anesthesia in ventilated dogs. Am J Vet Res 52:505–509, 1991.
8. Valverde A, Dyson DH, McDonell WN, Pascoe PJ. Use of epidural morphine in the dog for pain relief. Vet Comp Orthoped Traumatol 2:55–58, 1989.
9. Clark DM. An analysis of intraoperative and early postoperative mortality associated with cervical spinal decompressive surgery in the dog. J Am Anim Hosp Assoc 22:739–744, 1986.
10. Leicht P Wisborg T, Chraemmer-Jorgensen B. Does intravenous lidocaine prevent laryngospasm after extubation in children? Anesth Analg 64:1193–1196, 1985.
11. Cozanitis DA, Leijala M, Pesonen E, Zaki HI. Acute pulmonary oedema due to laryngeal spasm. Anaesthesia 37:1198–1199, 1982.
12. Lee KWT, Downes JJ. Pulmonary edema secondary to laryngospasm in children. Anesthesiology 59:347–349, 1983.
13. Glasser SA, Siler JN. Delayed onset of laryngospasm-induced pulmonary edema in an adult outpatient. Anesthesiology 62:370–371, 1985.
14. Kerr LY. Pulmonary edema secondary to upper airway obstruction in the dog: a review of nine cases. J Am Anim Hosp Assoc 25:207–212, 1989.
15. Abrahamsen EJ, Bohanon TC, Bednarski RM, et al. Bilateral arytenoid cartilage paralysis after inhalation anesthesia in a horse. J Am Vet Med Assoc 197:1363–1365, 1990.
16. Kollias-Baker CA, Pipers FS, Heard D, Seeherman H. Pulmonary edema associated with transient airway obstruction in three horses. J Am Vet Med Assoc 202:1116–1118, 1993.
17. Klein LV, Wilson DV. An unusual cause of increasing airway pressure during anesthesia. Vet Surg 18:239–241, 1989.
18. Weldon AD, Beck KA. Identifying a periesophageal hematoma as the cause of choke in a llama. Vet Med 88:1009–1011, 1993.
19. Komatsu H, Mitsuhata H, Hasegawa J, Matsumoto S. Decreased pressure of endotracheal tube cuff in general anesthesia without nitrous oxide. Masui 42:831–834, 1993.
20. Populaire C, Robard S, Souron R. An armoured endotracheal tube obstruction in a child. Can J Anaesth 36:331–332, 1989.
21. Quandt JE, Robinson EP, Walter PA, Raffe MR. Endotracheal tube displacement during cervical manipulation in the dog. Vet Surg 22:235–239, 1993.

ANESTHESIA FOR SPECIAL PATIENTS: OCULAR PATIENTS

Introduction

Other than traumatized patients, those most frequently presented for ophthalmic surgery are the young or the elderly. In elderly animals, altered left myocardial function and a variety of other metabolic derangements are common findings. Older patients are often receiving chronic drug therapy that can affect response to anesthesia. The requirement for deep general anesthesia when performing ophthalmic surgery increases risk. These factors taken together challenge the veterinarian's skill in providing safe anesthetic management. In large animals (e.g., horses and cattle) the most frequent problem is associated with depressed cardiopulmonary function as a result of the depth of anesthesia required for intraocular surgery and lateral recumbency. Whatever the exact cause, it seems that hypoxemia, hyper capnia (i.e., as a result of hypoventilation and/or venous admixture or ventilation perfusion mismatch; Chapter 6) and hypotension are most frequently cited as contributing factors to unsuccessful outcomes in patients undergoing ocular surgery. Because reduced blood flow is common during deep anesthesia, even successful management during the anesthetic/surgery period can be followed by postanesthetic rhabdomyolsis in large horses. Two primary objectives for safe, successful, surgery and anesthetic management of ophthalmic patients are maintenance of adequate cardiopulmonary function and normal intraocular pressure (IOP).

INTRAOCULAR PRESSURE

Aqueous humor is contained in the anterior and posterior chambers of the eye. Its dynamic movement and choroidal vascular volume are responsible in large part for maintaining normal IOP. Aqueous humor is the major transport system for oxygen and glucose and protein that nourish the eye.(1) The major route of travel for aqueous humor is from the posterior chamber to the anterior chamber to the jugular vascular system. The major portion of aqueous humor is formed in the ciliary body and actively secreted into the posterior chamber by the ciliary processes. It moves into the anterior chamber via the pupil. Intraocular hypertension is prevented by movement of aqueous humor out of the anterior chamber via Fontana's trabeculae and into the canal of Schlemm, where it enters the episcleral vasculature, finally reaching the jugular venous circulation. The canal of Schlemm as well as choroid blood volume are responsible in large part for maintaining normal IOP.

Intraocular pressure normally ranges from 10 to 26 mm Hg in dogs, 12 to 32 mm Hg in cats and 23 to 28 mm Hg in horses.(2–4) Pressures exceeding these values should be considered abnormal. Coughing or straining can result in a pressure increase of greater than 40 mm Hg. Tracheal intubation can increase IOP without any outward clinical signs (e.g., coughing, gagging). Maintenance of IOP in the normal range is essential for ocular health and successful intraocular surgery. Marked decreases in arterial pressure, as may occur in deep anesthesia, can reduce IOP drastically. Obstruction of ocular outflow induced by coughing, retching, or manual restraint of the head and neck can dramatically increase IOP. A sudden rise in IOP of patients with an ocular penetrating wound or when the anterior chamber is open can easily result in extrusion of vitreous and permanent loss of vision. Some physiologic factors and drugs associated with alterations in IOP are presented in Table 24A–1.

CARDIOPULMONARY FUNCTION

The degree of cardiopulmonary depression induced by general anesthesia is directly related to anesthetic depth and regimen. Surgical anesthesia with halothane or isoflurane will decrease IOP. The depth of anesthesia providing complete eyeball immobility required for delicate intraocular surgery often results in pronounced hypotension. Administration of mannitol (1–2 g/kg over 15–20 minutes) will result in a transient increase in plasma volume that may reverse hypotension while decreasing IOP. A dose of 0.25 g/kg does not appear to have any beneficial effect.(5) Histologically, pulmonary edema has been identified in dogs anesthetized with methoxyflurane and receiving mannitol.(6, 7) Osmotic diuresis following mannitol administration can result in hypokalemia and should be used with caution in patients with heart failure, hypokalemia, and renal failure. Mannitol therapy is no longer used routinely except prior to surgery to relieve glaucoma. The urethra should be catheterized to prevent overdistension of the bladder. Strict asepsis should be adhered to in order to avoid postoperative cystitis. The anesthetic depth required for complete eyeball immobility can be decreased when a nondepolarizing neuromuscular relaxant (e.g., pancuronium or atracurium; Table 24A–1) is used (Chapter 13). Decreased anesthetic depth will allow for more normal cardiovascular function.

THE OCULOCARDIAC REFLEX (OCR)

The OCR occurs most often in younger patients. This reflex is more likely to occur when there is inadequate relaxation of the extraocular muscles and hypercapnia is present. Dysrhythmias associated with the OCR include atrioventricular block, bradycardia, bigeminy and ectopic beats.(1) If not corrected, these abnormal rhythms can terminate in cardiac arrest. The dysrhythmias are in response to manipulation of the eyeball and will persist until the stimulus is terminated. Stimuli that can activate the OCR include traction on the ocular muscles, enucleation, direct pressure on the globe, and other ocular manipulations. The afferent/efferent pathway of the OCR is trigeminal/vagal. Increased vagal tone (e.g., in the young or as a result of drug administration) may enhance the likelihood of initiating the OCR. The best prevention is gentle manipulation of the eyeball. Preoperative intramuscular atropine injection, gentle manipulation of the eyeball, and controlled ventilation will help decrease the incidence of OCR

activation. Intravenous atropine may induce dysrhythmias, but severe bradycardia may demand its use. Glycopyrrolate does not appear to be any more effective than atropine in relieving increased vagal tone. Retrobulbar blockade with lidocaine, although often effective in treating an episode of OCR, may be associated with a number of problems (Chapter 16). Possible complications include retrobulbar hemorrhage, undesirable proptosis of the globe, displacement of the vitreous humor if the eye has been penetrated, and increased IOP. When this block is performed, the needle may penetrate the meningeal sheath surrounding the optic nerve. Deposition of the local anesthetic in the cerebrospinal fluid can result in brain-stem anesthesia. If this occurs clinical signs include agitation, and respiratory and cardiac arrest.(1) Local and regional anesthetic techniques of the eye and orbit are presented in Chapter 16.

Should the OCR be triggered, eyeball manipulation should cease. Should bradycardia persist, intravenous atropine (0.02 mg/kg) should be given immediately. If this is ineffective, and bradycardia is judged to be life threatening, only then should lidocaine be injected cautiously into the retrobulbar muscles to inhibit afferent stimuli transmission to the CNS.

General Anesthesia

Safe effective anesthesia in ocular patients requires maintenance of near normal IOP, prevention of the activation of the OCR, control of hemorrhage, and complete immobilization of the eyeball. Stable IOP is provided with deep anesthesia. Tracheal intubation in the dog and cat should be delayed until the depth of anesthesia prevents coughing, gagging, vomiting, and straining. These responses to intubation will increase venous pressure, causing an increase in IOP. Nasotracheal intubation, commonly used in the awake foal for induction of anesthesia with an inhalant anesthetic should be avoided. The heavy restraint required for nasotracheal intubation and the gagging and coughing that often occur during intubation increase IOP.

Horses scheduled for enucleation of an eye in which vision has been lost should be approached from the unblind side. If sudden contact is made with the horse on the blind side, it may react unpredictably. A safe approach from the blind side requires words of assurance and gentle hand contact. Once contact has been made, it should be maintained until the intended procedure has been completed. Horses seldom cough during intubation. An exception may be seen in horses afflicted with heaves or with strangles.

With a penetrating wound it is especially important to prevent coughing that can cause extrusion of the lens and vitreous humor, and possible retinal detachment with permanent loss of vision of the involved eye. The anesthetic technique and drug protocol should be designed to rapidly achieve balanced anesthesia while preventing increases in IOP.

Table 24A–1.   Factors Altering Intraocular Pressure

Altering Factors	Change	Comments
Blockade of aqueous outflow	↑	Caused by acute venous congestion and increased choroidal congestion
Acute increase in arterial pressure	↑	Sudden increase in blood pressure causes only a transient increase in IOP
Hypoventilation, airway obstruction, hypercapnia, choroidal vessel dilation	↑	
Hyperventilation, hypocapnia	↓	
Endotracheal intubation	↑	Resulting from coughing, straining, or vomiting; prevented with laryngeal lidocaine spray
Eyeball pressure	↑	Face mask, orbital tumors, ocular muscle traction, retrobulbar traction
Anesthetic Drugs		
Barbiturates	↓	May depress central centers controlling IOP or promote aqueous outflow
Propofol	↓	May prevent the increase in IOP associated with tracheal intubation, appears to suppress the increase in IOP induced by depolarizing muscle relaxants
Etomidate	↑	Etomidate-induced myoclonus appears to be responsible in large part for the increase in IOP
Ketamine	↑ or ↓	Controversial. In patients properly premedicated (e.g., a benzodiazepine) there probably is little or no effect.
Alpha$_2$ agonists	↓	Induced bradycardia, may promote initiation of the OCR. Decreases IOP directly.
Benzodiazepines	↓	The decrease in IOP appears to be in response to a central relaxing action of these drugs on the ocular muscles.
Acepromazine	↓	Decreases arterial blood pressure, suppresses retching and vomiting
Opioids	↓	Sudden increases can occur with retching and vomiting and should be preceded by administration of a tranquilizer
Muscle relaxants		
Depolarizing		
Succinylcholine	↑	Increase is transient. minimal effect when given in stage III anesthesia.
Nondepolarizing		
Pancuronium	↓	Either decrease or have no effect. IOP may during intubation of lightly anesthetized patients
Vecuronium		
Atracurium		
Other drugs		
Acetazolamide	↓	Carbonic anhydrase inhibitor. Decreases formation of aqueous humor. Acts within 2 minutes after IV injection. May produce metabolic acidosis and compensatory hyperventilation
Hypertonic Solutions (Mannitol)	↓	Increase plasma osmotic pressure decreasing formation of aqueous humor and IOP
Phenylephrine	↑ or ↓	Depends on dose. 1.5 mg IV or 5 mg SQ should not be exceeded. For topical application, 1 drop of 2.5% per hour should not be exceeded.
Epinephrine	↑ or ↓	Depends on dose. A topical dose of 0.5 mg in humans has been recommended

Preanesthetic Medication

Preanesthetic medication should relieve anxiety, suppress coughing, prevent vomiting, and provide analgesia in the perioperative period. The drugs selected should have minimal effect on normal IOP. Preanesthetics most frequently used are anticholinergics, tranquilizers, sedatives, and opioids (Table 24A–1).

The cornea is one of the most enervated tissues in the body, and corneal or intraocular surgery may cause intense pain. Control of pain to improve the animal's comfort and minimize self-trauma is essential to a successful outcome. Topical anesthesia can be used to perform a number of diagnostic or therapeutic procedures including tonometry, third eyelid examination, corneal scraping, flushing of the nasolacrimal duct, conjunctival biopsy and electroretinography, and grid keratotomy. Proparicaine (0.5%) is the most commonly used topical anesthetic (Chapters 12 and 16). Analgesia occurs within several seconds and may persist for 10 to 20 minutes following topical application. Tear production and the blink reflex are often impaired during this time. Excessive application in small animals or into an open ocular wound should be avoided to prevent systemic toxicosis. Topical anesthetics should not be used to control ocular pain over a long period of time because they can damage corneal epithelium and delay healing.

Tear production decreases during general anesthesia in most species. Although the administration of an anticholinergic has been shown to decrease tearing, general anesthesia with inhalants will nearly abolish production. This effect is less dramatic in horses. Ocular lubrications to prevent corneal drying are commonly administered in small animals but are not entirely necessary in the horse.

ANTICHOLINERGICS

Atropine or glycopyrrolate can be used to decrease salivary and airway secretions and relieve bradycardia in dogs, cats, and cattle. Neither drug is widely used in horses except when confronted with vagally mediated bradycardia as a result of preanesthetic medication (e.g., xylazine) or to prevent or relieve vagal tone in response to activation of the OCR. Although activation of the OCR is not a common problem in the mature horse, it may be encountered in foals and young horses up to one year of age. In mature horses, bradycardia resulting from intravenous xylazine can be relieved with atropine 2 to 6 mg IV, total dose. Atropine (0.02–0.04 mg/kg IV) may not effectively abolish bradycardia resulting from activation of the OCR. In dogs and cats, atropine (0.04 mg/kg IM or SQ) or glycopyrrolate (0.02 mg/kg IM or SQ) administered 20 minutes prior to surgery may prevent activation of the OCR. Controversy exists with regard to the routine preanesthetic administration of an anticholinergic in ophthalmic patients. Their use is advocated when opioids are used but discouraged prior to parotid duct transposition surgery, as it makes

cannulation more difficult. The effects of systemically administered anticholinergics in glaucomatous patients is unclear. However, they appear to have little or no effect on IOP when administered systemically. Topical administration, however, is associated with mydriasis, filtration angle closure, and increases in IOP. Reportedly, tachycardia and dysrhythmias are not as frequently encountered with glycopyrrolate as with atropine. When atrioventricular blockade accompanies bradycardia that is unresponsive to atropine, either isoprenaline or epinephrine can be administered to prevent progression to asystole. Beta-adrenergic drugs should be used with caution in patients anesthetized with halothane.

TRANQUILIZERS, SEDATIVES, AND OPIOIDS

Xylazine is an effective sedative in horses and cattle but may cause vomiting in dogs and cats and should not be used as premedication in patients of the latter two species having penetrating wounds of the eye or scheduled for intraocular surgery. Similarly, vomiting may occur in response to premedication with an opioid in dogs and cats. Gagging and vomiting can usually be prevented if the opioid is administered after the onset of action of a tranquilizer (e.g., acetylpromazine 0.1–0.2 mg/kg IV). A phenothiazine tranquilizer may prevent vomiting during the postoperative period while the opioid promotes a pain-free recovery and stable blood pressure. In horses and other species, acepromazine premedication has been shown to decrease IOP. Diazepam (0.2–0.4mg/kg IV) or midazolam (0.1–0.2 mg/kg IV or IM) may be safely used in the dog and cat scheduled for ocular surgery. Benzodiazepines enhance ocular muscle relaxation and promote smooth recovery.

Because horses often react violently to pain when emerging from anesthesia, appropriate measures should be taken to protect the operated eye and to ensure a pain-free, smooth recovery. A padded head stall can be used to protect the eye. A small dose of xylazine (0.1–0.2 mg/kg IV) combined with butorphanol (0.02–0.04 mg/kg IV) will promote a smoother recovery.

It should be appreciated that xylazine's inhibiting action on central parasympathetic tone to the iris or perhaps stimulation of alpha$_2$-adrenoceptors located in the iris can result in mydriasis in some species.(8) In rabbits, cats, and monkeys, it has been reported that xylazine decreases IOP by suppressing sympathetic neuronal function and decreasing aqueous flow.(9) Topical administration of the more selective alpha$_2$-adrenergic agonist medetomidine also causes mydriasis and decreases IOP.(10, 11) More recently it has been reported that topical medetomidine decreases IOP in rabbits.(11) The results of these studies demonstrate that alpha$_2$-adrenoceptor agonists mediate mydriasis and decrease IOP in several species.(12)

Of interest is the finding that systemically injected xylazine causes acute reversible lens opacity in rats and mice. Topical application of xylazine results in cataract formation in the treated eye, whereas the contralateral eye is unaffected. The exact mechanism of xylazine-induced lens opacity is unknown. Speculations imply that the transient lens opacification is a result of transcorneal water loss and alteration of aqueous humor composition due to corneal exposure. This physiologic side effect of xylazine should be considered prior to its use in animals undergoing ocular physiologic studies.(13) Lens opacification has not been reported following medetomidine administration. Prolonged sedation or anesthesia of mice, rats, and hamsters can also result in transient lens opacification because of the lack of blinking and subsequent evaporation of fluids from the shallow anterior chamber.

Most anesthetics except for ketamine induce miosis. The opioids have different effects on pupil size in different species. For example morphine causes miosis in dogs and rabbits and mydriasis in cats, rats, mice, and monkeys. Opioid preanesthetic medication in dogs may prevent mydriasis necessary for cataract surgery. The pupil should be dilated and immobile for cataract extraction. Although pupil size is commonly utilized to help assess anesthetic depth, the pupil is rarely accessible during ocular surgery and normal pupillary reflexes are often altered by a variety of drug effects.

In summary, the use of xylazine given alone in low doses or in combination with an opioid should be considered in healthy horses and cattle undergoing intraocular surgery. The use of acepromazine, diazepam, or midazolam to promote smooth emergence in small animals may in fact increase patient activity if they are experiencing severe pain. In dogs and cats recovering from ocular surgery where severe pain is anticipated, the use of a tranquilizer to smooth recovery is made more effective when combined with a strong analgesic (e.g., an opioid).

Induction of Anesthesia

All commonly used anesthetics tend to decrease IOP (Table 24A–1). Gentle handling and restraint of the patient is important to avoid excitement and struggling. Tight-fitting leashes will result in increased jugular venous pressure and should not be used for restraint during induction. When using a nose cone for administration of oxygen or inducing anesthesia, direct pressure on or around the eye should be avoided.(14) This is extremely important in patients with preexisting high IOP, corneal laceration, or a penetrating wound. Struggling is a common problem associated with face mask inhalant induction, which should only be attempted in deeply sedated patients.

Preanesthetic drugs that induce analgesia, sedation, and/or tranquilization will decrease the incidence of excitement during the induction period and thus decrease the probability of increasing IOP. In appropriately premedicated dogs and cats, a thiobarbiturate, propofol, or ketamine may be used to induce anesthesia. A tranquilizer (e.g., acepromazine, diazepam, midazolam, or droperidol) opioid (e.g., oxymorphone, meperidine, fentanyl, or morphine) combination can be used for induction but may require concomitant anticholinergic administration. Induction may be completed with a low dose of thiobarbiturate, ketamine, or an inhalant. Thiobarbiturates or propofol decrease cardiac output, lower blood pressure, relax extraocular muscles, and promote aqueous outflow. Ketamine may increase or have no effect on IOP when given alone but when combined with a benzodiazepine has been shown to actually decrease IOP.(15) Dissociative anesthetics in combination with a tranquilizer are useful for ocular examination as long as globe integrity is present. Etomidate-induced myoclonus may produce hazardous increases in IOP in patients with penetrating eye injuries and should not be used alone for induction in this group of patients. Lidocaine given intravenously (1.0 mg/kg) or by topical application to the larynx following the onset of unconsciousness may be helpful in suppressing the cough reflex during tracheal intubation.

Maintenance of Anesthesia

The inhalants halothane, isoflurane, and methoxyflurane all decrease arterial blood pressure. The decrease is proportionate to the depth of anesthesia and is reflected in a proportionate decrease in IOP. Decreases in IOP may range from 35 to 55%.(15) The depth of anesthesia required to ensure eye immobility for delicate intraocular surgery in the horse and cow will cause hypotension and may decrease tissue blood flow, which can lead to postanesthetic myopathy. In order to avoid this untoward effect, fluid loading and inotropic drug (e.g., dobutamine) administration may be required in large animals undergoing long periods of ophthalmic surgery. In all species high-flow inhalation anesthetic techniques are recommended over low-flow techniques so that the alveolar concentration more nearly reflects vaporizer concentration output, thus ensuring an adequate depth of anesthesia. Unexpected nystagmus and sudden body movement are more likely to occur with low-flow techniques unless depth of anesthesia is closely and continuously monitored, which is sometimes made difficult during ophthalmic surgery. Eye reflexes and jaw tone cannot be conveniently monitored because the patient's head is usually covered by surgical drapes. The surgeon can provide information on the depth of anesthesia by indicating abrupt changes in eye position or movement of the eyelids. Respiration rate, HR, BP, and the ECG should be monitored continuously. In small animals a guarded endotracheal tube to prevent kinking should be used and all connections must be well secured before draping of the head is begun.

Nitrous oxide is not commonly used in ocular patients. Its administration is contraindicated following air injection into the anterior chamber of a closed eye. Nitrous oxide will diffuse into an intraocular bubble faster than air can diffuse out, causing air bubble expansion and increased IOP. During retinal reattachment surgery where an expandable gas such as sulfur hexafluoride is injected into the vitreous to expand the globe, nitrous oxide will rapidly diffuse into the bubble, increasing IOP. When nitrous oxide is discontinued at the end of surgery, the air bubble within the vitreous and IOP will rapidly decrease. It is suggested that if nitrous oxide is used it should be discontinued 15 to 20 minutes prior to injection of an intraocular gas into a closed eye. Nitrous oxide should not be used for at least 5 days after intraocular air injection should a subsequent anesthetic be necessary.(16)

Renal tubular necrosis has been reported in dogs after flunixin meglumine administration and methoxyflurane anesthesia (Chapters 11 and 23). Although it is not approved by the FDA for use in these species, flunixin meglumine is commonly used as a preoperative analgesic and antiinflammatory drug in small animal ocular patients. Its use with methoxyflurane is discouraged.(16)

Nondepolarizing muscle relaxants (i.e., pancuronium, vecuronium, atracurium) are commonly used in the dog and cat to assure complete immobility of the eye. In birds these drugs are required to induce mydriasis because birds have striated musculature of the iris rather than smooth muscle as in mammals (Chapter 20). Intracameral injections of d-tubocurare have been used to induce mydriasis in birds undergoing intraocular surgery.(16) When combined with a strong analgesic, muscle relaxants provide balanced anesthesia while decreasing anesthetic requirement and the level of cardiopulmonary depression. This is an important consideration in many elderly small animal patients. Muscle relaxants are not widely used in the horse and cow because of the problems associated with prolonged reduced muscle strength and its influence on larger animals' ability to stand at recovery. Struggling during the recovery period can cause an increase in IOP. Rapid reversal of nondepolarizing muscle relaxants with antiacetylcholinesterase drugs such as neostigmine may result in undesirable increases in visceral vagal stimulation, causing bradycardia and increased intestinal spastic motility. For this reason if a nondepolarizing muscle relaxant is to be used in large animals, more rapidly metabolized drugs such as atracurium are less likely to require reversal with an anticholinesterase drug and are preferred. Because of the large dose of atracurium required in mature horses, drug expense may become a factor.

Succinylcholine, a depolarizing muscle relaxant, cannot be routinely recommended for ocular surgical patients because it causes muscle fasciculation that can increase IOP. In an early report, it was shown that while succinylcholine causes an increase of 5.3 mm Hg in IOP when given in stage I anesthesia, IOP was not increased when the drug was given in stage III anesthesia.(17) Cholinergic agents and/or cholinesterase inhibitors are often employed in the treatment of glaucomatous patients to increase aqueous outflow. Anticholinesterase drugs can deplete plasma pseudocholinesterase concentrations and interfere with metabolism of succinylcholine, prolonging paralysis. Consequently it has been recommended that cholinesterase inhibitors be discontinued 2 to 4 weeks prior to succinylcholine administration.(16)

Considerable controversy surrounds the sequential use of nondepolarizing and depolarizing muscle relaxants in ocular surgical patients. In people, a small dose (0.1 of the ED_{95} dose) of a nondepolarizing drug (e.g. pancuronium, atracurium, vecuronium) is commonly given intravenously followed in 2 or 3 minutes by an immobilizing dose of succinylcholine. This drug sequence is designed to minimize muscle fasciculations and attenuate the increase in IOP caused by succinylcholine. With this technique, the trachea is easily intubated and there is no coughing or gagging. However, the act of intubation can still cause an increase in IOP even though coughing or gagging is not induced and fasciculations are not evident. (1) The use of peripheral muscle relaxants requires controlled ventilation for prevention of hypercapnia and its accompanying increase in IOP. Prolonged intraocular surgery will require either repeated dosing or a continuous infusion of the muscle relaxant. Additional dosing of longer-acting nondepolarizing muscle relaxants such as pancuronium is discouraged when surgery is nearing completion. At completion of surgery, the patient must be weaned from the ventilator and if spontaneous ventilation does not ensue, antagonism of the nondepolarizing muscle relaxants' paralytic action is necessary for timely recovery. Intravenous atropine (0.02 mg/kg IV) followed by neostigmine (0.02–0.04 mg/kg IV) is commonly used. These drugs are not associated with increases in IOP.

Recovery

A smooth recovery is essential for a successful outcome following ophthalmic surgery. Floundering in the cage or recovery stall can easily disrupt the surgical repair, leading to complete loss of vision in the operated eye. A padded hood will provide some protection for the horse. The cow seldom experiences a rough recovery, but a protective hood should be used if available. The tranquility of a quiet darkened large animal recovery stall and a low-lighted cage for small animals will promote smooth emergence.

References

1. Donlon JV. Anesthesia of the eye, ear, nose and throat. In: Miller RD, ed. Anesthesia. New York: Churchill Livingstone, 1986: 1839–1852.
2. Miller PE, Pickett JP. Comparison of the human and canine Schiotz tonometry conversion tables in clinically normal dogs. J Am Vet Med Assoc 201:1021–1025, 1992.
3. Miller PE, Pickett JP. Comparison of the human and canine Schiotz tonometry conversion tables in clinically normal cats. J Am Vet Med Assoc 201:1017–1020, 1992.
4. Miller PE, Majors LJ. Evaluation of two applanation tonometers in horses. Am J Vet Res 51:935, 1990.
5. Gilroy BA. Intraocular and cardiovascular effects of low dose mannitol in the dog. Vet Surg 15:342–344, 1986.
6. Brock KA, Thurmon JC. Pulmonary edema associated with mannitol administration. Can Pract 6:31–33, 1979.
7. Brock KA, Thurmon JC, Benson GJ, et al. Selected hemodynamic and renal effects of intravenous infusion of hypertonic mannitol

in dogs anesthetized with methoxyflurane in oxygen. J Am Anim Hosp Assoc 21:207–214, 1985.

8. Hsu WH, Lee P, Betts DM. Xylazine induced mydriasis in rats and its antagonism by alpha-adrenergic agents. J Vet Pharmacol Ther 4:97–101, 1981.
9. Burke JA, Potter DE. The ocular effects of xylazine in rabbits, cats and monkeys. J Ocul Pharmacol 2:9–12, 1986.
10. Jin Y, Wilson S, Elco EE, Yorio T. Ocular hypotension effects of medetomidine and its analogs. J Ocul Pharmacol 7:285–296, 1991.
11. Potter DE, Ogidigben MJ. Medetomidine-induced alterations of intraocular pressure and contraction of the nictitating membrane. Invest Ophthalmol Vis Sci 32:2799–2805, 1991.
12. Ogidigben MJ, Potter DE. Comparative effects of alpha-2 and DA2 agonists on intraocular pressure in pigmented and nonpigmented rabbits. J Ocul Pharmacol 9:187–199, 1993.
13. Calderone L, Grimes P, and Shalev M. Acute reversible cataract

induction by xylazine and by ketamine-xylazine anesthesia in rats and mice. Exp Eye Res 42:331–337, 1986.
14. Ludders JW. Anesthesia for ophthalmic surgery. Anesthetic considerations for surgery. In: Slatter D, ed. Slatter's textbook of small animal surgery, 2nd ed. Philadelphia: WB Saunders, 1991: 2276–2278.
15. Cunningham AJ. Intraocular pressure—physiology and implications for anesthetic management. Can Anesth Soc J 32:195–208, 1986.
16. Collins BK, Gross ME, Moore CP, Branson KR. Physiologic, pharmacologic, and practical considerations for anesthesia of domestic animals with eye disease. J Am Vet Med Assoc 207:220–230, 1995.
17. Craythorne NWB, Rottenstein HS, Dripps RD. The effect of succinylcholine on intraocular pressure in adults during general anesthesia. Anesthesiology 21:59–63, 1960.

chapter 24B

CESAREAN SECTION PATIENTS

Obstetric Anesthesia

The ideal anesthetic protocol for cesarean section would provide ample analgesia, muscle relaxation, and sedation or narcosis for optimal operating conditions and safety without unduly endangering either mother or fetus. Anesthetics, analgesics, tranquilizers, and sedatives must of necessity cross the blood-brain barrier. Because the physicochemical properties that allow drugs to cross the blood-brain barrier also enable their placental transfer, it is not possible to anesthetize the mother selectively while sparing the fetus. Drug-induced fetal depression and hence decreased viability is equal to that of the mother. Cesarean section is commonly an emergency procedure. Frequently, the physical condition of the mother and fetus is less than optimal because veterinary assistance has been delayed. Thus, the veterinarian is faced with the dilemma of having to anesthetize the mother, who may already be compromised, without adversely affecting the fetus.

No anesthetic or anesthetic protocol is ideal for all parturients. Selection of an anesthetic protocol should be based upon safety to the mother and fetus, patient comfort, convenience to the surgeon, allowing rapid completion of the procedure, and familiarity with the anesthetic technique. Further, the choice of an anesthetic protocol must be based upon knowledge of the physiologic alterations induced by pregnancy and labor,

the pharmacology of the drugs when administered in the perinatal period and their direct and indirect effects on the fetus and neonate, the benefits and risks of the techniques chosen, and the significance of obstetric complications in anesthetic management. Regardless of the technique used, drugs should be chosen and administered to minimize fetal depression. Decreasing time from induction to delivery, will decrease fetal exposure to anesthetic drugs and minimize the period of anesthetic-induced maternal cardiopulmonary depression. Surgical expediency decreases maternal recumbency time and is of major importance in the larger species. With prolonged uterine isolation prior to fetal delivery, placental perfusion decreases, resulting in fetal hypoxemia, acidosis and distress.

Physiologic Alterations Induced by Pregnancy

Metabolic demands of gestation and parturition are met by altered physiologic function (Table 24B–1). Most of the data describing physiologic alterations of pregnancy have been obtained from women and ewes. Although minimal work has been done in other species, the changes should be comparable, even if not of equal magnitude. Birth weight expressed as percent of maternal weight for people, sheep, dogs, and cats is 5.7, 11.4, 16.1, and 13.2%, respectively.(1) This suggests that the physiologic burden and therefore physiologic alterations may in fact be greater in animals than in women.

CARDIOVASCULAR ALTERATIONS AND THEIR CLINICAL IMPLICATIONS

During pregnancy, plasma estrogens decrease peripheral vascular resistance, resulting in an increase in cardiac output while systolic and diastolic blood pressures remain unchanged. Blood volume increases by approximately 40%; plasma volume increases more than red cell mass, resulting in decreased hemoglobin concentration and packed cell volume.(2) Increased heart rate and stroke volume cause cardiac output to increase during pregnancy 30 to 50% above normal near term.(3, 4) During labor and immediately postpartum, cardiac output increases an additional 10 to 25% as a result of blood being extruded from the contracting uterus.(5) Cardiac output during labor is also influenced by the parturient's body position, pain, and apprehension.(2) During labor, systolic pressure increases by 10 to 30 mm Hg. While central venous pressure does not change during pregnancy because of increased venous capacity, it increases slightly (4 to 6 cm H_2O) during labor and has been reported to increase by 50 cm H_2O during painful fetal extraction.(6) Compression of the posterior vena cava and aorta by the enlarged uterus and its contents can occur during dorsal recumbency. This can cause decreased venous return and cardiac output with resultant decreased uterine and renal blood flow. Although this does not appear to be as serious a problem in dogs and cats, time spent restrained or positioned in dorsal recumbency should be kept to a minimum.(7, 8)

Table 24B–1. Physiologic Alterations Induced by Pregnancy

Variable	
Heart rate	↑
Cardiac output	↑
Blood volume	↑
Plasma volume	↑
Packed cell volume, hemoglobin, plasma protein	↓
Arterial blood pressure	o
Central venous pressure	o, ↑ during labor
Minute volume of ventilation	↑
Oxygen consumption	↑
pHa and PaO_2	o
$PaCO_2$	↓
Total lung and vital capacity	o
Functional residual capacity	↓
Gastric emptying time and intra-gastrical pressure	↑
Gastric motility and pH of gastric secretions	↓
Gastric Cl^- and enzyme concentration	↑
SGOT, LDH, and BSP, retention time	↑
Plasma cholinesterase	↓
Renal plasma flow and GFR	↑
BUN and creatinine	↓
Na^+ and water balance	o

o, no change.

Because cardiac work is increased during pregnancy and a parturition, cardiac reserve is decreased. Pulmonary congestion and heart failure may occur in patients with previously well-compensated heart disease. In such patients, pain and anxiety should be controlled. However, care must be taken to avoid excessive cardiac depression and decompensation induced by excessive doses of sedatives or anesthetics. The use of ecbolic agents during or after parturition can adversely affect cardiovascular function. Oxytocin in large or repeated doses induces peripheral vasodilation and hypotension, which can adversely affect both mother and fetus through decreased tissue perfusion. Ergot derivatives induce vasoconstriction and hypertension.(9)

PULMONARY ALTERATIONS AND THEIR CLINICAL IMPLICATIONS

During pregnancy, increased serum concentration of progesterone increases the sensitivity of the respiratory center to arterial carbon dioxide tension (P_aCO_2). As a result of increased minute volume of ventilation, P_aCO_2 decreases and is near 30 torr at parturition. This respiratory alkalosis does not affect arterial pH because of long-term renal compensation. Ventilation may be further increased during labor by pain, apprehension, and anxiety. Oxygen consumption increases by 20% owing to the developing fetus, placenta, uterine muscle, and mammary tissue. Arterial oxygen tension remains unchanged.(2)

Pregnancy also affects the mechanics of ventilation. Airway conductance is increased and total pulmonary resistance is decreased as a result of progesterone-induced relaxation of bronchial smooth muscle. Lung compliance is unaffected. Functional residual capacity (FRC) is decreased by anterior displacement of the diaphragm and abdominal organs by the gravid uterus (Chapter 6). In addition, FRC decreases further during labor due to increased pulmonary blood volume subsequent to intermittent uterine contraction. Due to the decrease in FRC, airway closure at end exhalation develops in approximately one third of human parturients during tidal ventilation.(2) Total lung capacity and vital capacity are unaltered.

Because FRC is decreased, hypoventilation induces hypoxemia and hypercapnia more readily in pregnant than nonpregnant patients. Hypoxemia is exacerbated by increased oxygen consumption during labor. Thus, oxygen administration prior to induction to denitrogenate the lung is advisable if the patient will tolerate it. Induction of anesthesia must be smooth and rapid. Excitation and struggling associated with excessive restraint and poor technique must be avoided. Intubation should be accomplished quickly and ventilation supported to ensure adequate oxygenation. Adequacy of ventilation and oxygenation may be assessed by observing rate of respiration, excursion of the chest wall and/or reservoir bag, and color of mucous membranes, by implementation of pulse oximetry, and by

determination of P_aCO_2 and P_aO_2. Close monitoring is essential.

Induction of anesthesia with inhalation agents is more rapid in pregnant than nonpregnant patients. The rate of equilibration between inspired and alveolar anesthetic partial pressure is increased by the increased alveolar ventilation and decreased FRC. Additionally, increased progesterone and endorphins decrease anesthetic requirements. MAC (minimum alveolar anesthetic concentration that prevents purposeful movement in response to a noxious stimulus in 50% of patients) values are reduced by 25% for halothane, 32% for methoxyflurane, and 40% for isoflurane in pregnant compared to nonpregnant ewes (Chapters 2 and 11). Thus, anesthetic induction may be extremely rapid, requiring as little as one fourth to one fifth the time required for nonpregnant patients.(10) Care must be taken to prevent overanesthetization of pregnant patients. Likewise, there is an increased sensitivity to local anesthetic agents (Chapter 12). As a result, the dose of local anesthetic for epidural or spinal anesthesia can be reduced by approximately one third in the pregnant patient as compared to the nonparturient (Chapter 16).

GASTROINTESTINAL ALTERATIONS AND THEIR CLINICAL IMPLICATIONS

Physical displacement of the stomach by the gravid uterus, decreased gastric motility, and increased serum progesterone delay gastric emptying. Acid, chloride, and enzyme concentrations in gastric secretions are increased. Lower esophageal sphincter tone is decreased, and intragastric pressure is increased. Pain and anxiety during labor decrease gastric motility further.(2)

As a result of altered gastric function, the risk of regurgitation (both active and passive) and aspiration is greater in the parturient. Because increased gastric acidity and decreased gastric muscular tone may be present, metoclopramide (Reglan) and cimetidine (Tagamet) may be given as preanesthetics.(11) Frequently, patients presented for cesarean section have been fed or the time of the last feeding is unknown. Parturients should be regarded as having a full stomach. Tracheal intubation should be performed rapidly upon induction of general anesthesia to gain control of the airway and prevent aspiration of foreign material. Incidence of vomiting is increased by hypotension, hypoxia, and toxic reactions to local anesthetics. Smooth induction of general anesthesia and prevention of hypotension during epidural anesthesia will decrease the incidence of vomiting. Because silent regurgitation can occur when intragastric pressure is high, a cuffed endotracheal tube is desirable. Passive regurgitation can be induced by positive pressure ventilation with a face mask or by manipulation of abdominal viscera. Atropine may increase gastroesophageal sphincter tone, thereby helping to prevent regurgitation (6), but may also inhibit the actions of metoclopramide (0.2–0.4 mg/kg, IM) that increase gastric motility and emptying by sensitizing gastric smooth muscle to acetylcholine.(11) Cimetidine is an H_2 antagonist that decreases gastric secretions and increases pH. The recommended preanesthetic dose is 6–11 mg/kg administered IM or PO.(11)

HEPATIC AND RENAL ALTERATIONS AND THEIR CLINICAL IMPLICATIONS

Pregnancy induces minor alterations in hepatic function. Plasma protein concentration decreases slightly, but total plasma protein is increased due to the increase in blood volume. Bilirubin concentration is unaltered. Serum enzyme concentrations are slightly increased, and sulfobromophthalein sodium (BSP) retention is increased. Plasma cholinesterase concentration decreases. In spite of these alterations, overall liver function is generally well maintained and adequate.(2)

Renal plasma flow and glomerular filtration rate are increased by approximately 60% in pregnant patients. As a result, blood urea nitrogen and creatinine concentrations are lower than in nonpregnant patients.(6) Sodium and water balance are unaffected.

Decreased plasma cholinesterase may result in prolonged action of succinylcholine in pregnant patients, particularly if they have been exposed recently to organophosphate parasiticides (e.g., anthelmintic, flea collars, or dips). Normal or slightly elevated blood urea nitrogen or creatinine levels may indicate renal pathology or compromise in parturient patients. It would appear wise in such patients to avoid drugs with known nephrotoxic potential, such as methoxyflurane, aminoglycoside antibiotics, and nonsteroidal antiinflammatory drugs.

UTERINE BLOOD FLOW ALTERATION AND ITS CLINICAL IMPLICATIONS

Fetal and maternal homeostasis and neonatal survival are dependent upon maintenance of the uteroplacental circulation. Uterine blood flow is directly proportional to perfusion pressure and inversely proportional to uterine vascular resistance. Obstetric anesthesia may decrease uterine blood flow and thereby contribute to reduce fetal viability. In addition, uterine vascular resistance is indirectly increased by uterine contractions and hypertonia (oxytocic response). Arterial hypotension is induced by hypovolemia, anesthetic-induced cardiovascular depression, or sympathetic blockade. Vasoconstriction is induced by endogenous sympathetic discharge or by exogenous sympathomimetics having alpha$_1$-adrenergic effects, such as epinephrine, norepinephrine, methoxamine, phenylephrine, or metaraminol.(2, 12, 13) Hypotension induced by adjunctive drugs and increased uterine tone induced by ecbolics should be avoided.

SUMMARY

Because cardiac reserve diminishes during pregnancy, cardiac decompensation or failure can occur. Likewise, pregnant patients are prone to hypoventilation, hypoxia, and hypercapnia as a result of altered pulmonary function. Inhalation and local anesthetic requirement is decreased, thus increasing the likelihood of a relative overdose and excessive depression. Finally, vomition or regurgitation and aspiration can occur if induction is not followed immediately by rapid control of the airway. Because of the physiologic alterations induced by pregnancy, parturients are a greater anesthetic risk than healthy nonparturient patients.

Perinatal Pharmacology

Alterations in physiologic function induced by pregnancy will variably affect the uptake, distribution, and final disposition of anesthetic agents and adjuncts. The concentration of free (nonionized, unbound) drug in maternal plasma, which is the portion of the administered dose exerting maternal and fetal effects, depends upon several complex processes that occur simultaneously. These include uptake from the site of administration, protein binding, distribution to maternal tissues, biotransformation by maternal liver, excretion, placental transfer, and fetal distribution and metabolism. Because quantitative studies of drug disposition in pregnant patients are sparse, the effects of pregnancy upon drug disposition are largely unknown.(14) The effects of pregnancy on drug biotransformation and excretion are variable and not fully understood. Inhalation anesthetic dose (MAC) is reduced (Chapters 2 and 11). Hepatic biotransformation of barbiturates appears to be decreased in pregnancy.(14) As a result of decreased plasma cholinesterase concentrations, succinylcholine and procaine metabolism is decreased, although usually not significantly.(14) The increase in renal blood flow and glomerular filtration should favor renal excretion of drugs.

The placenta was once regarded as a relative barrier to passage of drugs from mother to fetus. It is now recognized as being quite permeable to anesthetics and anesthetic adjuncts. Any drug administered to the mother will cross the placenta at a rate unique to each drug and induce its effect upon the fetus. These effects will be proportionate to those observed in the mother. Factors that determine placental transfer of drugs and their distribution into and ultimate removal from fetal tissues include physiochemical properties of the compound; the anatomic features of the maternal circulation, placenta, and fetus; and the hemodynamic and pharmacokinetic events that occur within them.(14)

Medications administered at parturition affect the fetus either directly as a result of placental transfer or indirectly through their effects on the mother. Placental transfer of drugs can occur by several mechanisms but by far the most important is simple diffusion. The placenta does not appear to metabolize anesthetics or anesthetic adjuncts. The amount of drug crossing the placenta and entering the fetal circulation is described by the Fick equation:

$$Q/t = K\, A(C_m - C_f)/D$$

where Q/t = amount of diffused substance per unit time.

K = diffusion constant of a given substance.

A = surface area available for diffusion.

D = thickness of the membrane (placental).

C_m = concentration of the substance in the maternal, blood perfusing the placenta (uterine artery, concentration).

C_f = concentration of drug in fetal blood perfusing the placenta (umbilical artery concentration).

Surface area and thickness of the placenta are determined by the type of placenta present in a given species. The common domestic farm animals have thick epitheliochorial placentas with relatively small areas for diffusion because of their cotyledonary or patchy diffuse distribution. The dog and cat have thinner endotheliochorial placentas with somewhat larger zonary areas of implantation. Women and rodents have the thinnest type of placenta, the hemochorial.(15, 16) Thus, the placental diffusion barrier, although not of great significance, is greatest in ruminants, pigs, and horses, intermediate in the dog and cat, and least in rodents and women.

The diffusion constant K is unique to each drug and affected by the conditions present at the time of its administration. The diffusion constant is determined by molecular weight, degree to which the drug is bound to maternal plasma proteins, lipid solubility, and degree of ionization. Drugs with low molecular weight (MW < 500), a low degree of protein binding, high lipid solubility, and poor ionization have high K values and diffuse rapidly across the placenta. Those with high molecular weights (MW > 1000) that are highly protein bound, have low lipid solubility, and are highly ionized cross the placenta slowly. Most anesthetics and anesthetic adjuncts have high K values because of their low molecular weight, high lipid solubility, low degree of ionization, and low degree of protein binding. The muscle relaxant drugs are an exception because they are highly ionized and of low lipid solubility. Thus, their K value is low, and although they can be recovered from fetal blood, they are generally regarded as having minimal placental transfer and negligible direct fetal affects.(14, 17) The degree to which a drug is ionized in the body is determined by its pK_a and the pH of the patient's body fluids. The pK_a is the pH at which the ionized and nonionized forms of the drug exist in equal proportions and is unique to each drug (Chapter 2). Drugs that are weak acids will be less highly ionized as pH decreases.(17) For example, thiopental is a weak acid with a pK_a of 7.6. Thus, when administered to a patient with pH of 7.4, 61% of the drug is nonionized and

active. In acidemic patients with pHs less than 7.4, a greater proportion of the administered dose will be nonionized. Therefore, acidemia decreases the required anesthetic dose of thiopental and other barbiturates. As the degree of ionization decreases, so does the fraction of the dose that is protein bound, so more nonionized drug is available to exert its anesthetic effect. Weakly basic drugs such as opioids and local anesthetics are more highly ionized at pHs below their pK_a.(18) In addition to the effect upon degree of ionization and thus the fraction of the dose in active form, distribution of drug between mother and fetus is influenced by their blood pH and drug pK_a. Normally, the fetal pH is 0.1 unit less than that of the mother. Thus, weakly basic drugs such as opiates and local anesthetics will be found in higher concentration in fetal tissues and plasma than in those of the mother because of "ion trapping." The nonionized form can cross the placenta, but, owing to the maternal-fetal pH difference, ionization occurs in the fetus. This decreases the concentration of fetal nonionized drug, maintaining the maternal-fetal concentration gradient and increasing the nonionized drug transfer across the placenta to the fetus.(19)

Maternal blood concentration of drug depends upon total dose, site and route of administration, rate of distribution and uptake of the drug by maternal tissues, and maternal metabolism and excretion. Thus, drugs with rapidly declining plasma concentration after administration of a fixed dose (e.g., thiopental, propofol, or succinylcholine) result in a short period of exposure of the fetus and placenta to high maternal blood drug concentration. This can be contrasted to the sustained maternal blood levels of drugs administered by continuous infusion and inhalation anesthetics, which result in continuous placental transfer of drug to the fetus.(14, 19)

Fetal drug concentration is the result of passive diffusion across the placenta and is altered by fetal redistribution, metabolism, and protein binding. The concentration of drug in the umbilical vein is not that which is available to the fetal target organs (brain, heart, and other vital organs). As much as 85% of umbilical venous blood initially passes through the fetal liver, where drug may be sequestered or metabolized. In addition, umbilical venous blood containing drug enters the inferior vena cava via the ductus venosus and mixes with drug-free blood returning from the lower extremities and pelvic viscera (Fig. 24B–1). In this way the fetal circulation buffers vital fetal tissues from sudden high drug concentrations. Binding of drug to fetal proteins may limit the amount of available drug and thus reduce toxicity.(14, 17) Fetal metabolism of drugs is not as efficient as in the adult because the fetal liver microsomal enzyme system is not as active as in later life. Drug concentrations and effects can be considerably greater and of longer duration than in the mother. Fetal drug toxicity can be enhanced by fetal or maternal metabolism to more toxic metabolites and by drug interaction.(19)

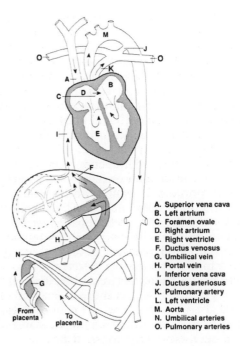

A. Superior vena cava
B. Left artrium
C. Foramen ovale
D. Right artrium
E. Right ventricle
F. Ductus venosus
G. Umbilical vein
H. Portal vein
I. Inferior vena cava
J. Ductus arteriosus
K. Pulmonary artery
L. Left ventricle
M. Aorta
N. Umbilical arteries
O. Pulmonary arteries

From placenta   To placenta

Fig. 24B–1. The direction of blood flow in the fetal vascular system is indicated by arrows. The darkened vascular segments represent umbilical blood and its path of flow into the liver and inferior vena cava via the ductus venosus. Blood flow through the foramen ovale and ductus arteriosus provides a direct path to the arterial system, bypassing the lungs. In the neonate, the ductus arteriosus and foramen ovale closed shortly after birth. This functional closure results in blood flowing through the neonate's lungs, where it is arterialized as in the adult. Time required for anatomic closure of the foramen ovale in the foal may be as much as 12 months. Two months may be required for permanent closure of the foramen ovale.

Clinical Implications

Anesthetic and anesthetic adjunct drugs should be carefully chosen and properly administered to avoid undue maternal and fetal depression and to maximize neonatal vigor and viability. No agent should be used unless distinctly indicated. Drugs that induce sedation and/or tranquilization include the barbiturates, phenothiazines, butyrophenones, benzodiazepines, and alpha$_2$-adrenoceptor agonists. All of these agents rapidly cross the placenta, resulting in neonatal depression. Barbiturates cause neonatal respiratory depression, sleepiness, and decreased activity. Suckling activity is decreased and has been reported to be depressed for 4 days in the human neonate.(19)

Phenothiazine and butyrophenone tranquilizers are frequently used as preanesthetic agents and are often used in conjunction with opiates (Chapter 8). Phenothiazines potentiate opioid-induced depression but add little to analgesia. They induce hypotension via alpha-adrenergic blockade as well as central nervous depression. This results in respiratory depression and decreased ability to regulate body temperature. Their duration of action is long, up to 8 hours.(6, 19) The use of tranquilizer-sedative drugs should be restricted to the markedly apprehensive or excited parturient and

then only in doses sufficient to induce a calming effect without undue generalized depression. There is little indication for the routine use of these agents in the parturient patient.(19)

Diazepam, when used to induce maternal sedation, can induce neonatal lethargy, hypotonus, and hypothermia.(14) It has been suggested that these effects can be minimized by administering less than 0.14 mg/kg IV.(19) Residual benzodiazepine-induced lethargy and muscle relaxation in either the mother or neonate can be antagonized with flumazenil, a specific benzodiazepine antagonist administered to effect. A ratio of 1:13 (flumazenil:diazepam or midazolam) is a reasonable initial dose.(20)

Xylazine is a potent sedative-hypnotic with significant analgesic properties. However, this drug rapidly crosses the placenta and induces both maternal and fetal respiratory and circulatory depression. When used in conjunction with ketamine, there are significant and potentially life-threatening cardiopulmonary changes resulting in decreased tissue perfusion in healthy dogs.(21) Thus, use of xylazine or xylazine-ketamine combinations probably should be avoided in patients presented for cesarean section. Similar effects have been reported for ketamine-acepromazine in the cat. Opioids rapidly cross the placenta and can cause neonatal respiratory and neurobehavioral depression that may last up to 24 hours.(19, 22, 23) In addition, fetal elimination may require 2 to 6 days. It appears that depression is proportional to degree of analgesia; equianalgesic doses of opioids induce equal degrees of depression. Thus, the choice of an opioid is based upon the duration of action desired. The most commonly used opioids are fentanyl, meperidine, and oxymorphone, in order of increasing duration of action.(19) Recently, agents having opiate agonist and antagonist activity have been used to induce analgesia. These agents include butorphanol and buprenorphine (Chapter 8). They reportedly induce less respiratory depression than pure opiate agonists. In addition, a narcotics license is not required for use of these agents. One of the advantages of opioid agonists is that direct antagonists are available to reverse their action. Of the antagonist agents, naloxone (0.04 mg/kg) appears to be one of the most effective. It is a pure antagonist without opiate agonist action. Because nalorphine and levallorphan possess opiate activity of their own, they can increase depression induced by other nonopiate agents (e.g., barbiturates, phenothiazines, and inhalation agents). Because all opioid antagonists rapidly cross the placenta, maternal administration before delivery has been advocated to reverse opioid-induced neonatal depression. This technique deprives the mother of analgesia at the time when it is needed most. Therefore, these agents should be administered directly to the neonate. Finally, because naloxone has a shorter duration of action than most opioid agonists, renarcotization may occur when naloxone is metabolized and excreted. Thus, both mother and neonates should be carefully monitored after opioid reversal with naloxone for recurring signs of narcosis.(19) Should this occur, additional naloxone should be given.

The most commonly used intravenous induction agents are the ultra-short-acting barbiturates thiopental or methohexital (Chapter 9). When these are administered in low doses (less than 4 mg/kg) to women, fetal depression is minimal.(19) Ketamine can be given intravenously to induce anesthesia for intubation rather than a barbiturate. In women, doses of less than 1 mg/kg induced minimal neonatal depression.(19, 24) Alternatively, thiopental (2–3 mg/kg) and ketamine (0.5 mg/kg) have been coadministered to induce anesthesia in parturient women. Because effective induction doses for these agents are higher in dogs and cats than humans, some neonatal depression is more likely to be associated with their use.

Some other injectable short-acting nonbarbiturate induction drugs are currently in use in the United Kingdom and Europe. These agents are not yet approved for use in the United States but may become available in the future. Saffan is a combination of two progesteronelike steroids (alphaxalone, 9 mg/mL, and alphadolone, 3 mg/mL) (Chapter 9). This agent can be administered intravenously or intramuscularly to cats. Anesthetic induction is smooth and rapid. Cardiovascular depression is proportionate to dose and similar to that of equivalent doses of thiopental or methohexital. Saffan induces less respiratory depression than barbiturates. Saffan is compatible with the commonly used preanesthetics, muscle relaxants, and inhalation anesthetics.(24) Because of its short duration of action, the agent is best suited for induction of anesthesia for cesarean section. Saffan has been shown to cross the placenta. Its use in the dog is limited because the solubilizing agent causes severe histamine release. However, it has been used to induce anesthesia in dogs pretreated with antihistamines.(25)

The hypnotics propofol and etomidate can induce hypnosis or basal narcosis sufficient to allow intubation as can the barbiturates (Chapter 9). Their proper use is as an induction agent for intubation and/or as part of a balanced anesthetic protocol where they are accompanied by an analgesic agent. Etomidate is a short-acting nonbarbiturate hypnotic. In dosages suitable for anesthetic induction, etomidate induced rapid safe anesthesia with no significant cardiovascular effects in dogs.(26, 27) In women, induction and recovery occur more rapidly with etomidate than with thiopental. Fetal tissue perfusion is enhanced, as shown by more rapid initiation of neonatal spontaneous breathing and greater fetal vitality at delivery than with thiopental.(28) Etomidate is rapidly redistributed and metabolized by hepatic microsomal enzymes and by plasma esterases. Etomidate frequently causes pain on intravenous injection in nonpremedicated patients. In addition, myoclonus or involuntary movements can occur upon injection, but can be prevented by premedication with benzodiazepines and/or opioids. The induction

dose of etomidate in the unpremedicated dog and cat is 1.5 to 3.0 mg/kg IV.(29) Etomidate is an alternative induction agent for patients with unstable cardiovascular function, hypovolemia or in those with increased intracranial pressure (Chapter 23). Based on its rapid elimination profile in the cat, etomidate may be suitable for repeated intravenous administration in low doses in this species.(30) However, repeated administration of etomidate may result in acute hemolysis as has been reported in the dog.(31)

Propofol induces rapid induction of basal narcosis for intubation and inhalation anesthesia (Chapter 9). Recovery from propofol is prompt and smooth owing to rapid redistribution and metabolism. Metabolism occurs primarily in the liver, but extrahepatic metabolism also cocurs. Because of the extensive distribution and metabolism of propofol, recovery is very rapid. Although propofol rapidly crosses the placenta, it is rapidly cleared from the neonatal circulation. The pharmacologic effects of propofol on cardiovascular and respiratory function are nearly identical to but slightly greater than those of thiopental; arterial pressure and vascular resistance decrease. Cerebral blood flow, oxygen consumption, perfusion pressure, and intracranial pressure decrease as with thiopental. Apnea is common on induction. The advantages of propofol are fast onset and rapid smooth termination of action without residual sedation or depression. The drug does not accumulate in the body, so it can be administered repeatedly or by infusion without saturation of body tissues and prolonged recovery. In the dog and cat the induction dose of propofol is 8 mg/kg IV in unpremedicated patients. Supplemental doses are 0.5 to 2.0 mg/kg IV. Propofol should be approved for veterinary use in the near future.

Skeletal muscle relaxants cross the placenta to a very limited degree and induce little effect on the neonate when used in reasonable clinical doses (17); thus, these drugs are very useful in balanced anesthesia techniques for cesarean section.(32, 33) The most commonly used agents are succinylcholine and pancuronium. Succinylcholine, because of its rapid onset and short duration of action, is especially useful when combined with an ultra-short-acting barbiturate for induction or where muscle relaxation of short duration is desired. Pancuronium can be used to induce muscle relaxation of longer duration (45 minutes). Gallamine may also be used; however, because this drug appears to cross the placenta more readily than the other muscle relaxants and because it offers no distinct advantages, its use in obstetrics has diminished.(19)

Atracurium and vecuronium are nondepolarizing muscle relaxants that are rapidly metabolized in the liver. Atracurium is metabolized by Hofmann elimination and has a short duration of action similar to that of succinylcholine. These agents have fewer cardiovascular side effects than the other muscle relaxants.

Inhalation anesthetics readily cross the placenta with rapid fetal and maternal equilibration. Thus, the degree of neonatal depression is proportional to the depth of anesthesia induced in the mother. Deep levels of maternal anesthesia cause maternal hypotension, decreased uterine blood flow, and fetal acidosis. The less soluble agents halothane, isoflurane, enflurane, or desflurane are preferable to highly soluble agents such as methoxyflurane because induction and recovery of mother and neonate are more rapid. Nitrous oxide can be used to potentiate the more potent volatile agents, thus decreasing the total amount of volatile agent administered. If nitrous oxide is administered at 60%, fetal depression is minimal and neonatal diffusion hypoxia does not occur upon delivery.(19, 32, 33)

Administration of oxygen to the mother is not associated with a significant decrease in uterine blood flow or fetal acidosis.(19) Fetal red blood cells have a lower 2, 3-diphosphoglycerate (2, 3-DPG) concentration than adult red blood cells (Chapters 5 and 6). This anion competes with oxygen for the binding site on the hemoglobin molecule. Thus, fetal hemoglobin can carry more oxygen at low oxygen tensions than adult hemoglobin. Physiologically, this is important in that it ensures a higher level of hemoglobin saturation at the normally low oxygen partial pressures (Po_2 of umbilical vein equals 30 torr)(34, 35) to which the fetus is exposed. Maternal oxygen administration can result in a significant increase in fetal oxygen content. Therefore, oxygen administration is indicated regardless of the anesthetic protocol. Inspired oxygen concentrations of 50% or more during general anesthesia result in more vigorous neonates because of improved oxygenation.(19)

The total effect of carbon dioxide on the fetus is not clear, but passive hyperventilation of the dam results in hypocapnia with decreased uterine artery blood flow. This decreased placental perfusion causes fetal hypoxia, hypercapnia, and acidosis. Maternal active hyperventilation may have the same effect. With adequate arterial oxygenation, a modest increase in P_aCO_2 is well tolerated by the fetus.(19)

Local anesthetic agents are frequently used in combination with other agents or as the sole anesthetic agent for regional techniques. Esters of paraaminobenzoic acid, such as procaine or tetracaine, are metabolized by maternal and fetal pseudocholinesterase. Thus, there is little accumulation of these agents in the fetus. Amide derivatives (e.g., lidocaine, mepivacaine, bupivacaine, and etidocaine) are metabolized by hepatic microsomal enzymes. After absorption from the site of injection, blood levels decrease slowly but can reach significant levels in the fetus. Neonatal blood concentrations in excess of 3 μg/mL of lidocaine or mepivacaine cause neonatal depression at delivery. These concentrations rarely occur after epidural administration but can occur with excessive volumes of drug used for local infiltration.(19) Use of these agents can indirectly affect the fetus. Sympathetic blockade resulting in maternal hypotension and decreased uteroplacental perfusion may occur after epidural injection. This can be controlled by judicious administration of intravenous fluids to offset increased capacity of the vascular tree.(19) In addition to intravenous fluids, vasopressors can be used to treat maternal hypotension resulting from sympathetic blockade. Because ephedrine acts centrally and has minimal arterial vasoconstrictor properties while increasing venous tone and thereby preload, it is used to treat maternal hypotension, thus restoring uterine blood flow. Mephentermine acts in a similar manner. Other agents with alpha-adrenergic activity increase maternal blood pressure by increasing systemic vascular resistance. This results in decreased uterine blood flow, and fetal deterioration often occurs. In addition, these agents stimulate hypertonic uterine contractions, further decreasing uteroplacental perfusion.(19, 33)

Anticholinergic agents such as atropine or glycopyrrolate should be administered to most parturient patients (24, 32) to decrease salivation and inhibit excessive vagal tone that may occur when traction is applied to the uterus. Many parturients have recently eaten, increasing the likelihood of regurgitation, which is enhanced by hypoxia or hypotension. The influence of anticholinergics upon vomition is controversial.(6, 33) In women, atropine has not been shown to decrease the incidence of vomition at parturition.(33) Glycopyrrolate increases gastric pH, thus decreasing severity of Mendelson's syndrome should regurgitation and aspiration of vomitus occur.(34) Additionally, because glycopyrrolate does not readily cross the placenta, it does not effect the fetus to the same extent as atropine. Therefore, it may be a more appropriate anticholinergic.

Anesthetic Techniques for Cesarean Section

Satisfactory anesthesia for cesarean section can be induced by a number of methods. Cesarean section can be accomplished either by regional or general anesthesia. Advantages of general anesthesia include speed and ease of induction, reliability, reproducibility, and controllability. General anesthesia provides optimum operating conditions with a relaxed immobile patient. Tracheal intubation ensures control of the maternal airway, thereby preventing aspiration of vomitus or regurgitated rumen contents. In addition, it provides a route for maternal oxygen administration, thereby improving fetal oxygenation. When general anesthesia is properly administered, maternal cardiopulmonary function is well maintained.(24, 33) In addition, most veterinarians are more confident of their ability to induce general anesthesia safely than to induce regional anesthesia successfully. General anesthesia is not without disadvantages, however, because it induces greater neonatal depression than regional anesthesia. If the anesthetic plane is too light, maternal catecholamine release can result in hypertension and decreased uteroplacental perfusion, leading to both maternal and fetal stress and deterioration of cardiopulmonary function.(12, 13, 22) Aspiration and problems of airway management with general anesthesia are more likely to occur when the trachea is not properly intubated.

Aspiration and inability to successfully intubate the trachea are the leading causes of maternal mortality associated with cesarean section in women.(24, 33) Fortunately, dogs, cats, and horses are relatively easy to intubate because of their anatomic features. However, ruminants and swine are relatively difficult to intubate, and this presents problems for most veterinarians on the farm. General anesthesia is essential in mares and may be more appropriate than regional anesthesia in selected clinical situations in other species. These include maternal hypovolemia, prolonged dystocia in which the mother is exhausted and the fetus is severely stressed, maternal cardiac disease or failure, morbid obesity, cases in which the mother is so aggressive or fractious as to preclude regional anesthesia, brachyce-phalic dogs with upper airway obstruction, and instances in which the veterinarian is inexperienced in regional anesthetic techniques.

Many different techniques for induction of general anesthesia for cesarean section in dogs and cats have been shown to be satisfactory (Table 24B–2).(36) Regional anesthesia for cesarean section is a well-established technique.(32) Local infiltration or field block may be used, but it has several disadvantages when compared to the epidural technique. Infiltration requires larger amounts of anesthetic agent, which are absorbed and depress the fetus. Muscle relaxation and analgesia are not as profound or as uniform as with

Table 24B–2. Drugs Used to Induce Anesthesia for Cesarean Section in Dogs and Cats

Species	Drug or Technique	Dosage	Comment
Elective cesarean section			
Dogs	1. Lidocaine (epidural)	1 mL/3–5 kg	Assistant required for restraint. Oxygen administered by face mask. Glycopyr-rolate given as needed.
	Oxymorphone	0.05–0.2 mg/kg	
	2. Droperidol-fentanyl (Innovar-Vet)	1 mL/20–30 kg IV	Supplemental dose of droperidol-fentanyl or fentanyl may be needed. Inhalant given in low dosage until delivery. N$_2$O probably should not be given prior to umbilical vein clamp to prevent diffusion hypoxia in the neonate when initial breathing of room air ensues.
	Glycopyrrolate	0.01 mg/kg, as needed to effect	
	Isoflurane*	0.5–1.0%	
	Halothane*	0.35–0.75%	
	3. Propofol	5–8 mg/kg IV to effect	
Cats	1. Ketamine	1–3 mg/kg IV to effect	Fetal depression occurs with excessive doses. Lidocaine (0.25 mL) applied to arytenoid cartilages reduces likelihood of laryngospasm.
	Isoflurane*	0.5–1.0%	
	Halothane*	0.35–0.75%	
	2. Propofol	5–8 mg/kg IV to effect	
Emergency cesarean section			
Dogs	1. Diazepam	0.2 mg/kg IV	Opioids used to keep dose of inhalant low. Large doses may result in excessive "ion trapping." Patient may decompensate with excessive dose of inhalant.
	Ketamine	5.5 mg/kg IV	
	Isoflurane*	0.5–1.0%	
	Oxymorphone	0.05–0.1 mg/kg IV	
	2. Diazepam	0.2 mg/kg IV	Supplemental doses of oxymorphone may be needed.
	Oxymorphone	0.05–0.1 mg/kg IV	
	3. Diazepam	0.2 mg/kg IV	
	Etomidate	1.5–3.0 mg/kg IV	
Cats	1. Diazepam	0.2 mg/kg IV	Topical lidocaine to larynx facilitates intubation.
	Ketamine	1–2 mg/kg IV	
	Oxymorphone	0.05 mg/kg IV	
	Isoflurane*	0.05–1.0%	
	2. Diazepam	0.2 mg/kg IV	
	Etomidate	1.5–3.0 mg/kg IV	

Techniques listed for emergencies are also suitable for elective cesarean sections.
*Inhalant anesthetics are used in low concentrations, and only if necessary, before the fetuses are delivered.

epidural techniques. Therefore, field block is often supplemented with heavy sedation or tranquilization, contributing to profound maternal and fetal depression. For these reasons, this type of approach is often abandoned for either general or epidural anesthesia.

Because the spinal cord terminates at the level of the sixth lumbar vertebra in the dog and cat, subarachnoid (true spinal) injection of the anesthetic agent is not common when made at the lumbosacral junction. Because the spinal cord terminates at the midsacrum in swine and ruminants, subarachnoid injection can occur at the lumbosacral junction. Spinal anesthesia (epidural or subarachnoid) has the advantages of simplicity of technique, minimal exposure of the fetus to drugs, less intraoperative bleeding, and, because the mother remains awake, minimal risk of aspiration.(37) In addition, muscle relaxation and analgesia are optimal. Disadvantages include hypotension secondary to sympathetic blockade. Nausea and vomiting can occur during the procedure as a result of hypotension and visceral manipulation.(38) Because the dam remains conscious, movement of the forelimbs and head often occurs. This precludes the use of spinal technique in highly excited or fractious patients and in mares, because they become hysterical when they are unable to stand. Finally, the successful induction of epidural anesthesia requires that the veterinarian be well acquainted with the technique. However, the skill required is well within the reach of anyone wishing to utilize this approach and can be readily acquired with minimal practice of the techniques. The hypotension induced by epidural anesthesia can be readily offset by concurrent fluid and catecholamine administration. Lactated Ringer's solution, normal saline, or half-strength saline mixed with equal volumes of 5% dextrose solution can be administered at approximately 20 mL/kg over 15 to 20 minutes to maintain arterial blood pressure (Chapter 19). When hypotension is severe, ephedrine may be administered (0.15 mg/kg IV). As with general anesthesia, anticholinergic agents are indicated to prevent bradycardia.

Spinal anesthesia will induce recumbency, which may not be desirable in large ruminants because of adverse effects on cardiopulmonary function. If the veterinarian prefers, standing cesarean section in cattle may be performed using either a proximal or distal paralumbar block (Chapter 16). In cows that are in poor condition, exhausted, or in shock, the distal technique is preferred because it does not induce a scoliosislike position and the cow is more likely to remain standing throughout the procedure. These techniques may also be used in sheep and goats; however, most veterinarians find it convenient to place small ruminants in lateral recumbency for cesarean section. Therefore, spinal techniques are preferable to regional techniques in sheep and goats.

Spinal techniques work well in sows. The technique is well established and not difficult to perform. When utilizing this technique, it is sometimes necessary to restrain the sow's head and forelimbs. If this is done, usually by placing a rope around the upper jaw, it is important that the head not be placed in extension (Chapter 20). If pigs are sedated and restrained in lateral recumbency with the head extended, the soft palate may occlude the airway and the patient may suffocate. This occurrence has been observed in sows and gilts undergoing cesarean section with spinal anesthesia without additional sedatives or tranquilizers. Because cesarean section in swine is often viewed as a last-ditch effort by producers, it is often delayed until the sow's condition has deteriorated severely. Often, the sow has been traumatized by repeated efforts to manually extract the piglets and has received large repeated doses of oxytocin. Thus a high percentage of sows presented for cesarean section are hypovolemic and hypotensive. Success or failure is often predicated on restoring effective circulating blood volume before anesthesia and surgery. Fluids can be readily administered to sows via indwelling catheters placed percutaneously into the ear veins. Prior to anesthetic administration, 1 to 3 liters of lactated Ringer's solution or another balanced electrolyte solution can be given rapidly. This will restore circulating volume and offset hypotension induced by spinal techniques. Fluid administration can be continued throughout surgery to maintain a patent vein for administration of other supportive therapy as indicated. As with general anesthesia, anticholinergic agents should be used to prevent vagal bradycardia.

Care of the Newborn

After delivery, the head is cleared of membranes and the oropharynx of fluid. The umbilical vessels should be milked toward the fetus to empty them of blood, clamped approximately 2 to 5 cm from the body wall, and severed from the placenta. The neonate can then be gently rubbed with a towel to dry it and stimulate breathing. It may also be helpful to gently swing the neonate in a headdown position to help clear the respiratory tree of fluid. The head and neck should be supported to avoid a whiplash action and prevent injury.

When general anesthesia is used in ruminants or horses, an alternate method of managing the neonate may be used to good advantage. After uterine incision, the fetal head is delivered through the incision, the oropharynx is cleared of fluid, and the trachea is intubated with a cuffed tube. The fetus can then be delivered and the umbilicus severed. Because the uteroplacental and umbilical circulation is preserved until the airway is secured, hypoxia is prevented. Once the fetus is delivered, ventilation can be supported if necessary via an Ambu bag.

Doxapram can be used to stimulate breathing in the neonate. In the pup, the dosage is 1 to 5 mg (approximately 1 to 5 drops from a 20- to 22-gauge needle). In the kitten, the dosage is 1 to 2 mg (1 to 2 drops) administered topically to the oral mucosa or injected intramuscularly or subcutaneously.(36) Newborns are susceptible to chilling and should be kept warm.(36) After completion of surgery and recovery from anesthesia, the young can be introduced to their mother. If regional anesthesia was used, they can be placed with their mother as soon as the surgery is complete.

References

1. Dawes GS. Foetal and neonatal physiology. Chicago: Year Book, 1968: 15.
2. Shnider SM. The physiology of pregnancy. Annual Refresher Course Lectures. Park Ridge, IL: American Society of Anesthesiologists, 1978: 1251–1258.
3. Kerr MG. Cardiovascular dynamics in pregnancy and labor. Br Med Bull 24:19, 1968.
4. Ueland K, Parer JT. Effects of estrogens on the cardiovascular system of the ewe. Am J Obstet Gynecol 96:400, 1966.
5. Ueland K, Hansen JM. Maternal cardiovascular dynamics. II. Posture and uterine contractions. Am J Obstet Gynecol 103:1–7, 1969.
6. James EM III. Physiologic Changes during Pregnancy. Annual Refresher Course Lectures. Park Ridge, IL: American Society of Anesthesiologists, 1980: 1251–1255.
7. Marx CE. Physiology of pregnancy—High risk implications. Annual Refresher Course Lectures. Park Ridge, IL, American Society of Anesthesiologists. 1979: 1251–1254.
8. Kerr MC, Scott DB. Inferior vena caval occlusion in late pregnancy. In: Marx C, ed. Clinical anesthesia, vol. 10-2. Philadelphia: FA Davis, 1973: 38.
9. Lipton B, Hershey SC, Baez S. Compatibility of oxytocics with anesthetic agents. JAMA 179:410–416, 1962.
10. Palahniuk RJ, Shnider SM, Eger EI III, Lopez-Manzanara P. Pregnancy decreases the requirements of inhaled anesthetic agents. Anesthesiology 41:82–83, 1974.
11. Paddleford RR. Anesthesia for Cesarean section in the dog. Opinions in small animal anesthesia. In: Haskins SC, Klide Am, eds. Vet Clin North Am, Small Animal Practice Series, Philadelphia: WB Saunders, 1992: 481–484.
12. Wright RC, Shnider SM, Levinsan G, et al. The effect of maternal stress on plasma catecholamines and uterine blood flow in the ewe [Abstract]. Annual Meeting of the Society of Obstetric Anesthesia and Perinatology, 1978: 17.
13. Morishema HO, Yeh M-N, James LS. The effects of maternal pain and hyperexcitability upon the fetus—possible benefits of maternal sedation [Abstract]. Scientific Session of American Society of Anesthesiologists Annual Meeting, Atlanta, Georgia, 1977.
14. Alper MH. Perinatal pharmacology. Annual Refresher Course Lectures. Park Ridge, IL: American Society of Anesthesiologists, 1979: 1261–1267.
15. Ramsey EM. The placenta of laboratory animals and man. New York: Holt. Rinehart & Winston, 1975: 73, 142, 154, 160.
16. Nalbandav AV. Reproductive Physiology. San Francisco: WH Freeman, 1958: 196.
17. Einster M. Perinatal pharmacology. Annual Refresher Course Lectures. Park Ridge, IL: American Society of Anesthesiologists, 1980: 1261–1264.
18. Collins VI. Principles of anesthesiology, 2nd ed. Philadelphia: Lea & Febiger, 1976: 199.
19. Gutsche B. Perinatal pharmacology. Annual Refresher Course Lectures. Park Ridge, IL: American Society of Anesthesiologists, 1978: 1291–1299.
20. Tranquilli WJ, Lemke K, Williams LL, et al. Flumazenal efficacy in reversing diazepam or midazolam overdose in dogs. J Vet Anaesth 19:65–68, 1992.
21. McDonnell W, Van Corder I. Cardiopulmonary effects of xylazine/ketamine in dogs [Abstract]. Annual Scientific Meeting American College of Veterinary Anesthesiologists, Las Vegas, Nevada, 1982.
22. Palahniuk RJ. Obstetric anesthesia in the healthy parturient. Annual Refresher Course Lectures. Park Ridge, IL: American Society of Anesthesiologists, 1979: 1271–1274.
23. Hodgkinson R, Bhatt M, Wang CN. Double-blind comparison of the neurobehavior of neonates following the administration of different doses of meperidine to the mother. Can Anaesth Soc J 25:405, 1978.
24. Hall LW. Althesin in the large animal. Postgrad Med J 48(suppl 2):55–58, 1972.
25. Corbet HR. The use of saffan in the dog. Aust Vet Pract 7(4):184–188, 1977.
26. Nagel ML, Muir WW, Nguyen K. Comparison of the cardiopulmonary effects of etomidate and thiamylal in dogs. Am J V Res 40(2):193–196, 1979.
27. Muir WW, Swanson CR. Principles, techniques, and complications of feline anesthesia and chemical restraint. In: Sherding R, ed. The Cat: Diseases and Clinical Management. New York, Churchhill Livingstone, 1989: 81–116.
28. Downing JW, Buley RJR, Brock-Utney JG, Houlton PC. Etomidate for induction of anesthesia at caesarean section: comparison with thiopentone. Br J Anaesth 51:135–140, 1979.
29. Tranquilli WJ. Anesthesia for cesarian section in the cat. Opinions in small animal anesthesia. In: Haskins SC, Klide AM, eds. Vet Clin North Am, Small Animal Practice Series. 1992: Philadelphia: WB Saunders, 484–486.
30. Wertz EM, Benson GJ, Thurmon JC, et al. Pharmacokinetics of etomidate in the cat. Am J Vet Res 5(2):281–285, 1990.
31. Ko JCH, Thurmon JC, Benson GJ, Tranquilli WJ. Acute hemolysis with etomidate-propylene glycol infusion in the dog. J Vet Anaesth. 20:92–94, 1993.
32. Gibbs CP. Anesthesia for cesarean section: general. Annual Refresher Course Lectures. Park Ridge, IL: American Society of Anesthesiologists, 1981: 2181–2185.
33. Datta S, Alper MH: Anesthesia for cesarean section. Anesthesiology 53:142–160, 1980.
34. Goodjier WJ, Levy W. Anesthetic management of the cesarean section. In: Short CE, ed. Veterinary Clinics of North America, vol. 3, no. 1, Philadelphia: WB Saunders, 1973: 85.
35. Guyton AC. Textbook of medical physiology, 4th ed. Philadelphia: WB Saunders, 1971: 78.
36. Hellyer PW. Anesthesia for cesarian section. Anesthetic considerations for surgery. In: Slatter D, ed. Slatter's Textbook of Small Animal Surgery, 2nd ed. Philadelphia: WB Saunders, 1991: 2300–2303.
37. Ratra CK, Badola RP, Bhargava KP. A study of factors concerned with emesis during spinal anesthesia. Br J Anaesth 44:1208–1211, 1972.
38. Dow TJB, Brock-Utney JG, Rubin J, et al. The effect of atropine on the lower esophageal sphincter during pregnancy. Obstet Gynecol 51:426–430, 1978.

TRAUMA PATIENTS

David D. Martin

Evaluation of the Trauma Patient

Proper care of the trauma victim requires advanced planning, an ordered protocol, and efficient use of time and resources. When a team approach is taken in the emergency room with each member of the team given preassigned duties, rapid evaluation and treatment are possible. Upon the patient's arrival, airway, breathing, circulation, and neurologic status should be quickly assessed. Assessment of circulation, ventilatory, and neurologic function should be made repeatedly during the initial treatment period. A trauma score can be used in an attempt to quantify the patient's prognosis upon arrival and during the initial treatment period (Table 24C–1).(1) A high score is consistent with a good prognosis, whereas a low score is indicative of severe trauma and a poorer prognosis. Severely traumatized patients are subject to a variety of complications that may manifest themselves in the first few days following the traumatic incident. These complications may not be directly related to the initial traumatic damage, but reflect overall tissue destruction, immune suppression, and metabolic imbalances. These complications may be septic, nonseptic, or both.(2, 3)

A global activation of many cytokine mediators of the inflammatory response resulting in a generalized increase in vascular permeability, neutrophil infiltration, and capillary microemboli has been termed the systemic inflammatory response syndrome (SIRS). Early signs of SIRS or septic shock include brick-red mucous membranes, tachycardia, high cardiac output (in euvolemic patients), normal or low blood pressure, and low vascular resistance. Definitions of SIRS for dogs and cats based upon the presence of various key clinical signs have been proposed and are presented in Table 24C–2.(4) All organs may be affected. In cats lung function due to rapid fluid accumulation appears to be most often disrupted early in the course of SIRS. In dogs, the order of organ dysfunction is commonly gastrointestinal tract, followed by liver, kidney, and then lung. Patients suffering from noncardiogenic pulmonary edema may have this condition exacerbated by rapid crystalloid fluid administration. Persistent microcirculatory perfusion failure may lead to sludging of blood and increased cellular and platelet aggregation. Along with the release of inflammatory mediators, these conditions result in enhanced coagulation and propagation of the inflammatory response. Toxic oxygen

829

Table 24C–1. Method to Determine Prognosis in Severely Traumatized Animals

	Trauma	Value	Points	Score
A.	**Respiratory Rate/Minute:**	10 to 20	4	
	Number of respirations	20 to 30	**3**	
	in 15 s, multiply by four	>30	2	
		<5	1	A ____
B.	**Respiratory Effort:**	Normal	1	
	Shallow or labored		0	B ____
C.	**Systolic Blood Pressure:**	>90	4	
	Systolic cuff pressure/either	70 to 90	3	
	by auscultation or palpation	50 to 69	2	
		<50	1	C ____
D.	**Capillary Refill:**			
	Normal/refill in 2 s		2	
	Delayed more than 2 s		1	
	None/no refill		0	D ____
E.	**CNS Function Scale:**			
	1. Eye opening:			
	Spontaneously		4 ____	
	To voice		3 ____	
	To pain		2 ____	
	Will not open		1 ____	
	2. Mentation:			
	Alert		4 ____	
	Stuporous		3 ____	
	Comatose		2 ____	
	3. Motor responses:			
	Obeys commands		5 ____	
	Purposeful movement (pain)		4 ____	
	Withdraws (pain)		3 ____	
	Flexion (pain)		2 ____	
	No response		1 ____	E ____
	A low score is indicative of severe trauma and poor prognosis.			
			Total Score	

metabolites can cause further cellular damage, persistent edema, and increased oxygen diffusion distance between cells and capillaries. If oxygen delivery to tissues is chronically impaired, the systemic inflammatory state can result in multiple organ dysfunction (MODS), traditionally defined as irreversible shock. Successful management of animals with septic shock or SIRS depends on anticipation, not reaction.(3) Appropriate antibiotic administration, aggressive cardiovascular support, and monitoring of the susceptible organs must be undertaken during the first 24 to 72 hours following insult. Early intervention and cardiovascular

resuscitation to supernormal levels is recommended (Table 24C–3). A list of 20 parameters to be assessed twice daily has been proposed to improve the clinical management of the patient with SIRS (Table 24C–4). An algorithm depicting SIRS management is given in Figure 24C–1.(3) Therapeutic agents and doses used in the treatment of various metabolic derangements associated with SIRS are given in Tables 24C–5, 6, and 7.

When anesthetizing such patients, the primary goal is to optimize tissue perfusion and oxygen delivery to all vital organ systems while achieving unconsciousness, an appropriate degree of analgesia, and muscle relax-

Table 24C–2. Proposed Definitions of Systemic Inflammatory Response Syndrome in Dogs and Cats

Proposed for Dogs

The presence of two or more of the following clinical conditions:
- Body temperature > 40° C or < 38° C.
- Heart rate > 120 beats/min in calm, resting dog.
- Hyperventilation of P_aCO_2 < 30 mm Hg.
- White blood count > 18,000/mL or < 5000/mL or > 5% immature (band) forms

Proposed for Cats

The presence of two or more of the following clinical conditions:
- Body temperature > 40° C or < 38° C.
- Heart rate > 140 beats/min in calm, resting cat.
- Respiratory rate > 20 breaths/min or P_aCO_2 < 28 mm Hg.
- White blood cell count > 18,000/mL or < 5000/mL or > 5% immature (band) forms.

(From Hardie, E.M. Life Threatening Bacterial Infection. Compend Cont Educ 17(6):763–777, 1995.)

Table 24C–3. Cardiovascular Resuscitation Goals for Animals with Systemic Inflammatory Response Syndrome

Variable	Goal
Mixed venous oxygen tension, P_vO_2 (mm Hg)	>40
Pulmonary artery pressure (mm Hg)	>25/10
Pulmonary wedge pressure (mm Hg)	<18
Systemic vascular resistance (dyne × s/cm^{-5} × m^2)	>1450
Pulmonary vascular resistance (dyne × s/cm^{-5} × m^2)	45–250
Oxygen extraction (%)	22–30
Cardiac index (L/min × m^2)	>4.5
Oxygen delivery (mL/min × m^2)	>600
Oxygen consumption (mL/min × m^2)	>170

(From Hardie, E.M. Life Threatening Bacterial Infection. Compend Cont Educ 17(6):763–777, 1995.)

ation. The patient should be stabilized and anesthetics selected that will not magnify preexisting pathology. In some circumstances where patients are presented in an unconscious state, securing the airway, oxygen administration, and ensuring analgesia may be all that is required.

Shock and Stabilization of the Traumatized Patient

As a general rule, anesthesia should not be undertaken until the patient's vital organ functions have been stabilized. In cases with a history of severe trauma, the patient should always be considered a likely candidate for developing some type of shock. Shock is defined as a state of generalized inadequate tissue perfusion. Hypotension usually accompanies shock, but shock can occur with normal blood pressure and hypotension can

occur without shock, as is often the case with anesthetic overdose. Shock may result from blood loss, poor cardiac function, sepsis, and interruption of blood flow. Anaphylactic and neurogenic shock are characterized by relative hypovolemia and hypotension resulting from acute increases in vascular capacitance. Hypovolemic and neurogenic shock are typically observed in the acutely traumatized patient, whereas septic shock (SIRS) develops after the initial insult. Clinical signs of hemorrhagic shock most commonly encountered in the acutely traumatized patient include pallor, cyanosis, disorientation, tachycardia, cold extremities, cardiac dysrhythmias, pump failure, tachypnea, hypotension, oliguria, disseminated intravascular coagulation (DIC), and progressive metabolic acidosis.(1)

With acute blood loss, normal homeostatic reflexes vigorously defend blood pressure in an attempt to maintain vital organ function. As hemorrhage ensues, plasma renin levels elevate, antidiuretic hormone increases, and the sympathetic nervous system activates to produce tachycardia and arteriolar vasoconstriction (Chapter 5). These mechanisms can maintain blood pressure until about 40% of normal blood volume is lost.(1) Thus, an animal can be severely hypovolemic but normotensive. Once blood loss exceeds 40% of blood volume, compensatory organ mechanisms fail over time and shock becomes "irreversible." Prolonged poor tissue perfusion results in vital organ ischemia, loss of cell membrane integrity, and cell death.(1) If the trauma involves crushing of tissues or severe burns,

Table 24C–4. SIRS Treatment Checklist*

☐	1. Fluid balance
☐	2. Blood pressure/perfusion
☐	3. Cardiac function/rhythm
☐	4. Albumin
☐	5. Oncotic pull
☐	6. Oxygenation/ventilation
☐	7. Glucose
☐	8. Electrolytes/acid-base balance
☐	9. Mentation/intracranial pressure
☐	10. Coagulation
☐	11. RBC/hemoglobin
☐	12. Renal function/urine output
☐	13. Immune state/WBC/antibiotic ±
☐	14. GI motility/integrity
☐	15. Drug metabolism/dosages
☐	16. Nutrition
☐	17. Pain control
☐	18. Nursing mobility/catheter care
☐	19. Bandage/wound care
☐	20. Tender loving care

*The importance of each will vary from patient to patient. (From Purvis, D., and Kirby, R. Systemic Inflammatory Response Syndrome: Septic Shock. Vet Clin North Am: Small Anim Pract 24(6):1225–1247, 1994.

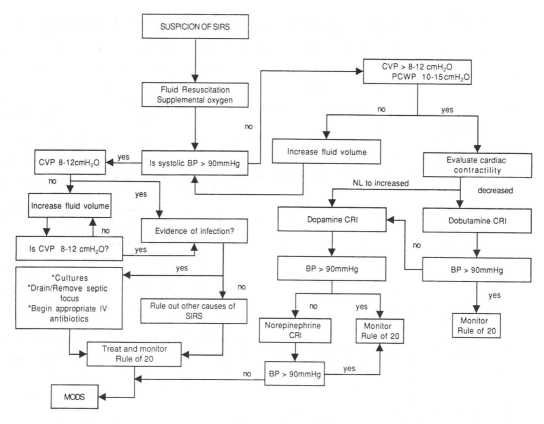

Fig. 24C–1. Algorithm depicting SIRS patient management. CVP, central venous pressure; PCWP, pulmonary capillary wedge pressure; NL, normal; CRI, continuous rate infusion; BP, blood pressure (implies systolic); MODS, multiple organ dysfunction syndrome; SIRS, systemic inflammatory response syndrome; septic shock. (From Purvis, D., and Kirby, R. Systemic Inflammatory Response Syndrome: Septic Shock. Vet Clin North Am. Small Anim Pract 24(6):1225–1247, 1994.)

shock is accompanied by increased capillary permeability and rapid translocation of fluids. In addition, toxic factors from exogenous sources (microbial toxins) and endogenous sources (e.g., fat emboli, K^+ release, lysosomal enzymes, and myocardial depressant factor) are simultaneously released, resulting in further organ malfunction (MODS).(5) The primary treatment of hemorrhagic shock is aggressive fluid therapy. Large-bore intravenous catheters should be placed in each cephalic vein and/or jugular veins, and warm, crystalloid solutions and/or blood rapidly infused. If necessary, fluids can also be given rapidly into the intraosseous space of the tibia or femur. When rapid infusion of large volumes of crystalloids decreases serum total solids concentration to below 3.5 g/dL, simultaneous colloid solution administration is advantageous in maintaining intravascular volume (Chapters 5 and 19).(6) There is increasing evidence that hypertonic saline may be beneficial in the early treatment of hypovolemic and hemorrhagic shock in animals.(7) Intravenous administration of small volumes (4 to 6 mL/kg) of 7.5% hypertonic saline results in beneficial cardiovascular effects in hypovolemic dogs and cats.(8–10) Although the basic mechanisms are not understood completely, increases in pressure and cardiac output appear to be mediated primarily by rapid increases in plasma vol-

ume.(9) A second potential benefit of hypertonic saline administration is minimizing the risk of cerebral edema in head trauma patients.(11, 12) Massive blood loss will eventually require transfusion of whole blood or packed red blood cells to replace oxygen transport capacity. Trend monitoring of hematocrit, total solids, central venous pressure, and urine output are helpful in guiding resuscitation efforts (Chapter 15).

Spinal shock is a common sequela to spinal cord injury or blunt trauma, which can cause a mechanical disruption of sympathetic nervous system outflow. The patient's extremities will feel warm (peripheral vasodilation), and even though hypotension is present, heart rate is slow because of sympathetic denervation. These patients are relatively hypovolemic; that is, intravascular capacity greatly exceeds intravascular volume. Organ perfusion may or may not be adequate, and vascular resistance is drastically reduced. These patients are more susceptible to hypothermia because they are unable to constrict peripheral vasculature. Fluids should be given to increase vascular volume. If arterial pressure is low and the pulse cannot be palpated, mixed inotropic/vasoconstrictor-type drugs should be given to increase blood flow to vital organs. Intravenous ephedrine, epinephrine, mephentermine, or metaraminol are good choices in these patients (Tables 24C–6 and

Table 24C–5. **Therapeutic Agents Used to Treat Metabolic Derangements Associated with SIRS**

Metabolic Derangement	Dose Regimen	Use and/or Frequency
Hypovolemia		
Hypertonic crystalloids		
7.5% NaCl solution	4 mL/kg, IV	Once
(70 mL 23.4% NaCl in 180 mL 0.9% NaCl or 6% dextran 70)		
Colloids		
Plasma	Maximum: 20 mL/kg/24 h IV	As needed
Hetastarch 120	Maximum: 20 mL/kg/first 24 h, then 10 mL/kg/24 h IV (slow infusion)	As needed
Dextran 70	Maximum: 20 mL/kg/first 24 h, then 10 mL/kg/24 h IV (slow infusion)	As needed
3% Albumin (12 mL 25% human albumin in 488 mL lactated Ringer's solution)	20 mL/kg IV	Resuscitation
Isotonic crystalloids		
Lactated Ringer's solution	90–270 mL/kg IV 10–20 mL/kg/h IV	Resuscitation To meet ongoing needs
Altered Clotting Function		
Heparin (low dosage)	75–100 units/kg SQ	Every 6–8 h
Heparin-activated plasma (incubate 5–10 units/kg heparin with 1 unit fresh plasma for 30 minutes)	10 mL/kg IV	Every 3 h, based on clotting function
Metabolic Dysfunction		
KCl	0.125–0.25 mEq/kg/h IV; do not exceed 0.5 mEq/kg/h	As needed
Glucose	50–500 mg/kg/h IV	As needed
NaHCO$_3$	Base excess × 0.3 × body weight in kg = mEq needed to correct deficit, IV (slow infusion)	As needed (pH 7.1 or less)
Gastrointestinal Tract Dysfunction		
Cimetidine	5–10 mg/kg IV, IM, PO	Every 6–8 h
Ranitidine	2 mg/kg IV, IM, PO	Every 8–12 h
Omeprazole	0.7 mg/kg PO	Every 24 h
Misoprostol	3 μg/kg PO	Every 24 h
Sucralfate	250 mg (cats) PO 500 mg (dogs < 20 kg) PO 1 gram (dogs > 20 kg) PO	Every 8–12 h Every 8–12 h Every 8–12 h
Kaolin/pectin	1–2 mL/kg PO	Every 6–8 h
Metoclopramide	0.2–0.5 mg/kg SQ	Every 6–8 h
Renal Dysfunction		
Mannitol	0.25–1 g/kg IV	Once (slow bolus)
Furosemide	1–2 mg/kg IV	If no effect, repeat in 2 h and increase dose by 1 mg/kg
Dopamine	1–3 μg/kg/min IV	As needed until urine production consistently >2 mL/kg/h

IV, intravenously; SQ, subcutaneously; IM, intramuscularly; PO, orally.
(From Hardie, E.M. Life Threatening Bacterial Infection. Compend Cont Education 17(6):763–777, 1995.)

834 ANESTHESIA MANAGEMENT

Table 24C–6. Vasoconstrictor and Mixed Inotropic/Vasoconstrictor Drugs

Drug (Trade Name)	Catecholamine Receptor Activation				Drug Dose and Infusion Schemes
	α_1	α_2	β_1	β_2	
Phenylephrine (Neo-Synephrine)	+++	+	– little at high dose	–	*Bolus:* 0.15 mg/kg IV *Infusion:* 0.5–1.0 µg/kg/min
Methoxamine (Vasoxyl)	++	+	–	–	*Bolus:* 0.1–0.8 mg/kg IV (cardiac arrest) *Bolus:* 0.01–0.04 mg/kg IV (vasopressor)
Ephedrine	+	+	+ Direct and indirect (NE release) effects	+	*Bolus:* 0.1–0.25 mg/kg IM; 0.03–0.07 mg/kg IV
Metaraminol (Aramine)	+	+	+ Similar to ephedrine effects initially*	+	*Bolus:* 30–100 µg/kg IM *Infusion:* 20–50 µg/kg/min
Mephenteramine (Wyamine)	+	+	+ Similar to ephedrine effects	+	*Bolus:* 0.2–0.6 mg/kg IM
Norepinephrine (Levophed)	+++	+++	+	little	*Infusion:* 0.01–0.03 µg/kg/min up to a maximum 0.1 µg/kg/min to effect.

NE, Norepinephrine; +, positive effect; –, no effect.
*Metaraminol replaces NE in storage vesicles in the nerve terminal. It has only 1/10 the potency of NE at alpha receptors and may eventually produce hypotensive effect.

Table 24C–7. Positive Inotropic Drugs

Drug (Trade Name)	Catecholamine Receptor Activation					Noncatecholamine Mechanism	Drug Dose and Infusion Schemes
	α_1	α_2	β_1	β_2	Dopamine		
Epinephrine (Adrenalin)	+++	+++	++	++	–	No	0.01–0.03 µg/kg/min (vasopressor) 0.1–0.2 mg/kg IV (cardiac arrest)
Isoproterenol (Isuprel)	–	–	+++	+++	–	No	0.01–0.1 µg/kg/min; used primarily to increase heart rate; may cause hypotension
Dobutamine (Dubutrex)	little	little	+++	++ Direct and minimal indirect effects	–	No*	2–10 µg/kg/min
Dopamine (Intropin)	++ (high dose)	+	++ (low dose)	+ (low dose) Direct and indirect actions	+++	No*†	2–5 µg/kg/min; "renal dose" 5–10 µg/kg/min; β effects 10–20 µg/kg/min; vasoconstriction
Dopexamine	–	–	little	+++	++	No*	1–10 µg/kg/min
Ephedrine	+	+	+ Both direct and indirect effects	+	–	No†	0.1–0.25 mg/kg/min IM 0.03–0.07 mg/kg IV
Milrinone	–	–	– Phosphodiesterase inhibitor, ↑ cAMP in heart, peripheral vasodilator, ↑ inotropy additive to other types	–	–	Yes	50–75 µg/kg IV bolus; oral administration possible

cAMP, cyclic adenosine monophosphate; +, positive effect; –, no effect; ↑, increased.
*Blocks reuptake of norepinephrine.
†Promotes release of norepinephrine from nerve terminal.

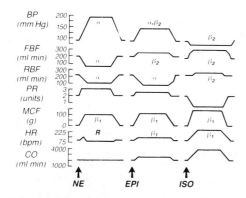

Fig. 24C–2. Differences in cardiovascular effects of intravenously administered norepinephrine (NE), epinephrine (EPI), and isoproterenol (ISO). Schematics represent relative effects on blood pressure (BP), femoral blood flow (FBF), renal blood flow (RBF), peripheral vascular resistance (PR), myocardial contractile force (MCF), heart rate (HR), and cardiac output (CO). Primary responses are noted as either alpha-, beta$_1$-, or beta$_2$-receptor-mediated; R, reflex-mediated. Differences in cardiovascular effects of these catecholamines are due to variation in alpha and beta selectivity for each agonist and dose.

24C–7).(13) Not all inotropic/vasoconstrictor drugs produce equivalent hemodynamic action. Hemodynamic differences induced by norepinephrine, epinephrine, and isoproterenol are illustrated in Figure 24C–2. These differences are mediated by variations in adrenergic receptor activation and dose. Indirect-acting agents such as ephedrine enhance release of endogenous norepinephrine from sympathetic neuronal terminals and also induce direct vasoconstrictive effects.

Traumatized patients may often present in near cardiopulmonary collapse or cardiac arrest. Causes of acute circulatory failure in patients with a history of severe trauma include severe myocardial ischemia, malignant dysrhythmias, hypoxemia associated with severe lung damage, hemorrhagic shock, acid-base or electrolyte abnormalities, profound vagal tone such as is associated with the oculocardiac reflex, and electrocution. When cardiovascular collapse occurs during attempts to stabilize severely traumatized patients, CPR should be instituted immediately. For details on performing CPR refer to Chapter 25.

Preanesthetic Evaluation

TRAUMA OF THE HEAD

The hallmark of closed head injury is loss of consciousness associated with increased intracranial pressure and brain ischemia (Chapter 23). With severe lacerations of the head, severe blood loss and shock may also be present. If airway obstruction is evident, a tracheostomy may be necessary to ensure airway patency. Time is of the essence, as unchecked intracranial hemorrhage can have devastating effects. In general, severe closed head injury resulting in stupor or coma has a poor prognosis. Anesthetic agents that increase cerebral blood flow (e.g., halothane, N$_2$O, ketamine) should not be used in these patients. Because barbiturates produce rapid induction

and decrease cerebral metabolism (CMRO$_2$) and blood flow, they may be the preferred agents for patients with severe head injury.(14) Following acute brain injury, large doses of glucocorticosteroids (1–3 mg/kg dexamethasone) may be helpful in controlling cerebral edema.(15) Hyperventilation with an Ambu bag or anesthetic machine prevents potentially dangerous increases in brain blood flow by reducing P$_a$CO$_2$ values to 25 to 35 mm Hg. This procedure decreases intracranial pressure and the likelihood of cerebral edema formation. The use of hyperosmotic solutions may help to minimize intracranial pressure. Mannitol is an ideal drug for preventing or treating increased intracranial pressure and cerebral edema associated with global ischemia caused by cardiogenic shock or cardiac arrest. However, it is *not* recommended for immediate use in patients with suspected intracranial hemorrhage (head trauma). Hemorrhage or leaking of hyperosmotic solutions into extravascular neural tissue runs the risk of increasing interstitial fluid volume and intracranial pressure. Cervical trauma may also injure the innervation (phrenic nerve) to respiratory muscles such that O$_2$ therapy, tracheal intubation, and mechanical ventilation may be necessary (Chapter 17). Spinal injury may also cause autonomic dysfunction, resulting in gastric bloat, bradycardia, and electrolyte imbalances. Thermoregulation may also be seriously impaired.

THORACIC AND ABDOMINAL TRAUMA

Penetrating trauma of the thorax and abdomen is usually obvious. Blunt trauma presents a greater diagnostic challenge, as external examination may reveal nothing. A chest radiograph is essential following any type of thoracic trauma and will often require anesthesia. Lung contusions, broken ribs, and flail chest are common. Severe hypoxia often results from extensive lung contusions, and ventilatory support or oxygen therapy may be required. Pulmonary lesions tend to worsen within 24 to 36 hours after injury.(16) Chest tubes are often necessary for evacuation of air or fluids (pneumothorax and hemothorax) and will require local, regional (intercostal nerve block) (Chapter 16), or general anesthesia for placement. Lung contusions will usually resolve in 2 to 5 days.(1) Medical management of pulmonary contusions includes oxygen, corticosteroid, analgesic, and antibiotic administration, and diuretic therapy when pulmonary edema is present. When contusions are severe, anesthesia, intubation, and low-pressure mechanical ventilation may be necessary.(16)

In small animals, thoracic and abdominal injuries are commonly associated with blunt trauma rather than penetrating objects. Common cardiac injuries include tamponade, contusion, and rupture. Patients with pericardial effusion and cardiac tamponade will manifest jugular vein distention, muffled heart sounds, and hypotension (Beck's triad) in addition to tachycardia and narrowed pulse pressure. Intravenous fluid administration, inotropic drugs (Table 24C–7), and immediate pericardial tap and drainage (pericardiocentesis) may be necessary to maintain an adequate cardiac output. It is best to avoid controlled positive pressure ventilation in patients with tamponade. Patients with myocardial contusions will often develop ventricular dysrhythmias. These require correct diagnosis and appropriate therapy with antiarrhythmic agents prior to and during the surgical period (Chapter 5). Myocardial rupture usually results in death at the scene of the accident.

In the urban environment, the incidence of abdominal injury in dogs and cats has been reported to involve 13% of all trauma cases treated.(17) Blunt abdominal trauma can result in damage to several vital organs including ruptured spleen and/or liver, bowel perforation, kidney and urinary bladder rupture, and the perforation of large abdominal vessels. In cases with a history of severe abdominal trauma, hypovolemic shock caused by organ or vessel rupture and/or septic shock resulting from septicemia are common sequelae. Abdominal vascular injuries can be assessed by peritoneal lavage. Although not organ specific, this technique is helpful in diagnosing the unstable patient with history of severe abdominal injury. Abdominal compression may reduce abdominal hemorrhage. Urinary catheterization will help to evaluate urinary tract injury and renal function.

THERMAL/BURN TRAUMA

Although extensive treatment of the severely burned patient is uncommon, several factors important to intensive care management should be kept in mind. As is true with any trauma patient, initial treatment involves attention to airway, breathing and circulation. If the patient is apneic, is in stridor, the face is burned, or the history indicates inhalation of steam, smoke, or toxic fumes, the trachea should be intubated immediately following sedation.(1) Inhalation of carbon monoxide can result in severe hypoxia. Arterial P_aO_2 may be normal, but oxygen blood content can be drastically reduced because carbon monoxide has 200 times more affinity for hemoglobin than oxygen. After intubation, the animal should be placed in an oxygen cage or ventilated mechanically with oxygen. After the airway has been secured, the burn patient will require large volumes of fluid. Fluid loss due to increased capillary permeability, protein loss into the interstitial tissues, and evaporative losses can be extensive, especially within the first 12 to 24 hours after the accident.(1) It has been suggested that only crystalloid solutions be administered during this time, as colloid solutions would likely rapidly extravasate. Volume replacement should be closely monitored by measuring urine output and hemodynamic variables regularly. Burn patients are hypermetabolic and will often have increased temperatures, increased catabolism, and increased oxygen requirements. Tachypnea and tachycardia are common, and parenteral nutrition is usually necessary to overcome metabolic losses. Parenteral solutions commonly administered to fulfill nutritional requirements include 50% dextrose, 20% lipid, 8.5% amino acid with electrolytes, vitamin B complex, and lactated Ringer's.

Providing anesthesia for burned and crushed patients presents some unique problems but selection of anesthetics is not critical if done on a rational patient by patient basis. Opioids (e.g., fentanyl patches; Duragesic) should be considered with any technique to enhance pre- and postoperative analgesia (Chapters 4 and 8). Ventilation may be necessary if lung damage occurred. Burn patients may not respond normally to muscle relaxants.(18) Within 24 hours of injury, succinylcholine administration is associated with a rapid increase in serum potassium concentration, which can cause cardiac arrest. In contrast, burn patients demonstrate increased resistance to nondepolarizing muscle relaxants (e.g., pancuronium and vecuronium) (Chapter 13). The principles of treatment for patients with electric burns are similar to those for patients with thermal burns. If the burn is located in the oral cavity, severe swelling of pharyngeal tissues may complicate efforts to intubate. The extent of burn is often misleading. Small cutaneous lesions may overlie extensive areas of devitalized tissue and muscle (Fig. 24C–3). Accordingly, these patients should be carefully observed for myoglobinemia and renal failure as well as neurologic deficits.(1)

Anesthetic Management of the Trauma Patient

All classes of anesthetic agents may be used in the trauma patient; however, dosage requirement is usually reduced. Endogenous release of enkephalins, endorphins, and other amino peptides to reduce pain and stress may produce mild sedation and analgesia, reducing subsequent anesthetic agent requirement. Patient management to protect the airway, provide ventilatory support, and provide a stable surgical field usually necessitates inducing general anesthesia in most trauma patients. Premedicants are discouraged to decrease the likelihood of drug interaction overdose caused by altered potency, distribution, or clearance of drugs (Chapters 2 and 3). Nevertheless, premedicants may prove advantageous in some circumstances.

PREMEDICATION

During the preoperative period, vagal influences on cardiopulmonary function and excess secretions can be controlled by atropine or glycopyrrolate administration. Anticholinergics are not routinely recommended for use in the trauma patient because they often increase heart rate and myocardial oxygen consumption while decreasing the threshold for cardiac dysrhythmias.(19) Because the stomach may be full, measures to prevent aspiration before induction need to be considered. Aspiration of acid gastric contents (pH < 2.5) will usually result in pneumonitis and increased morbidity and mortality. Several steps can be taken to minimize this occurrence including glycopyrrolate administration to increase pH of gastric contents (20), positioning of the animal to reduce gastric pressure, immediate intubation

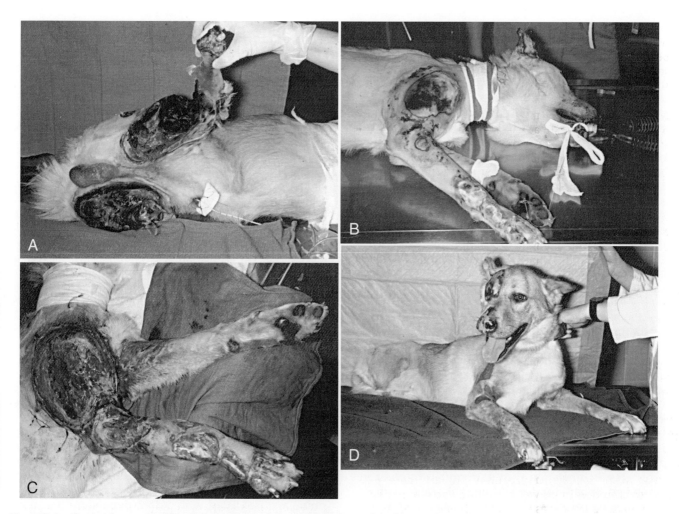

Fig. 24C–3. Dog with extensive burn lesions on the hind and forelimbs produced by touching a high-voltage electric transformer (A and B). Extensive skin burns will usually overlie areas of devitalized subcutaneous tissue and muscle (C). Treatment consisted of multiple surgeries and long-term analgesic and fluid therapy to control pain and stress. Adequate pain control, proper fluid therapy, and attention to nutrition in patients with severe burns are prerequisites for a successful outcome (D).

of the unconscious patient, the availability of suction to clear the pharynx of gastric reflux.(15)

When stabilization is necessary prior to surgery, analgesics and/or sedatives can be given to help alleviate pain, fear, and apprehension. Some clinicians have utilized the application of partial (cats and small dogs) or full (large dogs) fentanyl patches (Duragesic; 25 μg/h release rate) that provide continual release for transcutaneous absorption of fentanyl over several days. To insure adequate blood levels and analgesia, these patches should be applied at least 12 hours prior to induction of anesthesia. Although control studies are not yet available, it should be assumed that anesthetic induction and maintenance dose requirements will be lessened in patients who have had fentanyl patches applied long enough for effective blood concentrations to be achieved. Sedative doses of barbiturates are contraindicated in patients that are excited, delirious, or in pain because small doses often enhance these actions.(15) If an analgesic is needed for immediate pain

relief, either butorphanol (0.2 mg/kg IV) or oxymorphone (0.05 mg/kg IV) may be given in small incremental doses. When further CNS depression is desirable, diazepam (0.2 mg/kg IV) or midazolam (0.2 mg/kg IV or IM) can be combined with the opioid. Benzodiazepines are not usually administered alone because they can induce unpredictable behavior in both dogs and cats. In depressed dogs, however, low doses have resulted in profound CNS depression.(21) If shock and/or severe blood loss are not of concern, acepromazine (0.05 mg/kg) can be combined with butorphanol or oxymorphone to induce neuroleptanalgesia. In cats demerol (1 to 2 mg/kg IM) has proven to be a good short-duration sedative-analgesic.

INDUCTION

Barbiturates may decrease myocardial contractility and depress baroreceptor reflexes.(22) They are respiratory depressants and poor analgesics. When given intravenously, they can cause venodilation and usually decrease venous return, cardiac output, and blood pressure. In the presence of moderate blood loss, however, thiopental has been shown to increase renal blood flow.(23) Thiopental exerts less myocardial depression and provokes fewer dysrhythmias than thiamylal. The degree of myocardial depression induced is a function of dose and rate of injection which together determine peak blood concentration following intravenous injection.(24) Barbiturates are highly bound to proteins, and normal pharmacokinetics are influenced by the patient's acid-base status, albumin content, and concurrent drug administration (Chapters 2 and 9). (19) Trauma victims are often acidotic and hypoproteinemic, so the induction dose requirement may be greatly decreased and should be anticipated by the clinician. Because barbiturates are arrhythmogenic when given rapidly, they should be used cautiously in patients with preexisting arrhythmias. In the severely hypovolemic, hypotensive patient or when severe cardiac disease and/or preexisting arrhythmias are present, other agents or induction combinations may prove safer. If barbiturates are used, simultaneous administration of adjuvant drugs such as diazepam (0.2 mg/kg) or lidocaine (2.0 mg/kg) will decrease barbiturate requirement and the incidence of arrhythmias.(25) Propofol induces similar hemodynamic depressive effects to those of thiopental. Accordingly, propofol is not recommended as a primary induction agent in trauma patients unless cardiovascular stability has been reinstated.

Unlike injectable agents, inhalation agents are retrievable should an adverse response (other than cardiac arrest) result. Inhalation agents are equally hypotensive compared to barbiturates and are only safer as induction agents because homeostatic mechanisms have longer to compensate for the depressant effects of the anesthetic during induction. Halothane, enflurane, isoflurane, and methoxyflurane all induce dose-dependent cardiopulmonary depression (Chapter 11). Isoflurane is least depressant to cardiac output at equipotent (e.g., 1.5 MAC) concentrations. If the traumatized dog or cat is alert and likely to struggle, induction with an inhalation agent alone is not recommended.

Ketamine is one of the few anesthetic agents with indirect cardiovascular stimulant properties. In healthy patients, it raises blood pressure secondary to increased sympathetic activity, heart rate, and cardiac output (Chapter 10).(26) However, it also induces a direct myocardial depressant effect in patients whose sympathetic system is maximally stressed by hemorrhagic shock.(27) This is often the case in severely traumatized patients. In patients with hypertrophic or restrictive cardiomyopathy (e.g., cats with idiopathic cardiomyopathy and normal left ventricular contractility), ketamine is contraindicated because it may induce tachycardia and decrease preload further.(19) In contrast, in large- or giant-breed dogs suffering from cardiogenic shock and myocardial failure as defined by poor contractility (dilated cardiomyopathy), ketamine may be a good choice for inducing anesthesia. When given alone,

ketamine does not provide good muscle relaxation and spontaneous movement is common. Because of their propensity to increase intracranial pressure, dissociatives are not recommended for patients with severe closed head injury or open eye injury.

Benzodiazepines enhance muscle relaxation and sedation when combined with ketamine, barbiturates, or opioids. Diazepam (0.2 mg/kg IV) and ketamine (2 to 3 mg/kg IV) can be given in rapid sequence to induce anesthesia in either the traumatized dog or cat. If the patient is not sufficiently depressed after diazepam-ketamine administration, delivery of low concentrations of halothane or isoflurane (0.5 to 1.0%) by face mask will complete the induction. Ventricular arrhythmias occurring during light halothane anesthesia can often be converted to sinus rhythm by simply increasing halothane concentration.(28) However, in patients with questionable cardiopulmonary reserve, this method of abolishing arrhythmias may be an unwise approach to the problem. Because isoflurane is less arrhythmogenic and faster acting than halothane, it is the preferred agent in any trauma victim exhibiting arrhythmias or suspected of having severe myocardial contusions.(29, 30)

Induction of anesthesia with opioids usually necessitates concomitant use of an adjunctive tranquilizer-sedative (neuroleptanalgesia) or inhalation agent. Because most opioid agonists have the potential to depress respiration and slow heart rate, intravenous administration should be preceded by preoxygenation and an anticholinergic should be available for rapid administration in the event that bradycardia is induced. In the dog, intravenously administered meperidine and morphine are associated with a dose-dependent histamine release, which can cause severe hypotension. In contrast, intravenous oxymorphone administration has not been associated with histamine release and has proven safe in critically ill patients. In depressed trauma victims, oxymorphone is commonly given intravenously in small increments (0.05 mg/kg) along with diazepam (0.2 mg/kg) until intubation is possible. Alternatively, midazolam (0.2 mg/kg) and oxymorphone (0.1 to 0.2 mg/kg) can be administered intramuscularly to induce neuroleptanalgesia.(19) Because opioids and benzodiazepines given together do not cause myocardial depression or vasodilation, they make a good induction combination in the hypovolemic, cardiogenic shock, septic shock, or dehydrated patient. Nevertheless, because opioid inductions are slower than those achieved with barbiturates or dissociatives, they are *not* recommended if rapid intubation of the airway is a necessity for patient survival.

For patients in shock with head trauma or with severe cardiac disease, perhaps the safest drug for inducing anesthesia while maintaining cerebral and hemodynamic homeostasis is etomidate. In doses of 0.5 to 2.0 mg/kg, etomidate produces minimal hemodynamic alterations and cardiac depression (Chapter 9).(31, 32) It has recently been shown that in dogs with experimentally induced hypovolemia, etomidate preserves hemodynamic function.(33) Adrenal cortical suppression may follow induction of anesthesia, but this is of limited concern when etomidate is given as a single bolus to a hemodynamically unstable patient for whom it may be life saving.(1) Etomidate is a safe induction agent for patients in compensated or decompensated (congestive) heart failure whether caused by acquired chronic atrioventricular valvular disease or myocardial failure (dilated cardiomyopathy).

MAINTENANCE

Along with proper monitoring, the first priority during maintenance of anesthesia is adequate oxygenation, which may require ventilating the lungs mechanically for normal gas exchange. Blood oxygen saturation can be easily monitored by pulse oximetry using a buccal mucosa, tongue, or ear site (Chapter 15). Preservation of hemodynamic stability is also essential. This is achieved by providing adequate intravascular volume, which can be monitored by placing central venous and arterial pressure catheters, use of inotropic agents if necessary (Table 24C–7) (13), and proper anesthetic dose. For trauma patients, there is a natural tendency to choose an anesthetic that is an adrenergic stimulant or is associated with little hypotensive affect when given to the healthy animal. However, there are limited data to suggest the superiority of stimulant drugs for maintenance of anesthesia during severe hypovolemic shock or in patients with severe CNS injury.(1) For example, in hypovolemic pigs, ketamine's overall cardiovascular effects are similar to those of thiopental.(27)

Opioids such as oxymorphone (0.1 mg/kg IV) or fentanyl (0.01 mg/kg IV) and ketamine can be given in small aliquots with diazepam or midazolam to maintain short periods of anesthesia. Ketamine should be repeated at an approximate dosage of 1 to 2 mg/kg IV every 20 to 30 minutes or as necessary to keep the patient anesthetized. Diazepam or midazolam can also be repeated (0.2 mg/kg IV) every 30 to 60 minutes or as necessary to provide adequate muscle relaxation. Recovery can be prolonged with repeated injections. Duration of anesthesia should be limited to less than 2 hours. Long recoveries may be problematic in cats because they metabolize benzodiazepines more slowly than dogs. Similarly, tiletamine plus zolazepam (Telazol) may be useful when given in low doses for minimal restraint. These injectable regimens are often supplemented with low concentrations of halothane or isoflurane (0.5 to 1.0%) if extension of anesthesia is necessary.

When administered to hypovolemic animals, nitrous oxide does not appear to offer any hemodynamic advantage over halothane.(34) Because trauma patients frequently have pulmonary contusions with increased venous admixture, causing large arterial-alveolar gradients, nitrous oxide is not routinely recommended. If blunt thoracic trauma is suspected and pneumo- or hemothorax is present, nitrous oxide is contraindicated. Similarly, in patients with a distended abdomen or diaphragmatic hernia resulting in respiratory compromise, nitrous oxide should be avoided. Nitrous oxide is a known stimulant of cerebral metabolism and causes increased cerebral blood flow and intracranial pressure.(35) Accordingly, nitrous oxide is not advocated for trauma patients with severe head or open eye injury.

Isoflurane is equally hypotensive to halothane and methoxyflurane but does not sensitize the myocardium to the arrhythmogenic effects of catecholamines to the same extent as halothane.(36) It is less depressant to the myocardium and a more potent vasodilator. Consequently, isoflurane is preferred in patients with congestive heart failure or with severe arrhythmias but not in patients in hypovolemic shock prior to volume replacement. When using an inhalation agent, myocardial depression and hypotension can be minimized by using as low a concentration as possible. In humans, it is common practice to administer a muscle relaxant to help prevent patient movement when using low inhalant concentrations. Unfortunately, human patients have recalled surgical events under these conditions.(1) Preanesthetic or intraoperative administration of an opioid or benzodiazepine tranquilizer with or without a muscle relaxant can help assure adequate CNS depression during low-dose inhalation anesthesia. In the hypovolemic anesthetized patient, fentanyl, oxymorphone, butorphanol, or diazepam is preferred for this purpose. Acepromazine is not a good choice in these circumstances because it may increase vascular capacity, rapidly reducing blood pressure. In hypovolemic patients, compensatory vasoconstriction is often necessary preoperatively to maintain normal pressure. On the other hand, if adequate volume replacement has been achieved prior to acepromazine administration, decreasing arterial resistance (alpha blockade) may improve perfusion to some vital organs (e.g., kidneys and intestines).

REGIONAL ANESTHESIA

Epidural or spinal blocks are contraindicated in trauma patients with severe hemorrhage. The profound sympathetic blockade induced by these techniques when using local anesthetics may result in acute hypotension. Epidural or intrathecal administration of opioids (0.1 mg/kg of morphine or oxymorphone diluted with 1 mL saline per 4.5 kg of body weight) or low doses of alpha$_2$-agonists may prove to be effective alternatives to local anesthetics in providing analgesia without sympathetic blockade.(37, 38) In the severely depressed or calm and stoic patient, superficial lacerations and wounds of the extremities can be managed with infiltration of local anesthetic or by performing peripheral nerve blocks.

Adjunctive regional therapy using a local anesthetic improves analgesia with lowering of inhalation agent requirement. Intercostal nerve blocks (0.5–1.0 mL per site) using 2% lidocaine or 0.5% bupivacaine can be used to control postoperative thoracotomy pain as well as pain associated with fractured ribs. Interpleural administration of local anesthetics is also effective for thoracotomy and cranial abdominal pain associated with pancreatitis, or diaphragmatic hernia repair. A bupivacaine dosage of 1.5 mg/kg in dogs or 0.75 mg/kg in cats diluted to 10 to 20 mL with 0.9% saline for volume to bathe the pleural surfaces can be used.

Intraoperative Support

FLUID SUPPORT

Several choices of fluids are available for use in the traumatized patient undergoing anesthesia and surgery. With hemorrhage there is a contraction of extracellular volume as the intravascular compartment is autotransfused with interstitial fluid (Chapter 19). Administration of a physiologic salt solution such as lactated Ringer's restores this depletion and also expands intravascular volume to help maintain cardiac output. In general patients should be administered 20 to 40 mL/kg intravenously prior to anesthetic induction. In general, patients in hypovolemic shock can be given one blood volume of isotonic electrolyte solution in the first hour. Many more animals have gotten into trouble following anesthetic drug injection, when underlying hypovolemia was unmasked as severe hypotension, than have developed problems when crystalloid fluids were administered unnecessarily at these rates.(19) Replacement solutions should be isotonic, but not all isotonic solutions are optimal. Although 5% dextrose in water and lactated Ringer's with 2.5% dextrose are isotonic, once glucose is metabolized the remaining fluid is hypotonic and contains either all (5% dextrose) or half (2.5% dextrose) free water, which rapidly leaves the vascular compartment.(12) In general, even optimal isotonic physiologic salt solutions remain intravascular for only 30 to 60 minutes before redistributing throughout the entire extracellular space.(39)

Plasma expanders such as colloid solutions maintain intravascular volume for 2 to 5 hours but may have associated complications (Table 24C–5). Dextran solutions can cause bleeding disorders and allergic reactions, and must be stored at stable temperatures (25° C) to prevent precipitate formation.(40, 41) Protein solutions can impair pulmonary function if they extravasate into damaged lung.(42) Hydroxyethyl starch (6% solution in normal saline) is a glucose polymer that has proven useful as a volume expander when the dose is limited to less than 20 mL/kg.(43) Because colloid solutions are hypertonic, they must be administered slowly to avoid rapid fluid shifts and volume overload.(11)

When extreme blood loss occurs, red cells must eventually be given. Fresh whole blood (less than 6 hours old) is preferable. After 1 day of storage, only 12% of the original platelets remain in human whole blood. Similar reductions may occur in stored blood of domestic animals. Regardless of its age, whole blood is preferred over packed red blood cells.(1) Fresh frozen plasma should be reserved for specific coagulation disorders.(44) In acute trauma, the large majority of

clotting disorders are secondary to large volume fluid replacement, resulting in dilutional thrombocytopenia. If possible, surgery and anesthesia should be delayed until the packed cell volume can be increased to above 20%. When ongoing losses and replacement are occurring simultaneously, the best method of assessing adequate blood volume replacement is to assess urine output ($1–2 \text{ mL} \cdot \text{kg}^{-1} \cdot \text{h}^{-1}$ is optimal), serial hematocrits, and total protein. Some questions remain with regard to optimum fluid management of severely traumatized patients in the perioperative period (45), including (a) the best methods of utilizing nonblood containing fluids in trauma resuscitation, (b) feasibility of systemic oxygen delivery (DO_2) and consumption goal oriented resuscitation in high-risk surgical patients, and (c) the effects of fluid therapy on cerebral hemodynamics.

With regards to nonblood fluid resuscitation, if membrane permeability is normal, fluids containing colloids (albumin, dextran, hydroxyethylstarch) expand plasma volume (PV) rather than interstitial fluid volume (IFV) or intracellular volume (ICV). Each gram of intravascular colloid holds approximately 20 mL of water (e.g., 16–17 mL of water per gram of hydroxyethylstarch). To estimate the effects of fluid infusion on PV the following equation can be used: $PV = \text{volume infused} \times (PV/V_d)$ where $V_d =$ distribution volume. In mature animals total body water (TBW) consists of 60% of the total body weight, intracellular volume (ICV) is 40%, extracellular volume (ECV) is 20%, interstitial fluid volume (IFV) is 16%, and plasma volume is 4% of total body weight. If an acute blood loss of 500 mL is to be replaced using the preceding formula and 5% dextrose, which contains no sodium, the remaining water after glucose metabolism distributes throughout the TBW. For a 70-kg dog where plasma volume of 500 mL is to be replaced, the volume of 5% dextrose infused is 500 mL = volume infused × (3 L/42 L), or approximately 7 liters. In contrast, 500 mL of blood loss can be replaced with lactated Ringer's (LRS), for which the V_d is equal to the ECV or only 20% of the body weight (3 L/14 L) with 2.3 liters of LRS. If hyperosmotic fluids such as hypertonic saline (HS) are used, increases in blood volume occur primarily by endogenous fluid PV expansion. These fluids come from the IFV initially and are transient in duration. The immediate effect of 7.5% HS is to increase plasma volume by 2 to 4 mL for each mL infused. Thus, 500 mL of PV may be replaced with only 150 to 200 ml of HS. However, following equilibration, 7.5% saline only increases PV by approximately 1.0 mL for each mL infused. It has been shown that small volumes of hyperosmotic solutions transiently restore hemodynamic function during shock, but because improved PV and flow decrease rather rapidly following resuscitation with hypertonic fluids, ongoing attention to maintenance of intravascular volume is necessary.(45) To prolong the initial improvement seen with hyperosmotic solutions beyond 30 to 60 minutes, continued infusion with a hypertonic solution, blood (if

PCV is below 20%), or conventional fluids, or the addition of colloids should be considered. One suggested protocol for volume resuscitation combines bolusing a synthetic colloid solution (7 mL/kg) with a replacement crystalloid solution (15 mL/kg). The dose of colloid solution should not exceed 20 mL/kg rate within the first 24 hours. Rapid fluid loading is often associated with dilutional thrombocytopenia, hypoglycemia, and/or hypokalemia, and fluids should be supplemented to maintain serum levels within normal ranges.(4)

Recent studies have documented that HS may have a negative inotropic effect whereas hyperosmotic dextrose produces a positive inotropic action in dogs.(46) Rapid (<30 s) administration of 2 to 4 mL of HS is also associated with an acute transient period of hypotension.(46) Infusion over a 3- to 4-minute period will diminish this initial response. Hypertonic saline likely exerts its beneficial effect in treating hemorrhagic or endotoxic shock by rapidly increasing preload whereas hyperosmotic dextrose solutions exert their beneficial effects by transiently increasing both preload and contractility.(46)

In high-risk traumatized patients who survive, it has been documented that average blood flow and DO_2 are greater than in those patients that did not survive.(47) Survival is correlated with a DO_2, that is at least 600 mL $O_2 \cdot min^{-1} \cdot m^{-2}$ (Table 24C–3). When Do_2 is maintained at this level complications are also reduced. In order to implement Do_2 goal-oriented fluid resuscitation, cardiac output, hemoglobin content, and oxygen-hemoglobin saturation must be continually monitored. Nevertheless, in many traumatized patients, improvement of overall systemic DO_2 may be less critical than the immediate restoration of adequate O_2 delivery to selected vital organ systems (Chapter 25).

With respect to the effects of fluid therapy on cerebral hemodynamics, it appears that in some subsets of traumatized patients (severe head injury), initial fluid therapy with 7.5% saline in 6% dextran improves patient survival (32%) when compared to those treated with conventional LRS (16%).(45) Concerns over adverse neurologic sequelae with hypertonic solutions have not proven valid with the exception of hyperosmotic resuscitation in canine experimental models of uncontrolled hemorrhage where hyperosmotic solutions actually increase bleeding tendency.(48)

Not uncommonly, trauma cases will present with nonrespiratory acidosis due to shock, hypothermia, and generalized stress (Chapter 18). Ventilation of the lungs to induce a mild respiratory alkalosis will help normalize blood pH for the short term. With time, improved tissue perfusion and renal and hepatic function should resolve the problem. Treatment with sodium bicarbonate or tromethamine (THAM) should be reserved for cases of severe nonrespiratory acidosis (Chapter 19). Studies in dogs suggest that rapid vigorous sodium bicarbonate therapy may in fact be detrimental in treating lactic acidosis, as it depresses both arterial pressure and cardiac output.(49) In patients with concurrent nonrespiratory and respiratory acidosis (as may occur during anesthesia), THAM may be the preferred alkalinizing agent because it does not increase P_aCO_2 as does bicarbonate therapy. Tromethamine (0.3 M) is contraindicated in anuria and uremic patients. Large doses can depress respiration due to pH change and rapid decreases in P_aCO_2. More important measures in treating metabolic acidosis are fluid resuscitation, adequate ventilation, and rewarming. It is possible for patients with normal liver function to develop metabolic alkalosis 6 to 24 hours after large volume replacement with lactated Ringer's solution.

INOTROPIC SUPPORT

Drugs commonly used to enhance myocardial contractility and increase cardiac output are listed in Table 24C–7.(13) Ephedrine has proven an effective alternative to dopamine or dobutamine when administered during inhalation anesthesia to enhance cardiac output.(50) A 0.1-mg/kg intravenous dose of ephedrine transiently increases arterial pressure, cardiac index, stroke volume, arterial oxygen content (C_aO_2), and oxygen delivery in dogs anesthetized with isoflurane (1.5 MAC). A dose of 0.25 mg/kg IV causes a greater and prolonged increase in arterial pressure while actually decreasing heart rate.(50) This presumably results from a reflex bradycardia associated with an acute increase in arterial pressure. The higher dose of ephedrine also increased hemoglobin concentration and C_aO_2, resulting in a 20 to 35% increase in oxygen delivery for at least 60 minutes. Increased hemoglobin concentration likely results from contraction of the spleen and increased circulating red blood cells. Splenic contraction results from either ephedrine's direct alpha-agonist effects or enhanced norepinephrine release. Because ephedrine can be administered as a convenient intravenous bolus with an onset of less than a minute, it is a useful drug for inotropic support of anesthetized patients. Dopamine and dobutamine are expensive, have short half-lives, and require constant infusion administration (Table 24C–7). With the latter drugs close monitoring to avoid intense alpha-receptor-mediated vasoconstriction (overdose) or development of arrhythmias is necessary. Dopexamine may be the preferred dopaminergic agent because it does not activate alpha receptors. In refractive cases, inotropic doses of dopamine and dobutamine may be supplemented with the coadministration of ephedrine to reduce vascular compliance and improve preload and stroke volume.(51)

TEMPERATURE AND RENAL SUPPORT

Hypothermia should be treated vigorously because it is associated with reduced kidney function, poor platelet activity, low glucose utilization, shivering and increased oxygen consumption by nonvital tissues, metabolic acidosis, and decreased metabolism of anesthetics.(1) Warming fluids and blood before administration helps maintain body temperature, reduces blood viscosity, and improves tissue blood flow. Warm water blankets and heat lamps may help prevent further heat loss but will not rewarm the patient because of inadequate body surface area contact. The operating room should not be cold.

To prevent acute oliguric renal failure every effort should be made to maintain normal renal function in severely traumatized patients. Unfortunately, there is no way to predict the degree of hypoperfusion that will result in renal failure in a given patient. Myoglobinemia must be treated by vigorous diuresis following muscle crush or electrocution. Once fluid volume and blood pressure have been normalized, furosemide (1 mg/kg) and dopamine (2–5 μg/kg/min) can be used together to increase renal blood flow and water and solute excretion. Maintaining a functional renal system is essential for a favorable outcome following massive tissue damage.(1)

Issues concerning perioperative renal function and renal physiology in traumatized patients remain.(52) It is not uncommon for severely traumatized critically ill patients to produce inadequate urine output. These patients are often given a "renal dose" of dopamine in an attempt to improve urine production and prevent oliguria. Dopaminergic receptors (DA_1 and DA_2) increase glomerular filtration rate (GFR) and inhibit proximal tubular reabsorption of sodium. This combination of effects results in increased sodium excretion in euvolemic patients, but this action is diminished with prolonged infusion. Furthermore, in critically ill patients dopamine's natriuretic action is not always apparent, as antinatriuretic factors (ADH, aldosterone) may be present to induce sodium conservation. It has also been demonstrated that with lower than normal levels of GFR, low doses of dopamine become less effective. This lack of response may be caused by exhaustion of the renal reserve system, where low renal blood flow may have already caused a shift of blood flow to the inner cortex in an adaptive response to loss of nephron renal function. Hence, dopamine's actions result in little additional urine production. Despite these problems, dopamine can increase urine output in oliguric patients and in patients that are adequately hydrated. Several studies have also shown that dopamine improves urine output in patients who have not responded to fluid expansion or furosemide alone. By increasing renal flow, dopamine may improve delivery of furosemide to its site of action in the nephron.(52)

It is not clear whether dopamine is advantageous in the treatment of oliguric renal failure. It appears that dopamine is no better than saline in protecting renal function. In fact, dopamine-induced natriuresis may cause intravascular volume depletion, making the kidney even more susceptible to ongoing ischemic injury. Questions remain as to the clinical implication of increasing renal perfusion when there is decreased systemic blood volume. The routine administration of dopamine in the severely traumatized patient should be carefully considered in the perioperative period.(52)

Urine flow, regardless of the quantity, indicates there is blood flow to the kidney, because without it, urine production would cease. Numerous studies have shown, however, that there is no correlation between the amount of urine volume produced and histologic evidence of acute tubular necrosis, GFR, creatinine clearance, BUN levels, and creatinine levels in burn patients, trauma patients, or shock states.(52, 53) The control of blood flow to the kidney, the fraction filtered, and the volume returned to the systemic circulation are all regulated by a variety of mechanisms in an attempt to preserve filtration function during compromised circulation. These compensatory mechanisms have limits, and excessive vasoconstriction may eventually decrease filtration. This shift from compensation to decompensation may be prevented or exacerbated by pharmacologic manipulations. The cortical to medullary redistribution of renal blood flow is designed to protect vulnerable medullary oxygen supply and demand balance at the expense of urine formation. Reduced GFR may reduce medullary tubular workload and oxygen consumption. Oliguria may be viewed in some circumstances (e.g., anesthesia) as a sign of normal protective compensatory mechanisms at work. Thus, oliguria can be both the result of acute renal failure and the consequence of normal compensatory mechanisms employed to prevent it.(52)

Traditionally, inadequate urine production or oliguria has been defined as a urine output of less than 0.5 $mL \cdot kg^{-1} \cdot h^{-1}$. Oliguria may, however, be reflective of a variety of factors independent of inadequate glomerular filtration. Thus, normal hourly urine output does not rule out impending renal failure any more than lower than normal hourly urine output predicts renal failure. Reduced urine output during the anesthetic period in euvolemic patients is usually of little consequence to long-term renal function. It is more likely to be the result of compensatory renal mechanisms than a consequence of acute tubular necrosis.(52)

References

1. Priano LL. Trauma. In Barash PG, Cullen BF, Stoelting RK, eds. Clinical anesthesia. Philadelphia: JB. Lippincott, 1989: 1365–1377.
2. Drobatz KJ, Powell S. Global approach to the trauma patient. Proceedings from Fourth International Veterinary Emergency and Critical Care Symposium, San Antonio, Texas, September 29–October 2, 1994: 32–36.
3. Purvis D, Kirby R. Systemic inflammatory response syndrome: septic shock. Vet Clin North Am Small Anim Pract; Emerg Med 24(6):1225–1247, 1994.
4. Hardie EM. Life threatening bacterial infection. Compen Cont Educ 17(6):763–777, 1995.
5. Stamp G. Metabolic responses to trauma. In: Zaslow I, ed. Trauma and Critical Care. Philadelphia: Lea & Febiger, 1984: 25–63.
6. Gallagher TJ, Banner MJ, Barnes PA. Large volume crystalloid resuscitation does not increase extravascular lung water. Anesth Analg 64:323, 1985.
7. Layon J, Duncan D, Gallagher TJ, et al. Hypertonic saline as a resuscitation solution in hemorrhagic shock. Anesth Analg 66:154, 1987.
8. Bitterman H, Triolo J, Lefer AM. Use of hypertonic saline in the treatment of hemorrhagic shock. Circ Shock 21:271–283, 1987.

9. Lopes OU, Velasco IT, Guertzenstein PG, et al. Hypertonic sodium restores mean circulatory filling pressure in severely hypovolemic dogs. Proceedings Suppl I. Hypertension. Inter-American Society. 1986: I195.
10. Muir WW, Sally J. Small volume resuscitation with hypertonic saline solution in hypovolemic cats. Am J Vet Res 50(11):1883, 1989.
11. Garvey MS. Fluid and electrolyte balance in critical patients. In: Kirby R, Stamp GL, eds. Veterinary clinics of north america:critical care. Philadelphia: WB Saunders, 1989: 1021–1058.
12. Layon AJ, Kirby RR. Fluids and electrolytes in the critically ill. In: Civetta JM, Taylor RM, Kirby RR, eds. Critical care. Philadelphia: JB Lippincott, 1988: 451–474.
13. Schwinn DA. Cardiovascular pharmacology. IARS 1994 Review Course Lectures, Supplement to Anesthesia and Analgesia, Orlando, Florida, March 5–9, 1994: 154–164.
14. Rockoff MA, Shapiro HM. Barbiturates following cardiac arrest: possible benefit or Pandora's box? Anesthesiology 49:385, 1978.
15. Evans T. Anesthesia and monitoring for trauma and critical care patients. In: Slatter DH, ed. Textbook of small animal surgery, 1985: 2702–2711.
16. Hackner SG. Emergency management of traumatic pulmonary contusions. Compend Cont Educ 17(5):677–686, 1995.
17. Kolata RJ, Kraut NJ, Johnston DE. Patterns of trauma in urban dogs and cats. A study of 1,000 cases. J Am Vet Med Assoc 164:499, 1974.
18. Martyn J. Clinical pharmacology and drug therapy in the burned patient. Anesthesiology 65:67, 1986.
19. Bednarski RM. Anesthesia and Pain Control. In: Kirby R, Stamp GL, eds. Veterinary Clinics of North America: Critical care. Philadelphia: WB Saunders 1989: 1223–1238.
20. Salem MR, Wong AY, Moni M, et al. Premedicant drugs and gastric juice pH and volume in pediatric patients. Anesthesiology 44:216, 1976.
21. Haskins SC, Farver TB, Patz BA. Cardiovascular changes in dogs given diazepam and diazepam-ketamine. Am J Vet Res 47:795–798, 1986.
22. Bernards C, Marvone B, Priano L. Effect of anesthetic induction agents on baroreceptor function. Anesthesiology 63:A31, 1985.
23. Priano LL. Renal hemodynamic alterations following administration of thiopental, diazepam, or ketamine in conscious hypovolemic dogs. Adv Shock Res 9:173, 1983.
24. Roberts JG. Intravenous anesthetic agents. In: Prys-Roberts C, ed. the circulation in anesthesia. Applied physiology and pharmacology. London, England: Blackwell Scientific Publications, 1980: 311–327.
25. Rawlings CA, Kolata RJ. Cardiopulmonary effects of thiopental/lidocaine combination during anesthetic induction in the dog. Am J Vet Res 44:144–149, 1983.
26. Haskins SC, Farver TB, Patz JD. Ketamine in dogs. Am J Vet Res 46:1855–1860, 1985.
27. Weiskopf RB, Bogetz MS, Roizen MF, et al. Cardiovascular and metabolic sequelae of inducing anesthesia with ketamine or thiopental in hypovolemic swine. Anesthesiology 60:214–219, 1984.
28. Muir WW, Hubble JAE, Flaherty S. Increasing halothane concentration abolishes anesthesia-associated arrhythmias in cats and dogs. J Am Vet Med Assoc 192(12):1730–1735, 1988.
29. Harvey RC, Short CE. The use of isoflurane for safe anesthesia in animals with traumatic myocarditis or other myocardial sensitivity. Canine pract 10:18, 1983.
30. Hubble JAE, Muir WW, Bednarski RM, et al. Change of inhalation anesthetic agents for management of ventricular premature depolarizations in anesthetized cats and dogs. J Am Vet Med Assoc 185:643–646, 1984.
31. Robertson S. Advantages of etomidate use as an anesthetic agent. Vet Clin North Am: Small Anim Pract; Opin Small Anim Anesth 22(2):277–280, 1992.
32. Gooding JM, Corssen G. Effect of etomidate on the cardiovascular system. Anesth Analg 56:717, 1977.
33. Pascoe PJ, Ilkiw JE, Haskins SC, Patz JD. Cardiopulmonary effects of etomidate in hypovolemic dogs. Am J Vet Res 53:2178–2182, 1992.
34. Weiskopf RB, Bogetz MS. Cardiovascular actions of nitrous oxide and halothane in hypovolemic swine. Anesthesiology 63:509, 1985.
35. Sakabe T, Kuramoto T, Inone S, et al. Cerebral effects of nitrous oxide in the dog. Anesthesiology 48:195, 1978.
36. Joas TA, Stevens WC. Comparison of the arrhythmic doses of epinephrine during forane, halothane, and fluroxene anesthesia in dogs. Anesthesiology 35:48–53, 1971.
37. Tung AS, Yaksh TL. The antinociceptive effects of epidural opiates in the cat: studies on the pharmacology and the effects of lipophilicity in spinal analgesia. Pain 12:343–356, 1982.
38. Valverde A, Dyson DH, McDonell WN et al. Epidural morphine reduces halothane MAC in the dog. Can J Anaesth, 36:629–632, 1989.
39. Cervera LA, Moss G. Crystalloid distribution following hemorrhage and hemodilution. J Trauma 14:506, 1974.
40. Giesecke AH Jr. Anesthesia for trauma surgery. In: Miller RD, ed. Anesthesia. New York: Churchill Livingstone, 1981: 1247–1264.
41. Giesecke AH, Jenkins MT. Fluid therapy. Clin Anesth 11:57, 1976.
42. Holcraft JW, Trunkey DD, Carpenter MA. Sepsis in the baboon: factors affecting resuscitation and pulmonary edema in animals resuscitated with Ringer's lactate verses plasmanate. J Trauma 17:600, 1977.
43. Munoz E, Raciti A, Dove DB, et al. Effect of hydroxyethyl starch versus albumin on hemodynamic and respiratory function in patients in shock. Crit Care Med 8:255, 1980.
44. Baldini M, Costea N, Dameshek W. The viability of stored human platelets. Blood 16:1669, 1960.
45. Prough DS. Controversies in perioperative fluid management. IARS 1994 Review Course Lectures, Supplement to Anesthesia and Analgesia, Orlando, Florida, March 5–9, 1994: 16–24.
46. Constable PD, Muir WW, Binkley PF. Hypertonic saline is a negative inotrope agent in normovolemic dogs. Am J Physiol 267:H667–H677, 1994.
47. Kovacic J. Management of life-threatening trauma. Vet Clin North Am: Small Anim Pract; Emerg Med 24(6):1057–1094, 1994.
48. Gross D, Landau EH, Klin B, Krausz MM. Treatment of uncontrolled hemorrhagic shock with hypertonic saline solution. Surg Gynecol Obstet 170:106–112, 1990.
49. Graf H, Leach W, Arrieff AI. Evidence for the detrimental effect of bicarbonate therapy on hypoxic lactic acidosis. Science 227:754, 1985.
50. Wagner AE, Dunlop CI, Chapman PL. Effects of ephedrine on cardiovascular function and oxygen delivery in isoflurane anesthetized dogs. Am J Vet Res 54(11):1917–1922, 1993.
51. Raffe M. Anesthetic management of the unstable trauma patient. Proceedings of 4th International Veterinary Emergency and Critical Care Symposium, San Antonio, Texas, 1994: 281–287.
52. Aronson S. Controversies: should anesthesiologists worry about the kidney? IARS 1995 Review Course Lectures, Supplement to Analgesia and Anesthesia, Honolulu, Hawaii, March 10–14, 1995: 68–73.
53. Kellen M, Aronson S, Roizen-Thisted R. Predictive and diagnostic tests of acute renal failure: a review. Anesth Analg 78:134–142, 1994.

chapter 24D

NEONATAL AND GERIATRIC PATIENTS

NEONATES	GERIATRIC PATIENTS

The frequency with which the veterinarian is asked to anesthetize very young and aged animals is increasing. This is the result of an increased interest in early neutering and spaying of dogs and cats, and owing to better health care, an increased population of aged pets. Pediatric dogs and cats are considered to be less than 12 weeks of age. The neonatal period varies among species, from 1 to 2 weeks in the foal to 6 weeks in calves, puppies, and pigs. Defining the geriatric period is difficult because of species, breed, and individual variation in life expectancy. Furthermore, there is little correlation between chronologic age and physiologic age. For the purposes of this discussion, geriatric patients are considered to be those who have attained 75% of their expected life span. Much of the information concerning the physiologic and pharmacologic characteristics of neonatal and geriatric patients has been derived in humans but is applicable in animals.

Neonates

Neonatal animals (Table 24D–1) gradually develop normal (adult) physiologic responses and function by 6 to 8 weeks. By 12 weeks the majority of circulatory, ventilatory, thermoregulation, hepatic and renal functions are well developed.(1–3) During the neonatal period, the immature cardiovascular system has limited ability to respond to stress. The neonatal heart has a relatively low contractile mass per gram of tissue. Increases in cardiac contractility are limited, and ventricular compliance is low.(4) There is limited ability to increase stroke volume. Cardiac output in neonates is therefore rate dependent. Slowing of the heart rate results in decreased cardiac output. The resting cardiac index is much higher in the neonate than the adult and is very close to maximal cardiac output, making the cardiac reserve minimal. An adult can increase cardiac output by 300%, whereas the neonate can only increase output by 30%.(5) Sympathetic stimulation results in minimal increases in rate and contractility because the sympathetic system itself is also not fully developed.(4)

In addition, the baroresponse, reflex tachycardia in response to hypotension, is immature. Sympathetic immaturity also manifests itself in poor vasomotor control and greater susceptibility to hypothermia. Bradycardia, most frequently caused by hypoxia or vagal stimulation, and hypovolemia are poorly tolerated. Rapid or excessive fluid administration may result in pulmonary edema.(6)

Neonates have a high oxygen consumption because of their high metabolic rate. Their minute ventilation is therefore higher than that of an adult and is achieved through higher breathing rates. High minute ventilation also raises the alveolar ventilation to a functional residual capacity (FRC) ratio above that of the adult. Closing volume (the volume at which alveoli close, resulting in arteriovenous shunting) is high in the neonate and within the lower range of the tidal volume. Last, the neonate's rib cage is pliable, resulting in less efficient ventilation and greater work of breathing. Neonates are especially susceptible to hypoxia during apnea or airway obstruction because of their high oxygen consumption, high closing volume, and low FRC. Because of their increased alveolar ventilation and centralized circulation, anesthetic induction and recovery occur quickly in neonates. Last, neonates are susceptible to fatigue with airway obstruction or pneumonia because of their compliant chest wall and immaturity of the muscles of ventilation.(6–8)

Neonates regulate their body temperature poorly and are susceptible to hypothermia because of their high body surface to mass ratio and limited ability to vasoconstrict to conserve heat. They are generally regarded as being more susceptible to the effects of drugs than adults. This increased sensitivity can be related to differences in the distribution, metabolism, and excretion of drugs by the neonate. These include lower binding of drugs to plasma proteins, increased volume of distribution of drugs that distribute in extracellular or total body fluid, increased permeability of the blood-brain barrier, and slower elimination, (i.e.,

Table 24D–1. Physiologic Characteristics of Neonates

Low myocardial contractile mass
Low ventricular compliance
High cardiac index
Low cardiac reserve
Fixed stroke volume
Cardiac output rate dependent
Immature sympathetic nervous system
Poor vasomotor control
High oxygen consumption and minute volume of ventilation
High closing volume
Thermoregulation limited
Permeable blood-brain barrier
Low body fat and muscle tissue
Low protein binding of drugs
High body water content, large extracellular fluid compartment
Immature hepatic microsomal enzyme system
Immature kidney function

longer half-life) of most drugs (Chapter 2).(9) Total body water of neonates comprises approximately 75% of body weight as opposed to 50 to 60% in the adult. In the 1-week-old foal, extracellular fluid accounts for 43% of body weight compared to 22% in the adult horse.(10) Furthermore, the extracellular fluid compartment is larger than the intracellular, unlike the adult.(11) The large extracellular fluid volume results in a greater apparent volume of distribution of drugs that are highly ionized in plasma or relatively polar (e.g., nonsteroidal antiinflammatory drugs, nondepolarizing neuromuscular blockers). Volume of distribution is also affected by lower protein binding and decreased rates of metabolism and excretion. Neonatal hypoalbuminemia, although common in the newborn, is species related, being least in the foal.(10) This may result in decreased amounts of drug being bound to albumen, making more drug available to diffuse into tissues. Last, body fat is low in the neonate as opposed to the adult, such that adipose tissue does not comprise a significant compartment for redistribution. Although these neonatal characteristics have variable effects on pharmacokinetics, the most important factor during early life is the deficiency of hepatic microsomal enzyme function during the first 4 weeks, and especially during the first week. The relative inability to metabolize drugs leads to prolonged tissue levels of drugs if adult dosages are used. In addition, renal function is not fully developed at birth and does not reach full function in most species until 1 to 2 months. This also contributes to prolonged tissue levels of drug. Glomerular filtration rate reaches adult values in 2 days in calves, and 2 to 4 days in foals, lambs, kids, and pigs, and requires at least 14 days in puppies. Tubular secretion reaches adult levels in 2 weeks in ruminants and may take up to 4 to 6 weeks in

puppies. In ruminants, renal function is adequate to excrete xenobiotics within 1 week, and is fully mature in 1 to 2 weeks.(10) The combined effect of slow hepatic microsomal metabolism (oxidation and glucuronide conjugation) and inefficient renal excretion considerably affects the elimination of lipid soluble drugs and their metabolites.

Drug toxicity in neonates is not uncommon. This apparent sensitivity to drugs is caused by several factors. The blood-brain barrier, because of the open tubocisternal endoplasmic reticulum of cerebral endothelial and choroid plexus epithelial cells, allows drugs greater access to the brain than occurs in the adult. Although little quantitative information is available concerning dosage rates and frequencies in neonates of the various species, dosage rates should be reduced for at least the first 4 weeks of life.(11)

Anesthetic management of neonatal and pediatric veterinary patients is determined by the nature of the procedure, the status of the patient, and the physiologic and pharmacologic characteristics of this age group. The choice of anesthetics and adjuncts does not differ greatly from those used in adults. There does not appear to be any specific contraindication to any drug on the basis of age alone. Successful anesthetic management depends on careful dosing and administration of drugs and adequate monitoring and support of cardiopulmonary function and body temperature. Anesthetics and adjuncts most commonly used in young patients include low doses of inhalants, opioids, benzodiazepines, dissociatives and alpha$_2$-adrenergic agonists.(12–15)

Geriatric Patients

Aging is an all-encompassing multifactorial process resulting in decreased capacity for adaptation and produces a decrease in functional reserve of the organ systems. Aging is not a disease itself but may be accompanied by the development of many age-related diseases. The aging process varies from individual to individual and from one organ system to another within a given patient. There is little correlation between chronologic and physiologic age. Physical status as defined by the American Society of Anesthesiologists (ASA) is not affected by age but rather by the number and severity of preexisting medical conditions (Chapter 2). The effect of age per se on perioperative morbidity and mortality is related to the decreased physiologic reserve of the various organ systems that occur with aging.

Pathophysiologic changes of organ systems associated with aging influence anesthetic management (Table 24D–2). Cardiovascular changes are multifactorial, reflecting not only age-related changes but also age-related disease and/or life-style that results in gradual deconditioning. Variable degrees of myocardial fiber atrophy result in decreased pump function and cardiac output. Heart rate may be affected should this involve pacemaker cells. Fibrosis of the endocardium

Table 24D–2. Physiologic Characteristics of Geriatric Patients

Decreased elasticity and compliance of the vasculature
Increased blood pressure
Increased left ventricular mass
Decreased responsiveness to catecholamines
Increased incidence of dysrhythmias
Increased incidence of conduction abnormalities
Cardiac output is preload dependent
Decreased ventilatory volumes
Decreased efficiency of pulmonary gas exchange
Decreased liver mass
Decreased total hepatic blood flow
Decreased renal mass
Decreased muscle mass
Increased body fat as a percent of total body weight
Decreased total body water
Decreased intracellular and blood volume
Decreased albumen
Decreased basal metabolic rate

and valves leads to decreased compliance. Valvular incompetence may accompany valvular fibrosis and calcification. The vascular tree gradually loses elasticity, resulting in decreased distensibility, increased impedance to left ventricular output, and progressive hypertrophy of the ventricle (Chapter 5). Maximum coronary perfusion decreases as coronary artery elasticity and caliber decrease. These factors can combine to cause hypertension.(16) With age, the maximum heart rate that can be generated decreases. In addition, the response to stress or to exogenously administered autonomic drugs is decreased. This appears to be due to a decreased number of adrenergic receptors in the heart and to a generalized decrease in adrenoceptor sensitivity to agonists in the heart, peripheral vasculature and kidney.(17, 18) This appears to explain the decreased maximum heart rate, increased preload, and decreased ejection fraction at maximum effort. Young adults increase cardiac output primarily through increased heart rate. In geriatric patients, increased cardiac output is achieved through increased stroke volume via increased end-diastolic volume. Thus, the geriatric patient is dependent on preload and is not as tolerant of volume depletion in the perioperative period.

Pulmonary changes associated with aging include decreased ventilatory volumes and efficiency of gas exchange. Vital capacity, total lung capacity, and maximum breathing capacity decrease as the intercostal and diaphragmatic muscles gradually waste and the thorax becomes more rigid and less compliant. Age-related parenchymal changes in the lung resemble those of emphysema. Functional alveoli and elasticity progressively decrease. As elasticity decreases, the ratio of residual volume and of FRC to total lung capacity

increase. Closing volume is increased, resulting in air trapping and ventilation perfusion mismatch (Chapter 6). As a result P_aO_2 decreases with age.(16)

Although an age-related decrease in central nervous function is not well established, aged patients have a decreased requirement for anesthetic agents as compared to young adults. This appears to be related to an age-related decrease in resistance to loss of consciousness. MAC decreases linearly with age, and requirement for local anesthetics, opioids, barbiturates, benzodiazepines, and other intravenous drugs is similarly reduced.(19–22) Factors thought to be involved in this increased sensitivity to anesthetics include the continual loss of neurons associated with aging, decreased receptors and affinity of the receptors for neurotransmitters, and decreased rate of synthesis of neurotransmitters.(16)

With aging there is a loss of kidney mass, primarily cortical tissue. As a result, glomerular filtration rate decreases, making the patient more susceptible to acute renal failure following nephrotoxic or ischemic episodes in the perioperative period. Tubular function is also decreased, and the renin-angiotensin system becomes less responsive in aged patients. Geriatric patients cannot maximally retain sodium or water under conditions of volume depletion. Thus, the ability to correct fluid, electrolyte, and acid-base disturbances and to tolerate hemodynamic insults is reduced. Because geriatric patients have difficulty excreting a salt and water load, vigorous fluid and electrolyte therapy may result in excessive intravascular and extravascular volume with subsequent congestive heart failure and peripheral edema. Drugs eliminated primarily by renal excretion will require dose modification.(23)

Hepatic clearance of drugs decreases with age as the mass of the liver decreases. In elderly people the liver mass as well as hepatic blood flow may be decreased by 40 to 50%. Microsomal and nonmicrosomal enzyme function appears to be well maintained. Metabolism of lipid soluble drugs, particularly anesthetics, is decreased because of the decreased mass of the liver and corresponding decreases in total hepatic blood flow. This, combined with the decreased filtration and excretory capacity of the kidney, results in a prolonged half-life and duration of effect of drugs.(23)

Age-related changes in body composition include a decrease in skeletal muscle, an increase in body fat as a percentage of total body weight, and a loss of intracellular water. A loss of total body water occurs as a result of decreased intracellular water and a reduction in blood volume (20–30%). Intravenous injection of anesthetic drugs into this contracted blood volume results in an increased plasma concentration. Because of the increased adipose content of the body, there is increased sequestration of fat-soluble drugs, which slows their elimination.

Protein binding of drugs is reduced in the elderly because of decreased concentrations of albumen in the blood, qualitative changes in the protein decrease binding to the available protein, coadministered drugs may compete for the binding sites, and certain diseases may inhibit plasma protein binding. As a result of decreased protein binding, drugs that are normally highly bound to protein may have an exaggerated clinical effect. Thiopental and etomidate are two examples of drugs that because of their altered pharmacokinetics have reduced dose requirements in aged patients. The benzodiazepines (e.g., diazepam and midazolam) and opioids are both pharmacokinetically and pharmacodynamically different in geriatric patients. That is, not only are their initial dose and effective plasma concentration lower (pharmacodynamics), but their elimination half-lives (pharmacokinetics) are prolonged.(16)

Basal metabolic rate decreases with age, as does ability to maintain body temperature. Geriatric patients tend to become more hypothermic than younger patients, delaying recovery. Shivering during recovery may increase oxygen consumption by 400 to 500%. This places severe demands on the cardiopulmonary system, which if not met, can result in arterial hypoxemia.

No one "ideal" anesthetic protocol can be recommended for all geriatric patients. An understanding of the pathophysiologic changes and the alterations of pharmacodynamics and pharmacokinetics that occur with aging is necessary when choosing an anesthetic protocol for a given geriatric patient. Rather than suggesting specific anesthetic protocols, attention to dose (decreased from young adults) and the "to effect" administration of anesthetics to achieve CNS depression commensurate with the anesthetic requirements of a specific surgical procedure are advocated (Table 24D–3). When possible, the use of local and regional anesthetic techniques in combination with sedation or neuroleptanalgesia may prove safer than general anesthesia. Appropriate management is based upon thorough evaluation and preoperative correction of abnormalities. Intensity of perioperative monitoring is dictated by the patient's condition and the procedure but in general will be greater than that in the younger adult.

Table 24D–3. Anesthetics Commonly Used in Small Animal Geriatric Patients

	Dose (mg/kg)	
Drug	Dog	Cat
Preanesthetics		
Anticholinergics		
Atropine*	0.01–0.02	0.01–0.02
Glycopyrrolate*	0.005–0.01	0.005–0.01
Sedatives and Analgesics		
Midazolam*	0.1–0.3	0.1–0.3
Diazepam†	0.2–0.4	0.2–0.4
Oxymorphone*	0.1–0.2	0.1–0.2
Butorphanol*	0.2–0.4	0.2–0.4
Buprenorphine*	0.005–0.01	0.005–0.01
Induction Drugs		
Fentanyl/Diazepam	0.1/0.2	—
Oxymorphone/Diazepam	0.1/0.2	0.1/0.2
Ketamine/Diazepam	3–5/0.2	3–5/0.2
Etomidate	0.5–1.5	0.5–1.5
Isoflurane (mask)	2–3%	2–3%
Maintenance		
Inhalant		
Isoflurane	1–2%	1–2%
Muscle relaxant		
Atracurium	0.1	0.1

*IM or IV administration is appropriate.
†Diazepam is not recommended for IM use and should be given slowly when administered IV.

REFERENCES

1. Baggot JD, Short CR. Drug disposition in the neonatal animal, with particular reference to the foal. Equine Vet J19:169–171, 1987.
2. Rossdale, PD. A clinician's view of prematurity and dysmaturity in Thoroughbred foals. Proc R Soc Med 69:631–632, 1976.
3. Robinson EP. Anesthesia of pediatric patients. Compend Cont Educ Pract Vet 5:1004, 1983.
4. Friedman WF. The intrinsic physiologic properties of the developing heart. Prog Cardiovasc Dis 15:87–111, 1972.
5. Friedman WF, George BL. Treatment of congestive heart failure by altering loading conditions of the heart. J Pediatr 106:697, 1985.
6. Berry FA. Neonatal anesthesia. In: Barash, PG, Cullen BF, Stoelting RK, eds. Clinical anesthesia. Philadelphia: JB Lippincott, 1989: 1253–1280.
7. Gillespie JR. Postnatal lung growth and function in the foal. J Reprod Fertil Suppl 23:667–671, 1975.
8. Pattle RE, Rossdale PD, Schock C, et al. The development of the lung and its surfactant in the foal and other species. J Reprod Fertil Suppl 23:651–657, 1975.
9. Baggot JD. Drug therapy in the neonatal animal. In: Principles of drug disposition in domestic animals: the basis of veterinary clinical pharmacology. Philadelphia: WB Saunders, 1992: 219–224.
10. Baggot JD. Drug therapy in the neonatal foal. Vet Clin North Am Equine Pract 10:87–107, 1994.
11. Jenkins WL. Disposition of anesthetic and anesthetic-related agents in ruminants. Vet Clin North Am Food Anim Pract 2:527–552, 1986.
12. Dunlop CI. Anesthesia and sedation of foals. Vet Clin North Am Equine Pract 10:67–85, 1994.
13. Faggella AM, Aronsohn MG. Anesthetic techniques for neutering 6- to 14-week-old kittens. J Am Vet Med Assoc 10:56–62, 1993.
14. Grandy JL, Dunlop CI. Anesthesia of pups and kittens. J Am Vet Med Assoc 198:1244–1249, 1991.
15. Tranquilli WJ, Thurmon JC. Management of Anesthesia in the foal. Vet Clin North Am Equine Pract 1:651–653, 1990.
16. McLeskey CH. Anesthesia for the geriatric patient. In: Barash PG, Cullen BF, Stoelting RK, eds. Clinical anesthesia. Philadelphia: JB Lippincott, 1989: 1301–1337.
17. Shocken DD, Roth GS. Reduced beta-adrenergic receptor concentrations in aging man. Nature 267:856, 1977.
18. Elliott HL, Sumner DJ, McLean K, et al. Effect of age on the responsiveness of vascular alpha-adrenoceptors in man. J Cardiovasc Pharmacol 4:388, 1982.

19. Arden JR, Holley FO, Stanski DR. Increased sensitivity to etomidate in the elderly: initial distribution versus altered brain response. Anesthesiology 65:19, 1986.
20. Homer TD, Stanski DR. The effect of increasing age on thiopental disposition and anesthetic requirement. Anesthesiology 62:714, 1985.
21. Reidenberg MM, Levy M, Warner H, et al. Relationship between diazepam dose, plasma level, age and central nervous system depression. Clin Pharmacol Ther 23:371, 1978.
22. Stanski DR, Greenblatt DJ, Lowenstein E. Kinetics of intravenous and intramuscular morphine. Clin Pharmacol Ther 24:52, 1978.
23. Evers BM, Townsend CM Jr, Thompson JC. Organ physiology of aging. Surg Clin North Am 74:23–39, 1994.

chapter 25

ANESTHETIC EMERGENCIES AND ACCIDENTS

A. T. Evans

INTRODUCTION	CARDIAC DYSRHYTHMIAS
EFFECTS OF ANESTHESIA	CARDIAC ARREST
HYPOXIA	TEMPERATURE MONITORING
ASPIRATION	MALIGNANT HYPERTHERMIA
RESPIRATORY INSUFFICIENCY	INJURIES DURING ANESTHESIA
CARDIOVASCULAR EMERGENCIES	EPIDURAL ANALGESIA
HEMORRHAGE	

Introduction

In many veterinary practices, after the induction of anesthesia, no one is assigned the task of anesthetist to monitor anesthesia and be vigilant to the occurrence of untoward events that might result in morbidity and mortality. Sometimes this practice leads to the development of anesthetic accidents or emergencies. As with most unwanted events, anticipation of possible problems and having a plan of action already mentally prepared will go a long way toward successful resolution of the problem (Chapter 2). Since the onset of general anesthesia upsets the physiologic equilibrium of the patient and can bring it closer to the threshold of harmful events, preparation to manage these problems is even more critical.

Effects of Anesthesia

Induction of general anesthesia will often decrease cardiac output, decrease blood pressure, affect peripheral perfusion, decrease alveolar ventilation, interfere with temperature regulation, and increase intracranial pressure. When the detrimental consequences of surgery are added to the impact of anesthesia, it is easy to understand how anesthetic emergencies or accidents develop.

Hypoxia

Apnea and airway obstructions leading to hypoxia commonly occur during induction of anesthesia. Brachycephalic breeds are prone to airway obstruction as a response to the relaxing effects of sedative preanesthetics or induction doses of anesthetics. Although among the brachycephalic breeds airway obstruction is more common in English bulldogs, any breed with redundant pharyngeal tissue or obstructive laryngeal disease is susceptible to airway blockade. A common scenario would be that a patient with few or no symptoms of respiratory obstruction becomes cyanotic after induction of anesthesia. Attempts at intubation reveal pharyngeal or laryngeal obstruction occluding the airway. Immediate reestablishment of a patent airway is accomplished using a laryngoscope blade or finger to retract the obstructing tissue. Additional anesthetic may be required to eliminate the gag reflex (Chapters 17 and 23).

If the airway impediment involves the nasal passages, the oral pathway must be kept open. Often a dog with a nasal tumor is anxious and difficult to restrain because of difficulty with breathing. In this situation a gauze muzzle is sometimes used to protect personnel from bites and injury. However, a muzzle applied to this patient could be a fatal mistake, as it would eliminate the patient's primary method of breathing.

Sometimes the perfect bandage or splint applied to the neck during anesthesia becomes potentially lethal during recovery. The problem arises if the bandage or splint is applied with the head and neck extended. Unfortunately, this is not the normal position for the animal's neck, and during recovery the patient attempts to flex the neck to a more normal position. This causes the bandage to apply pressure to the laryngeal area.

Any patient experiencing respiratory difficulties during induction of anesthesia can be expected to have problems during the recovery. It would be prudent to observe these patients through the recovery period to ensure preservation of a patent airway. Some patients require aggressive airway maintenance, in which the anesthetist holds the mouth open, pulls the tongue out, and even manually holds down the epiglottis.

The benefits of endotracheal intubation for most patients generally outweigh the disadvantages, so intubation is recommended for most anesthetized patients. The modern carefully placed endotracheal tube with a soft, high-volume atraumatic cuff does not harm the tracheal epithelium. Once the patient is intubated, the lungs can be protected from aspiration of foreign material, oxygen-enriched gases can be easily administered, ventilation can be controlled, and inhalation anesthetics can be precisely delivered. Laryngospasm occurs more often in certain species such as cats, pigs, and monkeys, and after administration of thiobarbiturates or as a response to direct stimulation of the glottic area. If laryngospasm is anticipated, 2% lidocaine applied to arytenoid cartilages prior to attempts to intubate will usually permit passage of the tube through the larynx. Diseases that affect the temporal mandibular joint or that cause atrophy of the masseter muscle can decrease the distance the mouth can be opened. Although intubation can be difficult under these circumstances, blind intubation can usually be successful when the head and neck are extended and the endotracheal tube carefully advanced into the pharyngeal area. By gently manipulating the larynx from the outside, coupled with careful movement of the tube through the larynx, the trachea can be intubated (Chapter 17).

Aspiration

Aspiration of foreign material into the trachea and bronchi usually occurs when the trachea is not intubated. Food is likely to be present in the stomach of dogs up to 10 hours after a meal depending on the consistency of the meal.(1, 2) The hydrogen ion concentration of the aspirated material will affect morbidity, as the Pao_2 of patients is lower when the aspirated material has a pH less than two.(3) When intraabdominal pressure is increased because of surgical manipulation or "bucking" (the sharp rhythmic contraction of abdominal and thoracic musculature) during anesthesia, gastric or esophageal contents are forced into the pharynx. Dogs with megaesophagus are particularly susceptible to regurgitation. To prevent aspiration, position the dog with the head lower than the esophagus and protect the airway with an endotracheal tube. Regurgitation is rare in dogs that are housed in a controlled environment (veterinary clinic) overnight prior to anesthesia and surgery. When regurgitation occurs, keep the head lower than the esophagus and use suction to empty the esophagus and stomach. Use forceps and gauze to clean out the pharyngeal area. Visually inspect the pharynx prior to extubation and closely monitor the patient for regurgitation during anesthesia recovery, particularly if sedatives and analgesics have been used. Sedative-analgesics will depress the animal's ability to protect the airway.

Bronchial spasms have been reported to be an uncommon result of aspiration of rumen contents.(4) Bronchial spasms can also occur as part of an allergic response to anesthetic administration. Atropine or the administration of halothane often relieves the spasm.(5)

Respiratory Insufficiency

Respiratory insufficiency is very common during the course of anesthesia. Causes include the administration of opioids and other sedatives prior to anesthesia, the relative overdose of induction agents, positioning for surgery, respiratory effects of inhalants, surgical trauma, and the excessive use of opioids during recovery. The use of opioids with or without tranquilizers prior to induction of anesthesia to provide sedation and analgesia often results in a patient that is well sedated but has depressed ventilation. High doses of mu-receptor agonists such as oxymorphone and morphine are more likely to produce respiratory depression than the kappa-receptor agonist butorphanol. In addition, the decreased responsiveness to increased carbon dioxide tensions ($Paco_2$) during methoxyflurane, halothane, or isoflurane anesthesia tends to promote an increase in $Paco_2$, although surgical stimulation and duration of anesthesia often ameliorates this effect.(6, 7) In addition to the depressant effects of inhalants on responsiveness to increased $Paco_2$, subanesthetic doses depress the peripheral chemoreceptors such that hypoxia does not stimulate a ventilation response (Chapters 6 and 11).(8, 9) Hypoxia often occurs during recovery from anesthesia, and a slow ventilatory response to low Pao_2 could be ominous. Oxygen should be administered by mask until the patient is able to maintain a normal Pao_2 while breathing room air (Table 25–1).

Apnea is common during the course of routine anesthesia. It occurs during induction following the administration of thiobarbiturates or propofol, during maintenance of anesthesia with ketamine, as a result of controlled ventilation, and as a consequence of deep inhalation anesthesia. Generally, in addition to depression of ventilatory response, apnea during induction of anesthesia with thiobarbiturates or propofol is caused by a relative overdose or a fast bolus injection.(10) Ketamine and diazepam in a 50:50 mixture by volume

Table 25–1. Management of Complications Associated with Anesthesia

Complication	Treatment	Trade Name	Dosage	Side Effects
Excitement, delirium	Acepromazine	PromAce	0.05–0.2 mg/kg IV, IM	Prolonged recovery
	Diazepam	Valium	0.25–0.5 mg/kg IV	Hypothermia
	Midazolam	Versed	0.05–0.2 mg/kg IV, IM	
Hypoventilation	Oxygen	—	—	Respiratory depression
	Ventilation	—	—	Resisting mask
Laryngospasm	Lidocaine spray	Xylocaine 2%	—	
	Lidocaine jelly	—		
Dyspnea	Oxygen		—	
	Tracheostomy	Portex*		
	Ventilation			Hyperventilation
Pneumothorax	Oxygen			
	Chest tubes	—	—	Infection
	Ventilation			Hyperventilation
Cardiac dysrhythmias:				
Tachycardia	LRS	—	10–20 mL/kg per hour	Bradycardia
	Propranolol	Inderal	0.05–0.1 mg/kg IV	Hypotension
	Increase anesthesia	—	—	Bradycardia
Bradycardia	Atropine	—	0.02 mg/kg IV	Tachycardia
	Glycopyrrolate	Robinul V	0.005 mg/kg IV	
Ventricular dysrhythmias	Lidocaine	Xylocaine	Dogs: 0.5 mg/kg IV	Bradycardia
			Cats: 0.2 mg/kg IV	Convulsions
	Procainamide	Pronestyl	10–20 mg/kg IM	Hypotension
			10–20 mg/kg IV per hour	
Hypotension	Fluids (LRS)	—	10–20 mL/kg IV	
	Dopamine	Intropin	3–5 µg/kg per minute	Dysrhythmias
	Dobutamine	Dobutrex	3–5 µg/kg per minute	Tachycardia, hypertension
Blood or fluid loss	Fluids (LRS)	—	40–90 mL/kg IV per hour	Pulmonary edema
	Blood	—	20–40 mL/kg IV	Allergic reaction
Hypothermia	Warmed fluids		5–10 mL/kg IV per hour	Overhydration
	H₂O heating pad	Gaymar†		
Hypoglycemia	Dextrose 5%	—	1–2 mL/kg IV	Hyperosmolality
Metabolic acidosis	Sodium bicarbonate	—	1–2 mEq/kg IV every 10 minutes	Metabolic alkalosis, hypokalemia, hyperosmolality
Hyperkalemia	Sodium bicarbonate	—	0.5–1.0 mEq/kg IV	As above
	0.9% Sodium chloride	—	10–40 mL/kg per hour	
	Calcium chloride	—	10 mg/kg IV	Tachycardia
Hyperpyrexia	Oxygen			
	Fluids (LRS)		5–10 mL/kg IV	
	Tranquilizers	PromAce	0.1 mg/kg IM	
	Dantrolene sodium		2–4 mg/kg IV	
Prolonged recovery	Doxapram	Dopram V	1–2 mg/kg IV	Excitement
	Yohimbine	Yobine	0.5 mg/kg IV	
Postoperative pain	Morphine sulfate		0.1–1.0 mg/kg IM	Respiratory depression
	Buprenorphine	Buprenex	0.01 mg/kg IV, IM	Slow recovery
	Butorphenol	Torbugesic	0.2–0.4 mg/kg IM	Slow recovery

is commonly used for anesthesia in cats. Apnea often occurs, especially when anesthesia is maintained with supplemental isoflurane. This combination of drugs, each of which is a respiratory depressant alone, can combine to effect a persistent respiratory depression. If, as a response to respiratory depression, assisted or controlled ventilation is employed, the Pa_{CO_2} will be lowered below the highest arterial or alveolar P_{CO_2} at which the cat will remain apneic (apneic threshold) (Chapter 11).

Decreased functional residual capacity (FRC) during anesthesia can increase hypoxia by lowering alveolar ventilation-perfusion ratios (V_A/Q) and expanding atelectatic areas (Chapter 6). This occurs because the

FRC is close to or less than the closing volume (CV) of the lung. The CV is the volume of the lung at which small airways begin to close. When the tidal volume is less than the CV, small airways remain closed throughout the breathing cycle and atelectasis increases. If the CV of some airways remains within the tidal volume range, then there is some air exchange during inspiration and expiration, though not the normal amount. This partial ventilation decreases the ventilation perfusion ratio (V_A/Q). These lung changes are prevalent in older animals and during anesthesia. Intermittent positive pressure breathing (IPPB) and positive end-expiratory pressure (PEEP) can be used to diminish the hypoxia that occurs from changes in FRC. During anesthesia with a circle rebreathing system, slightly closing the pop-off valve so that it requires 5 or 10 cm H_2O pressure to open the valve will add 5 or 10 cm of H_2O PEEP.

Cardiovascular Emergencies

Cardiovascular emergencies are sometimes caused by the patient being "too deep." Anesthetics in a dose-related fashion can affect the various components of the cardiovascular system's response to stress. Usually a loss of blood results in an increase in cardiac output and adjustments in vascular reactivity so that organ perfusion is maintained. The response is initiated and controlled by various reflexes (Chapter 5). The dose-related alterations in cardiovascular function decrease cardiac contractility, relax vascular smooth muscle, and alter baroreceptor reflex. Cardiac contractility is diminished through depression of the isometric twitch strength of cardiac muscle. This is determined by analyzing the peak developed force and the maximum rate of rise of the developed force. Both halothane and isoflurane depress the twitch strength, with halothane being slightly more depressant. Vascular smooth muscle is relaxed by the inhalation anesthetics, and this also contributes to the hypotension observed during anesthesia. Deep halothane anesthesia causes vasodilation in vascular beds.(11) Alteration of the baroreceptor reflex by halothane and isoflurane can make it difficult to detect hypovolemia and hypotension during anesthesia. Normally the baroreceptor reflex responds to a decrease in pulse pressure and slope of the systolic pressure rise by invoking an increase in heart rate, vasoconstriction, and cardiac output. Halothane and isoflurane depress the heart rate response to hypotension, making it difficult to recognize during anesthesia. Maintaining a moderate depth of anesthesia will lessen the detrimental effects of the anesthetic on the cardiovascular system and eliminate this as a cause of mishap. Deep anesthesia can be prevented by maintaining the vaporizer setting near the minimum alveolar concentration (MAC) of the anesthetic being used (Chapters 2 and 11).

Hemorrhage

The incidence of life-threatening hemorrhage during surgical procedures is low. Acute hemorrhage as a result of laceration of a large vein or artery is immediately recognized and corrective measures initiated. However, blood oozing during nasal exploratories or from venous sinuses during spinal surgery might become life threatening because the oozing is usually controlled by the use of surgical suction. The volume of blood aspirated by the suction line is deceptively large and commonly not noticed by the surgeon, who is concentrating on surgery. Signs of serious blood loss include decreasing packed cell volume when given large quantities of fluid, weak pulse, lower blood pressure, deeper anesthesia, and pale mucous membranes (Chapters 15 and 19). Other avenues of fluid loss during surgery include evaporation from pleural and peritoneal surfaces, continued formation of ascites and pleural effusions, loss of fluid into the bowel, and third space losses. Third space losses are represented for the most part as a generalized increase in extracellular tissue water. This fluid is effectively lost from the general circulation and should be considered when replacing fluid lost from hemorrhage. Lost fluids or blood can be replaced by either crystalloids or colloids or both. Examples of crystalloids are lactated Ringer's solution (LR), 0.9% NaCl, and hypertonic NaCl solutions ranging from 1.8 to 10% (Chapter 19). LR is the most commonly used crystalloid and is administered in a 3:1 ratio to correct blood loss. Small volumes of hypertonic salt solution extract water from the interstitial space and move it into the plasma volume. The transient increase in blood volume is a result of osmotic forces, which diminish as equilibrium is reached. In most situations, hypertonic solutions alone do not seem to have a distinct advantage over isotonic crystalloid solutions.(12) The obvious advantage of crystalloid solutions is the low price. Colloid solutions such as whole blood, plasma, and dextrans can be used as a substitute for crystalloids. The use of colloids has the advantage of sustaining colloid osmotic pressure while preserving plasma volume but has the disadvantage of being expensive. The best treatment for acute hemorrhage greater than 20% of body weight is replacement 1:1 with whole blood. Smaller amounts of surgical hemorrhage can be attended with LR or colloids rather than whole blood (Table 25-1).

Cardiac Dysrhythmias

Cardiac dysrhythmias occur as a result of preexisting medical conditions, administration of premedications, anesthesia induction and maintenance agents, and surgical stimulation. Dysrhythmias require treatment if they reduce cardiac output, cause sustained tachycardia, or are likely to initiate dangerous ventricular dysrhythmias (Chapter 5).

Canine gastric dilation/volvulus or multiple trauma precipitate dysrhythmias, which may require treatment prior to induction of anesthesia.(13, 14) Dysrhythmias following gastric dilation/volvulus presumably have their origin from acid-base imbalance, electrolyte disturbances, ischemic myocardium, circulating cardiac stimulatory substances, and/or autonomic nervous system imbalance. Treatment involves correcting the physiologic abnormalities and administering lidocaine, procainamide, or quinidine, either singly or in combination (Chapter 23). Premature ventricular contractions (PVCs) and ventricular tachycardia as a repercussion of a traumatic myocardium have also been curtailed with lidocaine and quinidine. Often surgery can be delayed until the dysrhythmias have subsided. Several of the popular drugs used as preanesthetic medication can predispose the patient to conduction abnormalities. Atropine or glycopyrrolate can cause sinus tachycardia and increase myocardial work. Phenothiazine tranquilizers predispose the heart to sinus bradycardia, sinus arrest, and occasional first and second degree heart block. Xylazine has been implicated as causing bradycardias and decreasing the epinephrine threshold for VPCs. The mu-receptor agonist opioids (morphine, oxymorphone), will also precipitate a slow heart rate (Chapter 8).

The anesthesia induction agents thiamylal, thiopental, and ketamine have been reported to increase the likelihood of dysrhythmias from epinephrine during halothane anesthesia (Chapter 9).(15, 16) This phenomenon has also been described for thiopental and isoflurane.(17) Although it is an unlikely sequela following epinephrine interaction, dogs anesthetized with thiamylal and maintained with halothane can spontaneously develop ventricular fibrillation.

Other factors responsible for the development of the dysrhythmias during the surgical period include altered $Paco_2$, Pao_2, pH, reflexes from surgical manipulation, central nervous system disturbances, and cardiac disease. Because most perioperative dysrhythmias do not seriously affect cardiac output, treatment can be discrete. Changing to a different inhalation anesthetic or increasing the depth of anesthesia may eliminate the

dysrhythmia.(18, 19) Other treatments for controlling ventricular dysrhythmias include giving a small dose (0.01 mg/kg) of acepromazine intravenously, correcting blood gas abnormalities, or administering a small quantity (0.5 mg/kg) of intravenous lidocaine (Table 25–1).

Cardiac Arrest

Successful treatment of cardiac arrest requires early diagnosis. The brain is the organ most susceptible to hypoxia-ischemia, as serious injury develops after only 4 or 5 minutes of cardiac arrest. Once the diagnosis of cardiac arrest has been confirmed, all efforts must be toward developing effective blood flow and reestablishing a heartbeat. CPR with external cardiac massage appears to be ineffective in protecting the brain from injury and should only be part of the initial resuscitation protocol and not be continued for long periods of time.(20)

Diagnosis of cardiac arrest is made when the signs listed in Table 25–2 are present. When the thoracic heartbeat or peripheral pulse cannot be palpated, the systolic blood pressure is generally less than 50 mm Hg. In this circumstance, the heart may actually have a weak beat, but cardiac output is probably very low and true cardiac arrest imminent. A nonpalpable weak heartbeat along with a regular electric rhythm has been termed *electric mechanical dissociation* (EMD) (Fig. 25–1). This type of functional cardiac arrest occurs with overdose of anesthesia and from many other causes such as hypovolemia, acute cardiogenic decompensation, severe acidosis, or hypoxemia. It is important to look for correctable causes of EMD during the first moments of resuscitation to improve the odds of success. Other forms of cardiac arrest include asystole and ventricular fibrillation (Fig. 25–2). Three types of cardiac arrest can be differentiated with an electrocardiogram or by direct observation of the heart. Apnea usually precedes cardiac arrest, but if sudden ventricular fibrillation occurs, the patient may continue to breathe for a few seconds after blood flow stops. Other signs of cardiac arrest include surgical incisions not bleeding and a darkening of the blood in the surgical field. The jaw tone, which is used to monitor anesthetic depth, will be

Table 25–2. Signs of Cardiac Arrest

1. No palpable heart beat
2. No palpable pulse
3. Apnea
4. Lack of surgical hemorrhage
5. Cyanosis
6. No muscle tone
7. Dilated pupils (later)

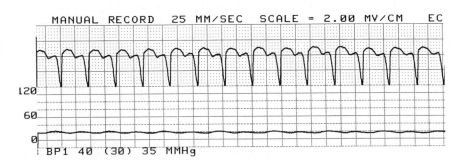

Fig. 25–1. Electric mechanical dissociation is displayed above the corresponding arterial blood pressure. The ECG has a rhythmic though bizarre pattern. Note that blood pressure is 40 mm Hg systolic, 30 mm Hg diastolic, with a mean pressure of 35 mm Hg. This low pressure cannot be palpated at peripheral sites.

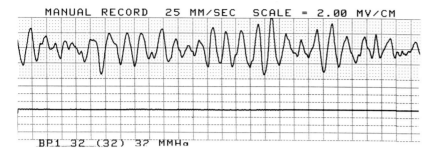

Fig. 25–2. The uncoordinated bizarre ECG pattern of ventricular fibrillation in the top tracing is displayed with corresponding blood pressure. The blood pressure is displayed as a flat line below the ECG and represents residual intravascular pressure during cardiac arrest.

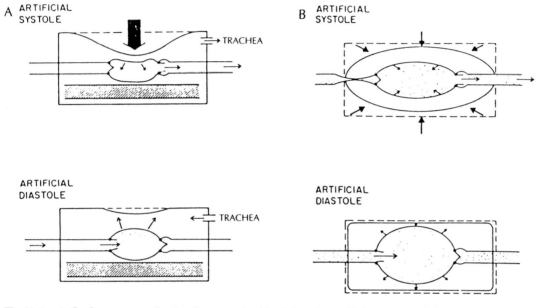

Fig. 25–3. A, Cardiac pump mechanism for generating blood flow during CPR. During artificial systole, central chest compression squeezes the heart against the spine, forcing blood out. Air is vented from the thorax via the trachea (top left). During artificial diastole, chest resiliency creates negative pressure for filling. The site of application of force (broad arrow) is critical. For simplicity only one pumping chamber is shown. B, The thoracic pump generates intrathoracic pressure, which is vented by arterial outflow to peripheral tissues. During artificial diastole, release of intrathoracic pressure allows for filling. Site of application of force is not important. (From Babbs, C.F. New Versus Old Theories of Blood Flow During CPR. Crit Care Med 8:191, 1980)

absent. After several minutes of cardiac arrest, the pupils will dilate.

When any or all of these signs are present, the traditional ABCD protocol for treatment of cardiac arrest must be started immediately. *A* refers to *airway* and reminds the resuscitator that a patent airway is a necessity. Always confirm a patent airway for an animal previously intubated for general anesthesia. Endotracheal intubation is the best method of insuring a patent airway. The goal of *B, breathing,* is to supply high concentrations of oxygen to the alveoli and to eliminate carbon dioxide. Although external thoracic massage results in some alveolar gas exchange, the recommendations for breathing rate have been revised downward from 10 to 12 per minute to 4 or 5.(21) The volume of inspired gas required to produce an inspiratory pressure of 15 to 20 cm water should be sufficient to cause

the thorax to move in a normal pattern. If an overdose of inhalation anesthetic has contributed to the cardiac arrest, the breathing rate should initially remain higher than 4 or 5 breaths per minute in order to help remove the remaining anesthetic. *C* refers to *cardiac massage,* which can be either external (thoracic) or internal cardiac massage.

External thoracic massage is thought to produce cardiac output by one or a combination of two methods. The thoracic pump theory holds that blood moves out of the thoracic cavity during the compression half of the cardiopulmonary resuscitation (CPR) stroke due to a buildup of internal thoracic pressure (Fig. 25–3). This mechanism is thought to occur primarily in animals larger than 15 to 20 kg body weight. Evidence for the thoracic pump theory includes the phenomenon of cough CPR in humans and artificial cough CPR in dogs.(22, 23) The cardiac pump theory explains blood flow in smaller animals or animals with a narrow side-to-side thoracic width and refers to actual mechanical compression of the myocardium by the thoracic wall during CPR systole (Fig. 25-4). Blood flow in some patients is produced by a combination of the cardiac and thoracic pump mechanisms. Whatever the reason for forward blood flow, it appears that external thoracic massage is not very protective of the brain, as CPR performed for more than 3 or 4 minutes often results in

significant neurologic injury.(24) It has even been proposed that neurologic insult during the first few minutes of cardiac arrest when external CPR is being used is worse than the neurologic injury resulting from no CPR at all.

One explanation for the inadequacy of external CPR is that the brain is perfused with a small trickle flow of blood carrying glucose substrate but little oxygen.(25) This combination of substrate and low oxygen results in anaerobic metabolism, with the production of large

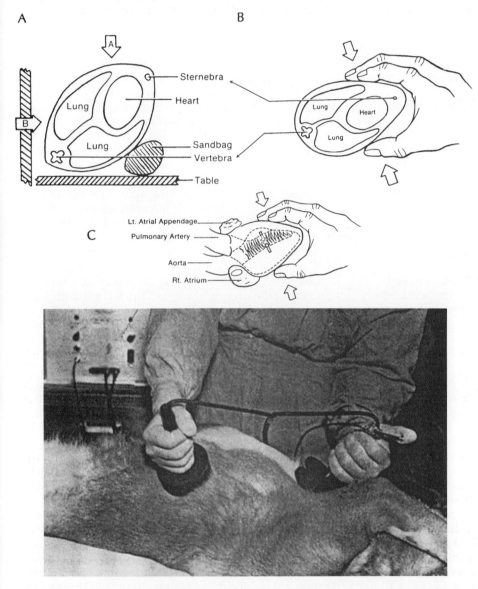

Fig. 25–4. A, Diagram illustrating the techniques of external cardiac compression in most animals (5 to 60 kg in body weight). Rhythmic downward force A is applied with the heel of the hand to the left lateral thorax (80 times per minute) in the area of the costochondral junction at the level of the sixth rib. The patient is stabilized by the technique of external cardiac compression in small animals (less than 5 kg in body weight). B, The fingers and thumb of one hand are used to compress the right and left hemithorax at the costochondral junction at the level of the sixth rib. The compression rate in smaller animals should approach 120/min. C, Diagram illustrating a technique of internal cardiac compression in small animals. The palmar surfaces of the fingers and thumb of one hand are used to compress the ventricular free walls toward the interventricular septum. D, Placement of external defibrillator electrodes over the manubrium and on the left precordial region. (A to C from Ross, J.N., and Breznock, E.M. Resuscitation. In: Veterinary Critical Care, Edited by F.P. Sattler, R.P. Knowles, and W.G. Whittick. Philadelphia: Lea & Febiger, 1981. D from Ott, B.S. Closed Chest Cardiac Resuscitation. Small Anim Clin 2:572, 1962.)

amounts of lactate and other metabolic byproducts. Conversely, if resuscitation is not attempted for the first 4 to 5 minutes, metabolism will slow as the glucose substrate is exhausted. The brain is still deteriorating during this time, though not as fast as during active external CPR. Because traditional external thoracic massage is apparently ineffective, various maneuvers have been proposed to improve blood flow during CPR. Interposed abdominal compression has been proposed as a way of improving cardiac output during CPR.(26) This method involves manually compressing the abdomen in counterpoint to the rhythm of the chest compression. The physiologic reason for improvement of blood flow is that compression of the abdominal aorta responds like an intraaortic balloon pump and that pressure on the abdominal veins primes the right heart and pulmonary vasculature in preparation for the next thoracic compression.(27)

In one study in people this method of augmenting external CPR has improved survivals, but comparable clinical studies are not available in animals.(28) Interposed abdominal compression in dogs involves placing one hand over the other and compressing the abdomen counterpoint to thoracic compressions. Another way of improving blood flow during CPR is to simultaneously ventilate at the time of thoracic compression. Simultaneous compression-ventilation (SCV-CPR) has improved carotid blood flow during resuscitation of animals.(29) Opposing evidence has also been presented that shows that the mitral valve of dogs may in fact close as a response to rhythmic increases in intrathoracic pressure.(30) In spite of this evidence to the contrary, SCV-CPR probably improves blood flow during CPR of large dogs when the thoracic pump is the primary reason for flow. Open thoracic or internal CPR is more effective at perfusing the heart and brain during the critical beginning minutes of CPR.(31) Higher blood pressures and cardiac outputs can be achieved with internal CPR. Most veterinary practices are well equipped to perform internal CPR because controlled ventilation and thoracotomy can be performed. The limiting factor will probably be the surgical experience of the attending veterinarian.

Whichever method of CPR is chosen, there are some guidelines for CPR technique that when followed can improve success (Figure 25–4). The patient should be in right lateral recumbency with the resuscitator standing at the animal's back. With the animal in this position, there won't be movement of the patient on the table during resuscitation and access to the left ventricle for intracardiac injections is possible. The thoracic or cardiac compression rate should be 80 to 100 per minute.(32) Various patterns of compressions have been recommended depending on the mechanism of blood flow. If the cardiac pump is the primary mechanism of blood flow, the compression time versus relaxation time is not as important as during the thoracic pump method of blood flow. That is, the blood will be expelled from the ventricles of the heart at peak compression and it

won't matter how long the peak pressure is maintained. With larger patients, the thoracic pump probably contributes to blood flow and therefore depends on intrathoracic pressure to move blood out of the heart. As long as intrathoracic pressure is applied, blood will be squeezed from the heart. Therefore, the recommendations for compression pattern with the thoracic pump include a slight hesitation at the moment of peak force. Realistically, with a compression rate of 80 to 100 per minute, it may be difficult to hesitate at the moment of peak thoracic compression.

The recommendations for D, definitive or drug therapy, start with the immediate use of epinephrine. Other alpha- and beta-adrenergic drugs have been used, but none have proven to be superior to the traditional use of epinephrine for cardiac arrest.(33) Epinephrine should be given early in the treatment protocol, preferably into a central vein. Because access to a central vein may be difficult, epinephrine may alternatively be administered into a peripheral vein, intrabronchially, or directly into the ventricle. For intrabronchial administration, use a flexible plastic catheter wedged into a distal bronchus.(34) For intracardiac placement, use a 22-gauge needle inserted at the left thoracic fourth interspace and costochondral junction. A long spinal needle may be needed for larger dogs. For intravenous use, a dose of 0.05 to 0.1 mg/kg is used, whereas bronchial administration requires 0.05 to 0.1 mg/kg diluted to 2 to 3 mL volume with saline. The dose for intracardiac epinephrine is 0.025 to 0.05 mg/kg. Even though intracardiac epinephrine seems appealing as a way of efficiently delivering the drug to the heart, the technical difficulty of positioning the needle in the chamber of the left ventricle when the heart cannot be palpated along with the potential for myocardial injury makes this technique the least advantageous. Since the goal of CPR is to revive the patient's heart as soon as possible, early administration of epinephrine is crucial and should be given immediately after diagnosis of cardiac arrest.

Lidocaine is used after resuscitation if ventricular dysrhythmias are compromising cardiac output. The use of lidocaine during ventricular fibrillation to improve the results of electric defibrillation is being reevaluated. In nonischemic models of CPR, the use of lidocaine apparently increases the energy required for electric defibrillation, although pentobarbital anesthesia used in the experimental studies may in part explain the difference.(35, 36) Lidocaine is usually given as a bolus intravenously at a dose of 0.5 mg/kg. Metabolic acidosis from hypoxia and ischemia and respiratory alkalosis as a result of ventilation during treatment of cardiac arrest commonly occur during resuscitation.(37) The immediate use of bicarbonate or THAM is controversial, as metabolic acidosis is slow to develop during CPR and is somewhat neutralized by an ensuing respiratory alkalosis (Chapters 18 and 19). Respiratory alkalosis occurs as a result of external thoracic compression and controlled ventilation during CPR. Generally sodium bicarbonate or THAM will not be required immediately after the onset of cardiac arrest unless an existing nonrespiratory acidosis contributed to the arrest. In addition, acid-base abnormalities do not necessarily correlate with successful resuscitation.(38) Atropine or glycopyrrolate are important drugs to administer during CPR because reflex bradycardia may have contributed to the initial cardiac arrest. In addition, bradycardia often occurs after a heartbeat has been established. Atropine at 0.02 to 0.04 mg/kg or glycopyrrolate at a dose of 0.01 mg/kg intravenously will protect against bradycardia.

Few studies in veterinary medicine document the most common form of cardiac arrest. Because coronary artery disease is a major form of heart disease in people, ventricular fibrillation is the common expression of cardiac arrest.(39) In dogs and cats, electric mechanical dissociation is apparently more common than ventricular fibrillation.(40) Epinephrine should be administered to all dogs and cats with cardiac arrest irrespective of the form of arrest. Epinephrine has been shown to increase cerebral and myocardial blood flow through mechanisms of prevention of arterial collapse and by producing vasoconstriction, which prevents sequestration of blood in noncritical areas.(41)

Asystole, or flat-line electrocardiogram, is the next most common form of cardiac arrest, with ventricular fibrillation the least common. It is fortuitous that ventricular fibrillation is the least common expression of cardiac arrest, as most veterinary practices do not have on their premises a direct current defibrillator. If a direct current defibrillator is available, clip the hair from a small area from each side of the thorax. After applying electrode gel to each paddle, firmly apply the paddles to the thorax (Fig. 25–4) and administer a shock of approximately 2 to 5 joules (watt/seconds) per kg. Sequential discharges of increasing energy may be more effective at converting fibrillation.(42) Internal defibrillation requires a smaller electric discharge, a total of 10 to 50 joules.

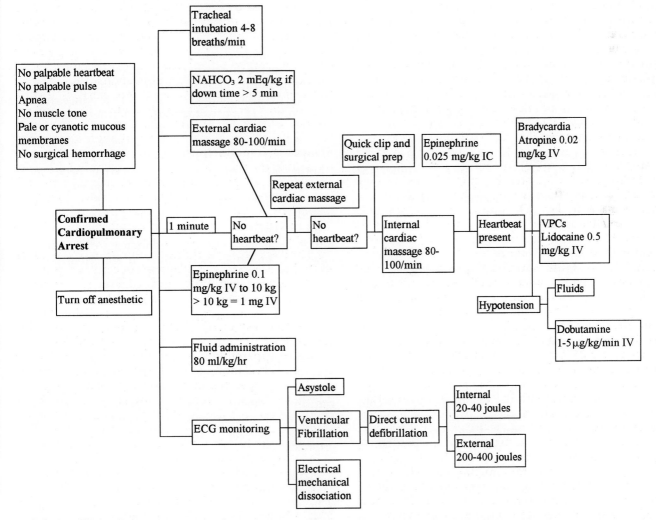

Fig. 25–5.   An algorithm for CPR. This simplified protocol for CPR is used to resuscitate animals that have the potential for surviving cardiac arrest. Because early restoration of brain perfusion is the most important goal to be achieved, a quick decision for internal cardiac massage is required (ECG, electrocardiogram; IC, intracardiac; NaHCO₃, sodium bicarbonate; VPCs, ventricular premature contractions).

After administration of epinephrine, and after attention to airway (A) and breathing (B) of the CPR protocol, begin external thoracic massage. It seems reasonable to start external CPR even though success rates are low with this method. Some animals respond positively to one or two doses of epinephrine and 1 or 2 minutes of external CPR. These appear to be primarily animals in EMD or asystole. If there is no response after 2 minutes, it also seems reasonable to begin the more productive internal CPR.(43) Unfortunately, many practitioners may not feel confident about performing a thoracotomy when they have little or no previous experience with this procedure. There is little to lose, however, when the patient is in cardiac arrest and hasn't responded to initial resuscitation attempts.

Emergency thoracotomy can be accomplished quickly in an arrested animal. Clip the hair from the left thorax at the fifth interspace. Spray or wipe the area with an antiseptic solution and incise the skin starting 1 inch from the spine to within 1 inch of the sternum. With surgical scissors continue incision through the various tissue layers, avoiding the internal thoracic artery near the sternum. Bluntly penetrate the pleura, extend the incision, and spread the ribs. Reach into the thorax and begin cardiac massage at a rate of 80 to 100 compressions per minute. Depending on its size, the heart can be massaged with fingers, one hand, or two hands.(44) Epinephrine can now be easily administered into the left ventricle as required. If the resuscitation is successful and mental alertness improves, the subject can be anesthetized to complete closure of the thoracic incision. The thorax should be flushed with warm sterile physiologic saline and closed in a routine manner. Infection is rare after emergency thoracotomy in people and from clinical experience uncommon in dogs.(45) An algorithm for patients with confirmed cardiac arrest is presented in Figure 25–5.

Temperature Monitoring

Intraoperative hypothermia is a common sequela of general anesthesia in small animals. Body temperature is governed by input from the hypothalamus, other parts of the brain, skin surface, spinal cord, and deep central tissues. This information is integrated, predominately in the hypothalamus, and compared with threshold temperatures for heat and cold. The response to temperature aberrations is based on mean body temperature, which is a weighted average of input from the various afferent sensing sites. The responses to cold include vasoconstriction, nonshivering thermogenesis, shivering, piloerection, puffing of feathers, and lowering of body temperature. Warm thermoregulatory effector mechanisms consist of vasodilation, sweating, panting, and salivation. Hypothermia results if heat production is less than heat loss. Heat loss is generally through convection and radiation from the skin and surgical incision. Inhalation anesthetics lower the threshold for response to hypothermia in people to about 34.5° C (46), and presumably the same trend occurs in animals.

Accidental surgical hypothermia can be limited in people by maintaining ambient temperature of at least 21° C for adults and 26° C in premature infants. It would be reasonable to include small animals in the size range of infants, but most veterinarians would find 26° C too warm for ambient temperature. Accidental hypothermia can be limited by cocooning using warm water blankets (47) and warming intravenous crystalloid fluids if large amounts are used. Other factors contributing to hypothermia involve the use of high-flow anesthesia systems and long surgeries. The moderate hypothermia that occurs during routine surgery in small animal veterinary practices is probably not harmful. If hypothermia is a concern, central temperatures are best monitored by observing esophageal temperature. The use of electric heating pads for prevention of hypothermia is discouraged because of the inconsistent temperatures they produce (Chapters 2 and 15).(48)

From clinical experience, accidental hyperthermia develops during warm ambient temperatures, in animals with thick hair coats, and with the use of warm water blankets. Because dogs and cats use panting as a method of reducing body temperature, the use of a circle anesthesia system, which traps expired heat, can contribute to hyperthermia. Increased production of carbon dioxide during hyperthermia also contributes to the temperature increase within the circle machine, as removal of carbon dioxide by sodasorb produces heat as a byproduct. In most situations, hyperthermia subsides after recovery from anesthesia.

Malignant Hyperthermia

Another rare form of hyperthermia has been documented in animals. The term *malignant hyperthermia* was used in 1966 to describe a syndrome of people that included muscle rigidity, tachycardia, and fever. The use of volatile anesthetics and succinylcholine caused affected subjects to undergo an increase of aerobic and anaerobic metabolism, resulting in abnormal production of heat, carbon dioxide, and lactate. As a consequence, the whole body's acid-base balance was affected. Pigs inbred for muscle development such as landrace, pietrain, or Poland china, provide an animal model for studying this syndrome (Chapters 2, 13, 20, and 22).

One theory of how malignant hyperthermia evolves describes a scenario of decreased control of intracellular calcium that results in a release of free unbound ionized calcium. Metabolism then increases to provide the ATP to drive the calcium pumps to maintain intracellular homeostasis. Rigidity occurs when unbound calcium approximates the contractile threshold. Dantrolene (2 mg/kg IV), the drug used to prevent the onset of malignant hyperthermia, blocks sarcoplasmic reticulum calcium release without altering reuptake (Table 25–1) (Chapter 5).(49) Malignant hyperthermia has been suspected in several species besides the pig, including dogs, cats, and horses.(50-52) Susceptible patients should be anesthetized with nitrous oxide, barbiturates, opiates, tranquilizers, and nondepolarizing muscle relaxants. It is best to avoid the potent inhalation anesthetics and the depolarizing muscle relaxants.

Injuries During Anesthesia

Prevention of patient injuries during the anesthetic period is the responsibility of the veterinary surgeon anesthetist. It must be remembered that the anesthetized patient will not be able to respond to noxious tissue-damaging stimuli in the same manner as an unanesthetized animal. The veterinary anesthetist must carefully observe the animal's position on the surgery table, the position of the eyes in relationship to the surface of the table, and any prominent bony protuberances that might be under pressure during the surgery. In addition, observe the position of the limbs, particularly when they are in the abducted position, to see if any nerves might be under unnecessary strain or tension (Chapters 2, 20, 21, and 22).

A common injury during small animal anesthesia occurs when the animal is supine (ventral-dorsal) with the legs tied to the surgery table. If the ties are tight enough to inhibit venous drainage of distal legs, the feet will become edematous. Another problem during anesthesia involves corneal dehydration. Anesthetics reduce or eliminate the palpebral and corneal reflex and reduce tear formation, making artificial tears an important component of anesthesia protocol (Chapter 24). Potential injury is also possible from careless endotracheal intubation technique. Most new endotracheal tubes are too long for small dogs and cats. When they are advanced into the trachea, there is danger of bronchial intubation. New tubes should be correctly sized to the patient by comparing the length of the tube with the distance from the muzzle to the thoracic inlet when the head and neck are in the natural position (not extended or flexed). Overinflation of the cuff, causing tracheal epithelial injury, may not be as common as in the past owing to increased use of low-pressure cuffs (Chapters 14 and 17).

High atmospheric pressure–induced injury, or volotrauma, is always a possibility when semiclosed or high-oxygen-flow anesthesia systems are used. When an oxygen flow rate of greater than 4 to 6 mL/kg is used, the pop-off valve must always be open unless assisted or controlled ventilation is applied. Another technique for providing a safety valve is to inflate the cuff of the endotracheal tube to a pressure of 15 to 20 cm water so that if the pop-off valve were accidently closed, the pressure in the airway would not exceed this value. That is, as airway pressure exceeded 15 to 20 cm water, a hissing or gurgling sound from air passing the cuff would be noticed.

Epidural Analgesia

The use of epidural anesthetics and analgesics for relief of pain gained new popularity after reports of successful use of epidural opioids and alpha$_2$-agonists.(53–55) The technique is easy to perform (56), has close to a 90% success rate (57), and gives the veterinary practitioner another option with which to provide intra- and postoperative analgesia. Potential complications of epidural injection include accidental intravascular injection and neurologic injury. The chance of intravascular injection can be diminished by always aspirating before injecting the recommended volume of analgesic (Chapter 16).

The hanging drop technique is a good method of confirming correct position of the spinal needle within the epidural space. Once the needle contacts the ligamentum flavum, a drop of solution is placed on the hub of the needle. As the needle is advanced into the epidural space, the solution is drawn into the space. If the animal is positioned in a head down orientation for the epidural technique, however, accidental intravenous position of the needle may not be recognized because the negative venous blood pressure will suck in the hanging drop, giving a false positive sign. If intravascular puncture occurs, in addition to intravenous injection of the agent, epidural hemorrhage may develop. Hemorrhage severe enough to cause neurologic signs is rare, though, and may occur only if there are concurrent coagulopathies. Epidural opioids can cause delayed respiratory depression, retention of urine, pruritus, and dysphoria.(58) These complications are rare in dogs and cats.

References

1. Miyabayashi MS, Morgan JP. Gastric emptying in the normal dog. Vet Rad 25:187, 1984.
2. Hinder RA, Kelly KA. Canine gastric emptying of solids and liquids. Am J Physiol 233:335, 1977.
3. Awe WC, Fletcher WS, Jacob SW. The pathophysiology of aspiration pneumonitis. Surgery 60:232, 1966.
4. Hall LW, Clarke KW. Veterinary anaesthesia, 9th ed. London: Balliere Tindall, 1991.
5. Klide AM, Aviado DM. Mechanism for the reduction in pulmonary resistance induced by halothane. J Pharmacol Exp Ther 158:28, 1967.
6. Hickey RF, Severinghaus JW. In: Hornbein TF, ed. Regulation of breathing. Lung biology in health and disease, vol. 17, chap. 21, part II. New York: Marcel Dekker, 1981.
7. Dunlop CI, Steffey EP, Miller MF, Woliner MJ. Temporal effects of halothane and isoflurane in laterally recumbent ventilated male horses. Am J Vet Res 48:1250, 1987.
8. Weiskopf RB, Raymond LW, Severinghaus JW. Effects of halothane on canine respiratory responses to hypoxia with and without hypercarbia. Anesthesiology. 41:350, 1974.
9. Hirshman CA, McCullough RE, Cohen PJ. Hypoxic ventilatory drive in dogs during thiopental, ketamine, or pentobarbital anesthesia. Anesthesiology 43:628, 1975.
10. Goodman NW, Black AMS, Carter JA. Some ventilatory effects of propofol as sole anesthetic agent. Br J Anaesth 59:1497, 1987.
11. Longnecker DE, Harris PD. Microcirculatory actions of general anesthetics. Fed Proc 39:1580, 1980.
12. Prough DS, Johnston WE. Fluid resuscitation in septic shock: no solution yet. Anesth Analg 69:699, 1989.
13. Muir WW III, Lipowitz AJ. Cardiac dysrhythmias associated with gastric dilatation-volvulus in the dog. J Am Vet Med Assoc 172:683, 1978.
14. Macintire DK, Snider TG III. Cardiac arrhythmias associated with multiple trauma in dogs. J Am Vet Med Assoc 184:541, 1984.
15. Bednarski RM, Majors LJ, Atlee JL. Potentiation by thiamylal and thiopental of halothane-epinephrine induced ventricular arrhythmias in dogs. Am J Vet Res 46:1829, 1985.
16. Koehntop DE, Liao JC, VanBergen FH. Effects of pharmacologic alterations of adrenergic mechanisms by cocaine, tropoline,

aminophylline, and ketamine on epinephrine-induced arrhythmias during halothane-nitrous oxide anesthesia. Anesthesiology 46:83, 1977.

17. Atlee JL, Roberts JL. Thiopental and epinephrine-induced dysrhythmias in dogs anesthetized with enflurane or isoflurane. Anesth Analg 65:437, 1986.
18. Hubbell JAE, Muir WW III, Bednarski RM, Bednarski LS. Change of inhalation anesthetic agents for management of ventricular premature depolarizations in anesthetized cats and dogs. J Am Vet Med Assoc 185:643, 1984.
19. Muir WW III, Hubbell JAE, Flaherty S. Increasing halothane concentration abolishes anesthesia-associated arrhythmias in cats and dogs. J Am Vet Med Assoc 192:1730, 1988.
20. Wingfield WE, Van Pelt DR Respiratory and cardiopulmonary arrest in dogs and cats: 265 cases (1986–1991). J Am Vet Med Assoc 200:1993, 1992.
21. Sanders AB, Ewy GA, Taft TV. Resuscitation and arterial blood gas abnormalities during prolonged cardiopulmonary resuscitation. Ann Emerg Med 13:676, 1984.
22. Criley JM, Blaufuss AN, Kissel GL. Cough induced cardiac compression. J Am Med Assoc 236:1246, 1976.
23. Neimann JT, et al. Mechanical "cough" cardio-pulmonary resuscitation during cardiac arrest in dogs. Am J Cardiol 55:199, 1985.
24. Kern KB, et al. Neurologic outcome following successful cardiopulmonary resuscitation in dogs. Resuscitation 14:149, 1986.
25. White BC, Wiegenstein JG, Winegar CD. Brain ischemic anoxia mechanisms of injury. J Am Med Assoc 251:1586, 1984.
26. Ralston SH, Babbs CF, Niebauer MJ. Cardiopulmonary resuscitation with interposed abdominal compression in dogs. Anesth Analg 61:645, 1982.
27. Babbs CF. Interposed abdominal compression-CPR: a case study in cardiac arrest research. Ann Emerg Med 22:24, 1993.
28. Sack JB, Kesselbrenner MB, Bregman D. Survival from in-hospital cardiac arrest with interposed abdominal counterpulsation during cardiopulmonary resuscitation. J Am Med Assoc 267:379, 1992.
29. Chandra N, et al. Augmentation of carotic flow during cardiopulmonary resuscitation by ventilation at high airway pressure simultaneous with chest compression. Am J Cardiol 48:1053, 1981.
30. Halperin GR, et al. Cyclic elevation of intrathoracic pressure can close the mitral valve during cardiac arrest in dogs. Circulation 78:754, 1988.
31. Sanders AB, et al. Improved resuscitation from cardiac arrest with open-chest massage. Ann Emerg Med 13:672, 1984.
32. Feneley MP, et al. Influence of compression rate on initial success of resuscitation and 24 hour survival after prolonged manual cardiopulmonary resuscitation in dogs. Circulation 77:240, 1988.
33. Van Pelt DT, Wingfield WE. Controversial issues in drug treatment during cardiopulmonary resuscitation. J Am Vet Med Assoc 200:1938, 1992.
34. Mazkereth R, et al. Epinephrine blood concentrations after peripheral bronchial versus endotracheal administration of epinephrine in dogs. Crit Care Med 20:1582, 1992.
35. Echt DS, Black JN, Barbey JT. Evaluation of antiarrhythmic drugs on defibrillation energy requirements in dogs. Circulation 79:1106, 1989.
36. Kerber RE, et al. Effect of lidocaine and bretylium on energy requirements for transthoracic defibrillation: experimental studies. J Am Coll Cardiol 7:397, 1986.
37. Sanders AB, Ewy GA, Taft TV. Resuscitation and arterial blood gas abnormalities during prolonged cardiopulmonary resuscitation. Ann Emerg Med 13:676, 1984.
38. Federiuk CS, et al. The effect of bicarbonate in resuscitation from cardiac arrest. Ann Emerg Med 20:1173, 1991.
39. White RD. Cardiopulmonary resuscitation. In: Miller RD, ed. Anesthesia, 3rd ed. New York: Churchill Livingstone, 1990.
40. Rush JE, Wingfield WE. Recognition and frequency of dysrhythmias during cardiopulmonary arrest. J Am Vet Med Assoc 200:1932, 1992.
41. Michael JR, et al. Mechanisms by which epinephrine augments cerebral and myocardial perfusion during cardiopulmonary resuscitation in dogs. Circulation 69:822, 1984.
42. Gold JH, et al. Transthoracic defibrillation of 100-kg calves with sequentially applied pulses. Am J Physiol 243:H982, 1982.
43. Haskins SC. Internal cardiac compression. J Am Vet Med Assoc 200:1945, 1992.
44. Barnett WM, et al. Comparison of open-chest cardiac massage techniques in dogs. Ann Emerg Med 15:408, 1986.
45. Altemeier WA, Todd J. Studies on the incidence of infection following open-chest cardiac massage for cardiac arrest. Ann Surg 158:596, 1963.
46. Sessler DI, Olofsson CI, Rubinstein EH, Beebe JJ. The thermoregulatory threshold in humans during halothane anesthesia. Anesthesiology. 68:836, 1988.
47. Haskins SC. Hypothermia and its prevention during general anesthesia in cats. Am J Vet Res 42:856, 1981.
48. Swaim SF, Lee AH, Hughes KS. Heating pads and thermal burns in small animals. J Am Anim Hosp Assoc 25:156, 1989.
49. Gronert GA. Malignant Hyperthermia. Anesthesiology 60:395, 1981.
50. Bagshaw RJ, Cox RH, Knight DH, Detweiler DK. Malignant hyperthermia in a greyhound. J Am Vet Med Assoc 172:61, 1978.
51. Bellah JR, Robertson SR, Buergelt CD, McGavin D. Suspected malignant hyperthermia after halothane anesthesia in a cat. Vet Surg 18:483, 1989.
52. Waldron-Mease EW, Klein LV, Rosenberg H, Leitch M. Malignant hyperthermia in a halothane-anesthetized horse. J Am Vet Med Assoc 179:896, 1981.
53. Behar M, Olshwang D, Magoroa J, Davison JT. Epidural morphine in the treatment of pain. Lancet 1:527, 1979.
54. Bonath KH, Saleh AS. Long term pain treatment in the dog by peridural morphine. Proceedings 2nd International Congress of Veterinary Anesthesia, Sacramento, CA, 1985.
55. Leblanc PH, et al. Epidural injection of xylazine for perineal analgesia in horses. J Am Vet Med Assoc 193:1405, 1988.
56. Klide AM, Soma LR Epidural analgesia in the dog and cat. J Am Vet Med Assoc 153:165, 1968.
57. Heath RB. Lumbosacral epidural management. Vet Clin North Am Small Anim Pract 22: 1992.
58. Cousins MJ, Mather LM. Intrathecal and epidural administration of opioids. Anesthesiology 61:276, 1984.

section **IX**

EUTHANASIA

chapter 26

EUTHANASIA*

*The major portion of this chapter is the Report of the American Veterinary Medical Association Panel on Euthanasia. This Report was published in the J.A.V.M.A., 173:59, 1978. Panel members were:

L.E. McDonald, DVM, PhD (Chairman), College of Veterinary Medicine, University of Georgia, Athens, GA 30602

N.H. Booth, DVM, PhD, College of Veterinary Medicine, University of Georgia, Athens, GA 30602

W.V. Lumb, DVM, PhD, College of Veterinary Medicine and Biomedical Sciences, Colorado State University, Fort Collins, CO 80523

R.W. Redding, DVM, PhD, School of Veterinary Medicine, Auburn University, Auburn, AL 36830

D.C. Sawyer, DVM, PhD, College of Veterinary Medicine, Michigan State University, East Lansing, MI 48824

Lois Stevenson, Science Writer and Columnist, 49 Rock Rd West, Green Brook, NJ 08812

W.M. Wass, DVM, PhD, College of Veterinary Medicine, Iowa State University, Ames, IA 50011

Introduction

The term *euthanasia* is derived from the Greek terms *eu* meaning "good" and *thanatos* meaning "death." (1, 2) A "good death" would be one that occurs without pain and distress. In the context of this report, euthanasia is the act of inducing humane death in an animal. Euthanasia techniques should result in rapid unconsciousness followed by cardiac or respiratory arrest and ultimate loss of brain function. In addition, the technique should minimize any stress and anxiety experienced by the animal prior to unconsciousness. Stress may be minimized by technical proficiency and humane handling of the animals to be euthanatized.

Emotional uneasiness, discomfort, or distress experienced by people involved with euthanasia of animals may be minimized by assuring that the person performing the euthanasia procedure is technically proficient. Uninformed observers may mistakenly relate any movement of animals with consciousness and lack of movement with unconsciousness. Although these are not adequate criteria, euthanasia techniques that preclude movement of animals are those aesthetically acceptable to most people.

Pain must be defined before criteria for painless death can be established. Pain is that sensation (perception) that results from nerve impulses reaching the cerebral cortex via specific nociceptive neural pathways. The term *nociceptive* is derived from *noxious stimuli,* those that threaten to, or actually do, destroy tissue. The stimuli initiate nerve impulses by acting on a specific set of receptors, called *nociceptors.* Nociceptors respond to mechanical, thermal, or chemical stimuli. Endogenous chemical substances such as hydrogen ions, serotonin, histamine, bradykinin, and prostaglandins as well as electric currents are capable of generating nerve impulses by nociceptors (Chapter 4).

Nerve impulse activity generated by nociceptors is conducted to the spinal cord or the brain stem via nociceptor primary afferent fibers. In the spinal cord or brain stem, nerve impulses are transmitted to two sets of neural networks. One set is related to nociceptive reflexes that are mediated spinally, and the second set consists of ascending pathways to the reticular formation, thalamus, and cerebral cortex for sensory processing (Chapter 7). The transmission of nociceptive neural activity is highly variable. Under certain conditions, both the nociceptive reflexes and the ascending pathways may be suppressed, as, for example, in deep surgical anesthesia. In another set of conditions, nociceptive reflex actions may occur, but the activity in the ascending pathways is suppressed; thus, the noxious stimuli are not perceived as pain, as, for example, in a light plane of surgical anesthesia. It is incorrect to use the term *pain* for stimuli, receptors, reflexes, or pathways because the term implies perception, whereas all of the others may be active without consequential pain perception.(3-7)

Pain is divided into two broad categories: (a) sensory-discriminative, which indicates the site of origin and the stimulus giving rise to the pain; and (b) motivational-affective, in which the severity of the stimulus is perceived and the animal's response is determined. Sensory-discriminative processing of nociceptive impulses is most likely to be accomplished by subcortical and cortical mechanisms similar to those utilized for processing of other sensory-discriminative input that provides the individual with information about the intensity, duration, location, and quality of the stimulus. Motivational-affective processing involves the ascending reticular formation for behavioral and cortical arousal. It also involves thalamic input to the forebrain and the limbic system for perceptions such as discomfort, fear, anxiety, and depression. The motivational-affective neural networks also have strong inputs to the hypothalamus and the autonomic nervous system for reflex activation of the cardiovascular, pulmonary, and pituitary-adrenal systems (Chapters 4 and 5). Responses activated by these systems feed back to the forebrain and enhance the perceptions derived via motivational-affective inputs. On the basis of neurosurgical experience in human beings, it is possible to separate the sensory-discriminative components from the motivational-affective components of pain.(4)

For pain to be experienced, the cerebral cortex and subcortical structures must be functional. An unconscious animal cannot experience pain because the cerebral cortex is not functioning. If the cerebral cortex is nonfunctional because of hypoxia, depression by drugs, electric shock, or concussion, pain is not experienced. Therefore, the choice of the euthanasia agent or method is of less importance if it is to be used on an animal that is anesthetized or unconscious, provided that the animal does not regain consciousness prior to death.

An understanding of the continuum that represents stress and distress is essential for evaluating techniques that minimize any distress experienced by an animal being euthanatized. Stress has been defined as the effect of physical, physiologic, or emotional factors (stressors) that induce an alteration in an animal's homeostasis or adaptive state.(8) The response of an animal to stress represents the adaptive process that is necessary to restore the baseline mental and physiologic state. These responses may involve changes in an animal's neuroendocrinologic system, autonomic nervous system, and mental state that may lead to overt behavioral changes. An animal's response varies according to its experience, age, species, breed, and current physiologic and psychologic state.(9)

Stress and the resulting responses have been divided into three phases.(10) Eustress results when harmless stimuli initiate adaptive responses that are beneficial to the animal. Neutral stress results when the animal's response to stimuli causes neither harmful nor beneficial effects to the animal. Distress results when an animal's response to stimuli interferes with its well-being and comfort (Chapter 4).

As with many other procedures involving animals, some methods of euthanasia require physical handling of the animal. The amount of control and kind of restraint needed will be determined by the animal species, breed, size, state of domestication, presence of painful injury or disease, degree of excitement, and method of euthanasia. Proper handling is vital to minimize pain and distress in animals, to assure safety of the person performing euthanasia, and, frequently, to protect other animals and people.

Personnel who perform euthanasia must have appropriate certification and/or training and experience with the techniques to be used, to assure that animal pain and distress are minimized during euthanasia. This training and experience should include familiarity with

Table 26–1. Agents and Methods of Euthanasia by Species (Refer to Table 26–4 for Unacceptable Agents and Methods)

Species	Acceptable (Refer to Table 26–2 and Text for Details)	Conditionally Acceptable (Refer to Table 26–3 and Text for Details)
Amphibians	Inhalant anesthetics, CO, CO_2, barbiturates, tricaine methanesulfonate, double pithing, benzocaine	Pithing, gunshot, penetrating captive bolt, stunning and decapitation, decapitation and pithing
Birds	Inhalant anesthetics, CO, CO_2, barbiturates	N_2, Ar, cervical dislocation, decapitation
Cats	Inhalant anesthetics, CO, CO_2, barbiturates	N_2, Ar
Dogs	Inhalant anesthetics, CO, CO_2, barbiturates	N_2, Ar, electrocution, penetrating captive bolt
Fish	Tricaine methanesulfonate, benzocaine, barbiturates	Stunning and decapitation, decapitation
Horses	Barbiturates, chloral hydrate, chloral hydrate/$MgSO_4$/pentobarbital	Penetrating captive bolt, gunshot, electrocution
Marine mammals	Barbiturates, etorphine hydrochloride	Succinylcholine chloride and potassium chloride, gunshot
Mink, fox, and other animals produced for fur	Inhalant anesthetics, CO, CO_2, barbiturates	N_2, Ar, electrocution followed by cervical dislocation
Nonhuman primates	Barbiturates	Inhalant anesthetics, CO, CO_2, N_2, Ar
Rabbits	Inhalant anesthetics, CO, CO_2, barbiturates	N_2, Ar, cervical dislocation, decapitation, penetrating captive bolt
Reptiles	Barbiturates, inhalant anesthetics, CO_2	Gunshot, penetrating captive bolt, stunning and decapitation, decapitation and pithing
Rodents and other small animals	Inhalant anesthetics, CO, CO_2, microwave irradiation, barbiturates	N_2, Ar, cervical dislocation, decapitation
Ruminants	Barbiturates	Penetrating captive bolt, gunshot, electrocution, chloral hydrate
Swine	Barbiturates, CO_2	Inhalant anesthetics, CO, penetrating captive bolt, gunshot, electrocution, chloral hydrate
Zoo animals	Inhalant anesthetics, CO_2, CO, barbiturates	N_2, Ar, penetrating captive bolt, gunshot

the normal behavior of the species being euthanatized and how handling and restraint affects that behavior, and an understanding of the mechanism by which the selected technique induces unconsciousness and death. Prior to being assigned full responsibility for performing euthanasia, all personnel must have demonstrated proficiency in the use of the technique in a closely supervised environment. References provided at the end of this chapter may be useful for training personnel.(11-13) An in-depth discussion of euthanasia procedures is beyond the scope of this chapter; however, several excellent euthanasia procedural manuals are particularly applicable to animal care and control agencies.(11, 13, 14)

Selection of the most appropriate method of euthanasia in any given situation depends on the species of the animal involved, available means of animal restraint, skill of personnel, number of animals, and other considerations. This chapter deals primarily with domestic animals, but the same general considerations should be applied to all species. Table 26–1 lists acceptable and conditionally acceptable methods of euthanasia, categorized by species. Tables 26–2 and 26–3 provide summaries of characteristics for acceptable and conditionally acceptable methods of euthanasia. Table 26–4 provides a summary of unacceptable euthanasia agents and methods.

General Considerations

In evaluating methods of euthanasia, several criteria were used: (a) ability to induce loss of consciousness and death without causing pain, distress, anxiety, or apprehension; (b) time required to induce unconsciousness; (c) reliability; (d) safety of personnel; (e) irreversibility; (f) compatibility with requirement and purpose; (g) emotional effect on observers or operators; (h)

Table 26–2. Summary of Acceptable Agents and Methods of Euthanasia – Characteristics and Modes of Action (Refer to Text for Details)

Agent	Classification	Mode of Action	Rapidity	Ease of Performance	Safety for Personnel	Species Suitability	Efficacy and Comments
Barbiturates	Hypoxia owing to depression of vital centers	Direct depression of cerebral cortex, subcortical structures, and vital centers; direct depression of heart muscle	Rapid onset of anesthesia	Animal must be restrained; personnel must be skilled to perform IV injection	Safe except for human abuse potential; DEA-controlled substance	Most species	Highly effective when appropriately administered; acceptable IV and IP in small animals
Inhalant anesthetics	Hypoxia due to depression of vital centers	Direct depression of cerebral cortex and subcortical structures and vital centers	Moderately rapid onset of anesthesia; some excitation may occur during induction	Easily performed with closed container; can be administered to large animals by means of a mask	Must be properly scavenged or vented to minimize exposure to personnel	Amphibians, birds, cats, dogs, fur-bearing animals, rabbits, reptiles, rodents and other small animals, zoo animals	Highly effective provided that subject is sufficiently exposed
Carbon dioxide	Hypoxia due to depression of vital centers	Direct depression of cerebral cortex, subcortical structures, and vital centers; direct depression of heart muscle	Moderately rapid	Used in closed container	Minimal hazard	Small laboratory animals, birds, cats, small dogs, mink, zoo animals, amphibians	Effective, but time required may be prolonged in immature and neonatal animals

Table 26–2.   Summary of Acceptable Agents and Methods of Euthanasia—Characteristics and Modes of Action (Refer to Text for Details) (continued)

Agent	Classification	Mode of Action	Rapidity	Ease of Performance	Safety for Personnel	Species Suitability	Efficacy and Comments
Carbon monoxide (bottled gas only)	Hypoxia	Combines with hemoglobin, preventing its combination with oxygen	Moderate onset time; insidious, so animal is unaware of onset	Requires appropriately operated equipment for gas production	Extremely hazardous, toxic, and difficult to detect	Most small species including dogs, cats, rodents, mink, chinchillas, birds, reptiles, amphibians, and zoo animals	Effective; acceptable only when equipment is properly designed and operated
Microwave	Brain enzyme inactivation	Direct inactivation of brain enzymes by rapid heating of brain	Very rapid	Requires training and highly specialized equipment	Safe	Mice and rats	Highly effective for special needs
Tricaine methane-sulfonate	Hypoxia due to depression of vital centers	Depression of CNS	Very rapid, depending on dose	Easily used	Safe	Fish and amphibians	Effective but expensive
Benzocaine	Hypoxia due to depression of vital centers	Depression of CNS	Very rapid, depending on dose	Easily used	Safe	Fish and amphibians	Effective but expensive

Table 26–3. Summary of Conditionally Acceptable Agents and Methods of Euthanasia – Characteristics and Modes of Action (Refer to Text for Details)

Agent	Classification	Mode of Action	Rapidity	Ease of Performance	Safety	Species Suitability	Efficacy and Comments
Cervical dislocation	Hypoxia due to disruption of vital centers	Direct depression of brain	Moderately rapid	Requires training and skill	Safe	Poultry, birds, laboratory mice, and rats less than 1 kg	Irreversible. Violent muscle contractions can occur after cervical dislocation
Decapitation	Hypoxia due to disruption of vital centers	Direct depression of brain	Moderately rapid	Requires training and skill	Guillotine poses potential employee injury hazard	Laboratory rodents, small rabbits, birds, amphibians, and reptiles	Irreversible. Violent muscle contractions can occur after decapitation
Penetrating captive bolt	Physical damage to brain	Direct concussion of brain tissue	Rapid	Requires skill, adequate restraints, and proper placement of captive bolt	Safe	Ruminants, horses, swine, dogs, rabbits, zoo animals, reptiles	Instant unconsciousness but motor activity may continue
Gunshot	Hypoxia due to disruption of vital centers	Direct concussion of brain tissue	Rapid	Requires skill and appropriate firearm	May be dangerous	Large domestic and zoo animals, reptiles, and wildlife	Instant unconsciousness but motor activity may continue
Electrocution	Hypoxia	Direct depression of brain and cardiac fibrillation	Can be rapid	Not easily performed in all instances	Hazardous to personnel	Used primarily in foxes, sheep, swine, and mink	Violent muscle contractions occur at same time as unconsciousness
Pithing	Hypoxia caused by disruption of vital centers, physical damage to brain	Trauma of brain and spinal cord tissue	Rapid	Easily performed but requires skill	Safe	Some poikilotherms	Effective, but death not immediate unless double pithed
Nitrogen, argon	Hypoxic hypoxemia	Reduced partial pressure of oxygen available to blood	Rapid	Use closed chamber with rapid filling	Safe if used with ventilation	Cats, small dogs, birds, rodents, mink, rabbits and other small species of zoo animals	Effective except in young and neonates; an effective agent, but other methods preferable; not acceptable in most animals less than 4 months old

Table 26–4. Summary of Unacceptable Agents and Methods of Euthanasia (Refer to Text for Details)

Agent	Comments
Exsanguination	Because of the anxiety associated with extreme hypovolemia, exsanguination should be done only in sedated, stunned, or anesthetized animals.
Decompression	Decompression is not a recommended method for euthanasia of animals because of the numerous disadvantages. (a) Many chambers are designed to produce decompression at a rate 15 to 60 times faster than that recommended as optimum for animals, resulting in pain and distress caused by expanding gases trapped in body cavities. (b) Immature animals are tolerant of hypoxia, and longer periods of decompression are required before respiration ceases. (c) Accidental recompression, with recovery of injured animals, can occur. (d) Bloating, bleeding, vomiting, convulsions, urination, and defecation, which are aesthetically unpleasant, may occur in the unconscious animal. For more information, see Reference 1.
Rapid freezing	Rapid freezing as a sole means of euthanasia is not considered to be humane. If it is used, animals should be anesthetized prior to freezing.
Air embolism	Air embolism may be accompanied by convulsions, opisthotonos, and vocalization. If used, it should be done only in anesthetized animals.
Drowning	Drowning as a means of euthanasia is inhumane.
Strychnine	Strychnine causes violent convulsions and painful muscle contractions.
Nicotine, magnesium sulfate, potassium chloride, all curariform agents (neuromuscular blocking agents)	When used alone, these drugs all cause respiratory arrest before unconsciousness, so the animal may perceive pain after it is immobilized.
Chloroform	Chloroform is a known hepatotoxin and suspected carcinogen, and therefore hazardous to human beings.
Cyanide	Cyanide poses an extreme danger to personnel, and the manner of death is aesthetically objectionable.
Stunning	Stunning may render an animal unconscious, but is not a method of euthanasia. If used, it must be followed by a method to ensure death (see text).

compatibility with subsequent evaluation, examination, or use of tissue; (i) drug availability and human abuse potential; (j) age and species limitations; and (k) ability to maintain equipment in proper working order.

The definition of *euthanasia* used in this chapter may not apply when needed control over the animal makes it difficult to assure death without pain and distress. The slaughter of animals for food, fur, or fiber and techniques commonly used to control wild and feral animal populations may represent such situations. Although we recognize these interactions with animals, we do not believe the term *euthanasia* is appropriate in some of these cases.

Animals for food should be slaughtered as specified by the U.S. Department of Agriculture.(15) Painless death can be achieved by properly stunning animals, followed immediately by exsanguination. Preslaughter handling of animals should be as stress-free as possible. Electric prods or other devices to encourage movement

of animals should not be used. Chutes and ramps should be properly designed to enable animals to be moved and restrained without undue stress.(16, 17) Animals must not be restrained in a painful position before slaughter.

The ethical considerations that must be made when euthanatizing healthy and unwanted animals raise both professional and societal issues.(18, 19) These issues are complex and warrant thorough consideration by both the profession and all those concerned with the welfare of animals. Any recommendations on euthanasia should be carried out in accordance with applicable federal, state, and local laws governing drug acquisition and storage, occupational safety, and methods used for euthanasia and disposal of animals.

Euthanasia of neonatal or prenatal animals or uncommonly encountered species may be necessary. Whenever such situations arise, a veterinarian or other experienced professional should use professional judgment and knowledge of clinically acceptable techniques in selecting an appropriate euthanasia technique. Essential to the application of professional judgment is the consideration of the animal's size and its species-specific physiologic and behavioral characteristics. In all circumstances, the euthanasia method should be selected and used with the highest ethical standards and social conscience.

It is imperative that death be verified after euthanasia and before disposal of the animal. To a casual observer, an animal in deep narcosis following administration of an injectable or inhalant agent may appear dead, but may eventually recover. Death should be confirmed by examining the animal for cessation of vital signs. Professional judgment should be used, considering the animal species and method of euthanasia, to determine the means of confirming death.

Animal Behavioral Considerations

The facial expressions and body postures that indicate various emotional states of animals have been described.(20–22) Behavioral and physiologic responses to noxious stimuli include distress vocalization, struggling, attempts to escape, defensive or redirected aggression, salivation, urination, defecation, evacuation of anal sacs, pupillary dilation, tachycardia, sweating, and reflex skeletal muscle contractions causing shivering, tremors, or other muscular spasms. Some of these responses can occur in unconscious as well as conscious animals. Fear can cause immobility or "playing dead" in certain species, particularly rabbits and chickens. This immobility response should not be interpreted as unconsciousness when the animal is, in fact, conscious.

The need to minimize animal distress, including fear, anxiety, and apprehension, must be considered in determining the method of euthanasia. Distress vocalizations, fearful behavior, and release of certain odors or pheromones by a frightened animal may cause anxiety and apprehension in other animals. Therefore, whenever possible, other animals should not be present when euthanasia is performed, especially euthanasia of the same species. This is particularly important when vocalization or release of pheromones may occur during induction of unconsciousness. Gentle restraint, preferably in a familiar environment, careful handling, and talking during euthanasia often have a calming effect on companion animals. However, some of these methods may not be effective with wild animals or animals that are injured or diseased. When struggling during capture or restraint may cause pain, injury, or anxiety to the animal or danger to the operator, the use of tranquilizers, analgesics, and/or immobilizing drugs should be considered (Chapters 20 to 22).

Human Behavioral Considerations

Moral and ethical imperatives associated with individual animal or mass euthanasia should be consistent with acceptable humane practice. Grief at the loss of an animal's life is the most common reaction.(23) There are three circumstances in which we are most aware of the effects of euthanasia on people. The first of these is the clinical setting. The owner will have had to make the decision about whether and when to euthanatize, and, although many owners rely heavily on their veterinarian's judgment, others may have misgivings about their own decision. This is particularly apt to be the case if the owner feels responsible for allowing an animal's medical or behavioral problem to go unattended so that euthanasia became necessary. Counseling services for grieving owners are now available in some communities (24), and telephone counseling is available at some veterinary schools.(25) Owners are not the only people affected by euthanasia of animals. Veterinarians and their staffs may also be attached to patients they have known and treated for many years.

The second circumstance in which people are affected by euthanasia is at humane societies and animal control facilities where unwanted, homeless, diseased, and injured animals must be euthanatized in large numbers. Distress may develop among personnel directly involved in performing euthanasia repetitively. Constant exposure to, or participation in, euthanasia procedures can cause a psychologic state characterized by a strong sense of work dissatisfaction or alienation, which may be expressed by absenteeism, belligerence, or careless and callous handling of animals.(26) This is one of the principal reasons for turnover of employees directly involved with repeated animal euthanasia. This should be recognized as a bona fide personnel problem related to animal euthanasia, and management measures should be instituted to decrease or eliminate the potential for this problem. Specific coping strategies can make the task more tolerable. Some of these strategies are: adequate training programs so that the method of euthanasia is performed competently; peer support in the workplace, focusing on animals that are successfully adopted or returned to owners; devoting some work time to educational activities; and providing time off when workers feel stressed.

The third setting in which people are affected by euthanasia of animals is in the laboratory. Researchers, technicians, and students may become attached to an animal that must be euthanatized.(27) The same considerations given to pet owners or shelter employees should be afforded to those working in such facilities.

Human attitudes and responses should be considered whenever animals are euthanatized, including animals in zoos, at sites of roadside or racetrack accidents, and in cases of stranded marine animals. However, these considerations should not outweigh the primary responsibility of using the most rapid and painless euthanasia method possible under the circumstances.

Modes of Action of Euthanatizing Agents

Euthanatizing agents cause death by three basic mechanisms: (a) hypoxia, direct or indirect; (b) direct depression of neurons vital for life function; and (c) physical disruption of brain activity and destruction of neurons vital for life.

Agents that induce death by direct or indirect hypoxia can act at various sites and can cause unconsciousness at different rates. For death to be painless and distress-free, unconsciousness should precede loss of motor activity (muscle movement). This means that agents that induce muscle paralysis without unconsciousness are absolutely condemned as sole agents for euthanasia (e.g., curare, succinylcholine, gallamine, strychnine, nicotine, magnesium or potassium salts, pancuronium, decamethonium, vecuronium, atracurium, pipecuronium, and doxacurium). With other techniques that induce hypoxia, some animals may have motor activity following unconsciousness, but this is reflex activity and is not perceived by the animal.

The second group of euthanatizing agents depress nerve cells of the brain, inducing unconsciousness followed by death. Some of these agents "release" muscle control during the first stage of anesthesia, resulting in a so-called "excitement or delirium phase," during which there may he vocalization and some muscle contraction. These responses do not appear to be purposeful. Death follows unconsciousness and is attributable to hypoxemia following direct depression of respiratory centers and/or cardiac arrest.

Physical disruption of brain activity, caused by concussion, direct destruction of the brain, or electric depolarization of the neurons, induces rapid unconsciousness. Death occurs because of destruction of midbrain centers controlling cardiac and respiratory activity or by adjunctive methods (e.g., exsanguination) used to kill the animal. Exaggerated muscular activity can follow unconsciousness; although this may disturb some observers, the animal is not experiencing pain or distress.

Inhalant Agents

Any gas that is inhaled must reach a certain concentration in the alveoli before it can be effective; therefore, euthanasia with any of these agents takes some time. The suitability of a particular agent depends on whether an animal experiences distress between the time it begins to inhale the agent and the time it loses consciousness. Some agents may induce convulsions, but these generally follow unconsciousness. Agents inducing convulsions prior to unconsciousness are unacceptable for euthanasia.

Certain considerations are common to all inhalant agents: (a) In most cases, onset of unconsciousness is more rapid, and euthanasia more humane, if the animal is rapidly exposed to a high concentration of the agent. (b) The equipment used to deliver and maintain this high concentration must be in good working order. Leaky or faulty equipment may lead to slow, distressful death and/or be hazardous to other animals and to personnel. (c) Most of these agents are hazardous to the health of personnel because of the risk of explosions (e.g., ether), narcosis (e.g., halothane), hypoxemia (e.g.,

nitrogen, carbon monoxide), addiction (e.g., nitrous oxide), or health effects resulting from chronic exposure (e.g., nitrous oxide, carbon monoxide). (d) Alveolar concentrations rise slowly in an animal with decreased ventilation, making agitation more likely during induction. Other noninhalant methods of euthanasia should be considered for such animals. (e) Neonatal animals appear to be resistant to hypoxia, and because all inhalant agents ultimately cause hypoxia, neonatal animals take longer to die than adults. Therefore, these agents should not be used in neonates unless the animal can be exposed long enough to ensure death. Glass et al.(28) reported that newborn dogs, rabbits, and guinea pigs survived a nitrogen atmosphere much longer than adults. Dogs, at 1 week of age, survived for 14 minutes compared with 3 minutes at the age of 4 weeks or as adults. Guinea pigs survived for 4.5 minutes at 1 day of age, compared with 3 minutes at 8 days and as adults. Rabbits survived for 13 minutes at 6 days of age, 4 minutes at 14 days, and 1.5 minutes at 19 days and as adults. Until more reliable data are available, the authors recommend that inhalant agents not be used alone in pups and kittens less than 16 weeks of age. Inhalants may be used to induce unconsciousness, followed by use of some other method to kill the animal. (f) Rapid gas flows can produce a noise that frightens animals. If high flows are required, the equipment should be designed to minimize noise. (g) Animals placed together in chambers should be of the same species and, if needed, should be restrained so that they will not hurt themselves or others. Chambers should be kept clean to minimize odors that might distress animals subsequently euthanatized.

INHALANT ANESTHETICS

Inhalant anesthetics (e.g., ether, halothane, methoxyflurane, isoflurane, and enflurane) have been used to euthanatize many species.(29) Ether has high solubility in blood and induces anesthesia slowly, is irritating to the eyes and nose, and poses serious risks associated with its flammability. Although ether is acceptable for euthanasia, other agents may be preferable. Methoxyflurane also has high solubility, and the slow anesthetic induction with its use may be accompanied by agitation. It is more acceptable than ether, but other agents may be preferable. Halothane induces anesthesia rapidly and is the most effective inhalant anesthetic for euthanasia. Enflurane is less soluble in blood than is halothane, but, because of its lower vapor pressure and lower potency, induction rates may be similar to those for halothane. At deep anesthetic planes, animals often seizure. It is an effective agent for euthanasia, but the seizure activity may be disturbing to personnel. Isoflurane is the least soluble of the potent inhalant anesthetics commonly used by veterinarians and it should induce anesthesia more rapidly. However, it has a slightly pungent odor and animals often hold their breath, delaying the onset of unconsciousness. Isoflurane also may require more drug to kill an animal, compared with halothane.

Although isoflurane is acceptable as a euthanasia agent, halothane is preferred.

With inhalant agents, the animal is placed in a closed receptacle containing cotton or gauze soaked with the anesthetic.(30) The anesthetic also may be introduced from a vaporizer, but this usually results in longer induction time. Vapors are inhaled until respiration ceases and death ensues. Because the liquid state of most inhalant anesthetics is irritating, animals should be exposed only to vapors. Also, sufficient air or oxygen must be provided during the induction period to prevent hypoxemia.(30) In the case of small rodents placed in a large container, there will be sufficient oxygen in the chamber to prevent hypoxemia. Larger species placed in small containers may need supplemental air or oxygen.

Nitrous oxide (N_2O) may be used with the other inhalants to speed the onset of anesthesia, but it alone does not induce anesthesia in animals, even at 100% concentration. If N_2O is used as a sole euthanasia agent, hypoxemia develops before respiratory or cardiac arrest, and animals may become distressed prior to unconsciousness.

Occupational exposure to inhalant anesthetics constitutes a human health hazard. Spontaneous abortion and congenital abnormalities have been associated with exposure of women to trace amounts of inhalation anesthetic agents in early stages of pregnancy.(31) In human exposure to inhalant anesthetics, the concentration of ether, halothane, methoxyflurane, enflurane, and isoflurane should be less than 2 ppm, and less than 25 ppm for nitrous oxide.(32) There are no controlled studies proving that such concentrations of anesthetics are "safe," but these concentrations were established because they were shown to be attainable under hospital conditions. Effective procedures must be used to protect personnel from anesthetic vapors.

Advantages. (a) Inhalant anesthetics are particularly valuable for euthanasia of smaller animals (under about 7 kg) or in animals in which venipuncture may be difficult. (b) Halothane, enflurane, isoflurane, methoxyflurane, and N_2O are nonflammable and nonexplosive under ordinary environmental conditions.

Disadvantages. (a) Struggling and anxiety may develop during induction of anesthesia because anesthetic vapors may be irritating and can induce excitement. (b) Ether is flammable and explosive, and should not be used near an open flame or other ignition sources. Explosions have occurred when animals, euthanatized with ether, were placed in an ordinary (not explosion-proof) refrigerator or freezer and when bagged animals were placed in an incinerator. (c) Nitrous oxide will support combustion. (d) Personnel and animals can be injured by exposure to these agents. (e) There is a potential for human abuse of some of these drugs, especially N_2O.

Recommendations. In order of preference, halothane, enflurane, isoflurane, methoxyflurane, and ether, with or without nitrous oxide, are acceptable for euthanasia

of small animals (under about 7 kg). Nitrous oxide should not be used alone, pending further scientific studies on its suitability for animal euthanasia. Although acceptable, these agents are generally not used in larger animals because of their cost and difficulty of administration.

CARBON DIOXIDE

Room air contains 0.04% carbon dioxide (CO_2), which is heavier than air and nearly odorless. Inhalation of CO_2 in concentrations of 7.5% increases the pain threshold, and higher concentrations of CO_2 have a rapid anesthetic effect.(33–37)

Leake and Waters (35) reported the experimental use of CO_2 as an anesthetic agent in dogs. At concentrations of 30 to 40% CO_2 in oxygen, anesthesia was induced within 1 to 2 minutes, usually without struggling, retching, or vomiting. The signs of effective CO_2 anesthesia are those associated with deep surgical anesthesia, such as loss of withdrawal and palpebral reflexes.(38)

In cats, inhalation of 60% CO_2 results in loss of consciousness within 45 seconds and respiratory arrest within 5 minutes.(39) Carbon dioxide has been used to euthanatize groups of small laboratory animals, including mice, rats, guinea pigs, chickens, and rabbits (3, 40–44), and to render swine unconscious before humane slaughter.(15, 45, 46) Several investigators have suggested that inhalation of high concentrations of CO_2 may be distressing to animals (45–48) because of mucosal irritation and ventilatory stimulation. However, the degree of distress appears to be mild, and it is unlikely that it is any more unpleasant than inhalation of volatile anesthetics.(49)

The combination of 40% CO_2 and approximately 3% CO has been used experimentally for euthanasia of dogs.(47) Carbon dioxide has been used in specially designed chambers to euthanatize cats (50, 51) and other small laboratory animals.(30, 40, 49)

Studies in day-old chickens have shown that CO_2 is an effective euthanatizing agent. Inhalation of CO_2 caused little distress to the birds, suppressed nervous activity, and induced death within 5 minutes.(41) Because respiration begins during embryonic development, the unhatched chicken's environment may normally have a CO_2 concentration as high as 14%. Thus, CO_2 concentration for euthanasia of newly hatched chickens and neonates of other species should be especially high. A CO_2 concentration of 60 to 70% with a 5-minute exposure time appears to be optimal.(41) A similar technique was used in mink and, although 70% carbon dioxide induced unconsciousness, it did not kill the animals.(52) These and other diving animals may have physiologic mechanisms for coping with high concentrations of CO_2. It is necessary, therefore, to have a high enough concentration of CO_2 to kill the animal by hypoxemia following the induction of anesthesia with CO_2.

Carbon dioxide is used for preslaughter anesthesia of swine. The undesirable side effect of CO_2, as used in commercial slaughterhouses, is that swine experience a stage of excitement with vocalization for about 40 seconds before they lose consciousness.(45, 46, 53) For that reason, CO_2 preslaughter anesthesia may appear less humane than other techniques.

Advantages. (a) The rapid depressant and anesthetic effects of CO_2 are well established. (b) Carbon dioxide may be purchased in cylinders or in solid state as "dry ice." (c) Carbon dioxide is inexpensive, nonflammable, and nonexplosive, and poses minimal hazard to personnel when used with properly designed equipment. (d) Carbon dioxide does not result in accumulation of tissue residues in food producing animals. (e) Carbon dioxide euthanasia does not distort cellular architecture.(54)

Disadvantages. (a) Because CO_2 is heavier than air, incomplete filling of a chamber may permit tall or climbing animals to avoid exposure and to survive. This appears to be very distressful to the animals. (b) Some species may have extraordinary tolerance for CO_2.

Recommendations. Carbon dioxide is acceptable for euthanasia. Compressed CO_2 gas in cylinders is preferable to dry ice because the inflow to the chamber can be regulated precisely. If dry ice is used, animal contact must be avoided to prevent freezing or chilling. Carbon dioxide generated by other methods such as from a fire extinguisher or from chemical means (e.g., Alka-Seltzer) is unacceptable. With an animal in the chamber, an optimal flow rate should displace at least 20% of the chamber volume per minute.(55) Unconsciousness may be induced more rapidly by exposing animals to a CO_2 concentration of 70% or more by prefilling the chamber. It is important to verify that an animal is dead before removing it from the chamber. If an animal is not dead, CO_2 narcosis must be followed with another method of euthanasia. Larger animals, such as rabbits, cats, and swine, appear to be more distressed by CO_2 euthanasia; therefore, other methods of euthanasia are preferable.

NITROGEN, ARGON

Nitrogen (N_2) and argon (Ar) are colorless, odorless gases that are inert, nonflammable, and nonexplosive. Nitrogen comprises 78% of atmospheric air, whereas Ar is present at less than 1% of atmospheric air. Euthanasia is induced by placing the animal in a closed container into which N_2 or Ar is rapidly introduced or prefilled at atmospheric pressure. Nitrogen/Argon displaces oxygen in the container, thus inducing death by hypoxemia.

In studies by Herin et al. (56) dogs become unconscious within 76 seconds when N_2 concentration of 98.5% was achieved in 45 to 60 seconds. The electroencephalogram (EEG) became isoelectric (flat) in a mean of 80 seconds, and arterial blood pressure was undetectable at a mean of 204 seconds. Although all dogs hyperventilated prior to unconsciousness, the investigators concluded that this method induced death without pain. Following loss of consciousness, vocalization, gasping, convulsions, and muscular tremors

occurred in some dogs. At the end of a 5-minute exposure period, all dogs were dead.(56) These findings were similar to those for rabbits (57) and mink.(52, 58)

With N_2 flowing at a rate of 39% of chamber volume per minute, rats collapsed in approximately 3 minutes and stopped breathing in 5 to 6 minutes. Regardless of flow rate, signs of panic and distress were evident before the rats collapsed and died.(55) Insensitivity to pain under such circumstances is questionable.(59)

Tranquilization with acepromazine, in conjunction with N_2 euthanasia of dogs, was investigated by Quine et al.(60) Using ECG and EEG recordings, they found that these animals had much longer survival times than animals not given acepromazine before the administration of N_2. In one dog, the ECG activity continued for 51 minutes. Quine (61) also addressed the issue of distress associated with exposure to N_2 by removing cats and dogs from the chamber following unconsciousness and allowing them to recover. When these animals were put back into the chamber, they did not appear afraid or apprehensive.

When Ar was used to euthanatize chickens, exposure to a chamber prefilled with Ar, with an oxygen concentration of under 2%, led to EEG changes and collapse in 9 to 12 seconds. Birds removed from the chamber at 15 to 17 seconds failed to respond to comb pinching. Continued exposure led to convulsions at 20 to 24 seconds. Somatosensory-evoked potentials were lost at 24 to 34 seconds, and the EEG became isoelectric at 57 to 66 seconds. The onset of convulsions appeared after the loss of consciousness (collapse and loss of response to comb pinch), so this would appear to be a humane method of euthanasia in chickens.(62)

Advantages. (a) Nitrogen and Ar are readily available as compressed gases. (b) Hazards to personnel are minimal.

Disadvantages. (a) Unconsciousness is preceded by hypoxemia and ventilatory stimulation, which may be distressing to the animal. (b) Reestablishing a low concentration of O_2 (i.e., 6% or greater) in the chamber before death will allow immediate recovery.

Recommendations. Nitrogen and Argon can be distressful in some species (e.g., rats); therefore, this technique is acceptable only if oxygen concentrations below 2% are achieved rapidly and the animal is heavily sedated or anesthetized. With heavy sedation or anesthesia, it should be recognized that death may be delayed. In dogs, cats, and chickens, this appears to be a humane method of euthanasia. Although N_2 and Ar are effective, other methods of euthanasia are preferable.

CARBON MONOXIDE

Carbon monoxide (CO) is a colorless, odorless gas that is nonflammable and nonexplosive until concentrations exceed 10%. It combines with hemoglobin to form carboxyhemoglobin and blocks the uptake of oxygen by erythrocytes, leading to fatal hypoxemia.

In people, the most common symptoms of early CO toxicosis are headache, dizziness, and weakness. As concentrations of carboxyhemoglobin increase, these signs may be followed by decreased visual acuity, tinnitus, nausea, progressive depression, confusion, and collapse.(63) Because CO stimulates motor centers in the brain, unconsciousness may be accompanied by convulsions and muscular spasms.

Carbon monoxide is a cumulative poison.(64) Distinct signs of CO toxicosis are not evident until the concentration is 0.05% in air, and acute signs do not develop until the concentration is approximately 0.2%. In human beings, exposure to 0.32% CO and 0.45% CO for 1 hour will induce unconsciousness and death, respectively.(65) Carbon monoxide is extremely hazardous for personnel because it is highly toxic and difficult to detect. Chronic exposure to low concentrations of carbon monoxide may be a health hazard, especially with regard to cardiovascular disease and teratogenic effects.(66–68) An efficient exhaust or ventilatory system is essential to prevent accidental exposure of human beings.

In the past, mass euthanasia has been accomplished by using three methods for generating CO: (a) chemical interaction of sodium formate and sulfuric acid; (b) exhaust fumes from idling gasoline internal combustion engines; and (c) commercially compressed CO in cylinders. The first two techniques are associated with a number of problems, such as production of other gases, inadequate concentrations of carbon monoxide achieved, inadequate cooling of the gas, and maintenance of the equipment; therefore, the only recommended source is compressed CO in cylinders.

In a study by Ramsey and Eilmann, (69) 8% CO caused guinea pigs to collapse in 40 seconds to 2 minutes, and death occurred within 6 minutes. Carbon monoxide has been used to euthanatize mink (52, 58) and chinchillas. These animals collapsed in 1 minute, breathing ceased in 2 minutes, and the heart stopped beating in 5 to 7 minutes.

In a study evaluating the physiologic and behavioral characteristics of dogs exposed to 6% CO in air, Chalifoux and Dallaire (70) could not determine the precise time of unconsciousness. Electroencephalographic recordings revealed 20 to 25 seconds of abnormal cortical function prior to unconsciousness. It was during this period that agitation and vocalization occurred. It is not known whether animals experience distress; however, human beings in this phase reportedly are not distressed.(64) Subsequent studies have shown that tranquilization with acepromazine significantly decreases behavioral and physiologic responses of dogs euthanatized with CO.(71)

In a comparative study, CO (gasoline engine exhaust) and 70% CO_2 + 30% O_2 were used to euthanatize cats. Euthanasia was divided into 3 phases. Phase I was the time from initial contact to onset of clinical signs (e.g., yawning, staggering, or trembling). Phase II extended from the end of phase I until recumbency, and phase III from the end of phase II until death.(33) The study revealed that signs of agitation before unconsciousness were greatest with CO_2 + O_2. Convulsions occurred during phases II and III with both methods. However, when the euthanatizing chamber was prefilled with CO (i.e., "exhaust fumes"), convulsions did not occur in phase III. Time to complete immobilization was greater with CO_2 + O_2 (approximately 90 seconds) than with CO alone (approximately 56 seconds).(33) In neonatal pigs, excitation was more likely to precede unconsciousness if the animals were exposed to a rapid rise in CO concentration. This agitation was decreased at lower flow rates, or when CO was combined with N_2O.(72)

Advantages. (a) Carbon monoxide induces unconsciousness without pain and with minimal discernible discomfort. (b) Hypoxemia induced by CO is insidious, so the animal appears to be unaware. (c) Death occurs rapidly if concentrations of 4–6% are used.

Disadvantages. (a) Safeguards must be taken to prevent exposure of personnel. (b) Any electric equipment exposed to CO (e.g., lights and fans) must be explosion-proof.

Recommendations. Carbon monoxide used for individual animal or mass euthanasia is acceptable for small animals, including dogs and cats, provided that commercially compressed CO is used and the following precautions are taken: (a) Personnel using CO must be instructed thoroughly in its use and must understand its hazards and limitations. (b) The CO source and chamber must be located in a well-ventilated environment, preferably out of doors. (c) The chamber must be well lit and have viewports that allow personnel direct observation of the animals. (d) The CO flow rate should be adequate to rapidly achieve a uniform CO concentration of at least 6% after animals are placed in the chamber, although some species (e.g., neonatal pigs) are less likely to become agitated with a gradual rise in CO concentration.(72) (e) If the chamber is inside a room, CO monitors must be placed in the room to warn personnel of hazardous concentrations.

Noninhalant Pharmaceutical Agents

Intravenous administration is the most rapid and reliable method of performing euthanasia with injectable euthanasia agents. It is the most desirable method when it can be performed without causing fear or distress in the animal. Sedation of aggressive, fearful, wild, or feral animals should be accomplished prior to intravenous administration of the euthanasia agent.

When intravenous administration is considered impractical or impossible (e.g., in animals weighing ≤ 7 kg), intraperitoneal administration of a nonirritating euthanasia agent is acceptable, provided that it does not contain neuromuscular blocking agents. Intrahepatic administration has also been described for use in cats.(73) Intracardiac administration is not considered acceptable in awake animals, owing to the difficulty and unpredictability of performing the injection accurately.

Intracardiac injection is acceptable only when performed on heavily sedated, anesthetized, or comatose animals. Intramuscular, subcutaneous, intrathoracic, intrapulmonary, intrarenal, intrasplenic, intrathecal, and other nonvascular injections are not acceptable methods of administering injectable euthanasia agents. When injectable euthanasia agents are administered other than intravenously, animals may be slow to pass through stages I and II of anesthesia.

BARBITURIC ACID DERIVATIVES

Barbiturates depress the central nervous system in descending order, beginning with the cerebral cortex, with unconsciousness progressing to anesthesia. With an overdose, deep anesthesia progresses to apnea, owing to depression of the respiratory center, which is followed by cardiac arrest (Chapter 9).

All barbituric acid derivatives used for anesthesia are acceptable for euthanasia. Induction of unconsciousness by barbiturates results in minimal or transient pain associated with needle puncture, therefore satisfying the basic criterion for classifying an agent as acceptable for euthanasia. Barbiturates have rapid onset of action, which is a desirable characteristic for a euthanasia agent. Desirable barbiturates are those that are potent, long acting, stable in solution, and inexpensive. Sodium pentobarbital fits these criteria and is the most widely used, although others such as secobarbital are acceptable.

Advantages. (a) A primary advantage of barbiturates is speed of action. This effect depends on the dose, concentration, and rate of injection. (b) Barbiturates induce euthanasia smoothly, with minimal discomfort to the animal. (c) Barbiturates are less expensive than many other injectable euthanasia agents.

Disadvantages. (a) Intravenous injection is necessary for best results, necessitating trained personnel. (b) Each animal must be restrained. (c) Current federal drug regulations require strict accounting for the barbiturates, and they must be used under the supervision of personnel registered with the U.S. Drug Enforcement Administration (DEA). (d) An aesthetically objectional terminal gasp may occur in unconscious animals.

Recommendations. The advantages of using barbiturates for euthanasia in small animals far outweigh the disadvantages. The intravenous injection of a barbituric acid derivative is the preferred method for euthanasia of dogs, cats, other small animals, and horses. Intraperitoneal injection may be used in situations where these approaches would cause less distress than intravenous injection.

PENTOBARBITAL COMBINATIONS

Several euthanasia products are formulated to include a barbituric acid derivative (usually sodium pentobarbital) with added local anesthetic agents or agents that metabolize to pentobarbital. Although some of these additives are slowly cardiotoxic, this pharmacologic effect is inconsequential. These combination products are listed by the DEA as Schedule III drugs, making them somewhat simpler to obtain, store, and administer than Schedule II drugs such as sodium pentobarbital. The pharmacologic properties and recommended use of combination products presently available (which combine sodium pentobarbital with lidocaine or phenytoin) are interchangeable with those of pure barbituric acid derivatives. A combination of pentobarbital with a neuromuscular blocking agent is not an acceptable euthanasia agent.

CHLORAL HYDRATE

Chloral hydrate depresses the cerebrum slowly; therefore, restraint may be a problem in some animals. Death is caused by hypoxemia resulting from progressive depression of the respiratory center and may be preceded by gasping, muscle spasms, and vocalization.

Recommendations. Chloral hydrate is acceptable for euthanasia of large animals only when administered intravenously, preferably after sedation to decrease the aforementioned undesirable side effects. Chloral hydrate is not acceptable for dogs, cats, and other small animals because the side effects may be severe and are aesthetically objectionable.

COMBINATION OF CHLORAL HYDRATE, MAGNESIUM SULFATE, AND SODIUM PENTOBARBITAL

A commercially available combination of chloral hydrate, magnesium sulfate, and sodium pentobarbital has been used for anesthesia of large animals, and is an acceptable large animal euthanasia agent when an overdose is administered intravenously.

T-61

T-61 is an injectable nonbarbiturate, nonnarcotic mixture of three drugs used for euthanasia. These drugs provide a combination of general anesthetic, curariform, and local anesthetic actions. T-61 has been withdrawn from the market and is no longer manufactured or commercially available in the United States, although it is available in Canada. T-61 should be used only intravenously, because there is some question as to the differential absorption and onset of action of the active ingredients when administered by other routes.(1)

UNACCEPTABLE INJECTABLE AGENTS

The injectable agents listed in Table 26–4 (strychnine, nicotine, caffeine, magnesium sulfate, potassium chloride, and all neuromuscular blocking agents), when used alone, are unacceptable and are absolutely condemned for use as euthanasia agents.

Physical Methods

Physical methods of euthanasia include captive bolt, gunshot, cervical dislocation, decapitation, electrocution, microwave irradiation, exsanguination, stunning, and pithing. However, some of these procedures—namely exsanguination, stunning, and pithing—are not recommended as a sole means of euthanasia, but are adjuncts when used in association with other agents or methods. Some consider physical methods of euthanasia aesthetically displeasing. However, some of these methods cause less fear and anxiety, and may be more rapid, painless, humane, and practical than other forms of euthanasia when properly used by skilled personnel with well-maintained equipment.

Physical methods are appropriate in three general situations: (a) easily handled small animals with anatomic features compatible with the method used; (b) large farm, wild, or zoo animals; and (c) in research when other methods might invalidate experimental results or interfere with subsequent use of tissues or body fluids.

Given that most physical methods involve trauma, there is inherent risk for animals and human beings; therefore, extreme care and caution should be used. Skill and experience of the personnel are of paramount importance when using physical methods. If the method is not accomplished correctly, animals may be injured and may have varying degrees of consciousness, resulting in pain and distress. Before using physical methods, inexperienced persons should be trained by experienced persons and should practice on carcasses or anesthetized animals to be euthanatized until they are proficient in performing the method properly and humanely. In general, physical methods are recommended for use only after other acceptable means have been excluded; in sedated or unconscious animals when practical; and when scientifically or clinically justified. Consequently, the panel considers all physical methods, except microwave irradiation, conditionally acceptable.

PENETRATING CAPTIVE BOLT

A penetrating captive bolt is used for euthanasia in ruminants, horses, and swine and has recently been developed for use in laboratory rabbits and dogs.(74) Its mode of action is concussion and trauma to the cerebral hemisphere and brain stem.(75, 76) Captive bolts are powered by gunpowder or compressed air. Animals must be adequately restrained to ensure proper placement of the captive bolt. The correct placement of the captive bolt on the animal's head is critical. It is imperative that a cerebral hemisphere and the brain stem are sufficiently disrupted by the projectile to induce sudden unconsciousness and subsequent death. Accurate placement of captive bolts for various species has been described.(75–78) A multiple projectile has been suggested as a more effective technique, especially on large cattle.(75) A nonpenetrating captive bolt only stuns animals and therefore should not be used as a sole means of euthanasia (see "Stunning").

Advantage. The penetrating captive bolt is an effective method for use in slaughterhouses and in research facilities when the use of drugs is inappropriate.

Disadvantages. (a) It is aesthetically displeasing. (b) Death may not occur.

Recommendations. Use of the penetrating captive bolt is a practical method of euthanasia for horses, ruminants, and swine when chemical agents cannot be used. It is strongly recommended that other adjunctive measures (e.g., exsanguination) be used to ensure rapid death. Except for unusual circumstances, there are more acceptable methods of euthanasia for dogs and rabbits. The nonpenetrating captive bolt is not recommended as a method of euthanasia.

GUNSHOT

In some circumstances, gunshot may be the only practical method of euthanasia. It should be performed by highly skilled personnel using a firearm appropriate for the situation. For captive animals, the firearm should be aimed so that the projectile enters the brain, causing instant unconsciousness.(30, 78–80) For wildlife and other freely roaming animals, the preferred target area should be the head or neck.

Advantages. (a) Unconsciousness is instantaneous if the projectile destroys most of the brain. (b) Under field conditions, gunshot may be the only effective method available.

Disadvantages. (a) It may be dangerous to personnel. (b) It is aesthetically unpleasant. (c) Under field conditions, it may be difficult to hit the vital target area.

Recommendations. When other methods cannot be used, an accurately delivered gunshot is an acceptable method of euthanasia. When the animal can be appropriately restrained, the penetrating captive bolt is preferred to gunshot. Gunshot should not be used for routine euthanasia of animals in animal control situations, such as municipal pounds or shelters.

CERVICAL DISLOCATION

Cervical dislocation is used to euthanatize poultry, other small birds, mice, and immature rats and rabbits. For mice and rats, the thumb and index finger are placed on either side of the neck at the base of the skull or, alternatively, a rod is pressed at the base of the skull. With the other hand, the base of the tail or hind limbs are quickly pulled, causing separation of the cervical vertebrae from the skull. For immature rabbits, the head is held in one hand and the hind limbs in the other. The animal is stretched and the neck is hyperextended and dorsally twisted to separate the first cervical vertebra from the skull.(40, 77) In poultry, cervical dislocation by stretching is a common method for mass euthanasia, but unconsciousness may not be instantaneous.(81)

Advantages. (a) Cervical dislocation is a technique that may induce rapid unconsciousness.(82) (b) It does not chemically contaminate tissue. (c) It is rapidly accomplished.

Disadvantages. (a) Cervical dislocation may be aesthetically displeasing to personnel. (b) Data suggest that electric activity in the brain persists for 13 seconds following cervical dislocation.(82) (c) Its use is limited to poultry, other small birds, mice, and immature rats and rabbits.

Recommendations. When properly executed, manual cervical dislocation is a humane technique for euthanasia of poultry, other small birds, mice, rats weighing under 200 g, and rabbits weighing under 1 kg. In heavier rats and rabbits, the greater muscle mass in the cervical region makes manual cervical dislocation physically more difficult; accordingly, it should be performed only with mechanical dislocators or by individuals who have demonstrated proficiency euthanatizing heavier animals.

Until additional information is available to better define the nature of the persistent EEG activity (82), this technique should be used in research settings only when scientifically justified by the user and approved by the Institutional Animal Care and Use Committee. Those responsible for the use of this technique must determine that personnel who perform cervical dislocation techniques have been properly trained to do so.

DECAPITATION

Decapitation is most often used to euthanatize rodents and small rabbits. It provides a means to recover tissues and body fluids that are chemically uncontaminated. It also provides a means of obtaining anatomically undamaged brain tissue for study.(54) Guillotines that are designed to accomplish decapitation in a uniformly instantaneous manner are commercially available.

Advantages. (a) Decapitation is a technique that may induce rapid unconsciousness.(82–84) (b) It does not chemically contaminate tissues. (c) It is rapidly accomplished.

Disadvantages. (a) The handling and restraint required to perform this technique may be distressful to animals.(85) (b) Data suggest that electric activity in the brain persists for 13 or 14 seconds following decapitation.(82, 86) (c) Personnel performing this technique should recognize the inherent danger of the guillotine and take adequate precautions to prevent personal injury. (d) Decapitation may be aesthetically displeasing to personnel performing or observing the technique.

Recommendation. Until additional information is available to better define the nature of the persistent EEG activity (82, 86), this technique should be used in research settings only when scientifically justified by the user and approved by the Institutional Animal Care and Use Committee. Decapitation of amphibians, fish, and reptiles is addressed elsewhere in this chapter. Those responsible for the use of this technique must determine that personnel who perform decapitation techniques have been properly trained to do so.

ELECTROCUTION

Electrocution, using alternating current, as a form of euthanasia has been used in species such as dogs, cattle, sheep, swine, foxes, and mink.(79, 87–92) Electrocution induces death by cardiac fibrillation, which causes cerebral hypoxia.(89, 91, 93) However, animals do not lose consciousness for 10 to 30 seconds or more after onset of cardiac fibrillation. It is imperative that animals be unconscious before being electrocuted. Therefore, euthanasia by electrocution must be a two-step procedure. First, an animal must be rendered unconscious by any acceptable means, including electric stunning (electronarcosis; Chapter 9). If electric stunning or narcosis is used, the electric current must pass through the brain (see "Adjunctive Methods").

Advantages. (a) Electrocution is humane if the animal is first rendered unconscious. (b) It does not chemically contaminate tissues. (c) It is economic.

Disadvantages. (a) Electrocution may be hazardous to personnel. (b) It is not a useful method for mass euthanasia because so much time is required per animal. (c) It is not a useful method for dangerous, intractable animals. (d) It is aesthetically objectionable because of violent extension and stiffening of the limbs, head, and neck. (e) It may not result in death in small animals (< 5 kg) because ventricular fibrillation and circulatory collapse do not always persist after cessation of current flow.

Recommendation. Electric stunning and euthanasia by electrocution require special skills and equipment that will assure passage of sufficient current through the brain to induce unconsciousness followed by electrically induced cardiac fibrillation. Although the method is conditionally acceptable if the aforementioned requirements are met, its disadvantages far outweigh its advantages in most applications. Techniques that apply electric current from head to tail or head to foot are unacceptable.

MICROWAVE IRRADIATION

Heating by microwave irradiation is used primarily by neurobiologists to fix brain metabolites in vivo while maintaining the anatomic integrity of the brain.(94) Microwave instruments have been specifically designed or modified for use in euthanasia of laboratory mice and rats. The instruments differ in design from kitchen units and may vary in the maximal power output from 1.3 to 10 kW. All units direct their microwave energy to the head of the animal. The power required to rapidly halt brain enzyme activity depends on the efficiency of the unit, the ability to tune the resonant cavity, and the size of the rodent head.(95) There is considerable variation among instruments in the time required to induce unconsciousness and euthanasia. A 10-kW, 2450-MHz instrument operated at a power of 9 kW will increase the brain temperature of 18- to 28-g mice to 79° C in 330 ms and the brain temperature of 250- to 420-g rats to 94° C in 800 ms.(96)

Advantages. (a) Unconsciousness is achieved in less than 100 ms, and death in less than one second. (b) This is the most effective method to fix brain tissue in vivo for subsequent assay of enzymatically labile chemicals.

Disadvantages. (a) Instruments are expensive. (b) Only animals the size of mice and rats can be euthanatized with commercial instruments that are currently available.

Recommendations. Microwave irradiation is a humane method to euthanatize small laboratory rodents if instruments that induce rapid unconsciousness are used. Only instruments that are designed for this use and have appropriate power and microwave distribution can be used. Microwave ovens designed for domestic and institutional kitchens are absolutely unacceptable for euthanasia.

ADJUNCTIVE METHODS

Stunning and pithing, when properly done, induce unconsciousness but do not ensure death. Therefore, these methods should be used in conjunction with other procedures such as pharmacologic agents, exsanguination, or decapitation to kill the animal.

Exsanguination. Exsanguination can be used to ensure death subsequent to stunning, electric stunning, or to otherwise unconscious animals. Because anxiety is associated with extreme hypovolemia, exsanguination must not be used as a sole means of euthanasia.(97) Animals may be exsanguinated to obtain blood products, but only when they are sedated, stunned, or anesthetized.(98)

Stunning. Animals may be stunned by a blow to the head, use of a nonpenetrating captive bolt, and electric current. With stunning, evaluation of unconsciousness is difficult, but it is usually associated with a loss of the menace or blink response, pupillary dilation, and a loss of coordinated movements. Specific changes in the electroencephalogram and a loss of visually evoked responses are also thought to indicate unconsciousness.(38, 99)

Blow to head. Stunning (9, 100–102) by a blow to the head is used primarily in small laboratory animals with thin craniums. A single sharp blow must be delivered to the central skull bones with sufficient force to produce immediate depression of the central nervous system. When this is properly done, unconsciousness is rapid.

Nonpenetrating captive bolt. A nonpenetrating captive bolt may be used to induce unconsciousness in ruminants, horses, and swine. The signs of effective stunning by captive bolt are immediate collapse and a several-second period of tetanic spasm, followed by slow hind limb movements of increasing frequency.(38) Other aspects regarding use of nonpenetrating captive bolt are similar to use of a penetrating captive bolt (see "Captive Bolt" for additional information).

Electric stunning. Alternating electric current has been used for stunning in species such as dogs, cattle, sheep, goats, hogs, and chickens.(87, 88, 103–105) Experiments in dogs have shown the necessity of directing the electric current through the brain in order to induce rapid loss of consciousness. In the dog, when electricity passes only between fore- and hind limbs or neck and feet, it causes the heart to fibrillate but does not induce sudden unconsciousness.(93) For electric stunning of any animal, an apparatus that applies electrodes to opposite sides of the head or in another way directs electric current immediately through the brain is necessary to induce rapid unconsciousness (Chapter 9). Attachment of electrodes and animal restraint can pose problems with this form of stunning. The signs of effective electric stunning are extension of the limbs, opisthotonos, downward rotation of the eyeballs, and tonic spasm changing to clonic spasm, with eventual muscle flaccidity. Electric stunning should be followed promptly by electrically induced fibrillation of the heart, exsanguination, or other appropriate methods to ensure death (see "Electrocution" for additional information).

Water jet stunning. A stunning and slaughter method for swine using water under high pressure has been described recently.(106)

Pithing. In general, pithing is used as an adjunctive procedure to ensure death in an animal that has been rendered unconscious by other means. For some species, such as frogs, with anatomic features that facilitate easy access to the central nervous system, pithing may be used as a sole means of euthanasia, but anesthetic overdose is a more suitable method.

Special Considerations

EQUINE EUTHANASIA

Pentobarbital or a pentobarbital combination is the best choice for equine euthanasia. Because a large volume of solution must be injected, a catheter should be placed in the jugular vein. To facilitate catheterization of an excitable or fractious animal, a tranquilizer, such as acepromazine, or an alpha$_2$-adrenergic agonist can be administered, but these drugs may prolong the time to unconsciousness because of their effect on circulation. Opioid agonists or agonist/antagonists in conjunction with alpha$_2$-adrenergic agonists may further facilitate restraint (Chapters 8 and 20).

In certain emergency circumstances, it may be difficult to restrain a dangerous horse or other large animal for intravenous injection and the animal might cause injury to itself or to bystanders before a sedative could take effect. In such cases, which might include euthanasia of a horse with a serious injury at a racetrack, the animal can be given an immobilizing agent such as succinylcholine, but an anesthetic must be administered as soon as the animal can be controlled. After the animal is anesthetized, an overdose of the anesthetic can be used to accomplish euthanasia. Succinylcholine alone or without sufficient anesthetic must not be used for euthanasia.

PRECAUTIONS CONCERNING USE OF EUTHANATIZING AGENTS IN ANIMALS INTENDED FOR HUMAN OR ANIMAL FOOD

In euthanasia of animals intended for human or animal food, agents that result in tissue residues cannot be used unless they are approved by the U.S. Food and Drug Administration.(107) Carbon dioxide is the only chemical currently used in euthanasia of food animals (primarily swine) that does not lead to tissue residues. Carcasses of animals euthanatized by barbituric acid derivatives or other chemical agents may contain potentially harmful residues. These carcasses should be disposed of in a manner that will prevent them from being consumed by human beings or animals.

EUTHANASIA OF NONCONVENTIONAL SPECIES: ZOO, WILD, AQUATIC, AND POIKILOTHERMIC ANIMALS

Compared with objective information on companion, farm, and laboratory animals, euthanasia of species such as zoo, wild, aquatic, and poikilothermic animals has been studied less, and guidelines are more limited. In selecting a means of euthanasia for these species, factors and criteria in addition to those previously discussed must be considered. The means selected will depend on the species, size, safety aspects, location of the animals to be euthanatized, and experience of personnel. Whether the animal to be euthanatized is in the wild, in captivity, or roaming free is a major consideration. Anatomic differences must be considered. For example, amphibians, fish, reptiles, and marine mammals differ anatomically from domestic species (Chapters 20F and 21). Veins may be difficult to locate. Some species have a carapace. For physical methods, access to the central nervous system may be difficult because the brain may be small and difficult to locate by inexperienced persons.

Zoo animals. For captive zoo mammals and birds with related domestic counterparts, many of the means described previously are appropriate. However, to minimize injury to persons or animals, additional precautions such as handling and physical or chemical restraint are important considerations (Chapters 20, 21, and 22).(108)

Wildlife. For wild and feral animals, many of the recommended means of euthanasia for captive animals are not feasible. In field circumstances, wildlife biologists generally do not use the term *euthanasia,* but use terms such as *killing, collecting,* or *harvesting,* recognizing that a distress-free death may not be possible (Chapters 21 and 22).

For many field studies, the only practical means of animal collection are those involving direct killing of the animal.(12, 109–113) Under these conditions, methods must be as age- species- or taxonomic/class-specific as possible. Commonly used methods include gunshot and kill trapping. Gunshot is the most effective or only way to collect some species. When shooting is used as the means of animal collection, the firearm and ammunition should be appropriate for the species and purpose of the study. Personnel should be sufficiently skilled to be able to accurately hit preferred target organs for the particular species of animal. Personnel should be experienced in the proper and safe use of firearms and must comply with laws and regulations governing their possession and use. For killing larger wildlife with gunshot, preferred target areas are the head or neck.

Kill traps are practical and effective for animal collection when used in a manner that minimizes the potential for attraction and collection of nontarget species. Traps should be checked at least once daily. In those instances when an animal is wounded or captured but not dead, the animal must be killed quickly and humanely.

Amphibians, fish, and reptiles. When euthanasia of poikilothermic animals is performed, the differences in their metabolism, respiration, and tolerance to cerebral hypoxia may preclude some procedures that would be acceptable in homeothermic animals. Additionally, it is often more difficult to ascertain when an animal is dead. Euthanasia of amphibians, fishes, and reptiles has been addressed.(12, 30, 114)

Sodium pentobarbital (60 mg/kg of body weight) or other barbiturates can he administered intravenously, intraabdominally, intrapleurally, or intraperitoneally in most cold-blooded animals, depending on anatomic features.

Tricaine methanesulfonate (TMS, MS-222) may be administered by a variety of routes to induce euthanasia. For aquatic animals, including amphibians, this chemical may be placed in the water. Large fish may be removed from the water, a gill cover lifted, and a concentrated solution from a syringe flushed over the gills. This is an effective but expensive means of euthanasia, and is not hazardous to personnel. Benzocaine hydrochloride, a compound similar to TMS, may be used as a bath or in a recirculation system for euthanasia of fish (113, 115) or amphibians (Chapters 20 and 21).(12)

Species such as snakes, lizards, turtles, frogs, and toads may be killed by overexposure to gaseous anesthetics such as halothane or methoxyflurane in a chamber or via face mask. Carbon dioxide gas may be used for terrestrial animals. Some reptiles can stop or reduce their breathing for long periods without overt ill effects, and may not die even after prolonged exposure (Chapter 20).

It has been suggested that, when using physical methods of euthanasia in poikilothermic species, cooling to 4° C will decrease metabolism and facilitate handling, but there is no evidence that it raises the pain threshold. Line drawings of the head of various amphibians and reptiles, with recommended locations for captive bolt or firearm penetration, are available.(12)

Most amphibians, fishes, and reptiles can be euthanatized by cranial concussion (stunning) followed by decapitation or some other physical method. Decapitation with heavy shears or guillotine is effective in some species that have appropriate anatomic features. It has been assumed that stopping blood supply to the brain by decapitation causes rapid unconsciousness. Recently, this view has been questioned because the central nervous system of reptiles and amphibians is tolerant to hypoxic and hypotensive conditions.(12) Consequently, decapitation should be followed by pithing.

Severing the spinal cord behind the head by pithing is an effective method of killing some poikilotherms. Inasmuch as death may not be immediate unless both the brain and spinal cord are pithed, double pithing is recommended. Pithing of the spinal cord should be followed by decapitation and pithing of the brain or some other appropriate procedure. The anatomic features of some species preclude effective use of this method. Pithing requires dexterity and skill, and should be done only by trained personnel.

Snakes and turtles, immobilized by cooling, have been killed by subsequent freezing. However, this method is not recommended.(12) Formation of ice crystals on the skin and in tissues of an animal may cause pain or distress. Quick freezing of deeply anesthetized animals is acceptable. Crocodilians and other large reptiles can be shot through the brain.(30)

Marine mammals. For smaller pinnipeds and cetaceans, barbiturates or potent opioids (e.g., etorphine hydrochloride [M-99] and carfentanil) are recommended. An accurately placed gunshot may also be an acceptable method for euthanasia of stranded marine mammals.(30) For beached whales or other large cetaceans or pinnipeds, succinylcholine chloride in conjunction with potassium chloride, administered intravenously or intraperitoneally, has been used.(116) This method, which is not a method of euthanasia as defined here, should be used only as a last resort. Although it leads to complete paralysis of the respiratory musculature and death due to hypoxemia, it may be more humane than allowing the stranded animal to suffocate over a period of hours or days.

EUTHANASIA OF ANIMALS RAISED FOR FUR PRODUCTION

Animals raised for fur are usually killed individually at the location where they are raised. Although any handling of these species constitutes a stress, it is possible to minimize this by euthanatizing animals in or near their cages. For the procedures described here, please refer to the previous sections for a more detailed discussion.

Carbon monoxide. In the case of the smaller species (e.g., mink), CO appears to be an adequate method for euthanasia. Compressed CO is delivered from a tank into an enclosed cage that can be moved adjacent to holding cages. Using the apparatus outside reduces the risk to human beings; however, people using this method should still be made aware of the dangers of CO. Animals introduced into a chamber containing 4% CO lost consciousness in 64 ± 14 seconds and were dead within 215 ± 45 seconds.(52) In a study involving electroencephalography of mink being euthanatized with 3.5% CO, the animals were comatose in 21 ± 7 seconds.(117) Only one animal should be introduced into the chamber at a time, and death should be confirmed in each case.

Carbon dioxide. Carbon dioxide (CO_2) is also a good euthanasia method for the smaller species and is less dangerous than CO for personnel operating the system. Using compressed CO_2 from a tank is likely to be more reliable and efficient than using solid CO_2. When exposed to 100% CO_2, mink lose consciousness in 19 ± 4 seconds and are dead in 153 ± 10 seconds. When 70% CO_2 is used with 30% O_2, the animals are unconscious in 28 seconds, but they are not dead after a 15-minute exposure.(52) Therefore, if animals are first stunned by 70% CO_2, they should be killed by exposure to 100% CO_2 or by some other means. As with carbon monoxide, only one animal should be introduced into the chamber at a time.

Barbiturate overdose. Barbiturate overdose is an acceptable procedure for euthanasia of many species of animals raised for fur. The drug is injected intraperitoneally and the animal slowly loses consciousness. It is important that the death of each animal be confirmed following barbiturate injection. Barbiturates will contaminate the carcass; therefore the skinned carcass cannot be used for animal food.

Electrocution. Electrocution has been used for killing foxes and mink.(89) The electric current must pass through the brain to induce unconsciousness (electronarcosis; Chapter 9) before electricity is passed through the rest of the body. Use of a nose-to-tail or nose-to-foot (89) method may kill the animal by inducing cardiac fibrillation, but the animal may be conscious for a period before death; therefore, these techniques are unacceptable (electroimmobilization; Chapter 9). Electric stunning may be followed by cervical dislocation in mink and other small animals. It is recommended that cervical dislocation be done within 20 seconds of electric stunning.(118)

Addendum

This chapter summarizes contemporary scientific knowledge on euthanasia in animals and calls attention to the lack of scientific reports assessing pain, discomfort, and distress in animals being euthanatized. Many reports on various methods of euthanasia are either anecdotal, testimonial narratives or unsubstantiated opinions and are therefore not cited in this chapter. We strongly endorse the need for well-designed experiments to more fully determine the extent to which each procedure meets the criteria used for judging the methods of euthanasia.

Each means of euthanasia has advantages and disadvantages. It is impractical to address every potential circumstance in which animals are to be euthanatized. Therefore, the use of professional judgment is imperative.

Failure to list or recommend a means of euthanasia in this report does not categorically condemn its use. There may occasionally be special circumstances or situations in which other means may be acceptable. For research animals, these exceptions should be carefully considered by the attending veterinarian and the Institutional Animal Care and Use Committee. In other settings, professional judgment should be used.

The references cited in this chapter do not represent a comprehensive bibliography on all methods of euthanasia. Persons interested in additional information on a particular aspect of animal euthanasia are encouraged to contact the Animal Welfare Information Center, National Agricultural Library, 10301 Baltimore Boulevard, Beltsville, Maryland 20705.

We are fully committed to the concept that, whenever it becomes necessary to kill any animal for any reason whatsoever, death should be induced as painlessly and quickly as possible. It has been our charge to develop workable guidelines for addressing this need, and it is our sincere desire that these guidelines be used conscientiously by all animal care providers.

References

1. Smith AW, Houpt KA, Kitchell RL, et al. Report of the AVMA panel on euthanasia. J Am Vet Med Assoc 188:252–268, 1986.
2. Webster's ninth new collegiate dictionary. Springfield, MA: Merriam-Webster Inc., 1990.
3. Breazile JE, Kitchell RL. Euthanasia for laboratory animals. Fed Proc 28:1577–1579, 1969.
4. Kitchell RL, Erickson HH, Carstens E, et al., eds. Animal pain: perception and alleviation. Bethesda, MD: American Physiological Society, 1983.
5. Kitchell RL, Johnson RD. Assessment of pain in animals. In: Moberg GP, ed. Animal stress. Bethesda, MD: American Physiological Society, 113–140, 1983.
6. Willis WD. The pain system. The neural basis of nociceptive transmission in the mammalian nervous system. Basel: S Karger, 1985:346.
7. Zimmerman M. Neurobiological concepts of pain, its assessment and therapy. In: Bromm B, ed. Pain measurement in man. Neurophysiological correlates of pain. Amsterdam: Elsevier, 1984:15–35.
8. Kitchen H, Aronson AL, Bittle JL, et al. Panel report on the colloquium on recognition and alleviation of animal pain and distress. J Am Vet Med Assoc 191:1186–1191, 1987.
9. National Research Council. Recognition and alleviation of pain and distress in laboratory animals. Washington, DC: National Academy Press, 1992.
10. Breazile JE. Physiologic basis and consequences of distress in animals. J Am Vet Med Assoc 191:1212–1215, 1987.
11. Grier RL, Clovin TL. Euthanasia guide (for animal shelters). Ames, IA: Moss Creek Publications, 1990.
12. Cooper JE, Ewbank R, Platt C, et al. Euthanasia of amphibians and reptiles. London: UFAW/WSPA, 1989.
13. Greyhavens T. Handbook of pentobarbital euthanasia. Salem, OR: Humane Society of Willamette Valley.
14. Operational guide for animal care and control agencies. Denver: American Humane Association, 1988.
15. Humane slaughter regulations. Fed Reg 44:68809–68817, 1979.
16. Grandin T. Observations of cattle behavior applied to design of cattle-handling facilities. Appl Anim Ethol 6:19–31, 1980.
17. Grandin T. Pig behavior studies applied to slaughter-plant design. Appl Anim Ethol 9:141–151, 1982.
18. Tannenbaum J. Issues in companion animal practice. In: Veterinary ethics. Baltimore: Williams & Wilkins, 1989:208–225.
19. Rollin BE. Ethical question of the month. Can Vet J 33:7–8, 1992.
20. Beaver B. Veterinary aspects of feline behavior. St. Louis: CV Mosby, 1980:217.
21. Houpt KA. Domestic animal behavior for veterinarians and animal scientists. Ames, IA: Iowa State University Press, 1991:408.
22. Hart BL. The behavior of domestic animals. New York: WH Freeman, 1985:390.
23. Hart LA, Hart BL, Mader B. Humane euthanasia and companion animal death: caring for the animal, the client, and the veterinarian. J Am Vet Med Assoc 197:1292–1299, 1990.
24. Neiburg HA, Fischer A. Pet loss, a thoughtful guide for adults and children. New York: Harper & Row, 1982.
25. Hart LA, Mader B. Pet loss support hotline: the veterinary students' perspective. Calif Vet January-February:19–22, 1992.
26. Arluke A. Coping with euthanasia: a case study of shelter culture. J Am Vet Med Assoc 198:1176–1180, 1991.
27. Wolfle TL. Laboratory animal technicians: their role in stress reduction and human-companion animal bonding. Vet Clin North Am Small Anim Pract 15:449–454, 1985.
28. Glass HG, Snyder FF, Webster E. The rate of decline in resistance
29. to anoxia of rabbits, dogs, and guinea pigs from the onset of viability to adult life. Am J Physiol 140:609–615, 1944.
29. Booth NH. Inhalant anesthetics. In: Booth NH, McDonald LE, eds. Veterinary pharmacology and therapeutics, 6th ed. Ames, IA: Iowa State University Press, 1988:181–211.
30. Humane killing of animals. Preprint of 4th ed. South Mimms, Potters Bar, Herts, England: Universities Federation for Animal Welfare, 1988:16–22.
31. Occupational exposure to waste anesthetic gases and vapors. No. 77-140. Washington, DC: Department of Health, Education, and Welfare (National Institute for Occupational Safety and Health), 1977.
32. Lecky JH, ed. Waste anesthetic gases in operating room air: a suggested program to reduce personnel exposure. Park Ridge, IL: The American Society of Anesthesiologists, 1983.
33. Simonsen HB, Thordal-Christensen AA, Ockens N. Carbon monoxide and carbon dioxide euthanasia of cats: duration and animal behavior. Br Vet J 137:274–278, 1981.
34. Klemm WR. Carbon dioxide anesthesia in cats. Am J Vet Res 25:1201–1205, 1964.
35. Leake CD, Waters, RM. The anesthetic properties of carbon dioxide. Curr Res Anesthesiol Analg 8:17–19, 1929.
36. Mattsson JL, Stinson JM, Clark CS. Electroencephalographic power-spectral changes coincident with onset of carbon dioxide narcosis in rhesus monkey. Am J Vet Res 33:2043–2049, 1972.
37. Woodbury DM, Rollins LT, Gardner MD, et al. Effects of carbon dioxide on brain excitability and electrolytes. Am J Physiol 192:79–90, 1958.
38. Blackmore DK, Newhook JC. The assessment of insensibility in sheep, calves, and pigs during slaughter. In: Eikelenboom G, ed. Stunning of animals for slaughter. Boston: Martinus Nijhoff Publishers, 1983.
39. Glen JB, Scott WN. Carbon dioxide euthanasia of cats. Br Vet J 129:471–479, 1973.
40. Hughes HC. Euthanasia of laboratory animals. In: Melby, Altman, eds. Handbook of laboratory animal science, vol. 3. Cleveland, OH: CRC Press, 553–559, 1976.
41. Jaksch W. Euthanasia of day-old male chicks in the poultry industry. Int J Stud Anim Prob 2:203–213, 1981.
42. Kline BE, Peckham V, Hesit HE. Some aids in handling large numbers of mice. Lab Anim Care 13:84–90, 1963.
43. Kotula AW, Brewniak EE, Davis LL. Experimentation with in-line carbon dioxide immobilization of chickens prior to slaughter. Poult Sci 40:213–216, 1961.
44. Stone WS, Amiraian K, Duell C, et al. Carbon dioxide anesthetization of guinea pigs to increase yields of blood and serum. Proc Care Panel 11:299–303, 1961.
45. Hoenderken R. Electrical and carbon dioxide stunning of pigs for slaughter. In: Eikelenboom G, ed. Stunning of animals for slaughter. Boston: Martinus Nijhoff Publishers, 1982:59–63.
46. Gregory NG, Moss BW, Leeson RH. An assessment of carbon dioxide stunning in pigs. Vet Rec 121:517–518, 1987.
47. Carding AH. Mass euthanasia of dogs with carbon monoxide and/or carbon dioxide: preliminary trials. J Small Anim Pract 9:245–259, 1968.
48. Britt DP. The humaneness of carbon dioxide as an agent of euthanasia for laboratory rodents. In: Euthanasia of unwanted, injured or diseased animals or for educational or scientific purposes. UFAW, 1987:19–31.
49. Blackshaw JK, Fenwick DC, Beattie AW, et al. The behaviour of chickens, mice and rats during euthanasia with chloroform, carbon dioxide and ether. Lab Anim 22:67–75, 1988.
50. Euthanasia (carbon dioxide). In: Report and accounts 1976–1977. South Mimms, Potters Bar, Herts, England: Universities Federation for Animal Welfare, 1977:13–14.
51. Hall LW. The anaesthesia and euthanasia of neonatal and juvenile dogs and cats. Vet Rec 90:303–306, 1972.
52. Hansen NE, Creutzberg A, Simonsen HB. Euthanasia of mink (Mustela vison) by means of carbon dioxide (CO₂), carbon monoxide (CO) and nitrogen (N₂). Br Vet J 147:140–146, 1991.
53. Laursen AM. Choosing between CO₂ and electrical stunning of pigs. A preliminary examination of stress and ethics. In:

Eikelenboom G, ed. Stunning of animals for slaughter. Boston: Martinus Nijhoff Publishers, 1983:64–72.

54. Feldman DB, Gupta BN. Histopathologic changes in laboratory animals resulting from various methods of euthanasia. Lab Anim Sci 26:218–221, 1976.

55. Hornett TD, Haynes AP. Comparison of carbon dioxide/air mixture and nitrogen/air mixture for the euthanasia of rodents. Design of a system for inhalation euthanasia. Anim Technol 35:93–99, 1984.

56. Herin RA, Hall P, Fitch JW. Nitrogen inhalation as a method of euthanasia in dogs. Am J Vet Res 39:989–991, 1978.

57. Noell WK, Chinn HI. Time course of failure of the visual pathway in rabbits during anoxia. Fed Proc 8:119, 1949.

58. Vinter FJ. The humane killing of mink. London: Universities Federation for Animal Welfare, 1957.

59. Stonehouse RW, Loew FM, Quine JP, et al. The euthanasia of dogs and cats: a statement of the humane practices committee of the Canadian Veterinary Medical Association. Can Vet J 19:164–168, 1978.

60. Quine JP, Buckingham W, Strunin L. Euthanasia of small animals with nitrogen; comparison with intravenous pentobarbital. Can Vet J 29:724–726, 1988.

61. Quine JP. Euthanasia by hypoxia using nitrogen. A review after four years of operation involving 20,500 animals [Letter]. Can Vet J 21:320, 1980.

62. Raj ABM, Gregory NG, Wotton SB. Changes in the somatosensory evoked potentials and spontaneous electroencephalogram of hens during stunning in Argon-induced anoxia. Br Vet J 147:322–330, 1991.

63. Lowe-Ponsford FL, Henry JA. Clinical aspects of carbon monoxide poisoning. Adverse Drug React Acute Poisoning Rev 8:217–240, 1989.

64. Haldane J. The action of carbonic oxide in man. J Physiol 18:430–462, 1895.

65. Bloom JD. Some considerations in establishing divers' breathing gas purity standards for carbon monoxide. Aerosp Med 43:633–636, 1972.

66. Norman CA, Halton DM, Is carbon monoxide a workplace teratogen? A review and evaluation of the literature. Ann Occup Hyg 34:335–347, 1990.

67. Fechter LD. Neurotoxicity of prenatal carbon monoxide exposure. Research report. Health Effects Institute, 1987:3–22.

68. Wojtczak-Jaroszowa J, Kubow S. Carbon monoxide, carbon disulfide, lead and cadmium–four examples of occupational toxic agents linked to cardiovascular disease. Med Hypotheses 30:141–150, 1989.

69. Ramsey TL, Eilmann HJ. Carbon monoxide acute and chronic poisoning and experimental studies. J Lab Clin Med 17:415–427, 1932.

70. Chalifoux A, Dallaire A. Physiologic and behavioral evaluation of CO euthanasia of adult dogs. Am J Vet Res 44:2412–2417, 1983.

71. Dallaire A, Chalifoux A. Premedication of dogs with acepromazine or pentazocine before euthanasia with carbon monoxide. Can J Comp Med 49:171–178, 1985.

72. Lambooy E, Spanjaard W. Euthanasia of young pigs with carbon monoxide. Vet Rec 107:59–61, 1980.

73. Grier RL, Schaffer CB. Evaluation of intraperitoneal and intrahepatic administration of a euthanasia agent in animal shelter cats. J Am Vet Med Assoc 197:1611–1615, 1990.

74. Dennis MB, Dong WK, Weisbrod KA, et al. Use of captive bolt as a method of euthanasia in larger laboratory animal species. Lab Anim Sci 38:459–462, 1988.

75. Blackmore DK. Energy requirements for the penetration of heads of domestic stock and the development of a multiple projectile. Vet Rec 116:36–40, 1985.

76. Daly CC, Whittington PE. Investigation into the principal determinants of effective captive bolt stunning of sheep. Res Vet Sci 46:406–408, 1989.

77. Clifford DH. Preanesthesia, anesthesia, analgesia, and euthanasia. In: Fox JG, Cohen BJ, Loew FM, eds. Laboratory animal medicine. New York: Academic Press, 528–563, 1984.

78. Australian Veterinary Association. Guidelines on humane slaughter and euthanasia. Aust Vet J 64:4–7, 1987.

79. Carding T. Euthanasia of dogs and cats. Anim Reg Stud 1:5–21, 1977.

80. Longair JA, Finley GG, Laniel M-A, et al. Guidelines for euthanasia of domestic animals by firearms. Can Vet J 32:724–726, 1991.

81. Gregory NG, Wotton SB Comparison of neck dislocation and percussion of the head on visual evoked responses in the chicken's brain. Vet Rec 126:570–572, 1990.

82. Vanderwolf CH, Buzak DP, Cain RK, et al. Neocortical and hippocampal electrical activity following decapitation in the rat. Brain Res 451:340–344, 1988.

83. Derr RF. Pain perception in decapitated rat brain. Life Sci 49:1399–1402, 1991.

84. Holson RR. Euthanasia by decapitation: evidence that this technique produces prompt, painless unconsciousness in laboratory rodents. Neurotoxicol Teratol 14:253–257, 1992.

85. Urbanski HF, Kelly SF. Sedation by exposure to gaseous carbon dioxide-oxygen mixture: application to studies involving small laboratory animal species. Lab Anim Sci 41:80–82, 1991.

86. Mikeska JA, Klemm WR. EEG evaluation of humaneness of asphyxia and decapitation euthanasia of the laboratory rat. Lab Anim Sci 25:175–179, 1975.

87. Warrington R. Electrical stunning, a review of the literature. Vet Bull 44:617–628, 1974.

88. Lambooy E, van Voorst N. Electrocution of pigs with notifiable diseases. Vet Q 8:80–82, 1986.

89. Loftsgard G, Braathen S, Helgebostad A. Electrical stunning of mink. Vet Rec 91:132–134, 1972.

90. Hatch RC. Euthanatizing agents. In: Booth NH, McDonald LE, eds. Veterinary pharmacology and therapeutics, 6th ed. Ames, IA: Iowa State University Press, 1988:1143–1148.

91. Croft PG, Hume CW. Electric stunning of sheep. Vet Rec 68:318–321, 1956.

92. Roberts TDM. Electrocution cabinets. Vet Rec 95:241–242, 1974.

93. Roberts TDM. Cortical activity in electrocuted dogs. Vet Rec 66:561–567, 1954.

94. Stavinoha WB. Study of brain neurochemistry utilizing rapid inactivation of brain enzyme activity by heating and microwave irradiation. In: Black CL, Stavinoha WB, Maruyama Y, eds. Microwave irradiation as a tool to study labile metabolites in tissue. Elmsford, NY: Pergamon Press, 1983:1–12.

95. Stavinoha WB, Frazer J, Modak AT. Microwave fixation for the study of acetylcholine metabolism. In: Jenden DJ, ed. Cholinergic mechanisms and psychopharmacology. New York: Plenum, 169–179, 1978.

96. Ikarashi Y, Maruyama Y, Stavinoha WB. Study of the use of the microwave magnetic field for the rapid inactivation of brain enzymes. Jpn J Pharmacol 35:371–387, 1984.

97. Blackmore DK. Differences in behaviour between sheep and cattle during slaughter. Res Vet Sci 37:223–226, 1984.

98. Gregory NG, Wotton SB. Time to loss of brain responsiveness following exsanguination in calves. Res Vet Sci 37:141–143, 1984.

99. Blackmore DK. Non-penetrative percussion stunning of sheep and calves. Vet Rec 105:372–375, 1979.

100. Canadian Council on Animal Care. Guide to the care and use of experimental animals, vol. I. Ontario, Canada: Canadian Council on Animal Care, 1980.

101. Green C. Euthanasia. In: Animal anaesthesia. London: Laboratory Animals Ltd, 1979:237–241.

102. Clifford DH. Preanesthesia, anesthesia, analgesia, and euthanasia. In: Fox JG, Cohen BJ, Loew FM, eds. Laboratory animal medicine. Orlando, FL: Academic Press, 1984:527–562.

103. Gregory NG, Wotton SB. Effect of slaughter on spontaneous and evoked activity of the brain. Br Poult Sci 27:195–205, 1986.

104. Anil MH, McKinstry JL. Reflexes and loss of sensibility following head-to-back electrical stunning in sheep. Vet Rec 128:106–107, 1991.

105. Eikelenboom G, ed. Stunning of animals for slaughter. Boston: Martinus Nijhoff Publishers, 1983.

106. Schatzmann U, Leuenberger T, Fuchs P, et al. Jet injection: the possibility of using a high pressure water jet for the stunning of slaughter pigs. Fleischwirtschaft 71:899–901, 1991.

107. Booth NH. Drug and chemical residues in the edible tissues of animals. In: Booth NH, McDonald LE, eds. Veterinary pharmacology and therapeutics, 6th ed. Ames, IA: Iowa State University Press, 1149–1205, 1988.

108. Fowler ME, ed. Zoo and wild animal medicine. Philadelphia: WB Saunders, 1986.

109. Acceptable field methods in mammalogy: preliminary guidelines approved by the American Society of Mammalogists. J Mammal 68(suppl 4):1–18, 1987.

110. American Ornithologists' Union Report of committee on use of wild birds in research. Auk 105(suppl 1):1A-41, 1988A

111. American Society of Ichthyologists and Herpetologists, Herpetologist League, Society for the Study of Amphibians and Reptiles. Guidelines for the use of live amphibians and reptiles in field research. J Herpetol 21(suppl 4):1–14, 1987.

112. American Society of Ichthyologists and Herpetologists, American Fisheries Society, American Institute of Fisheries Research Biologists. Guidelines for use of fishes in field research. Copeia Suppl 1–12, 1987.

113. Cailliet GM. Fishes: a field guide and laboratory manual on their structure, identification, and natural history. Belmont, CA: Wadsworth, 1986.

114. Zwart P, deVries HR, Cooper JE. Tijdschr Diergeneeskd 114:557–565, 1989.

115. Brown LA. Anesthesia in fish. Vet Clin North Am Small Anim Pract 18:317–330, 1988.

116. Hyman J. Euthanasia in marine animals. In: Dierauf LA, ed. CRC handbook of marine mammal medicine: health, disease, and rehabilitation. Boca Raton, FL: CRC Press, 1990:265–266.

117. Lambooy E, Roelofs JA, Van Voorst N. Euthanasia of mink with carbon monoxide. Vet Rec 116:416, 1985.

118. Recommended code of practice for the care and handling of mink. Ottawa, Canada: Agriculture Canada, 1988:17.

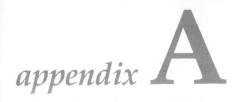

appendix A

SOURCES OF SELECTED DRUGS*

Generic Name	Trade Name	Source†
Acepromazine Maleate	Promace	12
Adrenocorticosteroids		
Prednisolone Na succinate	Solu-Delta Cortef	37
Dexamethasone Na phosphate	Azium	31
Alfentanil hydrochloride	Alfenta	16
Alphaxalone-Alphadolone	Saffan	14
Aminophylline	Aminophylline	1
Atipamezole	Antisedan	25
4-Aminopyridine	4-AP	33
Atropine sulfate	Atropine	11
Atracurium besylate	Tracrium	7
Azaperone	Stresnil	26
Bretylium tosylate	Bretylol	1
Bupivacaine hydrochloride	Marcaine	40
Buprenorphine hydrochloride	Buprenex	23
Butrophanol tartrate	Torbugesic	12
Calcium chloride solution	—	4
Calcium gluconate	Cal-Dextro	12
Carbon dioxide	—	—
Carfentanil citrate	Wildnil	39
Carisoprodol	Soma	38
Alpha-Chloralose	Chloretone	33
Cimetidine	Tagamet	34
Dantrolene sodium	Dantrium	23
Desflurane	Suprane	3
Detomidine	Dormosedan	25
Dextran	(Dextran-70)	5
	(Dextran-40)	1
Diazepam	Valium	29
Dibucaine hydrochloride	Nupercaine	8
Digoxin	Lanoxin	7
Diprenorphine hydrochloride	M50-50	18
Dobutamine hydrochloride	Dobutrex	19
Dopamine hydrochloride	Intropin	10
Doxacurium chloride	Nuromax	7
Doxapram hydrochloride	Dopram-V	28
Droperidol	Inapsine	16
Edrophonium chloride	Reversol	24
Enflurane	Ethrane	3
Ephedrine sulfate	Ephedrine	1
Epinephrine hydrochloride	Adrenalin	11
Ethyl chloride	Fluro-Ethyl	13
Etidocaine hydrochloride	Duranest	4
Etomidate hydrochloride	Amidate	1
Etorphine hydrochloride	M-99	18
Etorphine-Acepromazine	Immobilon-LA	27

DRUGS (continued)

Generic Name	Trade Name	Source†
Etorphine-Methotrimeprazine	Immobilon-SA	27
Fentanyl citrate	Sublimaze	16
Fentanyl citrate-droperidol	Innovar-Vet	26
Fentanyl transdermal	Duragesic	16
Fentanyl-azeperone	Fentaz	16
Flumazenil	Romazicon	29
Flunixin meglumine	Banamine	31
Furosemide	Lasix	15
Gallamine triethiodide	Flaxedil	9
Glycopyrrolate	Robinul	28
Guaifenesin	Gecolate	36
Halothane	Fluothane	41
Heparin	Heparin	37
Hexafluorenium bromide	Mylaxen	38
Hyaluronidase	Wydase	41
Hydroxyethyl starch	Hespan	10
Hypertonic saline	—	5
Idazoxine	—	27
Isoflurane	Isoflo	35
Isoproterenol hydrochloride	Isuprel	40
Ketamine hydrochloride	Ketaset	12
Lactated Ringer's solution	—	5
Levarterenol bitartrate	Levophed	40
Lidocaine hydrochloride	Xylocaine	4
Mannitol	Osmitrol	1
Medetomidine	Domitor	25
Meperidine hydrochloride	Demerol	40
Mephentermine sulfate	Wyamine	41
Mepivacaine hydrochloride	Carbocaine	40
Metaraminol bitartrate	Aramine	21
Methadone hydrochloride	Dolophine	19
Methohexital sodium	Brevane	19
Methotrimeprazine hydrochloride	Levoprome	17
Methoxamine hydrochloride	Vasoxyl	7
Methoxyflurane	Metofane	1
Metoclopramide	Reglan	28
Metocurine iodide	Metubine	19
Metomidate hydrochloride	Hypnodil	16
Midazolam hydrochloride	Versed	29
Milrinone lactate	Primacor	30
Misoprostol	Cytotec	32
Morphine sulfate	Astramorph	4
Nalorphine hydrochloride	Nalline	23
Naloxone hydrochloride	Narcan	10
Naltrexone hydrochloride	ReVia	10
Neostigmine methylsulfate	Prostigmin	29
Nitrous oxide	—	—
Oxygen	—	—
Omeprazole	Prilosec	4
Oxymorphone hydrochloride	Numorphan	10
Pancuronium bromide	Pavulon	24
Pentazocine lactate	Talwin-V	30
Pentobarbital	Beuthanasia	31
Pentobarbital sodium	Nembutal	1
Phenobarbital sodium	Phenobarbital	41
Phenoxybenzamine hydrochloride	Dibenzyline	34
Phentolamine mesylate	Regitine	8
Phenylephrine hydrochloride	Neo-Synephrine	40
Phenytoin sodium	Dilantin	11
Pipecuronium bromide	Arduan	24
Procainamide hydrochloride	Procainamide	11
Procaine hydrochloride	Novocain	40

DRUGS (continued)

Generic Name	Trade Name	Source†
Proparacaine hydrochloride	Alcaine	2
Propofol	Diprivan	42
Propranolol hydrochloride	Inderal	41
Protamine sulfate	Lyphomed	19
Pyridostigmine bromide	Regonol	24
Sevoflurane	Ultane	1
Sodium bicarbonate	—	1
Succinylcholine chloride	Anectine	7
Sufentanil citrate	Sufenta	16
Tetracaine hydrochloride	Pontocaine	40
Thiopental Sodium	Pentothal	1
Thiamylal Sodium	Biotal	6
Tiletamine-Zolazepam	Telazol	12
Tolazoline hydrochloride	Priscoline	8
Tromethamine	THAM	1
Tubocurarine	Tubocurarine	1
Urethane	Urethane	21
Vecuronium bromide	Norcuron	24
Xylazine hydrochloride	Rompun	22
Yohimbine	Yobine	20

* See list of drug companies and corresponding manufacturer number codes. Only one company is listed as a specific drug source, even though several companies may market the same drug but under a different trade name.

† Inclusion of a specific drug in this list does not imply author or publisher endorsement.

COMPANIES

1.
Abbott Laboratories
1 Abbott Park Road
Abbott Park, IL 60064-3500
(708) 937-6100
(800) 323-9100

2.
Alcon Laboratories Inc.
62101 S. Freeway
Fort Worth, TX 76134
(817) 293-0450

3.
Anaquest
110 Allen Road
Liberty Center, NJ 07938
(990) 647-9200

4.
Astra Pharmaceutical Products
50 Otis Street
Westborough, MA 01581
(508) 366-1100

5.
Baxter General Health Care
1 Pky. N. Ste. 100
Deerfield, IL 60015
(708) 940-1935
Fax (800) 423-2311

6.
Bio-Ceutic Laboratories Inc.
2621 North Belt Highway
P.O. Box 999
St. Joseph, MO 64502
(816) 233-2571
Fax (816) 233-4767
(800) 821-7467

7.
Burroughs-Welcome Co.
3030 Cornwallis Road
Research Triangle Park,
NC 27709
(919) 248-3000
Fax (919) 248-8375
(800) 722-9292

8.
Ciba-Geigy Corporation
444 Saw Mill River Road
Ardsley, NY 10502
(914) 479-5000
Fax (914) 478-3480
(799) 431-1874

9.
Davis and Geck
One Cyanamid Plaza
Wayne, NJ 07470
(201) 831-2000

10.
DuPont Pharmaceuticals
1000 Stewart Avenue
Garden City, NY 11530
(516) 832-2210
Fax (516) 832-2255
(800) 543-8693

11.
Elkins-Sinn, Inc.
2 Easterbrook Lane
Cherry Hill, NJ 08034
(609) 424-3700
Fax (609) 424-8747

12.
Fort Dodge Laboratories
800 5th Street N.W.
Fort Dodge, IA 50501
(515) 955-4600

13.
Gebauer Chemical Company
9410 St. Catherine Avenue
Cleveland, OH 44104
(216) 271-5252
Fax (216) 271-5335
(800) 321-9348

14.
Glaxo Inc.
5 Moore Drive
Research Triangle Park,
NC 27709
(919) 248-2100
Fax (919) 248-2381

15.
Hoechst-Roussel Pharmaceutical, Inc.
Route 202-206 North
Summerville, NJ 08876
(908) 231-2000
Fax (908) 231-3225
(800) 235-2637

16.
Janssen Pharmaceutical
1125 Trenton Harborton Road
Titisville, NJ 08560
(609) 730-2000
Fax (609) 730-2323
(800) 253-3682

17.
Lederle Laboratories
One Cyanamid Plaza
Wayne, NJ 07470
(201) 831-2000
Fax (201) 831-3120
(800) 533-3753

18.
Lemmon Company
650 Cathill Road
P.O. Box 904
Sellersville, PA 18960
(215) 723-5544
Fax (215) 721-9669

19.
Lilly, Eli and Company
640 East McArty Street
Indianapolis, IN 42685
(317) 276-2000
Fax (317) 276-2095

20.
Lloyds Laboratories
P.O. Box 86
Shenandoah, IA 51601
(712) 246-4000

21.
Merck and Company
126 East Lincoln Avenue
P.O. Box 2000
Rahway, NJ 07065
(908) 594-4000
Fax (908) 594-4662

22.
Miles Incorporation
Animal Health Products
12707 West 63rd Street
P.O. Box 390
Shawnee, KS 66201
(913) 631-4800
Fax (913) 962-2803
(800) 255-6517

23.
Norwich-Eaton Pharmaceuticals
P.O. Box 2468
Greenville, SC 29602
(803) 277-5535
Fax (803) 299-2303

24.
Organon, Inc.
375 Mount Pleasant Avenue
West Orange, NJ 07052
(201) 325-4500
Fax (201) 325-4589
(800) 631-1253

25.
Pfizer, Charles and Company, Inc.
235 East 42nd Street
New York, NY 10017
(212) 573-2323
Fax (212) 573-7851
(800) 533-4535

26.
Pitman-Moore, Inc.
(Johnson & Johnson/Mallinckrodt Medical)
1425 Lower Ferry Road
Trenton, NJ 06608
(609) 771-1629
Fax (609) 771-4453

27.
Rickett Colman Pharmaceuticals
Dansom Lane
Kingston-upon-Hull
England HU8 7DS

28.
Robins, A.H. Company
P.O. Box 8299
Philadelphia, PA 19101-1245
(215) 688-4400
Richmond, VA 23261

29.
Roche Laboratories
(Division of Hoffmann-La Roche Inc.
340 Kingsland Street
Nutley, NJ 07110
(201) 235-5000
Fax (201) 235-7605
(800) 526-6367

30.
Sanofi-Winthrop Pharmaceuticals
90 Park Avenue
New York, NY 10016
(212) 907-3500

31.
Schering-Plough Animal Health
110 Allen Road
Liberty Corner, NJ 07938
(201) 822-7000
Fax (908) 604-1640

32.
Searle
5200 Old Orchard Road
Skokie, IL 60077
(708) 982-7000

33.
Sigma Chemical Co.
P.O. Box 14508
St. Louis, MO 63178
(314) 771-5750

34.
SmithKline Beecham Pharmaceuticals
P.O. Box 7929
Philadelphia, PA 19103
(215) 751-4000

35.
Solvay Animal Health
1201 Northland Drive
Mendota, MN 55120
(612) 681-9555
Fax (612) 681-9425
(800) 524-1645

36.
Summit Hill Laboratories
Navesink, NJ 07752
(908) 291-3600
Fax (908) 872-1389

37.
Upjohn Company (The)
7000 Portage Road
Kalamazoo, MI 49001
(616) 323-4000
Fax (616) 329-8414
(800) 253-8600

38.
Wallace Laboratories
Half Acre Road
Cranbury, NJ 08512
(609) 655-6000

39.
Wildlife Pharmaceuticals Inc.
1401 Duff Drive, Suite 600
Fort Collins, CO 80524
(970) 484-6267
Fax (970) 482-6184
(800) 222-9453

40.
Winthrop Pharmaceuticals
(Division of Sterling Drug)
90 Park Avenue
New York, NY 10016
(212) 907-2000
Fax (212) 907-3626

41.
Wyeth-Ayerst Laboratories
555 East Lancaster Avenue
St. Davids, PA 19087
(215) 971-5557
Fax (215) 254-9157
(800) 999-9384

42.
Zeneca Pharmaceuticals
1800 Concord Pike
Wilmington, DE 19897
(302) 886-3000

Standard Values and Equivalents*

METRIC WEIGHTS

$$
\begin{aligned}
1 \text{ gram } (1 \text{ g}) &= \text{weight of 1 cc water at } 4° \text{ C} \\
1000 \text{ g} &= 1 \text{ kilogram (kg)} \\
0.1 \text{ g} &= 1 \text{ decigram (dg)} \\
0.01 \text{ g} &= 1 \text{ centigram (cg)} \\
0.001 \text{ g} &= 1 \text{ milligram (mg)} \\
0.001 \text{ mg} &= 1 \text{ microgram } (\mu\text{g})
\end{aligned}
$$

METRIC VOLUMES

1 liter (L) = 1 cubic decimeter or 1000 cubic centimeters (cc)
0.001 liter = 1 milliliter (ml)

SOLUTION EQUIVALENTS

1 part in	10 =	10.00 %	(1 ml contains	100	mg)
1 part in	50 =	2.00 %	(1 ml contains	20	mg)
1 part in	100 =	1.00 %	(1 ml contains	10	mg)
1 part in	200 =	0.50 %	(1 ml contains	5	mg)
1 part in	500 =	0.20 %	(1 ml contains	2	mg)
1 part in	1,000 =	0.10 %	(1 ml contains	1	mg)
1 part in	1,500 =	0.066 %	(1 ml contains	0.66 mg)	
1 part in	2,600 =	0.038 %	(1 ml contains	0.38 mg)	
1 part in	5,000 =	0.02 %	(1 ml contains	0.20 mg)	
1 part in	50,000 =	0.002 %	(1 ml contains	0.02 mg)	

The number of milligrams in 1 milliliter of any solution of known percentage strength is obtained by moving the decimal one place to the right.

APOTHECARIES' OR TROY WEIGHT

(Used in Prescriptions)

1 pound (lb)	= 12 ounces	= 5,760 grains
1 ounce ()	= 8 drams	= 480 grains
1 dram ()	= 60 grains	

Apothecaries' Volume

1 pint (O)	= 16 fluid ounces	
1 fluid ounce (fl.)	= 8 fluid dram	= 480 minims (min)
1 fluid dram (fl.)	= 60 minims	

*Systeme International (SI) units and conversions are shown later in this appendix.

AVOIRDUPOIS OR IMPERIAL WEIGHT

(Used in commerce in the United States and in the British Pharmacopeia)

Grain	= same as Troy grain		
Ounce (oz)	=		437.5 grains
Pound (lb)	= 16 oz	= 7000	grains
Ton	= 2000 lb		

IMPERIAL VOLUME

		Apothecaries' System
Minims (min)	=	0.96
Fluidrachm (fl dr)	= 60 min	= 0.96 fl
Fluidounce (fl oz)	= 8 drachms	= 0.96 fl
Pint (O)	= 20 fluidounces	= 1.2 O
Gallon (C)	= 8 pints	= 1.2 C

APPROXIMATE EQUIVALENT WEIGHTS

1 kilogram	= 2.2 Avoirdupois or Imperial pounds
1 kilogram	= 2.6 Apothecary or Troy pounds
1 gram	= 15 (15.4) grains
1 milligram	= 1/60 (1/64) grain
1 ounce	= 30 grams
(Avoirdupois or Imperial	= 28.350 grams)
(Apothecary or Troy	= 31.1035 grams)
1 dram	= 4 grams
1 grain	= 60 milligrams

APPROXIMATE VOLUMES

1 liter	= 1 quart
1 milliliter or cubic centimeter	= 15 minims
1 pint	= 500 cubic centimeters
1 fluid ounce	= 30 cubic centimeters
(Imperial	= 28.412 cubic centimeters)
(Apothecary	= 29.574 cubic centimeters)
1 fluid dram	= 4 cubic centimeters

EQUIVALENTS OF CENTIGRADE AND FAHRENHEIT
THERMOMETRIC SCALES

Centigrade Degree	Fahrenheit Degree	Centigrade Degree	Fahrenheit Degree
−17	+ 1.4	14	57.2
−16	3.2	15	59.0
−15	5.0	16	60.8
−14	6.8	17	62.6
−13	8.6	18	64.4
−12	10.4	19	66.2
−11	12.2	20	68.0
−10	14.0	21	69.8
− 9	15.8	22	71.6
− 8	17.6	23	73.4
− 7	19.4	24	75.2
− 6	21.2	25	77.0
− 5	23.0	26	78.8
− 4	24.8	27	80.6
− 3	26.6	28	82.4
− 2	28.4	29	84.2
− 1	30.2	30	86.0
0	32.0	31	87.8
+ 1	33.8	32	89.6
2	35.6	33	91.4
3	37.4	34	93.2
4	39.2	35	95.0
5	41.0	36	96.8
6	42.8	37	98.6
7	44.6	38	100.4
8	46.4	39	102.2
9	48.2	40	104.0
10	50.0	41	105.8
11	51.8	42	107.6
12	53.6	43	109.4
13	55.4	44	111.2
		45	113.0

GAS DENSITIES

(Wt of Unit Vol)

22.4 liters of any gas are equal to its molecular weight in grams at a pressure of 760 mm of mercury and 0° C

MOLECULAR WEIGHTS

Ethylene	=	28 g
Air	=	29 g
Oxygen	=	32 g
Cyclopropane	=	42 g
Nitrous oxide	=	44 g
Carbon dioxide	=	44 g
Ether	=	74 g
Chloroform	=	119 g

(From A.M.A.: *Fundamentals of Anesthesia*, 3rd ed. W. B. Saunders Co., Philadelphia, 1954.)

Special Symbols*

— Dash above any symbol indicates a *mean* value.
· Dot above any symbol indicates a *time derivative*.

FOR GASES

Primary Symbols
(Large Capital Letters)

Examples

V	= gas volume	V_A	= volume of alveolar gas
$\dot{V}$	= gas volume/unit time	$\dot{V}_{O_2}$	= O_2 consumption/min
P	= gas pressure	$P_{A_{O_2}}$	= alveolar O_2 pressure
$\bar{P}$	= mean gas pressure	$P_{A_{O_2}}$	= arterial partial pressure of oxygen
F	= fractional concentration in dry gas phase	$P_{C_{O_2}}$	= mean capillary O_2 pressure
		$F_{I_{O_2}}$	= fractional concentration of O_2 in inspired gas
f	= respiratory frequency (breaths/unit time)	D_{O_2}	= diffusing capacity for (O_2 (ml O_2/min/mm/Hg)
D	= diffusing capacity		
R	= respiratory exchange ratio	R	= $\dot{V}_{CO_2}/\dot{V}_{O_2}$

Secondary Symbols
(Small Capital Letters)

Examples

I	= inspired gas	F_ICO_2	= fractional concentration of CO_2 in inspired gas
E	= expired gas	V_E	= volume of expired gas
A	= alveolar gas	$\dot{V}_A$	= alveolar ventilation/min
T	= tidal gas	V_T	= tidal volume
D	= dead space gas	V_D	= volume of dead space gas
B	= barometric	P_B	= barometric pressure
STPD	= 0° C, 760 mm Hg, dry		
BTPS	= body temperature and pressure saturated with water vapor	V_D/V_T	= ratio of physiologic dead space to tidal volume
ATPS	= ambient temperature and pressure saturated with water vapor		

For Blood

Primary Symbols
(Large Capital Letters)   *Examples*

Q = volume of blood   Qc = volume of blood in pulmonary
                                                       capillaries

$\dot{Q}$ = volume flow of blood/unit time $\dot{Q}$c = blood flow through pulmonary
                                                        capillaries/min

C = concentration of gas in blood C_aO_2 = ml O_2 in 100 ml arterial blood
S = % saturation of Hb with O_2 or CO $S_{\bar{v}}CO_2$ = saturation of Hb with O_2 in mixed
                                                        venous blood

$\dot{V}/\dot{Q}$ = ventilation/perfusion ratios

Secondary Symbols
(small letters)   *Examples*

a = arterial blood P_aCO_2 = partial pressure of CO_2 in arterial
                                                        blood

v = venous blood $P_{\bar{v}}O_2$ = partial pressure of O_2 in mixed
                                                        venous blood

c = capillary blood P_cCO = partial pressure of CO in pulmonary
                                                        capillary blood

For Lung Volumes

VC = Vital Capacity   = maximal volume that can be expired
                                                   after maximal inspiration

IC = Inspiratory Capacity   = maximal volume that can be inspired
                                                   from resting expiratory level

IRV = Inspiratory Reserve Volume   = maximal volume that can be inspired
                                                   from end-tidal inspiration

ERV = Expiratory Reserve Volume   = maximal volume that can be expired
                                                   from resting expiratory level

FRC = Functional Residual Capacity   = volume of gas in lungs at resting
                                                   expiratory level

RV = Residual Volume   = volume of gas in lungs at end of
                                                   maximal expiration

TLC = Total Lung Capacity   = volume of gas in lungs at end of
                                                   maximal inspiration

SYSTEME INTERNATIONAL*

The following information on SI units and factors for conversion between SI and older conventional units is provided for the convenience of readers and authors.

Basic SI Units

Physical Quantity	Name	Symbol
Length	Meter	m
Mass	Kilogram	kg
Time	Second*	s
Electric current	Ampere	A
Thermodynamic temperature	Kelvin	K
Luminous intensity	Candela	cd
Amount of substance	Mole	mol

*Minute (min), hour (h), and day (d) will remain in use although they are not official SI units.

Prefixes for SI Units

Factor	Name	Symbol	Factor	Name	Symbol
10^{18}	Exa	E	10^{-18}	Atto-	a
10^{15}	Peta	P	10^{-15}	Femto	f
10^{12}	Tera-	T	10^{-12}	Pico-	p
10^{9}	Giga-	G	10^{-9}	Nano-	n
10^{6}	Mega-	M	10^{-6}	Micro-	μ
10^{3}	Kilo-	k	10^{-3}	Milli-	m
10^{2}	Hecto-	h	10^{-2}	Centi-	c
10^{1}	Deca-	da	10^{-1}	Deci-	d

Derived SI Units

Quantity	SI Unit	Symbol	Expression in Terms of SI Base Units or Derived Units
Frequency	Hertz	Hz	$1\ Hz = 1\ cycle/s\ (1\ s^{-1})$
Force	Newton	N	$1\ N = 1\ kg \cdot m/s^2\ (1\ kg \cdot mps^{-2})$
Work, energy, quantity of heat	Joule	J	$1\ J = 1\ N \cdot m$
Power	Watt	W	$1\ W = 1\ J/s\ (1\ J \cdot s^{-1})$
Quantity of electricity	Coulomb	C	$1\ C = 1\ A \cdot s$
Electric potential, potential difference, tension, electromotive force	Volt	V	$1\ V = 1\ W/A\ (1\ W \cdot A^{-1})$
Electric capacitance	Farad	F	$1\ F = 1\ A \cdot s/V\ (1\ A \cdot s \cdot V^{-1})$
Electric resistance	Ohm	Ω	$1\ \Omega = 1\ V/A\ (1\ V \cdot A^{-1})$
Flux of magnetic induction, magnetic flux	Weber	Wb	$1\ Wb = 1\ V \cdot s$
Magnetic flux density, magnetic induction	Tesla	T	$1\ T = 1\ Wb/m^2\ (1\ Wb \cdot m^{-2})$
Inductance	Henry	H	$1\ H = 1\ V \cdot s/A\ (1\ V \cdot s \cdot A^{-1})$
Pressure	Pascal	Pa	$1\ Pa = 1\ N/m^2\ (1\ N \cdot m^{-2})$ $= 1\ kg/m \cdot s^2\ (1\ kg \cdot m^{-1} \cdot s^{-2})$

The liter ($10^{-3}\ m^3 = dm^3$), though not official, will remain in use as a unit of volume as also will the dyne (dyn) as a unit of force (1 dyn = 10^{-5} N).

*Reprints of these tables are available on request from The Canadian Anaesthetists' Society Journal, 178 St. George Street, Toronto, Canada, M5R 2M7.

SI Unit	Old Unit	Conversion Factors	
		Old to SI (exact)	SI to Old (approx.)
kPa	mm Hg*	0.133	7.5
kPa	1 standard atmosphere† (approx: 1 Bar)	101.3	0.01
kPa	cmH₂O	0.0981	10
kPa	lbs/sq in	6.89	0.145

*e.g., systolic BP of 120 mm Hg = 16 kPa and diastolic BP of 80 mm Hg = 11 kPa
† = 760 mm Hg

BLOOD CHEMISTRY, UNITS AND CONVERSION FACTORS

Measurement	SI Unit	Old Unit	Conversion Factors	
			Old to SI (exact)	SI to Old (approx.)
Blood				
Acid-Base				
P$_{CO_2}$	kPa	mm Hg	0.133	7.5
P$_{O_2}$	kPa	mm Hg	0.133	7.5
Standard bicarbonate	mmol/liter	mEq/liter	Numerically equivalent	
Base excess	mmol/liter	mEq/liter	Numerically equivalent	
Glucose	mmol/liter	mg/100 ml	0.0555	18
Plasma				
Sodium	mmol/liter	mEq/liter	Numerically equivalent	
Potassium	mmol/liter	mEq/liter	Numerically equivalent	
Magnesium	mmol/liter	mEq/liter	0.5	2
Chloride	mmol/liter	mEq/liter	Numerically equivalent	
Phosphate (inorganic)	mmol/liter	mEq/liter	0.323	3.0
Creatinine	μmol/liter	mg/100 ml	88.4	0.01
Urea	mmol/liter	mg/100 ml	0.166	6.0
Serum				
Calcium	mmol/liter	mg/100 ml	0.25	4.0
Iron	μmol/liter	μg/100 mol	0.179	5.6
Bilirubin	μmol/liter	mg/100 ml	17.1	0.06
Cholesterol	mmol/liter	mg/100 ml	0.0259	39
Total proteins	g/liter	g/100 ml	10.0	0.1
Albumin	g/liter	g/100 ml	10.0	0.1
Globulin	g/liter	g/100 ml	10.0	0.1

BIOCHEMICAL CONTENT OF OTHER BODY FLUIDS

Measurement	SI Unit	Old Unit	Conversion Factors	
			Old to SI (exact)	SI to Old (approx.)
Urine				
Calcium	mmol/24 h	mg/24 h	0.025	40
Creatinine	mmol/24 h	mg/24 h	0.00884	113
Potassium	mmol/liter	mEq/liter	Numerically equivalent	
Sodium	mmol/liter	mEq/liter	Numerically equivalent	
Cerebrospinal fluid				
Protein	g/liter	mg/100 ml	0.01	100
Glucose	mmol/liter	mg/100 ml	0.0555	18

HEMATOLOGY

Measurement	SI Unit	Old Unit	Conversion Factors Old to SI	SI to Old
Hemoglobin (Hb)	g/dl	g/100 ml	Numerically equivalent	
Packed cell volume	No unit*	Percent	0.01	100
Mean cell Hb conc.	g/dl	Percent	Numerically equivalent	
Mean cell Hb	pg	μμg	Numerically equivalent	
Red cell count	Cells/liter	Cells/mm^3	10^6	10^{-6}
White cell count	Cells/liter	Cells/mm^3	10^6	10^{-6}
Reticulocytes	Percent	Percent	Numerically equivalent	
Platelets	Cells/liter	Cells/mm^3	10^6	10^{-6}

*Expressed as decimal fraction, e.g., normal adult male value 0.40 to 0.54.

pH AND nmol/liter OF H$^+$ ACTIVITY

pH	nmol/liter
6.80	158
6.90	126
7.00	100
7.10	79
7.20	63
7.25	56
7.30	50
7.35	45
7.40	40
7.45	36
7.50	32
7.55	28
7.60	25
7.70	20

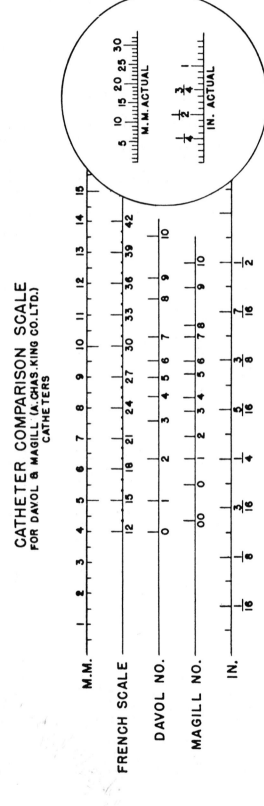

CATHETER COMPARISON SCALE
FOR DAVOL & MAGILL (A.CHAS.KING CO.LTD.)
CATHETERS

To compare catheter sizes, place a rule on one of the calibrations and check along the edge for the corresponding figures. The scale is enlarged eight times for easy reading. An actual-size scale is shown in the circle if measurements are required. (Courtesy of The British Oxygen Co., Ltd., London.) For an approximate conversion from French scale to internal diameter in millimeters, the French value can be divided by four.

INDEX

Page numbers in italic denote figures.